PEDIATRIC SOLID ORGAN TRANSPLANTATION

This book is dedicated to the memory of Amir H. Tejani, MD (1933–2002) whose inspiration and foresight led to the first edition of this textbook, *Pediatric Solid Organ Transplantation*, and to the founding of The International Pediatric Transplant Association (IPTA).

Pediatric Solid Organ Transplantation

SECOND EDITION

EDITED BY

Richard N. Fine

Dean, School of Medicine, MD
Distinguished Professor of Pediatrics
Stony Brook University School of Medicine
Stony Brook, New York 11794-8111
USA

Steven A. Webber

Professor of Pediatrics, MBChB, MRCP
University of Pittsburgh School of Medicine
Division of Cardiology
Children's Hospital
3705 Fifth Avenue
Pittsburgh, PA 15213
USA

Kim M. Olthoff

Associate Professor of Surgery, MD, FACS
Director, Liver Transplant Program
University of Pennsylvania and the Children's
    Hospital of Philadelphia
2 Dulles, 3400 Spruce Street
Philadelphia, PA 19104
USA

Deirdre A. Kelly

Professor of Paediatric Hepatology,
    MD, FRCPI, FRCP, FRCPCH
The Liver Unit
Birmingham Children's Hospital NHS Trust
Steelhouse Lane,
Birmingham, B4 6NH
UK

William E. Harmon

Professor of Pediatrics, MD
Division of Nephrology
Children's Hospital Boston
300 Longwood Avenue, Hunn-319
Boston, MA 02115
USA

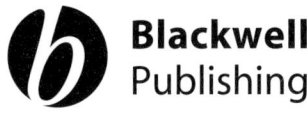

Blackwell
Publishing

First published 2000 Munksgaard, Copenhagen
Second edition 2007 Blackwell Publishing Ltd, Oxford

Library of Congress Cataloging-in-Publication Data
Pediatric solid organ transplantation. – 2nd ed. / edited by Richard N.
Fine . . . [et al.].
   p. ; cm.
  Includes bibliographical references and index.
  ISBN-13: 978-1-4051-2407-2 (alk. paper)
  ISBN-10: 1-4051-2407-5 (alk. paper)
1. Transplantation of organs, tissues, etc. in children. I. Fine,
Richard N.
  [DNLM: 1. Organ Transplantation. 2. Child. 3. Immunosuppression. 4. Infant.
WO 660 P356 2007]

RD120.77.C45P42 2007
617.9′540083–dc22

                                                     2006027961

ISBN-13: 978-1-4051-2407-2
ISBN-10: 1-4051-2407-5

A catalogue record for this title is available from the British Library

Set in 9.5/12pt Sabon by Graphicraft Ltd, Hong Kong
Printed and bound in Singapore by Utopia Press Pte Ltd

Commissioning Editor: Maria Khan
Development Editor: Rebecca Huxley
Production Controller: Debbie Wyer

For further information on Blackwell Publishing, visit our website:
http://www.blackwellpublishing.com

Contents

v

Preface to the Second Edition

Over six years has passed since the first edition of *Pediatric Solid Organ Transplantation* was published. This book remains the only textbook devoted to the field of pediatric transplantation. The concept for the first edition was that of the late Amir Tejani, an individual who relentlessly promoted the field of pediatric transplantation.

Transplantation of the major organs has now become routine in many countries across the globe, and some of the best results of transplantation are now being achieved in the youngest of recipients, including neonates and infants. In parallel with the growth and success of transplantation in children, the International Pediatric Transplant Association (IPTA), and its journal *Pediatric Transplantation*, have both flourished since the first edition of this book. Like the journal, this book is an official publication of the IPTA, and many of IPTA's members have contributed to this second edition.

In the second edition, the strengths of the first edition have been maintained, while new features have been added. The addition of three new co-editors has ensured that all facets of pediatric transplantation are represented in the editorial team. The organ specific sections have all been revised by experts (new and old) to keep the text up-to-date in this rapidly evolving field. Consistency has been applied to the content of all the organ specific sections to enhance the overall structure of the text. Section Two on Immunosuppression and its Complications has been expanded by four chapters to include sections on mechanisms of action, therapies for the sensitized patient, post-transplant lymphoproliferative disorders and organ toxicities of immunosuppressive therapy. A new section has been added (Section Eight) to emphasize the many special issues that effect survivors of pediatric transplantation. This new section focuses on topics related to quality of life; an issue of profound importance as the number of long-term survivors of pediatric solid organ transplantation continues to grow. A wide variety of topics ranging from growth and cognitive development to adherence and transition to adult care are covered in this important new section.

The editors wish to express their sincere appreciation to all the authors who contributed their time and expertise to this project. The end result reflects the sum of these excellent individual contributions. In addition, we would like to thank Kerrie Roberts who coordinated all the early stages of manuscript submission with endless forbearance and efficiency. We also would like to thank Rebecca Huxley and Maria Khan of Blackwell Publishing without whom this project would not have been possible. The final stages of production were carried out by Alice Nelson who assisted the editors in resolving the remaining issues and whose contribution to the final success of this publication is inestimable. The patience, collegiality and professionalism of these individuals has helped create a work that we hope will serve as the definitive reference for all those interested in improving the care and quality of life of children undergoing solid organ transplantation.

We believe Dr Tejani would be very pleased with this new edition of *Pediatric Solid Organ Transplantation*.

Richard N. Fine
Steven A. Webber
Kim M. Olthoff
Deirdre A. Kelly
William E. Harmon

January 2007

Preface to the First Edition

Pediatric solid organ transplantation has experienced exciting and substantial advances in the past decade consequent to continued improvement in clinical outcomes.

The data base of the North American Pediatric Renal Transplant Cooperative Study has demonstrated the value of a registry in changing clinical practice, and has stimulated the development of similar registries in other pediatric solid organ transplants such as liver and heart. The evolution of pediatric transplantation to its own independent status has been marked by several international meetings followed by the creation of the Journal of Pediatric Transplantation and, most recently, by the establishment of the International Pediatric Transplant Association (IPTA). Guided by the Pediatric Committee of the American Society of Transplantation, certification of programs in renal, hepatic and heart and lung transplants is now underway.

To provide a more cohesive approach to the teaching of pediatric transplantation in various subspecialities, the council of IPTA has initiated the compilation of this book.

In organizing the structure of the text, the Editors have recognized that there is a central core of information that is common to all clinical transplantation. Grouped together in the first two sections of the book, this core is intended to provide information about the immune system, rejection and tolerance, immunosuppressives and infections: issues common to all organs. Organ specific sections are structured in a common format designed to cover transplantation while maintaining the unique needs of the organ speciality.

The Editors wish to express their sincere appreciation to all the authors who contributed their time and expertise to this project. We are particularly grateful to the Associate Editors who contributed to the conception and realization of the book. It is our hope that this comprehensive text will strengthen intra-speciality cooperation, familiarize pediatric physicians and surgeons with the salient aspects of each other's respective areas and help improve the quality of life of children undergoing transplants.

Amir H. Tejani, MD
Professor of Pediatrics and Surgery
New York Medical College
Valhalla, New York

William E. Harmon, MD
Associate Professor of Pediatrics
Harvard Medical School
Boston, Massachusetts

Richard N. Fine, MD
Professor and Chairman
Department of Pediatrics
State University of New York
Stony Brook, New York

Contributors

Estella M. Alonso, MD
Professor of Pediatrics
Department of Pediatrics
Northwestern University School of Medicine
The Siragusa Transplantation Center
Children's Memorial Hospital
Chicago, IL

Carlos E. Araya, MD
Fellow
Division of Pediatric Nephrology
University of Florida College of Medicine
Gainesville, FL

Vincent T. Armenti, MD, PhD
Professor of Surgery
Abdominal Organ Transplant Program
Temple University School of Medicine
Philadelphia, PA

Sharon M. Bartosh, MD
Professor of Pediatrics
University of Wisconsin Children's Hospital
Madison, WI

Mark Bellinger, MD
Clinical Professor of Urology
University of Pittsburgh
Pittsburgh, PA

Mark R. Benfield, MD
Professor and Chief
Division of Pediatric Nephrology
University of Alabama at Birmingham
Birmingham, AL

Jean F. Botha, MD
University of Nebraska Medical Center
Omaha, NE

Gerard J. Boyle, MD
Department of Cardiology
Cleveland Clinic Foundation
Cleveland, OH

David M. Briscoe, MD
Associate Professor of Pediatrics
Havard Medical School
Boston, MA

Christoph E. Broelsch, MD, FACS
Professor of Surgery and Transplantation
Dept of General Surgery and Transplantation
University Hospital Essen
Germany

Gilbert J. Burckart, PharmD
Professor and Chairman, Department of Pharmacy
Director, Clinical Pharmacogenomics Laboratory
University of Southern California
Los Angeles, CA

Charles E. Canter, MD
Professor of Pediatrics
Washington University School of Medicine
St. Louis, MO

Richard E. Chinnock, MD
Department of Pediatrics
Loma Linda Medical Center
Loma Linda, CA

Arthur H. Cohen, MD
Emeritus Professor of Pathology and Medicine
UCLA School of Medicine and
Department of Pathology
Cedars-Sinai Medical Center
Los Angeles, CA

John M. Davison, MD
Emeritus Professor of Obstetrics and Gynaecology
Royal Victoria Infirmary
Newcastle upon Tyne
UK

Vikas R. Dharnidharka, MD
Associate Professor
Division of Pediatric Nephrology
University of Florida College of Medicine
Gainesville, FL

Paul S. Dickman, MD
Clinical Professor of Pathology, University of Arizona
Department of Pathology/Laboratory
Phoenix Children's Hospital
1919 East Thomas Road
Phoenix, AZ

René J. Duquesnoy, PhD
Professor of Pathology and Surgery
University of Pittsburgh Medical Center
Pittsburgh, PA

Udeme D. Ekong, MBBS, MRCP
Assistant Professor of Pediatrics
Department of Pediatrics
Northwestern University School of Medicine
The Siragusa Transplantation Center
Children's Memorial Hospital
Chicago, IL

Demetrius Ellis, MD
Professor of Pediatrics
University of Pittsburgh
Chief, Pediatric Nephrology
Children's Hospital of Pittsburgh
Pittsburgh, PA

Jean C. Emond, MD
Thomas S. Zimmer Professor and Vice Chairman
Department of Surgery
Columbia University
Center for Liver Disease and Transplantation
New York Presbyterian Hospital
New York, NY

Douglas G. Farmer, MD
Associate Professor of Surgery
Director, Intestinal Transplantation
Dumont-UCLA Transplant Center
Los Angeles, CA

Albert Faro, MD
Assistant Professor of Pediatrics
Washington University in St. Louis School of Medicine
St. Louis Children's Hospital
Division of Allergy and Pulmonary Medicine
St. Louis, MO

Thomas M. Fishbein, MD
Professor of Surgery
Director, Center for Intestinal Care and Transplant
Georgetown University Hospital
Children's National Medical Center
Washington, DC

Barbara A. Fivush, MD
Professor of Pediatrics
Chief, Division of Pediatric Nephrology
The Johns Hopkins University School of Medicine
Baltimore, MD

Michael Green, MD, MPH
Professor of Pediatrics and Surgery
University of Pittsburgh School of Medicine
Division of Infectious Diseases
Children's Hospital of Pittsburgh
Pittsburgh, PA

William E. Harmon, MD
Professor of Pediatrics
Division of Nephrology
Children's Hospital Boston
Harvard Medical School
Boston, MA

Erick Hernandez, MD
Assistant Professor of Clinical Pediatrics
Division of Pediatric Gastroenterology
Miller School of Medicine
University of Miami
Miami, FL

Ryutaro Hirose, MD
Associate Professor of Clinical Surgery
Dept of Surgery
University of California, San Francisco
Kidney Transplant Service
San Francisco, CA

Christer Holmberg, MD
Professor of Pediatrics
Hospital for Children and Adolescents
University of Helsinki
Helsinki
Finland

Charles B. Huddleston, MD
Professor of Surgery
Washington University School of Medicine
St. Louis Children's Hospital
St. Louis, MO

Elizabeth Ingulli, MD
Assistant Professor, Pediatrics
Division of Nephrology
Center for Immunology
University of Minnesota Medical School
Minneapolis, MN

Ronald Jaffe, MB.BCh
Professor of Pathology
University of Pittsburgh School of Medicine
Marjory K. Harmer Professor of Pediatric Pathology
Children's Hospital of Pittsburgh
Pittsburgh, PA

Hannu Jalanko, MD
Docent in Pediatrics
Head of Pediatric Nephrology and Transplantation
Hospital for Children and Adolescents
University of Helsinki
Helsinki
Finland

Dominique Jan, MD
Professor of Clinical Surgery
Department of Surgery
Columbia University
Center for Liver Disease and Transplantation
New York Presbyterian Hospital
New York, NY

Stanley C. Jordan, MD
Medical Director, Kidney Transplantation and
   Transplant Immunology
Center for Kidney Diseases and Transplantation
Comprehensive Transplant Center
Cedars-Sinai Medical Center
Professor of Pediatrics and Medicine
David Geffen School of Medicine at UCLA
Los Angeles, CA

Binita M. Kamath, MBBChir
Fellow
University of Pennsylvania
The Fred and Suzanne Biesecker Liver Center
Division of Gastroenterology and Nutrition
Children's Hospital of Philadelphia
Philadelphia, PA

Tomoaki Kato, MD
Assistant Professor of Clinical Surgery
Division of Liver and GI Transplantation
Miller School of Medicine
University of Miami
Miami, FL

Stuart S. Kaufman, MD
Medical Director, Pediatric Liver and Intestinal
   Transplantation
Georgetown University Transplant Institute and Children's
   National Medical Center
Washington, DC

Deirdre A. Kelly, MD, FRCPI, FRCP, FRCPCH
Professor of Paediatric Hepatology
The Liver Unit
Birmingham Children's Hospital NHS Trust
Steelhouse Lane
Birmingham
UK

Alan M. Krensky, MD
Shelagh Galligan Professor
Stanford University Medical Center
Stanford, CA

Steven J. Lobritto, MD
Medical Director, Pediatric Liver Transplantation
Associate Clinical Professor of Pediatrics and Medicine
Department of Surgery
Columbia University
Center for Liver Disease and Transplantation
New York Presbyterian Hospital
New York, NY

Janet McDonagh, MD
Senior Lecturer in Paediatric and Adolescent
   Rheumatology
Institute of Child Health
Birmingham Children's Hospital NHS Trust
Steelhouse Lane
Birmingham
UK

Ruth A. McDonald, MD
Associate Professor
Division of Nephrology
Children's Hospital and Regional Medical Center
University of Washington
Seattle, WA

Eithne F. MacLaughlin, MD
Associate Professor of Clinical Pediatrics
Keck School of Medicine of the University of Southern
    California
Division of Pulmonology
Children's Hospital Los Angeles
Los Angeles, CA

Massimo Malagó, MD
The Ilse Bagel Professor of Surgery and Transplantation
Department of General Surgery and Transplantation
University Hospital Essen
Germany

George B. Mallory, MD
Director, Lung Transplant Program
Associate Professor of Pediatrics
Baylor College of Medicine
Baylor University
Texas Children's Hospital
Houston, TX

Elaine S. Mansfield, MD
Senior Research Scientist
Department of Pediatrics
Stanford University School of Medicine
Stanford, CT

Cal S. Matsumoto, MD
Assistant Professor of Surgery
Center for Intestinal Care and Transplant
Georgetown University Hospital
Children's National Medical Center
Washington, DC

George V. Mazariegos, MD
Director, Pediatric Transplantation
Associate Professor of Surgery and Critical Care Medicine
University of Pittsburgh Medical Center
Thomas E. Starzl Transplantation Institute
Children's Hospital of Pittsburgh
Pittsburgh, PA

Marc L. Melcher, MD, PhD
Acting Assistant Professor
Stanford School of Medicine
Department of Surgery
University of California, San Francisco
San Francisco, CA

Eric N. Mendeloff, MD
Director, Congenital Heart Surgery and Pediatric
    Heart and Lung Transplantation
Medical City Children's Hospital
Dallas, TX

Marian G. Michaels, MD, MPH
Professor of Pediatrics and Surgery
University of Pittsburgh School of Medicine
Division of Infectious Diseases
Children's Hospital of Pittsburgh
Pittsburgh, PA

Shelley D. Miyamoto, MD
Director of Heart Failure and Cardiomyopathy Program
Department of Pediatrics, Division of Cardiology
University of Colorado Health Sciences
Cardiac Transplant Program
The Children's Hospital
Denver, CO

Michael J. Moritz, MD
Professor of Surgery
Lehigh Valley Hospital
Allentown, PA

W. Robert Morrow, MD
David Clark Chair in Pediatric Cardiology
Professor of Pediatrics
UAMS College of Medicine
Chief, Pediatric Cardiology
Arkansas Children's Hospital
Little Rock, AK

Pamela J. Murray, MD, MHP
Associate Professor of Pediatrics, Division Chief of
    Adolescent Medicine and Associate Professor of
    Obstetrics/Gynecology Reproductive Health Services
University of Pittsburgh School of Medicine
Pittsburgh, PA

Silvio Nadalin, MD
Department of General Surgery and Transplantation
University Hospital Essen
Germany

David C. Naftel, PhD
Professor of Surgery
University of Alabama Birmingham School of Medicine
Birmingham, AL

Nader Najafian, MD
Assistant Professor of Medicine
Transplantation Research Center
Brigham and Women's Hospital
Children Hospital Boston
Harvard Medical School
Boston, MA

John S. Najarian, MD
Professor of Surgery
Emeritus Professor and Chairman of Surgery
Emeritus Regents' Professor
Department of Surgery
University of Minnesota
Minneapolis, MN

William H. Neches, MD
Emeritus Professor of Pediatrics and Pediatric
    Cardiology
Children's Hospital of Pittsburgh
Pittsburgh, PA

Alicia M. Neu, MD
Associate Professor of Pediatrics
Clinical Director, Division of Pediatric Nephrology
Medical Director, Pediatric Dialysis and Kidney
    Transplantation
The Johns Hopkins University School of Medicine
Baltimore, MD

Vassilios E. Papalois, MD, PhD, FICS
Consultant Transplant and General Surgeon
Transplant Unit
St. Mary's Hospital
London
UK

Maria Parizhskaya, MD
Pathologist
Virginia Beach, VA

Uptal D. Patel, MD
Assistant Professor of Medicine and Pediatrics
Divisions of Nephrology and Pediatric Nephrology
Duke Children's Hospital and Health Center
Duke University
Durham, NC

Alice Peng, MD
Associate Director, Kidney Transplant Program
Center for Kidney Diseases and Transplantation
Comprehensive Transplant Center
Cedars-Sinai Medical Center
UCLA School of Medicine
Los Angeles, CA

Biagio A. Pietra, MD
Medical Director of Cardiac Transplant Program
Department of Pediatrics, Division of Cardiology
University of Colorado Health Sciences
Cardiac Transplant Program
The Children's Hospital
Denver, CO

Frank A. Pigula, MD
Assistant Professor
Department of Cardiothoracic Surgery
Boston Children's Hospital
Harvard Medical School
Boston, MA

Erik Qvist, MD
Assistant Professor of Pediatrics
Hospital for Children and Adolescents
University of Helsinki
Helsinki
Finland

Elizabeth B. Rand, MD
Associate Professor
Medical Director, Liver Transplant Program
Director Gastroenterology and Nutrition Fellowship Program
University of Pennsylvania
The Fred and Suzanne Biesecker Liver Center
Division of Gastroenterology and Nutrition
Children's Hospital of Philadelphia
Philadelphia, PA

Jorge Reyes, MD
Director, Transplant Services
Children's Hospital and University of Washington
    School of Medicine
Seattle, WA

John P. Roberts, MD
Department of Surgery
University of California, San Francisco
San Francisco, CA

Alan D. Salama, PhD, MRCP
Senior Lecturer and Honorary Consultant Physician
Renal Section, Division of Medicine
Imperial College London
Hammersmith Hospital
London
UK

Minnie M. Sarwal, MD, PhD, MRCP, DCH
Associate Professor of Nephrology
Department of Pediatrics
Stanford University School of Medicine
Stanford, CT

Mohamed H. Sayegh, MD
Professor of Medicine and Pediatrics
Transplantation Research Center
Brigham and Women's Hospital
Children Hospital Boston
Harvard Medical School
Boston, MA

Franz Schaefer, MD
Professor of Pediatrics
Head, Division of Pediatric Nephrology
Hospital for Pediatric and Adolescent Medicine
University of Heidelberg
Heidelberg
Germany

Ron Shapiro, MD
Professor of Surgery
Director, Kidney, Pancreas, and Islet Transplantation
Thomas E. Starzl Transplantation Institute
University of Pittsburgh
Director, Pediatric Renal Transplantation
Children's Hospital of Pittsburgh
Pittsburgh, PA

Eyal Shemesh, MD
Mt Sinai Medical Center
Assistant Professor of Psychiatry
Assistant Professor of Pediatrics
Recanati-Miller Transplant Institute, Psychiatry, Pediatrics
1 Gustave L. Levy Place
New York, NY

Rakesh Sindhi, MD
Associate Professor of Surgery
University of Pittsburgh Medical Center
Thomas E. Starzl Transplantation Institute
Children's Hospital of Pittsburgh
Pittsburgh, PA

Jodi M. Smith, MD
Acting Assistant Professor
Division of Nephrology
Children's Hospital and Regional Medical Center
University of Washington
Seattle, WA

Kyle Soltys, MD
Assistant Professor of Surgery
University of Pittsburgh Medical Center
Thomas E. Starzl Transplantation Institute
Children's Hospital of Pittsburgh
Pittsburgh, PA

Robert Squires, MD
Clinical Director of Gastroenterology
Children's Hospital of Pittsburgh
Pittsburgh, PA

Gina S. Sucato, MD, MPH
Assistant Professor of Pediatrics
Division of Adolescent Medicine
University of Pittsburgh School of Medicine
Pittsburgh, PA

Debra L. Sudan, MD
Professor of Surgery
University of Nebraska Medical Center
983285 Nebraska Medical Center
Omaha, NE

Manikkam Suthanthiran, MD
Stanton Griffis Distinguished Professor of Medicine
Division of Nephrology
Department of Medicine
Weill Medical College of Cornell University
and Department of Transplantation Medicine and
    Extracorporeal Therapy
New York Presbyterian Hospital
New York, NY

Stuart C. Sweet, MD, PhD
Assistant Professor of Pediatrics
Medical Director, Pediatric Lung Transplant Program
Medical Director, Lung Transplantation
Division of Allergy and Pulmonary Medicine
Department of Pediatrics
St. Louis Children's Hospital at Washington School of
    Medicine
St. Louis, MO

Robyn Temple-Smolkin, PhD
Postdoctoral Associate
University of Pittsburgh Medical Center
Pittsburgh, PA

Susan E. Thomas, MD
Clinical Associate Professor of Pediatrics
Medical Director, Pediatric Renal Transplant Program
C.S. Mott Children's Hospital
University of Michigan
Ann Arbor, MI

John F. Thompson, MD
Professor of Pediatrics
Division of Pediatric Gastroenterology
Miller School of Medicine
University of Miami
Miami, FL

Andreas G. Tzakis, MD, PhD
Professor of Surgery
Division of Liver and GI Transplantation
Miller School of Medicine
University of Miami
Miami, FL

Flavio Vincenti, MD
Professor of Clinical Medicine
University of California, San Francisco
Kidney Transplant Service
San Francisco, CA

Gary Visner, DO
Attending Physician
Children's Hospital of Philadelphia
University of Pennsylvania
Philadelphia, PA

Zoran Vukcevic, MD
Transplant Fellow
University of Pittsburgh Medical Center
Thomas E. Starzl Transplantation Institute
Department of Critical Care Medicine
Pittsburgh, PA

Steven A. Webber, MBChB, MRCP
Professor of Pediatrics
University of Pittsburgh School of Medicine
Pittsburgh, PA

Peter F. Whitington, MD
Professor of Pediatrics
Department of Pediatrics
Northwestern University School of Medicine
The Siragusa Transplantation Center
Children's Memorial Hospital
Chicago, IL

Marlyn S. Woo, MD
Medical Director, Cardiothoracic Transplant Program
Children's Hospital Los Angeles
Keck School of Medicine
University of Southern California
Los Angeles, CA

Adriana Zeevi, PhD
Professor of Pathology and Surgery
Director, Histocompatibility and Immunogenetics
    Laboratory
University of Pittsburgh Medical Center
Pittsburgh, PA

Immunology and Genetics

1

The Immune Response to Organ Allografts

Manikkam Suthanthiran

Organ transplantation has benefited significantly from advances in immunology and molecular biology. A relatively young scientific discipline, immunobiology of organ transplantation is the quientessential example of translational science that has resulted in truly life-saving remedies for those afflicted with irreparable end-organ failure. There are several commonalities in the immune response to cellular and solid organ allografts, and the essential principles are reviewed in this chapter.

T-CELL SURFACE PROTEINS, ANTIGEN RECOGNITION AND SIGNAL TRANSDUCTION

The antigen recognition complex is comprised of the clone specific T-cell antigen receptor (TCR) α and β heterodimer that is responsible for the recognition of the antigenic peptide displayed in the groove of major histocompatibility complex (MHC) encoded proteins, and the clonally invariant CD3 complex responsible for signal transduction (Table 1.1) [1–5]. Whereas the majority of peripheral blood T cells display TCR α and β heterodimer on their cell surface, a minority expresses TCR γ and δ chains.

The T-cell surface is also decorated with lineage specific and functional proteins that contribute to the immune synapse between the T cells and the antigen presenting cells (APCs). Peripheral blood T cells express either the CD4 protein or the CD8 protein on their cell surface and the CD4 and CD8 proteins bind nonpolymorphic domains of human leukocyte antigen (HLA) class II (DR, DP, DQ) and class I (A, B, C) molecules, respectively, and contribute to the associative recognition process termed MHC restriction. Kinetic models of the immune synapse suggest that a critical threshold of

Table 1.1 Cell-surface proteins important for T-cell activation.* (Reproduced from Suthanthiran *et al.* [52] with permission.)

T-cell surface	APC surface	Functional response	Consequence of blockade
LFA-1 (CD11a, CD18)	ICAM (CD54)	Adhesion	Immunosuppression
ICAM1 (CD54)	LFA-1 (CD11a, CD18)		
CD8, TCR, CD3	MHCI	Antigen recognition	Immunosuppression
CD4, TCR, CD3	MHCII		
CD2	LFA3 (CD58)	Costimulation	Immunosuppression
CD40L (CD154)	CD40		
CD5	CD72		
CD28	B7-1 (CD80)	Costimulation	Anergy
CD28	B7-2 (CD86)		
CTLA4 (CD152)	B7-1 (CD80)	Inhibition	Immunostimulation
CTLA4 (CD152)	B7-2 (CD86)		

APC, antigen-presenting cell; ICAM, intercellular adhesion molecule; LFA, leukocyte function-associated antigen; MHC, major histocompatibility complex.

* Receptor/counter-receptor pairs that mediate interactions between T cells and APCs are shown in this table. Inhibition of each protein-to-protein interaction, except the CTLA4–B7-1/B7-2 interaction results in an abortive *in vitro* immune response. Initial contact between T cells and APCs requires an antigen-independent adhesive interaction. Next, the T-cell antigen receptor complex engages processed antigen presented within the antigen-presenting groove of MHC molecules. Finally, costimulatory signals are required for full T-cell activation. An especially important signal is generated by B7-mediated activation of CD28 on T cells. Activation of CD28 by B7-2 may provide a more potent signal than activation by B7-1. CTLA4, present on activated but not resting T cells, imparts a negative signal.

TCR to MHC-peptide engagements is obligatory to stabilize the TCR/peptide physical contacts and the redistribution of cell surface proteins. An important consequence is the co-clustering of the TCR/CD3 complex with the T-cell surface proteins that include integrins such as leukocyte function-associated antigen 1 (LFA-1) and nonintegrins such as CD2 [6–8].

The immunologic synapse consists of a multiplicity of T-cell surface protein forms and clusters, thereby creating a platform for antigen recognition and generation of various crucial T-cell activation-related signals. The synapse begins to form when the initial adhesions between T-cell surface proteins and APC surface proteins are formed. These adhesions create intimate contact between T cells and APCs and

thereby provide an opportunity for T cells to recognize antigen. Antigen-driven T-cell activation, a tightly regulated, preprogrammed process, begins when T cells recognize intracellularly processed fragments of foreign proteins (approximately 8–16 amino acids) embedded within the groove of the MHC proteins expressed on the surface of APCs. Some recipient T cells directly recognize the allograft (i.e. donor antigen(s) presented on the surface of donor APCs), while other T cells recognize the donor antigen after it is processed and presented by self-APCs [9].

Following activation by antigen, the TCR/CD3 complex and co-clustered CD4 and CD8 proteins are physically associated with intracellular protein–tyrosine kinases (PTKs) of two different families, the src (including p59^{fyn} and p56^{lck}) and

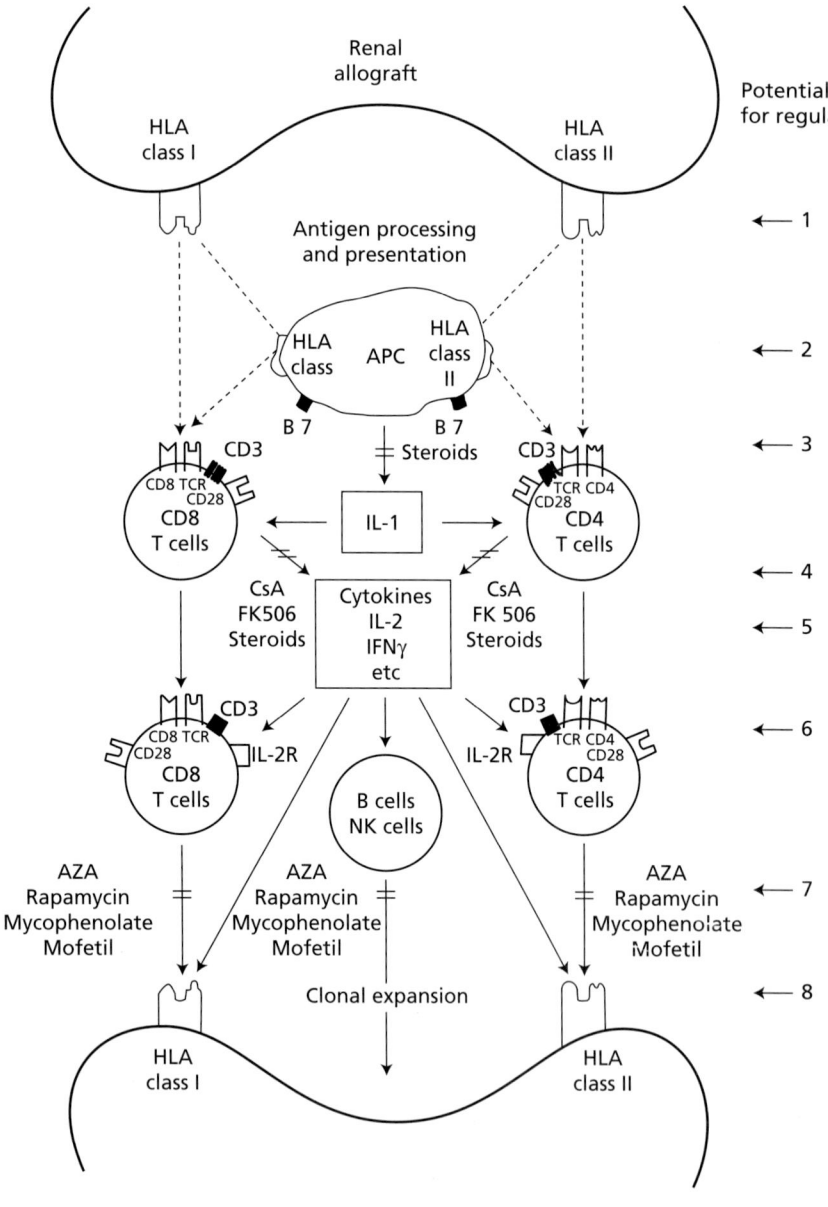

Fig. 1.1 The antiallograft response. Schematic representation of human leukocyte antigens (HLA), the primary stimuli for the initiation of the antiallograft response; cell surface proteins participating in antigenic recognition and signal transduction; contribution of the cytokines and multiple cell types to the immune response; and the potential sites for the regulation of the antiallograft response. Site 1: Minimizing histoincompatibility between the recipients and the donor (e.g. HLA matching). Site 2: Prevention of monokine production by antigen-presenting cells (e.g. corticosteroids). Site 3: Blockade of antigen recognition (e.g. OKT3 mAbs). Site 4: Inhibition of T-cell cytokine production (e.g. cyclosporin A [CsA]). Site 5: Inhibition of cytokine activity (e.g. anti-interleukin-2 [IL-2] antibody). Site 6: Inhibition of cell cycle progression (e.g. anti-IL-2 receptor antibody). Site 7: Inhibition of clonal expansion (e.g. azathioprine [AZA]). Site 8: Prevention of allograft damage by masking target antigen molecules (e.g. antibodies directed at adhesion molecules). HLA class I: HLA-A, B and C antigens; HLA class II: HLA-DR, DP and DQ antigens. IFNγ, γ-interferon; NK cells, natural killer cells. (Reproduced from Suthanthiran *et al.* [51] with permission.)

Table 1.2 Cellular elements contributing to the antiallograft response. (Reproduced from Suthanthiran *et al.* [52] with permission.)

Cell type	Functional attributes
T cells	The CD4+ T cells and the CD8+ T cells participate in the antiallograft response. CD4+ T cells recognize antigens presented by HLA class II proteins, and CD8+ T cells recognize antigens presented by HLA class I proteins. The CD3/TCR complex is responsible for recognition of antigen and generates and transduces the antigenic signal
CD4+ T cells	CD4+ T cells function mostly as helper T cells and secrete cytokines such as IL-2, a T-cell growth/death factor, and IFNγ, a proinflammatory polypeptide that can upregulate the expression of HLA proteins as well as augment cytotoxic activity of T cells and NK cells. Recently, two main types of CD4+ T cells have been recognized: CD4+ Th1 and CD4+ Th2. IL-2 and IFNγ are produced by CD4+ Th1 type cells, and IL-4 and IL-5 are secreted by CD4+ Th2 type cells. Each cell type regulates the secretion of the other, and the regulated secretion is important in the expression of host immunity
CD8+ T cells	CD8+ T cells function mainly as cytotoxic T cells. A subset of CD8+ T cells expresses suppressor cell function. CD8+ T cells can secrete cytokines such as IL-2, IFNγ, and can express molecules such as perforin, granzymes that function as effectors of cytotoxicity
APCs	Monocytes/macrophages and dendritic cells function as potent APCs. Donor's APCs can process and present donor antigens to recipient's T cells (direct recognition) or recipient's APCs can process and present donor antigens to recipient's T cells (indirect recognition). The relative contribution of direct recognition and indirect recognition to the antiallograft response has not been resolved. Direct recognition and indirect recognition might also have differential susceptibility to inhibition by immunosuppressive drugs
B cells	B cells require T-cell help for the differentiation and production of antibodies directed at donor antigens. The alloantibodies can damage the graft by binding and activating complement components (complement-dependent cytotoxicity) and/or binding the Fc receptor of cells capable of mediating cytotoxicity (antibody-dependent, cell-mediated cytotoxicity)
NK cells	The precise role of NK cells in the antiallograft response is not known. Increased NK cell activity has been correlated with rejection. NK cell function might also be important in immune surveillance mechanisms pertinent to the prevention of infection and malignancy

APCs, antigen presenting cells; IFN, interferon; IL, interleukin; NK, natural killer; TCR, T-cell antigen receptor.

ZAP-70 families. The CD45 protein, a tyrosine phosphatase, contributes to the activation process by dephosphorylating an autoinhibitory site on the p56^{lck} PTK. Intracellular domains of several TCR/CD3 proteins contain activation motifs that are crucial for antigen-stimulated signaling. Certain tyrosine residues within these motifs serve as targets for the catalytic activity of src family PTKs. Subsequently, these phosphorylated tyrosines serve as docking stations for the SH2 domains (recognition structures for select phosphotyrosine-containing motifs) of the ZAP-70 PTK. Following antigenic engagement of the TCR/CD3 complex, select serine residues of the TCR and CD3 chains are also phosphorylated.

The wave of tyrosine phosphorylation triggered by antigen recognition encompasses other intracellular proteins and is a cardinal event in initiating T-cell activation. Tyrosine phosphorylation of the phospholipase Cγ$_1$ activates this coenzyme and triggers a cascade of events that lead to full expression of T-cell programs: hydrolysis of phosphatidylinositol 4,5-biphosphate (PIP$_2$) and generation of two intracellular messengers, inositol 1,4,5-triphosphate (IP$_3$) and diacylglycerol [10]. IP$_3$, in turn, mobilizes ionized calcium from intracellular stores, while diacylglycerol, in the presence of increased cytosolic free Ca^{2+}, binds to and translocates protein kinase C (PKC) – a phospholipid/Ca^{2+}-sensitive protein serine/threonine

kinase – to the membrane in its enzymatically active form. Sustained activation of PKC is dependent on diacylglycerol generation from hydrolysis of additional lipids such as phosphatidylcholine.

The increase in intracellular free Ca^{2+} and sustained PKC activation promote the expression of several nuclear regulatory proteins (e.g. nuclear factor of activated T cells [NF-AT], nuclear factor kappa B [NF-κB], activator protein 1 [AP-1]) and the transcriptional activation and expression of genes central to T-cell growth (e.g. interleukin-2 [IL-2] and receptors for IL-2 and IL-15).

Calcineurin, a Ca^{2+}- and calmodulin-dependent serine/threonine phosphatase, is crucial to Ca^{2+}-dependent, TCR-initiated signal transduction [11]. Inhibition by cyclosporine and tacrolimus (FK506) of the phosphatase activity of calcineurin is considered central to their immunosuppressive activity [12,13].

Allograft rejection is contingent on the coordinated activation of alloreactive T cells and APCs (Fig. 1.1 and Table 1.2). Through the intermediacy of cytokines and cell-to-cell interactions, a heterogeneous contingent of lymphocytes, including CD4+ helper T cells, CD8+ cytotoxic T cells, antibody-forming B cells, and other proinflammatory leukocytes are recruited into the antiallograft response [14].

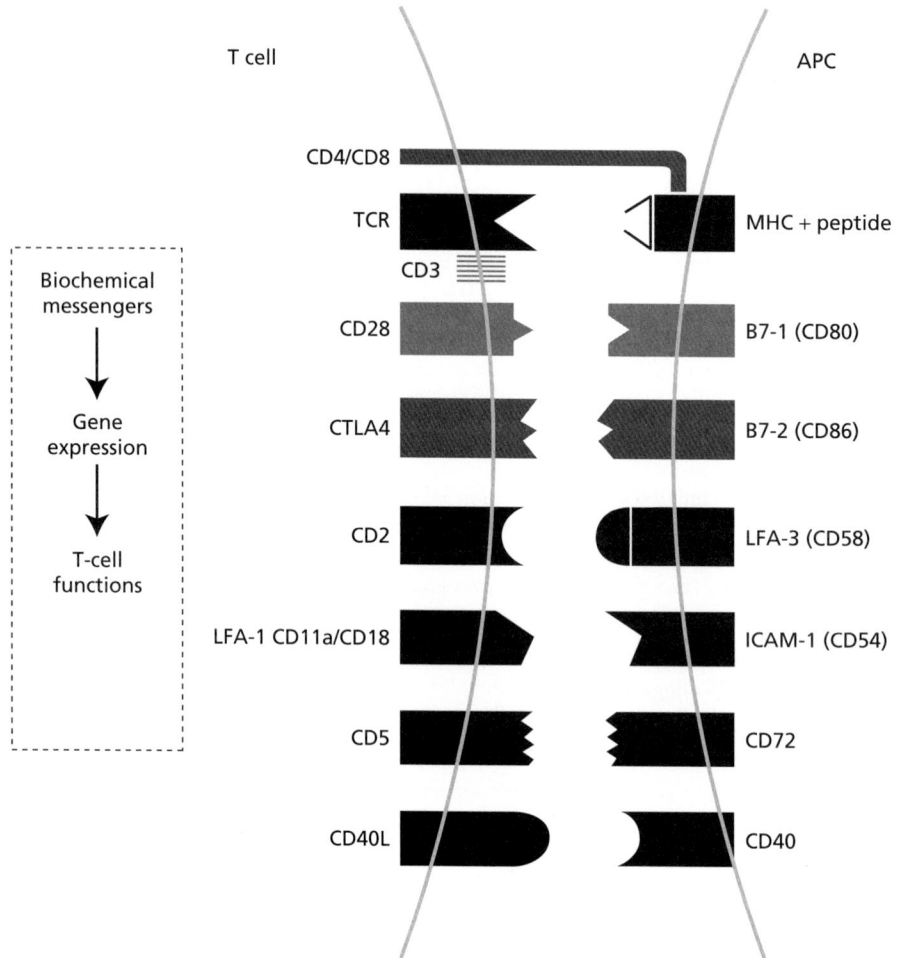

Fig. 1.2 T-cell/antigen-presenting cell contact sites. In this schema of T-cell activation, the antigenic signal is initiated by the physical interaction between the clonally variant T-cell antigen receptor (TCR) α, β-heterodimer and the antigenic peptide displayed by MHC on antigen-presenting cells (APCs). The antigenic signal is transduced into the cell by the CD3 proteins. The CD4 and the CD8 antigens function as associative recognition structures, and restrict TCR recognition to class II and class I antigens of MHC, respectively. Additional T-cell surface receptors generate the obligatory costimulatory signals by interacting with their counter-receptors expressed on the surface of the APCs. The simultaneous delivery to the T cells of the antigenic signal and the costimulatory signal results in the optimum generation of second messengers (such as calcium), expression of transcription factors (such as nuclear factor of activated T cells), and T-cell growth promoting genes (such as interleukin [IL]-2). The CD28 antigen as well as the CTLA4 antigen can interact with both the B7-1 and B7-2 antigens. The CD28 antigen generates a stimulatory signal, and the recent studies of CTLA4-deficient mice suggest that CTLA4, unlike CD28, generates a negative signal. CD, cluster designation; ICAM-1, intercellular adhesion molecule-1; LFA-1, leukocyte function-associated antigen 1; MHC, major histocompatibility complex. (Reproduced from Suthanthiran [48] with permission.)

COSTIMULATORY SIGNALS

Signaling of T cells via the TCR/CD3 complex (antigenic signal) is necessary, albeit insufficient, to induce T-cell proliferation; full activation is dependent on both the antigenic signals and the costimulatory signals (signal two) engendered by the contactual interactions between cell surface proteins expressed on antigen-specific T cells and APCs (Fig. 1.2; see Table 1.1) [15,16]. The interaction of the CD2 protein on the T-cell surface with the CD58 (leukocyte function-associated antigen 3 [LFA-3]) protein on the surface of APCs, and that of the CD11a/CD18 (LFA-1) proteins with the CD54 (intercellular adhesion molecule 1 [ICAM-1]) proteins [17], and/or the interaction of the CD5 with the CD72 proteins [8] aids in imparting such a costimulatory signal.

Recognition of the B7-1 (CD80) and B7-2 (CD86) proteins expressed upon CD4+ T cells generates a very powerful T-cell costimulus [18]. Monocytes and dendritic cells constitutively express CD86. Cytokines (e.g. granulocyte–macrophage colony-stimulating factor [GM-CSF] or γ-interferon [IFNγ]) stimulate expression of CD80 on monocytes, B cells, and dendritic cells. Many T cells express B7 binding proteins (i.e. CD28 proteins that are constitutively expressed on the surface of CD4+ T cells and CTLA-4 [CD152]), a protein whose ectodomain is closely related to that of CD28, and is expressed upon activated CD4+ and CD8+ T cells. CD28 binding of B7 molecules stimulates a Ca^{2+}-independent activation pathway that leads to stable transcription of the IL-2, IL-2 receptors, and other activation genes resulting in vigorous T-cell proliferation. For some time, the terms CD28 and the costimulatory receptor were considered synonymous by some, but the demonstration that robust T-cell activation occurs in CD28-deficient mice indicated that other receptor ligand systems contribute to signal two [19]. In particular the interaction between CD40 expressed upon APCs and CD40 ligand (CD154) expressed by antigen-activated CD4+ T cells has received great attention as a potent second signal [20].

The delivery of the antigenic signal and the costimulatory signal leads to stable transcription of the IL-2, several T-cell growth factor receptors, and other pivotal T-cell activation genes. The Ca^{2+}-independent costimulatory CD28 pathway is resistant to inhibition by cyclosporine or tacrolimus as compared to the calcium-dependent pathway of T-cell activation. In contrast, recognition of B7 proteins by CTLA-4, a protein primarily expressed on activated T cells, stimulates a negative signal to T cells and this signal is a prerequisite for peripheral T-cell tolerance [21].

The formulation that full T-cell activation is dependent on the costimulatory signal as well as the antigenic signal is significant, as T-cell molecules responsible for costimulation and their cognate receptors on the surface of APCs then represent target molecules for the regulation of the antiallograft response. Indeed, transplantation tolerance has been induced in experimental models by targeting a variety of cell-surface molecules that contribute to the generation of costimulatory signals.

INTERLEUKIN-2/INTERLEUKIN-15 STIMULATED T-CELL PROLIFERATION

T-cell proliferation occurs as a consequence of the T-cell activation-dependent production of IL-2 and the expression of multimeric high affinity IL-2 receptors on T cells formed by the noncovalent association of three IL-2 binding peptides (α, β, γ) [22–26]. IL-15 is a paracrine-type T-cell growth factor family member with very similar overall structural and identical T-cell stimulatory qualities to IL-2 [22]. The IL-2 and IL-15 receptor complexes share β and γ chains that are expressed in low abundance upon resting T cells; expression of these genes is amplified in activated T cells. The α-chain receptor components of the IL-2 and IL-15 receptor complexes are distinct and expressed upon activated, but not resting, T cells. The intracytoplasmic domains of the IL-2

receptor β and γ chains are required for intracellular signal transduction. The ligand-activated, but not resting, IL-2/IL-15 receptors are associated with intracellular PTKs [22,26–28]. Raf-1, a protein serine/threonine kinase that is prerequisite to IL-2/IL-15–triggered cell proliferation, associates with the intracellular domain of the shared β chain [29]. Translocation of IL-2 receptor-bound Raf-1 serine/threonine kinase into the cytosol requires IL-2/IL-15–stimulated PTK activity. The ligand-activated common γ chain recruits a member of the Janus kinase family, Jak 3, to the receptor complex that leads to activation of a member of the STAT family. Activation of this particular Jak-STAT pathway is prerequisite for proliferation of antigen-activated T cells. The subsequent events leading to IL-2/IL-15–dependent proliferation are not fully resolved; however, IL-2/IL-15–stimulated expression of several DNA binding proteins including bcl-2, c-jun, c-fos, and c-myc contributes to cell-cycle progression [30,31]. It is interesting and probably significant that IL-2, but not IL-15, triggers apoptosis of many antigen-activation T cells. In this way, IL-15–triggered events are more detrimental to the allograft response than IL-2. As IL-15 is not produced by T cells, IL-15 expression is not regulated by cyclosporine or tacrolimus.

IMMUNOBIOLOGY AND MOLECULAR FEATURES OF REJECTION

The net consequence of cytokine production and acquisition of cell-surface receptors for these transcellular molecules is the emergence of antigen-specific and graft-destructive T cells (see Fig. 1.1) [14]. Cytokines also facilitate the humoral arm of immunity by promoting the production of cytopathic antibodies. Moreover, IFNγ and tumor necrosis factor-α (TNFα) can amplify the ongoing immune response by up-regulating the expression of HLA molecules as well as costimulatory molecules (e.g. B7) on graft parenchymal cells and APCs. We and others have demonstrated the presence of antigen-specific cytotoxic T lymphocytes (CTL) and anti-HLA antibodies during, or preceding, a clinical rejection episode [32,33]. We have detected messenger RNA (mRNA) encoding the CTL-selective serine protease (granzyme B), perforin, and Fas-ligand attack molecules and immunoregulatory cytokines, such as IL-10 and IL-15, in human renal allografts undergoing acute rejection (reviewed in reference [34]). Indeed these gene-expression events can anticipate clinically apparent rejection. More recent efforts to develop a non-invasive method for the molecular diagnosis of rejection have proved rewarding. Using either peripheral blood [35] or urinary leukocytes [36] rejection-related, gene-expression events evident in renal biopsy specimens are also detected in peripheral blood or urinary sediment specimens. We suspect that a noninvasive, molecular-diagnostic approach to rejection may prove pivotal toward detection of insidious, clinically silent rejection episodes that, although rarely detected through standard measures, are steroid-sensitive but usually lead to chronic rejection [37].

The immune response directed at the allograft may not all be unidirectional and graft destructive; the immune repertoire appears to include both graft destructive immunity, as exemplified by the presence of granzyme B expressing cytopathic cells, and graft protective immunity, as exemplified by FoxP3$^+$CD25$^+$CD4$^+$ T-regulatory cells. Indeed, we and others have found that acute rejection of human allografts is associated not only with cytopathic cells but also with FoxP3$^+$ T-regulatory cells [38,39]. Emerging data also suggest that the outcome of an episode of acute rejection depends upon the balance between cytopathic cells and T-regulatory cells, with reversible acute rejection and renal graft salvage being associated with FoxP3 and T-regulatory cells [38].

TRANSPLANTATION TOLERANCE

There are many definitions of transplantation tolerance. We define clinical transplantation tolerance as an inability of the organ graft recipient to express a graft destructive immune response in the absence of exogenous immunosuppressive therapy. While this statement does not restrict either the mechanistic basis or the quantitative aspects of immune unresponsiveness of the host, tolerance is antigen-specific, induced as a consequence of prior exposure to the specific antigen, and is not dependent on the continuous administration of exogenous nonspecific immunosuppressants.

A classification of tolerance on the basis of the mechanisms involved, site of induction, extent of tolerance, and the cell primarily tolerized is provided in Table 1.3. Induction strategies for the creation of peripheral tolerance are listed in Table 1.4.

Table 1.3 Classification of tolerance.

A Based on the major mechanism involved
  1. Clonal deletion
  2. Clonal energy
  3. Suppression
B Based on the period of induction
  1. Fetal
  2. Neonatal
  3. Adult
C Based on the cell tolerized
  1. T cell
  2. B cell
D Based on the extent of tolerance
  1. Complete
  2. Partial, including split
E Based on the main site of induction
  1. Central
  2. Peripheral

Table 1.4 Potential approaches for the creation of tolerance.

A Cell depletion protocols
  1. Whole body irradiation
  2. Total lymphoid irradiation
  3. Panel of monoclonal antibodies
B Reconstitution protocols
  1. Allogeneic bone marrow cells with or without T-cell depletion
  2. Syngeneic bone marrow cells
C Combination of strategies A and B
D Cell-surface molecule targeted therapy
  1. Anti-CD4 mAbs
  2. Anti-ICAM-1 + anti-LFA-1 mAbs
  3. Anti-CD3 mAbs
  4. Anti-CD2 mAbs
  5. Anti-IL-2 receptor α (CD25) mAbs
  6. CTLA4Ig fusion protein
  7. Anti-CD40L mAbs
E Drugs
  1. Azathioprine
  2. Cyclosporine
  3. Rapamycin
F Additional approaches
  1. Donor-specific blood transfusions with concomitant mAb or drug therapy
  2. Intrathymic inoculation of cells/antigens
  3. Oral administration of cells/antigens

Several hypotheses, not necessarily mutually exclusive and at times even complementary, have been proposed for the cellular basis of tolerance. Data from several laboratories support the following mechanistic pathways – clonal deletion, clonal anergy, and immunoregulation – for the creation of a tolerant state.

Clonal deletion

Clonal deletion is a process by which self–antigen-reactive cells, (especially those with high affinity for the self-antigens), are eliminated from the organism's immune repertoire. This process is called central tolerance. In the case of T cells, this process takes place in the thymus, and the death of immature T cells is considered to be the ultimate result of high-affinity interactions between a T cell with productively rearranged TCR and the thymic nonlymphoid cells, including dendritic cells that express the self-MHC antigen. This purging of the immune repertoire of self-reactive T cells is termed negative selection and is distinguished from the positive selection process responsible for the generation of the T-cell repertoire involved in the recognition of foreign antigens in the context of self-MHC molecules. Clonal deletion, or at least marked depletion, of mature T cells as a consequence of apoptosis can also occur in the periphery (reviewed in reference [40]). The form of graft tolerance occurring as a consequence of mixed hematopoietic chimerism entails massive deletion of alloreactive clones [41]. Tolerance to renal allografts has been achieved in patients that have accepted a bone marrow graft from the same donor [42,43]. It is interesting that IL-2, the only T-cell growth factor that triggers T-cell proliferation as well as apoptosis, is an absolute prerequisite for the acquisition of organ graft tolerance through use of nonlymphoablative treatment regimens [44,45]. Tolerance achieved under these circumstances also involves additional mechanisms, including clonal anergy and suppressor mechanisms [46–48].

Clonal anergy

Clonal anergy refers to a process in which the antigen-reactive cells are functionally silenced. The cellular basis for the hyporesponsiveness resides in the anergic cell itself, and the current data suggest that the anergic T cells fail to express the T-cell growth factor, IL-2, and other crucial T-cell activation genes because of defects in the antigen-stimulated signaling pathway.

T-cell clonal anergy can result from suboptimal antigen-driven signaling of T cells, as mentioned earlier. The full activation of T cells requires at least two signals, one signal generated via the TCR/CD3 complex, and the second (costimulatory) signal initiated/delivered by the APCs. Stimulation of T cells via the TCR/CD3 complex alone – provision of antigenic signal without the obligatory costimulatory signal – can result in T-cell anergy/paralysis (Fig. 1.3 and Table 1.1).

B-cell activation, in a fashion analogous to T-cell activation, requires at least two signals. The first signal is initiated via the B-cell antigen receptor immunoglobulin, and a second costimulatory signal is provided by cytokines or cell surface proteins of T-cell origin. Thus, delivery of the antigenic signal alone to the B cells without the instructive cytokines or T-cell help can lead to B-cell anergy and tolerance.

Immunoregulatory (suppressor) mechanisms

Antigen-specific T or B cells are physically present and are functionally competent in tolerant states resulting from suppressor mechanisms. The cytopathic and antigen-specific cells are restrained by the suppressor cells or factors or express noncytopathic cellular programs. Each of the major subsets of T cells, the CD4 T cells and the CD8 T cells, has been implicated in mediating suppression. Indeed, a cascade involving MHC antigen-restricted T cells, MHC antigen-unrestricted T cells, and their secretory products have been reported to collaborate to mediate suppression. Recently, a subset of CD4+ T cells, the CD4+ CD25+ cells that express FoxP3, has been identified to mediate potent suppressive activity [49,50].

At least four distinct mechanisms have been advanced to explain the cellular basis for suppression: (i) An antiidiotypic regulatory mechanism in which the idiotype of the TCR of the original antigen-responsive T cells functions as an immunogen and elicits an antiidiotypic response. The elicited antiidiotypic regulatory cells, in turn, prevent the further responses of the idiotype-bearing cells to the original sensitizing stimulus; (ii) The veto process by which recognition by alloreactive T cells of alloantigen-expressing veto cells results in the targeted killing (veto process) of the original alloreactive T cells by the veto cells; (iii) Immune deviation, a shift in CD4+ T-cell programs away from Th1-type (IL-2, IFNγ expressing) toward the Th2-type (IL-4, IL-10 expressing) program; and (iv) The production of suppressor factors or cytokines. (e.g. the production of TGF-β by myelin basic protein-specific CD8 T cells or other cytokines with antiproliferative properties.) The process leading to full tolerance is infectious. Tolerant T cells recruit nontolerant T cells into the tolerant state [47]. The

Fig. 1.3 T-cell activation/anergy decision points. Several potential sites for the regulation of T-cell signaling are shown. The antigenic peptide displayed by major histocompatibility complex (MHC) (site 1), costimulatory signals (site 2), T-cell antigen receptor (TCR) (site 3), and cytokine signaling (site 4) can influence the eventual outcome. Altered peptide ligands, blockade of costimulatory signals, downregulation of TCR, and interleukin (IL)-10 favor anergy induction, whereas fully immunogenic peptides, delivery of costimulatory signals, appropriate number of TCRs, and IL-12 prevent anergy induction and facilitate full activation of T cells. (Reproduced from Suthanthiran [48] with permission.)

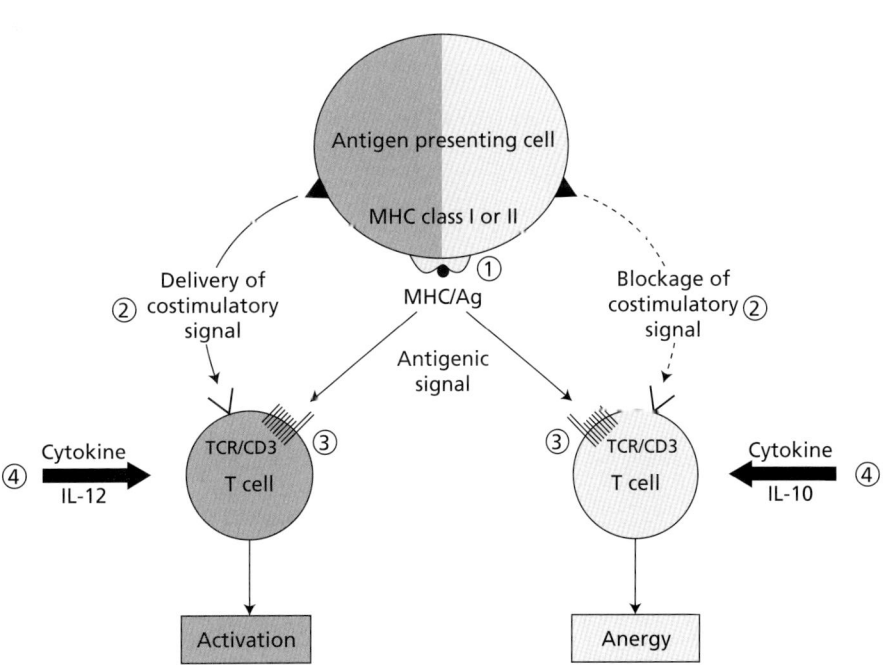

tolerant state also establishes a condition in which foreign tissues housed in the same microenvironment as the specific antigen to which the host has been tolerized are protected from rejection [47]. Tolerance is a multistep process [46–48].

Clearly more than one mechanism is operative in the induction of tolerance (see Fig. 1.3). The tolerant state is not an all-or-nothing phenomenon but is one that has several gradations. Of the mechanisms proposed for tolerance, clonal deletion might be of greater importance in the creation of self-tolerance, and clonal anergy and immunoregulatory mechanisms might be more applicable to transplantation tolerance. More recent data suggest both clonal depletion and immunoregulatory mechanisms are needed to create and sustain central or peripheral tolerance. From a practical viewpoint, a nonimmunogenic allograft (e.g. located in an immunologically privileged site or physically isolated from the immune system) might also be "tolerated" by an immuno-competent organ-graft recipient.

Authentic tolerance has been difficult to identify in human renal allograft recipients. Nevertheless, the clinical examples, albeit infrequent, of grafts functioning without any exogenous immunosuppressive drugs (either due to noncompliance of the patient or due to discontinuation of drugs for other medical reasons) does suggest that some long-term recipients of allografts develop tolerance to the transplanted organ and accept the allografts. The recent progress in our understanding of the immunobiology of graft rejection and tolerance and the potential to apply molecular approaches to the bedside hold significant promise for the creation of a clinically relevant tolerant state and transplantation without exogenous immuno-suppressants – the ultimate goal of the transplant physician.

ACKNOWLEDGMENTS

This chapter is adapted from an earlier chapter entitled "Immunobiology and immunopharmacology of renal allograft rejection" by M. Suthanthiran, C. Hartono and T.B. Strom. In: Schrier RW, ed. *Diseases of the Kidney and Urinary Tract*, 8th edn. Philadelphia, PA: Lippincott, Williams & Wilkins, 2006: 2540–52. The authors are grateful to Ms. Linda Stackhouse for her meticulous help in the preparation of this chapter.

REFERENCES

1 Unanue ER, Cerottini JC. Antigen presentation. *FASEB J* 1989;3:2496–502.
2 Jorgensen JL, Reay PA, Ehrich EW, *et al.* Molecular components of T cell recognition. *Annu Rev Immunol* 1992;10:835–73.
3 Germain RN. MHC-dependent antigen processing and peptide presentation: providing ligands for T lymphocyte activation. *Cell* 1994;76:287–99.
4 Acuto O, Cantrell D. T cell activation and the cytoskeleton. *Annu Rev Immunol* 2000;18:165–84.
5 Dustin ML, Cooper JA. The immunological synapse and the actin cytoskeleton: molecular hardware for T cell signaling. *Nature Immunol* 2000;1:23–9.
6 Brown MH, Cantrell DA, Brattsand G, *et al.* The CD2 antigen associates with the T-cell antigen receptor CD3 antigen complex on the surface of human T lymphocytes. *Nature* 1989;339:551–3.
7 Suthanthiran M. A novel model for the antigen-dependent activation of normal human T cells: transmembrane signaling by crosslinkage of the CD3/T cell receptor-alpha/beta complex with the cluster determinant 2 antigen. *J Exp Med* 1990;171:1965–79.
8 Beyers AD, Spruyt LL, Williams AF. Molecular associations between the T-lymphocyte antigen receptor complex and the surface antigens CD2, CD4, or CD8 and CD5. *Proc Natl Acad Sci USA* 1992;89:2945–9.
9 Shoskes DA, Wood KJ. Indirect presentation of MHC antigens in transplantation. *Immunol Today* 1994;15:32–8.
10 Nishizuka Y. Intracellular signaling by hydrolysis of phospholipids and activation of protein kinase C. *Science* 1992;258:607–14.
11 Clipstone NA, Crabtree GR. Identification of calcineurin as a key signalling enzyme in T-lymphocyte activation. *Nature* 1992;357:695–7.
12 O'Keefe SJ, Tamura J, Kincaid RL, *et al.* FK506- and CsA-sensitive activation of the IL-2 promoter by calcineurin. *Nature* 1992;357:692–4.
13 Liu J, Farmer JD Jr, Lane WS, *et al.* Calcineurin is a common target of cyclophilin-cyclosporin A and FKBP-FK506 complexes. *Cell* 1991;66:807–15.
14 Suthanthiran M, Strom TB. Renal transplantation. *N Engl J Med* 1994;334:365–76.
15 Schwartz RH. T cell anergy. *Sci Am* 1993;269:62–3; 66–71.
16 Suthanthiran M. Signaling features of T cells: implication for the regulation of the anti-allograft response. *Kidney Int Suppl* 1993;43:S3–11.
17 Dustin ML, Springer TA. T-cell receptor cross-linking transiently stimulates adhesiveness through LFA-1. *Nature* 1989;341:619–24.
18 Lenschow DJ, Walunas TL, Bluestone JA. CD28/B7 system of T cell costimulation. *Annu Rev Immunol* 1996;14:233–58.
19 Shahinian A, Pfeffer K, Lee KP, *et al.* Differential T cell co-stimulatory requirements in CD28-deficient mice. *Science* 1993;261:609–12.
20 Noelle RJ. CD40 and its ligand in host defense. *Immunity* 1996;4:415–9.
21 Oosterwegel MA, Greenwald RJ, Mandelbrot DA, *et al.* CTLA-4 and T cell activation. *Curr Opin Immunol* 1999;11:294–300.
22 Waldmann T, Tagaya Y, Bamford R. Interleukin-2, interleukin-15, and their receptors. *Int Rev Immunol* 1998;16:205–26.
23 Smith KA. Interleukin-2: inception, impact, and implications. *Science* 1988;240:1169–76.
24 Waldman TA. The interleukin-2 receptor. *J Biol Chem* 1991;266:2681–4.
25 Takeshita T, Asao H, Ohtani K. Cloning of the gamma chain of the human IL-2 receptor. *Science* 1992;257:379–82.
26 Hatakeyama M, Kono T, Kobayashi N, *et al.* Interaction of the IL-2 receptor with the src-family kinase p56[lck]: identification of novel intermolecular association. *Science* 1991;252:1523–8.

27 Fung MR, Scearce RM, Hoffman JA, *et al*. A tyrosine kinase physically associates with the beta-subunit of the human IL-2 receptor. *J Immunol* 1991;**147**:1253–60.

28 Remillard B, Petrillo R, Maslinski W, *et al*. Interleukin-2 receptor regulates activation of phosphatidylinositol 3-kinase. *J Biol Chem* 1991;**266**:14 167–70.

29 Maslinski W, Remillard B, Tsudo M, *et al*. Interleukin-2 (IL-2) induces tyrosine kinase-dependent translocation of active Raf-1 from the IL-2 receptor into the cytosol. *J Biol Chem* 1992;**267**:15 281–4.

30 Shibuya H, Yoneyama M, Ninomiya-Tsuji J, *et al*. IL-2 and EGF receptors stimulate the hematopoietic cell cycle via different signaling pathways: demonstration of a novel role for c-myc. *Cell* 1992;**70**:57–67.

31 Taniguchi T. Cytokine signalling through non-receptor protein tyrosine kinases. *Science* 1995;**260**:251–5.

32 Strom TB, Tilney NL, Carpenter CB, *et al*. Identity and cytotoxic capacity of cells infiltrating renal allografts. *N Engl J Med* 1975;**292**:1257–63.

33 Suthanthiran M, Garovoy MR. Immunologic monitoring of the renal transplant recipient. *Urol Clin North Am* 1983;**10**:315–25.

34 Strom TB, Suthanthiran M. Prospects and applicability of molecular diagnosis of allograft rejection. *Semin Nephrol* 2000;**20**:103–7.

35 Vasconcellos LM, Schachter AD, Zheng XX, *et al*. Cytotoxic lymphocyte gene expression in peripheral blood leukocytes correlates with rejecting renal allografts. *Transplantation* 1998;**66**:562–6.

36 Li B, Hartono C, Ding R, *et al*. Noninvasive diagnosis of renal-allograft rejection by measurement of messenger RNA for perforin and granzyme B in urine. *N Engl J Med* 2001;**344**:947–54.

37 Rush D, Nickerson P, Gough J, *et al*. Beneficial effects of treatment of early subclinical rejection: a randomized study. *J Am Soc Nephrol* 1998;**9**:2129–34.

38 Muthukumar T, Dadhania D, Ding R, *et al*. Messenger RNA for FOXP3 in the urine of renal allograft recipients. *New Engl J Med* 2005;**353**:2342–51.

39 Baan CC, van der Mast BJ, Klepper M, *et al*. Differential effect of calcineurin inhibitors. Anti-CD25 antibodies and rapamycin on the induction of FOXP3 in human T cells. *Transplantation* 2005;**80**:110–7.

40 Van Parijs L, Abbas AK. Homeostasis and self-tolerance in the immune system: turning lymphocytes off. *Science* 1998;**280**:243–8.

41 Wekerle T, Sayegh MH, Hill J, *et al*. Extrathymic T cell deletion and allogeneic stem cell engraftment induced with costimulatory blockade is followed by central T cell tolerance. *J Exp Med* 1998;**187**:2037–44.

42 Sayegh MH, Fine NA, Smith JL, *et al*. Immunologic tolerance to renal allografts after bone marrow transplants from the same donors. *Ann Intern Med* 1991;**114**:954–5.

43 Spitzer TR, Delmonico F, Tolkoff-Rubin N, *et al*. Combined histocompatibility leukocyte antigen-matched donor bone marrow and renal transplantation for multiple myeloma with end stage renal disease: the induction of allograft tolerance through mixed lymphohematopoietic chimerism. *Transplantation* 1999;**68**: 480–4.

44 Dai Z, Konieczny BT, Baddoura FK, *et al*. Impaired alloantigen-mediated T cell apoptosis and failure to induce long-term allograft survival in IL-2-deficient mice. *J Immunol* 1998;**161**: 1659–63.

45 Li Y, Li XC, Zheng XX, *et al*. Blocking both signal 1 and signal 2 of T-cell activation prevents apoptosis of alloreactive T cells and induction of peripheral allograft tolerance. *Nature Med* 1999;**5**:1298–302.

46 Li SC, Wells AD, Strom TB, *et al*. The role of T cell apoptosis in transplantation tolerance. *Curr Opin Immunol* 2000;**12**:522–7.

47 Waldmann H. Transplantation tolerance – where do we stand? *Nature Med* 1999;**5**:1245–8.

48 Suthanthiran M. Transplantation tolerance: fooling mother nature. *Proc Natl Acad Sci USA* 1996;**93**:12 072–5.

49 Sakaguchi S, Sakaguchi N, Shimizu J, *et al*. Immunologic tolerance maintained by CD25⁺CD4⁺ regulatory T cells: their common role in controlling autoimmunity, tumor immunity, and transplantation tolerance. *Immunol Rev* 2001;**182**:18–32.

50 Maloy KJ, Powrie F. Regulatory T cells in the control of immune pathology. *Nat Immunol* 2001;**2**:816–22.

51 Suthanthiran M, Hartono C, Strom TB. Immunobiology and immunopharmacology of renal allograft rejection. In: Schrier RW, ed. *Diseases of the Kidney and Urinary Tract*, 8th edn. Philadelphia, PA: Lippincott, Williams & Wilkin, 2006: 2540–52.

52 Suthanthiran M, Morris RE, Strom TB. Transplantation immunobiology. In: Walsh PC, Retik AB, Vaughn ED Jr, *et al*., eds. *Campbell's Urology*, 7th edn. Philadelphia, PA: W.B. Saunders, 1997:491–504.

2 Allorecognition Pathways

Nader Najafian and Mohamed H. Sayegh

Allorecognition is the ability of T cells to respond to foreign histocompatibility antigens of other members of the same species. The major histocompatibility complex (MHC) molecules were originally discovered by their ability to induce serologic responses and rejection of tumor and skin grafts in mice [1,2]. It is now clear that the MHC antigens are the primary antigens responsible for causing graft rejection and are generally associated with a brisk time course of rejection. Allograft rejection is a T-cell-dependent process [3]; animals that lack T cells do not reject an allograft. T lymphocytes initiate the immune response, which ultimately results in graft rejection. Allorecognition is the essential first step for triggering the cascade of events that results in rejection of the graft. Once activated, they secrete cytokines and chemokines to activate and attract various effector cells, such as CD8+ T cells and macrophages into the allograft. They are also able to interact with B cells which will secrete highly specific alloreactive antibodies. These cells in turn mediate the effector mechanisms of allograft destruction. Experimental and clinical data have confirmed that there are two distinct, nonmutually exclusive pathways of T-cell allorecognition: the "direct" and "indirect" pathways (Fig. 2.1) [4–6]. The "direct" pathway describes the ability of T cells through the T-cell receptor to engage and respond to *intact* allogeneic MHC molecules on the surface of antigen-presenting cells (APCs). This pathway is responsible for the vigorous *in vitro* response demonstrated in the primary allogeneic mixed lymphocyte reaction (MLR). *In vivo*, the direct pathway appears to be the principal route of T-cell sensitization leading to acute allograft rejection. The "indirect" pathway refers to the recognition of donor antigens presented as peptides in association with self-MHC by recipient APCs. This corresponds to the normal pathway of T-cell recognition of foreign or autoantigens in the context of self-MHC molecules such as the case in infections and autoimmune diseases. The following includes recent data about the role of allorecognition pathways in allograft rejection, both at the stage of priming of T cells and of effector phase of rejection. The importance of these pathways in developing tolerance-inducing strategies in organ transplantation is also reviewed.

DIRECT PATHWAY OF ALLORECOGNITION

Direct refers to cell recognition of a whole intact foreign MHC molecule on the surface of donor cells. Although the specific peptide (typically derived from endogenous proteins, including MHC antigens, see below) bound in the groove of the MHC molecule may be important in this recognition process, it does not restrict this response. The graft, which includes donor bone marrow-derived APCs, usually expresses several class I and II MHC molecules that differ from the recipient's MHC molecules, and which can directly stimulate recipients T cells. Donor APCs prime CD4+ and CD8+ T cells through the direct pathway. However, as these donor APCs are destroyed during the priming process, direct T-cell priming is likely to be time-limited. Thus, direct allorecognition may account for early acute cellular rejection. Consistent with this concept, direct alloreactivity was not detectable in the peripheral blood of a cohort of renal and lung allograft recipients with chronic allograft dysfunction several years after transplantation [7–9].

Two features of the direct pathway serve to define the strength of the allogeneic response [10]. First of all, the precursor frequency of T cells that directly recognize allo-MHC is unusually high, 100–1000 times higher than the response to nominal antigens [11]. Second, unlike the response to nominal antigens, the direct response to allo-MHC requires no previous exposure or priming (i.e. can be initiated by naïve T cells). Over the years, several theories have emerged to explain the molecular basis of the strength of the direct pathway of allorecognition.

Matzinger and Bevan [12] hypothesized that the high precursor frequency of alloreactive T cells is secondary to the high frequency of different allogeneic determinants presented on allogeneic APCs (determinant frequency theory). Formulated prior to our understanding of MHC-restricted peptide presentation, this model suggested that the each allo-MHC molecule was an "interaction antigen" and could form "binary complexes" with all other cell surface proteins on the membrane surface. The resulting complex of allo-MHC + X (where X is a cell surface protein) could interact with the T-cell receptor. Each allo-MHC could form a large

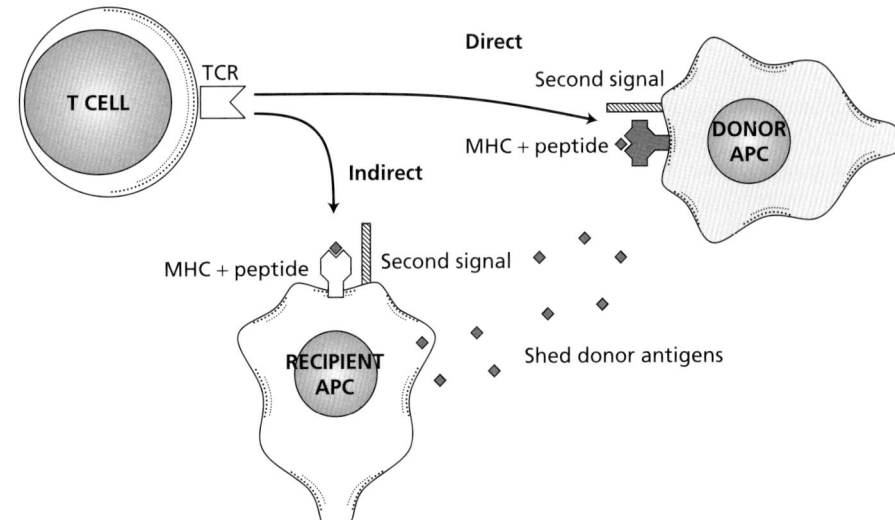

Fig. 2.1 Pathways of T-cell allorecognition. In the "direct" pathway, recipient T cells recognize intact allo-MHC + peptide complex on the surface of donor antigen-pesenting cells (APCs). In the "indirect" pathway, recipient T cells recognize processed allopeptides (derived primarily from MHC antigens) presented by recipient APCs.

number of different antigenic complexes with different cell surface receptors and create a high frequency of antigenic determinants. This theory predicts that the high precursor frequency of alloreactive T cells results from the ability of a single allogeneic APC to stimulate many T-cell clones because of the large number of different determinants created by allo-MHC and a cell surface receptor.

Bevan [13] later proposed an alternative theory to explain the phenomenon of alloreactivity. In this theory, alloreactive T cells recognize a determinant on the foreign MHC molecule itself, and the peptides being presented by the MHC is not of central importance. All the foreign MHC molecules (approximately 100 000) can serve to stimulate T cells with low-affinity receptors by creating a high density of foreign determinants (high determinant density theory). In contrast, the density of foreign determinants created by the presentation of a foreign peptide in the context of self-MHC would be quite low, as most of the self-MHC molecules would be presenting self-peptides. When the determinant density is high, as in the case of allogeneic APCs, even low-affinity T cells can be activated.

The determinant frequency and determinant density theories need not be mutually exclusive. In fact, experimental evidence now supports the notion that both the conformation of the MHC molecule itself and the peptide–MHC complex can determine alloreactivity [14–17].

Lechler *et al.* [18] used results from studies of specific HLA-DR primed T-cell clones to postulate that allorecognition is structurally heterogeneous and varies according to the responder and stimulator MHC types. In closely related MHC combinations, allorecognition would be caused by T cells recognizing novel endogenous peptides that have never been encountered by responder T cells. In more disparate MHC combinations, the alloresponse would be directed primarily against the residues on the allo-MHC itself, and the bound peptide would have a minimal role. T-cell recognition

of allo-MHC would thus be secondary to "molecular mimicry" by the allo-MHC of the three-dimensional complex of self-MHC + peptide. The "molecular mimicry" hypothesis may explain how a T cell positively selected to recognize foreign antigens in the context of self-MHC can now recognize and react to an intact allo-MHC molecule.

The concept of positive and negative selection in the thymus also helps to explain the strength of the alloimmune response [19]. During development, T cells with receptors of too high affinity are deleted (negative selection), whereas those with too low affinity are not selected. The end result of this selection is that TCRs of intermediate affinity exit the thymus and enter the periphery. Within an individual, clonal deletion occurs early in development. Potentially, autoreactive clones (with too high affinity for self) are deleted; failure of deletion of some clones may lead to autoimmunity. In the case of transplantation across an allelic difference, however, the recipient's T cells do not contact allo-MHC molecules during development in the thymus and thus escape the deletion (negative selection) imposed by interaction with self-MHC. Thus, the end result is the large number of donor MHC–peptide complexes on the graft to which a potential recipient has not been tolerized during ontogeny. Moreover, the relatively low affinity of any given TCR for its ligand suggest that each T cell could potentially recognize more than one MHC–peptide complex [20]. The high density of alloantigens on the surface of an allograft additionally contributes to the strong T-cell response.

STRUCTURE OF THE MHC MOLECULE AND ALLORECOGNITION

A key to our understanding of the molecular basis of allorecognition was the resolution of the X-ray crystal structure of the human class I MHC HLA-A2 molecule by Wiley and

Strominger [21]. The polymorphic sequences of the MHC molecule were found to be primarily within the peptide-binding groove, which contained not a single peptide but rather a heterogeneous population of peptides [22,23]. The implication of this important discovery was that a single MHC gene actually presented an array of thousands of different peptides within the peptide-binding groove [24–26]. MHC polymorphism thus serves to diversify the identity of different peptides that could bind within the peptide-binding site.

The concept that a number of different peptides could fit into the groove of a single MHC molecule is consistent with the high determinant frequency theory of Matzinger and Bevan. The high frequency of foreign determinants could reflect the diversity of "interaction antigens" created by a single allo-MHC molecule presenting a multitude of different cellular peptides.

ROLE OF ENDOGENOUS PEPTIDES IN ALLORECOGNITION

Emerging studies with T-cell clones have demonstrated that MHC-bound endogenous peptides are integral to T-cell allorecognition. For example, alloreactivity of T cells to class II MHC molecules is diminished after incubation of class II-bearing APCs with an exogenous influenza peptide, suggesting that the exogenous peptide blocked presentation of a particular endogenous peptide required for allorecognition [27]. Furthermore, several studies using CD4+ T-cell clones showed that reactivity to cells expressing the appropriate class II molecule depended on the type of cell expressing the class II antigens [28,29]. Alloreactivity required not only the appropriate allogeneic class II molecule but also the proper endogenous peptide expressed by the particular cell type.

The identification of mutant cell lines, such as T2 and RMA-S [30–32], that are defective in processing and transporting endogenous peptides further confirmed the necessity of MHC-bound peptides for allorecognition. When the human T2 cell line was transfected with the murine class I K^b gene, K^b was expressed on the cell surface in normal levels. However, all the K^b molecules lacked peptide. Most K^b-specific cytotoxic T lymphocyte (CTL) clones could not recognize the T2-K^b transfectants unless the cells were loaded with cytoplasmic peptides [33]. One clone was able to recognize empty K^b molecules, but the level of lysis was 10- to 100-fold lower than the level of lysis observed after peptide loading. Thus, it appears that the MHC-bound peptides create or stabilize the conformational determinants necessary for the interaction between the T-cell receptor (TCR) and MHC receptor. The resulting structural unit of recognition is a trimolecular complex formed by the TCR, the MHC molecule, and the MHC-bound peptide.

While numerous studies suggest that the majority of T cells recognize allo-MHC + peptide complex, there is evidence that some alloreactive T cells can recognize empty MHC molecules. Human T-cell clones specific for the human class I HLA-A2 antigen were able to respond to empty HLA-A2 molecules [34]. Further studies using the RMA-S cell line, which lacks the peptide transporter gene, have demonstrated that CTLs can lyse targets expressing empty class I molecules [35,36].

In addition to the importance of the presence of peptides bound to the peptide-binding groove, conformational changes of the MHC–peptide complex may also be important. Bluestone et al. [14,37] demonstrated that conformational changes induced by the peptide bound to the peptide-binding groove in class I MHC can alter T-cell alloreactivity. Thus, alloreactivity of some T-cell clones may be peptide dependent but not peptide specific. The conformational determinants created by MHC binding to peptide may determine whether or not the TCR can interact with the MHC molecule. Two different peptides may produce similar conformational determinants within the peptide-binding groove of the same MHC. This concept would predict the observation of cross-reactive allorecognition to unrelated peptides, which is supported by the literature.

INDIRECT PATHWAY OF ALLORECOGNITION

Indirect refers to T-cell recognition of nonself-MHC-derived peptides (allopeptides) in the context of self-MHC molecules expressed on recipient APCs. In this case, similar to the physiologic pathway of antigen recognition, the peptide sequence determines the response. Indirect presentation could occur through a number of mechanisms: soluble donor MHC molecules are shed from the graft, drain through the bloodstream or lymphatics to the recipient secondary lymphoid organs where they would be processed and/or presented by recipient APCs to recipient T cells. Alternatively, donor graft cells that migrate to recipient secondary secondary lymphoid organs could be endocytosed by recipient APCs. Third, recipient monocyte–macrophages entering the donor graft could endocytose donor antigens and present the peptides to recipient T cells. Interestingly, recent emerging data demonstrate that not only CD4+ T cells, as traditionally thought, but also CD8+ T cells can be primed through the indirect pathway of allorecognition and contribute to graft destruction [38].

Unlike the direct pathway, the indirect pathway requires previous priming to antigen. Moreover, the precursor frequency of T cells that can recognize a specific antigen through the indirect pathway is relatively low; 100–1000 times lower than that for directly alloreactive T cells. Until recently, most investigations in transplantation only addressed the direct pathway of allorecognition and very little was known about the contribution of the indirect pathway in graft rejection. The existence of the indirect pathway of allorecognition was originally suggested by Lechler and Batchelor [39,40] in the early 1980s based on rodent studies with passenger cell depleted kidney allografts. Subsequently, numerous studies have confirmed the ability of the indirect pathway of allorecognition to induce the complete gamut of alloresponses, including proliferation and cytokine production by CD4[+] T-helper cells [41], delayed-type hypersensitivity responses (42), CTL generation [43], and antidonor immunoglobulin G (IgG) formation by B cells [44]. Moreover, the indirect alloresponse was shown to comprise a significant proportion, approximately 10–15%, of the overall alloresponse in mice [45]. Using very sensitive EliSpot assays, this response was found to be directed primarily to MHC-derived peptides [45]. Several studies in rodents have clearly demonstrated a role for the indirect pathway in graft rejection [41,43,46–49]. In a vascularized cardiac allograft model, immunization of rats with donor class II MHC allopeptides also accelerated rejection with augmentation and acceleration of cellular and humoral responses [50]. More recently, the role of indirect allorecognition has been demonstrated in recipients of kidney, heart and lung transplants with biopsy-proven chronic rejection.

One feature of indirect allorecognition is the phenomenon of *immunodominance*. In mouse and human models of transplantation, recipient MHC-restricted T-cell responses were found to be invariably limited to a single or a few dominant epitopes on the donor MHC antigen [51–53]. These immunodominant epitopes represent allogeneic determinants that are efficiently processed and presented by host APCs to activate T cells. A *cryptic* epitope is a determinant that meets the structural requirements for MHC binding and can be potentially immunogenic to T cells. However, in the presence of the dominant epitope, the cryptic determinant does not effectively activate T cells. The precise mechanism of immunodominance is not definitively known, but competition for MHC binding may be responsible as removal of the dominant epitope often leads to unmasking of the cryptic determinants [54]. Immunodominance thus reflects a hierarchy of allogeneic determinants that are recognized by T cells via the indirect pathway. During graft rejection, recipient T cells are sensitized to a limited number of allogeneic determinants, despite the presence of numerous other foreign determinants.

A second feature of the indirect pathway is *epitope* or *antigen spreading*. This phenomenon refers to the observation that the hierarchy of allogeneic determinants of donor MHC peptides that are recognized through the indirect pathway can change during the course of rejection. For example, early in the course of rejection, T-cell responses are limited to a single or a few immunodominant determinants. In time, the alloresponse may shift to another allodeterminant on the same (intramolecular spreading) or different MHC molecule (intermolecular spreading). In a murine model of allogeneic skin grafts, the T-cell response was initially limited to one donor class I MHC peptide during acute rejection. However, 21 days post-transplant, T-cell reactivity to a formerly cryptic determinant on the same donor class I MHC molecule was detected [41,51]. This spreading of antigenic determinants may reflect differences in antigen processing from various anatomic sites or differences in T-cell trafficking during the rejection process. Epitope spreading may be prove essential for the amplification and progression of allograft rejection as the emergence of different allogeneic determinants leads to the recruitment of new alloreactive T-cell clones over time.

INDIRECT ALLORECOGNITION AND CHRONIC REJECTION

One theory to explain the contribution of direct versus indirect recognition in graft rejection suggests that direct allorecognition may mediate acute rejection as the donor graft contains a high density of passenger leukocytes, which display intact allo-MHC molecules. The corollary hypothesis is that direct allorecognition becomes less important as passenger leukocytes are replaced by self-APCs in time. Subsequently, the indirect pathway of allorecognition may predominate and lead to a smoldering form of rejection (i.e. chronic rejection) [4]. In fact, the strength of the T-cell response through the direct pathway of allorecognition may be so vigorous that it may be capable of inducing only acute and not chronic rejection [55]. The low precursor frequency of indirectly primed T cells is consistent with the hypothesis that small numbers of peptide-primed T cells mediate an indolent immune response, which reflects the natural history of chronic rejection. Because recipient monocytes migrating through the allograft can constantly endocytose donor antigen, priming through the indirect pathway could occur for as long as the graft is present in the host. Thus, while indirect alloreactive T cells may participate in acute rejection, they may have a predominant role in chronic rejection [56]. Consistent with this concept, several groups have now provided data correlating the indirect alloreactive T cells with the presence of chronic allograft dysfunction [57,58]. Recent clinical and experimental studies provide further support for the role of indirect recognition in chronic rejection [58,59]. Heart and liver transplant recipients undergoing chronic rejection display indirect alloreactivity to donor MHC peptides and epitope spreading to different determinants on donor MHC molecules [59]. Interestingly, the occurrence of epitope spreading was correlated with the frequency of chronic rejection [59] in heart and liver transplant patients. More recently, several studies demonstrated a correlation between indirect allorecognition of mismatched donor class I- and class II-derived peptides and the development of bronchiolitis obliterans syndrome (BOS) [9,60–62]. Experimentally, APC-depleted rat renal allografts are not acutely rejected but remain susceptible to chronic rejection [40]. Furthermore, long-surviving MHC-incompatible rat renal allografts that are parked in a primary recipient did not elicit acute rejection when retransplanted into a secondary recipient, but nevertheless succumbed to chronic rejection [63]. A mechanistic link between the indirect alloresponse and the morphologic changes of chronic rejection has been suggested by recent studies in which immunization of T cells with donor-derived MHC allopeptides accelerated and exacerbated the development of vasculitis in a rat cardiac allograft model [50]. In a murine cardiac transplant model, heart recipients who have only CD4+ T cells and an intact indirect pathway do not reject the allografts acutely, but develop chronic rejection [64]. Using a clinically relevant large animal model of cardiac transplantation in pigs, inbred miniature swine immunized with swine leukocyte antigen class I allopeptides developed significant obstructive coronary artery lesions after receiving donor MHC class I disparate hearts [65]. These results suggest that the indirect alloresponse may be a significant contributor to the development of transplant vasculopathy, the hallmark of chronic rejection of vascularized organs.

Another interesting observation to support an important role for indirect allorecognition in chronic rejection is the recent findings by Hornick *et al.* [66] in cardiac transplant recipients showing evidence of donor-specific hyporesposiveness of T cells reactive via the direct pathway in patients with chronic vasculopathy. Similarly, lung transplant recipients with BOS become hyporesponsive via the direct route but are sensitized via the indirect pathway [9]. Taken together, these experimental and clinical results have led to the formulation of a hypothesis linking indirect recognition and chronic rejection of vascularized organs (Fig. 2.2). Small numbers of indirectly primed T cells are targeted against a limited repertoire of immunodominant MHC peptides in the early post-transplant period. As the importance of the direct pathway wanes over time with the depletion of passenger leukocytes, the importance of the indirect pathway increases as T cells begin to recognize new epitopes (epitope spreading). Indirectly primed T cells produce cytokines, activate macrophages and provide help for B cells and precursor CTLs. The wall of intra-parenchymal graft vessels is targeted resulting in a low-grade inflammation and neointimal proliferation (i.e. transplant vasculopathy). Transplant vasculopathy leads to graft fibrosis and failure. This smoldering process occurs during a period in which immunosuppression is being reduced.

ENDOTHELIAL CELLS AND ALLORECOGNITION

Endothelial cells of donor origin are located at the interface between the recipient's blood and the allograft and have been implicated in graft rejection [5]. Graft endothelial cells express MHC class I and II molecules and have been shown recently to promote direct allorecognition by serving as APCs and as targets for T-cell-mediated cytotoxicity, although a more recent study suggested that vascular endothelium does not have an important role, at least in CD4+ direct allo-recognition [67]. In addition, endothelial cells may promote indirect allorecognition by a cross-talk mechanism, which

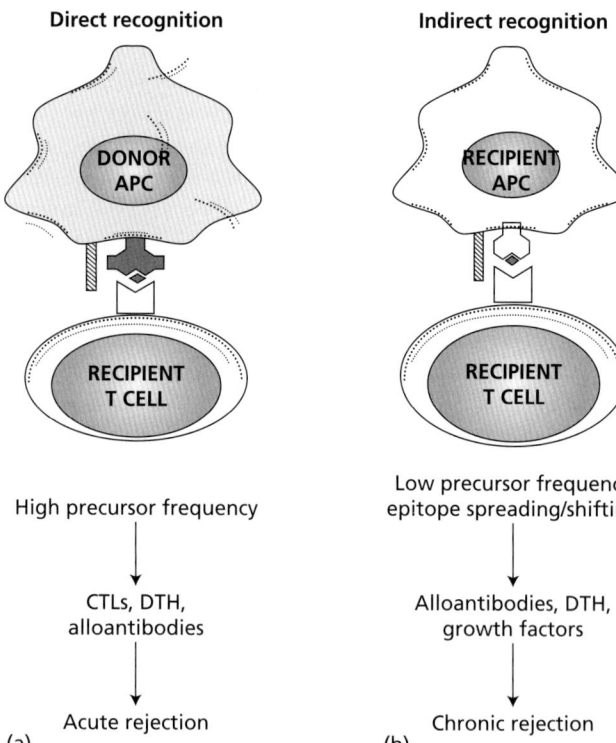

Fig. 2.2 A proposed link between indirect allorecognition (a) and chronic rejection (b). T cells that are primed to intact allo-MHC through the direct pathway are present in high frequency and induce cytotoxic T lymphocyte (CTL) formation, delayed-type hypersensitivity (DTH)-like responses, and alloantibody formation leading to acute cellular rejection. If acute rejection is suppressed, donor antigen-pesenting cells (APCs) are replaced by recipient APCs and T cells recognize donor antigens through the indirect pathway. Because present at a low precursor frequency, the indirectly primed T cells lead to a smoldering rejection with the production of alloantibodies, cytokines, chemokines and various growth factors (e.g. platelet-derived growth factor [PDGF], fibroblast growth factor [FGF], transforming growth factor β [TGF-β]). T cells are sensitized to different donor epitopes during the course of rejection (epitope spreading/shifting). Transplant vasculopathy, the hallmark of chronic rejection, results.

involves the recruitment and transformation of recipient monocytes by endothelial cells into highly efficient antigen-presenting dendritic cells capable of presenting allopeptides via the indirect pathway [5].

SITE OF ALLORECOGNITION

Finally, there has been recent interest in studying where T cells meet the transplant antigens [5]. The site of alloantigen recognition had until recently been believed to be in the allograft itself, but recent data seem to indicate that peripheral lymphoid organs are required for allograft rejection [68]. Whether unprimed T cells encounter antigens first outside of the allograft in peripheral lymphoid tissue or whether they migrate to secondary lymphoid organs after they encounter the alloantigens in the graft for further maturation and differentiation remains controversial. Interestingly, primed/effector/memory cells appear to mediate graft rejection independent of peripheral lymphoid organs, suggesting that they are activated by alloantigens in the graft itself [68].

ROLE OF ALLORECOGNITION IN THE EFFECTOR PHASE OF ALLOGRAFT REJECTION

Allorecognition is the initial first step for activation and priming of T cells and it has a role in effector mechanisms leading to allograft destruction. Transplant rejection has both cellular (delayed-type hypersensitivity [DTH] responses, cell-mediated cytotoxicity) and humoral components. Once fully activated via the direct or indirect pathway, T cells produce cytokines and chemokines which orchestrate various effector arms of the alloimmune response. Primed CD4+ T cells can provide help for production of alloantibody, and can also provide helper signals required for the induction of CD8+ CTLs [6,69], both of which can subsequently mediate graft injury. Moreover, CD4+ T cells capable of recognizing donor antigen on donor cells can directly mediate acute graft rejection [70], but there is some evidence that this outcome is frequency dependent [71]. Below a certain frequency threshold, primed T cells may not reject the transplanted organ but may alternatively be capable of inducing chronic injury that results in fibrosis and vasculopathy, characteristic of chronic allograft dysfunction [72]. Furthermore, directly primed Th1 cells and macrophages can mediate DTH reactions and contribute to the destruction of the graft. In that setting, it is hypothesized that some of the cytokines produced by T cells and macrophages may mediate apoptosis of graft cells. The pathology of a transplanted organ may also be dependent on the specific graft cell with which the primed T cells interact. It is tempting to speculate that direct recognition of donor endothelial cells by primed CD8+ T cells may participate in those acute rejections associated with pathologic evidence of vasculitis [73]. On the other hand, if intragraft donor parenchymal cells are the predominant targets of the direct alloresponse, acute rejection may appear as the classically described mononuclear cell infiltration with tubulitis. Analogous to T cells functioning through the direct pathway, indirectly primed CD4+ T cells preferentially differentiate into a proinflammatory type-1 cytokine-secreting phenotype [45], and provide helper signals to induce alloantibodies and cytotoxic CD8+ T cells capable of injuring the graft [43,44,46]. In addition, indirectly activated T cells are capable of mediating DTH [74], and DTH is associated with both acute and chronic graft injury [75,76]. One important question currently under investigation is whether indirectly primed, proinflammatory T cells can injure a graft even though they cannot interact with any antigen

expressed on the graft cells. At least in skin graft models, it is possible that recipient-derived vascular endothelial cells found on vessels feeding the graft may act as target of the indirectly primed immune response [77]. The frequency of activated cells may also influence the eventual outcome. Higher frequencies of indirectly primed CD4+ T cells seem to be associated with acute rejection, while lower frequencies may mediate fibrosis and vasculopathy [70].

In summary, the pattern of transplant rejection is not only influenced by the T-cell recognition pathway, but also by the frequency, the induced effector functions and the specific cellular targets of the alloreactive T cells.

ALLORECOGNITION PATHWAYS AND THE INDUCTION OF TOLERANCE

The primary goal of clinical transplantation is the induction of tolerance, which is defined as lack of a destructive alloimmune response to foreign tissue in the absence of maintenance immunosuppression [78]. Despite the increasing success in the induction of tolerance in rodent models, the ability to achieve tolerance in large animals and humans remains elusive and complex. Organ transplantation has been made possible by the development of powerful immunosuppressive drugs that can prevent the rejection process, but usually require lifelong administration, medication adherence and the risk for a wide range of unwanted side-effects [79]. While there has been great success in improving short-term allograft survival in recent years, chronic rejection remains the principal cause of late renal allograft failure and may even be accelerated by some immunosuppressive drugs. Immunologic tolerance would ideally prevent the side-effects of immunosuppression and would hopefully prevent chronic rejection, as demonstrated in several animal models [80]. The accumulating evidence from experimental data supports the notion that in order for any tolerance regimen to be successful, it must not only address T cells that are activated through the direct pathway [66], but also inactivate the indirect alloresponse, which is restricted to different determinants over time.

Two recent studies demonstrated that an intact indirect antigen recognition pathway is necessary for induction of tolerance [81] and the immunomodulatory effect of donor-specific transfusion (DST) in inducing transplantation tolerance *in vivo* [82]. This may be related to the requirement of indirect presentation for generation of regulatory T cells [83].

A recent study in humans provided the first evidence that regulatory T cells appear and persist in renal transplant patients and account for indirect pathway hyporeactivity in a proportion of renal transplant patients with stable allograft function [84]. A companion study showed that this is not the case for direct alloreactive T cells [85]. Therefore, while T-cell anergy and death are most likely the main regulatory mechanisms contributing to direct pathway hyporesponsiveness [86], regulatory T cells appear to have a role in regulation of indirect antidonor alloresponse in stable renal transplant patients [84]. The implications are that, because the indirect pathway appears to be the primary pathway during chronic rejection of allografts, modalities that are successful in tolerizing the indirect alloresponse to specific donor alloantigens (including expansion and infusion of regulatory CD4+CD25+ T cells) may be particularly successful in preventing chronic rejection of vascularized grafts.

CONCLUSIONS

In summary, T-cell sensitization to alloantigen is divided into two nonmutually exclusive pathways: the direct and indirect pathways of allorecognition. The direct pathway characterizes the brisk, vigorous T-cell response during acute rejection of allografts. The indirect pathway is likely to have the dominant role during chronic rejection and may be particularly important in the induction of transplant vasculopathy. On the other hand, the indirect pathway may be required for maintenance of a hyporesponsive state after tolerance induction regimens. Therefore, development of novel tolerance-inducing regimens will likely need to address both pathways of alloreactivity in order to be successful in clinical transplantation.

REFERENCES

1 Gorer P. The detection of a hereditary antigenic difference in the blood of mice by means of human group A serum. *J Genet* 1936;**32**:17.

2 Snell G. Methods for the study of histocompatibility genes. *J Genet* 1948;**49**:87.

3 Krensky AM, Weiss A, Crabtree G, Davis MM, Parham P. T-lymphocyte-antigen interactions in transplant rejection. *N Engl J Med* 1990;**322**:510–7.

4 Sayegh MH. Why do we reject a graft? Role of indirect allorecognition in graft rejection. *Kidney Int* 1999;**56**:1967–79.

5 Briscoe DM, Sayegh MH. A rendezvous before rejection: where do T cells meet transplant antigens? *Nat Med* 2002;**8**:220–2.

6 Heeger PS. T-cell allorecognition and transplant rejection: a summary and update. *Am J Transplant* 2003;**3**:525–33.

7 Baker RJ, Hernandez-Fuentes MP, Brookes PA, et al. Loss of direct and maintenance of indirect alloresponses in renal allograft recipients: implications for the pathogenesis of chronic allograft nephropathy. *J Immunol* 2001;**167**:7199–206.

8 Baker RJ, Hernandez-Fuentes MP, Brookes PA, Chaudhry AN, Lechler RI. The role of the allograft in the induction of donor-specific T cell hyporesponsiveness. *Transplantation* 2001;**72**:480–5.

9 Stanford RE, Ahmed S, Hodson M, Banner NR, Rose ML. A role for indirect allorecognition in lung transplant recipients with obliterative bronchiolitis. *Am J Transplant* 2003;**3**:736–42.

10 Garcia KC, Teyton L, Wilson IA. Structural basis of T cell recognition. *Annu Rev Immunol* 1999;**17**:369–97.

11 Sherman LA, Chattopadhyay S. The molecular basis of allorecognition. *Annu Rev Immunol* 199;**11**:385–402.

12 Matzinger P, Bevan MJ. Hypothesis: why do so many lymphocytes respond to major histocompatibility antigens? *Cell Immunol* 1977;**29**:1–5.

13 Bevan MJ. High determinant density may explain the phenomenon of alloreactivity. *Immunol Today* 1984;**5**:128.

14 Bluestone JA, Jameson S, Miller S, Dick R II. Peptide-induced conformational changes in class I heavy chains alter major histocompatibility complex recognition. *J Exp Med* 1992;**176**:1757–61.

15 Catipovic B, Dal Porto J, Mage M, Johansen TE, Schneck JP. Major histocompatibility complex conformational epitopes are peptide specific. *J Exp Med* 1992;**176**:1611–8.

16 Berkowitz N, Braunstein NS. T cell responses specific for subregions of allogeneic MHC molecules. *J Immunol* 1992;**148**:309–17.

17 Weber DA, Terrell NK, Zhang Y, et al. Requirement for peptide in alloreactive CD4+ T cell recognition of class II MHC molecules. *J Immunol* 1995;**154**:5153–64.

18 Lechler RI, Lombardi G, Batchelor JR, Reinsmoen N, Bach FH. The molecular basis of alloreactivity. *Immunol Today* 1990;**11**:83–8.

19 Jameson SC, Hogquist KA, Bevan MJ. Positive selection of thymocytes. *Annu Rev Immunol* 1995;**13**:93–126.

20 Brock R, Wiesmuller KH, Jung G, Walden P. Molecular basis for the recognition of two structurally different major histocompatibility complex/peptide complexes by a single T-cell receptor. *Proc Natl Acad Sci USA* 1996;**93**:13108–13.

21 Bjorkman PJ, Saper MA, Samraoui B, et al. Structure of the human class I histocompatibility antigen, HLA-A2. *Nature* 1987;**329**:506–12.

22 Bjorkman PJ, Saper MA, Samraoui B, et al. The foreign antigen binding site and T cell recognition regions of class I histocompatibility antigens. *Nature* 1987;**329**:512–8.

23 Madden DR, Gorga JC, Strominger JL, Wiley DC. The structure of HLA-B27 reveals nonamer self-peptides bound in an extended conformation. *Nature* 1991;**353**:321–5.

24 Hunt DF, Henderson RA, Shabanowitz J, et al. Characterization of peptides bound to the class I MHC molecule HLA-A2.1 by mass spectrometry. *Science* 1992;**255**:1261–3.

25 Hunt DF, Michel H, Dickinson TA, et al. Peptides presented to the immune system by the murine class II major histocompatibility complex molecule I-Ad. *Science* 1992;**256**:1817–20.

26 Rudensky A, Preston-Hurlburt P, Hong SC, Barlow A, Janeway CA Jr. Sequence analysis of peptides bound to MHC class II molecules. *Nature* 1991;**353**:622–7.

27 Eckels DD, Gorski J, Rothbard J, Lamb JR. Peptide-mediated modulation of T-cell allorecognition. *Proc Natl Acad Sci USA* 1988;**85**:8191–5.

28 Lombardi G, Sidhu S, Lamb JR, Batchelor JR, Lechler RI. Co-recognition of endogenous antigens with HLA-DR1 by alloreactive human T cell clones. *J Immunol* 1989;**142**:753–9.

29 Marrack P, Kappler J. T cells can distinguish between allogeneic major histocompatibility complex products on different cell types. *Nature* 1988;**332**:840.

30 Cerundolo V, Alexander J, Anderson K, et al. Presentation of viral antigen controlled by a gene in the major histocompatibility complex. *Nature* 1990;**345**:449–52.

31 Hosken NA, Bevan MJ. Defective presentation of endogenous antigen by a cell line expressing class I molecules. *Science* 1990;**248**:367–70.

32 Schumacher TN, Heemels MT, Neefjes JJ, *et al.* Direct binding of peptide to empty MHC class I molecules on intact cells and *in vitro. Cell* 1990;**62**:563–7.

33 Heath WR, Kane KP, Mescher MF, Sherman LA. Alloreactive T cells discriminate among a diverse set of endogenous peptides. *Proc Natl Acad Sci USA* 1991;**88**:5101–5.

34 Elliott TJ, Eisen HN. Cytotoxic T lymphocytes recognize a reconstituted class I histocompatibility antigen (HLA-A2) as an allogeneic target molecule. *Proc Natl Acad Sci USA* 1990; **87**:5213–7.

35 Ohlen C, Bastin J, Ljunggren HG, *et al.* Resistance to H-2-restricted but not to allo-H2-specific graft and cytotoxic T lymphocyte responses in lymphoma mutant. *J Immunol* 1990;**145**: 52–8.

36 Aosai F, Ohlen C, Ljunggren HG, *et al.* Different types of allospecific CTL clones identified by their ability to recognize peptide loading-defective target cells. *Eur J Immunol* 1991;**21**:2767–74.

37 Bluestone JA, Kaliyaperumal A, Jameson S, Miller S, Dick R II. Peptide-induced changes in class I heavy chains alter allorecognition. *J Immunol* 1993;**151**:3943–53.

38 Yewdell JW, Bennink JR. Immunodominance in major histocompatibility complex class I-restricted T lymphocyte responses. *Annu Rev Immunol* 1999;**17**:51.

39 Lechler RI, Batchelor JR. Restoration of immunogenicity to passenger cell-depleted kidney allografts by the addition of donor strain dendritic cells. *J Exp Med* 1982;**155**:31–41.

40 Lechler RI, Batchelor JR. Immunogenicity of retransplanted rat kidney allografts: effect of inducing chimerism in the first recipient and quantitative studies on immunosuppression of the second recipient. *J Exp Med* 1982;**156**:1835–41.

41 Benichou G, Takizawa PA, Olson CA, McMillan M, Sercarz EE. Donor major histocompatibility complex (MHC) peptides are presented by recipient MHC molecules during graft rejection. *J Exp Med* 1992;**175**:305–8.

42 Waaga AM, Chandraker A, Spadafora-Ferreira M, *et al.* Mechanisms of indirect allorecognition: characterization of MHC class II allopeptide-specific T helper cell clones from animals undergoing acute allograft rejection. *Transplantation* 1998;**65**:876–83.

43 Lee RS, Grusby MJ, Glimcher LH, Winn HJ, Auchincloss H Jr. Indirect recognition by helper cells can induce donor-specific cytotoxic T lymphocytes *in vivo. J Exp Med* 1994;**179**:865–72.

44 Steele DJ, Laufer TM, Smiley ST, *et al.* Two levels of help for B cell alloantibody production. *J Exp Med* 1996;**183**:699–703.

45 Benichou G, Valujskikh A, Heeger PS. Contributions of direct and indirect T cell alloreactivity during allograft rejection in mice. *J Immunol* 1999;**162**:352–8.

46 Auchincloss H Jr, Lee R, Shea S, *et al.* The role of "indirect" recognition in initiating rejection of skin grafts from major histocompatibility complex class II-deficient mice. *Proc Natl Acad Sci USA* 1993;**90**:3373–7.

47 Fangmann J, Dalchau R, Sawyer GJ, Priestley CA, Fabre JW. T cell recognition of donor major histocompatibility complex class I peptides during allograft rejection. *Eur J Immunol* 1992; **22**:1525–30.

48 Watschinger B, Gallon L, Carpenter CB, Sayegh MH. Mechanisms of allo-recognition: recognition by *in vivo*-primed T cells of specific major histocompatibility complex polymorphisms presented as peptides by responder antigen-presenting cells. *Transplantation* 1994;**57**:572–6.

49 Gallon L, Watschinger B, Murphy B, *et al.* The indirect pathway of allorecognition: the occurrence of self-restricted T cell recognition of allo-MHC peptides early in acute renal allograft rejection and its inhibition by conventional immunosuppression. *Transplantation* 1995;**59**:612–6.

50 Vella JP, Magee C, Vos L, *et al.* Cellular and humoral mechanisms of vascularized allograft rejection induced by indirect recognition of donor MHC allopeptides. *Transplantation* 1999;**67**:1523–32.

51 Benichou G, Fedoseyeva E, Lehmann PV, *et al.* Limited T cell response to donor MHC peptides during allograft rejection: implications for selective immune therapy in transplantation. *J Immunol* 1994;**153**:938–45.

52 Liu Z, Sun YK, Xi YP, *et al.* Contribution of direct and indirect recognition pathways to T cell alloreactivity. *J Exp Med* 1993;**177**:1643–50.

53 Najafian N, Salama AD, Fedoseyeva EV, Benichou G, Sayegh MH. Enzyme-linked immunosorbent spot assay analysis of peripheral blood lymphocyte reactivity to donor HLA-DR peptides: potential novel assay for prediction of outcomes for renal transplant recipients. *J Am Soc Nephrol* 2002;**13**:252–9.

54 Sercarz EE, Lehmann PV, Ametani A, *et al.* Dominance and crypticity of T cell antigenic determinants. *Annu Rev Immunol* 1993;**11**:729–66.

55 Braun MY, McCormack A, Webb G, Batchelor JR. Mediation of acute but not chronic rejection of MHC-incompatible rat kidney grafts by alloreactive CD4 T cells activated by the direct pathway of sensitization. *Transplantation* 1993;**55**:177–82.

56 Womer KL, Vella JP, Sayegh MH. Chronic allograft dysfunction: mechanisms and new approaches to therapy. *Semin Nephrol* 2000;**20**:126–47.

57 Vella JP, Vos L, Carpenter CB, Sayegh MH. Role of indirect allorecognition in experimental late acute rejection. *Transplantation* 1997;**64**:1823–8.

58 Vella JP, Spadafora-Ferreira M, Murphy B, *et al.* Indirect allorecognition of major histocompatibility complex allopeptides in human renal transplant recipients with chronic graft dysfunction. *Transplantation* 1997;**64**:795–800.

59 Ciubotariu R, Liu Z, Colovai AI, *et al.* Persistent allopeptide reactivity and epitope spreading in chronic rejection of organ allografts. *J Clin Invest* 1998;**101**:398–405.

60 SivaSai KS, Smith MA, Poindexter NJ, *et al.* Indirect recognition of donor HLA class I peptides in lung transplant recipients with bronchiolitis obliterans syndrome. *Transplantation* 1999;**67**:1094–8.

61 Reznik SI, Jaramillo A, SivaSai KS, *et al.* Indirect allorecognition of mismatched donor HLA class II peptides in lung transplant recipients with bronchiolitis obliterans syndrome. *Am J Transplant* 2001;**1**:228–35.

62 Lu KC, Jaramillo A, Mendeloff EN, *et al.* Concomitant allorecognition of mismatched donor HLA class I- and class II-derived peptides in pediatric lung transplant recipients with bronchiolitis obliterans syndrome. *J Heart Lung Transplant* 2003;**22**: 35–43.

63 Batchelor JR, Welsh KI, Maynard A, Burgos H. Failure of long surviving, passively enhanced kidney allografts to provoke T-dependent alloimmunity. I. Retransplantation of (AS X AUG)F1 kidneys into secondary AS recipients. *J Exp Med* 1979;**150**:455–64.

64 Yamada A, Laufer TM, Gerth AJ, *et al.* Further analysis of the T-cell subsets and pathways of murine cardiac allograft rejection. *Am J Transplant* 2003;**3**:23–7.

65 Lee RS, Yamada K, Houser SL, *et al.* Indirect recognition of allopeptides promotes the development of cardiac allograft vasculopathy. *Proc Natl Acad Sci USA* 2001;**98**:3276–81.

66 Hornick PI, Mason PD, Yacoub MH, *et al.* Assessment of the contribution that direct allorecognition makes to the progression of chronic cardiac transplant rejection in humans. *Circulation* 1998;**97**:1257–63.

67 Kreisel D, Krasinskas AM, Krupnick AS, *et al.* Vascular endothelium does not activate CD4$^+$ direct allorecognition in graft rejection. *J Immunol* 2004;**173**:3027–34.

68 Lakkis FG, Arakelov A, Konieczny BT, Inoue Y. Immunologic "ignorance" of vascularized organ transplants in the absence of secondary lymphoid tissue. *Nat Med* 2000;**6**:686–8.

69 Krieger NR, Yin DP, Fathman CG. CD4$^+$ but not CD8$^+$ cells are essential for allorejection. *J Exp Med* 1996;**184**:2013–8.

70 Pietra BA, Wiseman A, Bolwerk A, Rizeq M, Gill RG. CD4 T cell-mediated cardiac allograft rejection requires donor but not host MHC class II. *J Clin Invest* 2000;**106**:1003–10.

71 Jones ND, Turvey SE, Van Maurik A, *et al.* Differential susceptibility of heart, skin, and islet allografts to T cell-mediated rejection. *J Immunol* 2001;**166**:2824–30.

72 Ardehali A, Fischbein MP, Yun J, *et al.* Indirect alloreactivity and chronic rejection. *Transplantation* 2002;**73**:1805–7.

73 Kreisel D, Krupnick AS, Gelman AE, *et al.* Non-hematopoietic allograft cells directly activate CD8$^+$ T cells and trigger acute rejection: an alternative mechanism of allorecognition. *Nat Med* 2002;**8**:233–9.

74 Waaga AM, Gasser M, Kist-van Holthe JE, *et al.* Regulatory functions of self-restricted MHC class II allopeptide-specific Th2 clones *in vivo*. *J Clin Invest* 2001;**107**:909–16.

75 Sirak J, Orosz CG, Wakely E, VanBuskirk AM. Alloreactive delayed-type hypersensitivity in graft recipients: complexity of responses and divergence from acute rejection. *Transplantation* 1997;**63**:1300–7.

76 Carrodeguas L, Orosz CG, Waldman WJ, *et al.* Trans vivo analysis of human delayed-type hypersensitivity reactivity. *Hum Immunol* 1999;**60**:640–51.

77 Valujskikh A, Lantz O, Celli S, Matzinger P, Heeger PS. Cross-primed CD8$^+$ T cells mediate graft rejection via a distinct effector pathway. *Nat Immunol* 2002;**3**:844–51.

78 Salama AD, Remuzzi G, Harmon WE, Sayegh MH. Challenges to achieving clinical transplantation tolerance. *J Clin Invest* 2001;**108**:943–8.

79 Sayegh MH, Carpenter CB. Transplantation 50 years later: progress, challenges, and promises. *N Engl J Med* 2004;**351**:2761–6.

80 Sayegh MH, Carpenter CB. Tolerance and chronic rejection. *Kidney Int Suppl* 1997;**58**:S11–4.

81 Yamada A, Chandraker A, Laufer TM, *et al.* Recipient MHC class II expression is required to achieve long-term survival of murine cardiac allografts after costimulatory blockade. *J Immunol* 2001;**167**:5522–6.

82 Kishimoto K, Yuan X, Auchincloss H Jr, *et al.* Mechanism of action of donor-specific transfusion in inducing tolerance: role of donor MHC molecules, donor co-stimulatory molecules, and indirect antigen presentation. *J Am Soc Nephrol* 2004;**15**:2423–8.

83 Rulifson IC, Szot GL, Palmer E, Bluestone JA. Inability to induce tolerance through direct antigen presentation. *Am J Transplant* 2002;**2**:510–9.

84 Salama AD, Najafian N, Clarkson MR, Harmon WE, Sayegh MH. Regulatory CD25$^+$ T cells in human kidney transplant recipients. *J Am Soc Nephrol* 2003;**14**:1643–51.

85 Game DS, Hernandez-Fuentes MP, Chaudhry AN, Lechler RI. CD4$^+$CD25$^+$ regulatory T cells do not significantly contribute to direct pathway hyporesponsiveness in stable renal transplant patients. *J Am Soc Nephrol* 2003;**14**:1652–61.

86 Lechler RI, Garden OA, Turka LA. The complementary roles of deletion and regulation in transplantation tolerance. *Nat Rev Immunol* 2003;**3**:147–58.

3 Costimulation

Elizabeth Ingulli and David M. Briscoe

Allograft rejection is a complex process involving both innate and adaptive immune responses, and the activation of T cells, B cells, dendritic cells and macrophages. In addition, several other cell types, including those within the graft, contribute to graft destruction. Nevertheless, it is well-established that T-cell recognition of alloantigen is a primary event that initiates the alloimmune response. The nature of this activation response ultimately contributes to either graft acceptance or graft failure. Over the past two decades, knowledge of T-cell activation and its molecular basis have been expanded substantially, and the concept that costimulation is a key component of the alloimmune response is well established.

Bretscher and Cohn [1] in the late 1960s originally hypothesized that receptors on the cell surface of the lymphocyte transmit signals that result in either activation or cell death. Subsequently, Lafferty *et al.* [2] demonstrated that a specific signal, called the "allogeneic stimulus," could be given to a T cell by a bystander cell resulting in its activation. They hypothesized that "stimulator cells" derived from an allograft provided this signal [3]. A decade later, Jenkins and Schwartz [4] determined that T cells activated in the presence of antigen but in the absence of accessory signals failed to produce the cytokine interleukin 2 (IL-2) and proliferate. They also demonstrated that under these conditions the T cells remained alive but were unresponsive to additional antigen-specific signals. Antigen-specific signals are delivered through the T-cell receptor (TCR) upon contact with their specific peptide expressed within major histocompatibility complex (MHC) molecules that are displayed prominently on the cell surface of the antigen-presenting cell (APC). These signals are commonly called Signal 1. Accessory signals (called Signal 2) are delivered through interactions between cell surface receptors on T cells upon contact with *antigen-nonspecific* ligands that are also expressed on APCs or third party bystander cells. Because these assessory signals were shown to be critical for optimal and effective T-cell activation, they became known as costimulatory signals. Costimulation has thus been defined in the immunology literature as accessory signals that augment IL-2 production following antigen-specific activation of T cells. A lack of costimulation at the time of antigen presentation may eliminate a T cell from the pool of antigen-responsive lymphocytes, either by promoting lymphocyte death or by inducing a state of unresponsiveness called anergy.

Nevertheless, optimal T-cell activation, the development of T-cell effector functions and the generation of long-lasting memory T-cell depend upon the coordinated delivery of *numerous* signals between the APC and the naïve T cell. The term "costimulation" is now often loosely used to describe this complex and dynamic process involving the exchange of these various signals between APCs and T cells. In addition, costimulation occurs not only as a result of stimulatory signals, but also by a change in the delivery of inhibitory signals. Several accessory molecules can be induced to provide inhibitory signals that regulate T-cell responses in the course of immune activation. It is proposed that the relative effect and balance between stimulatory versus inhibitory signals may determine the ultimate outcome of an encounter with antigen. Indeed, the ability of the immune system to simultaneously generate alloreactive and regulatory immune responses following an encounter with an antigen creates a balance among cell populations that can elicit stimulation and those that can mediate regulation. A detailed discussion of how the immune system maintains this balance is beyond the scope of this chapter. The following sections review the various costimulatory pathways, their role in T-cell activation and their applicability to the field of solid organ transplantation. A schematic outline of several of those pathways is shown in Figure 3.1.

CD28/CTLA-4/B7-1/B7-2 PATHWAY

One of the most important and the most intensely studied costimulatory pathways involved in T-cell activation is the CD28/CTLA-4/B7-1/B7-2 pathway. The CD28 receptor is expressed on T cells and binds to the ligands B7-1 (CD80) and B7-2 (CD86) expressed on the surface of APCs. CD28 delivers signals to the T cells that enhance T-cell responses to antigen, promote IL-2 production and facilitate T-cell proliferation. In contrast, another T-cell surface molecule, CTLA-4, also binds B7-1 and B7-2, but it transmits signals that inhibit T-cell

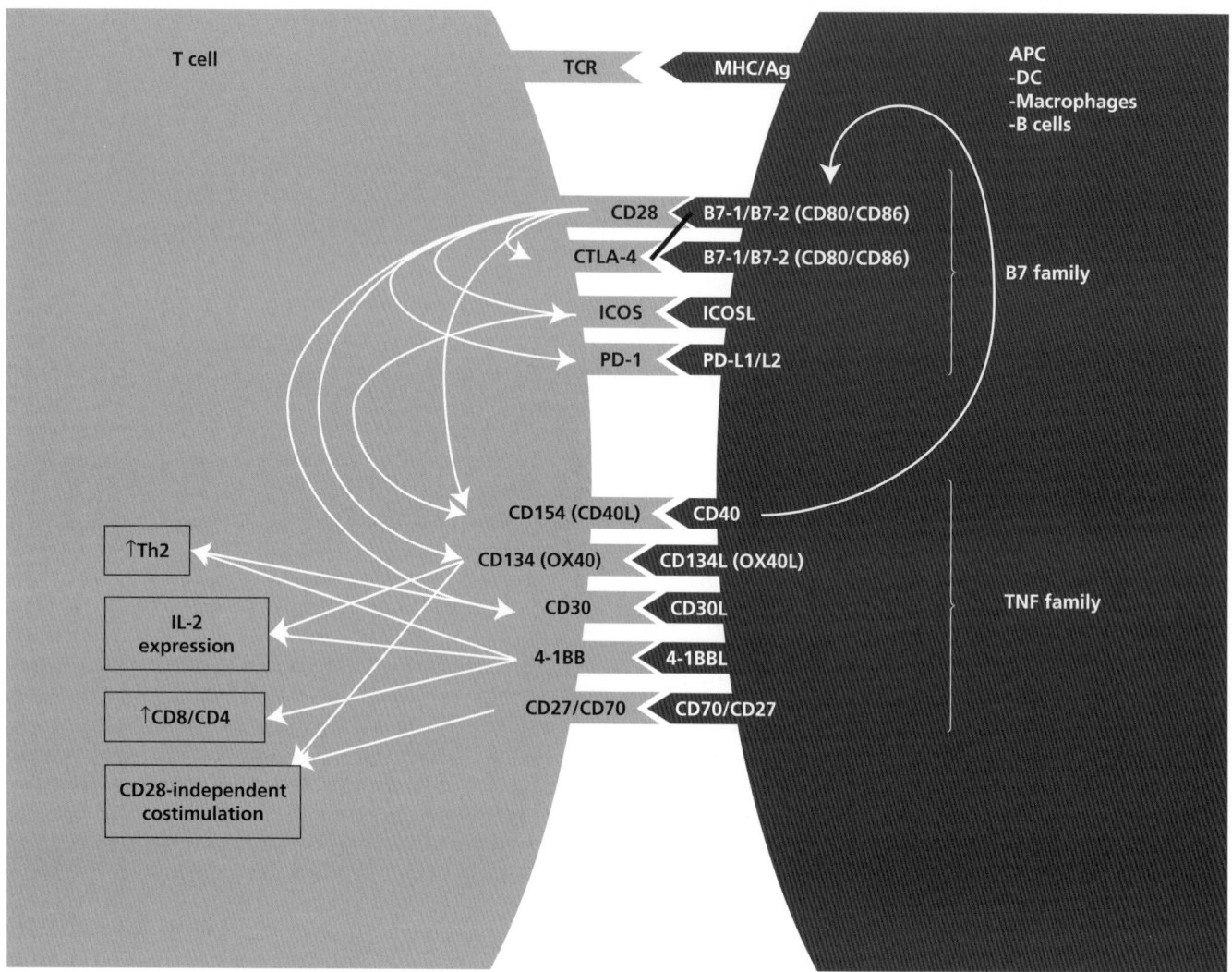

Fig. 3.1 Diagram depicting the primary (MHC/Ag–TCR) interaction between the antigen-presenting cell (APC) and the responding T cell and several modulating costimulatory pathways.

activation. CD28 and CTLA-4 are glycoprotein receptors of the immunoglobulin family and they share some homologies (approximately 30%) [5]. CD28 is constitutively expressed on most resting naïve CD4+ T cells and on approximately 50% of CD8 T cells, but expression of this receptor is increased upon TCR engagement [6]. In contrast, CTLA-4 is not constitutively expressed on naïve T cells, but its expression is tightly regulated and is induced upon T-cell activation and upon TCR engagement [7].

B7-1 and B7-2 are glycoproteins within the immunoglobulin family and are expressed on professional APCs, such as dendritic cells, B cells and macrophages. B7 molecules are induced by various inflammatory stimuli and have distinct patterns of expression. Importantly, the cell surface expression of B7 molecules is enhanced during the course of dendritic cell activation and maturation, facilitating optimal T-cell activation [8]. B7-2 is expressed early and B7-1 appears later

following stimulation of an APC [8,9]. Although both CD28 and CTLA-4 bind B7 molecules, CTLA-4 binds with higher affinity than CD28 [10]. In general, as CTLA-4 expression increases on a T cell, the binding affinity is thought to suppress interactions between CD28 and B7, and thus functions to suppress CD28-mediated costimulation. CTLA-4-mediated inhibition of T-cell activation is thus enhanced at late times following the binding of a T cell to an APC.

The CD28 pathway has been demonstrated to be critical in the primary activation and clonal expansion of naïve T cells. In the absence of TCR engagement, ligation of CD28 has no known immunologic effect but TCR/CD28 coligation has been found to lower the threshold requirement for T-cell activation as it amplifies TCR intracellular signaling [11]. The intracellular signaling cascade from both TCR/CD28-mediated events has profound synergistic effects upon T-cell clonal expansion [12], cytokine production and mRNA stability [13–15], and cell cycle progression [16,17]. CD28 signaling also promotes T-cell survival through enhanced expression of the anti-apoptotic protein, Bcl-XL [18]. The enhanced proliferation and survival of T cells following CD28-mediated activation also influences Th1 and Th2 cell differentiation [19,20], CD4-dependent cytotoxic T lymphocyte (CTL) responses [21] and CD4-dependent B-cell responses including germinal center formation and immunoglobulin (Ig) isotype switching [22,23]. In addition, CD28 signaling influences the expression of other costimulatory molecules (including some that will be discussed below) [24,25], thereby perpetuating further activation events.

In contrast to the stimulatory response achieved with CD28, ligation of CTLA-4 by B7 family molecules inhibits T-cell responses [26,27], in part by blocking CD28-mediated IL-2 production and T-cell proliferation [28–30]. However, CTLA-4 provides independent negative signals as demonstrated by the finding that CTLA-4 has effects in CD28-deficient animals [28,31]. In addition, studies using mice deficient for CTLA-4 have confirmed a major regulatory function for this molecule. In CTLA-4 knockout mice, T-cell proliferation is unrestrained and massive lymphoproliferation from unchecked costimulation occurs and results in autoimmune diseases and early death [32,33]. Regulatory T cells have been shown to contain large intracellular stores of CTLA-4, which is thought to influence their suppressive properties [34]. These data support the notion that CTLA-4 has a critical role in immune tolerance, and that agents that interfere with CTLA-4 signaling may augment T-cell activation and prevent tolerance induction [35]. In contrast, agents that inhibit CD28-mediated activation will limit the T-cell response to antigens (including alloantigens). Thus, agents that augment CTLA-4 signals and inhibit CD28-induced responses can augment regulation and regulatory immune functions.

ICOS–ICOS-L

Similar to CD28 but to a lesser degree, ligation of the costimulatory receptor ICOS (inducible T-cell costimulator) on T cells results in enhanced T-cell proliferation and cytokine production. In addition, ICOS-activated T cells provide help to B cells to generate antibodies. However, ICOS also has several properties that make it distinct from CD28. First, while CD28 is constitutively expressed on T cells, ICOS is not expressed on naïve T cells [36] but is inducible upon ligation of the TCR and following costimulation by CD28 [37–41]. Thus, while CD28-dependent costimulation occurs early and subsides in the later stages following T-cell activation, the inducible expression of ICOS shortly after T-cell activation suggests that it may be particularly important in providing later costimulatory signals to activated T cells. Indeed, consistent with this notion, ICOS expression is found on activated T cells and on memory T cells [36]. During the course of an immune response, ICOS levels have been found to remain high on subsets of T cells (especially Th2 cells) [24,42,43]. The fact that ICOS is upregulated following CD28 costimulation suggests that some of the functions previously ascribed to CD28 may in part be due to ICOS. For instance, while naïve T cells require CD28 signaling for their proliferation and IL-2 production, optimal activation of recently activated T cells may be independent of CD28 costimulation [43].

While ICOS is structurally related to CD28, it does not bind to B7 family molecules. Rather it interacts with ICOS-L, also known as B7H, GL50, B7RP-1 and B7-H2 [39,44–46]. ICOS-L does not bind to CD28 or CTLA-4 and is expressed by several cell types, including T cells, and cells in peripheral tissues, including endothelial cells [39,44,45]. The expression of ICOS-L in peripheral tissues (especially on endothelial cells) may be important for ICOS-mediated immune activation. ICOS-L is induced by inflammatory mediators and is expressed in association with inflammation in several diseases including allograft rejection [44].

As implied from its late expression pattern, ICOS stimulation has little effect on the initial stages of T-cell activation and proliferation. Rather it appears to affect cytokines produced by T cells after they are initially activated. This later ICOS stimulation thereby affects the development of T-cell effector function. For instance, ICOS ligation can enhance Th1 cytokines but has more profound effects on Th2 responses [42,43]. Furthermore, inhibition of ICOS–ICOS-L interactions skews the response in the Th1 direction [24]. In a model of allergic airway disease, ICOS blockade suppressed the production of Th2 cytokines [42,47]; and it is interesting to note that the pathology of inflammation in the lung was improved with late ICOS blockade [48]. ICOS costimulation has also been found to be important for humoral immunity [49,50], the regulation of IL-10 production and the development of regulatory T cells [51]. In the transplant setting, ICOS deficiency or blockade of ICOS can reduce Th1 cytokines and prolong cardiac allograft survival [52]. Sayegh et al. [53] demonstrated that the later upregulation of ICOS is of functional importance in allograft rejection. Blockade of ICOS–ICOS-L interactions was only found to inhibit allograft rejection when anti-ICOS treatment was administered late, as opposed to when treatment was given early [53]. This contrasts the effect of B7 antagonists, which are functional at early stages. In combination with other blocking agents (anti-CD154), inhibition of ICOS can prevent chronic allograft vasculopathy [52].

CD154–CD40

The interaction between CD40 and its ligand CD154 (also called CD40L, gp39, TRAP, T-BAM) is established to have a major role in cell-mediated immune responses, including allograft rejection. CD40 is an integral membrane glycoprotein member of the tumor necrosis factor (TNF) receptor family [54]. Its expression was initially thought to be limited to B cells and dendritic cells [55], but it is expressed on other cell types with a wide tissue distribution [56]. CD40 has a major role in the activation of B cells and antibody production but it has also been found to be important in the activation of dendritic cells, macrophages, endothelial cells, epithelial cells and fibroblasts [55]. The expression of CD40 is highly regulated by cytokines which ensures its ability to bind its ligand CD154, expressed by platelets and leukocytic infiltrates in the course of inflammatory reactions [57,58].

CD154 is a 39-kDa, type 2 membrane glycoprotein that is predominantly expressed on activated T cells and platelets, but is also expressed by B cells, dendritic cells, natural killer cells and endothelial cells [54,59,60]. CD40–CD154 interactions were first found to be important for human immunity when it was reported that mutations in CD154 which result in an inability of CD154 to bind CD40 cause a disease called the Hyper IgM (HIM) syndrome [61–65]. Patients with HIM syndrome have immunodeficiency with abnormalities in humoral and cellular immunity. The humoral immunodeficiency is associated with high serum levels of IgM and reduced levels of IgG, IgA and IgE. This defect is related to an inability of B cells to switch from IgM to IgG production. In addition, patients with HIM syndrome have been found to have defects in T-cell function and they do not mount appropriate cell-mediate immune responses.

The interaction between CD154 on activated CD4 T cells and CD40 on APCs is necessary for the generation of an effective T-cell activation, by enhancing the expression of the B7 family molecules on APCs [66] and by promoting dendritic cell maturation [67–69]. However, CD40 ligation on dendritic cells also has major effects on the adaptor function of the dendritic cell independent of enhancing CD28–B7 costimulation; for instance, through the production of pro-inflammatory mediators, such as IL-12 [70]. IL-12 is important in the generation of effector immune responses, IFNγ production and the development of cytolytic T-cell effector function [71,72]. Moreover, CD40 signaling has been shown to be important for promoting dendritic cell survival and antigen presentation [73–75]. Signaling through Toll-like receptors (TLR) synergize with CD40-induced responses to facilitate the maturation of dendritic cells [76–81] thereby promoting T-cell immunity. Blocking CD40-induced activation of dendritic cells inhibits the development of cytotoxic T-lymphocyte function [70], reduces autoimmunity [82–87] and promotes peripheral tolerance [88–91]. Blocking CD40–CD154 signaling has also been shown to induce regulatory T cells and populations of anergic CD4 cells with potent suppressive functions [92].

In summary, CD40 is an important costimulatory molecule expressed on many cell types. It functions in humoral and cellular immunity directly or indirectly via its ability to regulate the expression of accessory molecules and inflammatory mediators.

PD-1/PD-L

PD-1 (programmed death 1) is another member of the CD28/B7 family and was identified in cells undergoing activation induced cell death [93]; however, it does not appear to have a role in that process [94,95]. PD-1 expression is found in the thymus and is thought to have an important role in central tolerance [96,97]. Within secondary lymphoid tissues, a subpopulation of peripheral CD4 and CD8 T cells express PD-1 but its cell surface expression is increased upon activation [95]. The ligands for the PD-1 receptor are PD-L1 (B7-H1) and PD-L2 (B7 DC) [98–101] and the expression profile is low within secondary lymphoid tissue and higher in other tissues such as the placenta, heart, pancreas, lung and liver [98,99]. On APCs, the expression of PD-L1 and PD-L2 is only observed upon activation by inflammatory mediators [98–100].

Like CD28, PD-1 signaling occurs only when T- or B-cell receptors are cross-linked simultaneously [99]. The cytoplasmic tail of PD-1 has a immunoreceptor tyrosine-based switch motif (ITSM) which is characteristic of molecules that can transmit inhibitory signals [102]. Indeed, consistent with this structure, it has been found that TCR engagement, in association with coligation of PD-1, results in decreased cell proliferation, decreased cytokine production (i.e. IL-2) and failure to progress through the cell cycle [98–100]. PD-1 ligation also appears to inhibit B-cell activation [103]. Absence of PD-1 has been shown to induce a lymphoproliferation similar to that observed with CTLA-4 deficiency but to a lesser degree and with later onset [104]. The distribution of the ligand suggests that inhibition can occur not only during the primary response within secondary lymphoid tissues, but also within the periphery where the cells are reactivated thereby assisting in controlling self-reactivity. In rodent studies using knockout mice or antibody blocking studies, it has been found that inhibition of PD-1, or the lack of PD-1, leads to increases in B-cell numbers and a lupus-like syndrome with uncontrolled T-cell dependent B-cell activation, arthritis and glomerulonephritis suggesting a breakdown of peripheral tolerance [105]. Other studies have demonstrated an autoimmune phenomenon within the myocardium [106]. In the transplant setting, PD-1 signaling in the absence of CD28 signaling prolonged cardiac allograft survival [107] and in conjunction with anti-CD154 blockade prevented chronic allograft vasculopathy [108]. PD-1 blockade has also been shown to have an important role in exacerbating graft-versus-host disease [109].

COSTIMULATORY BLOCKADE AS A THERAPEUTIC APPROACH TO PREVENT ALLOGRAFT REJECTION

The first attempts to induce tolerance in the transplant setting by blocking the CD28/B7 pathway were successful in rodent models. CTLA4-Ig is a recombinant fusion protein containing the extracellular portion of CTLA-4 fused to the heavy chain of the immunoglobulin molecule. When administered, it targets APCs by binding to both B7-1 and B7-2 with high affinity and prevents CD28 signaling thereby limiting T-cell activation and proliferation [110]. However, CTLA4-Ig also prevents interactions between B7 and T-cell CTLA-4, which inhibit the immune response [31,111–113]. Several groups have shown that administration of CTLA4-Ig prevents acute allograft rejection and induces donor-specific tolerance in several animal models [10,114,115]. Blockade of B7 interactions with CTLA4-Ig has also been demonstrated to interrupt the progression of chronic allograft rejection [116]. However, preclinical studies in nonhuman primates demonstrated that CTLA4-Ig alone was less effective than that observed in small animal models [117,118] but when it was used in combination with low doses of immunosuppressive agents was quite a potent agent to promote graft survival [119–121]. Ongoing studies in humans are evaluating the efficacy of another anti-B7 agent, LEA29Y (belatacept), following transplantation [122]. Initial studies have been most promising and suggest that this agent is a potent immunosuppressant. This agent also has an advantage in that it is administered intraveneously once a month, thereby reducing major concerns regarding medication adherence. In animal models, the use of donor cells with anti-B7 costimulatory blockade promotes regulatory immune responses and tolerance. If B7 antagonists are approved for use, future studies addressing this possibility in humans may be forthcoming.

There has also been great interest in using a humanized antibody that blocks CD154–CD40 interaction to prevent allograft rejection, prevent alloantibody production and promote tolerance. Anti-CD154 antibodies have been shown to be effective in preventing acute allograft rejection and promote donor-specific tolerance in animal models [123–131]. Several strategies using CD154 blockade either alone or in combination with B7 blockade were shown to prevent chronic rejection and promote regulatory immune responses. However, this was not a universal observation and some groups found that while blockade of CD154 was efficacious in preventing acute rejection, it did not prevent the development of chronic rejection [132–135]. CD154 blockade has been tested in human kidney transplant recipients, but serious adverse effects of this therapy, including large vessel thrombosis, have precluded it from being used in additional clinical trials.

Despite all the promise with individual agents, recent studies have identified that multiple costimulatory pathways may need to be targeted simultaneously in order to achieve long-term graft survival [112,113,117,118,136–140]. Recently, several studies have identified that additional costimulatory molecules such as the OX40–OX40L pathway [141], and cytokines such as IL-15 [142], have the capacity to mediate significant costimulatory signals. Moreover, it is reported that the addition of donor-specific transfusions (DSTs) to existing costimulatory blockade regimens (CTLA4-Ig or anti-CD154)

is promising to induce long-lasting graft acceptance [133, 143–146]. Under these conditions, apoptosis and deletion of alloreactive clones in the periphery is achieved [126]. Further analysis is necessary to determine if the use of single costimulatory antagonist therapies alone can be used in humans. It is possible that the use of multiple agents to block several pathways simultaneously will have therapeutic potential. Nevertheless, it is exciting that these agents and protocols are currently being evaluated in clinical trials because they expand immune-modification strategies for organ transplant recipients and may promote long-term graft survival and perhaps true immune tolerance.

REFERENCES

1 Bretscher PA, Cohn M. Minimal model for the mechanism of antibody induction and paralysis by antigen. *Nature* 1968;**220**:444–8.

2 Lafferty KJ, Misko IS, Cooley MA. Allogeneic stimulation modulates the in vitro response of T cells to transplantation antigen. *Nature* 1974;**249**:275–6.

3 Lafferty KJ, Cooley MA, Woolnough J, Walker KZ. Thyroid allograft immunogenicity is reduced after a period in organ culture. *Science* 1975;**188**:259–61.

4 Jenkins MK, Schwartz RH. Antigen presentation by chemically modified splenocytes induces antigen-specific T cell unresponsiveness *in vitro* and *in vivo*. *J Exp Med* 1987;**165**:302–19.

5 Brunet JF, Denizot F, Luciani MF, *et al.* A new member of the immunoglobulin superfamily: CTLA-4. *Nature* 1987;**328**: 267–70.

6 Gross JA, Callas E, Allison JP. Identification and distribution of the costimulatory receptor CD28 in the mouse. *J Immunol* 1992;**149**:380–8.

7 Linsley PS, Bradshaw J, Greene J, Peach R, Bennett KL, Mittler RS. Intracellular trafficking of CTLA-4 and focal localization towards sites of TCR engagement. *Immunity* 1996;**4**:535–43.

8 Hathcock KS, Laszlo G, Pucillo C, Linsley P, Hodes RJ. Comparative analysis of B7-1 and B7-2 costimulatory ligands: expression and function. *J Exp Med* 1994;**180**:631–40.

9 Freeman GJ, Borriello F, Hodes RJ, *et al.* Murine B7-2, an alternative CTLA4 counter-receptor that costimulates T cell proliferation and interleukin 2 production. *J Exp Med* 1993;**178**:2185–92.

10 Linsley PS, Greene JL, Brady W, Bajorath J, Ledbetter JA, Peach R. Human B7-1 (CD80) and B7-2 (CD86) bind with similar avidities but distinct kinetics to CD28 and CTLA-4 receptors. *Immunity* 1994;**1**:793–801.

11 Viola A, Lanzavecchia A. T cell activation determined by T cell receptor number and tunable thresholds. *Science* 1996;**273**:104–6.

12 Kearney ER, Walunas TL, Karr RW, *et al.* Antigen-dependent clonal expansion of a trace population of antigen-specific CD4+ T cells *in vivo* is dependent on CD28 costimulation and inhibited by CTLA-4. *J Immunol* 1995;**155**:1032–6.

13 Jenkins MK, Taylor PS, Norton SD, Urdahl KB. CD28 delivers a costimulatory signal involved in antigen-specific IL-2 production by human T cells. *J Immunol* 1991;**147**:2461–6.

14 Fraser JD, Irving BA, Crabtree GR, Weiss A. Regulation of interleukin-2 gene enhancer activity by the T cell accessory molecule CD28. *Science* 1991;**251**:313–6.

15 Norton SD, Zuckerman L, Urdahl KB, Shefner R, Miller J, Jenkins MK. The CD28 ligand, B7, enhances IL-2 production by providing a costimulatory signal to T cells. *J Immunol* 1992;**149**:1556–61.

16 Bonnevier JL, Mueller DL. Cutting edge: B7/CD28 interactions regulate cell cycle progression independent of the strength of TCR signaling. *J Immunol* 2002;**169**:6659–63.

17 Appleman LJ, Berezovskaya A, Grass I, Boussiotis VA. CD28 costimulation mediates T cell expansion via IL-2-independent and IL-2-dependent regulation of cell cycle progression. *J Immunol* 2000;**164**:144–51.

18 Boise LH, Minn AJ, Noel PJ, *et al.* CD28 costimulation can promote T cell survival by enhancing the expression of Bcl-XL. *Immunity* 1995;**3**:87–98.

19 Rulifson IC, Sperling AI, Fields PE, Fitch FW, Bluestone JA. CD28 costimulation promotes the production of Th2 cytokines. *J Immunol* 1997;**158**:658–65.

20 Schweitzer AN, Borriello F, Wong RC, Abbas AK, Sharpe AH. Role of costimulators in T cell differentiation: studies using antigen-presenting cells lacking expression of CD80 or CD86. *J Immunol* 1997;**158**:2713–22.

21 Prilliman KR, Lemmens EE, Palioungas G, *et al.* Cutting edge: a crucial role for B7-CD28 in transmitting T help from APC to CTL. *J Immunol* 2002;**169**:4094–7.

22 Lane P, Burdet C, Hubele S, *et al.* B cell function in mice transgenic for mCTLA4-H gamma 1: lack of germinal centers correlated with poor affinity maturation and class switching despite normal priming of CD4⁺ T cells. *J Exp Med* 1994;**179**:819–30.

23 Ferguson SE, Han S, Kelsoe G, Thompson CB. CD28 is required for germinal center formation. *J Immunol* 1996;**156**:4576–81.

24 McAdam AJ, Chang TT, Lumelsky AE, *et al.* Mouse inducible costimulatory molecule (ICOS) expression is enhanced by CD28 costimulation and regulates differentiation of CD4⁺ T cells. *J Immunol* 2000;**165**:5035–40.

25 Walker LS, Gulbranson-Judge A, Flynn S, Brocker T, Lane PJ. Co-stimulation and selection for T-cell help for germinal centres: the role of CD28 and OX40. *Immunol Today* 2000;**21**:333–7.

26 Walunas TL, Lenschow DJ, Bakker CY, *et al.* CTLA-4 can function as a negative regulator of T cell activation. *Immunity* 1994;**1**:405–13.

27 Greenwald RJ, Boussiotis VA, Lorsbach RB, Abbas AK, Sharpe AH. CTLA-4 regulates induction of anergy *in vivo*. *Immunity* 2001;**14**:145–55.

28 Krummel MF, Allison JP. CD28 and CTLA-4 have opposing effects on the response of T cells to stimulation. *J Exp Med* 1995;**182**:459–65.

29 Walunas TL, Bakker CY, Bluestone JA. CTLA-4 ligation blocks CD28-dependent T cell activation. *J Exp Med* 1996;**183**:2541–50.

30 Brunner MC, Chambers CA, Chan FK, Hanke J, Winoto A, Allison JP. CTLA-4-Mediated inhibition of early events of T cell proliferation. *J Immunol* 1999;**162**:5813–20.

31 Lin H, Rathmell JC, Gray GS, Thompson CB, Leiden JM, Alegre ML. Cytotoxic T lymphocyte antigen 4 (CTLA4) blockade accelerates the acute rejection of cardiac allografts in CD28-deficient mice: CTLA4 can function independently of CD28. *J Exp Med* 1998;**188**:199–204.

32 Waterhouse P, Penninger JM, Timms E, *et al.* Lymphoproliferative disorders with early lethality in mice deficient in CTLA-4. *Science* 1995;**270**:985–8.

33 Tivol EA, Borriello F, Schweitzer AN, Lynch WP, Bluestone JA, Sharpe AH. Loss of CTLA-4 leads to massive lymphoproliferation and fatal multiorgan tissue destruction, revealing a critical negative regulatory role of CTLA-4. *Immunity* 1995;**3**:541–7.

34 Salomon B, Lenschow DJ, Rhee L, *et al.* B7/CD28 costimulation is essential for the homeostasis of the CD4⁺CD25⁺ immunoregulatory T cells that control autoimmune diabetes. *Immunity* 2000;**12**:431–40.

35 Fecteau S, Basadonna GP, Freitas A, Ariyan C, Sayegh MH, Rothstein DM. CTLA-4 up-regulation plays a role in tolerance mediated by CD45. *Nat Immunol* 2001;**2**:58–63.

36 Hutloff A, Dittrich AM, Beier KC, *et al.* ICOS is an inducible T-cell co-stimulator structurally and functionally related to CD28. *Nature* 1999;**397**:263–6.

37 Beier KC, Hutloff A, Dittrich AM, *et al.* Induction, binding specificity and function of human ICOS. *Eur J Immunol* 2000;**30**:3707–17.

38 Mages HW, Hutloff A, Heuck C, *et al.* Molecular cloning and characterization of murine ICOS and identification of B7h as ICOS ligand. *Eur J Immunol* 2000;**30**:1040–7.

39 Yoshinaga SK, Whoriskey JS, Khare SD, *et al.* T-cell co-stimulation through B7RP-1 and ICOS. *Nature* 1999;**402**:827–32.

40 Buonfiglio D, Bragardo M, Redoglia V, *et al.* The T cell activation molecule H4 and the CD28-like molecule ICOS are identical. *Eur J Immunol* 2000;**30**:3463–7.

41 Tezuka K, Tsuji T, Hirano D, *et al.* Identification and characterization of rat AILIM/ICOS, a novel T-cell costimulatory molecule, related to the CD28/CTLA4 family. *Biochem Biophys Res Commun* 2000;**276**:335–45.

42 Coyle AJ, Lehar S, Lloyd C, *et al.* The CD28-related molecule ICOS is required for effective T cell-dependent immune responses. *Immunity* 2000;**13**:95–105.

43 Kopf M, Coyle AJ, Schmitz N, *et al.* Inducible costimulator protein (ICOS) controls T helper cell subset polarization after virus and parasite infection. *J Exp Med* 2000;**192**:53–61.

44 Swallow MM, Wallin JJ, Sha WC. B7h, a novel costimulatory homolog of B7.1 and B7.2, is induced by TNFalpha. *Immunity* 1999;**11**:423–32.

45 Ling V, Wu PW, Finnerty HF, *et al.* Cutting edge: identification of GL50, a novel B7-like protein that functionally binds to ICOS receptor. *J Immunol* 2000;**164**:1653–7.

46 Wang S, Zhu G, Chapoval AI, *et al.* Costimulation of T cells by B7-H2, a B7-like molecule that binds ICOS. *Blood* 2000;**96**:2808–13.

47 Dong C, Juedes AE, Temann UA, *et al.* ICOS co-stimulatory receptor is essential for T-cell activation and function. *Nature* 2001;**409**:97–101.

48 Gonzalo JA, Tian J, Delaney T, *et al.* ICOS is critical for T helper cell-mediated lung mucosal inflammatory responses. *Nat Immunol* 2001;**2**:597–604.

49 McAdam AJ, Greenwald RJ, Levin MA, *et al.* ICOS is critical for CD40-mediated antibody class switching. *Nature* 2001;**409**:102–5.

50 Tafuri A, Shahinian A, Bladt F, *et al.* ICOS is essential for effective T-helper-cell responses. *Nature* 2001;**409**:105–9.

51 Akbari O, Freeman GJ, Meyer EH, *et al.* Antigen-specific regulatory T cells develop via the ICOS-ICOS-ligand pathway and inhibit allergen-induced airway hyperreactivity. *Nat Med* 2002;**8**:1024–32.

52 Ozkaynak E, Gao W, Shemmeri N, *et al.* Importance of ICOS-B7RP-1 costimulation in acute and chronic allograft rejection. *Nat Immunol* 2001;**2**:591–6.

53 Harada H, Salama AD, Sho M, *et al.* The role of the ICOS-B7h T cell costimulatory pathway in transplantation immunity. *J Clin Invest* 2003;**112**:234–43.

54 Quezada SA, Jarvinen LZ, Lind EF, Noelle RJ. CD40/CD154 interactions at the interface of tolerance and immunity. *Annu Rev Immunol* 2004;**22**:307–28.

55 van Kooten C, Bancchereau J. Functional role of CD40 and its ligand. *Int Arch Allergy Immunol* 1997;**113**:393–9.

56 Bourgeois C, Rocha B, Tanchot C. A role for CD40 expression on CD8+ T cells in the generation of CD8+ T cell memory. *Science* 2002;**297**:2060–3.

57 Jabara H, Laouini D, Tsitsikov E, *et al.* The binding site for TRAF2 and TRAF3 but not for TRAF6 is essential for CD40-mediated immunoglobulin class switching. *Immunity* 2002;**17**:265–76.

58 Ahonen C, Manning E, Erickson LD, *et al.* The CD40-TRAF6 axis controls affinity maturation and the generation of long-lived plasma cells. *Nat Immunol* 2002;**3**:451–6.

59 Henn V, Slupsky JR, Grafe M, *et al.* CD40 ligand on activated platelets triggers an inflammatory reaction of endothelial cells. *Nature* 1998;**391**:591–4.

60 Danese S, de la Motte C, Sturm A, *et al.* Platelets trigger a CD40-dependent inflammatory response in the microvasculature of inflammatory bowel disease patients. *Gastroenterology* 2003;**124**:1249–64.

61 Aruffo A, Farrington M, Hollenbaugh D, *et al.* The CD40 ligand, gp39, is defective in activated T cells from patients with X-linked hyper-IgM syndrome. *Cell* 1993;**72**:291–300.

62 Allen RC, Armitage RJ, Conley ME, *et al.* CD40 ligand gene defects responsible for X-linked hyper-IgM syndrome. *Science* 1993;**259**:990–3.

63 Korthauer U, Graf D, Mages HW, *et al.* Defective expression of T-cell CD40 ligand causes X-linked immunodeficiency with hyper-IgM. *Nature* 1993;**361**:539–41.

64 DiSanto JP, Bonnefoy JY, Gauchat JF, Fischer A, de Saint Basile G. CD40 ligand mutations in X-linked immunodeficiency with hyper-IgM. *Nature* 1993;**361**:541–3.

65 Fuleihan R, Ramesh N, Loh R, *et al.* Defective expression of the CD40 ligand in X chromosome-linked immunoglobulin deficiency with normal or elevated IgM. *Proc Natl Acad Sci USA* 1993;**90**:2170–3.

66 Yang Y, Wilson JM. CD40 ligand-dependent T cell activation: requirement of B7-CD28 signaling through CD40. *Science* 1996;**273**:1862–4.

67 Ridge JP, Di Rosa F, Matzinger P. A conditioned dendritic cell can be a temporal bridge between a CD4+ T-helper and a T-killer cell. *Nature* 1998;**393**:474–8.

68 Schoenberger SP, Toes RE, van der Voort EI, Offringa R, Melief CJ. T-cell help for cytotoxic T lymphocytes is mediated by CD40–CD40L interactions. *Nature* 1998;**393**:480–3.

69 Bennett SR, Carbone FR, Karamalis F, Flavell RA, Miller JF, Heath WR. Help for cytotoxic-T-cell responses is mediated by CD40 signalling. *Nature* 1998;**393**:478–80.

70 Filatenkov AA, Jacovetty EL, Fischer UB, Curtsinger JM, Mescher MF, Ingulli E. CD4 T cell-dependent conditioning of dendritic cells to produce IL-12 results in CD8-mediated graft rejection and avoidance of tolerance. *J Immunol* 2005;**174**:6909–17.

71 Schmidt CS, Mescher MF. Adjuvant effect of IL-12: conversion of peptide antigen administration from tolerizing to immunizing for CD8+ T cells *in vivo*. *J Immunol* 1999;**163**:2561–7.

72 Curtsinger JM, Schmidt CS, Mondino A, *et al.* Inflammatory cytokines provide a third signal for activation of naive CD4+ and CD8+ T cells. *J Immunol* 1999;**162**:3256–62.

73 Bancchereau J, Steinman RM. Dendritic cells and the control of immunity. *Nature* 1998;**392**:245–52.

74 Frleta D, Lin JT, Quezada SA, *et al.* Distinctive maturation of *in vitro* versus *in vivo* anti-CD40 mAb-matured dendritic cells in mice. *J Immunother* 2003;**26**:72–84.

75 Josien R, Li HL, Ingulli E, *et al.* TRANCE, a tumor necrosis factor family member, enhances the longevity and adjuvant properties of dendritic cells *in vivo*. *J Exp Med* 2000;**191**:495–502.

76 Sparwasser T, Koch ES, Vabulas RM, *et al.* Bacterial DNA and immunostimulatory CpG oligonucleotides trigger maturation and activation of murine dendritic cells. *Eur J Immunol* 1998;**28**:2045–54.

77 Brunner C, Seiderer J, Schlamp A, *et al.* Enhanced dendritic cell maturation by TNF-alpha or cytidine-phosphate-guanosine DNA drives T cell activation *in vitro* and therapeutic anti-tumor immune responses *in vivo*. *J Immunol* 2000;**165**:6278–86.

78 Jakob T, Walker PS, Krieg AM, Udey MC, Vogel JC. Activation of cutaneous dendritic cells by CpG-containing oligodeoxynucleotides: a role for dendritic cells in the augmentation of Th1 responses by immunostimulatory DNA. *J Immunol* 1998;**161**:3042–9.

79 Melief CJ, Van Der Burg SH, Toes RE, Ossendorp F, Offringa R. Effective therapeutic anticancer vaccines based on precision guiding of cytolytic T lymphocytes. *Immunol Rev* 2002;**188**:177–82.

80 Maxwell JR, Ruby C, Kerkvliet NI, Vella AT. Contrasting the roles of costimulation and the natural adjuvant lipopolysaccharide during the induction of T cell immunity. *J Immunol* 2002;**168**:4372–81.

81 Cho HJ, Hayashi T, Datta SK, *et al.* IFN-alpha beta promote priming of antigen-specific CD8+ and CD4+ T lymphocytes by immunostimulatory DNA-based vaccines. *J Immunol* 2002;**168**:4907–13.

82 Burkly LC. CD40 pathway blockade as an approach to immunotherapy. *Adv Exp Med Biol* 2001;**489**:135–52.

83 Becher B, Durell BG, Miga AV, Hickey WF, Noelle RJ. The clinical course of experimental autoimmune encephalomyelitis and inflammation is controlled by the expression of CD40 within the central nervous system. *J Exp Med* 2001;**193**:967–74.

84 Howard LM, Dal Canto MC, Miller SD. Transient anti-CD154-mediated immunotherapy of ongoing relapsing experimental autoimmune encephalomyelitis induces long-term inhibition of disease relapses. *J Neuroimmunol* 2002;**129**:58–65.

85 Davidson A, Wang X, Mihara M, *et al.* Co-stimulatory blockade in the treatment of murine systemic lupus erythematosus (SLE). *Ann NY Acad Sci* 2003;**987**:188–98.

86 Boumpas DT, Furie R, Manzi S, *et al.* A short course of BG9588 (anti-CD40 ligand antibody) improves serologic activity and decreases hematuria in patients with proliferative lupus glomerulonephritis. *Arthritis Rheum* 2003;**48**:719–27.

87 Kalunian KC, Davis JC Jr, Merrill JT, Totoritis MC, Wofsy D. Treatment of systemic lupus erythematosus by inhibition of T cell costimulation with anti-CD154: a randomized, double-blind, placebo-controlled trial. *Arthritis Rheum* 2002;**46**:3251–8.

88 Hawiger D, Inaba K, Dorsett Y, *et al.* Dendritic cells induce peripheral T cell unresponsiveness under steady state conditions *in vivo*. *J Exp Med* 2001;**194**:769–79.

89 Bonifaz L, Bonnyay D, Mahnke K, Rivera M, Nussenzweig MC, Steinman RM. Efficient targeting of protein antigen to the dendritic cell receptor DEC-205 in the steady state leads to antigen presentation on major histocompatibility complex class I products and peripheral CD8+ T cell tolerance. *J Exp Med* 2002;**196**:1627–38.

90 Steinman RM, Turley S, Mellman I, Inaba K. The induction of tolerance by dendritic cells that have captured apoptotic cells. *J Exp Med* 2000;**191**:411–6.

91 Scheinecker C, McHugh R, Shevach EM, Germain RN. Constitutive presentation of a natural tissue autoantigen exclusively by dendritic cells in the draining lymph node. *J Exp Med* 2002;**196**:1079–90.

92 Taylor PA, Friedman TM, Korngold R, Noelle RJ, Blazar BR. Tolerance induction of alloreactive T cells via *ex vivo* blockade of the CD40:CD40L costimulatory pathway results in the generation of a potent immune regulatory cell. *Blood* 2002;**99**:4601–9.

93 Ishida Y, Agata Y, Shibahara K, Honjo T. Induced expression of PD-1, a novel member of the immunoglobulin gene superfamily, upon programmed cell death. *EMBO J* 1992;**11**:3887–95.

94 Vibhakar R, Juan G, Traganos F, Darzynkiewicz Z, Finger LR. Activation-induced expression of human programmed death-1 gene in T-lymphocytes. *Exp Cell Res* 1997;**232**:25–8.

95 Agata Y, Kawasaki A, Nishimura H, *et al.* Expression of the PD-1 antigen on the surface of stimulated mouse T and B lymphocytes. *Int Immunol* 1996;**8**:765–72.

96 Nishimura H, Agata Y, Kawasaki A, *et al.* Developmentally regulated expression of the PD-1 protein on the surface of double-negative (CD4−CD8−) thymocytes. *Int Immunol* 1996;**8**:773–80.

97 Nishimura H, Honjo T, Minato N. Facilitation of beta selection and modification of positive selection in the thymus of PD-1-deficient mice. *J Exp Med* 2000;**191**:891–8.

98 Freeman GJ, Long AJ, Iwai Y, *et al.* Engagement of the PD-1 immunoinhibitory receptor by a novel B7 family member leads to negative regulation of lymphocyte activation. *J Exp Med* 2000;**192**:1027–34.

99 Latchman Y, Wood CR, Chernova T, *et al.* PD-L2 is a second ligand for PD-1 and inhibits T cell activation. *Nat Immunol* 2001;**2**:261–8.

100 Dong H, Zhu G, Tamada K, Chen L. B7-H1, a third member of the B7 family, co-stimulates T-cell proliferation and interleukin-10 secretion. *Nat Med* 1999;**5**:1365–9.

101 Tseng SY, Otsuji M, Gorski K, *et al.* B7-DC, a new dendritic cell molecule with potent costimulatory properties for T cells. *J Exp Med* 2001;**193**:839–46.

102 Sharpe AH, Freeman GJ. The B7-CD28 superfamily. *Nat Rev Immunol* 2002;**2**:116–26.

103 Nishimura H, Honjo T. PD-1: an inhibitory immunoreceptor involved in peripheral tolerance. *Trends Immunol* 2001;**22**:265–8.

104 Nishimura H, Minato N, Nakano T, Honjo T. Immunological studies on PD-1 deficient mice: implication of PD-1 as a negative regulator for B cell responses. *Int Immunol* 1998;**10**:1563–72.

105 Nishimura H, Nose M, Hiai H, Minato N, Honjo T. Development of lupus-like autoimmune diseases by disruption of the PD-1 gene encoding an ITIM motif-carrying immunoreceptor. *Immunity* 1999;**11**:141–51.

106 Nishimura H, Okazaki T, Tanaka Y, *et al.* Autoimmune dilated cardiomyopathy in PD-1 receptor-deficient mice. *Science* 2001;**291**:319–22.

107 Ozkaynak E, Wang L, Goodearl A, *et al.* Programmed death-1 targeting can promote allograft survival. *J Immunol* 2002;**169**:6546–53.

108 Gao W, Demirci G, Strom TB, Li XC. Stimulating PD-1-negative signals concurrent with blocking CD154 co-stimulation induces long-term islet allograft survival. *Transplantation* 2003;**76**:994–9.

109 Blazar BR, Carreno BM, Panoskaltsis-Mortari A, *et al.* Blockade of programmed death-1 engagement accelerates graft-versus-host disease lethality by an IFN-gamma-dependent mechanism. *J Immunol* 2003;**171**:1272–7.

110 Linsley PS, Brady W, Urnes M, Grosmaire LS, Damle NK, Ledbetter JA. CTLA-4 is a second receptor for the B cell activation antigen B7. *J Exp Med* 1991;**174**:561–9.

111 Yamada A, Kishimoto K, Dong VM, *et al.* CD28-independent costimulation of T cells in alloimmune responses. *J Immunol* 2001;**167**:140–6.

112 Markees TG, Phillips NE, Gordon EJ, *et al.* Long-term survival of skin allografts induced by donor splenocytes and anti-CD154 antibody in thymectomized mice requires CD4+ T cells, interferon-gamma, and CTLA4. *J Clin Invest* 1998;**101**:2446–55.

113 Zheng XX, Markees TG, Hancock WW, *et al.* CTLA4 signals are required to optimally induce allograft tolerance with combined donor-specific transfusion and anti-CD154 monoclonal antibody treatment. *J Immunol* 1999;**162**:4983–90.

114 Lenschow DJ, Zeng Y, Thistlethwaite JR, *et al.* Long-term survival of xenogeneic pancreatic islet grafts induced by CTLA4Ig. *Science* 1992;**257**:789–92.

115 Baliga P, Chavin KD, Qin L, *et al.* CTLA4Ig prolongs allograft survival while suppressing cell-mediated immunity. *Transplantation* 1994;**58**:1082–90.

116 Glysing-Jensen T, Raisanen-Sokolowski A, Sayegh MH, Russell ME. Chronic blockade of CD28-B7-mediated T-cell costimulation by CTLA4Ig reduces intimal thickening in MHC class I and II incompatible mouse heart allografts. *Transplantation* 1997;**64**:1641–5.

117 Kirk AD, Harlan DM, Armstrong NN, *et al.* CTLA4-Ig and anti-CD40 ligand prevent renal allograft rejection in primates. *Proc Natl Acad Sci USA* 1997;**94**:8789–94.

118 Onodera K, Chandraker A, Volk HD, *et al.* Distinct tolerance pathways in sensitized allograft recipients after selective blockade of activation signal 1 or signal 2. *Transplantation* 1999;**68**:288–93.

119 Adams AB, Shirasugi N, Durham MM, *et al.* Calcineurin inhibitor-free CD28 blockade-based protocol protects allogeneic islets in nonhuman primates. *Diabetes* 2002;**51**:265–70.

120 Levisetti MG, Padrid PA, Szot GL, *et al.* Immunosuppressive effects of human CTLA4Ig in a non-human primate model of allogeneic pancreatic islet transplantation. *J Immunol* 1997;**159**:5187–91.

121 Li Y, Zheng XX, Li XC, Zand MS, Strom TB. Combined costimulation blockade plus rapamycin but not cyclosporine produces permanent engraftment. *Transplantation* 1998;**66**:1387–8.

122 Larsen CP, Pearson TC, Adams AB, *et al.* Rational development of LEA29Y (belatacept), a high-affinity variant of CTLA4-Ig with potent immunosuppressive properties. *Am J Transplant* 2005;**5**:443–53.

123 Markees TG, Phillips NE, Noelle RJ, *et al.* Prolonged survival of mouse skin allografts in recipients treated with donor splenocytes and antibody to CD40 ligand. *Transplantation* 1997;**64**:329–35.

124 Jarvinen LZ, Blazar BR, Adeyi OA, Strom TB, Noelle RJ. CD154 on the surface of CD4+CD25+ regulatory T cells contributes to skin transplant tolerance. *Transplantation* 2003;**76**:1375–9.

125 Gordon EJ, Markees TG, Phillips NE, *et al.* Prolonged survival of rat islet and skin xenografts in mice treated with donor splenocytes and anti-CD154 monoclonal antibody. *Diabetes* 1998;**47**:1199–206.

126 Quezada SA, Fuller B, Jarvinen LZ, *et al.* Mechanisms of donor-specific transfusion tolerance: preemptive induction of clonal T-cell exhaustion via indirect presentation. *Blood* 2003;**102**:1920–6.

127 Elster EA, Xu H, Tadaki DK, *et al.* Treatment with the humanized CD154-specific monoclonal antibody, hu5C8, prevents acute rejection of primary skin allografts in nonhuman primates. *Transplantation* 2001;**72**:1473–8.

128 Benda B, Ljunggren HG, Peach R, Sandberg JO, Korsgren O. Co-stimulatory molecules in islet xenotransplantation: CTLA4Ig treatment in CD40 ligand-deficient mice. *Cell Transplant* 2002;**11**:715–20.

129 Kurtz J, Ito H, Wekerle T, Shaffer J, Sykes M. Mechanisms involved in the establishment of tolerance through costimulatory blockade and BMT: lack of requirement for CD40L-mediated signaling for tolerance or deletion of donor-reactive CD4+ cells. *Am J Transplant* 2001;**1**:339–49.

130 Camirand G, Caron NJ, Turgeon NA, Rossini AA, Tremblay JP. Treatment with anti-CD154 antibody and donor-specific transfusion prevents acute rejection of myoblast transplantation. *Transplantation* 2002;**73**:453–61.

131 Tung TH, Mackinnon SE, Mohanakumar T. Long-term limb allograft survival using anti-CD40L antibody in a murine model. *Transplantation* 2003;**75**:644–50.

132 Larsen CP, Pearson TC. The CD40 pathway in allograft rejection, acceptance, and tolerance. *Curr Opin Immunol* 1997;**9**:641–7.

133 Hancock WW, Sayegh MH, Zheng XG, Peach R, Linsley PS, Turka LA. Costimulatory function and expression of CD40 ligand, CD80, and CD86 in vascularized murine cardiac allograft rejection. *Proc Natl Acad Sci USA* 1996;**93**:13967–72.

134 Larsen CP, Alexander DZ, Hollenbaugh D, *et al.* CD40-gp39 interactions play a critical role during allograft rejection. Suppression of allograft rejection by blockade of the CD40-gp39 pathway. *Transplantation* 1996;**61**:4–9.

135 Honey K, Cobbold SP, Waldmann H. CD40 ligand blockade induces CD4+ T cell tolerance and linked suppression. *J Immunol* 1999;**163**:4805–10.

136 Linsley PS, Wallace PM, Johnson J, *et al.* Immunosuppression *in vivo* by a soluble form of the CTLA-4 T cell activation molecule. *Science* 1992;**257**:792–5.

137 Pearson TC, Alexander DZ, Winn KJ, Linsley PS, Lowry RP, Larsen CP. Transplantation tolerance induced by CTLA4-Ig. *Transplantation* 1994;**57**:1701–6.

138 Larsen CP, Elwood ET, Alexander DZ, *et al.* Long-term acceptance of skin and cardiac allografts after blocking CD40 and CD28 pathways. *Nature* 1996;**381**:434–8.

139 Sun H, Subbotin V, Chen C, *et al.* Prevention of chronic rejection in mouse aortic allografts by combined treatment with CTLA4-Ig and anti-CD40 ligand monoclonal antibody. *Transplantation* 1997;**64**:1838–43.

140 Elwood ET, Larsen CP, Cho HR, *et al.* Prolonged acceptance of concordant and discordant xenografts with combined CD40 and CD28 pathway blockade. *Transplantation* 1998;**65**:1422–8.

141 Demirci G, Amanullah F, Kewalaramani R, *et al.* Critical role of OX40 in CD28 and CD154-independent rejection. *J Immunol* 2004;**172**:1691–8.

142 Ferrari-Lacraz S, Zheng XX, Kim YS, Maslinski W, Strom TB. Addition of an IL-15 mutant/FCgamma2A antagonist protein protects islet allografts from rejection overriding costimulation blockade. *Transplant Proc* 2002;**34**:745–7.

143 Pearson TC, Alexander DZ, Hendrix R, *et al.* CTLA4-Ig plus bone marrow induces long-term allograft survival and donor specific unresponsiveness in the murine model. Evidence for hematopoietic chimerism. *Transplantation* 1996;**61**:997–1004.

144 Lin H, Bolling SF, Linsley PS, *et al.* Long-term acceptance of major histocompatibility complex mismatched cardiac allografts induced by CTLA4Ig plus donor-specific transfusion. *J Exp Med* 1993;**178**:1801–6.

145 Sayegh MH, Zheng XG, Magee C, Hancock WW, Turka LA. Donor antigen is necessary for the prevention of chronic rejection in CTLA4Ig-treated murine cardiac allograft recipients. *Transplantation* 1997;**64**:1646–50.

146 Parker DC, Greiner DL, Phillips NE, *et al.* Survival of mouse pancreatic islet allografts in recipients treated with allogeneic small lymphocytes and antibody to CD40 ligand. *Proc Natl Acad Sci USA* 1995;**92**:9560–4.

4 The HLA System and Histocompatibility Testing for Organ Transplantation

René J. Duquesnoy

The HLA (human leukocyte antigen) system has a crucial role in the humoral and cellular immune responses that cause transplant failures. Matching for HLA promotes the successful outcome of transplanted organs, in particular the kidney. Matching may enhance outcomes in thoracic transplantation but is rarely feasible in the clinical setting. The extensive polymorphism of HLA poses a major barrier to finding matched donors. The role of the tissue typing laboratory is to assess the degree of HLA compatibility between donor and recipient and determine the presence of donor-specific antibodies that might be harmful to the organ transplant. Although more effective immunosuppressive strategies have markedly increased transplant survival rates, the successful clinical management of the transplant patient requires an understanding of the HLA system.

This chapter provides a brief overview of the structure and function of HLA antigens in relation to issues of histocompatibility testing for transplantation. Several reviews provide more detailed information [1–3].

STRUCTURE AND FUNCTION OF HLA

HLA antigens are controlled by a series of highly polymorphic genes on the short arm of chromosome 6, referred to as the human major histocompatibility complex (MHC). These genes have been classified into two major categories. HLA-A, HLA-B and HLA-C encode for class I molecules consisting of a 45-kD glycopeptide chain complexed to a 12-kD β_2-microglobulin chain encoded by a nonpolymorphic gene on chromosome 15. The genes in the HLA-DR, HLA-DQ and HLA-DP regions encode for class II molecules consisting of a ~30-kD α chain and a ~28-kD β chain. These HLA class I and II alloantigens can induce transplant immunity at both humoral (antibody) and cellular (T lymphocyte) immune levels. The human MHC contains several other class I and II genes (e.g. HLA-G and HLA-DM) whose products do not seem important as transplantation antigens. An exception seems to be the recently discovered MICA locus, a polymorphic alloantigen system expression on endothelial cells, fibroblasts and monocytes [4].

Both class I and II HLA molecules contain four immunoglobulin-like domains and two of them form a peptide-binding groove consisting of two parallel α-helix amino acid chains on an eight β-pleated polypeptide sheet. Their primary role is to bind small antigenic peptides for presentation to the T-cell receptor (TCR) which then will lead to specific T-cell activation. Such antigenic peptides may generate from viruses and other microorganisms and they are essential in eliciting cellular immune responses to infections. HLA molecules with bound peptides appear on the surface of so-called antigen-presenting cells (APCs) by two general mechanisms. The endogenous pathway leads to the expression of class I molecules complexed with intracellularly produced peptides which are 8–9 amino acid residues long. Such complexes can activate CD8 T cells, including cytotoxic lymphocytes. In the exogenous pathway, APC take up and process external proteins to generate peptides 10–25 amino acid residues long that bind to class II molecules and this can lead to the activation of CD4 T lymphocytes, including T helper cells.

The considerable polymorphism of HLA is well-known. By serology for instance, at least 25 alleles have been reported for HLA-A, 60 alleles for HLA-B and 18 alleles for HLA-DR. Molecular typing has resulted in even greater numbers of HLA alleles and it is often very difficult to find perfectly HLA-matched unrelated donors for transplant recipients. The polymorphism of HLA is reflected by variations in amino acid sequences of HLA molecules. Differences in the amino acid composition of the peptide-binding site will alter the spectrum of antigenic peptides presented by HLA molecules and this will affect the repertoire of responding T cells. This concept may explain why many autoimmune diseases such as juvenile diabetes and rheumatoid arthritis are associated with specific HLA types.

HLA AND TRANSPLANT IMMUNITY

HLA compatibility affects transplant immunity in several ways (Table 4.1). First, HLA antigens can activate B cells to produce alloantibodies involved with humoral mechanisms

Table 4.1 Potential effects of human leukocyte antigen (HLA) on transplant immunity.

Humoral immunity
Against class I HLA antigens
    Complement-dependent antibodies
    Complement-independent antibodies
Against class II HLA antigens

Cellular immunity
Direct allorecognition
    Cytotoxic CD8 T cells
    Effector CD4 T cells
    Regulatory T cells
Indirect allorecognition
    Effector CD4 T cells

HLA-restricted immune responses
Antiviral immunity
    Cytotoxic CD8 T cells
Recurrent autoimmune disease
    Effector CD4 T cells

HLA-specific graft-versus-host disease
Mediated by donor T cells

of transplant rejection. Recent studies have established histopathologic evidence of humoral rejection with immunostains specific for complement components (especially C4d) and immunoglobulins [5–7]. Although class I antigens controlled by the HLA-A, HLA-B and HLA-C loci are the primary targets of alloantibodies, emerging evidence indicates antibody reactivity to class II antigens encoded by HLA-DR, HLA-DQ and even HLA-DP antigens may also result in graft loss [8–11]. Humoral immunity against HLA is now recognized as a major risk factor for chronic rejection and transplant failure [12,13]. Thus, post-transplant serum screening for HLA antibodies appears clinically useful for patients at risk for rejection-related transplant failure.

There are two general mechanisms for development of cellular immunity to HLA antigens (see Chapter 2). Direct recognition is the interaction of recipient T cells with incompatible HLA antigens on the surface of so-called professional APC from the donor. The general result is a strong T-cell response that recognizes differences in donor HLA antigens and the generation of allospecific effector T cells. These T cells infiltrate the graft and initiate transplant rejection [14–19]. It is thought that class I antigens mainly activate cytotoxic T cells while class II antigens activate helper and effector T cells that secrete inflammatory cytokines. On the other hand, an APC subset of dendritic cells can stimulate regulatory T cells that promote transplant tolerance [20,21]. Although most professional donor APC will disappear soon after transplantation, a small proportion may persist in the recipient.

This microchimerism seems pertinent to the long-term success of a transplant [22,23]. Relevant are the interactions between recipient alloreactive T cells and donor HLA antigens on epithelium and vascular endothelium [24–26].

Indirect allorecognition is a mechanism of T-cell activation induced by recipient APC that present donor HLA antigens released by the transplanted organ. The uptake and processing of such antigen is through the exogenous pathway of antigen processing and the class II HLA molecules on recipient APC present donor-derived peptides to recipient CD4 T cells. Indirect T-cell alloreactivity can be long-lasting because an *in situ* transplant is a continuous source of donor alloantigens. This mechanism may contribute to the development of chronic rejection [27–29].

Infections are a major hazard to transplant recipients and very often affect the transplanted tissues. T cells reactive to microbial peptides presented by self-HLA molecules on their APC develop in many patients with exposure prior to transplantation. These HLA-restricted T cells have been shown to promote rejection if the infected transplanted tissues express the same HLA antigens as the recipient. In this situation, HLA matching may promote nonalloimmune cellular immune mechanisms that cause inflammatory damage to the transplant. Several studies have shown an increased incidence of virus-induced injury of HLA matched transplants [30–34].

Thus, it appears that HLA matching can have a dualistic effect on transplant outcome, especially in liver transplantation [35,36]. On one hand, it reduces alloreactivity and graft rejection but, on the other hand, it can promote HLA-restricted immune mechanisms of graft injury secondary to infection or may also lead to recurrent autoimmune disease. An example is the increased incidence of recurrent glomerulonephritis in kidneys transplanted from HLA-matched living related donors [37]. These observations have been made with adult patients and it is not known how often HLA-restricted immune mechanisms affect pediatric transplants.

HLA is also involved in graft-versus-host disease (GVHD) whereby donor-derived lymphocytes react with HLA-incompatible recipient cells and induce inflammatory responses in host tissues such as the skin and gastrointestinal tract. This complication is frequent after bone marrow transplantation, but may also affect recipients of liver and other transplanted organs and even blood transfusions [38–41].

HLA ANTIGEN MATCHING FOR CLINICAL TRANSPLANTATION

Tissue typing for organ transplantation has four components: HLA and ABO matching, serum screening for HLA antibodies, cross-matching with donor cells and post-transplant monitoring (Table 4.2). ABO compatibility is necessary to avoid donor transplants that might be rejected by anti-ABO antibodies.

Table 4.2 Histocompatibility testing procedures for organ transplantation.

Procedure	Test design	Available methodologies	Clinical value of test results
Determine donor–recipient compatibility	Compare ABO and HLA types of patients and donors	Serology Molecular typing DNA sequencing	ABO and HLA matching reduces rejection and GVHD and increases graft survival
Analyze allosensitization status of patient	Serum screening against HLA-typed panels: Determine PRA Define HLA antibody specificity patterns	CDC and AHG Flow cytometry ELISA Flow beads Luminex	Identify high PRA patients Define acceptable HLA mismatched antigens Interpret cross-match results with potential donors
Perform cross-match	Test patient serum against cells from potential donors	CDC and AHG Flow cytometry	Prevent hyperacute rejection Reduce antibody-mediated vascular rejection
Monitor transplant recipients for HLA antibodies	Determine *de novo* donor-specific antibodies	CDC and AHG Flow beads ELISA Luminex	Associated with rejection Prognosticators of chronic rejection Risk factor for transplant failure

AHG, antihuman globulin; CDC, complement-dependent cytotoxicity; ELISA, enzyme-linked immunosorbent assay; GVHD, graft-versus-host disease; HLA, human leukocyte antigen; PRA, panel-reactive antibody.

Most HLA matching protocols consider the antigens controlled by three loci: HLA-A, HLA-B and HLA-DR. Zero-ABDR antigen mismatches have the highest graft survival rates and this has been implemented in many policies for deceased donor organ allocation. Nevertheless, a significant proportion of these transplants fail; some because of non-HLA related causes such as graft quality or disease recurrence, and others because of rejection caused by incompatible allelic variations of HLA-A, HLA-B and HLA-DR antigens not detectable by standard typing methods, and contributions of mismatches controlled by other loci such as HLA-C, HLA-DQ and HLA-DP [8,42,43].

Conversely, many mismatched transplants have long-term function with no evidence of rejection. Certain vascularized grafts can withstand antibody-mediated injury [44] with possible mechanisms including antigenic modulation [45], graft accommodation [46–48] and protection by anti-idiotypic antibodies [49–51]. Not every HLA mismatch induces antibody or effector T cells. Many reports describe different cellular mechanisms of long-term graft survival (even without immunosuppressive drugs) including hematolymphoid microchimerism [22,23], T-cell hyporesponsiveness [52] and apoptosis [53], regulatory cells [54] and immunologic tolerance [23]. Thus, in some yet undefined clinical situations, certain HLA mismatches are permissible.

Several investigators have attempted to determine mismatch permissibility by analyzing how specific donor and recipient HLA antigens affect graft survival [55–61]. The HLA type of the recipient may affect the immunogenicity of a mismatch [62]. An empirical analysis of graft survival in related donor kidneys identified certain immunogenic (also referred to as taboo mismatches [63]) and permissible donor–recipient antigen combinations. Subsequent studies with deceased donor transplant databases found superior graft survival for the permissible mismatch combinations [62,64] but conflicting results were noted in another registry analysis [65]. Another approach suggested noninherited maternal HLA antigens (NIMA) may result in mismatch permissibility through development of prenatal tolerance [66,67]. Registry analysis indicated one-haplotype mismatched related transplants mismatched for NIMAs had superior survival rates compared with those mismatched for noninherited paternal antigens [66,68,69], but again, these results were not validated in subsequent registry analyses [70–72]. Validation of mismatch permissibility models remains elusive.

The influence of HLA-DQ matching is less clear. Some studies found a beneficial effect [73–75] but others did not [76–78]. There is a similar controversy about the effect of HLA-DP matching [79–81].

STRUCTURALLY BASED HLA MATCHING

Although it is universally accepted that HLA compatibility has a major role in determining graft outcome, the ongoing debate about the utility of HLA matching seems to reflect the inadequacy of merely counting mismatched HLA-A, HLA-B and HLA-DR antigens. An alternative approach considers matching for serologically defined public epitopes shared by class I antigens belonging to so-called cross-reacting groups

(CREGs) [6–8]. Several studies have suggested CREG matching is associated with graft survivals that are better or comparable to those allocated on HLA antigen matching [10–18] but others have not found a beneficial effect of CREG matching [19–23]. The controversy about CREG matching is caused, in part, by the difficulty in defining the exact spectrum of public epitopes on all HLA antigens.

Many studies utilizing HLA-specific monoclonal antibodies have indicated that epitopes correspond to distinct amino acid residues or short sequences in HLA. These epitopes have been used as the basis for defining acceptable mismatches [82–86]. Retrospective registry analysis indicates that epitope matching could be used to provide compatible kidneys for highly sensitized patients [86]. Other structurally defined parameters such as peptide motif matching may also influence renal graft outcome [87–89].

HLAMatchmaker is a matching program that considers the structural basis of epitopes on class I HLA antigens [90]. Each HLA antigen can be viewed as a string of short sequences (triplets) involving polymorphic amino acid residues in antibody-accessible positions; they are considered key elements of epitopes that can induce the formation of specific antibodies. The patient's HLA phenotype represents the repertoire of self-triplets to which no antibodies can be made and HLAMatchmaker determines, for each mismatched HLA antigen, which triplets in corresponding sequence positions are different. HLAMatchmaker-based matching improves transplant outcome [91–95] and is useful for refractory thrombocytopenic patients requiring matched platelet transfusions [96]. The beneficial effect of triplet matching applies to both nonsensitized and sensitized patients and also for white and nonwhite patients.

SERUM SCREENING METHODS

Humoral allosensitization is the process of developing antibody reactive to HLA antigens. A transplant, blood transfusions and pregnancy are the primary causes of HLA sensitization. Serum screening for alloreactive antibodies against HLA-typed panels will provide an assessment of the degree of sensitization.

Several techniques are now available for serum screening [97]. Table 4.3 compares their features. The complement-dependent cytotoxicity (CDC) technique is "cell-based" because it uses HLA antigens expressed on the lymphocyte surface. There are two versions. One is a direct assay whereby the patient's antibodies exert a lymphocytotoxic effect through complement-dependent mechanisms of cell membrane lysis. The indirect technique utilizes an extra step with goat or rabbit antihuman globulin (AHG) to augment antibody reactivity and this test is more sensitive than CDC. The source of lymphocytes is an important consideration: T-cells express only class I antigens whereas B cells are used to detect class II-specific antibodies although they also express class I antigens. Serum treatment with dithiothreitol (DTT) is used to distinguish between immunoglobulin G (IgG) and IgM type antibodies.

Flow cytometric screening is the third cell-based assay for HLA antibody detection. This complement-independent antigen-binding uses also lymphocytes and is more sensitive than CDC and AHG. Three solid-phase techniques are clinically used: enzyme-linked immunosorbent assay (ELISA), flow beads and Luminex. Each represents a binding assay with solubilized HLA antigens coated on an artificial surface. Recent advancements have led to the use of single antigen preparations [98] that are more informative regarding antibody reactivity

Table 4.3 Comparisons of different screening methods for HLA antibodies.

	Cell-based assays	Solid phase assays
Method	CDC, AHG, flow cytometry	ELISA, flow beads, Luminex
Sensitivity	Lymphocytotoxicity is less sensitive	More sensitive
HLA antigens	HLA phenotypes	HLA phenotypes Single HLA antigens
HLA molecules	"Natural" configuration on cell surface	Isolated proteins on artificial surface
False-positive reactions	Non-HLA-specific reactivity Drugs Monoclonal antibody therapy	Reactions with cryptic epitopes on "denatured" HLA molecules Nonspecific antibody binding to artificial surface
False-negative reactions	No complement activation Low antigen density Weak antibody affinity	Loss of epitope expression Blocking of HLA epitopes by linking agents

AHG, antihuman globulin; CDC, complement-dependent cytotoxicity; ELISA, enzyme-linked immunosorbent assay; HLA, human leukocyte antigen.

with epitopes than HLA phenotypes representing mixtures of antigens encoded by different loci.

Although solid-phase assays are considered more sensitive than CDC and AHG, there is a potential disadvantage that HLA molecules have been put on an artificial surface rather than being in their natural configuration as membrane-bound proteins. Denaturing of the molecular structure may lead to the expression of "cryptic" epitopes responsible for false-positive reactions with patient sera. This is indicated by findings in some sensitized patients of circulating antibodies against self-HLA antigens. Conversely, denaturation may diminish epitope expression and this may cause false-negative reactions.

Cell-based assays may also show false-positive reactions resulting from antibodies against other antigens on the lymphocyte surface. This applies especially to patients receiving certain drugs or being treated with monoclonal antibodies against CD3, CD20 and other lymphocyte markers. A low HLA antigen expression on lymphocytes, anticomplement activity in certain sera and weak antibody affinity may cause false-negative reactions.

Given the shortcomings of each assay, serum screening should be performed with a combination of methods including lymphocytotoxicity. Consideration should be given to sensitization history, clinical status of the patient and reproducibility of screening results between two or more sera.

INTERPRETATION OF SERUM SCREENING RESULTS

The so-called panel-reactive antibody (PRA) represents a semiquantitative estimate of the degree of HLA sensitization. It is calculated as the percentage of an HLA panel that reacts with a serum. Patients with > 80% PRA are considered highly sensitized and for them it is difficult to find cross-match-negative donors. The use of several screening methods with different levels of sensitivity makes the determination of a PRA very complicated. Therefore, the degree of sensitization might better be assessed by a "virtual" PRA or percent reactive antigens (i.e. the cumulative frequency of HLA antigens that react with patient's serum as a probability estimate of a positive cross-match with a random donor). Conversely, the cumulative frequencies of self-antigens and acceptable antigens nonreactive with patient's serum can be used to calculate a probability of finding a donor (PFD) as an assessment of the transplantability of a sensitized patient [99].

The analysis of serum reactivity of transplant candidates has two goals. Most commonly used is the identification of unacceptable HLA antigens that should be avoided on donor organs. This system is designed to identify donors who must be excluded but it does not necessarily mean that all other HLA antigens would be compatible for a patient. The other goal is to determine HLA antigens that are acceptable mismatches.

This strategy represents a direct approach of finding a compatible donor for a sensitized patient [100,101].

Reactivity patterns with HLA phenotyped panels are primarily analyzed with 2×2 table statistical methods such as χ^2 to identify antigens and epitopes with significant correlations. Unfortunately, this approach has limited value for > 80% PRA sera. The use of single HLA antigens in ELISA and Luminex assays permits a better interpretation of antibody reactivity patterns. An important consideration is that each HLA antigen carries multiple epitopes that can be structurally defined by amino acid residues in polymorphic positions of the HLA molecule. Stereochemical modeling of crystallized HLA antigens has visualized these rather extreme structural polymorphisms.

Plate 4.1 (facing page 224) shows examples of three class I molecules, HLA-A2, HLA-B27 and HLA-Cw3, which can be downloaded from the Entrez Molecular Modeling Database of the National Center for Biotechnology Information website (http://www.ncbi.nlm.nih.gov/Structure) and viewed with the Cn3D structure and sequence alignment software program. The molecular surface around the bound peptide (see top view) has similar numbers of exposed polymorphic positions on the α1 helices of HLA-A and HLA-B antigens but more polymorphic positions are visible on the α2 helices of HLA-A antigens. The α helices of HLA-C antigens have much fewer polymorphic positions.

In contrast, HLA-C antigens have more polymorphic positions in the membrane-proximal region, which becomes visible upon side viewing. HLA-A antigens have also more surface-exposed polymorphic positions in that region than HLA-B antigens. It should be noted that the sequence positions in the membrane-proximal domain of HLA-B are all monomorphic.

Class II HLA antigens have similarly complex structural polymorphisms (not shown). This applies to all DRB, DQB and DPB chains. DQA chains have more structural polymorphisms than DPA chains whereas DRA chains are primarily monomorphic.

Considering the high number of HLA antigens (and alleles) and their extensive polymorphisms, one can expect that HLA antibody formation in transplant patients is extensive and complex. A better understanding of the epitope structure of HLA antigens is important not only for the characterization of HLA-specific antibodies but also will permit a more efficient, structurally based strategy to determine HLA compatibility.

HLAMATCHMAKER-BASED SERUM ANALYSIS

The structurally based HLAMatchmaker algorithm is useful in the interpretation of serum reactivity patterns in HLA sensitized patients. The number of amino acid triplet differences between patient and donor correlates with the degree of anti-HLA antibody formation induced by pregnancy and kidney transplantation [102]. Certain patients become highly sensitized following exposure to a single mismatched HLA antigen. The following two cases illustrate how HLAMatchmaker can explain this.

The first case is a patient who developed a serum PRA of approximately 90% resulting from class I antibodies after removal of a rejected kidney graft 7 months post-transplant [103]. This kidney was a one-antigen mismatch, namely HLA-B13, but patient's serum reacted not only with HLA-B13 but also with a large number of other HLA-A and HLA-B antigens. An HLAMatchmaker-based analysis showed antibody specificity to the 144tQl triplet unique to HLA-B13 and the 76En, 80rTa, 82aLr triplets shared between HLA-B13 and other HLA antigens such as HLA-A9, HLA-B17, HLA-B27 and many more. (The triplet notation system uses the amino acid letter code and the number represents the sequence position of the residue in upper-case letters. Neighboring residues are denoted in lower-case letters [90,104].) The 76En, 80rTa, 82aLr carrying antigens must be considered unacceptable mismatches although the patient might have never been exposed to them. The reason why they become unacceptable was that they share one or more epitopes with the immunizing HLA-B13.

The second example is a high anticlass II antibody activity following sensitization to a one HLA-DR antigen mismatch. This patient typed homozygous for HLA-DR7 and had rejected a kidney transplant with a HLA-DR11 mismatch. The patient's serum reacted with all DRB1 antigens except HLA-DR7. HLAMatchmaker identified a mismatched triplet 14ER on HLA-DR11 that is shared with all DRB1 antigens except HLA-DR7 which has 14QK. Thus, the high reactivity of this patient's serum might be caused by antibodies to a single epitope defined in this case by 14ER. This conclusion is consistent with descriptions of monoclonal antibodies reacting with all DRB1 antigens except HLA-DR7 [105]. Exposure to single HLA-DQ mismatches may also lead to antibody reactivity to all DQB1 antigens except self-DQB1 and corresponding structurally defined DQB1 epitopes can be readily identified.

It should be noted that HLA antibody responses are generally restricted to a limited number of epitopes [106,107]. High PRA sera often reflect the presence of antibodies against high-frequency epitopes. The HLAMatchmaker-based interpretation of serum reactivity incorporates the patient's HLA type, determined preferably by DNA methods at the four-digit allele level. HLA information of the immunizer (i.e. a previous transplant) will identify structurally defined epitopes the patient has been exposed to. This facilitates the interpretation of serum screening results and the determination of mismatch acceptability for prospective donors.

Increasing numbers of laboratories are now performing solid-phase screening with commercially available single HLA antigen kits. For practical reasons these kits contain only the more common alleles. HLAMatchmaker is useful in the interpretation of the reactivity patterns because this program can define epitopes shared by reactive antigens and determine the acceptability of other alleles not included in these kits.

DONOR–RECIPIENT CROSS-MATCHING

The cross-match test is a direct approach determining donor-specific antibody reactivity in a patient's serum. A positive cross-match is a contraindication for organ transplantation because of the risk for hyperacute rejection and the higher incidence of vascular and accelerated cellular rejection during the early post-transplant period. This applies particularly for kidney and heart transplants whereas the liver allograft seems more resistant to antibody-mediated injury.

Cross-matching has traditionally been based on complement-dependent lymphocytotoxicity techniques such as CDC and the more sensitive AHG. T-cell cross-matches (TXm) determine donor class I antigen reactivity whereas B-cell cross-matches (BXm) are performed to detect donor-reactive class II antibodies, although B cells also express class I antigens. Although TXm is considered the standard clinical procedure, there has been controversy about the clinical value of BXm. Many reports have addressed this issue and the collective data now indicate that TXm-negative, BXm-positive transplants are less successful [2].

Serum treatment with DTT is used to distinguish between IgG and IgM type antidonor antibody reactivity. IgM-type antibodies against donor HLA antigens tend to be disregarded in clinical practice because their effect on transplant outcome has not been clearly established [2].

Many laboratories use the flow cytometric cross-match (FCXm) which is considerably more sensitive than the complement-dependent lymphocytotoxicity cross-matches. The clinical significance of FCXm is controversial. Although FCXm-positive, CDC-Xm and/or AHG-Xm-negative transplants are often less successful, the FCXm test seems to be "too" sensitive and proficiency testing surveys have shown considerable interlaboratory variations [108]. A positive FCXm should not routinely be considered a contraindication to transplantation, but might be looked upon as a risk factor in the clinical management of a transplant recipient [2].

Most cross-matches are performed with current and recent sera drawn during the past 6 months. Inclusion of so-called historic sera (obtained more than 6 months prior to a cross-match) provides more complete information about HLA sensitization and several studies have shown that donor-specific HLA antibodies detectable only in historic sera increase the risk of transplant failure [109–111]. Such patients probably have memory B cells although the corresponding anti-HLA antibodies cannot be detected in current sera. Alternatively, the loss of anti-HLA antibody might be caused by the formation of anti-idiotypic antibodies that might protect a graft [50].

A proper interpretation requires information about the sensitization history and especially the anti-HLA antibody reactivity profiles of current and historic sera. A negative cross-match should correlate with the absence of donor-specific anti-HLA antibodies and the assays should have sufficient sensitivity and specificity.

Time constraints do not always permit prospective cross-matches for certain transplant candidates such as heart and lung. So-called virtual cross-matches can be performed for sensitized patients for whom detailed serum screening data can determine whether or not a potential donor is an acceptable HLA mismatch [3,112,113]. An actual cross-match can be carried out during or shortly after transplantation to verify the virtual cross-match and to assess the HLA-associated risk for transplant failure.

POST-TRANSPLANT MONITORING FOR HLA ANTIBODIES

The development of donor-specific anti-HLA antibodies represents a significant risk factor for transplant failure not only because of humoral rejection but also chronic rejection of kidney transplants [13,114,115]. Such antibodies correlate with C4d deposition in peritubular capillaries, a marker of humoral rejection [116]. Recent studies have also shown that *de novo* donor antibodies against donor class I and II HLA antigens precede bronchiolitis obliterans in lung transplant patients [117–120]. The development of donor-specific anti-HLA antibodies is also associated with heart transplant failures because of humoral rejection and coronary artery disease [121,122].

Prospective monitoring for anti-HLA antibodies following transplantation therefore seems useful in the diagnosis and prognosis of graft dysfunction and failure [123]. However, one must consider the concept that donor-specific anti-HLA antibodies may not be detectable in the serum of a transplant recipient because they would be absorbed by the graft. Indeed, allograft nephrectomy leads often to dramatic increases in the levels of antidonor HLA antibodies in patients with rejected kidney transplants [103,124]. With this caveat, monitoring for antidonor HLA antibodies is still feasible if one considers the expression of HLA epitopes in the graft. The more sensitive solid-phase assays such as ELISA and Luminex may identify antibodies to epitopes not readily accessible on donor HLA antigens expressed on the vascular endothelium and other graft tissues. For this reason, CDC-based methods would not be useful in the monitoring of antidonor HLA antibodies. Low tissue expression of certain HLA antigens may also lead to detectable levels of circulating anti-HLA antibodies. It is well-known that the expression of class II antigens is low, although under certain inflammatory conditions it can be upregulated. This may explain why antidonor HLA-DR and HLA-DQ antibodies are more often detected than antidonor HLA-A and HLA-B antibodies. Monitoring for antidonor HLA antibodies may also permit the application of therapeutic modalities to reduce antidonor antibodies such as plasmapheresis and intravenous IgG.

REFERENCES

1 Takemoto S, Port F, Claas F, Duquesnoy RJ. HLA matching for kidney transplantation. *Hum Immunol* 2004;**65**:1489–505.

2 Gebel H, Bray R, Nickerson P. Pre-transplant assessment of donor-reactive, HLA-specific antibodies in renal transplantation: contraindication vs. risk. *Am J Transplant* 2003;**3**:1488–500.

3 Reinsmoen N, Nelson K, Zeevi A. Anti-HLA antibody analysis and crossmatching in heart and lung transplantation. *Transpl Immunol* 2004;**13**:63–71.

4 Zwirner NW, Marcos CY, Mirbaha F, Zou Y, Stastny P. Identification of MICA as a new polymorphic alloantigen recognized by antibodies in sera of organ transplant recipients. *Hum Immunol* 2000;**61**:917–24.

5 Colvin RB. The renal allograft biopsy. *Kidney Int* 1996;**50**:1069–79.

6 Feucht HE, Schneeberger H, Hildebrand G, et al. Capillary deposition of C4d complement fragment and early renal graft loss. *Kidney Int* 1993;**43**:1333–42.

7 Feucht HE. Complement C4d in graft capillaries: the missing link in the recognition of humoral alloreactivity. *Am J Transplant* 2003;**3**:646–52.

8 al-Hussein KA, Shenton BK, Bell A, et al. Characterization of donor-directed antibody class in the post-transplant period using flow cytometry in renal transplantation. *Transpl Int* 1994;**7**:182–8.

9 Feucht HE, Opelz G. The humoral immune response towards HLA class II determinants in renal transplantation [Editorial]. *Kidney Int* 1996;**50**:1464–75.

10 Schoenemann C, Groth J, Leverenz S, May G. HLA class I and class II antibodies: monitoring before and after kidney transplantation. *Transplantation* 1998;**65**:1519–24.

11 Mahoney RJ, Taranto S, Edwards E. B-cell crossmatching and kidney allograft outcome in 9031 United States transplant recipients. *Hum Immunol* 2002;**63**:324–35.

12 McKenna RM, Takemoto S, Terasaki PI. Anti-HLA antibodies after solid organ transplantation. *Transplantation* 2000;**69**:319–26.

13 Terasaki PI. Humoral theory of transplantation. *Am J Transplant* 2003;**3**:665–73.

14 Mayer TG, Fuller AA, Fuller TC, Lazarovits AI, Boyle LA, Kurnick JT. Characterization of *in vivo*-activated allospecific T lymphocytes propagated from human renal allograft biopsies undergoing rejection. *J Immunol* 1985;**134**:258–64.

15 Zeevi A, Fung JJ, Zerbe TR, et al. Allospecificity of activated T-cells grown from endomyocardial biopsies from heart transplant patients. *Transplantation* 1986;**41**:620–6.

16 Fung JJ, Zeevi A, Markus B, Zerbe TR, Duquesnoy RJ. Dynamics of allospecific T lymphocyte infiltration in vascularized human allografts. *Immunol Res* 1986;**5**:149–63.

17 Moreau JF, Bonneville M, Peyrat MA, et al. T lymphocyte cloning from rejected human kidney allografts. *J Clin Invest* 1986;**78**:874–9.

18 Markus BH, Demetris AJ, Saidman S, et al. Alloreactive T lymphocytes cultured from liver transplant biopsies: associations of HLA specificity with clinicopathological findings. *Clin Transpl* 1988;**2**:70–5.

19 Zeevi A, Kaufman C, Duquesnoy RJ. Clinical relevance of lymphocyte analysis in cardiac and pulmonary transplantation.

In: Rose M, Yacoub M, eds. *Immunology of Heart and Lung Transplantation*, Edward Arnold, 1993:181–99.

20 Lechler RI, Ng WF, Steinman RM. Dendritic cells in transplantation: friend or foe? *Immunity* 2001;**14**:357–68.

21 Toby P, Coates H, Thomson AW. Dendritic cells: tolerance induction and transplant tolerance. *Am J Transplant* 2002;**2**:299–307.

22 Starzl TE, Demetris AJ, Murase N, Thomson AW, Trucco M, Ricordi C. Donor cell chimerism permitted by immunosuppressive drugs: a new view of organ transplantation. *Immunol Today* 1993;**14**:326–32.

23 Starzl TE, Zinkernagel R. Transplantation tolerance from a historical perspective. *Nat Rev Immunol* 2001;**1**:233–9.

24 Colson YL, Markus BH, Zeevi A, Duquesnoy RJ. Increased lymphocyte adherence to human arterial endothelial cell monolayers in the context of allorecognition. *J Immunol* 1990;**144**:2975–84.

25 Pober JS, Orosz CG, Rose ML, *et al*. Can graft endothelial cells initiate a host anti-graft response? *Transplantation* 1996;**61**:343–8.

26 Kirby JA, Cunningham AC. Intragraft antigen presentation: the contribution of bone-marrow derived, epithelial and endothelelial presenting cells. *Transpl Rev* 1997;**11**:127–40.

27 Liu Z, Colovai AI, Tugulea S, *et al*. Indirect recognition of donor HLA-DR peptides in organ allograft rejection. *J Clin Invest* 1996;**98**:1150–7.

28 Ciubotariu R, Liu ZR, Colovai AI, *et al*. Persistent allopeptide reactivity and epitope spreading in chronic rejection of organ allografts. *J Clin Invest* 1998;**101**:398–405.

29 Hornick P, Lechler R. Direct and indirect pathways of alloantigen recognition: relevance to acute and chronic allograft rejection. *Nephrol Dial Transplant* 1997;**12**:1806–10.

30 Blancho G, Josein R, Douillard D, Bignon JD, Cesbron JD, Soulillou JP. The influence of HLA A-B-DR matching on cytomegalovirus disease after renal transplantation. Evidence that HLA-DR7-matched recipients are more susceptible to cytomegalovirus disease. *Transplantation* 1992;**54**:871–4.

31 Kraat YJ, Christiaans MHL, Nieman FHM, Van den Berg-Loonen PM, Van Hooff JP, Bruggeman CA. Inreased frequency of CMV infection in HLA-DR7 matched renal allograft recipients. *Lancet* 1993;**341**:494–5.

32 Schnitzler MA, Woodward RS, Brennan DC, *et al*. Cytomegalovirus and HLA-A, B, and DR locus interactions: impact on renal transplant graft survival. *Am J Kidney Dis* 1997;**30**:766–71.

33 Manez R, Mateo R, Tabasco J, Kusne S, Starzl TE, Duquesnoy RJ. The influence of HLA donor-recipient compatibility on the recurrence of HBV and HCV hepatitis after liver transplantation. *Transplantation* 1995;**59**:640–2.

34 Manez R, White LT, Linden P, *et al*. The influence of HLA matching on cytomegalovirus hepatitis and chronic rejection after liver transplantation. *Transplantation* 1993;**55**:1067–71.

35 Markus BH, Duquesnoy RJ, Gordon RD, *et al*. Histocompatibility and liver transplatation: a dualistic effect of HLA? *Transplantation* 1988;**46**:372–7.

36 Donaldson P, Underhill J, Doherty D, *et al*. Influence of human leukocyte antigen matching on liver allograft survival and rejection: "the dualistic effect". *Hepatology* 1993;**17**:1008–15.

37 Andresdottir MB, Hoitsma AJ, Assmann KJ, Koene RA, Wetzels JF. The impact of recurrent glomerulonephritis on graft survival in recipients of human histocompatibility leucocyte antigen-identical living related donor grafts. *Transplantation* 1999;**68**:623–7.

38 Pageaux GP, Perrigault PF, Fabre JM, *et al*. Lethal acute graft-versus-host disease in a liver transplant recipient: relations with cell migration and chimerism. *Clin Transpl* 1995;**9**:65–9.

39 Gulbahce HE, Brown CA, Wick M, Segall M, Jessurun J. Graft-vs-host disease after solid organ transplant. *Am J Clin Pathol* 2003;**119**:568–73.

40 Ohto H, Anderson K. Survey of transfusion-associated graft-versus-host disease in immunocompetent recipients. *Transfus Med Rev* 1996;**10**:31–43.

41 Triulzi D, Duquesnoy R, Zeevi A, *et al*. Fatal transfusion-associated graft versus host disease in an immunocompetent recipient of a volunteer unit of red cells. *Transfusion* 2006;**46**:885–8.

42 Zou Y, Mirbaha F, Lazaro A, Zhang Y, Lavingia B, Stastny P. MICA is a target for complement-dependent cytotoxicity with mouse monoclonal antibodies and human alloantibodies. *Hum Immunol* 2002;**63**:30–9.

43 Sumitran-Holgerson S, Wilczek HE, Holgerson J, Soderstrom K. Identification of the nonclassical HLA molecules. MICA as targets for humoral immunity associated with irreversible rejection of kidney allografts. *Transplantation* 2002;**74**:268–77.

44 Andres G, Yamaguchi N, Brett J, Caldwell PRB, Godman G, Stern D. Cellular mechanisms of adaptation of grafts to antibody. *Transpl Immunol* 1996;**4**:1–17.

45 Chatenoud L, Bach J-F. Antigenic modulation: a major mechanism of antibody action. *Immunol Today* 1984;**5**:20–5.

46 Bach FH, Ferran C, Hechenleitner P, *et al*. Accomodation of vascularized xenografts: expression of "protective genes" by donor endothelial cells in a host Th2 cytokine environment. *Nat Med* 1997;**3**:196–204.

47 Platt JL. A perspecive of xenograft rejection and accommodation. *Immunol Rev* 1994;**141**:127–49.

48 Salama AD, Delikouras A, Pusey CD, *et al*. Transplant accomodation in highly sensitized patients: a potential role for Bcl-xL and alloantibody. *Am J Transplant* 2001;**1**:260–9.

49 Suciu-Foca N, Liu Z, Harris PE, *et al*. Indirect recognition of native HLA alloantigens and B-cell help. *Transplant Proc* 1995;**27**:455–6.

50 Reed E, Hardy M, Benvenisty A, *et al*. Effect of antiidiotypic antibodies to HLA on graft survival in renal-allograft recipients. *N Engl J Med* 1987;**316**:1450–5.

51 Phelan DL, Rodey GE, Anderson CB. The development and specificity of antiidiotypic antibodies in renal transplant recipients receiving single-donor blood transfusions. *Transplantation* 1989;**48**:57–60.

52 Reinsmoen NL. Post-transplant donor antigen-specific hyporeactivity in human transplantation. *Transpl Rev* 1995;**9**:17–28.

53 Kabelitz D. Apoptosis, graft rejection, and transplantation tolerance. *Transplantation* 1998;**65**:869–75.

54 Jiang S, Lechler RI. Regulatory T cells in the control of transplantation tolerance and autoimmunity. *Am J Transplant* 2003;**3**:516–24.

55 Hendriks GF, Schreuder GM, Claas FH, *et al*. HLA-DRw6 and renal allograft rejection. *Br Med J (Clin Res Ed)* 1983;**286**:85–7.

56 Dobbe C, Thorogood J, D'Amaro J, Lange PD, Persijn G, Giphart M. HLA-A1 in renal transplantation. *Transplantation* 1995;**59**:1053–5.

57 Dobbe CM, Thorogood J, de Lange P, *et al*. An unexpected effect of matching for HLA-A9 in renal transplantation [see comments]. *Transplantation* 1990;50:446–8.

58 Dyer PA, Martin S, Kippas R, Mallick NP, Gokal R, Johnson RWG. HLA-DR3 is a marker of graft failure in cadaveric renal transplantation. *Transplant Proc* 1985;11:2248–9.

59 Forsberg B, Ekberg H, Johnson U. Influence of recipient's HLA type on the outcome of renal transplantation. *Transplant Proc* 1992;24:2463–5.

60 Busson M, Gony J, Hors J. Is the strength of single HLA antigen variable in kidney transplant survival? *Transplantation* 1979;28:313–7.

61 Goulmy E, van der Poel JJ, Giphart MJ. The influence of HLA-A2 subtype mismatch on renal allograft survival. *Transplantation* 1992;53:1381–2.

62 Maruya E, Takemoto S, Terasaki PI. HLA matching: identification of permissible HLA mismatches. *Clin Transpl* 1993:511–20.

63 Doxiadis II, Smits JM, Stobbe I, *et al*. Taboo HLA mismatches in cadaveric renal transplantation: definition, analysis, and possible implications. *Transplant Proc* 1996;28:224.

64 van Rood JJ, Lagaaij EL, Doxiadis I, Roelen D, Persijn G, Claas F. Permissible mismatches, acceptable mismatches, and tolerance: new trends in decision making. *Clin Transpl* 1993:285–92.

65 Wujciak T, Opelz G. Evaluation of the permissible mismatch concept. *Transpl Int* 1996;9(Suppl 1):S8–10.

66 van Rood JJ, Claas F. Noninherited maternal HLA antigens: a proposal to elucidate their role in the immune response. *Hum Immunol* 2000;61:1390–4.

67 Van Rood JJ, Claas FHJ. Both self and non-inherited maternal HLA antigens influence the immune response. *Immunol Today* 2000;21:269–73.

68 Burlingham WJ, Grailer AP, Heisey DM, *et al*. The effect of tolerance of non-inherited maternal HLA antigens on the survival of renal transplants from sibling donors. *N Engl J Med* 1998;339:1657–64.

69 Smits JMA, Claas FHJ, Van Houwelingen HC, Persijn G. Do non-inherited maternal antigens (NIMAs) enhance renal allograft survival? *Transpl Int* 1998;82:82–8.

70 Opelz G. Analysis of the "NIMA" effect in renal transplantation. Collaborative Transplant Study. *Transplantation* 1990;63:1990–4.

71 Opelz G. The effect of tolerance to non-inherited maternal HLA antigens on the survival of renal transplant from sibling donors [Comment]. *N Engl J Med* 1999;340:1369–70.

72 Panajotopoulos N, Ianhez LE, Neuman J, Sabbaga E, Kalil J. Immunological tolerance in human transplantation. The possible existence of a maternal effect. *Transplantation* 1990;50:443–7.

73 Duquesnoy RJ, Annen KB, Marrari MM, Kauffman HM Jr. Association of MB compatibility with successful intrafamilial kidney transplantation. *N Engl J Med* 1980;302:821–5.

74 Matsuno N, Inoko H, Ando A, *et al*. Importance of DQB as indicator in living related kidney transplant. *Transplantation* 1990;49:208–13.

75 Tong JY, Hsia S, Parris GL, *et al*. Molecular compatibility and renal graft survival: the HLA DQB1 genotyping. *Transplantation* 1993;55:390–5.

76 Bushell A, Higgins RM, Wood KJ, Morris PJ. HLA-DQ mismatches between donor and recipient in the presence of HLA-DR compatibility do not influence the outcome of renal transplants. *Hum Immunol* 1989;26:179–85.

77 Fukuda Y, Kimura A, Hoshino H, *et al*. Significance of the HLA-DQ matching in one-haplotype identical kidney transplant pairs and the matching analysis by the polymerase chain reaction (PCR)-heteroduplex method. *Tissue Antigens* 1995;45:49–56.

78 Freedman BI, Thacker LR, Heise ER, Adams PL. HLA-DQ matching in cadaveric renal transplantation. *Clin Transpl* 1997;11:480–4.

79 Rosenberg WMC, Bushell A, Higgins RM, *et al*. Isolated HLA-DP mismatches between donors and recipients do not influence the function or outcome of renal transplants. *Hum Immunol* 1992;33:5–9.

80 Middleton D, Mytilineos D, Savage D, *et al*. Matching for HLA-DPB1 alleles in zero mismatched HLA-A, -B and -DR renal transplants. *Transplant Proc* 1992;24:2439–40.

81 Mytilineos J, Deufel A, Opelz G. Clinical relevance of HLA-DPB locus matching for cadaver kidney retransplants: a report of the Collaborative Transplant Study. *Transplantation* 1997;63:1351–4.

82 Park MS, Clark BD, Maruya E, Terasaki PI. HLA class I epitopes accounted for by single residues. *Clin Transpl* 1991:335–45.

83 Clark BD, Geer LI, Park MS, Terasaki PI. Association of high sensitization to the structure of HLA class I alleles. *Clin Transpl* 1991:347–62.

84 Akkoc N, Scornik J. Amino acid residues on HLA molecules critical for alloantibody binding. *Transplant Proc* 1991;23:389.

85 Laundy GJ, Bradley BA. The predictive value of epitope analysis in highly sensitized patients awaiting renal transplantation. *Transplantation* 1995;59:1207–13.

86 Duquesnoy RJ, Marrari M. Determination of HLA-A,B residue mismatch acceptability for kidneys transplanted into highly sensitized patients: a report of a collaborative study conducted during the 12th International Histocompatibility Workshop. *Transplantation* 1997;63:1743–51.

87 Takemoto S, Gjertson DW, Terasaki PI. HLA matching: a comparison of conventional and molecular approaches. *Clin Transpl* 1992:413–34.

88 Takemoto S, Terasaki PI, Maruya E, Park MS. Molecular matching for clinical kidney transplantation. *Transplant Proc* 1993;25:206.

89 Sada M, Hashimoto M, Kinoshita T, *et al*. Importance of HLA-DRB1 amino acid residue matching between recipient and donor in cadaveric renal transplantation. *Transplant Proc* 1995;27:698–700.

90 Duquesnoy RJ. HLAMatchmaker: a molecularly based algorithm for histocompatibility determination. I. Description of the algorithm. *Hum Immunol* 2002;63:339–52.

91 Duquesnoy RJ, Takemoto S, De Lange P, Doxiadis IIN, Schreuder GMT, Claas FHJ. HLAMatchmaker: a molecularly based algorithm for histocompatibility determination III. Effect of matching at the HLA-A,B amino acid triplet level on kidney transplant survival. *Transplantation* 2003;75:884–9.

92 Boehringer D, Reinhard T, Duquesnoy R, *et al*. Beneficial effect of matching at the HLA-A and B amino-acid triplet level on rejection free survival in panetrating keratoplasty. *Transplantation* 2004;77:417–21.

93 Laux G, Mytilineos J, Opelz G. Critical evaluation of the amino acid triplet-epitope matching concept in cadaver kidney transplanation. *Transplantation* 2004;77:902–7.

94 Duquesnoy R, Claas F. Is the application of HLAMatchmaker relevant in kidney transplantation? [Letter]. *Transplantation* 2005;**79**:250–1.

95 Haririan A, Fagoaga O, Daneshvar H, *et al.* Predictive value of HLA epitope matching using HLAMatchmaker for graft outcomes in a predominantly African-American renal transplant cohort. *Clin Transplant* 2006;**20**:226–33.

96 Nambiar A, Duquesnoy RJ, Adams S, *et al.* HLAMatchmaker-driven analysis of response to HLA matched platelet transfusions in alloimmunized patients. *Blood* 2006;**107**:1680–7.

97 Bray RA, Nickerson PW, Kerman RH, Gebel HM. Evolution of HLA antibody detection: technology emulating biology. *Immunol Res* 2004;**29**:41–54.

98 Pei R, Lee JH, Shih NJ, Chen M, Terasaki PI. Single human leukocyte antigen flow cytometry beads for accurate identification of human leukocyte antigen antibody specificities. *Transplantation* 2003;**75**:43–9.

99 Duquesnoy RJ, Howe J, Takemoto S. HLAMatchmaker: a molecularly based algorithm for histocompatibility determination. IV. An alternative strategy to increase the number of compatible donors for highly sensitized patients. *Transplantation* 2003;**75**:889–97.

100 Claas FH, Gijbels Y, von Veen A, *et al.* Selection of cross-match negative HLA-A and/or -B mismatched donors for highly sensitized patients. *Transplant Proc* 1989;**21**:665–6.

101 Claas FHJ, Witvliet M, Duquesnoy RJ, Persijn G, Doxiadis IIN. The acceptable mismatch program as a fast tool to transplant highly sensitized patients awaiting a post-mortal kidney: short waiting time and excellent graft outcome. *Transplantation* 2004;**78**:190–3.

102 Dankers MKA, Witvliet MD, Roelen DL, *et al.* The number of amino acid triplet differences between patient and donor is predicitve for the antibody reactivity against mismatched HLA antigens. *Transplantation* 2004;**128**;1236–9.

103 Adeyi O, Girnita A, Awadalla Y, *et al.* Serum analysis after kidney transplant nephrectomy reveals restricted antibody specificity patterns against donor HLA class I antigens. *Transpl Immunol* 2005;**14**:53–62.

104 Duquesnoy RJ, Marrari M. HLAMatchmaker: a molecularly based algorithm for histocompatibility determination. II. Verification of the algorithm and determination of the relative immunogenicity of amino acid triplet-defined epitopes. *Hum Immunol* 2002;**63**:353–63.

105 Bodmer J, Kennedy L, Aizawa M, *et al.* HLA-D region monoclonal antibodies. In: Albert E, Maur M, Mayr W, eds. *Histocompatibility Testing 1984*. Berlin: Springer-Verlag, 1984:217–36.

106 Duquesnoy RJ, White LT, Fierst JW, *et al.* Multiscreen serum analysis of highly sensitized renal dialysis patients for antibodies toward public and private class I HLA determinants. Implications for computer-predicted acceptable and unacceptable donor mismatches in kidney transplantation. *Transplantation* 1990;**50**:427–37.

107 Rodey GE, Revels K, Fuller TC. Epitope specificity of HLA class I alloantibodies: II. Stability of cross-reactive group antibody patterns over extended time periods. *Transplantation* 1997;**63**:885–93.

108 Duquesnoy RJ, Marrari M. Multilaboratory evaluation of serum analysis for HLA antibody and crossmatch reactivity by lymphocytotoxicity methods. Results of the ASHI/CAP Proficiency Testing Survey during 1993–2000. *Arch Pathol Lab Med* 2003;**127**:149–56.

109 Speiser DE, Loeliger CC, Siren MK, Jeannet M. Pretransplant cytotoxic donor T-cell activity specific to patient HLA class I antigens correlating with mortality after unrelated BMT. *Br J Haematol* 1996;**93**:935–9.

110 Noreen H, McKinley D, Gillingham K, Matas A, Segall M. Positive remote crossmatch: impact on short-term and long-term outcome in cadaver renal transplantation. *Transplantation* 2003;**75**:501–5.

111 Doxiadis IIN, Duquesnoy RJ, Claas HJ. Extending options for highly sensitized patients to receive a suitable kidney graft. *Curr Opin Immunol* 2005;**17**:536–40.

112 Appel J, Hartwig M, Cantu E, Palmer S, Reinsmoen N, Davis R. Role of flow cytometry to define unacceptable HLA antigens in lung transplant recipients with HLA-specific antibodies. *Transplantation* 2006;**81**:1049–57.

113 Zangwill S, Ellis T, Zlotcha J, *et al.* The virtual crossmatch – a screening tool for sensitized pediatric heart transplant recipients. *Pediatr Transplant* 2006;**10**:38–41.

114 Halloran P. The clinical importance of alloantibody-mediated rejection. *Am J Transplant* 2003;**3**:639–40.

115 Zhang Q, Liang L, Gjertson D, *et al.* Development of post-transplant antidonor HLA antibodies is associated with acute humoral rejection and early graft dysfunction. *Transplantation* 2005;**79**:591–8.

116 Mauiyyedi S, Colvin R. Humoral rejection in kidney transplantation: new concepts in diagnosis and treatment. *Curr Opin Nephrol Hypertens* 2002;**11**:609–20.

117 Jaramillo A, Smith M, Phelan D, *et al.* Development of ELISA-detected anti-HLA antibodies precedes the development of bronchiolitis obliterans syndrome and correlates with progressive decline in pulmonary function after lung transplantation. *Transplantation* 1999;**67**:1155–61.

118 Girnita A, McCurry K, Iacono A, *et al.* HLA-specific antibodies are associated with high-grade and persistent recurrent lung allograft rejection. *J Heart Lung Transplant* 2004;**23**:1135–41.

119 Girnita A, Duquesnoy R, Yousem S, *et al.* HLA-specific antibodies are risk factors for lymphocytic bronchiolitis and chronic lung allograft dysfunction. *Am J Transplant* 2005;**5**:131–8.

120 Ionescu D, Girnita A, Zeevi A, *et al.* C4d deposition in lung allografts is associated with circulating anti-HLA antibody. *Transpl Immunol* 2005;**15**:63–8.

121 Michaels P, Espejo M, Kobashigawa J, *et al.* Humoral rejection incardiac transplantation: risk factors, hemodynamic consequences and relationship to transplant coronary artery disease. *J Heart Lung Transplant* 2003;**22**:58–69.

122 Girnita A, Webber S, Zeevi A. Anti-HLA alloantibodies in pediatric solid organ transplantation. *Pediatr Transplant* 2006;**10**:145–53.

123 Takemoto S, Zeevi A, Feng S, *et al.* National conference to assess antibody-mediated rejection in solid organ transplantation. *Am J Transplant* 2004;**4**:1033–41.

124 Mohanakumar T, Waldrep JC, Phibbs M, Mendez-Picon G, Kaplan AM, Lee HM. Serological characterization of antibodies eluted from chronically rejected human renal allografts. *Transplantation* 1981;**32**:61–6.

5 Gene Polymorphisms and Pharmacogenomics

Robyn Temple-Smolkin, Gilbert J. Burckart and Adriana Zeevi

Pediatric transplant patients are treated with standard immuno-suppression regimens because few clinical or demographic risk factors have been identified that can reliably predict a child's chance of developing major post-transplant complications. The ability to predict the likelihood of a clinical event would allow clinicians to use a more rational approach to post-transplant pharmacologic therapy, tailoring the intensity of the immunosuppressive regimen and other treatments to the individual patient's needs. While human leukocyte antigen (HLA) incompatibility is one of the causes of the host immune response leading to acute and chronic rejection of the allograft, other gene polymorphisms might also affect allograft outcome. Several studies in a limited number of pediatric patients have reported correlations between graft rejection and polymorphisms in various cytokine genes, as well as other genes involved in tissue inflammation and drug disposition. Therefore, genetic variations of individual graft recipients may represent independent risk factors for prediction of clinical outcomes. An improved understanding of the consequences of these risk factors should allow for the development of individualized treatment protocols. In this chapter, the existing peer-reviewed literature with regard to genetic polymorphisms in pediatric solid organ transplant populations is surveyed and these findings are compared with selected adult studies.

GENE POLYMORPHISMS

A genetic polymorphism is defined as a variance in the sequence of a region of genomic DNA that occurs within a substantial number of individuals in a given population. These changes can either be silent, resulting in no biologic changes, or functional, with resultant alterations of gene expression, regulation or function. At the structural level, these polymorphisms can be single nucleotide base pair changes (SNP), sequence or tandem repeats, insertions or deletions. More than one polymorphism may be present for any given cytokine or pharmacogenetics gene, but not all the recognized polymorphisms will have an impact on gene expression. Based on *in vitro* and *in vivo* evaluation of cytokine production,

it has been possible to characterize individuals as "high" or "low" and sometimes "intermediate" producers for a given cytokine [1]. In healthy individuals, these polymorphisms may be of no clinical significance. However, in disease states (including the presence of an allograft) certain polymorphisms may predispose to adverse outcomes. Better understanding of these polymorphisms, their gene frequencies and patterns, and the role they may have in the outcome for a pediatric allograft recipient, may identify risk factors and therapy adjustments that can positively impact outcome.

ACUTE ALLOGRAFT REJECTION AND GRAFT FUNCTION

The immune response to a transplanted organ is complex and involves the production of proinflammatory cytokines that alter the graft vascular endothelial cells, mediate recruitment of leukocytes and impact the differentiation and maturation of effector cells. Cytokines are produced in response to allostimulation and can be found in rejecting organs. Cytokines may also promote an immunoregulatory response to an allograft and mediate allograft acceptance. Interindividual differences in production of cytokines may influence the relative risk for rejection and/or graft dysfunction. The most frequently studied cytokine is tumor necrosis factor α (TNFα), a pro-inflammatory cytokine implicated in both autoimmune diseases and acute rejection. An interleukin-10 (IL-10) promoter polymorphism has also been widely studied, as IL-10 has profound anti-inflammatory activity and may directly oppose the actions of TNFα in the allograft. Other commonly studied polymorphic cytokines are transforming growth factor β1 (TGF-β1), IL-6 and γ-interferon (IFNγ). Table 5.1 summarizes the pediatric studies that show a relationship to various clinical outcomes.

One study has demonstrated a significant association between IL-10 high genotype and protection from acute rejection at 1 year in a pediatric heart transplant cohort [2]. Furthermore, TNFα low genotype was also associated with protection from acute rejection at 1 year, while a combination

Table 5.1 Polymorphisms associated with pediatric allograft rejection and graft function.

Gene	Polymorphism(s)	Tx organ	No recipients/donors/controls	Clinical complications	Reference
TNFα	−308 G/A	Heart	93 R, 29 D	Acute rejection, R	Awad et al. [2]
IL-10	−1082 G/A, −819 C/T, −592 C/A	Heart	93 R, 29 D	Acute rejection, R	Awad et al. [2]
TNFα	−308 G/A	Liver	19 R, 37 C	Weaning off IS, R	Mazariegos et al. [5]
IL-10	−1082 G/A, −819 C/T, −592 C/A	Liver	19 R, 37 C	Weaning off IS, R	Mazariegos et al. [5]
TGF-β1	+869 C/T, +915 C/G	Heart	88 R	Renal failure, R	Di Filippo et al. [16]
IL-6	−174 G/C	Lung	93 R	BOS, R	Lu et al. [24]
IFNγ	+874 T/A	Lung	93 R	BOS, R	Lu et al. [24]

BOS, bronchiolitis obliterans syndrome; IFNγ, γ-interferon; IL, interleukin; IS, immunosuppression; R, rejection; TGF-β1, transforming growth factor β1; TNFα, tumor necrosis factor α; Tx, transplant.

of IL-10 high and TNFα low genotypes had the lowest risk for acute rejection. In two adult heart transplant studies, TNFα high, IL-10 low genotypes were associated with increased acute rejection while four other studies did not support these findings [3]. These discrepancies between various studies may result from differences between rejection criteria used (International Society of Heart and Lung Transplantation [ISHLT] ≥ 2 compared with ≥ 3A) and/or smaller population sizes with limited statistical power. IL-10 high gene polymorphism was also shown to be protective against acute refractory rejection in adult lung transplant recipients [4]. This combination of a low proinflammatory (TNFα) and high regulatory (IL-10) cytokine genotype was enriched in pediatric liver transplant patients off immunosuppression or on a minimal level of immunosuppression; while children resistant to immunosuppression weaning expressed TNFα high genotype [5]. The adult liver transplant experience is controversial; some publications support the notion of high TNFα as a risk factor for acute rejection while other studies failed to find an association. In a recent publication Warle et al. [6] carried out a meta-analysis on seven studies reporting cytokine gene polymorphism and acute rejection in liver transplant recipients. Although most of the individual studies lacked the statistical power to show a significant correlation, in the overall analysis the IL-10 polymorphism associated with low production (−1082A allele) was identified as a genetic risk factor for acute liver allograft rejection [6].

No studies have been reported in pediatric renal transplant patients regarding cytokine gene polymorphisms. In adult transplant recipients, high TNFα was correlated with acute rejection across various ethnic populations [7–10]. Lack of association of TNFα genotypes with acute renal rejection was also reported in a study that limited their follow-up to the first 30 days post-transplantation [11]. IL-10 high genotype in renal allograft has been associated with acute rejection [10,12], in contrast to its proposed protective function in heart, lung and liver allografts. This difference in outcome most likely is a result of IL-10 driven B-cell proliferation ultimately resulting in antibody-mediated renal graft damage. The opposite effect of the IL-10 high genotype in kidney allografts compared with other organs illustrates the importance of context when discussing a given cytokine's function.

TGF-β1 high genotype was associated with increased acute rejection in adult renal transplantation [13]. Interestingly, a small study recently associated donor TGF-β1 high genotype with acute renal rejection [14]. Other kidney transplant studies failed to show an association [15]. Pediatric heart and liver studies did not find an association between TGF-β1 and allograft acute rejection [2,5]; however, larger studies are necessary to confirm these results related to TGF-β1 polymorphism.

Renal failure is a common outcome for both renal and nonrenal transplant recipients. Although the causes are not completely understood, TGF-β1 may be an important factor as this cytokine promotes fibrosis by stimulating production of extracellular matrix proteins within the graft. In a recent study of renal dysfunction in pediatric heart recipients, TGF-β1 high genotype was associated with decreased renal function (based upon creatinine clearance) compared with low–intermediate genotype at each post-transplant time point from 6 months to 7 years [16]. Similar findings were reported in adult heart transplant studies [17], while Baan et al. [18] reported on increased renal dysfunction in patients with TGF-β1 low genotype.

The pediatric transplant literature related to cytokine genetic polymorphisms and allograft rejection is scant, but carries some important preliminary findings that are consistent with other reports in adult transplant populations. Studies to date in the pediatric heart and liver transplant population indicate that a high TNFα producer genotype may identify a subpopulation at higher risk for rejection. There are further suggestions of a protective effect conveyed by the high–intermediate IL-10 genotype in heart and liver, but perhaps not kidney, allograft recipients. TGF-β1 high was associated with renal dysfunction after pediatric heart transplantation. As is demonstrated by the current level of controversy in both the pediatric and adult literature, these pilot studies underscore the need for continued study of these polymorphisms in larger pediatric transplant populations.

CHRONIC ALLOGRAFT REJECTION

The initiation and progression of transplant coronary artery disease (TCAD) in cardiac recipients is partially mediated by immune processes. Polymorphisms of recipient and donor genes of cytokines and growth factors that affect endothelial and smooth muscle cell activation and proliferation may correlate with the development and severity of TCAD. Chronic transplant rejection is characterized by fibrosis and accelerated graft vasculopathy driven in part by the release of a number of growth factors, including vascular endothelial growth factor (VEGF) and platelet-derived growth factor (PDGF).

Calcineurin inhibitors and steroids have been implicated in the increased production of TGF-β1, a cytokine that has multiple complex functions including the regulation of PDGF expression (a fibroblast growth factor) and endothelin 1 (a smooth muscle mitogen and a powerful vasoconstrictor). The proinflammatory fibroproliferative cascade initiated by TGF-β1 may also have an important role in the development of chronic rejection and nephrotoxicity. A few studies have shown a relationship between cytokine and growth factor gene polymorphisms and the development of chronic rejection in adults while very limited similar studies have been carried out in pediatric solid organ transplant recipients.

One of the polymorphisms associated with TCAD is the SNP in the TGF-β1 gene at position +915 G/C changing the amino acid at codon 25 from Arg to Pro. In two studies involving adult heart transplant recipients expressing TGF-β1 high gene (homozygote GG at codon 25), patients were at higher risk for the development of TCAD but this could not be confirmed in other two studies [3]. In a cohort of 111 pediatric heart transplant recipients there was also a correlation between high TGF-β1 gene and the risk of TCAD (31 of 100 recipients expressing high TGF-β1 developed TCAD vs. none of 11 intermediate/low TGF-β1 expressing recipients; Zeevi, personal communication).

VEGF, a mitogen for endothelial cells, may also be important in the amplification of inflammatory responses to the allograft through its capacity to upregulate the expression of adhesion molecules (ICAM-1, VCAM-1 and E-selectin) on endothelial cells, thereby increasing leukocyte adhesion and transmigration to the site of inflammation [19]. Genetically controlled variations in VEGF production have been documented and associated with increased risk of renal allograft acute rejection [19]. The potential role of VEGF in TCAD has not been shown in pediatric or adult transplant recipients.

The main cause of long-term morbidity and mortality after lung transplantation is the development of chronic rejection referred to as bronchiolitis obliterans syndrome (BOS). Increased expression of proinflammatory cytokines (IL-6 and IFNγ) within the lung allograft have been associated with refractory acute cellular rejection and the development of BOS [20–22]. IFNγ high gene polymorphism is considered a risk factor for both lung fibrosis [23] and the development of BOS [24]. In addition, the proinflammatory cytokine IL-6 was also associated with an earlier development of BOS in lung transplant recipients while TGF-β1 was found to predict lung fibrosis [25] but not BOS [24]. Most of these studies were carried out in adult lung transplant recipients with the exception of a limited number of pediatric patients in a study reported by Lu *et al.* [24].

INFECTIOUS COMPLICATIONS

Transplantation, and the subsequent immunosuppression required to maintain the allograft, exposes pediatric patients to numerous opportunistic infections. However, no studies examining susceptibility of pediatric transplant patients to post-transplant infections and cytokine polymorphisms have been published at the time of this review. An adult renal transplant study demonstrated that low TNFα producers were at higher risk for post-transplant infections and further suggests that these patients would benefit from lowered immunosuppression as it also inhibits TNFα production [26].

Pediatric liver transplant patients with infection with the hepatitis C virus (HCV) have demonstrated accelerated onset and progression of clinical disease both in original and retransplanted grafts compared with nonimmunosuppressed individuals [27]. In adults, the presence of donor TNFα high genotype was associated with a more rapid and severe recurrence of HCV allograft hepatitis in seropositive recipients [28]. Increased recurrence of HCV was associated with proinflammatory cytokines (TNFα high and IL-10 low) [29] and with low production of TGF-β1, IL-10 and IFNγ [30,31]. In addition, the TGF-β1 high genotype has been associated with increased *in situ* expression and degree of hepatic fibrosis [30]. These investigations suggest that pediatric transplant patients acquiring a primary HCV infection may have more rapid progression to clinical disease and increased hepatic fibrosis if they possess a TNFα high, IFNγ low or TGF-β1 high genotype.

Post-transplant lymphoproliferative disorder (PTLD) is a serious complication following solid organ transplantation in pediatric recipients. Primary Epstein–Barr virus (EBV) infection after transplantation and the intensity of immunosuppression regimens are major risk factors for the development of PTLD [32]. However, only a small proportion of the patients who develop primary infection develop PTLD. EBV-specific cellular immune responses and proinflammatory Th1 cytokines (IFNγ and TNFα) have been shown to be important to prevent EBV reactivation and to control PTLD. A strong association with Th2 cytokines (IL-4 and IL-10) in PTLD lesions of lung and liver transplant recipients has been reported [33]. Furthermore, liver transplant recipients (adult and pediatric) who were at primary risk for EBV infection and expressed low IFNγ gene polymorphism (AA homozygous at +874) had a higher risk for developing PTLD than those patients who had high IFNγ gene polymorphism [34]. Similar findings were reported in a cohort of 12 renal transplant recipients [35].

PHARMACOGENETICS AND TRANSPLANTATION

Genetic polymorphisms have a profound effect on a patient's response to drug therapy and the importance of this field of genetic study is just beginning to be appreciated. As many as 500 different genes may be involved with the outcome of giving a classic pharmacologic moiety. Considering that each gene has multiple polymorphisms, the complexity of these interactions in producing the ultimate effect in a patient might be extremely complex. However, the effects of genetic polymorphisms are weighted and a small number of these will ultimately define most of the outcomes after drug administration.

The genetic factors affecting the biopharmaceutics of a transplant drug have a major impact on the therapeutic and toxicologic outcome after administration of an immunosuppressant. The simple explanation for this is that a drug has to enter the body (absorption) and reach the target site of action (distribution) before any effect can be achieved, and activation or termination of this action is through the processes of drug metabolism and elimination. This principle has already been demonstrated clearly for tacrolimus blood concentrations and CYP3A5 gene polymorphisms. The following discussion will focus on those known genetic polymorphisms that alter the biopharmaceutics of the immunosuppressant agents currently in use.

Drug absorption

The most significant drug absorption effects in transplant patients produced by genetic polymorphisms are currently believed to be on the drug transporter P-glycoprotein (P-gp), and on the drug-metabolizing enzyme CYP3A. Intestinal CYP3A and P-gp act synergistically as a barrier to oral drug absorption, with P-gp pumping the drug back into the gut and CYP3A metabolizing drug that does get absorbed. A strong substrate overlap between P-gp and CYP3A has been demonstrated [36], and the major immunosuppressive agents, including cyclosporine, tacrolimus, corticosteroids and sirolimus, are all substrates for both P-gp and CYP3A.

MDR1 polymorphisms and P-glycoprotein

P-gp is encoded by the human multidrug resistance gene (MDR1), and acts as an adenosine triphosphate (ATP) dependent pump expelling drugs to the outside of the cell and thereby reducing accumulation within the cell. P-gp has an important role in the absorption, distribution and elimination of drugs that are substrates for the pump. P-gp expression exhibits remarkable interindividual variability, which explains a substantial difference in the pharmacokinetics of P-gp sub-

strates, and this difference has recently been attributed to gene polymorphisms of MDR1. Recent studies have demonstrated that genetic polymorphisms lead to functional alterations and phenotypic variation in P-gp expression, and at least 28 polymorphisms of the MDR1 gene have been characterized [37–40]. These previous studies have focused on the functional outcomes of the SNPs C3435T, a silent mutation at a wobble position at exon 26, and G2677T, a missense mutation at exon 21. A study on tacrolimus dosing and MDR1 genotyping found a significant association between tacrolimus levels per dose/kilogram in pediatric heart transplant patients and both the MDR1 C3435T and G2677T polymorphisms at 6 and 12 months post-transplantation. Both the MDR1 3435 CC and the 2677 GG patients, who have the highest pump function, had a lower tacrolimus level per dose/kilogram, suggesting that these patients required more drug to achieve the same tacrolimus target levels than the CT/GT/TT patients [41]. Most adult studies have not demonstrated the association of MDR1 polymorphisms and tacrolimus dosing, but a recent report has associated MDR1 polymorphisms and cyclosporine dosing in liver transplant patients [42]. MDR1 polymorphisms have been associated previously with corticosteroid weaning in pediatric heart transplant patients [43], which could either be an effect on absorption or on drug resistance medicated by P-gp in T cells.

The potential prognostic effect of P-gp on clinical outcomes has been observed in several studies. In living-donor liver transplantation, intestinal MDR1 mRNA expression was found to predict both tacrolimus pharmacokinetics and patient survival [44]. In that study, high MDR1 mRNA expression was associated with a significantly poorer patient survival. These observations were extended to demonstrate that MDR1 and CYP3A5 polymorphisms predict tacrolimus dosing in pediatric heart transplant patients [41].

Cytochrome P450 3A5

CYP3A is the primary cytochrome P450 (CYP) subfamily in humans and is responsible for the phase I metabolism of more than 50% of drugs in use. Among the CYP3A subfamily, CYP3A4 and CYP3A5 are the most abundant and important enzymes. CYP3A4 is located in the liver, jejunum, colon and pancreas, while CYP3A5 is more commonly present in small intestine and stomach. Kuehl et al. [45,46] suggested that CYP3A5 contributes substantially to the CYP3A-dependent drug metabolism because of the high hepatic expression in approximately 30% of livers of Caucasian origin. They described two functional SNPs in CYP3A5 and provided a molecular explanation for the absence of the CYP3A5 protein from some people. The CYP3A5*3 (22893A → G) allele in intron 3 results in a truncated protein with partial loss of CYP3A5 activity. Subjects with the polymorphic *3 allele have lower hepatic expression and decreased hepatic CYP3A5 activity than subjects with at least one *1 allele. Previous studies in pediatric heart transplant [41] and adult lung transplant patients [4] have confirmed an association between the CYP3A5 *1/*3 genotype and a lower tacrolimus blood (level/dose) in comparison to the *3/*3 genotype over the first year post-transplantation. Multiple adult studies have confirmed this observation [47,48].

Drug distribution

Drug distribution is critical for access to tissues where a pharmacologic or toxicologic effect is to be exerted. The limitation to drug distribution is best represented in the brain, where the blood–brain barrier limits access to the brain by many pharmacologic substances. P-gp activities in the endothelial cells of the blood vessels of the brain are responsible for this limitation in distribution.

The increased distribution of tacrolimus to the brain in an mdr1 knockout mouse model has been previously demonstrated [49]. The neurotoxicity of tacrolimus is not associated with blood concentrations of the drug, but tremors, encephalopathy and seizures are frequently observed in patients on tacrolimus. The association between MDR1 gene polymorphisms and tacrolimus neurotoxicity has been suggested in a small series of liver transplant patients [50].

Drug metabolism and excretion

The metabolism and elimination of a drug has a critical role in either activating a pharmacologic entity or in curtailing its pharmacologic and toxicologic effects. Immunosuppressant agents are well recognized as targets for drug interactions involving drug metabolism. Members of the CYP3A subfamily of cytochrome P450 enzymes are involved with the metabolism of a large number of substrates. CYP3A4 has more than 20 identified single nucleotide polymorphisms [51], and CYP3A4*1B carriers require more tacrolimus to achieve target trough concentrations than CYP3A4*1 homozygotes [52].

Transplant rejection and adverse drug effects

P-gp is involved in a number of cellular processes beyond the simple transport of xenobiotics out of cells. Therefore, MDR1 polymorphisms may be associated with both rejection and adverse drug effects in ways that are not presently understood.

Transplant rejection

A relationship between the MDR1 3435 CC/CT genotype and the incidence of acute persistent rejection in adult lung transplant patients has been reported [53]. P-gp has both systematic effects on drug disposition and local effects on intracellular drug concentration. Either or both of these two actions of P-gp may be involved with resistance to immunosuppressant therapy in lung transplant patients. One possibility is that P-gp

substrates, such as tacrolimus and corticosteroids, were not absorbed well in the MDR1 3435 C allele carriers. The second possibility is that T-lymphocytes with enhanced P-gp function were also more resistant to drug therapy, or were resistant to apoptosis [49]. This situation would result in persistent problems with rejection in the CC/CT patients in comparison to the TT patients. Both of these mechanisms would be logical explanations of the incidence of acute persistent rejection in the MDR1 3435 CC/CT lung transplant patients.

Adverse drug effects – nephrotoxicity

Hebert et al. [54] have associated an MDR1 genotype with chronic renal dysfunction in liver transplant patients. A relationship between the highest serum creatinine in the first postoperative year in lung transplant patients and an MDR1 exon 26 polymorphism has also been observed [51]. While these initial reports are not conclusive, the involvement of P-gp in renal function and the prolonged administration of a P-gp blocker such as cyclosporine may prove to be contributing factors to this frequent adverse effect of calcineurin antagonists.

CONCLUSIONS

There are many challenges in associating a genetic polymorphism with a patient outcome, such as acute rejection or graft function. The presence of a polymorphism may not equal a functional change in the protein (phenotypic change) as most quantitative effects of the polymorphisms are based upon in vitro rather than in vivo tests. This identifies a need for the careful preliminary investigation of a given gene's functionality in multiple genetic backgrounds. The frequency of gene polymorphisms within patient populations can vary greatly within racial groups, a variable that must be considered when a polymorphism is associated with an outcome. African-American renal transplant patients have a significantly higher probability of a high IL-6 and low IL-10 alleles, resulting in an increased expression of the costimulatory molecule CD80 on antigen-presenting cells and potentially a factor in increased risk of allograft loss [55]. This study was confirmed and extended to include observation of increased IFNγ low frequency in Asians compared to Caucasians [56]. Expression levels of various cytokines can influence immunologic responses and therefore may have significant impact on clinical outcomes such as allograft rejection or chronic graft dysfunction. Furthermore, the contribution of an individual gene polymorphism can be obscured by multiple other factors that are capable of masking the true impact of the change. Transplant recipients have additional risk factors, such as age, level of HLA mismatch and viral infection, which necessitate multivariate statistical analyses.

Another limitation with gene association studies and their clinical significance is the consistency in the definition of outcome measures. It is very difficult to compare findings from various centers if the diagnosis and definition of acute and chronic rejection are different. Small, often single-center, studies lack the statistical power to perform multivariate analyses. Individual center patient demographics do not typically allow adequate analysis of contribution of race and gender. Many of the existing pediatric studies focus on acute rejection, possibly because of absence of extended clinical follow-up. Large multicenter long-term studies using mechanism-driven investigations with clearly defined clinical endpoints should be performed to further investigate the role of genetic polymorphism in solid organ transplantation outcomes.

Although the current data are incomplete and sometimes conflicting, the overriding hypothesis emerging from this research is that an HLA-driven immune response to an allograft is modulated in the presence or absence of certain cytokine, growth factor or drug disposition polymorphisms. Knowing the impact of these genetic polymorphisms on various clinical outcomes may improve the care and post-transplant management of pediatric solid organ transplant recipients. It may soon be possible to identify those patients with a given profile who will require more aggressive immunosuppression to prevent rejection while other recipients may have the genetic makeup that will allow graft acceptance with minimal immunosuppression and drug toxicity. Our challenge is to identify these risk factors, understand their clinical significance and translate these findings into improved care for pediatric transplant patients.

REFERENCES

1 Bidwell J, Keen L, Gallagher G, et al. Cytokine gene polymorphism in human disease: on-line databases. Genes Immun 1999;1:3–19.

2 Awad MR, Webber S, Boyle G, et al. The effect of cytokine gene polymorphisms on pediatric heart allograft outcome. J Heart Lung Transplant 2001;20:625–30.

3 Holweg CT, Weimar W, Uitterlinden AG, et al. Clinical impact of cytokine gene polymorphisms in heart and lung transplantation. J Heart Lung Transplant 2004;23:1017–26.

4 Zheng HX, Burckart GJ, McCurry K, et al. Interleukin-10 production genotype protects against acute persistent rejection after lung transplantation. J Heart Lung Transplant 2004;23:541–6.

5 Mazariegos GV, Reyes J, Webber SA, et al. Cytokine gene polymorphisms in children successfully withdrawn from immunosuppression after liver transplantation. Transplantation 2002;73:1342–5.

6 Warle MC, Metselaar HJ, Hop WC, et al. Cytokine gene polymorphisms and acute liver graft rejection: a meta-analysis. Liver Transpl 2004;11:19–26.

7 Poli F, Boschiero L, Giannoni F, et al. Tumour necrosis factor-α gene polymorphism: implications in kidney transplantation. Cytokine 2000;12:1778–83.

8 Lee H, Clark B, Gooi HC, et al. Influence of recipient and donor IL-1α, IL-4, and TNFα genotypes on the incidence of acute renal allograft rejection. J Clin Pathol 2004;57:101–3.

9 Hahn AB, Kasten-Jolly JC, Constantino DM, et al. TNF-α, IL-6, IFN-γ, and IL-10 gene expression polymorphisms and the IL-4 receptor alpha-chain variant Q576R: effects on renal allograft outcome. Transplantation 2001;72:660–5.

10 Pelletier R, Pravica V, Perrey C, et al. Evidence for a genetic predisposition towards acute rejection after kidney and simultaneous kidney-pancreas transplantation. Transplantation 2000;70:674–80.

11 Marshall SE, McLaren AJ, Haldar NA, et al. The impact of recipient cytokine genotype on acute rejection after renal transplantation. Transplantation 2000;70:1485–91.

12 Sankaran D, Asderakis A, Ashraf S, et al. Cytokine gene polymorphisms predict acute graft rejection following renal transplantation. Kidney Int 1999;56:281–8.

13 McDaniel DO, Barber WH, Nguyan C, et al. Combined analysis of cytokine genotype polymorphism and the level of expression with allograft function in African-American renal transplant patients. Transpl Immunol 2003;11:107–19.

14 Ligeiro D, Sancho MR, Papoila A, et al. Impact of donor and recipient cytokine genotypes on renal allograft outcome. Transplant Proc 2004;36:827–9.

15 Ochsner S, Guo Z, Binswanger U, et al. TGF-β1 gene expression in stable renal transplant recipients: influence of TGF-β1 gene polymorphism and immunosuppression. Transplant Proc 2002;34:2901–3.

16 Di Filippo S, Zeevi A, McDade KK, et al. Impact of TGF-β1 gene polymorphisms on late renal function in pediatric heart transplantation. Hum Immunol 2005;66:133–9.

17 Lacha J, Hubacek JA, Potmesil P, et al. TGF-β1 gene polymorphism in heart transplant recipients: effect on renal function. Ann Transplant 2001;6:39–43.

18 Baan CC, Balk AH, Holweg CT, et al. Renal failure after clinical heart transplantation is associated with the TGF-β1 codon 10 gene polymorphism. J Heart Lung Transplant 2000;19:866–72.

19 Shahbazi M, Fryer AA, Pravica V, et al. Vascular endothelial growth factor gene polymorphisms are associated with acute renal allograft rejection. J Am Soc Nephrol 2002;13:260–4.

20 Iacono A, Dauber J, Keenan R, et al. Interleukin 6 and interferon-γ gene expression in lung transplant recipients with refractory acute cellular rejection: implications for monitoring and inhibition by treatment with aerosolized cyclosporine. Transplantation 1997;64:263–9.

21 Ross DJ, Moudgil A, Bagga A, et al. Lung allograft dysfunction correlates with γ-interferon gene expression in bronchoalveolar lavage. J Heart Lung Transplant 1999;18:627–36

22 Scholma J, Slebos DJ, Boezen HM, et al. Eosinophilic granulocytes and interleukin-6 level in bronchoalveolar lavage fluid are associated with the development of obliterative bronchiolitis after lung transplantation. Am J Respir Crit Care Med 2000;162:2221–5.

23 Awad M, Pravica V, Perrey C, et al. CA repeat allele polymorphism in the first intron of the human interferon-γ gene is associated with lung allograft fibrosis. Hum Immunol 1999;60:343–6.

24 Lu KC, Jaramillo A, Lecha RL, et al. Interleukin-6 and interferon-γ gene polymorphisms in the development of bronchiolitis obliterans syndrome after lung transplantation. Transplantation 2002;74:1297–302.

25 El-Gamel A, Awad MR, Hasleton PS, *et al.* Transforming growth factor-β (TGF-β1) genotype and lung allograft fibrosis. *J Heart Lung Transplant* 1999;**18**:517–23.

26 Sahoo S, Kang S, Supran S, *et al.* Tumor necrosis factor genetic polymorphisms correlate with infections after renal transplantation. *Transplantation* 2000;**69**:880–4.

27 McDiarmid SV, Conrad A, Ament ME, *et al. De novo* hepatitis C in children after liver transplantation. *Transplantation* 1998;**66**:311–8.

28 Rosen HR, Lentz JJ, Rose SL, *et al.* Donor polymorphism of tumor necrosis factor gene: relationship with variable severity of hepatitis C recurrence after liver transplantation. *Transplantation* 1999;**68**:1898–902.

29 Mas VR, Fisher RA, Maluf DG, *et al.* Polymorphisms in cytokines and growth factor genes and their association with acute rejection and recurrence of hepatitis C virus disease in liver transplantation. *Clin Genet* 2004;**65**:191–201.

30 Ben-Ari Z, Pappo O, Druzd T, *et al.* Role of cytokine gene polymorphism and hepatic transforming growth factor β1 expression in recurrent hepatitis C after liver transplantation. *Cytokine* 2004;**27**:7–14.

31 Tambur AR, Ortegel JW, Ben-Ari Z, *et al.* Role of cytokine gene polymorphism in hepatitis C recurrence and allograft rejection among liver transplant recipients. *Transplantation* 2001;**71**:1475–80.

32 Webber SA, Green M. Post-transplantation lymphoproliferative disorders: advances in diagnosis, prevention and management in children. *Prog Pediatr Cardiol* 2000;**11**:145–57.

33 Nalesnik M, Jaffe R, Reyes J, *et al.* Posttransplant lymphoproliferative disorders in small bowel allograft recipients. *Transplant Proc* 2000;**32**:1213.

34 Zeevi A, Green M, Row D, *et al.* Association of low IFN-γ and high IL-10 cytokine genotype with PTLD in pediatric solid organ transplant recipients. In: First IPTA Congress on Pediatric Transplantation, 2000; Venice, 2000.

35 VanBuskirk AM, Malik V, Xia D, *et al.* A gene polymorphism associated with posttransplant lymphoproliferative disorder. *Transplant Proc* 2001;**33**:1834.

36 Wacher VJ, Wu CY, Benet LZ. Overlapping substrate specificities and tissue distribution of cytochrome P450 3A and P-glycoprotein: implications for drug delivery and activity in cancer chemotherapy. *Mol Carcinog* 1995;**13**:129–34.

37 Hoffmeyer S, Burk O, von Richter O, *et al.* Functional polymorphisms of the human multidrug-resistance gene: multiple sequence variations and correlation of one allele with P-glycoprotein expression and activity *in vivo. Proc Natl Acad Sci USA* 2000;**97**:3473–8.

38 Hitzl M, Drescher S, van der Kuip H, *et al.* The C3435T mutation in the human *MDR1* gene is associated with altered efflux of the P-glycoprotein substrate rhodamine 123 from CD56+ natural killer cells. *Pharmacogenetics* 2001;**11**:293–8.

39 Cascorbi I, Gerloff T, Johne A, *et al.* Frequency of single nucleotide polymorphisms in the P-glycoprotein drug transporter MDR1 gene in white subjects. *Clin Pharmacol Ther* 2001;**69**:169–74.

40 Ito S, Ieiri I, Tanabe M, *et al.* Polymorphism of the ABC transporter genes, MDR1, MRP1 and MRP2/cMOAT, in healthy Japanese subjects. *Pharmacogenetics* 2001;**11**:175–84.

41 Zheng H, Webber S, Zeevi A, *et al.* Tacrolimus dosing in pediatric heart transplant patients is related to CYP3A5 and MDR1 gene polymorphisms. *Am J Transplant* 2003;**3**:477–83.

42 Bonhomme-Faivre L, Devocelle A, Saliba F, *et al.* MDR-1 C3435T polymorphism influences cyclosporine a dose requirement in liver-transplant recipients. *Transplantation* 2004;**78**:21–5.

43 Zheng H, Webber S, Zeevi A, *et al.* The MDR1 polymorphisms at exons 21 and 26 predict steroid weaning in pediatric heart transplant patients. *Hum Immunol* 2002;**63**:765–70.

44 Hashida T, Masuda S, Uemoto S, *et al.* Pharmacokinetic and prognostic significance of intestinal MDR1 expression in recipients of living-donor liver transplantation. *Clin Pharmacol Ther* 2001;**69**:308–16.

45 Zhang H, Yang G, Yang X. Prospective study of combination of interferon-alpha with ribavirin for treatment of chronic hepatitis C in children. *Zhonggua Shi Yan Xue Ye Xue Za Zhi* 2001;**15**:81–2.

46 Kuehl P, Zhang J, Lin Y, *et al.* Sequence diversity in CYP3A promoters and characterization of the genetic basis of polymorphic CYP3A5 expression. *Nat Genet* 2001;**27**:383–91.

47 Tsuchiya N, Satoh S, Tada H, *et al.* Influence of CYP3A5 and MDR1 (ABCB1) polymorphisms on the pharmacokinetics of tacrolimus in renal transplant recipients. *Transplantation* 2004;**78**:1182–7.

48 Haufroid V, Mourad M, Van Kerckhove V, *et al.* The effect of CYP3A5 and MDR1 (ABCB1) polymorphisms on cyclosporine and tacrolimus dose requirements and trough blood levels in stable renal transplant patients. *Pharmacogenetics* 2004;**14**:147–54.

49 Johnstone RW, Cretney E, Smyth MJ. P-glycoprotein protects leukemia cells against caspase-dependent, but not caspase-independent, cell death. *Blood* 1999;**93**:1075–85.

50 Yamauchi A, Ieiri I, Kataoka Y, *et al.* Neurotoxicity induced by tacrolimus after liver transplantation: relation to genetic polymorphisms of the ABCB1 (MDR1) gene. *Transplantation* 2002;**74**:571–2.

51 Zheng HX, Zeevi A, Lamba J, *et al.* Tacrolimus nephrotoxicity is predicted by MDR1 Exon21 gene polymorphism while dosing is predicted by cytochrome P4503A5 polymorphism in adult lung transplant patients. *Am J Transplant* 2003;**3**(Suppl 5):426.

52 Hesselink DA, van Schaik RH, van der Heiden IP, *et al.* Genetic polymorphisms of the CYP3A4, CYP3A5, and MDR-1 genes and pharmacokinetics of the calcineurin inhibitors cyclosporine and tacrolimus. *Clin Pharmacol Ther* 2003;**74**:245–54.

53 Zheng HX, Zeevi A, McCurry K, *et al.* The impact of pharmacogenomic factors on acute persistent rejection in adult lung transplant patients. *Transpl Immunol* 2005;**14**:37–42.

54 Hebert MF, Dowling AL, Gierwatowski C, *et al.* Association between MDR1 (multidrug resistance transporter) genotype and post liver transplantation renal dysfunction in patients receiving calcineurin inhibitors. *Pharmacogenetics* 2003;**13**:661–74.

55 Hutchings A, Guay-Woodford L, Thomas JM, *et al.* Association of cytokine single nucleotide polymorphisms with B7 costimulatory molecules in kidney allograft recipients. *Pediatr Transplant* 2002;**6**:69–77.

56 Hoffmann SC, Stanley EM, Cox ED, *et al.* Ethnicity greatly influences cytokine gene polymorphism distribution. *Am J Transplant* 2002;**2**:560–7.

6 Genomics and Proteomics as Research Tools

Elaine S. Mansfield and Minnie M. Sarwal

Research in solid organ transplantation has elucidated some of the mechanisms of acute rejection based on analysis of selected genes [1–4]. While these serve as the backbone for further studies, characterization of the interactions and coordinate expression of whole gene families in the immunologic cascade are required for full understanding of events leading to organ rejection. The enormous redundancy of the immune system suggests that several molecular pathways contribute to the heterogeneity of clinical graft outcome [5]. The lack of individual patient therapeutic responses results in inadequate or over-immunosuppression, resulting in undesirable confounding clinical outcomes, from rejection to malignancy [6]. More importantly, mechanisms of early regulatory responses leading to chronic rejection remain to be defined. One possible method of implementing preventative measures early requires high-throughput screening methods to identify and test candidate genes.

MICROARRAYS OR "GENE CHIPS"

A DNA microarray is a high-density array of oligonucleotide probes or polymerase chain reaction (PCR) products (also known as cDNA or copy-DNA) immobilized onto a solid support such as a glass slide. The immobilized DNA selectively retrieves genes or sequences of interest when the array is hybridized to a mixture of complementary sequences. Signal intensity is generally proportional to the relative abundance of messenger (mRNA) in the sample because hybridization is concentration driven. Currently, over 50 000 genes can be spotted on a single slide; smaller dedicated arrays may be custom-designed to focus on individual metabolic pathways [7]. DNA arrays are hybridized with a labeled nucleic acid sample to measure parallel expression for each of the thousands of represented genes. The parallelism inherent in this analytic technique makes this technology exceptionally powerful, especially with the human genomic sequence from the Human Genome Mapping Project [8]. Expression data have been collected in various expression systems using the "gene discovery" approach, based on analysis

of genes most relevant to the biologic question approached, or the "expression profiling" approach, in which a generally restricted and functionally well-characterized set of genes is used to obtain information on the expression profile for a clinical sample series, to develop prognostic and therapeutic information.

Microarrays, also popularly called "gene chips" have been widely used in oncology where they have been extensively applied to the classification of distinct molecular subtypes [9–11]. DNA microarrays or gene chips reveal global patterns of gene expression [12–14]. This powerful tool has the potential to unravel the complex immunologic circuits that interplay in various immune responses, such as acute rejection, vascular rejection, chronic rejection, infection and drug toxicity. In transplantation biology, for example, sets of genes have been found to be differentially regulated in patients undergoing rejection compared to those without rejection [15,16]. These results may lead to a better understanding of the molecular staging of rejection, and hence suggest appropriate intervention strategies to improve treatment and minimize the occurrence of allograft rejection.

Expression analysis of colony filters containing cDNA clones began in the early 1980s with qualitative differential screening of duplicate membranes, hybridized in parallel with a mix of labeled radioactive cDNA mixtures isolated from two different samples (see Plate 6.1a; facing page 224). This method was instrumental in the isolation of the T-cell receptor and CTLA genes [17,18]. This is the high-density filter or macroarray that is used for analysis of experiments of moderate scope and small sample numbers. Imaging plate systems were used next for quantitative expression analysis such as enzyme-linked immunosorbent assay (ELISA) assays [19]. DNA arrays in the 1990s evolved towards miniaturization, aiming to increase the number of genes available for analysis in a single experiment. Concomitantly also reducing sample usage for hybridization, DNA arrays could also be produced on nylon membranes. However, because of the intrinsic fluorescence of nylon supports, enzymatic detection [20,21] or radioactive labeling were required, both of which are relatively insensitive. Optical detection methods (fluorescence), allowing for two-color labeling, and use of glass slides were introduced with improved results [12,14].

As more genomic sequence information and sophisticated bioinformatics tools have become available, arrays have further migrated from cDNA to oligonucleotide arrays because of greater versatility. Both expression profiling and genotyping studies can be conducted using these arrays while cDNA probes are generally too long to detect alternatively spliced mRNA variants. However, cDNA arrays can be much more readily adapted and customized to include new probe sets than arrays generated by photolithographic methods such as the Affymetrix array system [22]. To overcome this limitation, new methods of DNA synthesis or attachment of presynthesized probes are being used more widely in arrays. These improvements permit longer oligonucleotide probes to be spotted on gene chips [23]. This improves both hybridization consistency and batch consistency and helps overcome other limitations originally associated with cDNA arrays [24,25]. Probe construction is simplified because no PCR amplification and clean up is required, and hybridization is improved because probes can be better melting temperature (Tm) balanced. In addition, the arrays can be made at a lower cost. Thus, cDNA-based studies are increasingly migrating to long-oligonucleotide probe-based arrays. This approach can also be designed to bridge intron–exon junctions so splice variants can be detected [26,27].

A technology that promises to revolutionize the DNA gene chip world is the use of micro-well plate-sized "array of microarrays" in a standard 8×12 cm plate format (see Plate 6.1b, facing page 224). In these plates, multiple individual samples can be simultaneously processed using automated methods for sample handling. Standard laboratory robots perform all the steps in sample preparation: amplification, labeling, washing and hybridization. To keep sample cost as low as possible, competitive hybridization is eliminated and experiments conducted using only a single dye. Most single-color microarray applications make use of internal control probes to normalize expression results. Expression signals are normalized to invariant "housekeeping" genes and spiked controls, a method commonly used in quantitative reverse transcriptase polymerase chain reaction (RT-PCR) based expression assays. Another array method for multiplex genomic sample screening across a smaller number of genes is the 96-well Microfluidic Card methodology (TaqMan® Low Density Array; Applied Biosystems, Inc.), which Kirk [28] has used to assay a group of immune-specific genes that can be rapidly interrogated in the card by PCR. Each miniaturized well contains probes and primer pairs for a single gene. Microfluidic distribution of template and PCR reagents to the wells is robotically controlled. Cost savings in this platform are realized by the dramatic reduction in reaction volume per well and time saved optimizing within-well multiplex PCR tests. There is tremendous potential for microwell plate-based methods in the rapid and economic high-throughput screening of transplant patients, if the footprint of genes specific to different etiologies of graft dysfunction is discovered.

GENOMIC STUDIES IN TRANSPLANTATION

Allograft injury by infiltrating cells of the host immune system underlies the complex process of acute rejection, resulting in clinical heterogeneity of graft dysfunction etiology and treatment response. Single molecule analysis by PCR has shown a strong correlation between acute rejection biopsy diagnosis and expression of cytotoxic genes, such as granulysin, granzyme, perforin and fas in tissue biopsy [4,29], blood [4,30], as well as urine analysis in renal rejection [31] and broncholalveolar lavage analysis in lung rejection [32]. Microarray analysis offers simultaneous interrogation of thousands of genes with current versions of these chips having almost the entire human genome present for expression scanning [26]. This results in a mixture of genes, where interrelated expression studies might infer common cellular and biologic pathways in rejection. These studies have been conducted on solid organ transplants such as lung [33], liver [34–36], heart [37], intestine [38] and kidney [4,39]. Recently, molecular heterogeneity in treatment response and graft outcome was demonstrated by genomic profiling of kidney transplant biopsies, across approximately 12 500 unique genes [5]. Clear evidence of tubulitis was demonstrated in a subset of biopsies, with immune quiescence and excellent graft recovery (see Plate 6.2a, facing page 224). A redundancy of molecular pathways are differentially regulated in acute renal allograft rejection and suggest explanations for anemia [40], steroid resistance [4,41], poor graft outcomes [5] and infection [36]. Acute rejection expression overlaps with the innate immune response to infection as evidenced by cluster analysis and by differential expression of several transforming growth factor γ (TGF-γ) modulated genes including RANTES, MIC-1, several cytokines, chemokines and cell adhesion molecules [25]. Differential and confounding genomic responses may also relate to baseline immunosuppression [5]. In fact, marked elevation in the baseline expression of certain cytokine genes was seen in pediatric recipients on a steroid-free protocol [42,43], compared with stable pediatric recipients on steroid-based immunosuppression, suggesting that a higher baseline value of T-cell activation seen in stable non-rejecting steroid-free recipients may be a noninjurious mechanism for graft accommodation rather than acute rejection. The most highly differentially expressed genes selected in the class prediction analysis contain significant enrichment for ion transporters, major histocompatibility complex (MHC) antigens (both class I and II), apoptotic genes as well as T- and B-cell specific genes. Interestingly, more B-cell-specific genes were observed than T-cell-specific genes despite the fact that histologic data were inconsistent with humeral rejection within the patient set. This observation is confirmed by global functional gene-family

Table 6.1 Useful genomics websites.

Website	HTML
Cluster and Treeview	http://rana.lbl.gov/EisenSoftware.htm
Xcluster	http://genetics.stanford.edu/~sherlock/cluster.html#formats
BRB ArrayTools (NIH informatics tools)	http://linus.nci.nih.gov/BRB-ArrayTools.html
KEGG Kyoto gene classification database	http://www.genome.ad.jp/kegg/
GoMiner gene classification	http://discover.nci.nih.gov/gominer/index.jsp
Argon Laboratories metabolic pathways	http://wit.mcs.anl.gov/WIT2/
DRAGON microarray bioinformatics tools	http://pevsnerlab.kennedykrieger.org/dragon.htm
DAVID: EASE functional analysis	http://apps1.niaid.nih.gov/david/
ExPAS biochemical pathways	http://www.expasy.org/cgi-bin/search-biochem-index
GenMAPP metabolic pathways	http://www.genmapp.org/
GeneCards human gene database	http://bioinformatics.weizmann.ac.il/cards/
Gene Ontology (GO) Consortium	http://www.geneontology.org/
Stanford Microarray Database (SMD)	http://genome-www5.stanford.edu/
SOURCE gene database	http://source.stanford.edu
SAM: Significance Analysis of Microarrays	http://www-stat.stanford.edu/~tibs/ElemStatLearn/
PAM: Prediction Analysis of Microarrays	http://www-stat.stanford.edu/%7Etibs/PAM/Rdist/index.html
R: Statistics for Microarray Analysis	http://ihome.cuhk.edu.hk/~b400559/arraysoft_rpackages.html
Protein Data Bank	http://www.rcsb.org/pdb
NCBI Entrez tutorials	http://www.ncbi.nlm.nih.gov/Education/index.html
The Wellcome Trust Sanger Institute	http://www.sanger.ac.uk/
European Molecular Biology Lab	http://www.ebi.ac.uk/embl
Swiss Institute of Bioinformatics	http://www.expasy.ch/
Protein Information Resource (PIR)	http://pir.georgetown.edu
National Library of Medicine (NLM)	http://www.nlm.nih.gov/
EMBL Genome Browser	http://www.ensembl.org/
NIH list of genome sites	http://linus.nci.nih.gov/pilot/links.htm
UK list of genome sites	http://www.hgmp.mrc.ac.uk/GenomeWeb/ UK genome sites

analysis of the full transcriptisome using the publicly available program Database for Annotation, Visualization, and Integrated Discovery (DAVID); http://www.david.niaid.nih.gov) [44]. It is evident from this analysis that many immune related gene families are overrepresented in each class of rejection (Table 6.1).

Genomic studies underscore the complex molecular processes underlying rejection. It is likely that most of what is understood about classic pathways employing γ-interferon driven CD8, macrophage and natural killer (NK) cell activation is seen across many acute rejection episodes and across organs. A subset of these rejections is predestined to respond poorly to therapy, and may be utilizing a humoral mechanism for injury [45] or employing antigen-presenting cell (APC) help from B cells [5]. Identification of these rejections and stratifying treatment (steroids vs. antibody vs. plasmapharesis) may be a valuable result of genomic analysis. Survival analysis of graft function recovery and graft loss following kidney rejection revealed a significant association with B-cell cluster density in a "learning" data set of 67 biopsies, as well as in an additional "test" data set of 31 acute rejection biopsies [5]. On the other hand, genomic studies also suggest that there is a group of pathologically suggestive cellular infiltrates that

may not represent an injurious alloimmune response [5]. The ability to titrate immunosuppression intensification for transplant patients by means of genomic criteria would lead to a substantial improvement in the management of transplant recipients.

Specific genes associated with clinical graft events or outcomes might be considered as potential targets for individualized drug therapy for rejection. For example, CD4[+] acute rejections have a higher incidence of steroid resistance; and complement deposition in the graft may be indicative of antibody-mediated injury [5,46,47]. Because of the strong association between CD20[+] lymphocyte infiltration and graft loss, a trial of rejection treatment with anti-CD20 monoclonal antibody (Rituxan®) might be indicated in this setting [5,25]. Strong cell cycle signature in acute rejections with immunological quiescence and good outcomes (AR-111 [5]) suggests that spontaneous tubular cell regeneration (demonstrated by proliferating cell nuclear antigen [PCNA] staining [5]) could signify the recovery phase of the injury response. Thus, cell cycle G1/S phase inhibitors such as rapamycin might inhibit repair. Using the array class prediction tool, Predictive Analysis of Microarrays (PAM) [48], a group of only 97 genes with greater than fivefold difference in expression levels were

49

identified across clinically relevant acute rejection subgroups (see Plate 6.2b, facing page 224). The most highly differentially expressed genes in this group were ion transporters, MHC antigens (both class I and II), and T- and B-cell-specific genes. Interestingly, more B-cell-specific genes than T-cell-specific genes were represented in the informative gene set, again supporting the importance of dissecting the role of B cells in aggressive rejections.

Despite multiple reports of single gene analyses and chronic allograft injury, mechanisms and predictors of progressive alloimmune scarring are not described. Scherer et al. [49] analyzed 6 month protocol biopsies to ascertain a set of genes that may predict the development of chronic allograft nephropathy (CAN) 1 year post-transplantation. Some of the identified genes have a role in cellular remodeling, fibrogenesis (fibroblast growth factor-2 [FGF-2], TGF-β) and immune activation (prolactin receptor), although levels of the genes were variable and did not correlate with injury progression. Hoffmann et al. [50] have recently shown that the study of donor genomic DNA restriction fragment length polymorphisms may be informative and reflect the recipient's immune response to chronic injury. A study of renal allograft biopsies could not identify triggers for chronic allograft nephropathy after the graft had established injury [5]. Extensive homogeneity of genomic responses are seen at this time and the signature of increased fibrogenesis may be simply reflecting the current injury mechanism.

PROTEOMICS IN TRANSPLANTATION

Gene chips provide information about mRNA expression levels that may not correlate with protein expression levels [51]. Post-translational modifications that modify protein activity such as phosphorylation cannot be measured using these arrays. Thus, array results provide an incomplete view of the functional significance of the differentially expressed genes. Techniques for protein analysis such as western blotting, two-dimensional polyacrylamide gel electrophoresis, radio-ligand receptor binding, chromatographic separation and detection, as well as mass spectrometry are methods of identifying protein levels or function [52]. Enabling technologies such as consistent antibody library production and cost-effective slide production methods are expanding the field (see Plate 6.3, facing page 224).

Proteomics is a rapidly evolving field with potential clinical applications. Proteomic analysis of body fluids identifies peptide patterns correlating with disease states [9]. An early application of protein-based expression analysis identified altered expression of stromal-derived growth factor (SDF-1) as a potential novel predictive marker of poor graft outcomes following acute renal transplant rejection [53]. Tissue sources for biomarker studies currently include urine for bladder and renal cell carcinomas [54], cerebrospinal fluid

for neurodegenerative disorders, synovial fluid for rheumatologic diseases, and breast or seminal fluid aspirates for cancer detection [54–56]. Proteomics promises to provide information regarding the heterogeneity of disease states, yielding information regarding disease processes and potential response to treatments [57]. Advancements in mass spectroscopy and nuclear magnetic resonance (NMR) have significantly improved the validity and reproducibility of proteomic assays. In addition, novel bioinformatics algorithms and database tools enable rapid identification of diagnostic protein expression patterns.

Because of the complex heterogeneity of transplant rejection, an ideal diagnostic test would have to be developed from a combination of multiple biomarkers, using a combination of transcription and translation techniques. A similar approach has been taken by Dos Remedios et al. [58] in characterizing transcriptional and post-translational changes in end-stage heart failure. Another promising animal study applying proteomics to transplantation was recently reported by Pan et al. [59] examining orthotopic liver transplants (OLT) in different donor and recipient rat strains in which no immunosuppression was used following transplant. Serum protein expression profiles were different in naive than in post-transplanted animals; among these proteins, haptoglobin (Hp), which is known to inhibit T-cell proliferation, was found to be upregulated following OLT in recipients tolerating the grafts. In addition, the transcriptional expression level and intracellular localization of Hp correlated with rejection [59]. This study suggests that haptoglobin may have a role in modulating spontaneous tolerance of liver transplantation and that the serum protein expression map could be used to discover other potential protein targets in transplant acceptance [59].

A surface-enhanced laser desorption ionization (SELDI) mass spectrometry platform was used in two studies screening urine samples from renal transplant patients with the objective of identifying non-invasive biomarkers for acute rejection [60,61]. Clarke et al. [60] used specialized sample preparation chips to enrich for hydrophobic proteins while comparing 17 transplant recipients with acute rejection with urine from 15 patients with no rejection and identified two proteins of unknown function of high predictive value. The system's pattern recognition software (Biomarker Pattern Software; Ciphergen, Inc.) correctly classified 91% of the study samples with a sensitivity of 83% and specificity of 100% using these two peptide products. In a subsequent study, Schaub et al. [61] analyzed 55 urine samples from post-transplant patients with and without acute rejection (AR) and included controls with acute tubular necrosis, glomerulopathies, lower urinary tract infection and cytomegalovirus viremia. None of these conditions were found to be confounding variables in a profile of AR characterized by the presence of three predominant peptide peaks present in 94% of the AR patients (17/18), only 18% of non-AR patients (4/22) and none of the normal controls. More importantly, sequential urine protein profiles were analyzed in the AR patients and diagnostic peaks were found to correlate with the clinical course of AR. In six patients, whose graft function returned to baseline with normal subsequent protocol biopsies, time-matched urine samples reverted to the normal pattern. In contrast, five patients who experienced further episodes of acute clinical rejection all retained the rejection pattern throughout the study [61].

An alternative proteomics approach has been applied to identify proteins upregulated in the heart during rejection [62] using 33 sequential cardiac biopsies (from four patients) comparing those with rejection ($n = 16$) to no rejection ($n = 17$). Proteins were analyzed by two-dimensional gel electrophoresis, over 100 proteins were found to be upregulated 2- to 50-fold during rejection and selected candidates sequenced. Of the 100 gene candidates, 13 were identified to be cardiac-specific or heat shock proteins. These included αβ-crystallin and tropomyosin which were validated by ELISA assays in the sera of 17 patients followed for 3 months post-transplants. Mean levels of both proteins were significantly higher in sera with biopsy-proven rejection ($P = 0.022$) compared with no rejection [62]. Kaiser et al. [63] used proteomic screening to monitor the clinical follow-up of patients after allogeneic hematopoietic stem cell transplantation in a phase 1 diagnostic study with the aim of identifying early indicators of graft-versus-host disease (GVHD). More than 1000 different polypeptides could be detected in individual samples using proteomic research based on platform capillary electrophoresis and mass spectrometry. Urine from 40 hematopoietic stem cell transplant patients (35 allogeneic, 5 autologous) and five patients with sepsis was collected and analyzed in a longitudinal study (100 days). Eighteen patients developed GVHD after allogeneic transplantation and a pattern characteristic of GVHD identified discrimination of GVHD from patients without complications with 82% specificity and 100% sensitivity. Moreover, including 13 sepsis-specific polypeptides was found to distinguish sepsis from GVHD and to reduce false-positives, giving a profile with a specificity of 97% and a sensitivity of 100% [63]. Two of the serum peptides identified were found to be derived from peptide from leukotriene A4 hydrolase and a peptide derived from serum albumin.

Cells, tissues and capture (affinity substrates) can be used in proteomic arrays. An antibody capture system has been used to characterize cellular immune responses using peptide-MHC microarrays [64]. Antigen-specific T-cell population dynamics can be used to understand the development and physiology of the immune system and its responses in health and disease. Multiple antigen-specific populations of T-cell lymphocytes (e.g. CD4$^+$, CD8$^+$ or any other abundant cell surface marker) can be captured using their ligand specificity with a high-density array of peptide-MHC complexes printed on a film-coated glass surface similar to those used in DNA gene chips. The initial feasibility study demonstrated the ability of the array to detect a rare population of antigen-specific T cells following vaccination of a normal mouse [64]. Tissue microarray (TMA) technology, where blocks of tissue from pathology cores are arrayed, have been applied to the analysis of prognostic markers in a series of 553 breast carcinomas in biopsy material [65]. In this application, a single sample from each tumor was sufficient to identify associations between molecular alterations and clinical outcome and, contrary to expectation, tissue heterogeneity did not negatively influence the predictive power of the TMA results [65].

CONVERGENCE OF GENOMICS AND PROTEOMICS

Immune tolerance, defined as the ability to completely wean patients from immunosuppressive therapy without immune-mediated injury to the graft, is a common goal of transplant research [66–68]. An interim step includes immunosuppression minimization protocols [69], including elimination of either corticosteroids [42] or calcineurin inhibitors [70]. Organ transplantation trials are progressing with due caution in the quest for transplant tolerance [71]. Knowledge gained from these efforts may help in the development of innovative strategies and new immunosuppressive agents [72]. These studies have seen recent advances in both genomics and proteomics. One such study analyzed genomic-wide transcription profiles of double-negative regulatory T cells (DN-Treg) and functionally inactive naturally occurring mutant cell lines derived from them [73]. In vivo studies using mouse allogeneic cardiac grafts demonstrated all animals preinfused with the DN-Treg clones survived over 100 days, while allograft survival was equivalent following infusion of mutant clones and untreated controls (19.5 ± 11.1 days vs. 22.8 ± 10.5 days). The identified gene expression signature comparing the DN-Treg cells and inactive clones identified over 1000 highly differentially expressed genes (significance analysis of microarrays [SAM] $P < 0.025$%) with increased expression of cell proliferation and survival, immune regulating and chemotaxis-related genes together with decreased expression of genes for antigen presentation, apoptosis, as well as several protein phosphatases involved in signal transduction [73]. Large-scale analysis of the functions of gene products will impact our understanding of the biochemistry of proteins, processes and pathways that are involved in graft acceptance or rejection [74]. For example, proteomic analysis using immunoaffinity purification is now extensively used to separate MHC complexes from their peptide epitomes [75]. The specific alloantigens of the peptides are sequenced by tandem mass spectrometry. Proteomic studies also show promise in the generation of individualized tolerizing vaccines in an emerging field known as reverse genomics which uses proteomics-determined specificity of autoantibodies found in patient profiles to develop and select DNA tolerizing vaccines

Table 6.2 Key genes associated with AR 1 biopsies as ascertained by genomic microarray analysis.

AR1 functional category	Genes	Total	EASE score	Fisher exact	Example genes
Defense/immune response	47	747	1.36E-30	1.73E-31	IL2RB, IL6R, IGLL1, LTB, LTF
MHC class II receptor activity	10	18	2.09E-15	1.44E-17	HLA-C, -DM, -DP, -DQa, CD74
Antigen processing/presentation	11	28	1.1E-14	1.54E-16	MHC class I and II genes
Signal transduction	34	1971	0.00000146	0.000000629	ITGA2, ITGB2, STAT1, -3, -6
Humoral immune response	9	144	0.0000256	0.00000326	CD53, CSF1R, UBD
Complement activation	4	29	0.00177	0.0000971	DAF, BF, C1s, SERPING1
MHC class I receptor activity	3	16	0.0062	0.000219	HLA-C, HLA-E, B2M
Innate immune response	6	175	0.0155	0.00362	CXCL9, LYZ, SPP1, NMI
Cell adhesion	10	549	0.0394	0.0172	CD9, CD69, TSPAN-1, VCAM1
Chemokine activity	3	43	0.041	0.00416	CCL5, CXCL9, CXCL10
Mitochondrion	20	476	0.0000159	0.00000489	ACAT1, ATP5B, DLD, GATM
Regulation of coagulation	3	9	0.00653	0.000215	ANXA5, ANXA7, KLKB1
Energy pathways	8	160	0.00704	0.00185	ATP5B, ATP5G3, ME2, OXCT1
Regulation of translation	5	60	0.00969	0.0015	EEF1A1, EIF4A2, HRSP12
Actin polymerization	3	13	0.0136	0.000702	CXCL12, DSTN, PFN2
Membrane fusion	3	23	0.0404	0.00392	CALM, CDH17, CLTB, GCA
Calcium ion binding	12	499	0.0608	0.0309	CDH17, RGN, EFHD1, CLTB
Cell motility	8	253	0.0639	0.0263	ATP1A1, CD9, C4A, TM4SF8
Negative regulation of cell cycle	4	71	0.0767	0.0176	RAP1A, RB1, RBL2, CDK2AP1
Defense/immune response	20	747	0.00000174	0.000000483	CCL13, CD6, CD79, APOH
Cell proliferation	17	899	0.000899	0.000351	CDC20, CCNA2, -B1, -B2, IL1B
Regulation of cell cycle	10	337	0.000926	0.000228	CKS1B, CKS2, CDC20
Response to wounding	8	250	0.00271	0.000616	GAGE8, IL1B, IL9, LBP
Nuclear division	6	137	0.00369	0.000609	CDC20, NEK2, PTTG1
Acute phase response	3	20	0.00978	0.000447	LBP, ORM2, SERPINA3
Chemokine binding	3	24	0.0102	0.000485	CCL13, CCR5, CX3CR1
Humoral immune response	5	144	0.0233	0.00483	ADA, BATF, IL1B, PAX5

MHC, major histocompatibility complex.

[76]. These synthetic vaccines are simple rings of DNA containing a specific antigen-encoding gene region and a promoter–terminator sequence required for expression in mammalian cells. Studies performed using animal models for multiple sclerosis and autoimmune diabetes support the feasibility of the reverse genomics approach [76].

The large complex data sets generated by typical genomics or proteomics studies require sophisticated data analysis. Three broad steps are involved in data analysis: data normalization, data filtering and pattern identification. Data must first be normalized in order to compare expression levels effectively. Data are then reduced by eliminating genes expressed below a defined threshold value. Finally, clustering and visualization programs are used to generate gene expression patterns. Such patterns infer possible biologic or clinical relevance. These tools can be applied to proteomic studies once the data are reduced into tabular form and many are available from public sources (Table 6.2).

Hierarchical clustering, the most commonly used form of unsupervised data analysis, uses standard statistical algorithms to link genes or proteins having similar gene expression patterns, forming clusters [77]. This method iteratively joins the two closest clusters, which effectively groups both genes and samples according to their similarity in expression profiles. Cluster analysis of microarray data produces coherent patterns of gene expression that are easily visualized but provides little information about statistical significance. A statistical method, SAM, was therefore developed to be specifically adapted for the analysis of gene chip data [78] and can be applied to unsupervised and supervised data analysis of either DNA microarray or proteomic data.

An important emerging application in genomic and proteomic screens is the ability to classify and predict the diagnostic sample classes (categories) based on gene signatures [10]. This is particularly challenging because of the large number of genes from which to predict classes and the relatively small number of samples. It is also important to identify genes or peptides that are most characteristic of and therefore contribute most to identified sample groups. Methods that have been implemented to discover and simplify sample classification include clustering methods, compound covariate prediction, fuzzy logic, sunken centroid gene list filtering and neural networks.

CONCLUSIONS

Gene chips now have an important role in molecular medicine research. Global gene expression studies provide valuable insights into molecular signatures of acute allograft rejection. Different molecular classes of acute allograft rejection that correlate with therapeutic response and survival, while appearing clinically and pathologically homogenous, have been identified. This suggests the possibility of using patient-specific treatment. Global gene expression monitoring or proteomic profiling may provide the opportunity for therapeutic approaches and programs based on the needs of individual patients. Biomarkers discovered from global expression monitoring may help predict how much immunosuppression an individual patient needs. Novel mass spectrometric, affinity and display techniques offer tools for the large-scale analysis of proteomes and represent alternative screening approaches for informative biomarkers. Other analytical methods such as protein interaction studies, cell separation and gene inactivation experiments add functional confirmation and biologic significance to the gene expression-based studies currently underway. The orchestration of genes in the post-transplant setting may be informative in monitoring rejection susceptibility, assessing risk, stratifying cases of acute rejection and in the prediction of long-term graft outcomes.

ACKNOWLEDGMENTS

We gratefully acknowledge the contributions of Szu-Chuan Hseish, Sheryl Shah and Meixia Zhang to laboratory projects summarized in this review. Support for this work was funded by grants from the NIH (NIH5P3-05 and NIH3P3-05S1), Clinical Center for Immunological Studies at Stanford University (CCIS), Packard Foundation and Roche Pharmaceuticals.

REFERENCES

1 Raasveld MH, Weening JJ, Kerst JM, Surachno S, ten Berge RJ. Local production of interleukin-6 during acute rejection in human renal allografts. *Nephrol Dial Transplant* 1993;**8**:75–8.

2 Hariharan S, Alexander JW, Schroeder TJ, First MR. Impact of first acute rejection episode and severity of rejection on cadaveric renal allograft survival. *Clin Transplant* 1996;**10**:538–41.

3 Ozdemir BH, Bilezikci B, Haberal AN, Demirhan B, Gungen Y. Histologic evaluation, HLA-DR expression, and macrophage density of renal biopsies in OKT3-treated acute rejection: comparison with steroid response in acute rejection. *Transplant Proc* 2000;**32**:528–31.

4 Sarwal MM, Jani A, Chang S, *et al*. Granulysin expression is a marker for acute rejection and steroid resistance in human renal transplantation. *Hum Immunol* 2001;**62**:21–31.

5 Sarwal M, Chua MS, Kambham N, *et al*. Molecular heterogeneity in acute renal allograft rejection identified by DNA microarray profiling. *N Engl J Med* 2003;**349**:125–38.

6 Soulillou J, Giral M. Controlling the incidence of infection and malignancy by modifying immunosuppression. *Transplantation* 2001;**72**(Suppl):S89–93.

7 Alizadeh A, Eisen M, Davis RE, *et al*. The lymphochip: a specialized cDNA microarray for the genomic-scale analysis of gene expression in normal and malignant lymphocytes. *Cold Spring Harb Symp Quant Biol* 1999;**64**:71–8.

8 Lander ES, Linton LM, Birren B, *et al*. Initial sequencing and analysis of the human genome. *Nature* 2001;**409**:860–921.

9 Golub TR, Slonim DK, Tamayo P, *et al*. Molecular classification of cancer: class discovery and class prediction by gene expression monitoring. *Science* 1999;**286**:531–7.

10 Alizadeh AA, Eisen MB, Davis RE, *et al*. Distinct types of diffuse large B-cell lymphoma identified by gene expression profiling. *Nature* 2000;**403**:503–11.

11 Alizadeh AA, Staudt LM. Genomic-scale gene expression profiling of normal and malignant immune cells. *Curr Opin Immunol* 2000;**12**:219–25.

12 Schena M, Shalon D, Davis RW, Brown PO. Quantitative monitoring of gene expression patterns with a complementary DNA microarray. *Science* 1995;**270**:467–70.

13 Brown FG, Nikolic-Paterson DJ, Metz C, Bucala R, Atkins RC, Lan HY. Up-regulation of macrophage migration inhibitory factor in acute renal allograft rejection in the rat. *Clin Exp Immunol* 1999;**118**:329–36.

14 Brown PO, Botstein D. Exploring the new world of the genome with DNA microarrays. *Nat Genet* 1999;**21**(Suppl):33–7.

15 Akalin E, Hendrix RC, Polavarapu RG, *et al*. Gene expression analysis in human renal allograft biopsy samples using high-density oligoarray technology. *Transplantation* 2001;**72**:948–53.

16 Morgun A, Shulzhenko N, Silva ID, *et al*. Differentially expressed genes in cardiac transplant biopsies and in mixed lymphocyte culture. *Transplant Proc* 2002;**34**:471–3.

17 Hedrick SM, Cohen DI, Nielsen EA, Davis MM. Isolation of cDNA clones encoding T cell-specific membrane-associated proteins. *Nature* 1984;**308**:149–53.

18 Brunet JF, Denizot F, Golstein P. A differential molecular biology search for genes preferentially expressed in functional T lymphocytes: the CTLA genes. *Immunol Rev* 1988;**103**:21–36.

19 Gress TM, Hoheisel JD, Lennon GG, Zehetner G, Lehrach H. Hybridization fingerprinting of high-density cDNA-library arrays with cDNA pools derived from whole tissues. *Mamm Genome* 1992;**3**:609–19.

20 Chen JJ, Wu R, Yang PC, *et al*. Profiling expression patterns and isolating differentially expressed genes by cDNA microarray system with colorimetry detection. *Genomics* 1998;**51**:313–24.

21 Bertucci F, Bernard K, Loriod B, *et al*. Sensitivity issues in DNA array-based expression measurements and performance of nylon microarrays for small samples. *Hum Mol Genet* 1999;**8**:1715–22.

22 Chee M, Yang R, Hubbell E, *et al*. Accessing genetic information with high-density DNA arrays. *Science* 1996;**274**:610–4.

23 Ben-Dor A, Bruhn L, Friedman N, Nachman I, Schummer M, Yakhini Z. Tissue classification with gene expression profiles. *J Comput Biol* 2000;**7**:559–83.

24 Mansfield ES, Hernandez-Boussard, T, Sarwal, M. Arrays amaze: unraveling the transcriptisome in transplantation. *ASHI Quarterly* 2003;**27**:11–5.

25 Mansfield ES, Sarwal MM. Arraying the orchestration of allo-graft pathology. *Am J Transplant* 2004;**4**:853–62.

26 Li J, Spletter ML, Johnson JA. Dissecting tBHQ induced ARE-driven gene expression through long and short oligonucleotide arrays. *Physiol Genomics* 2005;**21**:43–58.

27 Pan Q, Shai O, Misquitta C, *et al.* Revealing global regulatory features of Mammalian alternative splicing using a quantitative microarray platform. *Mol Cell* 2004;**16**:929–41.

28 Kirk AD. What's new: what's hot in basic science: American Transplant Congress 2004. *Am J Transplant* 2004;**4**:1741–6.

29 D'Errico A, Corti B, Pinna AD, *et al.* Granzyme B and perforin as predictive markers for acute rejection in human intestinal transplantation. *Transplant Proc* 2003;**35**:3061–5.

30 Simon T, Opelz G, Wiesel M, Ott RC, Susal C. Serial peripheral blood perforin and granzyme B gene expression measurements for prediction of acute rejection in kidney graft recipients. *Am J Transplant* 2003;**3**:1121–7.

31 Kotsch K, Mashreghi MF, Bold G, *et al.* Enhanced granulysin mRNA expression in urinary sediment in early and delayed acute renal allograft rejection. *Transplantation* 2004;**77**:1866–75.

32 Bittmann I, Muller C, Behr J, Groetzner J, Frey L, Lohrs U. Fas/FasL and perforin/granzyme pathway in acute rejection and diffuse alveolar damage after allogeneic lung transplantation: a human biopsy study. *Virchows Arch* 2004;**445**:375–81.

33 Gimino VJ, Lande JD, Berryman TR, King RA, Hertz MI. Gene expression profiling of bronchoalveolar lavage cells in acute lung rejection. *Am J Respir Crit Care Med* 2003;**168**:1237–42.

34 Yagi T, Iwagaki H, Urushihara N, *et al.* Participation of IL-18 in human cholestatic cirrhosis and acute rejection: analysis in living donor liver transplantation. *Transplant Proc* 2001;**33**:421–5.

35 Flohe S, Speidel N, Flach R, Lange R, Erhard J, Schade FU. Expression of HSP 70 as a potential prognostic marker for acute rejection in human liver transplantation. *Transpl Int* 1998;**11**:89–94.

36 Mueller AR, Platz KP, Gebauer B, *et al.* Changes at the extra-cellular matrix during acute and chronic rejection in human liver transplantation. *Transpl Int* 1998;**11**(Suppl 1):S377–82.

37 Alpert S, Lewis NP, Ross H, Fowler M, Valantine HA. The relationship of granzyme A and perforin expression to cardiac allograft rejection and dysfunction. *Transplantation* 1995;**60**:1478–85.

38 Tian L, Guo W, Yuan Z, *et al.* Association of the CD134/CD134L costimulatory pathway with acute rejection of small bowel allograft. *Transplantation* 2002;**74**:133–8.

39 Flechner SM, Kurian SM, Head SR, *et al.* Kidney transplant rejection and tissue injury by gene profiling of biopsies and peripheral blood lymphocytes. *Am J Transplant* 2004;**4**:1475–89.

40 Chua MS, Barry C, Chen X, Salvatierra O, Sarwal MM. Molecular profiling of anemia in acute renal allograft rejection using DNA microarrays. *Am J Transplant* 2003;**3**:17–22.

41 Mauiyyedi S, Pelle PD, Saidman S, *et al.* Chronic humoral rejection: identification of antibody-mediated chronic renal allograft rejection by CD4 deposits in peritubular capillaries. *J Am Soc Nephrol* 2001;**12**:574–82.

42 Sarwal MM, Yorgin PD, Alexander S, *et al.* Promising early outcomes with a novel, complete steroid avoidance immunosuppression protocol in pediatric renal transplantation. *Transplantation* 2001;**72**:13–21.

43 Sarwal MM, Vidhun JR, Alexander SR, Satterwhite T, Millan M, Salvatierra O Jr. Continued superior outcomes with modification and lengthened follow-up of a steroid-avoidance pilot with extended daclizumab induction in pediatric renal transplantation. *Transplantation* 2003;**76**:1331–9.

44 Dennis G Jr, Sherman BT, Hosack DA, *et al.* DAVID: Database for annotation, visualization, and integrated discovery. *Genome Biol* 2003;**4**:P3.

45 Collins AB, Schneeberger EE, Pascual MA, *et al.* Complement activation in acute humoral renal allograft rejection: diagnostic significance of C4d deposits in peritubular capillaries. *J Am Soc Nephrol* 1999;**10**:2208–14.

46 Racusen LC, Halloran PF, Solez K. Banff 2003 meeting report: new diagnostic insights and standards. *Am J Transplant* 2004;**4**:1562–6.

47 Racusen LC. The Banff schema and differential diagnosis of allograft dysfunction. *Transplant Proc* 2004;**36**:753–4.

48 Tibshirani R, Hastie T, Narasimhan B, Chu G. Diagnosis of multiple cancer types by shrunken centroids of gene expression. *Proc Natl Acad Sci USA* 2002;**99**:6567–72.

49 Scherer A, Krause A, Walker JR, Korn A, Niese D, Raulf F. Early prognosis of the development of renal chronic allograft rejection by gene expression profiling of human protocol biopsies. *Transplantation* 2003;**75**:1323–30.

50 Hoffmann S, Park J, Jacobson LM, *et al.* Donor genomics influence graft events: the effect of donor polymorphisms on acute rejection and chronic allograft nephropathy. *Kidney Int* 2004;**66**:1686–93.

51 Goodstadt L, Ponting CP. Sequence variation and disease in the wake of the draft human genome. *Hum Mol Genet* 2001;**10**:2209–14.

52 Halloran PF. Immunosuppression in the post-adaptation period. *Transplantation* 2000;**70**:3–5.

53 Shah S, Mansfield E, Kambham N, Hsieh S, Liu R, Sarwal M. Intragraft expression of SDF-1 is a novel predicitve marker of poor graft outcomes following acute renal transplant rejection. In: American Transplant Congress, 2004: Boston, MA. 2004.

54 Kommu S, Sharifi R, Edwards S, Eeles R. Proteomics and urine analysis: a potential promising new tool in urology. *BJU Int* 2004;**93**:1172–3.

55 Petricoin EF, Ornstein DK, Liotta LA. Clinical proteomics: applications for prostate cancer biomarker discovery and detection. *Urol Oncol* 2004;**22**:322–8.

56 Johann DJ Jr, McGuigan MD, Patel AR, *et al.* Clinical proteomics and biomarker discovery. *Ann N Y Acad Sci* 2004;**1022**:295–305.

57 Richards J, Le Naour F, Hanash S, Beretta L. Integrated genomic and proteomic analysis of signaling pathways in dendritic cell differentiation and maturation. *Ann N Y Acad Sci* 2002;**975**:91–100.

58 Dos Remedios CG, Liew CC, Allen PD, Winslow RL, Van Eyk JE, Dunn MJ. Genomics, proteomics and bioinformatics of human heart failure. *J Muscle Res Cell Motil* 2003;**24**:251–60.

59 Pan TL, Wang PW, Huang CC, Goto S, Chen CL. Expression, by functional proteomics, of spontaneous tolerance in rat ortho-topic liver transplantation. *Immunology* 2004;**113**:57–64.

60 Clarke W, Silverman BC, Zhang Z, Chan DW, Klein AS, Molmenti EP. Characterization of renal allograft rejection by urinary proteomic analysis. *Ann Surg* 2003;**237**:660–4; discussion 664–5.

61 Schaub S, Rush D, Wilkins J, *et al.* Proteomic-based detection of urine proteins associated with acute renal allograft rejection. *J Am Soc Nephrol* 2004;**15**:219–27.

62 Borozdenkova S, Westbrook JA, Patel V, *et al.* Use of proteomics to discover novel markers of cardiac allograft rejection. *J Proteome Res* 2004;**3**:282–8.

63 Kaiser T, Kamal H, Rank A, *et al.* Proteomics applied to the clinical follow-up of patients after allogeneic hematopoietic stem cell transplantation. *Blood* 2004;**104**:340–9.

64 Soen Y, Chen DS, Kraft DL, Davis MM, Brown PO. Detection and characterization of cellular immune responses using peptide-MHC microarrays. *PLoS Biol* 2003;**1**:E65.

65 Torhorst J, Bucher C, Kononen J, *et al.* Tissue microarrays for rapid linking of molecular changes to clinical endpoints. *Am J Pathol* 2001;**159**:2249–56.

66 Ansari MJ, Sayegh MH. Clinical transplantation tolerance: the promise and challenges. *Kidney Int* 2004;**65**:1560–3.

67 Luke PP, Jordan ML. Contemporary immunosuppression in renal transplantation. *Urol Clin North Am* 2001;**28**:733–50.

68 Oluwole SF, Oluwole OO, DePaz HA, Adeyeri AO, Witkowski P, Hardy MA. CD4+CD25+ regulatory T cells mediate acquired transplant tolerance. *Transpl Immunol* 2003;**11**:287–93.

69 Kirk AD, Mannon RB, Swanson SJ, Hale DA. Strategies for minimizing immunosuppression in kidney transplantation. *Transpl Int* 2005;**18**:2–14.

70 Flechner SM, Kurian SM, Solez K, *et al. De novo* kidney transplantation without use of calcineurin inhibitors preserves renal structure and function at two years. *Am J Transplant* 2004;**4**:1776–85.

71 Kirk AD. Ethics in the quest for transplant tolerance. *Transplantation* 2004;**77**:947–51.

72 Hardinger KL, Koch MJ, Brennan DC. Current and future immunosuppressive strategies in renal transplantation. *Pharmacotherapy* 2004;**24**:1159–76.

73 Lee BP, Mansfield EM, Hsieh SC, *et al.* Expression profiling of murine double negative regulatory T cells suggest mechanisms for prolonged cardiac allograft survival. *J Immunol* 2005;**174**:4535–44.

74 Meri S, Baumann M. Proteomics: posttranslational modifications, immune responses and current analytical tools. *Biomol Eng* 2001;**18**:213–20.

75 Shoshan SH, Admon A. MHC-bound antigens and proteomics for novel target discovery. *Pharmacogenomics* 2004;**5**:845–59.

76 Liu MA. DNA vaccines: a review. *J Intern Med* 2003;**253**:402–10.

77 Eisen MB, Spellman PT, Brown PO, Botstein D. Cluster analysis and display of genome-wide expression patterns. *Proc Natl Acad Sci USA* 1998;**95**:14863–8.

78 Tusher VG, Tibshirani R, Chu G. Significance analysis of microarrays applied to the ionizing radiation response. *Proc Natl Acad Sci USA* 2001;**98**:5116–21.

7 Tolerance: A Review of its Mechanisms in the Transplant Setting

Alan D. Salama

The last 50 years have seen immense effort spent on trying to understand the mechanisms underlying transplantation tolerance, so that they may be applied in a clinical setting. Tolerance would allow for the long-lasting function of a graft in the absence of immunosuppression, thus eliminating the exposure of patients to the adverse effects induced by these nonspecific agents. It might also mean an end to the increased incidence of infections, malignancies and various metabolic side-effects, which result in problems such as growth retardation and an increased risk of death from cardiovascular causes. The first description of successful experimental transplantation tolerance was by Billingham *et al.* [1], in 1953, who demonstrated that *in utero* exposure of a fetus to alloantigens from a particular donor resulted in unresponsiveness of the adult animal towards the same donor antigens. The difficulty with these experiments was that in order to achieve tolerance manipulation of embryos was required, a situation that could not be easily translated to the clinical arena. However, having provided the proof that such an acquired state could be induced at all, many others were inspired to study mechanisms of tolerance induction in adults with fully developed immune systems.

Using numerous animal models and novel experimental strategies in patients, we have understood some but not all of the key elements that underlie tolerance and how we may be able to achieve them, at least in a restricted setting. We have learned once again that rodents are not humans and that there are much bigger hurdles to overcome if tolerance is to become a clinical reality for all transplant recipients. We are currently missing a vital tool, which is the ability to measure the tolerant state, and without this we are hampered by being unable to monitor what we have achieved at all but the basic level. It has recently been suggested that we should not try to achieve complete or true tolerance, but should accept a lesser state, "prope tolerance," in which a small (less toxic) dose of some immunosuppressive is administered, so as to maintain graft function [2]. Perhaps this is a more realistic ambition and, at least in the first instance, it is an interim goal that we should be able to achieve.

SELF AND TRANSPLANTATION TOLERANCE

The immune system has evolved to distinguish "self" from "nonself." In this way, it is set up to efficiently eliminate all invading foreign molecules, while not reacting adversely to the multitude of "self" molecules, which make up the complex human organism. This process occurs during a period of immunologic development, when the vast array of our own molecules are presented to the immune system so as to educate it as to what is what, and teach it "friend from foe." Thus, tolerance is a state in which a nondestructive immune response occurs to a particular antigen. It is more than mere unresponsiveness to that antigen, as there are complex mechanisms of regulation within the adaptive immune response that dictate the outcome of the antigen–immune cell encounter. When this mechanism goes wrong, either through a deficiency in immunologic schooling or a breakdown of the regulatory mechanisms, a destructive immune response is mounted towards our own molecules, and autoimmunity ensues. The fact that clinically relevant autoimmune diseases occur in only a small minority of people is a testament to the highly efficient way in which the immune system regulates and monitors itself.

Tolerance to alloantigens follows the same rules, except that the mechanisms come into play from the time of transplantation when the new foreign antigens are first introduced to the immune system. Without intervention, the alloantigens are recognized as foreign and the immune response aimed at removing and destroying these molecules initiated, ultimately resulting in graft rejection. However, if the immune system can be re-educated towards the alloantigens, which would then be treated as "self," a tolerant state would be induced, reproducing the process that occurs during immunologic development. Thus, in a transplanted individual with an already developed mature immune system, regulating the adaptive immune response towards the new alloantigens and inducing a long-lasting state of immune acceptance towards them is the goal of transplant biologists.

Immune responsiveness towards the transplanted organ relies on the recognition of alloantigens by lymphocytes, in

56

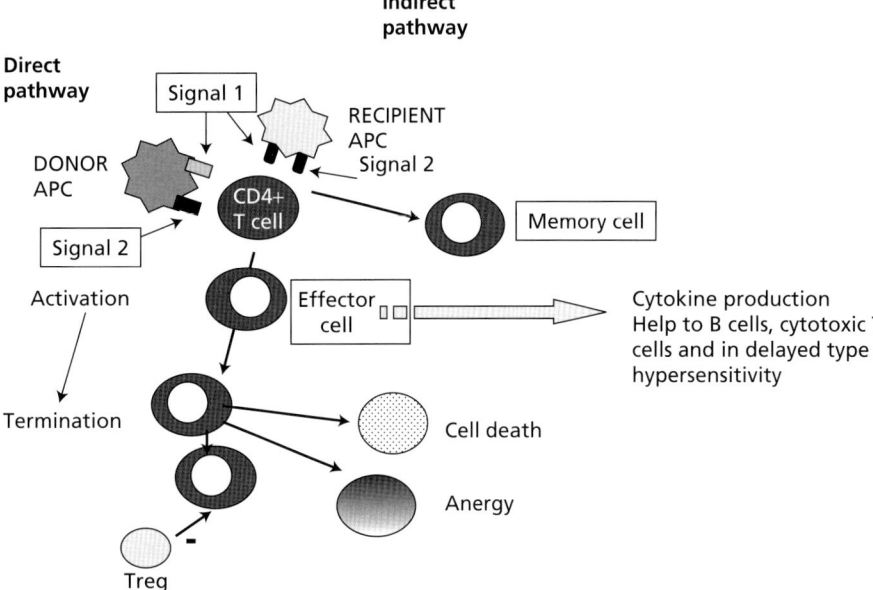

Fig. 7.1 The alloreactive T-cell response. Upon antigen engagement and in the presence of adequate costimulatory signals, the alloreactive T cell becomes activated, proliferates and can subsequently undergo a number of different fates, such as differentiation to an effector or memory cell. Effector functions are terminated through a process of apoptosis, through regulation by other cells or soluble factors, or by anergy following inadequate stimulation. The majority of alloreactive T cells will proliferate, produce cytokines and provide help to other limbs of the immune response then die through activation-induced cell death (AICD).

particular the CD4⁺ T cells that orchestrate the rest of the immune response. CD4⁺ T cells may recognize alloantigen through two distinct pathways. In the direct pathway, the T cell recognizes the intact allo-MHC molecule on the donor antigen-presenting cells (APCs), while in the indirect pathway, the allo-MHC is degraded, processed and presented by self (recipient) APC (Fig. 7.1). These pathways have different relative contributions in mediating transplant rejection, with the direct pathway predominating during the early post-transplant period, while the indirect pathway contributes in both the early and late post-transplant periods (Fig. 7.2). Moreover, the indirect pathway has been implicated in mediating chronic rejection, in part through epitope spreading.

Immunologic education and central T-cell tolerance

During immunologic development the T lymphocytes are matured and educated in the thymus while the B lymphocytes undergo a similar process in the bone marrow.

The first and perhaps most critical step in preventing the maturation of autoreactive lymphocytes is the early elimination of such self-reactive cells, a process termed clonal deletion. T cells developing in the thymus that react most strongly with antigens presented by self-MHC are eliminated (negative selection), while those with lesser avidity continue to develop and are subsequently exported to the periphery (positive

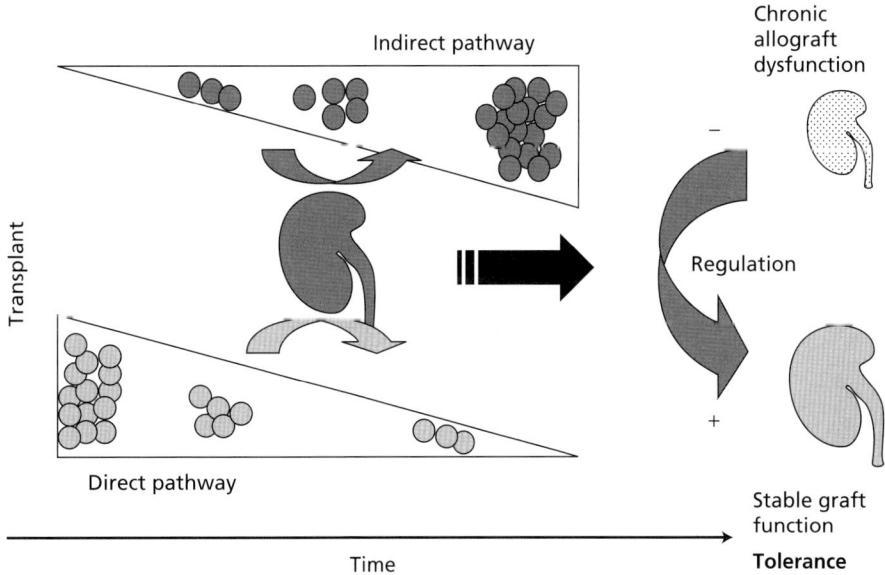

Fig. 7.2 The immune response to a kidney graft. Cartoon representing the balance between direct and indirect pathways of alloimmunity and their relative contributions to rejection and tolerance at different stages following transplantation. Low effector cell numbers and greater regulatory factors favor graft acceptance and tolerance, while the converse results in rejection.

selection). Thus, additional mechanisms are required to keep in check those T cells that have been selected in the thymus but exhibit low avidity autoreactivity [3,4]. The double positive (CD4$^+$CD8$^+$) thymocytes whose T-cell receptors (TCR) do not engage with self-MHC molecules die; while those T cells that bind to self-MHC molecules survive as a result of expression of the antiapoptotic protein Bcl-2 [5]. However, even following TCR engagement, negative or positive selection may ensue [6]. The selection depends on the particular peptide bound to the MHC molecule, its concentration, the TCR affinity for the MHC–peptide complex, and other secondary costimulatory signals provided to the T cell [7–10]. This allows those cells with the strongest avidity for self-MHC and antigen to undergo apoptosis [11], so that the only cells emigrating from the thymus are of low to intermediate affinity for self-MHC and antigen, and are positive for either CD4 or CD8. This has been termed the affinity-avidity model of thymic selection.

Obviously, for clonal deletion to occur within the thymus, the antigen has to be presented on the surface of APC within the thymus and this underlies tolerance to many antigens, even those with restricted tissue expression [12–14]. Not surprisingly, attempts have been made to induce tolerance through intrathymic antigen injection. Intrathymic inoculation of both auto- and alloantigens has been reported to induce tolerance, with T-cell tolerance being easier to achieve than B cell, and Th1 responses easier than Th2 [15–17], although this has not been a universal finding [18,19]. The critical role of the thymus in tolerance induction has been identified by investigators who cotransplanted donor thymic tissue alongside the donor organ graft and demonstrated the development of donor-specific tolerance [20].

Despite negative selection, autoreactive T and B cells do migrate into the periphery and have been identified in normal individuals as well as patients with clinical autoimmunity [21,22]. These cells are generally prevented from initiating damage by a number of different regulatory mechanisms, each of which contribute towards tolerance to a variable degree, depending on the experimental system studied. Data on these mechanisms in human disease remains sparse but is beginning to emerge.

Mechanisms of peripheral T-cell tolerance

Deletion and apoptosis

One fate of activated T cells is programmed cell death termed activation-induced cell death (AICD). This is mediated by the interaction of Fas (CD95) with its ligand (Fas-L or CD95L) on T cells, and can occur in developing thymocytes as well as mature T cells [23]. Interleukin-2 (IL-2) acting on its receptor and activating the STAT5 signaling pathway potentiates the upregulation of Fas-L and downregulates Bcl-2 expression on T cells, thus sensitizing them to AICD [24,25]. Augmented AICD can promote tolerance through elimination of allo-

reactive lymphocytes [26–28]. Central to this process are IL-15 acting as growth and survival factors for T cells, and IL-2 sensitizing them through the STAT5 pathway to AICD [24,25,29].

Anergy

Successful T-cell activation requires the presentation of peptide on the appropriate MHC molecule to the TCR, termed "signal 1," and costimulatory signals, termed "signal 2" [30], the most significant of which are the B7–CD28 and CD40–CD154 interactions [31]. T cells stimulated by low or high antigen doses or in a costimulation deficient manner may be rendered *anergic*, that is hyporesponsive to further antigenic stimulation. In some models, these cells are capable of certain effector functions, such as production of γ-interferon (IFNγ), but cannot produce IL-2 (the major T-cell growth factor) or undergo autocrine proliferation. Thus, antigen presentation by professional APC, carrying the full complement of costimulatory molecules, stimulate T-cell proliferation, whereas tolerance is achieved using nonprofessional APC, lacking such molecules [32]. Anergy underlies the donor-specific hyporesponsiveness that is found in the direct alloreactive pathway, after the graft has been *in situ* for some time [33]. Experimentally, anergic T cells persist *in vivo* for a number of weeks or while antigen is still administered. However, while the anergic state is not overcome by supplementation with T-cell growth factors, derived from activated bystander cells [34], *in vitro* anergy can be reversed by the addition of exogenous IL-2 [31]. Thus, peripheral tolerance can be maintained through anergy so long as the antigen is still present and available to the T cells despite other ongoing immune responses.

This situation is somewhat complicated by the recent recognition of a myriad of other costimulatory molecules, from both the B7 (immunoglobulin) and tumor necrosis factor (TNF) superfamilies [35,36] which can induce T-cell activation in the absence of B7 signaling. Although initially thought of as representing multiple redundant pathways, it now appears that some molecules act on particular cellular compartments and at particular time points [35]. Furthermore, it is apparent that memory T cells, CD8$^+$ T cells and natural killer (NK) cells rely less on B7–CD28 interactions in order to achieve full activation.

Anergic cells may themselves act to attenuate the responsiveness of other T cells, by downregulating the costimulation molecules on dendritic cells and thus inhibiting effective antigen presentation [37]. This appeared to be dependent on cell–cell contact mechanisms, and represents one end of the spectrum of regulatory cells.

Regulation or suppression

The regulation of effector T cells by a subset of professional regulatory T cells (Treg) is an important mechanism for maintaining tolerance, which has recently become better understood and attracted much attention [38,39]. Early evidence for their role came from numerous animal models in which certain T-cell subsets were shown to attenuate autoimmune phenomena, suppress tumour growth [38] and prolong graft survival [40]. Subsequent studies have confirmed the existence of these cells in alloimmune rodent models and in human transplant recipients [41–43].

We now appreciate that a number of cell populations can act as regulatory cells. The most studied being a population of thymus-derived Treg that express CD4CD25, CTLA4 and GITR [44], and termed "natural" Treg, which constitute approximately 10% of the CD4 population. Further characterization of the regulatory population has been attempted but no unique cell surface marker has been satisfactorily identified [41–43,45,46]. However, these cells are characterized by the expression of the foxp3 transcription factor [47–49]. Deficiency of foxp3 or neonatal thymectomy results in a loss of these Treg and is manifested by various autoimmune phenomena [50]. This is mirrored in a human condition, in which foxp3 is absent, termed immune dysregulation, polyendocrinopathy, enteropathy and X-linked inheritance (IPEX) [51], a rare and aggressive autoimmune disease characterized by diabetes, enteropathy, eczema, thyroid and haematologic abnormalities, lymphadenopathy and premature death. Conversely, overexpression of foxp3 in naïve T cells renders them regulatory [49].

A second population of regulatory cells develop in the periphery, in a thymic-independent manner, following antigen encounter under particular circumstances, and following exposure to certain cytokines including transforming growth factor β (TGF-β) [52,53] and are termed "adaptive" Treg. These cells also appear to express foxp3, although their expression of other cell surface markers is more variable.

The mechanisms of action of Treg are only partly understood. In certain model systems and *in vivo*, altered cytokine profiles may underlie the inhibitory effects, with predominant IL-10, IL-5, TGF-β and IL-4 production depending on the system studied [41]. *In vitro* cell contact appears to be essential as suppression is prevented when regulatory and effector cells are physically separated [54] and cytokine effects appear to be unimportant [55]. In addition, other regulatory cell phenotypes have been additionally described, such as CD8+CD25+ and CD8+CD28− T cells [56,57]. The significance of these cells in tolerance induction in part depends on the model system studied and the methods used for inducing tolerance. However, it is apparent that such cells constitute an important mechanism underlying peripheral tolerance towards alloantigens.

Alteration in cytokine environment

It is now well established that T-cell effector responses in rodents and humans can be separated according to the cytokine profile that the T cells secrete [58]. Th1 cells produce IFNγ, IL-2, lymphotoxin and tumor necrosis factor (TNFα), and are involved in cell-mediated responses and some antibody-mediated responses, whereas Th2 cells produce IL-4, IL-5, IL-10 and IL-13 and provide help for B cells to produce IgM, IgA and particularly IgE antibodies. Differentiation along the Th1 pathway is under the influence of IL-12, IFNγ and IFNα, whereas IL-4 appears to be the essential Th2 pathway differentiation cytokine. Regulation to Th1 and Th2 responses is tightly controlled by the transcription factors, T-bet and GATA3, respectively [59–61]. Th1 cytokines antagonize some of the effects of Th2 cytokines and vice versa. In allograft rejection, Th1 responses appear to be dominant while Th2 cytokine deviation may confer protection from rejection in both rodents and humans [62–64]. However, it should be noted that the situation is not so clear-cut as STAT4-deficient (Th2 predominant) and STAT6-deficient animals (Th1 predominant) reject their allografts with a similar tempo to their wild-type counterparts [65], as do IFNγ-deficient recipients [66]. The requirement for Th1 cytokines for tolerance induction through activation induced death is only found when the T-cell clone size is large [67]. The deviation of a T-cell cytokine response to a single antigen may result in infectious tolerance towards other related antigens or coadministered antigens [68]. Cytokine deviation may also in part underlie the tolerogenic effects of altered peptide ligands which can provoke alterations in the responding T-cell cytokine profile, from a Th1 to a Th2 response, with protection from disease [69]. One additional factor regulating the cytokine profile is costimulation through particular molecules. B7 molecules on APC interacting with CD28 on T cells are intimately involved with T-cell IL-2 production and the regulation of responsiveness to IL-12, through the upregulation of the IL-12 β2 receptor subunit. They therefore have a role in deviation towards Th1 responses. Hence, by antagonising the B7–CD28 interaction, it is possible to generate predominant Th2 responses in alloimmunity [62].

Whether Th2 cytokine deviation is an adequate regulatory mechanism to inhibit Th1 immune responsiveness is in part dependent on the strength and size of the immune response, and related to the degree of MHC gene mismatch. Some evidence for this process regulating responses in human transplantation has recently been demonstrated [64]. An important caveat to the proposed skewing of the cytokine response is that deviation from a Th1 to a Th2 profile may not always be benign [70].

Immunologic ignorance

In some cases, tolerance is maintained to antigens without deletion or anergy of the antigen-reactive T cells. In this instance the T cells do not interact with but ignore the antigen under normal circumstances, because they do not encounter the antigen-bearing cells or because those cells do not possess the appropriate machinery in the form of costimulatory molecules or antigen concentration to activate the T cells [71]. However, under circumstances where the APC or T cells change their phenotype, allowing the T-cell activation threshold to be reduced, or where they express greater quantities of antigen, the T-cell antigen recognition can occur and the cells can be activated to mediate tissue damage. It remains unclear whether levels of alloantigen expression would be low enough to promote ignorance as a physiological mechanism of nonresponsiveness.

IMMUNOLOGIC CHANGES FOLLOWING TRANSPLANTATION

Following transplantation, there is a high frequency of direct pathway alloreactive T cells that predominates. These can react with the donor passenger leukocytes, which constitutively express the class II MHC molecules, and are responsible for the acute transplant rejection, necessitating the high levels of early post-transplant immunosuppression. With time, the loss of passenger leukocytes from the graft leaves only class II MHC expression on nonprofessional APCs, such as the resident graft parenchymal cells (Fig. 7.2). As the memory T cells passage through the graft, the interaction with costimulatory deficient parenchymal cells induces anergy in the direct pathway T cells [33]. Concurrently, uptake and processing of donor MHC by recipient APC promotes presentation of alloantigen to the indirectly reactive T cells. Continuous shedding of donor antigen may allow for the epitope spreading and expansion of the indirect alloreactive pathway. Therefore, in order to promote long-term graft acceptance and tolerance, the direct pathway needs to be kept in check long enough to allow the hyporesponsiveness that occurs "naturally" to take place and downregulation of the indirect pathway needs to be induced.

CLINICAL TOLERANCE

Based on the mechanisms of immune regulation, investigators have attempted to manipulate the alloimmune response so as to induce donor-specific transplant tolerance. This has mainly been attempted in rodent models and claims of transplant tolerance are generally based on grafts surviving for over 100 days with donor-specific hyporesponsiveness, as evidenced by acceptance of a second graft from the original donor strain and rejection of third party grafts. How this translates with regard to longevity of human transplants is impossible to know. Moreover, many reports fail to document whether chronic rejection is present in their long-term surviving grafts. Issues relating to durability are important, as clinical tolerance maybe fragile and liable to break down, for example following an infectious episode [72]. Indeed, some reports of

human transplant tolerance have subsequently been revised following later graft loss [73,74]. Thus, many of these reports represent what can be achieved in model systems, and would need to be replicated in nonhuman primates before applicability to humans can be inferred.

Examples of tolerance in clinical organ transplantation exist, but are uncommon and have generally occurred fortuitously. Patients who have stopped their maintenance immunosuppression rarely keep their grafts, but there are a small number who have maintained a well-functioning transplant [75]. The basis of this immunosuppression-free unresponsiveness remains poorly understood. The essential requirements, and importantly a means of confirming the attainment of the tolerant state, must be first worked out. Other examples of successful clinical transplant tolerance are in patients who received total lymphoid irradiation as induction therapy for their transplants [73,74], and in patients who received combined bone marrow and kidney transplants from the same donor for hematologic diseases complicated by renal failure, and have not required long-term immunosuppression [76,77]. Finally, using a combination of antilymphocyte therapy and limited post-transplant immunosuppression, Starzl et al. [78] have recently reported on a cohort of patients, some of whom required only weekly dosing with immunosuppressive agents 1 year post-transplantation. Although not true drug-free tolerance, this "prope" tolerance appears to be further along the road than our current situation, and may be a more realistic goal for the immediate future [2].

The use of bone marrow transplantation in order to induce tolerance has been extensively studied in animal models and to a lesser extent in patients [79]. Establishing mixed chimeric immune systems, with components from the donor and recipient bone marrow, allows the re-education of the immune system with deletion and anergy of alloreactive T cells, resulting in tolerance towards the host tissues as well as the foreign graft. Interestingly, the tolerance may outlast the chimerism, suggesting that the graft itself has some tolerogenic capacity [79]. More recent approaches based on nonmyeloablative regimens have been attempted in small numbers of patients (including children), using hemopoietic stem cells, total (or targeted) lymphoid irradiation, conventional immunosuppression [80] and additional intrathymic alloantigen inoculation in some [81]. These have reported varying degrees of success, but longer term follow-up is required. Development of such clinically applicable nonmyeloablative regimens that induce lasting chimerism in HLA-mismatched patients are required [82].

An alternative approach to bone marrow chimerism involves the use of in vitro manipulated or immature donor dendritic cells (DC) that have the capacity to induce peripheral and central tolerance [83,84]. However, there is no evidence that manipulated DCs can be used successfully to induce tolerance in higher animals.

Clinical manipulation of donor-specific regulatory cell

populations has not yet been achieved, although interestingly this may underlie the beneficial effect of donor-specific transfusion that had previously been reported [85]. However, *in vitro* expansion of regulatory cell populations has been reported and may form a potential therapy for subgroups of patients who demonstrate evidence of ongoing immune activation and graft damage.

Other strategies that have successfully been utilized to achieve tolerance in animal transplant models are the use of costimulatory blockade or T-cell depleting agents, in the presence or absence of donor antigens (given in the form of donor-specific transfusions or donor bone marrow). However, they do not, at least in the way that they have been currently used, reproducibly achieve tolerance in primates [86–88]. This may reflect the predominance of memory cells, generated to infectious agents, in outbred primates and humans compared to laboratory rodents [89]. Based on the impressive tolerizing potential in small animal models, B7 and CD154 T-cell costimulatory blockade strategies are being tested clinically [90,91]. Such an approach was applied with some success to bone marrow transplant recipients [92], and trials using CTLA4-Ig in renal transplantation are ongoing, but trials with one preparation of anti-CD154 were abandoned as a result of adverse reactions.

Although the B7–CD28 and CD40–CD154 pathways have dominated the drive for therapeutic costimulatory blockade, they have not proven to be as successful in patients as they were in animal models, and the suggestion that we would be less dependent on conventional immunosuppressive agents has not be fulfilled [93]. In part this is because of the alternative mechanisms that allow full T-cell activation, through other costimulatory molecules, such as ICOS, CD134, CD70, CD30, 4-1BB [94]. In particular, it has become apparent that certain immunologic compartments, such as alloreactive CD8+ T cells, memory CD4+ T cells and NK cells, are less reliant on B7–CD28 and CD40–CD154 signaling for their activation, but may depend on these alternative pathways. Our understanding of how these newly recognized costimulatory molecules impact on each other, as well as their relation to the B7 and CD40 pathways is still unfolding (Table 7.1) [35,95]. For example, CD8-mediated T-cell rejection has been a hurdle in many tolerogenic strategies that has only been overcome using a potent T-cell depletion strategy. However, recent data on the effects of 4-1BB [96], ICOS [97] and CD70 suggest that these molecules exert a preferential role on CD8+ T cells. In contrast, the CD134–CD134L pathway has been demonstrated to be of prime importance in memory T-cell activation and in the absence of B7–CD28 signaling [95,98]. Thus, understanding how these new pathways can be manipulated to attenuate alloimmune responses is critical and should lead to new (but more complex) immunotherapeutics.

In alloimmune responses, many of the peptides presented by APC are themselves derived from degraded allo-MHC molecules. Interestingly, certain peptides corresponding to the

Table 7.1 Predominant roles and targets of the costimulatory pathways in alloimmune responses.

Costimulatory pathway	Target cell/phase of immune response
CD28–B7	Initiation phase, CD4+, CD8+ T cells
ICOS–B7h	Effector phase, CD4+, CD8+ T cells
CD154–CD40	Initiation phase, CD4+, CD8+ T cells, B cells
CD134–CD134L	Maintenance phase, CD4+ T cells*
CD27–CD70	CD8+ T cells, NK cells, B cells*
4-1BB–4-1BBL	Maintenance phase, CD8+ T cells*

* More prominent effects in the absence of CD28–B7 signaling.

nonpolymorphic regions of class I or II MHC molecules have been shown in animal models to induce transplant tolerance (in association with a course of cyclosporine), in part through alterations in cytokine profiles as well as via deletional mechanisms, with induction of apoptosis [69,99,100]. The usefulness of these peptides in human transplantation remains to be confirmed, because use of altered peptide ligands in human autoimmune disease disappointingly failed to show significant beneficial effects.

Blockade of costimulatory pathways, induction of regulatory cell populations or use of other tolerogenic strategies may only work under circumstances in which the alloimmune response is of a manageable size for all the alloreactive T cells to be tolerized. Reduction of the alloreactive T-cell repertoire, with depleting or deletional (central or peripheral T-cell apoptosis) mechanisms may therefore have a crucial role allowing regulatory mechanisms to function in maintaining a tolerant state [101]. However, more recent data have demonstrated that tolerance based on costimulatory blockade and deletional mechanisms may be problematic. Induction of lymphopenia leads to homeostatic proliferation with the expansion of memory T cells, themselves resistant to tolerance induction by costimulatory blockade [102]. An alternative protocol that has capitalized on the roles of certain cytokines in regulating T-cell death, utilized agonistic IL-2 and antagonistic IL-15 chimeric molecules and resulted in tolerance in highly stringent models [27]. Interestingly, inducing alloreactive effector T cell death did not seem to lead to loss of alloreactive regulatory cell populations as these are relatively resistant to apoptosis [103] and the AICD-promoting effects of IL-2 [27]. Such a combination therefore augments regulatory mechanisms while attenuating effector responses through deletion.

The newer immunosuppressive drugs may also have a role by inducing T-cell apoptosis and deletion, and may thus be required at least for a limited period following transplantation. Agents such as rapamycin during the induction phase, along with anti-T-cell antibodies such as humanized non-mitogenic anti-CD3 [104] or Campath-1 [105] may therefore facilitate tolerance induction [106], although data confirming this are still lacking.

The effect of conventional immunosuppressive drugs on tolerizing strategies needs further investigation, because the initial suggestion that certain drugs would impair the generation of tolerance in some models [106,107] have not proven founded in others [108]. For example, calcineurin inhibitors do not impair long-term graft survival if given with certain costimulatory blockade regimens, such as multiple rather than single doses of anti-CD154 [109]. Whether some agents are more for permissive in generating regulatory cells remains unclear, but is of considerable interest [110]. Short-term follow-up data demonstrating that withdrawal of conventional immunosuppressants following specific induction therapy can be achieved successfully, at least in a subset of patients, are highly encouraging [78].

PEDIATRIC ISSUES

Despite concerns that children may have vigorous immune responses and that they may be "high risk" transplant recipients, recent registry reports have identified young children as outstanding transplant recipients, sometimes with the best long-term graft survival rates of all ages of recipients [111,112]. Although there is no consensus of the relative risks and benefits of including children in tolerance protocols, there is no reason to expect that they would be any less likely to be excellent candidates. Indeed, certain approaches to tolerance induction may be particularly relevant to pediatric organ transplantation [113]. The neonate and young infant may be particularly suited to strategies that lead to central deletional tolerance. A trial of intrathymic inoculation of donor-specific bone marrow at the time of pediatric heart transplantation is in progress, with some preliminary evidence for enhanced graft accommodation [114].

CONCLUSIONS

Clinical transplantation tolerance is not yet around the corner, although our increasing understanding of the biology of alloimmune responses is allowing us to get ever closer to defining the strategies that will realistically allow or prevent clinical donor-specific hyporesponsiveness. More tangible is a state of "operational tolerance," which may require limited use of conventional immunosuppression in association with other biologic induction strategies. Defining the optimum protocols remains a significant challenge.

REFERENCES

1 Billingham RE, Brent L, Medewar PB. Actively acquired tolerance of foreign cells. *Nature* 1953;**172**:603–6.
2 Calne RY. Prope tolerance: the future of organ transplantation: from the laboratory to the clinic. *Transplantation* 2004;**77**: 930–2.
3 Kappler JW, Roehm N, Marrack P. T cell tolerance by clonal elimination in the thymus. *Cell* 1987;**49**:273–80.
4 Kappler JW, Staerz U, White J, Marrack PC. Self-tolerance eliminates T cells specific for Mls-modified products of the major histocompatibility complex. *Nature* 1988;**332**:35–40.
5 Egerton M, Scollay R, Shortman K. Kinetics of mature T cell development in the thymus. *Proc Nat Acad Sci USA* 1990;**87**: 2579–82.
6 Anderson G, Jenkinson EJ. Thymus organ cultures and T-cell receptor repetoire development. *Immunology* 2000;**100**:405–10.
7 Ashton-Rickardt PG, Bandeira A, Delaney JR, *et al.* Evidence for a differential avidity model of T cell selection in the thymus. *Cell* 1994;**76**:651–63.
8 Turka LA, Linsley PS, Paine R, Schieven GL, Thompson CB, Ledbetter JA. Signal transduction via CD4, CD8 and CD28 in mature and immature thymocytes: implications for thymic selection. *J Immunol* 1991;**146**:1428–36.
9 Degermann S, Surh CD, Glimcher LH, Sprent J, Lo D. B7 expression on thymic medullary epithelium correlates with epithelium-mediated deletion of vβ5+ thymocytes. *J Immunol* 1994;**152**:3254–63.
10 Sebzda E, Wallace VA, Mayer J, Yeung RSM, Mak TW, Ohashi PS. Positive and negative thymocyte selection induced by different concentrations of a single peptide. *Science* 1994; **263**:1615–8.
11 Sprent J, Lo D, Er-Kai G, Ron Y. T cell selection in the thymus. *Immunol Rev* 1988;**101**:172–90.
12 Farr AG, Rudensky A. Medullary thymic epithelium: a mosaic of epithelial "self"? *J Exp Med* 1998;**188**:1–4.
13 Sospedra M, Ferrer-Francesch X, Dominguez O, Juan M, Foz-Sala M, Pujol-Borrell R. Transcription of a broad range of self-antigens in human thymus suggests a role for central mechanisms in tolerance toward peripheral antigens. *J Immunol* 1998;**161**:5918–29.
14 Salama AD, Chaudhry AN, Ryan JJ, *et al.* In Goodpasture's disease CD4+ T cells escape thymic deletion and react to the autoantigen α3(IV)NC1. *J Am Soc Nephrol* 2001;**12**:1908–15.
15 Husby S, Mestecky J, Moldoveanu Z, Holland S, Elson CO. Oral tolerance in humans. T cell but not B cell tolerance after antigen feeding. *J Immunol* 1994;**152**:4663–70.
16 Ohtsuru I, Matsuo H, Fukudome T, Sueaga A, Tsujihata M, Nagataki S. "Split tolerance" induction by intrathymic injection of acetylcholine receptor in a rat model of autoimmune myasthenia gravis; implications for the design of specific immunotherapies. *Clin Exp Immunol* 1995;**102**:462–7.
17 Shirwan H, Mhoyan A, Kakoulidis TP, Yolcu ES, Ibrahim S. Prevention of chronic rejection with immunoregulatory cells induced by intrathymic immune modulation with class I allo-peptides. *Am J Transplant* 2003;**3**:581–9.
18 Chaib E, Brons IG, Papalois A, Calne RY. Does intrathymic injection of alloantigen-presenting cells before islet allo-transplantation prolong graft survival? *Transpl Int* 1994;**7**(Suppl 1):S423–5.
19 Abbate M, Kalluri R, Corna D, *et al.* Experimental Goodpasture's syndrome in Wistar-Kyoto rats immunized with alpha3 chain of type IV collagen. *Kidney Int* 1998;**54**:1550–61.
20 Barth RN, Yamamoto S, LaMattina JC, *et al.* Xenogeneic thymokidney and thymic tissue transplantation in a pig-to-baboon model. I. Evidence for pig-specific T-cell unresponsiveness. *Transplantation* 2003;**75**:1615–24.

21 Naquet P, Ellis J, Tibensky D, *et al*. T cell autoreactivity to insulin in diabetic and related non-diabetic individuals. *J Immunol* 1988;**140**:2569–78.

22 Hafler DA, Weiner HL. Immunologic mechanisms and therapy in multiple sclerosis. *Immunol Rev* 1995;**144**:75–107.

23 Ju S-T, Panka DJ, Cui H, *et al*. Fas(CD95)/FasL interactions required for programmed cell death after T-cell activation. *Nature* 1995;**373**:444–8.

24 Van Parijs L, Refaeli Y, Lord JD, Nelson BH, Abbas AK, Baltimore D. Uncoupling IL-2 signals that regulate T cell proliferation, survival, and Fas-mediated activation-induced cell death. *Immunity* 1999;**11**:281–8.

25 Li XC, Demirci G, Ferrari-Lacraz S, *et al*. IL-15 and IL-2: a matter of life and death for T cells *in vivo*. *Nat Med* 2001; **7**:114–8.

26 Zhou T, Song L, Yang P, Wang Z, Lui D, Jope RS. Bisindolylalemide VIII facilitates FAS-mediated apoptosis and inhibits T cell-mediated autoimmune diseases. *Nat Med* 1999;**5**:42–8.

27 Zheng XX, Sanchez-Fueyo A, Sho M, Domenig C, Sayegh MH, Strom TB. Favorably tipping the balance between cytopathic and regulatory T cells to create transplantation tolerance. *Immunity* 2003;**19**:503–14.

28 Li XC, Ima A, Li Y, Zheng XX, Malek TR, Strom TB. Blocking the common gamma-chain of cytokine receptors induces T cell apoptosis and long-term islet allograft survival. *J Immunol* 2000;**164**:1193–9.

29 Van Parijs L, Abbas AK. Homeostasis and self-tolerance in the immune system: turning lymphocytes off. *Science* 1998;**280**: 243–8.

30 Bretscher P, Cohn M. A theory of self-nonself discrimination. *Science* 1970;**169**:1042–9.

31 Schwartz RH. Costimulation of T lymphocytes: the role of CD28, CTLA4, and B7/BB1 in interleukin-2 production and immunotherapy. *Cell* 1992;**71**:1065–8.

32 Ridge JP, Fuchs EJ, Matzinger P. Neonatal tolerance revisited: turning on newborn T cells with dendritic cells. *Science* 1996;**271**:1723–6.

33 Ng WF, Hernandez-Fuentes M, Baker R, Chaudhry A, Lechler RI. Reversibility with interleukin-2 suggests that T cell anergy contributes to donor-specific hyporesponsiveness in renal transplant patients. *J Am Soc Nephrol* 2002;**13**:2983–9.

34 Pape KA, Merica R, Mondino A, Khoruts A, Jenkins MK. Direct evidence that functionally impaired CD4+ T cells persist *in vivo* following induction of peripheral tolerance. *J Immunol* 1998;**160**:4719–29.

35 Salama AD, Sayegh MH. Alternative T-cell costimulatory pathways in transplant rejection and tolerance induction: hierarchy or redundancy? *Am J Transplant* 2003;**3**:509–11.

36 Yamada A, Salama AD, Sayegh MH. The role of novel T cell costimulatory pathways in autoimmunity and transplantation. *J Am Soc Nephrol* 2002;**13**:559–75.

37 Vendetti S, Chai JG, Dyson J, Simpson E, Lombardi G, Lechler R. Anergic T cells inhibit the antigen-presenting function of dendritic cells. *J Immunol* 2000;**165**:1175–81.

38 Sakaguchi S, Fukuma K, Kuribayashi K, Masuda T. Organ-specific autoimmune diseases induced in mice by elimination of a T cell subset. *J Exp Med* 1985;**161**:72–87.

39 Shevach EM. Regulatory T cells in autoimmunity. *Ann Rev Immunol* 2000;**18**:423–49.

40 Hall BM, Pearce NW, Gurley KE, Dorsch SE. Specific unresponsiveness in rats with prolonged cardiac allograft survival after treatment with cyclosporine. III. Further characterization of the CD4+ suppressor cell and its mechanisms of action. *J Exp Med* 1990;**171**:141–57.

41 Kingsley CI, Karim M, Bushell AR, Wood KJ. CD25+CD4+ regulatory T cells prevent graft rejection: CTLA-4- and IL-10-dependent immunoregulation of alloresponses. *J Immunol* 2002;**168**:1080–6.

42 Hara M, Kingsley CI, Niimi M, *et al*. IL-10 is required for regulatory T cells to mediate tolerance to alloantigens *in vivo*. *J Immunol* 2001;**166**:3789–96.

43 Salama AD, Najafian N, Clarkson MR, Harmon WE, Sayegh MH. Regulatory CD25+ T cells in human kidney transplant recipients. *J Am Soc Nephrol* 2003;**14**:1643–51.

44 Shimizu J, Yamazaki S, Takahashi T, Ishida Y, Sakaguchi S. Stimulation of CD25+CD4+ regulatory T cells through GITR breaks immunological self-tolerance. *Nat Immunol* 2002;**3**: 135–42.

45 Baecher-Allan C, Brown JA, Freeman GJ, Hafler DA. CD4+CD25 high regulatory cells in human peripheral blood. *J Immunol* 2001;**167**:1245–53.

46 Stephens LA, Barclay AN, Mason D. Phenotypic characterization of regulatory CD4+CD25+ T cells in rats. *Int Immunol* 2004;**16**:365–75.

47 Fontenot JD, Gavin MA, Rudensky AY. Foxp3 programs the development and function of CD4+CD25+ regulatory T cells. *Nat Immunol* 2003;**4**:330–6.

48 Khattri R, Cox T, Yasayko SA, Ramsdell F. An essential role for Scurfin in CD4+CD25+ T regulatory cells. *Nat Immunol* 2003;**4**:337–42.

49 Hori S, Nomura T, Sakaguchi S. Control of regulatory T cell development by the transcription factor Foxp3. *Science* 2003;**299**:1057–61.

50 Taguchi O, Nishizuka Y. Self tolerance and localized autoimmunity. Mouse models of autoimmune disease that suggest tissue-specific suppressor T cells are involved in self tolerance. *J Exp Med* 1987;**165**:146–56.

51 Wildin RS, Smyk-Pearson S, Filipovich AH. Clinical and molecular features of the immunodysregulation, polyendocrinopathy, enteropathy, X linked (IPEX) syndrome. *J Med Genet* 2002;**39**:537–45.

52 Chen W, Jin W, Hardegen N, *et al*. Conversion of peripheral CD4+CD25− naïve T cells to CD4+CD25+ regulatory T cells by TGF-beta induction of transcription factor Foxp3. *J Exp Med* 2003;**198**:1875–86.

53 Walker MR, Kasprowicz DJ, Gersuk VH, *et al*. Induction of FoxP3 and acquisition of T regulatory activity by stimulated human CD4+CD25− T cells. *J Clin Invest* 2003;**112**:1437–43.

54 Thornton AM, Shevach EM. CD4+CD25+ immunoregulatory T cells suppress polyclonal T cell activation *in vitro* by inhibiting interleukin 2 production. *J Exp Med* 1998;**188**:287–96.

55 Piccirillo CA, Letterio JJ, Thornton AM, *et al*. CD4+CD25+ regulatory T cells can mediate suppressor function in the absence of transforming growth factor beta1 production and responsiveness. *J Exp Med* 2002;**196**:237–46.

56 Cosmi L, Liotta F, Lazzeri E, *et al*. Human CD8+CD25+ thymocytes share phenotypic and functional features with CD4+CD25+ regulatory thymocytes. *Blood* 2003;**102**:4107–14.

63

57 Stephens LA, Mason D. CD25 is a marker for CD4$^+$ thymocytes that prevent autoimmune diabetes in rats, but peripheral T cells with this function are found in both CD25$^+$ and CD25$^-$ subpopulations. *J Immunol* 2000;**165**:3105–10.

58 Mosmann TR, Coffman RL. TH1 and TH2 cells: different patterns of lymphokine secretion lead to different functional properties. *Annu Rev Immunol* 1989;**7**:145–73.

59 Szabo SJ, Kim ST, Costa GL, Zhang X, Fathman CG, Glimcher LH. A novel transcription factor, T-bet, directs Th1 lineage commitment. *Cell* 2000;**100**:655–69.

60 Das J, Chen CH, Yang L, Cohn L, Ray P, Ray A. A critical role for NF-κB in GATA3 expression and Th2 differentiation in allergic airway inflammation. *Nat Immunol* 2001;**2**:45–50.

61 Rao A, Avni O. Molecular aspects of T-cell differentiation. *Br Med Bull* 2000;**56**:969–84.

62 Sayegh MH, Akalin E, Hancock WW, *et al*. CD28-B7 blockade after alloantigenic challenge *in vivo* inhibits Th1 cytokines but spares Th2. *J Exp Med* 1995;**181**:1869–74.

63 Waaga AM, Gasser M, Kist-van Holthe JE, *et al*. Regulatory functions of self-restricted MHC class II allopeptide-specific Th2 clones *in vivo*. *J Clin Invest* 2001;**107**:909–16.

64 Kist-van Holthe JE, Gasser M, Womer K, *et al*. Regulatory functions of alloreactive Th2 clones in human renal transplant recipients. *Kidney Int* 2002;**62**:627–31.

65 Kishimoto K, Dong VM, Issazadeh S, *et al*. The role of CD154–CD40 versus CD28–B7 costimulatory pathways in regulating allogeneic Th1 and Th2 responses *in vivo*. *J Clin Invest* 2000;**106**:63–72.

66 Nagano H, Mitchell RN, Taylor MK, Hasegawa S, Tilney NL, Libby P. Interferon-gamma deficiency prevents coronary arteriosclerosis but not myocardial rejection in transplanted mouse hearts. *J Clin Invest* 1997;**100**:550–7.

67 Kishimoto K, Sandner S, Imitola J, *et al*. Th1 cytokines, programmed cell death, and alloreactive T cell clone size in transplant tolerance. *J Clin Invest* 2002;**109**:1471–9.

68 Tian J, Lehmann PV, Kaufman DL. Determinant spreading of T helper cell 2 (Th2) responses to pancreatic islet autoantigens. *J Exp Med* 1997;**186**:2039–43.

69 Murphy B, Kim KS, Buelow R, Sayegh MH, Hancock WW. Synthetic MHC class I peptide prolongs cardiac survival and attenuates transplant arteriosclerosis in the Lewis→Fischer 344 model of chronic allograft rejection. *Transplantation* 1997;**64**:14–9.

70 Coles AJ, Wing M, Smith S, *et al*. Pulsed monoclonal antibody treatment and autoimmune thyroid disease in multiple sclerosis. *Lancet* 1999;**354**:1691–5.

71 Ohashi PS, Oehen S, Buerki K, *et al*. Ablation of "tolerance" and induction of diabetes by virus infection in viral antigen transgenic mice. *Cell* 1991;**65**:305–17.

72 Williams MA, Tan JT, Adams AB, *et al*. Characterization of virus-mediated inhibition of mixed chimerism and allospecific tolerance. *J Immunol* 2001;**167**:4987–95.

73 Strober S, Benike C, Krishnaswamy S, Engleman EG, Grumet FC. Clinical transplantation tolerance twelve years after prospective withdrawal of immunosuppressive drugs: studies of chimerism and anti-donor reactivity. *Transplantation* 2000;**69**:1549–54.

74 Strober S, Dhillon M, Schubert M, *et al*. Acquired immune tolerance to cadaveric renal allografts: a study of three patients treated with total lymphoid irradiation. *N Engl J Med* 1989;**321**:28–33.

75 Burlingham WJ, Grailer AP, Fechner JH Jr, *et al*. Microchimerism linked to cytotoxic T lymphocyte functional unresponsiveness (clonal anergy) in a tolerant renal transplant recipient. *Transplantation* 1995;**59**:1147–55.

76 Sayegh MH, Fine NA, Smith JL, Rennke HG, Milford EL, Tilney NL. Immunologic tolerance to renal allografts after bone marrow transplants from the same donors. *Ann Intern Med* 1991;**114**:954–5.

77 Spitzer TR, Delmonico F, Tolkoff-Rubin N, *et al*. Combined histocompatibility leukocyte antigen-matched donor bone marrow and renal transplantation for multiple myeloma with end stage renal disease: the induction of allograft tolerance through mixed lymphohematopoietic chimerism. *Transplantation* 1999;**68**:480–4.

78 Starzl TE, Murase N, Abu-Elmagd K, *et al*. Tolerogenic immunosuppression for organ transplantation. *Lancet* 2003;**361**:1502–10.

79 Sykes M. Mixed chimerism and transplant tolerance. *Immunity* 2001;**14**:417–24.

80 Millan MT, Shizuru JA, Hoffmann P, *et al*. Mixed chimerism and immunosuppressive drug withdrawal after HLA-mismatched kidney and hematopoietic progenitor transplantation. *Transplantation* 2002;**73**:1386–91.

81 Trivedi HL, Vanikar AV, Modi PR, *et al*. Allogeneic hematopoietic stem-cell transplantation, mixed chimerism, and tolerance in living related donor renal allograft recipients. *Transplant Proc* 2005;**37**:737–42.

82 Auchincloss HJ. In search of the elusive holy grail: the mechanisms and prospects for achieving clinical transplantation tolerance. *Am J Transplant* 2001;**1**:6–12.

83 Thomson AW, Lu L. Dendritic cells as regulators of immune reactivity: implications for transplantation. *Transplantation* 1999;**68**:1–8.

84 Lechler R, Ng WF, Steinman RM. Dendritic cells in transplantation: friend or foe? *Immunity* 2001;**14**:357–68.

85 Bushell A, Karim M, Kingsley CI, Wood KJ. Pretransplant blood transfusion without additional immunotherapy generates CD25$^+$CD4$^+$ regulatory T cells: a potential explanation for the blood-transfusion effect. *Transplantation* 2003;**76**:449–55.

86 Kenyon NS, Chatzipetrou M, Masetti M, *et al*. Long-term survival and function of intrahepatic islet allografts in rhesus monkeys treated with humanized anti-CD154. *Proc Natl Acad Sci USA* 1999;**96**:8132–7.

87 Kirk AD. Transplantation tolerance: a look at the nonhuman primate literature in the light of modern tolerance theories. *Crit Rev Immunol* 1999;**19**:349–88.

88 Knechtle SJ, Fechner JH Jr, Dong Y, *et al*. Primate renal transplants using immunotoxin. *Surgery* 1998;**124**:438–46; discussion 446–7.

89 Adams AB, Williams MA, Jones TR, *et al*. Heterologous immunity provides a potent barrier to transplantation tolerance. *J Clin Invest* 2003;**111**:1887–95.

90 Sayegh MH, Turka LA. The role of T-cell costimulatory activation pathways in transplant rejection. *N Engl J Med* 1998;**338**:1813–21.

91 Kishimoto K, Dong VM, Sayegh MH. The role of costimulatory molecules as targets for new immunosuppressives in transplantation. *Curr Opin Urol* 2000;**10**:57–62.

92 Guinan EC, Boussiotis VA, Neuberg D, *et al*. Transplantation of anergic histoincompatible bone marrow allografts. *N Engl J Med* 1999;**340**:1704–14.

93 Schwartz RS. The new immunology: the end of immunosuppressive drug therapy? *N Engl J Med* 1999;**340**:1754–6.

94 Watts TH, DeBenedette MA. T cell co-stimulatory molecules other than CD28. *Curr Opin Immunol* 1999;**11**:286–93.

95 Demirci G, Amanullah F, Kewalaramani R, *et al*. Critical role of OX40 in CD28 and CD154-independent rejection. *J Immunol* 2004;**172**:1691–8.

96 Wang J, Guo Z, Dong Y, *et al*. Role of 4-1BB in allograft rejection mediated by CD8+ T cells. *Am J Transplant* 2003;**3**:543–51.

97 Harada H, Salama AD, Sho M, *et al*. The role of the ICOS–B7h T cell costimulatory pathway in transplantation immunity. *J Clin Invest* 2003;**112**:234–43.

98 Yuan X, Salama AD, Dong V, *et al*. The role of the CD134–CD134 ligand costimulatory pathway in alloimmune responses *in vivo*. *J Immunol* 2003;**170**:2949–55.

99 Murphy B, Magee CC, Alexander SI, *et al*. Inhibition of allorecognition by a human class II MHC-derived peptide through the induction of apoptosis. *J Clin Invest* 1999;**103**:859–67.

100 Krensky AM, Clayberger C. HLA-derived peptides as novel immunosuppressives. *Nephrol Dial Transplant* 1997;**12**:865–8.

101 Li XC, Strom TB, Turka LA, Wells AD. T cell death and transplantation tolerance. *Immunity* 2001;**14**:407–16.

102 Wu Z, Bensinger SJ, Zhang J, *et al*. Homeostatic proliferation is a barrier to transplantation tolerance. *Nat Med* 2004;**10**:87–92.

103 Banz A, Pontoux C, Papiernik M. Modulation of Fas-dependent apoptosis: a dynamic process controlling both the persistence and death of CD4 regulatory T cells and effector T cells. *J Immunol* 2002;**169**:750–7.

104 Woodle ES, Xu D, Zivin RA, *et al*. Phase I trial of a humanized, Fc receptor nonbinding OKT3 antibody, huOKT3gamma1 (Ala-Ala) in the treatment of acute renal allograft rejection. *Transplantation* 1999;**68**:608–16.

105 Calne R, Moffatt SD, Friend PJ, *et al*. Campath IH allows low-dose cyclosporine monotherapy in 31 cadaveric renal allograft recipients. *Transplantation* 1999;**68**:1613–6.

106 Li Y, Li XC, Zheng XX, Wells AD, Turka LA, Strom TB. Blocking both signal 1 and signal 2 of T-cell activation prevents apoptosis of alloreactive T cells and induction of peripheral allograft tolerance. *Nat Med* 1999;**5**:1298–302.

107 Larsen CP, Elwood ET, Alexander DZ, *et al*. Long-term acceptance of skin and cardiac allografts after blocking CD40 and CD28 pathways. *Nature* 1996;**381**:434–8.

108 Kawai T, Cosimi AB, Colvin RB, *et al*. Mixed allogeneic chimerism and renal allograft tolerance in cynomolgus monkeys. *Transplantation* 1995;**59**:256–62.

109 Sho M, Sandner SE, Najafian N, *et al*. New insights into the interactions between T-cell costimulatory blockade and conventional immunosuppressive drugs. *Ann Surg* 2002;**236**:667–75.

110 Game DS, Hernandez-Fuentes MP, Lechler RI. Everolimus and basiliximab permit suppression by human CD4+CD25+ cells *in vitro*. *Am J Transplant* 2005;**5**:454–64.

111 Cecka JM, Gjertson DW, Terasaki PI. Pediatric renal transplantation: a review of the UNOS data. United Network for Organ Sharing. *Pediatr Transplant* 1997;**1**:55–64.

112 Harmon WE, McDonald RA, Reyes JD, *et al*. Pediatric transplantation, 1994–2003. *Am J Transplant* 2005;**5**:887–903.

113 Guenther DA, Madsen JC. Advances in strategies for inducing central tolerance in organ allograft recipients. *Pediatr Transplant* 2005;**9**:277–81.

114 Webber SA, Boyle GJ, Law YM, *et al*. A clinical trial of intrathymic inoculation of donor bone marrow with pediatric heart transplantation. *Pediatr Transplant* 2003;**7**(Suppl. 4):92.

Immunosuppression and its Complications

8 Mechanisms of Action of Immunosuppressive Agents

Alan M. Krensky

The classic approach to prolongation of organ transplantation is to block the immune response known as "rejection". So-called "immunosuppression" can involve any or all of the effector responses. In general, most current immunosuppressives were identified empirically, but newer agents are being developed based upon an understanding of the humoral and cellular pathways [1]. Although the incidence of acute forms of rejection has been substantially reduced by current protocols, chronic rejection still gives rise to ultimate graft loss, while drug toxicities may lead to premature death with functioning grafts [2]. This chapter highlights what is known about the mechanisms of action of the major immunosuppressives: (i) glucocorticoids; (ii) antiproliferative and antimetabolic agents; (iii) calcineurin inhibitors; and (iv) biologics – antibodies and antibody-derived reagents.

GLUCOCORTICOIDS

The use of glucorticoids as immunosuppressives in the 1960s helped to make clinical organ transplantation a reality [3]. Prednisone, prednisolone and other glucocortoicoids are generally used in combination with other immunosuppressives, but recent protocols are aimed at steroid sparing because of the multiple side-effects of glucocorticoids [4,5]. Steroids have a myriad of effects and their toxicities are intimately and inextricably connected to their therapeutic efficacy.

Despite the 50 years of use of glucocorticoids, their mechanism of action is still incompletely understood. Glucorticoid responses are immensely complex, based upon their interaction with glucorticoid-binding proteins (nonsignaling) and receptors (signaling) both inside and outside cells [6]. Glucocorticoids in the blood are either bound to specific serum protein, cortisol-binding globulin, or in a free, pharmacologically active form (Fig. 8.1). Unbound glucocorticoids diffuse freely across cell membranes where they interact with specific glucocorticoid receptors. When glucocorticoids bind to their receptors in cells they have many effects. Glucocorticoid receptors within the cell cytoplasm are bound to heat shock proteins. The heat shock protein is released when the steroid binds its receptor and a series of signal transduction pathways are activated as both the receptor and heat shock protein are phosphorylated. The receptor-steroid complex translocates to the nucleus where it binds to steroid response elements in the promoters of a large number of genes. The receptor-steroid complex may either activate or repress gene expression and a hierarchy of effects are made possible by the number of response elements and the context of other transcription factors and transcriptional machinery.

In this manner, glucocorticoids decrease expression (and/or release) of several cytokines and growth factors, including interleukins IL-1, IL-2, IL-3, IL-4, IL-6, insulin-like growth factor-α, tumor necrosis factor (TNF), γ-interferon (IFNγ), IL-8, RANTES, macrophage chemotactic and activating factor (MCAF) and platelet-activating factor (PAF), as well as some of their receptors, such as IL-2R [7]. Proteases, such as elastases, collagenases and plasminogen activator, involved in antigen presentation and movement of cells through the extracellular matrix, are also decreased in expression. Major histocompatibility complex (MHC) class II expression is decreased. Glucocorticoids inhibit vasodilatation and decrease vascular permeability. For example, they induce expression of neural endopeptidase, which degrades neuropeptides such as substance P and bradykinin which mediate vasodilatation. They effect the shape, contractility and adhesiveness of endothelial cells by inhibiting the expression of adhesion molecules and chemokines (chemoattractant cytokines). The immense complexity of steroid transcriptional effects at the cellular level are all multiplied by the respective downstream signaling pathways. In sum, the effects are dramatically immunosuppressive. To complicate matters further, steroids have nontranscriptional effects; for example, glucocorticoids affect translation and extracellular release of IL-1 and TNF [8,9].

The cellular effects of these events include poor antigen presentation by dendritic and other antigen-presenting cells, poor proliferative responses by T lymphocytes and dampening of effector responses by T lymphocytes [10,11]. In general, the glucocorticoid effect is on cellular immunity, particularly decreasing Th1 responses, and favoring humoral (and Th2) responses [12,13].

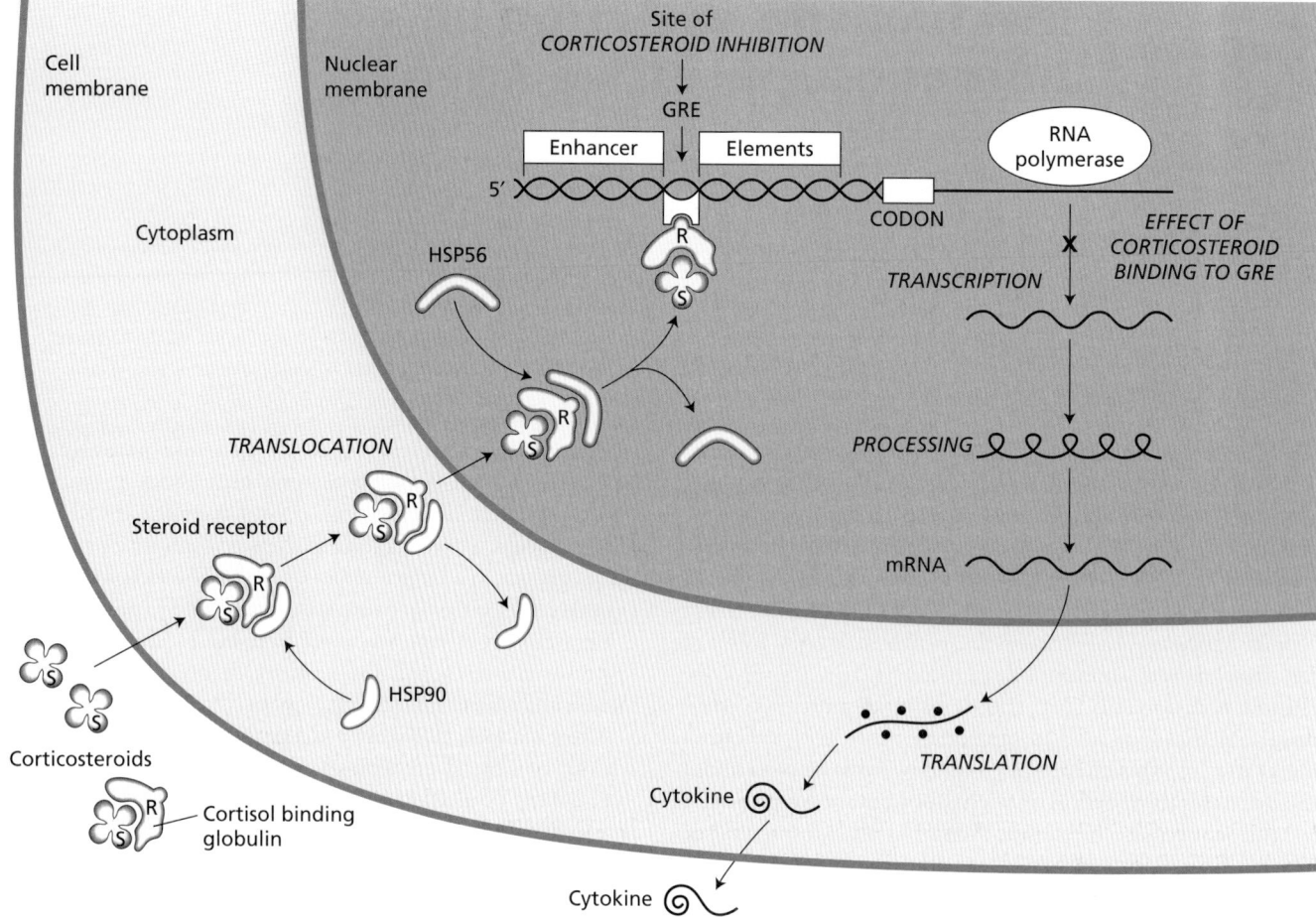

Fig. 8.1 Mechanism of action of glucocorticoids. Free corticosteroids in the bloodstream (not bound to cortisol-binding globulin) diffuse into the cell cytoplasm where they bind steroid receptors. After a series of processing events involving binding to heat shock protein chaperones and phosphorylation changes, the steroid receptor complex binds to the glucocorticoid receptor element in the promoter/enhancer of many different genes. The result is changes in expression of many proteins associated with the therapeutic and side-effects of steroid therapy.

ANTIPROLIFERATIVE AGENTS

The earliest immunosuppressives applied to transplant rejection were inhibitors of purine and pyrimidine biosynthesis [3,14]. Purine and pyrimidine biosynthesis occurs by two routes: the *de novo* and salvage pathways (Fig. 8.2). Both pathways are present in all cell types but T and B lymphocytes are profoundly susceptible to interruption of the *de novo* synthesis pathway. This susceptibility is at least partly a result of the high turnover rates and need for rapid proliferation of these immune cells in the adaptive immune response underlying transplant rejection.

Azathioprine is an imidazolyl derivative of 6-mercaptopurine (6-MP) with superior efficacy and less toxicity than its parent compound (6-MP) [14]. Glutathione and other sulfhydryl containing molecules (nucleophiles) nonenzymatically cleave azathioprine into 6-MP and a methylnitroimidazole moiety inside cells (Fig. 8.2). 6-MP in turn is converted into a series of additional metabolites that inhibit *de novo* purine synthesis. 6-thio-IMP, a fraudulent nucleotide, gets converted to 6-thio-GMP and then 6-thio-GTP, which when incorporated into DNA, halts gene translation. This inhibits cell proliferation which is fundamental to early stages of immune responses by both T and B lymphocytes. Numerous other metabolites, including the methylnitroimidazole moiety, have been shown to interrupt other pathways involved in the generation of adenosine triphosphate (ATP), cyclic adenosine monophosphate (cAMP) and guanosine triphosphate (GTP), all fundamental for normal cell function.

More recently, mycophenolate mofetil, the 2-morphlinoethyl ester of mycophenolic acid (MPA), has largely supplanted azathioprine in this drug class [15,16]. Mycophenolate mofetil is rapidly hydrolyzed to MPA, a selective, noncompetitive and reversible inhibitor of inosine monophosphate dehydrogenase (IMPDH), an important enzyme in the *de novo* guanine nucleotide biosynthesis pathway (Fig. 8.3). Once again, because of

Fig. 8.2 Mechanism of action of azathioprine (AZ). Azathioprine is cleaved to release active 6-mercaptopurine (6-MP) which in turn is converted to a series of metabolic intermediates that inhibit *de novo* purine synthesis. Thio-IMP (inosine monophosphate), Thio-GMP (guanine monophosphate) and Thio-GTP (guanine triphosphate) lead to a halt in gene translation and cell proliferation. A, adenine; AMP, adenosine monophosphate; AR, adenosine ribose; G, guanine; GR, guanine ribose; HX, hypoanthine; IMP, inosine monophosphate; IR, inoasine ribose; PRA, phosphoribosyl amine; PRPP, 5-phosphoribosyl-1-pyrophosphate; X, xanthine; XMP, xanthine monophosphate; XR, xanthine ribose.

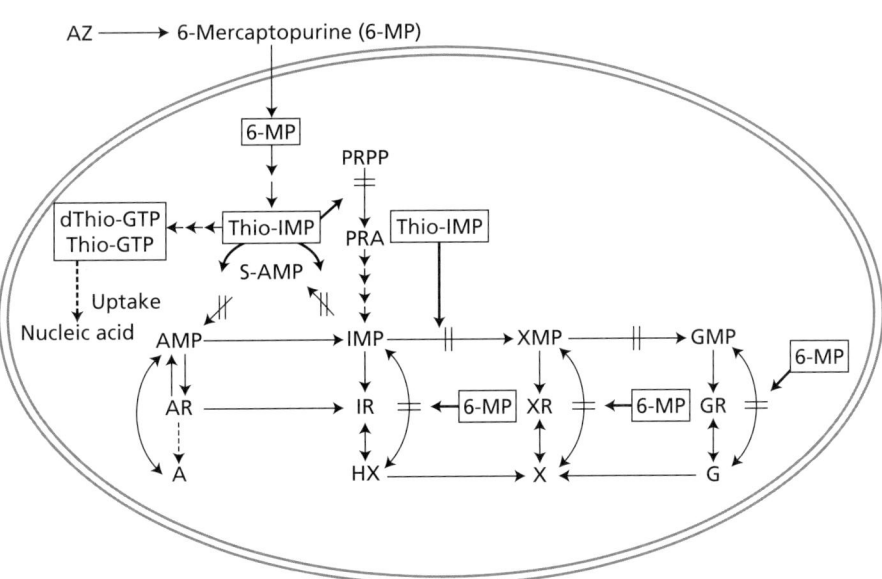

the high sensitivity of B and T lymphocytes to inhibition of this pathway, MPA selectively inhibits lymphocyte proliferation and effector functions related to cell adhesion, migration and antibody formation. The addition of guanosine or deoxyguanosine to cells can reverse the effect.

A new class of antiproliferative agents binds to and inhibits the kinase, mammalian target of rapamycin (mTOR), a key enzyme in cell cycle progression [17,18]. Sirolimus (rapamycin), a macrocyclic lactone from *Streptomyces hygroscopicus*,

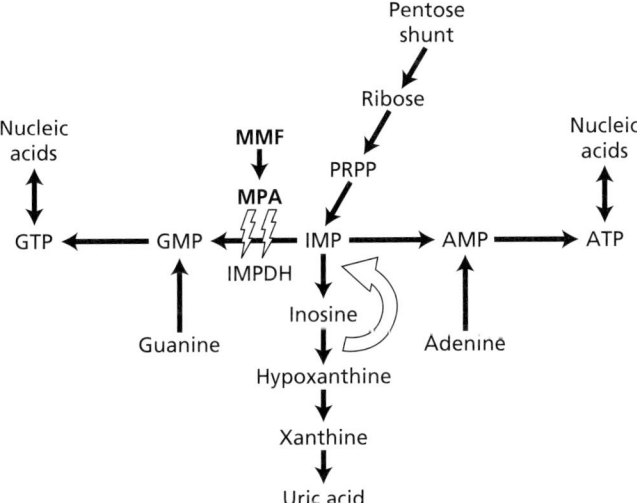

Fig. 8.3 Mechanism of action of mycophenolate mofetil (MMF). MMF is rapidly hydrolyzed to mycophenolic acid (MPA), inhibiting the *de novo* pathway of purine biosynthesis (left side of schematic). The right side of the schematic shows the salvage pathway. B and T lymphocytes rely primarily on the *de novo* pathway as their source of purine for DNA and RNA synthesis. AMP, adenosine monophosphate; ATP, adenosine triphosphate; GMP, guanosine monophosphate; GTP, guanosine triphosphate; IMPDH, inosine monophosphate dehydrogenase.

inhibits transplant rejection by blocking the cell cycle at transition from G1 to S phase (Fig. 8.4). Of particular interest, the immunosuppressive (and tolerizing) effect of this drug appears long-lasting (months) for reasons that are still unclear. Sirolimus binds an immunophilin, FKB-12, but its mechanism of action is different from other immunophilin binders that block calcineurin activity, cyclosporine and tacrolimus.

CALCINEURIN INHIBITORS

The potent immunosuppressive activity of cyclosporine, first noted in the 1970s, revolutionized organ transplantation [19]. This cyclic undecapeptide from a soil fungus *Tolypocladium inflatum* was the prototype for drugs that are now known to target intracellular signaling pathways downstream of the IL-2 receptor (Fig. 8.4) [20]. Both cyclosporine and tacrolimus bind to immunophilins and "gain function" after binding, now able to interact with calcineurin, blocking its phosphatase activity. Calcineurin is required for movement of nuclear factor of activated T lymphocytes (NFAT) and other transcription factors into the nucleus from the T-cell cytoplasm. NFAT, in turn, is required for induction of IL-2 and other cytokine genes necessary for T-cell growth and differentiation. Remarkably, cyclosporine and tacrolimus are structurally unrelated and bind different immunophilins to accomplish this inhibition. Cyclosporine binds cyclophilins while tacrolimus (previously FK506) binds the FK506 binding protein (FKBP). The ultimate downstream effects are remarkably similar although toxicities differ somewhat between the two drugs (see Chapter 9). Although immunophilins are peptidyl-prolyl *cis-trans* isomerases involved in the folding of a variety of cytosolic proteins, this activity is not related to the antiproliferative and immunosuppressive activities of the two drugs.

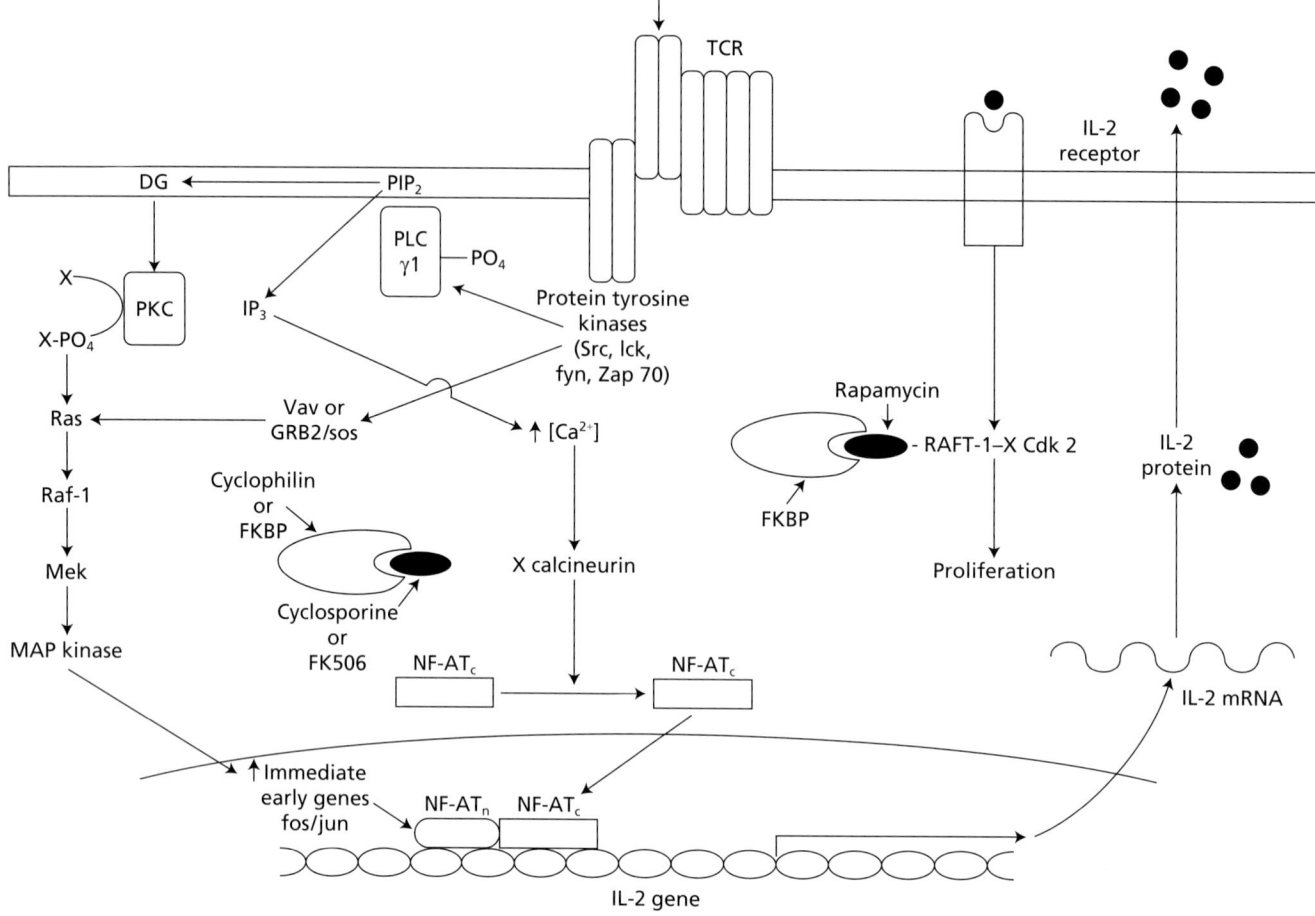

Fig. 8.4 Cytoplasmic and nuclear events in T-cell activation, with sites of action of cyclosporine, FK506 (tacrolimus) and rapamycin (sirolimus). Specific antigen triggers the T-cell receptor (TCR) complex, activating phospholipase C (PLC), tyrosine kinases, protein kinase C (PKC) and calcium ion flux [1]. These cell surface biochemical events trigger the pathways shown, resulting in transcription of activation-associated genes in the T-cell nucleus. Cyclosporine binds cyclophilin and FK506 binds FKBP to block calcineurin-mediated translocation of nuclear factor of activated T lymphocytes (NF-AT) to the nucleus. Rapamycin blocks interleukin 2 (IL-2) receptor-mediated T-cell proliferation downstream of cyclin-dependent kinase 2 (Cdk 2) by binding the target of rapamycin (TOR, referred to in the figure as RAFT-1, rapamycin and FKPB12 target 1). DG, diacylglycerol; IP_3, inositol 1,4,5-triphosphate; PIP_2, phosphatidylinositol 4,5-biphosphate. From Pattison JM, Sibley RK, Krensky AM. Mechanisms of allograft rejection. In: Neilson ED, Couser WG, eds. *Immunologic Renal Diseases*. Philadelphia: Lippincott-Raven, 1997; 331–54 with permission.

A second hypothesis explaining the mechanism of action of cyclosporine involves increased expression of transforming growth factor β (TGF-β) [21]. This multifunctional cytokine inhibits T-cell growth and differentiation *in vitro*. The mechanism of inhibition appears to involve other transcription factors binding to the IL-2 promoter, such as Oct-1, or perhaps inhbition of c-*myc* by the retinoblastoma (Rb) protein. TGF-β expression is also increased by glucocoticoids.

FTY720

FTY720 is the first of a new class of small molecules that function as sphingosine 1-phosphate receptor (S1P-R) agonists [22]. FTY720 is a synthetic structural analog of a naturally occurring protein from ascomycete *Isaria sinclarii*, a fungus that parasitizes insects and plants. FTY720 appears to work by an entirely novel mechanism; it inhibits T-cell immunity by affecting homing. FTY720 appears to sequester lymphocytes in lymph nodes and Peyer patches, keeping inflammatory cells out of the circulation and out of inflammatory "infiltrates." At the same time, it has no direct effects on either T- or B-cell functions, as measured by mixed lymphocyte response, IL-2 production, T-cell proliferation, cytotoxicity or antibody production *in vitro*.

BIOLOGICS

Biologics, antibodies or agents derived from antibodies, have shown increasing efficacy as immunotherapeutics by either

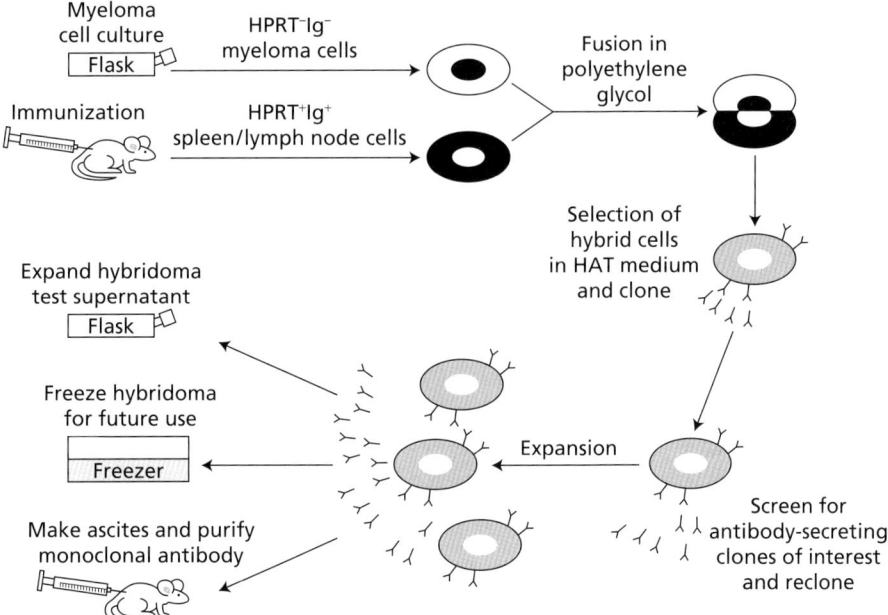

Fig. 8.5 Generation of monoclonal antibodies. Kohler and Milstein [25] received the Nobel Prize for generation of monoclonal antibodies. Briefly, mice are immunized and B cells from the spleen or lymph nodes are harvested and fused with a B-cell myeloma selected for the inability to grow in hypoxanthine, aminopterin, thymidine (HAT) containing medium. Only B-cell myeloma cells that fuse with normal mouse B cells can survive in HAT supplemented media. After the hybridoma lines are expanded in culture, cells secreting antibodies of interest are identified and cloned. Monoclonal antibodies can be used directly from the supernatants of cell line cultures or purified from supernatants or ascites fluid from mice injected intraperitoneally with the hybridoma. Ig, immunoglobulin. From Krensky AM. Transplantation immunobiology. In: Barratt TM, Avner ED, Harmon WE, eds. *Pediatric Nephrology*, 4th edn. Baltimore: Lippincott Williams & Wilkins, 1999; 1289–1307 with permission.

depleting the T-cell pool or as specific inhibitors of T-cell activation and/or differentiation. Polyclonal antibodies are generated by repeated injections of human thymocytes (antithymocyte globulin, ATG) or lymphocytes (antilymphocyte globulin, ALG) into animals, such as horses, rabbits, sheep or goats, followed by purification of the serum immunoglobulin fraction [23,24]. Although highly effective as immunosuppressives, these preparations vary in both efficacy and toxicity from batch to batch. The development of hybridoma technology by Kohler and Milstein [25] made possible the production of essentially unlimited amounts of a single antibody of defined specificity (Fig. 8.5). These monoclonal antibodies overcame issues of variability but are more limited in their target specificity and antiantibody responses. First generation murine antihuman antibodies have largely been replaced by chimeric or "humanized" monoclonal antibodies with much more limited antigenicity, improved half-lives and better efficacy. Both polyclonal and monoclonal antibodies have a place in modern immunosuppressive therapy.

Polyclonal antibodies

ATG and ALG contain cytotoxic antibodies against numerous T-cell surface antigens, including CD2, CD3, CD4, CD8, CD11a, CD18, CD25, CD44, CD45 and human leukocyte antigen (HLA) class I and II molecules [26]. The antibodies both deplete circulating lymphocytes by direct cytoxicity (complement and cell-mediated) and inhibit lymphocyte function by binding to cell surface molecules involved in adhesion, activation, proliferation and differentiation [27].

Monoclonal antibodies

The major monoclonal antibodies in clinical use are against OKT3 and IL-2 receptors but newer reagents aimed at other targets (Campath-1 and costimulatory molecules) are also under investigation (Fig. 8.6) [28].

OKT3

Monoclonal antibodies directed against a trimeric molecule associated with the T-cell receptor on the surface of human T lymphocytes have been effective immunosuppressives since first introduced in the 1980s [29–31]. The original agent, muromonab-CD3, or OKT3, was a mouse antihuman ε chain of CD3. The antibody binds to the ε chain of CD3, interrupting antigen recognition, T-cell signaling and proliferation. The T-cell receptor complex is internalized after binding antibody, preventing subsequent antigen recognition. In addition, T cells are depleted from the peripheral circulation by extravasation

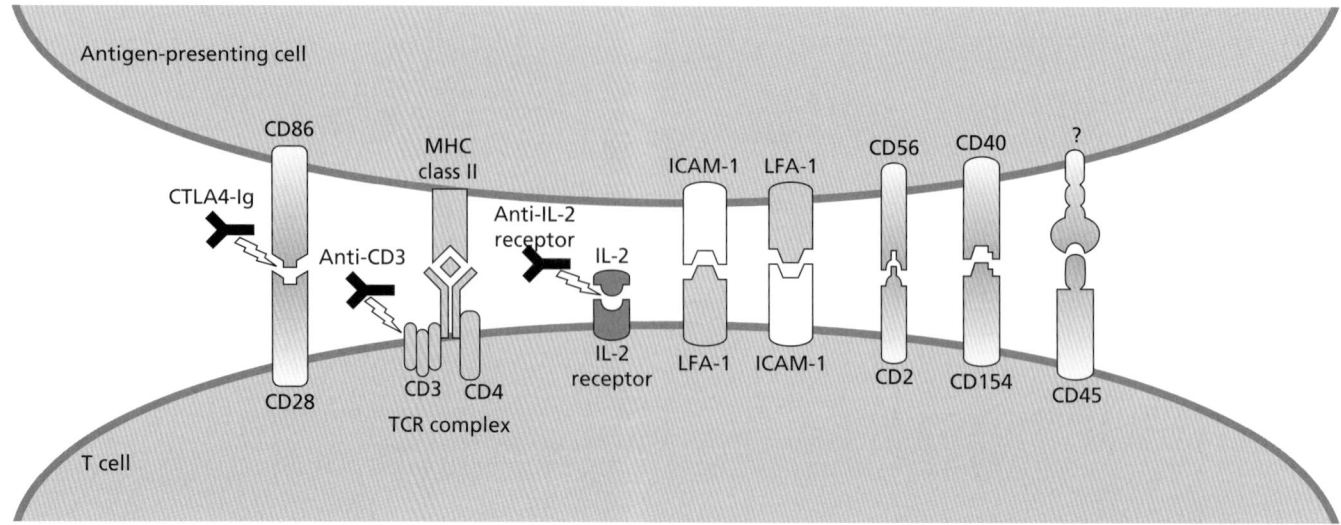

Fig. 8.6 Cell surface targets for biologic therapeutics. Selected cell surface molecules and their ligands on T lymphocytes and antigen-presenting cells are depicted in this figure. ICAM-1, intercellular adhesion molecule 1 (CD54); IL, interleukin; LFA-1, lymphocyte function-associated antigen 1 (CD11a, CD18); MHC, major histocompatibility complex; TCR, T-cell receptor.

from the bloodstream to peripheral lymphoid organs such as lymph nodes and spleen, and cell lysis by antibody and complement and/or activation induced cell death. T cells remaining in the periphery have reduced function as measured by production of cytokines, such as IL-2. Remarkably, IL-4 and IL-10 production is not reduced. Anti-OKT3 antibodies are routinely used in induction therapy and/or treatment of acute rejection. Most recently, genetically altered anti-CD3 antibodies have been developed to prevent the development of antiantibodies. These "humanized" reagents are not recognized by the human immune system, do not bind human Fc receptors and may have less "cytokine release" associated with use [32,33].

Anti-IL-2 receptor

Another important monoclonal antibody class is directed against the IL-2 receptor (IL-2R), blocking the effect of this important T-cell growth factor and targeting activated T lymphocytes [34,35]. Daclizumab is a genetically engineered, humanized IgG1 monoclonal antibody that specifically binds to the α chain of the IL-2R [36]. Basiliximab is a human–mouse chimeric IgG1 monoclonal antibody obtained from human heavy and light chain constant regions and mouse heavy and light chain variable regions [37]. Daclizumab has a somewhat lower affinity for the IL-2R than does basiliximab but a longer half-life. Although the exact mechanism of anti-IL-2R monoclonal antibody therapy is incompletely understood, there is significant depletion of T lymphocytes, especially activated T lymphocytes, from peripheral blood. In addition, circulating T lymphocytes show decreased IL-2R chain expression, indicating poor responsiveness to this important growth and differentiation factor. These reagents are recommended for prophylaxis against acute rejection and are commonly used in induction therapy.

Campath-1

Campath-1H is a humanized monoclonal antibody against CD52, a glycoprotein expressed on lymphocytes, monocytes, macrophages and natural killer cells [38,39]. This monoclonal antibody causes extensive depletion of peripheral blood cells. The resultant prolonged B- and T-cell depletion allows minimization of other drug use. Clinical investigation of this reagent is in progress.

Antilymphocyte function-associated antigen 1

Efalizumab is a humanized IgG1 monoclonal antibody directed against the CD11a chain of lymphocyte function-associated antigen 1 (LFA-1) [40,41]. Binding of this antibody to the LFA-1 molecule blocks its interaction with its ligand, intercellular adhesion molecule 1 (ICAM-1), inhibiting T-cell adhesion, activation and trafficking. This agent has been approved for use in psoriasis but its utility in transplantation is still under investigation.

Costimulatory blockade

T-cell activation requires two signals: one signal is via the antigen-specific T-cell receptor and the other is an antigen-nonspecific "costimulatory" signal provided by the interaction of molecules such as CD28 on the T cell and CD80 and/or CD86 on the antigen-presenting cell (APC) [42]. Monoclonal antibodies recognizing CD80 or CD86 block the mixed lymphocyte response and have been shown to block a variety of animal models of transplantation and autoimmunity. Recently humanized antibodies h1F1 and h3D1 need to be used in tandem because either CD80 or CD86 alone are sufficient to stimulate T cells via CD28 [29]. These reagents are currently under clinical evaluation after some success in nonhuman primate renal transplantation.

CTLA4-Ig is a novel reagent that competitively inhibits CD28 signaling [43]. CTLA4 is a CD28 homolog with stronger affinity than CD28 for its ligands. CTLA4-Ig consists of the ligand-binding region of CTLA4 engineered to the constant region of human IgG1. Many animal studies confirmed the utility of this reagent in organ transplantation and autoimmunity. A new reagent, LEA29Y, is a second generation reagent with two amino acid changes that increase affinity to both CD80 and CD86, with a reported 10-fold increase in potency. This reagent is also currently undergoing clinical evaluation.

A second costimulatory pathway involves the interaction of CD40 on activated T lymphocytes with CD40 ligand (CD154) on APCs, B lymphocytes and/or vascular endothelium [43]. Two humanized anti-CD154 monoclonal antibodies have been evaluated in clinical trials but have been on hold because of thromboembolic events. It is also theoretically possible to target this costimulatory pathway with anti-CD40 antibodies. Among the actions of anti-CD154 antibody treatment is blockade of CD80 and CD86 expression after immune activation.

CONCLUSIONS

A great deal of progress has been made in understanding the molecular mechanisms underlying the effects of immunosuppressives in clinical use. In addition, an understanding of the immune response to alloantigens and transplants has allowed the rational design of new drugs, largely biologics, some of which have proven useful clinically (anti-CD3 and anti-IL-2R) while others are under evaluation (e.g. CTLA4-Ig, Campath-1). Information gleaned about the molecular mechanisms have clarified that the major side-effects of the currently used drugs seem inexorably related to their mechanism of action. Therefore, sparing protocols, trying to eliminate the use of glucocorticoids or calcineurin inhibitors, have become popular approaches to reducing toxicity while maintaining immunosuppressive efficacy [44,45].

REFERENCES

1 Krensky AM, Weiss A, Crabtree G, Davis MM, Parham P. T-lymphocyte-antigen interactions in transplant rejection. *N Engl J Med* 1990;**322**:510–7.

2 Braun WE. Renal transplantation: basic concepts and evolution of therapy. *J Clin Apheresis* 2003;**18**:141–52.

3 Murray JE, Merrill JP, Harrison JH, Wilson RE, Dammin GJ. Prolonged survival of human-kidney homografts by immunosuppressive drug therapy. *N Engl J Med* 1963;**268**:1315–23.

4 Hricik DE, O'Toole MA, Schulak JA, Herson J. Steroid-free immunosuppression in cyclosporine-treated renal transplant recipients: a meta-analysis. *J Am Soc Nephrol* 1993;**4**:1300–5.

5 Ahsan N, Hricik D, Matas A, *et al.* Prednisone withdrawal in kidney transplant recipients on cyclosporine and mycophenolate mofetil: a prospective randomized study. Steroid Withdrawal Study Group. *Transplantation* 1999;**68**:1865–74.

6 Buckbinder L, Robinson RP. The glucocorticoid receptor: molecular mechanism and new therapeutic opportunities. *Curr Drug Targets Inflamm Allergy* 2002;**1**:127–36.

7 Pan J, Ju D, Wang Q, *et al.* Dexamethasone inhibits the antigen presentation of dendritic cells in MHC class II pathway. *Immunol Lett* 2001;**76**:153–61.

8 Kovalovsky D, Refojo D, Holsboer F, Arzt E. Molecular mechanisms and Th1/Th2 pathways in corticosteroid regulation of cytokine production. *J Neuroimmunol* 2000;**109**:23–9.

9 Elenkov IJ. Glucocorticoids and the Th1/Th2 balance. *Ann N Y Acad Sci* 2004;**1024**:138–46.

10 Abe M, Thomson AW. Influence of immunosuppressive drugs on dendritic cells. *Transpl Immunol* 2003;**11**:357–65.

11 Almawi WY, Melemedjian OK, Rieder MJ. An alternate mechanism of glucocorticoid anti-proliferative effect: promotion of a Th2 cytokine-secreting profile. *Clin Transplant* 1999;**13**:365–74.

12 Elenkov IJ, Chrousos GP. Stress hormones, Th1/Th2 patterns, pro/anti-inflammatory cytokines and susceptibility to disease. *Trends Endocrinol Metab* 1999;**10**:359–68.

13 Franchimont D. Overview of the actions of glucocorticoids on the immune response: a good model to characterize new pathways of immunosuppression for new treatment strategies. *Ann N Y Acad Sci* 2004;**1024**:124–37.

14 Elion GB. The George Hitchings and Gertrude Elion Lecture. The pharmacology of azathioprine. *Ann N Y Acad Sci* 1993;**685**:400–7.

15 Sollinger HW. Mycophenolate mofetil. *Kidney Int Suppl* 1995;**52**:S14–7.

16 Sollinger HW. Mycophenolates in transplantation. *Clin Transplant* 2004;**18**:485–92.

17 Sehgal SN. Sirolimus: its discovery, biological properties, and mechanism of action. *Transplant Proc* 2003;**35**(Suppl):7S–14S.

18 Ettenger RB, Grimm EM. Safety and efficacy of TOR inhibitors in pediatric renal transplant recipients. *Am J Kidney Dis* 2001;**38**(Suppl 2):S22–8.

19 Kahan BD. Cyclosporine. *N Engl J Med* 1989;**321**:1725–38.

20 Brown EJ, Schreiber SL. A signaling pathway to translational control. *Cell* 1996;**86**:517–20.

21 Khanna A, Li B, Stenzel KH, Suthanthiran M. Regulation of new DNA synthesis in mammalian cells by cyclosporine. Demonstration of a transforming growth factor beta-dependent mechanism of inhibition of cell growth. *Transplantation* 1994;**57**:577–82.

22 Gabardi S, Cerio J. Future immunosuppressive agents in solid-organ transplantation. *Prog Transplant* 2004;**14**:148–56.

23 Shield CF, Edwards EB, Davies DB, Daily OP. Antilymphocyte induction therapy in cadaver renal transplantation: a retrospective, multicenter United Network for Organ Sharing Study. *Transplantation* 1997;**63**:1257–63.

24 Wechter WJ, Brodie JA, Morrell RM, Rafi M, Schultz JR. Antithymocyte globulin (ATGAM) in renal allograft recipients: multicenter trials using a 14-dose regimen. *Transplantation* 1979;**28**:294–302.

25 Kohler G, Milstein C. Continuous cultures of fused cells secreting antibody of predefined specificity. *Nature* 1975;**256**:495–7.

26 Bonnefoy-Berard N, Vincent C, Revillard JP. Antibodies against functional leukocyte surface molecules in polyclonal anti-lymphocyte and antithymocyte globulins. *Transplantation* 1991;**51**:669–73.

27 Hardinger KL, Schnitzler MA, Miller B, *et al*. Five-year follow up of thymoglobulin versus ATGAM induction in adult renal transplantation. *Transplantation* 2004;**78**:136–41.

28 Dhanireddy KK, Xu H, Mannon RB, Hale DA, Kirk AD. The clinical application of monoclonal antibody therapies in renal transplantation. *Expert Opin Emerg Drugs* 2004;**9**:23–37.

29 Kung P, Goldstein G, Reinherz EL, Schlossman SF. Monoclonal antibodies defining distinctive human T cell surface antigens. *Science* 1979;**206**:347–9.

30 Cosimi AB, Colvin RB, Burton RC, *et al*. Use of monoclonal antibodies to T-cell subsets for immunologic monitoring and treatment in recipients of renal allografts. *N Engl J Med* 1981;**305**:308–14.

31 Ortho Multicenter Transplant Study Group. A randomized clinical trial of OKT3 monoclonal antibody for acute rejection of cadaveric renal transplants. *N Engl J Med* 1985;**313**:337–42.

32 Gaston RS, Deierhoi MH, Patterson T, *et al*. OKT3 first-dose reaction: association with T cell subsets and cytokine release. *Kidney Int* 1991;**39**:141–8.

33 Schroeder TJ, First MR, Mansour ME, *et al*. Antimurine antibody formation following OKT3 therapy. *Transplantation* 1990;**49**:48–51.

34 Taniguchi T, Minami Y. The IL-2/IL-2 receptor system: a current overview. *Cell* 1993;**73**:5–8.

35 Soulillou JP, Cantarovich D, Le Mauff B, *et al*. Randomized controlled trial of a monoclonal antibody against the interleukin-2 receptor (33B3.1) as compared with rabbit antithymocyte globulin for prophylaxis against rejection of renal allografts. *N Engl J Med* 1990;**322**:1175–82.

36 Vincenti F, Kirkman R, Light S, *et al*. Interleukin-2-receptor blockade with daclizumab to prevent acute rejection in renal transplantation. Daclizumab Triple Therapy Study Group. *N Engl J Med* 1998;**338**:161–5.

37 Nashan B, Moore R, Amlot P, Schmidt AG, Abeywickrama K, Soulillou JP. Randomised trial of basiliximab versus placebo for control of acute cellular rejection in renal allograft recipients. CHIB 201 International Study Group. *Lancet* 1997;**350**:1193–8.

38 Kirk AD, Hale DA, Mannon RB, *et al*. Results from a human renal allograft tolerance trial evaluating the humanized CD52-specific monoclonal antibody alemtuzumab (Campath-1H). *Transplantation* 2003;**76**:120–9.

39 Knechtle SJ, Fernandez LA, Pirsch JD, *et al*. Campath-1H in renal transplantation: the University of Wisconsin experience. *Surgery* 2004;**136**:754–60.

40 Hourmant M, Le Mauff B, Le Meur Y, *et al*. Administration of an anti-CD11a monoclonal antibody in recipients of kidney transplantation: a pilot study. *Transplantation* 1994;**58**:377–80.

41 Le Mauff B, Hourmant M, Le Meur Y, *et al*. Anti-LFA-1 adhesion molecule monoclonal antibody in prophylaxis of human kidney allograft rejection. *Transplant Proc* 1995;**27**:865–6.

42 Rothstein DM, Sayegh MH. T-cell costimulatory pathways in allograft rejection and tolerance. *Immunol Rev* 2003;**196**:85–108.

43 Kirk AD, Harlan DM, Armstrong NN, *et al*. CTLA4-Ig and anti-CD40 ligand prevent renal allograft rejection in primates. *Proc Natl Acad Sci USA* 1997;**94**:8789–94.

44 Vincenti F. A decade of progress in kidney transplantation. *Transplantation* 2004;**77**(Suppl):S52–61.

45 Vincenti F. Immunosuppression minimization: current and future trends in transplant immunosuppression. *J Am Soc Nephrol* 2003;**14**:1940–8.

Induction and Maintenance Immunosuppression

William E. Harmon

SPECIAL ISSUES ABOUT PEDIATRICS

Children develop end-stage organ failure at a much lower frequency than adults and the diseases that result in organ failure are substantially different [1]. Children have unique medical and surgical requirements both before and following transplantation and they suffer some complications, such as post-transplant lymphoproliferative disorder (PTLD) at substantially different rates to adults [2]. Importantly, infants and young children cannot swallow pills and they metabolize medications at substantially different rates from adults; thus, they frequently require special formulations and schedules [3–6]. If these issues are addressed directly and carefully, the outcome of organ transplantation in children can be the same or even better than that seen in adults [1].

PROTOCOLS FOR SPECIFIC ORGAN SYSTEMS

Chronic dialysis and kidney transplantation are both excellent treatments for end-stage renal disease (ESRD). Kidney transplantation was recognized as the better form of treatment for children with ESRD two decades ago [7]. Both peritoneal dialysis, delivered as continued ambulatory peritoneal dialysis (CAPD) or continuous cycling peritoneal dialysis (CCPD), and hemodialysis lead to a deceleration of growth. Data from the dialysis component of the North American Pediatric Renal Transplant Cooperative Study (NAPRTCS) registry [8] show that the overall height deficit of −1.8 standard deviations (SD) became more negative, reaching a value of −2.16 SD at 24 months after initiation of dialysis. Additionally, children do not tolerate being "dependent" on the any modality and maintenance dialysis induces loss of self-esteem and emotional maladjustment [9]. Cognitive achievement testing may diminish with prolonged time on dialysis [10]. In contrast, the mobility and freedom from dietary restrictions afforded by a functioning renal transplant enable children to live nearly normal lives. Although renal transplantation has not lived up to the promise of normal growth for all children, dramatic short-term improvements in height can be seen in many, and final adult height is improving after transplantation [11–14]. Most importantly, successful transplantation permits the child to attend school and to develop normally. School function testing improves dramatically following transplantation [15,16]. Importantly, young children now have the best long-term outcomes of all ages of transplant recipients, verifying the utility of transplantation in this age group [17]. For all of these reasons, successful renal transplantation remains the primary goal of programs that care for children with ESRD. In general, the majority of children who receive kidney transplants are treated with antibody induction and chronic triple immunosuppression, typically corticosteroids, mycophenolate mofetil (MMF) and a calcineurin inhibitor [18].

The consequences of end-stage heart, lung, liver and intestine failure in children are even more serious than ESRD because of the lack of long-term artificial organ support. Thus, heart, lung, liver and intestine transplants are considered to be more acutely "life-saving." The results of pediatric transplants in these areas have improved recently and generally they are equivalent or better than the results in adults [1]. There is less registry information about these other organ systems, although steroid withdrawal is more common in heart and liver transplant recipients than in kidney recipients and antibody induction treatment and use of sirolimus is currently less frequent.

INDUCTION IMMUNOSUPPRESSION

Retrospective data from the NAPRTCS registry had consistently shown a beneficial effect of prophylactic anti-T-cell antibody in pediatric renal transplant graft survival. In a review of living donor (LD) transplants, 5-year graft survival was 81% in 1041 patients who received T-cell antibody therapy compared with 75% in 1399 patients who did not. Similar figures for deceased donor (DD) kidneys were 66% in 1423 T-cell antibody treated patients, compared with 56% in 1034 patients who did not receive T-cell antibody [19]. Major problems of these analyses include the fact that all of the analyses were retrospective and could be subject to confounding variables such as center effect and that several different types of T-cell antibody were used. In the early years, a polyclonal antibody was used, the most common of which was prepared from horse serum and designated as MALG (Minnesota antilymphocyte globulin) [20]. A monoclonal antibody called OKT3, which was derived from mouse mammary cells and which was directed at subsets of T cells, was subsequently employed [21]. More recently, standardized polyclonal antibodies, Atgam (Abbott) [22] and Thymoglobulin (Genzyme) [23,24] have been used most commonly. Currently, the majority of pediatric kidney transplant recipients are treated with some form of induction antibody [18], but there have been no controlled trials that have verified the benefits of this. In fact, a large controlled trial of OKT3 induction versus induction with intravenous cyclosporine in pediatric kidney transplantation showed no benefit to antibody induction [25].

Polyclonal lymphocyte depleting antibodies

Two polyclonal antibodies currently available are Atgam (Upjohn) and Thymoglobulin (Genzyme). Atgam, because of the sclerosing nature of the preparation, is given intravenously through a central catheter for 10–15 days. The dose used is 15 mg/kg, and calcineurin inhibitors are generally withheld during the administration of the antibody. Thymoglobulin is provided through a peripheral vein at a dose of 1.5–2 mg/kg. A recent report suggests daily monitoring of CD3$^+$ subsets to guide therapy: the daily dose is given only when the CD3$^+$ count exceeds 20 cells/mm^3 [24]. Thymoglobulin has been studied in small groups of pediatric renal transplant recipients and was found to be effective [23]. Comparison of efficacy of removal of circulating T cells suggested that Thymoglobulin may have some benefit over Atgam [22], but no direct controlled comparisons of clinical outcomes have been performed. In a historical comparison of Atgam and Thymoglobulin in pediatric kidney transplant recipients at a single center, the incidence of acute rejection was noted to be lower in the Thymoglobulin-treated recipients [26], but this result may also be because it was provided to the more recent cohort and the outcomes of kidney transplantation have generally improved with time [18].

Monoclonal lymphocyte depleting antibodies

OKT3

The monoclonal antibody, OKT3, is administered as a bolus injection into a peripheral vein daily for 10–14 days at a dose of 5 mg for older children and 2.5 mg for children weighing less than 30 kg. Calcineurin inhibitors are also withheld during the use of OKT3. The major problems with these induction therapies include the "first-dose reaction" [27,28], neurologic problems [29] and the potential for the development of superimposed infections, such as cytome-galovirus (CMV) or Epstein–Barr virus (EBV) disease. Although retrospective analysis of pediatric kidney transplantation continued to show a clear benefit for the use of prophylactic induction antibody [30], a recent prospective randomized trial of OKT3 induction showed no clear advantage [25]. Currently, very few pediatric transplant recipients receive OKT3 as induction therapy [30].

Campath

There have been multiple uncontrolled pilot trials of Campath (alemtuzumab, Berlex) in adult renal transplant recipients. In 1999, Calne et al. [31,32] reported the use of two doses of Campath combined with low-dose cyclosporine monotherapy in 31 consecutive renal transplant recipients. Cyclosporine was begun 48 hours post-transplantation and doses were adjusted to maintain levels of 75–125 ng/mL. Of the 31 patients, one died of heart failure with a functioning graft and one had recurrent immunoglobulin A (IgA) nephropathy. Twenty-nine grafts were functioning at the time of the report and six of these had rejection episodes (19%). All rejections responded to intravenous steroids and three of the patients had prednisone and azathioprine added; the rest remained on cyclosporine monotherapy. One patient had systemic CMV infection and one had reactivation of abdominal tuberculosis. In 2003, Knechtle et al. [33] reported on 29 primary renal transplant recipients who received Campath induction therapy (23 LD, 6 DD). Sirolimus was started on day 1 and adjusted to a level of 8–12 ng/mL. All patients were alive at the time of the report and 28 had functioning grafts. One patient lost the graft as a result of rejection at 2 months post-transplantation. There were no systemic infections and no malignancies. However, eight patients had rejection episodes (28%). Five of the rejections were noted to be acute humoral rejections with positive CD4 staining and these were noted to be prevalent in younger adult recipients. Biopsies of long-term survivors showed no evidence of chronic allograft nephropathy. Twenty-two patients remained on sirolimus monotherapy. In 2003, Kirk et al. [34] reported on seven living donor kidney recipients who received perioperative Campath and no subsequent immunosuppression. All seven patients had acute rejection episodes between days 14 and 28. All seven patients were successfully treated and eventually weaned to sirolimus monotherapy, but one had oral prednisone reinstituted for recurrent focal segmental glomerulosclerosis (FSGS). There were no serious infections in the patients and all seven had normal renal function at the time of the report.

There have been other uncontrolled studies of Campath in kidney and pancreas transplantation in adults and, in general, it has been tolerated without an increase in serious infections. In one small series of three high-risk pediatric kidney transplant recipients, Campath was well tolerated, but some of the children had acute rejections episodes. Campath induction has been used more extensively in pediatric small bowel transplantation. In a review of intestinal transplantation at the University of Miami, Nishida *et al.* [35] reviewed 54 children receiving grafts between 1994 and 2000. Although there were multiple protocols and this was not a clinical trial, they concluded that the introduction of Campath was associated with improved patient and graft survival and was not associated with an increased rate of opportunistic infections.

Monoclonal nondepleting antibodies

IL2-r antibodies

There are two two high-affinity chimeric or humanized antibodies that act on the inducible α chain of the interleukin-2 receptor (IL-2r) on the surface of the activated lymphocyte: basilizimab (Simulect, Novartis) and daclizumab (Zenapax, Roche). Basiliximab is generally given as two-dose regimen (generally 10 mg for children less than 40 kg and 20 mg for those more than 40 kg) on days 0 and 4 post-transplantation [36]. A pharmacologic study showed that basiliximab clearance in children and adults is reduced by approximately half compared with adults and was independent of age, weight or body surface area [37]. One study has noted that pediatric recipients receiving basiliximab may have significantly elevated levels of cyclosporine and may require reduced doses to avoid toxicity [38]. Daclizumab is generally given in a regimen of 1 mg/kg intravenously on the day of transplantation and every 14 days thereafter for a total of five doses [39]. Higher doses may be required for saturation of IL-2r in younger children [11]. Both antibodies are generally well tolerated without substantial side-effects. Both antibodies have been studied extensively in children and have been shown to be safe and effective [11,36,38,40–42]. The precise mechanism of the antibodies is not known, but is presumed to be saturation of the IL-2r and subsequent competitive antagonism of IL-2-dependent proliferation. A novel 6-month regimen of daclizumab has been reported as part of a steroid-avoidance pilot study and appears to be well tolerated [11]. There are no comparative studies between the two antibodies. Up to 65% of pediatric renal transplant recipients are now receiving an IL-2r antibody as induction therapy [30].

Costimulation blockade

Antigen recognition alone is not sufficient for full T-cell activation. T cells require two distinct signals for full activation [43]. The first signal is provided by the engagement of the T-cell receptor (TCR) with the major histocompatibility complex (MHC) plus peptide complex on antigen-presenting cells (APCs) called allorecognition, in the case of transplantation; and the second "costimulatory" signal is provided by engagement of one or more T-cell surface receptors with their specific ligands on APCs [44–46]. Signaling through the TCR alone

without a costimulatory signal can lead to a prolonged state of T-cell anergy [47]. The best-characterized and perhaps most important costimulatory signal is that provided by interaction of CD28 on T cells with either B7-1 or B7-2 on APCs [43]. The CD28/CTLA4-B7-1/B7-2 T-cell costimulatory pathway is a unique and complex pathway that regulates T-cell activation [43,48]. After activation, T cells express another CD28 family member, CTLA-4 (CD152), which has a higher affinity for B7-1 and B7-2 and functions to provide a "negative" signal resulting in physiologic termination of T-cell responses [49–51]. Furthermore, recent evidence suggests that CTLA-4 negative signaling pathway may be required for induction of acquired tolerance *in vivo* [52,53]. Indeed, it has been hypothesized that CTLA-4 may function as a "master switch" for peripheral T-cell tolerance [45].

Ligation of CD28 by B7-1 or B7-2 is blocked by CTLA4-Ig, a recombinant fusion protein that contains the extracellular domain of CTLA-4 fused to an IgG heavy chain tail. The administration of CD28-B7 blockade prevents acute allograft rejection and induces donor-specific tolerance in several animal models [54–58]. In addition, CD28-B7 blockade prevents development [59–61] and interrupts progression [62,63] of chronic allograft rejection in transplant models.

CTLA4-Ig is currently undergoing human phase I–II testing in autoimmune diseases. A phase I trial with CTLA4-Ig in patients with psoriasis vulgaris has been recently reported [64–66]. Other trials in rheumatoid arthritis and multiple sclerosis are underway. A slightly modified version of CTLA4-Ig is known as LEA29Y or belatacept. Recently, a new trial of belatacept, designed to spare calcineurin inhibitors in adult kidney transplant recipients, was performed with encouraging preliminary results [67]. In this study, 218 patients were randomized into three groups: one group received intensive belatacept, another received less intensive belatacept and the control group received cyclosporine as primary immunosuppression. Belatacept is typically administered intravenously on a once-per-month schedule. All three groups received induction therapy with basiliximab, MMF and corticosteroids. At 6 months, the incidence of rejection was 6–8% in all groups. At 12 months glomerular filtration rate (GFR) was significantly higher (62–66 mL/min/1.73 m^2) and the incidence of chronic allograft nephropathy was significantly lower (20–29%) in the belatacept groups than in the cyclosporine group (53 mL/min/1.73 m^2 and 44%, respectively). Of concern, however, was the occurrence of three episodes of PTLD in the belatacept group [68], two of which were related to primary EBV infection. The authors noted that two of the episodes occurred after the subjects had been changed from belatacept to other immunosuppressive agents. Nonetheless, the concern about its use in children who are at higher risk of PTLD should be balanced against its potential benefit of improving adherence. Because belatacept is provided intravenously on an infrequent schedule, the usual adherence issues entailed with repetitive oral administration of immunosuppressive medications should be avoided. Additional studies of belatacept with less concomitant nonspecific immunosuppression are ongoing [68].

MAINTENANCE IMMUNOSUPPRESSION

Prednisone

The NAPRTCS reports show that until recently, up to 96% of children with a functioning kidney graft were maintained on prednisone [18,19]. Chronic treatment with corticosteroids is less common in pediatric liver and heart transplantation, but probably as frequent in pediatric lung transplantation. The numerous mechanisms of action of steroids lead to side-effects and toxicities. The important concern in children is growth retardation. Studies have shown that doses in excess of 8.5 mg/day will impair normal growth [69]. Other side-effects include increased susceptibility to infection, impaired wound healing, aseptic necrosis of the bone, cataracts, glucose intolerance, hypertension, cushingoid facies and acne [70]. The preparations commonly used are prednisolone, its 11-keto metabolite, prednisone, and methylprednisone. Although the half-lives of these preparations are very short, they can be administered once daily because their effect on inhibition of lymphocyte production persists for 24 hours [71]. The dosage is usually high in the immediate post-transplant period, approximately 2 mg/kg/day, with a gradual reduction to approximately 0.2–0.3 mg/kg/day within a 6-month to 1-year period. Because of the multiple side-effects of maintenance steroid therapy, attempts have been made to withdraw steroids altogether, reported both in adult and pediatric kidney transplantation [72]. Unfortunately, the majority of these attempts have failed because of the development of acute rejection episodes [73–75]. The use of alternate-day steroid therapy, which appears to reduce the growth inhibiting effect without unduly increasing rejection episodes [76,77], seems reasonable, but only a minority of pediatric renal transplant recipients is receiving steroids in that manner [30]. Recently, an uncontrolled pilot trial of prolonged IL-2r antibody administration to permit steroid avoidance has shown very promising results, with low acute rejection rates and striking reduction in post-transplant complications [78]. This steroid-avoidance protocol is currently undergoing a controlled trial against conventional immunosuppression, under the auspices of the Cooperative Clinical Trials in Pediatric Transplantation (CCTPT) program of the National Institute of Allergy and Infectious Disease (NIAID), in order to define the risks and benefits of this approach. Also, a previous CCTPT multicenter double-blind randomized controlled trial of corticosteroid withdrawal in pediatric kidney transplantation enrolled 274 subjects before it was halted [79]. Unfortunately, although the acute rejection rate during the first 6 months was very low, the incidence of PTLD in this trial was unacceptably high.

Nonetheless, those children who had corticosteroids successfully withdrawn had no higher rates of late rejection and equivalent long-term graft survival compared with the control group who were receiving chronic low-dose corticosteroids. Taken together, it seems reasonable to propose that, with modern immunosuppression techniques, pediatric renal transplant recipients will likely not require chronic corticosteroid treatment in the future. The majority of pediatric liver and heart transplant recipients are successfully withdrawn from corticosteroids. Reasons for different requirements for immunosuppression for different types of pediatric organ transplant recipients are not known.

Antiproliferative agents

Azathioprine

Azathioprine was the first immunosuppressive agent approved for organ transplantation use. For several decades virtually all organ transplant recipients received azathioprine, but other agents have supplanted its use during the past decade [18]. For pediatric patients, azathioprine is given in the dosage of 1–2 mg/kg/day. Higher doses should be closely monitored for myelosuppression. In 1989 and 1990, 80% of pediatric patients in the NAPRTCS registry were receiving azathioprine, but as more familiarity is established with MMF the use of azathioprine has diminished substantially and is currently in less that 10% of pediatric kidney transplant patients in the USA [30]. One serious side-effect of chronic azathioprine use is the occurrence of skin cancers [80]. Azathioprine has been used in combination with all other immunosuppressants except MMF.

Mycophenolate mofetil

As of 1996, the NAPRTCS registry noted that only 6.5% of patients were being maintained on MMF [19] but the most recent figures show that it is used in about two-thirds of pediatric kidney transplant recipients [30]. There are mixed results concerning its advantages over azathioprine [81–84]. A well-controlled study, however, concluded that it was safe and effective for use in pediatric renal transplantation [85]. A major difficulty in widespread use of the drug in children has been the gastrointestinal disturbance, especially in young children [3]. Both nausea and vomiting are common, but in some patients the drug has to be withdrawn because of intolerable diarrhea. An advantage over azathioprine is that the drug is less likely to induce leukopenia. Current recommended dosage of MMF for pediatric patients is 1200 mg/m^2/day, divided into two, three or four doses [86]. It is possible that therapeutic monitoring should be employed, but clear standards are not yet available to guide treatment [87–92]. MMF has been used in combination with all other immunosuppressants except azathioprine.

Calcineurin inhibitors

Cyclosporine

Cyclosporine was first used in renal transplantation by Calne et al. [93] in 1978. The initial experience was followed by controlled trials in the USA, Canada and Europe, all of which showed a significant improvement in graft survival over existing therapies. The drug was licensed in the USA in 1983, and has been used in all types of solid organ transplantation for over 20 years. There have been no controlled trials in children, but over the years of use a large body of information regarding its dosing and side-effects has accumulated [30].

For induction purposes cyclosporine is given intravenously in a dosage of 165 mg/m^2/day for children under 6 years of age, and 4.5 mg/kg/day in children over 6 years. The dosage for younger children is calculated in square meter format because they metabolize the drug differently. The drug is preferably given in a continuous infusion over a 24-hour period starting intraoperatively. If practicality precludes a continuous infusion, the drug should be administered in three divided doses daily but over as long an interval as possible. If possible, induction therapy using cyclosporine should be continued only for 48 hours and then converted to oral cyclosporine. The recommended starting oral dosage for children under the age of 6 years is 500 mg/m^2/day, administered in three divided doses; for children over the age of 6 years it is 15 mg/kg/day, administered in two divided doses. These doses are higher than those prescribed for adults as experience over the last 10 years has determined that the drug is metabolized more rapidly in children [5]. A calcium-channel blocker is typically given with cyclosporine to reduce nephrotoxicity [94].

Because of its irregular absorption and inherent nephrotoxicity, dosage adjustments of cyclosporine are constantly necessary [95]. Data from the NAPRTCS shows that at 1 year post-transplant the mean cyclosporine dose can vary from 5.6 to 8 mg/kg [19]. It has also been demonstrated that higher maintenance doses are associated with diminished chronic graft rejection [5]. Among cadaver kidney recipients, the rate of rejection was 16% in those receiving doses higher than 8 mg/kg at 1 year post-transplant, compared with 24% in those receiving less than 6 mg/kg/day [96]. The difficulty of maintaining constant dosing has led to several methods of measuring cyclosporine blood levels [97]. Either high-pressure liquid chromatography (HPLC) or fluorescence polarization immunoassay (FPIA) techniques are used. Drug adequacy is considered to be in the range of 100–200 ng/mL HPLC whole blood trough level, or 200–450 ng/mL TDX whole blood levels for patients more than 3 months post-transplant. Higher levels are necessary in the first 3 months. More recent data suggest that measuring the level 2 hours after receiving the dose may lead to more accurate dosing, assess the true area under the curve and avoid toxicity [98–100].

Treatment with cyclosporine is associated with nephrotoxicity, hypertension and hepatotoxicity. A major concern in children is hypertrichosis and facial dysmorphism [101]. Hyperkalemia is common in patients on cyclosporine [102], and also responds to dose reduction. The mechanism is possibly caused by diminished tubular excretion. Renal handling of uric acid is also altered, leading to hyperuricemia [103]. Hypomagnesemia is also observed as a result of altered tubular function [104]. Tremor, convulsion and parasthesia have been recorded in patients on cyclosporine [105]. These side-effects may be multidrug-induced rather than from cyclosporine alone; however, they are often seen with high blood levels. Both hypertension and hyperlipidemia are observed in patients on cyclosporine. A worrisome side-effect in children is gingival hypertrophy [106], seen more often with higher doses and in the presence of poor dental hygiene [107]. The most recent data from the NAPRTCS registry shows that less than 50% of renal transplant recipients are currently receiving cyclosporine as initial immunosuppression [30]. Cyclosporine has been used in combination with all other immunosuppressants except tacrolimus. However, because of the potential increased risk of PTLD, the use of a combination of a calcineurin inhibitor, rapamycin and corticosteroids should probably be avoided, especially in high-risk children [108].

Tacrolimus

Tacrolimus (Prograf, Astellas) was introduced as an immunosuppressant for kidney transplantation in the mid-1990s [109–111]. Recent data from the NAPRTCS show that more than 50% of children are being maintained on tacrolimus at 31 days post-transplantation [30]. The overwhelming majority of pediatric liver and intestine recipients are maintained on tacrolimus.

One method of initiatiation of tacrolimus is to provide 0.1 mg/kg/24 hours as a continuous infusion, with a switch to oral therapy within 2–3 days. However, because of the good absorption of the oral preparation and the concern about nephrotoxicity, many programs begin treatment via oral or nasogastric tube very early post-transplant rather than providing it intravenously. Initial oral doses should not exceed 0.15 mg/kg twice daily and should be reduced to 0.1 mg/kg as maintenance dose. Blood monitoring is necessary as with cyclosporine, and target whole blood trough levels, measured by an enzyme-linked immunosorbent assay (ELISA), should be maintained at 5–20 ng/L. Blood levels can also be measured by HPLC and the resulting levels are approximately 10% lower than with the more commonly used ELISA methods. Because of the concern of dose-related complications, especially the incidence of PTLD, tacrolimus levels are more commonly maintained at the lower level of recommendations, with some recipients even lower after the first post-transplant year. Diarrhea, which is common particularly in infants, may lead to increased tacrolimus levels [112].

Because of the similar mechanism of action, virtually all of the side-effects of cyclosporine therapy are also seen with tacrolimus [110]. The nephrotoxic effect is similar [113]. The hypertrichosis and the dysmorphic features noted with cyclosporine, however, are not seen with tacrolimus [114]. Neurologic side-effects are common and may be seen more frequently than with cyclosporine [115,116]. A concern for the use of tacrolimus in pediatric renal transplantation was the development of post-transplant diabetes mellitus (PTDM), because in an early Japanese renal study one-third of the patients developed hyperglycemia requiring insulin therapy [117], which has also been reported from other single-center reports [118,119]. The mechanism may be related to a diminished insulin secretion in association with the insulin resistance related to steroid use [120]. The incidence of PTLD was much higher with the use of tacrolimus than with other immunosuppresants during early experience [111,121]. However, a more recent retrospective analysis showed that the use of tacrolimus was not a risk factor for development of PTLD, likely because of the lower doses more recently utilized [122]. Tacrolimus has been used in combination with all other immunosuppressants except cyclosporine. However, as noted with cyclosporine, the combination of a calcineurin inhibitor, rapamycin and corticosteroids should be used with caution in children at high risk for developing PTLD [108].

Choice of calcineurin inhibitor

Calcineurin inhibitors have been mainstays of immunosuppression for pediatric transplantation for the past decade and likely account for the continuing improvement in graft survival rates [17,123,124]. The choice between the two calcineurin inhibitors has often been based on a center preference. An open-label randomized trial of the two drugs with steroids and azathioprine in pediatric renal transplant recipients was recently completed [125]. Tarolimus-treated patients had a lower rate of acute rejection (37%) than cyclosporine-treated patients (59%), although both rates in that study were higher than current standards [30] and not all episodes were biopsy-proven. One-year graft survival rates were similar, although the GFR was higher in the tarolimus group. Hypomagnesium, diarrhea and PTDM were higher in the tarolimus group and hypertrichosis and gum hyperplasia were higher in the cyclosporine group. In a retrospective analysis of NAPRTCS data of the two drugs given with MMF and steroids [114], there was no difference in early rejection rate (29%), risk of rejection or risk of graft loss. At 2 years, graft survival was not different (tacrolimus 91%, cyclosporine 95%). Tacrolimus-treated patients were less likely to require antihypertensives and had higher GFR at 2 years. Early concern about the higher risk of PTLD associated with tacrolimus use [111,121] seems no longer to be true, probably related to lower levels of tacrolimus used in current practice [122]. The majority of pediatric kidney, liver and intestine transplant recipients are currently receiving

tacrolimus because of its efficacy and lack of cosmetic side-effects, which is particularly important for adolescent transplant recipients. One unfortunate consequence of chronic calcineurin inhibitor use is nephrotoxicity and chronic renal insufficiency (CRI). One recent review demonstrated an incidence of CRI of 11.8% and an incidence of ESRD of 4.3% 10 years after pediatric heart transplantation [126].

TOR inhibitors

Sirolimus

Rapamycin (sirolimus, Rapamune®; Wyeth) is the newest immunosuppressive agent used for kidney transplantation. It is the product of a fungus that was discovered on Easter Island (Rapa Nui) in 1969. It was first investigated for anti-fungal properties and its immunosuppressant properties were first discovered in 1988. It was approved by the FDA in 1999. A similar compound which may be an analog, SDZ-RAD, is currently undergoing clinical trials but the pediatric component of that study was halted because of concern about potential complications in immature subjects. Rapamycin is classified as a TOR inhibitor. TOR is a cytosolic enzyme that regulates differentiation and proliferation of lymphocytes. TOR is activated as a result of the cascade of reactions in lymphocytes by the proliferation of cytokines, it initiates production of messenger RNAs that trigger cell-cycle progression from G_1 to S phase. The TOR inhibitors bind to the immunophilin FKBP12 and inhibit the actions of TOR [127–132]. The TOR inhibitors may be particularly important in long-term immunosuppression because they stimulate T-cell apoptosis. TOR inhibitors also inhibit mesenchymal proliferation, which may prove to be important in graft vascular disease [133,134]. Also, because the mechanism of action of rapamycin is different from other currently available immunosuppressants, it can be used in combination with all of them. Rapamycin has been found to be effective in combination with calcineurin inhibitors [135–139], in a calcineurin-inhibitor sparing protocol [140] and in a steroid-free protocol [141]. The role of rapamycin or SDZ-RAD in pediatric transplantation is undergoing study [6,142,143].

Rapamycin is available as an oral preparation, either as a solid or liquid. Rapamycin was shown to have a prolonged half-life in adults, which allowed a single daily dose in adults [137–139]. However, pharmacokinetic studies in children have demonstrated a much shorter half-life, as short as 12 hours [6,144]. Thus, children may require twice daily schedules in order to maintain therapeutic levels. Retrospective analysis of early trials of rapamycin have suggested a relationship between blood levels and risk of rejection [145]. Current suggestions for therapeutic levels remain speculative and range from 25 ng/mL in the early post-transplant period without calcineurin inhibitors [6,140] to 5–10 ng/mL later in the course of transplantation.

The major side-effects of rapamycin are hyperlipidemia, thrombocytopenia and leucopenia, and possibly delayed wound healing [137]. The former complications can respond to lipid lowering drugs or dose reduction. The latter complication may require suspension of the drug until the wound heals completely.

IMMUNOSUPPRESSION COMBINATIONS

Most pediatric renal transplant recipients are treated with triple immunosuppression [30]. When the number of drugs was limited, the number of possible combinations was small. However, there are at least 20 possible combinations of the six available drugs, and when the induction antibodies are added there are over 60 possible reported protocols [146]. No "best" protocol for children has been established, although most clinical trials are currently directed at eliminating either steroids or calcineurin inhibitors, or both.

There are many possible targets for immunosuppression strategies for children [147]. One promising new protocol of steroid avoidance has been recently reported [11]. This approach consists of 6 months of anti-IL-2r antibody, tacrolimus and MMF. Short-term patient and graft survival rates have been excellent and growth rates have been very good. Major complications have included bone marrow suppression and nephrotoxicity. A randomized controlled trial of steroid withdrawal was successful in preventing acute and delayed rejections [79] but the initial immunosuppression of IL-2r antibody induction, followed by initial immunosuppression of corticosteroids, sirolimus and a calcineurin inhibitor was too robust, leading to an unacceptably high rate of PTLD in young children [108]. Other protocols currently under investigation include calcineurin inhibitor avoidance or withdrawal [148], or costimulation blockade [67], with the eventual goal of avoiding both corticosteroids and calcineurin inhibitors [68]. One other approach is to use robust induction therapy with Campath, followed by eventual monotherapy with tacrolimus [149,150]. Clearly, there is no single, defined approach to immunosuppression for children, but the eventual goal is to permit long-term graft acceptance with the fewest possible chronic medications.

TREATMENT OF REJECTION

There have been no controlled trials of treatment of acute organ transplant rejection in children. In general, the initial treatment of a rejection episode is with pulse intravenous corticosteroids, typically lasting 3 consecutive days with 10–30 mg/kg for each dose. This regimen may be followed by a slow taper of oral prednisone, but some centers do not routinely used the oral taper. Severe, recurrent or steroid-resistant rejection episodes are most often treated with lymphocyte-depleting antibodies, including OKT3, Atgam or Thymoglo-bulin (see above), although Campath is also being studied for this indication [151,152]. Antibody-mediated rejection may be treated with plasmapheresis, infusion of intravenous immunoglobulin (IVIG) or rituximab in addition to these other treatments, but the efficacy of these approaches is unknown [153–157]. Another novel and unproven approach is the use of photopheresis [158,159].

CONCLUSIONS

Children currently have excellent outcomes of most types of organ transplants. However, long-term success has limited by the complications of lifetime immunosuppression. The current medications used to prevent graft loss are toxic and have substantial complications. In addition, the need to continue to use these medications on a continuing daily basis requires adherence that few recipients, especially adolescents, can accomplish. The future of immunosuppression for children depends on our ability to develop nontoxic long-term medications that are safe, effective and simple to administer. Of course, the ultimate solution is transplant-specific tolerance.

REFERENCES

1 Harmon WE, McDonald RA, Reyes JD, et al. Pediatric transplantation, 1994–2003. Am J Transplant 2005;5:887–903.
2 Dharnidharka VR, Tejani AH, Ho PL, Harmon WE. Post-transplant lymphoproliferative disorder in the United States: young Caucasian males are at highest risk. Am J Transplant 2002;2:993–8.
3 Bunchman T, Navarro M, Broyer M, et al. The use of mycophenolate mofetil suspension in pediatric renal allograft recipients. Pediatr Nephrol 2001;16:978–84.
4 Hoppu K, Koskimies O, Holmberg C, Hirvisalo EL. Pharmacokinetically determined cyclosporine dosage in young children. Pediatr Nephrol 1991;5:1–4.
5 Harmon WE, Sullivan EK. Cyclosporine dosing and its relationship to outcome in pediatric renal transplantation. Kidney Int Suppl 1993;43:S50–5.
6 Schachter AD, Meyers KE, Spaneas LD, et al. Short sirolimus half-life in pediatric renal transplant recipients on a calcineurin inhibitor-free protocol. Pediatr Transplant 2004;8:171–7.
7 Fine RN. Renal transplantation for children: the only realistic choice. Kidney Int Suppl 1985;17:S15–7.
8 Warady BA, Hebert D, Sullivan EK, Alexander SR, Tejani A. Renal transplantation, chronic dialysis, and chronic renal insufficiency in children and adolescents. The 1995 Annual Report of the North American Pediatric Renal Transplant Cooperative Study. Pediatr Nephrol 1997;11:49–64.
9 Trachtman H, Hackney P, Tejani A. Pediatric hemodialysis: a decade's (1974–1984) perspective. Kidney Int Suppl 1986;19:S15–22.
10 Brouhard BH, Donaldson LA, Lawry KW, et al. Cognitive functioning in children on dialysis and post-transplantation. Pediatr Transplant 2000;4:261–7.

11 Sarwal MM, Yorgin PD, Alexander S, *et al.* Promising early outcomes with a novel, complete steroid avoidance immunosuppression protocol in pediatric renal transplantation. *Transplantation* 2001;**72**:13–21.

12 Ingelfinger JR, Grupe WE, Harmon WE, Fernbach SK, Levey RH. Growth acceleration following renal transplantation in children less than 7 years of age. *Pediatrics* 1981;**68**:255–9.

13 Fine RN, Ho M, Tejani A, North American Pediatric Renal Trasplant Cooperative Study. The contribution of renal transplantation to final adult height: a report of the North American Pediatric Renal Transplant Cooperative Study (NAPRTCS). *Pediatr Nephrol* 2001;**16**:951–6.

14 Fine RN. Growth following solid-organ transplantation. *Pediatr Transplant* 2002;**6**:47–52.

15 Mendley SR, Zelko FA. Improvement in specific aspects of neurocognitive performance in children after renal transplantation. *Kidney Int* 1999;**56**:318–23.

16 Fennell EB, Fennell RS, Mings E, Morris MK. The effects of various modes of therapy for end stage renal disease on cognitive performance in a pediatric population: a preliminary report. *Int J Pediatr Nephrol* 1986;**7**:107–12.

17 Colombani PM, Dunn SP, Harmon WE, Magee JC, McDiarmid SV, Spray TL. Pediatric transplantation. *Am J Transplant* 2003;**3**(Suppl 4):53–63.

18 Benfield MR, McDonald RA, Bartosh S, Ho PL, Harmon W. Changing trends in pediatric transplantation: 2001. Annual Report of the North American Pediatric Renal Transplant Cooperative Study. *Pediatr Transplant* 2003;**7**:321–35.

19 Feld LG, Stablein D, Fivush B, Harmon WE, Tejani A. Renal transplantation in children from 1987–1996: The 1996 Annual Report of the North American Pediatric Renal Transplant Cooperative Study. *Pediatr Transplant* 1997;**1**:146–62.

20 Simmons RL, Canafax DM, Fryd DS, *et al.* New immunosuppressive drug combinations for mismatched related and cadaveric renal transplantation. *Transplant Proc* 1986;**18**(Suppl 1):76–81.

21 Norman DJ. Mechanisms of action and overview of OKT3. *Ther Drug Monit* 1995;**17**:615–20.

22 Brophy PD, Thomas SE, McBryde KD, Bunchman TE. Comparison of polyclonal induction agents in pediatric renal transplantation. *Pediatr Transplant* 2001;**5**:174–8.

23 Ault BH, Honaker MR, Osama Gaber A, *et al.* Short-term outcomes of Thymoglobulin induction in pediatric renal transplant recipients. *Pediatr Nephrol* 2002;**17**:815–8.

24 Peddi VR, Bryant M, Roy-Chaudhury P, Woodle ES, First MR. Safety, efficacy, and cost analysis of thymoglobulin induction therapy with intermittent dosing based on CD3+ lymphocyte counts in kidney and kidney-pancreas transplant recipients. *Transplantation* 2002;**73**:1514–8.

25 Benfield MR, Tejani A, Harmon WE, *et al.* A randomized multicenter trial of OKT3 mAbs induction compared with intravenous cyclosporine in pediatric renal transplantation. *Pediatr Transplant* 2005;**9**:282–92.

26 Khositseth S, Matas A, Cook ME, Gillingham KJ, Chavers BM. Thymoglobulin versus ATGAM induction therapy in pediatric kidney transplant recipients: a single-center report. *Transplantation* 2005;**79**:958–63.

27 Norman DJ, Chatenoud L, Cohen D, Goldman M, Shield CD. Consensus statement regarding OKT3-induced cytokine-release syndrome and human antimouse antibodies. *Transplant Proc* 1993;**25**(Suppl 1):89–92.

28 Robinson ST, Barry JM, Norman DJ. The hemodynamic effects of intraoperative injection of muromonab CD3. *Transplantation* 1993;**56**:356–8.

29 Shihab FS, Barry JM, Norman DJ. Encephalopathy following the use of OKT3 in renal allograft transplantation. *Transplant Proc* 1993;**25**(Suppl 1):31–4.

30 Seikaly M, Ho PL, Emmett L, Tejani A. The 12th Annual Report of the North American Pediatric Renal Transplant Cooperative Study: renal transplantation from 1987 through 1998 (updated at www.naprtcs.org). *Pediatr Transplant* 2001;**5**:215–31.

31 Calne R, Moffatt SD, Friend PJ, *et al.* Campath IH allows low-dose cyclosporine monotherapy in 31 cadaveric renal allograft recipients. *Transplantation* 1999;**68**:1613–6.

32 Calne R, Moffatt SD, Friend PJ, *et al.* Prope tolerance with induction using Campath 1H and low-dose cyclosporin monotherapy in 31 cadaveric renal allograft recipients. *Nippon Geka Gakkai Zasshi J Jpn Surg Soc* 2000;**101**:301–6.

33 Knechtle SJ, Pirsch JD, Fechner HJ Jr, *et al.* Campath-1H induction plus rapamycin monotherapy for renal transplantation: results of a pilot study [see comment]. *Am J Transplant* 2003;**3**:722–30.

34 Kirk AD, Hale DA, Mannon RB, *et al.* Results from a human renal allograft tolerance trial evaluating the humanized CD52-specific monoclonal antibody alemtuzumab (Campath-1H). *Transplantation* 2003;**76**:120–9.

35 Nishida S, Levi D, Kato T, *et al.* Ninety-five cases of intestinal transplantation at the University of Miami. *J Gastrointest Surg* 2002;**6**:233–9.

36 Offner G, Broyer M, Niaudet P, *et al.* A multicenter, open-label, pharmacokinetic/pharmacodynamic safety, and tolerability study of basiliximab (Simulect) in pediatric de novo renal transplant recipients. *Transplantation* 2002;**74**:961–6.

37 Kovarik JM, Offner G, Broyer M, *et al.* A rational dosing algorithm for basiliximab (Simulect) in pediatric renal transplantation based on pharmacokinetic-dynamic evaluations. *Transplantation* 2002;**74**:966–71.

38 Strehlau J, Pape L, Offner G, Nashan B, Ehrich JH. Interleukin-2 receptor antibody-induced alterations of ciclosporin dose requirements in paediatric transplant recipients [Comment]. *Lancet* 2000;**356**:1327–8.

39 Ciancio G, Burke GW, Suzart K, *et al.* Daclizumab induction, tacrolimus, mycophenolate mofetil and steroids as an immunosuppression regimen for primary kidney transplant recipients. *Transplantation* 2002;**73**:1100–6.

40 Swiatecka-Urban A, Garcia C, Feuerstein D, *et al.* Basiliximab induction improves the outcome of renal transplants in children and adolescents. *Pediatr Nephrol* 2001;**16**:693–6.

41 Vester U, Kranz B, Testa G, *et al.* Efficacy and tolerability of interleukin-2 receptor blockade with basiliximab in pediatric renal transplant recipients. *Pediatr Transplant* 2001;**5**:297–301.

42 Zamora I, Berbel O, Simon J, Sanahuja MJ. [Anti-CD25 monoclonal antibody against polyclonal antibodies in pediatric renal transplantation.] *Nefrologia* 2002;**22**:66–70.

43 Sayegh MH, Turka LA. The role of T cell costimulatory activation in transplant rejection. *N Engl J Med* 1998;**338**:1813–21.

44 Linsley PS, Ledbetter JA. The role of the CD28 receptor during T cell responses to antigen. *Ann Rev Immunol* 1993;**11**:191–212.

45 Bluestone JA. Is CTLA-4 a master switch for peripheral T cell tolerance? *J Immunol* 1997;**158**:1989–93.

46 Thompson CB. Distinct roles for the costimulatory ligands B7-1 and B7-2 in T helper cell differentiation. *Cell* 1995;**81**:979–82.

47 Janeway CA, Bottomly K. Signals and signs for lymphocyte responses. *Cell* 1994;**76**:275–85.

48 Reiser H, Stadecker MJ. Costimulatory B7 molecules in the pathogenesis of infectious and autoimmune diseases. *N Engl J Med* 1996;**335**:1369–77.

49 Linsley PS, Brady W, Urnes M, Grosmaire LS, Damle NK, Ledbetter JA. CTLA-4 is a second receptor for the B cell activation antigen B7. *J Exp Med* 1991;**174**:561–9.

50 Walunas TL, Lenschow DJ, Bakker CY, et al. CTLA-4 can function as a negative regulator of T cell activation. *Immunity* 1994;**1**:405–13.

51 Walunas TL, Bakker CY, Bluestone JA. CTLA-4 ligation blocks CD28-dependent T cell activation. *J Exp Med* 1996;**183**:2541–50.

52 Perez V, Parijs LV, Biuckians A, Zheng X, Strom T, Abbas A. Induction of peripheral T cell tolerance *in vivo* required CTLA-4 engagement. *Immunity* 1997;**6**:411–7.

53 Greenwald RJ, Boussiotis VA, Lorsbach RB, Abbas AK, Sharpe AH. CTLA-4 regulates induction of anergy *in vivo*. *Immunity* 2001;**14**:145–55.

54 Turka LA, Linsley PS, Lin H, et al. T-cell activation by the CD28 ligand B7 is required for cardiac allograft rejection *in vivo*. *Proc Natl Acad Sci USA* 1992;**89**:11102–5.

55 Lin H, Bolling SF, Linsley PS, et al. Long-term acceptance of major histocompatibility complex mismatched cardiac allografts induced by CTLA4Ig plus donor-specific transfusion. *J Exp Med* 1993;**178**:1801–6.

56 Pearson TC, Alexander DZ, Winn KJ, Linsley PS, Lowry RP, Larsen CP. Transplantation tolerance induced by CTLA4-Ig. *Transplantation* 1994;**57**:1701–6.

57 Pearson T, Alexander D, Hendrix R, et al. CTLA4-Ig plus bone marrow induces long-term allograft survival and donor specific unresponsiveness in the murine model: evidence for hematopoietic chimerism. *Transplantation* 1995;**61**:997–1004.

58 Sayegh MH, Akalin E, Hancock WW, Russell ME, Carpenter CB, Turka LA. CD28-B7 blockade after alloantigenic challenge *in vivo* inhibits Th1 cytokines but spares Th2. *J Exp Med* 1995;**181**:1869–74.

59 Russell ME, Hancock WW, Akalin E, et al. Chronic cardiac rejection in the Lewis to F344 rat model: Blockade of CD28-B7 costimulation by CTLA4Ig modulates T cell and macrophage activation and attenuates arteriosclerosis. *J Clin Invest* 1996;**97**:833–8.

60 Azuma H, Chandraker A, Nadeau K, et al. Blockade of T cell costimulation prevents development of experimental chronic allograft rejection. *Proc Natl Acad Sci USA* 1996;**93**:12439–44.

61 Chandraker A, Russell ME, Glysing-Jensen T, Willett TA, Sayegh MH. T cell costimulatory blockade in experimental chronic cardiac allograft rejection: effects of cyclosporine and donor antigen. *Transplantation* 1997;**63**:1053–8.

62 Chandraker A, Azuma H, Nadeau K, et al. Late blockade of T cell costimulation interrupts progression of experimental chronic allograft rejection. *J Clin Invest* 1998;**101**:2308–18.

63 Kim KS, Denton MD, Chandraker A, et al. CD28-B7-mediated T cell costimulation in chronic cardiac allograft rejection: differential role of B7-1 in initiation versus progression of graft arteriosclerosis. *Am J Pathol* 2001;**158**:977–86.

64 Abrams JR, Lebwohl MG, Guzzo CA, et al. CTLA4Ig-mediated blockade of T cell costimulation in patients with psoriasis vulgaris. *J Clin Invest* 1999;**103**:1243–52.

65 Abrams JR, Kelley SL, Hayes E, et al. Blockade of T lymphocyte costimulation with cytotoxic T lymphocyte-associated antigen 4-immunoglobulin (CTLA4Ig) reverses the cellular pathology of psoriatic plaques, including the activation of keratinocytes, dendritic cells, and endothelial cells. *J Exp Med* 2000;**192**:681–94.

66 Sayegh MH. Finally, CTLA4Ig graduates to the clinic. *J Clin Invest* 1999;**103**:1223–5.

67 Vincenti F, Larsen C, Durrbach A, et al. Costimulation blockade with belatacept in renal transplantation. *N Engl J Med* 2005;**353**:770.

68 Dharnidharka VR. Costimulation blockade with belatacept in renal transplantation. *N Engl J Med* 2005;**353**:2085.

69 Potter D, Belzer FO, Rames L, Holliday MA, Kountz SL, Najarian JS. The treatment of chronic uremia in childhood. I. Transplantation. *Pediatrics* 1970;**45**:432–43.

70 Baqi N, Tejani A. Maintenance immunosuppression regimens. In: Tejani AH, Fine RN, eds. *Pediatric Renal Transplantation*. New York: Wiley-Liss, 1994: 201–10.

71 Danovitch GB. *Handbook of Kidney Transplantation*, 2nd edn. Boston: Little, Brown and Company, 1996.

72 Ingulli E, Tejani A. Steroid withdrawal after renal transplantation. In: Tejani AH, Fine RN, eds. *Pediatric Renal Transplantation*. New York: Wiley-Liss, 1994: 221–38.

73 Ingulli E, Sharma V, Singh A, Suthanthiran M, Tejani A. Steroid withdrawal, rejection and the mixed lymphocyte reaction in children after renal transplantation. *Kidney Int Suppl* 1993;**43**:S36–9.

74 Reisman L, Lieberman KV, Burrows L, Schanzer H. Follow-up of cyclosporine-treated pediatric renal allograft recipients after cessation of prednisone. *Transplantation* 1990;**49**:76–80.

75 Hymes LC, Warshaw BL. Tacrolimus rescue therapy for children with acute renal transplant rejection. *Pediatr Nephrol* 2001;**16**:990–2.

76 Broyer M, Guest G, Gagnadoux MF. Growth rate in children receiving alternate-day corticosteroid treatment after kidney transplantation. *J Pediatr* 1992;**120**:721–5.

77 Jabs K, Sullivan EK, Avner ED, Harmon WE. Alternate-day steroid dosing improves growth without adversely affecting graft survival or long-term graft function. A report of the North American Pediatric Renal Transplant Cooperative Study. *Transplantation* 1996;**61**:31–6.

78 Sarwal MM, Vidhun JR, Alexander SR, Satterwhite T, Millan M, Salvatierra O Jr. Continued superior outcomes with modification and lengthened follow-up of a steroid-avoidance pilot with extended daclizumab induction in pediatric renal transplantation. *Transplantation* 2003;**76**:1331.

79 Benfield MR, Munoz R, Warshaw BL, et al. A randomized controlled double blind trial of steroid withdrawal in pediatric renal transplantation. A study of the Cooperative Clinical Trials in Pediatric Transplantation (Abstract). *Am J Transplant* 2005;**5**(Suppl 11):402.

80 Buell JF, Gross TG, Woodle ES. Malignancy after transplantation. *Transplantation* 2005;80(Suppl):S254.

81 Benfield MR, Symons JM, Bynon S, *et al.* Mycophenolate mofetil in pediatric renal transplantation [Comment]. *Pediatr Transplant* 1999;3:33–7.

82 Butani L, Palmer J, Baluarte HJ, Polinsky MS. Adverse effects of mycophenolate mofetil in pediatric renal transplant recipients with presumed chronic rejection. *Transplantation* 1999;68:83–6.

83 Jungraithmayr T, Staskewitz A, Kirste G, *et al.* Pediatric renal transplantation with mycophenolate mofetil-based immunosuppression without induction: results after three years. *Transplantation* 2003;75:454–61.

84 Filler G, Gellermann J, Zimmering M, Mai I. Effect of adding mycophenolate mofetil in paediatric renal transplant recipients with chronical cyclosporine nephrotoxicity. *Transplant Int* 2000;13:201–6.

85 Staskewitz A, Kirste G, Tonshoff B, *et al.* Mycophenolate mofetil in pediatric renal transplantation without induction therapy: results after 12 months of treatment. German Pediatric Renal Transplantation Study Group. *Transplantation* 2001;71:638–44.

86 Ettenger R, Cohen A, Nast C, Moulton L, Marik J, Gales B. Mycophenolate mofetil as maintenance immunosuppression in pediatric renal transplantation. *Transplant Proc* 1997;29:340–1.

87 Oellerich M, Shipkova M, Schutz E, *et al.* Pharmacokinetic and metabolic investigations of mycophenolic acid in pediatric patients after renal transplantation: implications for therapeutic drug monitoring. German Study Group on Mycophenolate Mofetil Therapy in Pediatric Renal Transplant Recipients. *Ther Drug Monit* 2000;22:20–6. [Erratum appears in *Ther Drug Monit* 2000;22:500.]

88 Filler G, Feber J, Lepage N, Weiler G, Mai I. Universal approach to pharmacokinetic monitoring of immunosuppressive agents in children. *Pediatr Transplant* 2002;6:411–8.

89 Shipkova M, Armstrong VW, Weber L, *et al.* Pharmacokinetics and protein adduct formation of the pharmacologically active acyl glucuronide metabolite of mycophenolic acid in pediatric renal transplant recipients. *Ther Drug Monit* 2002;24:390–9.

90 Weber LT, Schutz E, Lamersdorf T, *et al.* Therapeutic drug monitoring of total and free mycophenolic acid (MPA) and limited sampling strategy for determination of MPA-AUC in paediatric renal transplant recipients. The German Study Group on Mycophenolate Mofetil (MMF) Therapy. *Nephrol Dial Transplant* 1999;14(Suppl 4):34–5.

91 Weber LT, Schutz E, Lamersdorf T, *et al.* Pharmacokinetics of mycophenolic acid (MPA) and free MPA in paediatric renal transplant recipients: a multicentre study. The German Study Group on Mycophenolate Mofetil (MMF) Therapy. *Nephrol Dial Transplant* 1999;14(Suppl 4):33–4.

92 Weber LT, Shipkova M, Armstrong VW, *et al.* The pharmacokinetic–pharmacodynamic relationship for total and free mycophenolic acid in pediatric renal transplant recipients: a report of the German study group on mycophenolate mofetil therapy. *J Am Soc Nephrol* 2002;13:759–68.

93 Calne RY, Rolles K, White DJ, *et al.* Cyclosporin A initially as the only immunosuppressant in 34 recipients of cadaveric organs: 32 kidneys, 2 pancreases, and 2 livers. *Lancet* 1979;2:1033–6.

94 Suthanthiran M, Haschemeyer RH, Riggio RR, *et al.* Excellent outcome with a calcium channel blocker-supplemented immunosuppressive regimen in cadaveric renal transplantation: a potential strategy to avoid antibody induction protocols [see comments]. *Transplantation* 1993;55:1008–13.

95 Tejani A, Sullivan EK. Higher maintenance cyclosporine dose decreases the risk of graft failure in North American children: a report of the North American Pediatric Renal Transplant Cooperative Study. *J Am Soc Nephrol* 1996;7:550–5.

96 Tejani A, Sullivan EK, Fine RN, Harmon W, Alexander S. Steady improvement in renal allograft survival among North American children: a five year appraisal by the North American Pediatric Renal Transplant Cooperative Study. *Kidney Int* 1995;48:551–3.

97 Kahan BD. Cyclosporine [see comments]. *N Engl J Med* 1989;321:1725–38.

98 David-Neto E, Araujo LP, Feres Alves C, *et al.* A strategy to calculate cyclosporin A area under the time–concentration curve in pediatric renal transplantation. *Pediatr Transplant* 2002;6:313–8.

99 Belitsky P, Dunn S, Johnston A, Levy G. Impact of absorption profiling on efficacy and safety of cyclosporin therapy in transplant recipients. *Clin Pharmacokinet* 2000;39:117–25.

100 Dunn SP. Neoral monitoring 2 hours post-dose and the pediatric transplant patient. *Pediatr Transplant* 2003;7:25–30.

101 Crocker JF, Dempsey T, Schenk ME, Renton KW. Cyclosporin A toxicity in children. *Transplant Rev* 1993;7:72.

102 Foley RJ, Hamner RW, Weinman EJ. Serum potassium concentrations in cyclosporine- and azathioprine-treated renal transplant patients. *Nephron* 1985;40:280–5.

103 Chapman JR, Griffiths D, Harding NG, Morris PJ. Reversibility of cyclosporin nephrotoxicity after three months' treatment. *Lancet* 1985;1:128–30.

104 Allen RD, Hunnisett AG, Morris PJ. Cyclosporin and magnesium [Letter]. *Lancet* 1985;1:1283–4.

105 Beaman M, Parvin S, Veitch PS, Walls J. Convulsions associated with cyclosporin A in renal transplant recipients. *Br Med J* 1985;290:139–40.

106 Thomas DW, Baboolal K, Subramanian N, Newcombe RG. Cyclosporin A-induced gingival overgrowth is unrelated to allograft function in renal transplant recipients. *J Clin Periodontol* 2001;28:706–9.

107 Seymour RA, Jacobs DJ. Cyclosporin and the gingival tissues. *J Clin Periodontol* 1992;19:1–11.

108 McDonald RA, McIntosh M, Stablein D, *et al.* Increased incidence of PTLD in pediatric renal transplant recipients enrolled in a randomized controlled trial of steroid withdrawal: a study of the CCTPT [Abstract]. *Am J Transplant* 2005;5(Suppl 11):418.

109 Shapiro R, Jordan ML, Scantlebury VP, *et al.* The superiority of tacrolimus in renal transplant recipients: the Pittsburgh experience. *Clin Transpl* 1995:199–205.

110 McKee M, Segev D, Wise B, *et al.* Initial experience with FK506 (tacrolimus) in pediatric renal transplant recipients. *J Pediatr Surg* 1997;32:688–90.

111 Ellis D. Clinical use of tacrolimus (FK-506) in infants and children with renal transplants. *Pediatr Nephrol* 1995;9:487–94.

112 Eades SK, Boineau FG, Christensen ML. Increased tacrolimus levels in a pediatric renal transplant patient attributed to chronic diarrhea. *Pediatr Transplant* 2000;4:63–6.

113 Shapiro R, Jordan M, Fung J, *et al*. Kidney transplantation under FK 506 immunosuppression. *Transplant Proc* 1991;**23**:920–3.

114 Neu AM, Ho PL, Fine RN, Furth SL, Fivush BA. Tacrolimus vs. cyclosporine A as primary immunosuppression in pediatric renal transplantation: a NAPRTCS study. *Pediatr Transplant* 2003;**7**:217–22.

115 Eidelman BH, Abu-Elmagd K, Wilson J, *et al*. Neurologic complications of FK 506. *Transplant Proc* 1991;**23**:3175–8.

116 Neu AM, Furth SL, Case BW, Wise B, Colombani PM, Fivush BA. Evaluation of neurotoxicity in pediatric renal transplant recipients treated with tacrolimus (FK506). *Clin Transpl* 1997;**11**:412–4.

117 Japanese FK506 Study Group. Morphological characteristics of renal allografts showing renal dysfunction under FK506 therapy: is graft biopsy available to reveal the morphological findings corresponding with FK506 nephropathy? *Transplant Proc* 1993;**25**:624.

118 Furth S, Neu A, Colombani P, Plotnick L, Turner ME, Fivush B. Diabetes as a complication of tacrolimus (FK506) in pediatric renal transplant patients. *Pediatr Nephrol* 1996;**10**:64–6.

119 Greenspan LC, Gitelman SE, Leung MA, Glidden DV, Mathias RS. Increased incidence in post-transplant diabetes mellitus in children: a case–control analysis. *Pediatr Nephrol* 2002;**17**:1–5.

120 Filler G, Neuschulz I, Vollmer I, Amendt P, Hocher B. Tacrolimus reversibly reduces insulin secretion in paediatric renal transplant recipients. *Nephrol Dial Transplant* 2000;**15**:867–71.

121 Ciancio G, Siquijor AP, Burke GW, *et al*. Post-transplant lymphoproliferative disease in kidney transplant patients in the new immunosuppressive era. *Clin Transpl* 1997;**11**:243–9.

122 Dharnidharka VR, Ho PL, Stablein DM, Harmon WE, Tejani AH. Mycophenolate, tacrolimus and post-transplant lymphoproliferative disorder: a report of the North American Pediatric Renal Transplant Cooperative Study. *Pediatr Transplant* 2002;**6**:396–9.

123 Tejani A, Ho PL, Emmett L, Stablein DM, North American Pediatric Renal Transplant Cooperative Study. Reduction in acute rejections decreases chronic rejection graft failure in children: a report of the North American Pediatric Renal Transplant Cooperative Study (NAPRTCS). *Am J Transplant* 2002;**2**:142–7.

124 Tejani A, Stablein DM, Donaldson L, *et al*. Steady improvement in short-term graft survival of pediatric renal transplants: the NAPRTCS experience. *Clin Transpl* 1999:95–110.

125 Trompeter R, Filler G, Webb NJ, *et al*. Randomized trial of tacrolimus versus cyclosporin microemulsion in renal transplantation. *Pediatr Nephrol* 2002;**17**:141–9.

126 Lee CK, Christensen LL, Magee JC, Ojo AO, Leichtman AM, Bridges ND. Chronic renal failure in a 10-year national cohort of pediatric heart transplant recipients. *J Heart Lung Transplant* 2005;**24**(2S):S114.

127 Sehgal SN, Molnar-Kimber K, Ocain TD, Weichman BM. Rapamycin: a novel immunosuppressive macrolide. *Med Res Rev* 1994;**14**:1–22.

128 Kim HS, Raskova J, Degiannis D, Raska K Jr. Effects of cyclosporine and rapamycin on immunoglobulin production by preactivated human B cells. *Clin Exp Immunol* 1994;**96**:508–12.

129 Ferraresso M, Tian L, Ghobrial R, Stepkowski SM, Kahan BD. Rapamycin inhibits production of cytotoxic but not noncytotoxic antibodies and preferentially activates T helper 2 cells that mediate long-term survival of heart allografts in rats. *J Immunol* 1994;**153**:3307–18.

130 Aagaard-Tillery KM, Jelinek DF. Inhibition of human B lymphocyte cell cycle progression and differentiation by rapamycin. *Cell Immunol* 1994;**156**:493–507.

131 Dumont FJ, Staruch MJ, Koprak SL, Melino MR, Sigal NH. Distinct mechanisms of suppression of murine T cell activation by the related macrolides FK-506 and rapamycin. *J Immunol* 1990;**144**:251–8.

132 Wood MA, Bierer BE. Rapamycin: biological and therapeutic effects, binding by immunophilins and molecular targets of action. *Perspect Drug Disc Design* 1994;**2**:163–84.

133 Marx SO, Jayaraman T, Go LO, Marks AR. Rapamycin-FKBP inhibits cell cycle regulators of proliferation in vascular smooth muscle cells. *Circ Res* 1995;**76**:412–7.

134 Cao W, Mohacsi P, Shorthouse R, Pratt R, Morris RE. Effects of rapamycin on growth factor-stimulated vascular smooth muscle cell DNA synthesis. Inhibition of basic fibroblast growth factor and platelet-derived growth factor action and antagonism of rapamycin by FK506. *Transplantation* 1995;**59**:390–5.

135 El-Sabrout R, Weiss R, Butt F, *et al*. Rejection-free protocol using sirolimus-tacrolimus combination for pediatric renal transplant recipients. *Transplant Proc* 2002;**34**:1942–3.

136 Montgomery SP, Mog SR, Xu H, *et al*. Efficacy and toxicity of a protocol using sirolimus, tacrolimus and daclizumab in a nonhuman primate renal allotransplant model. *Am J Transplant* 2002;**2**:381–5.

137 Kahan BD, Camardo JS. Rapamycin: clinical results and future opportunities. *Transplantation* 2001;**72**:1181–93.

138 Kahan BD, Julian BA, Pescovitz MD, Vanrenterghem Y, Neylan J. Sirolimus reduces the incidence of acute rejection episodes despite lower cyclosporine doses in caucasian recipients of mismatched primary renal allografts: a phase II trial. Rapamune Study Group. *Transplantation* 1999;**68**:1526–32.

139 Kahan BD, Podbielski J, Napoli KL, Katz SM, Meier-Kriesche HU, Van Buren CT. Immunosuppressive effects and safety of a sirolimus/cyclosporine combination regimen for renal transplantation. *Transplantation* 1998;**66**:1040–6.

140 Kreis H, Cisterne JM, Land W, *et al*. Sirolimus in association with mycophenolate mofetil induction for the prevention of acute graft rejection in renal allograft recipients. *Transplantation* 2000;**69**:1252–60.

141 Mital D, Podlasek W, Jensik SC. Sirolimus-based steroid-free maintenance immunosuppression. *Transplant Proc* 2002;**34**:1709–10.

142 Vester U, Kranz B, Wehr S, Boger R, Hoyer PF, Group RBS. Everolimus (Certican) in combination with neoral in pediatric renal transplant recipients: interim analysis after 3 months. *Transplant Proc* 2002;**34**:2209–10.

143 Van Damme-Lombaerts R, Webb NA, Hoyer PF, *et al*. Single-dose pharmacokinetics and tolerability of everolimus in stable pediatric renal transplant patients. *Pediatr Transplant* 2002;**6**:147–52.

144 Sindhi R, Webber S, Goyal R, Reyes J, Venkataramanan R, Shaw L. Pharmacodynamics of sirolimus in transplanted children receiving tacrolimus. *Transplant Proc* 2002;**34**:1960.

145 MacDonald A, Scarola J, Burke JT, Zimmerman JJ. Clinical pharmacokinetics and therapeutic drug monitoring of sirolimus. *Clin Ther* 2000;**22**(Suppl B):B101–21.

146 Harmon WE, Stablein DM, Sayegh MH. Trends in immuno-suppression strategies in pediatric kidney transplantation. *Am J Transplant* 2003;**3** (Suppl 5):285.

147 Sho M, Samsonov DV, Briscoe DM. Immunologic targets for currently available immunosuppressive agents: what is the optimal approach for children? *Semin Nephrol* 2001;**21**:508–20.

148 Harmon W, Myers K, Ingelfinger J, *et al.* Safety and efficacy of a calcineurin-inhibitor avoidance regimen in pediatric renal transplantation. *J Am Soc Nephrol* 2006;**17**:1735–45.

149 Tan HP, Kaczorowski D, Basu A, *et al.* Steroid-free tacrolimus monotherapy after pretransplantation Thymoglobulin or Campath and laparoscopy in living donor renal transplantation. *Transplant Proc* 2005;**37**:4235.

150 Shapiro R, Basu A, Tan H, *et al.* Kidney transplantation under minimal immunosuppression after pretransplant lymphoid depletion with Thymoglobulin or Campath. *J Am Coll Surg* 2005;**200**:505.

151 Csapo Z, Benavides-Viveros C, Podder H, Pollard V, Kahan BD. Campath-1H as rescue therapy for the treatment of acute rejection in kidney transplant patients. *Transplant Proc* 2005;**37**:2032.

152 Schneeberger S, Kreczy A, Brandacher G, Steurer W, Margreiter R. Steroid- and ATG-resistant rejection after double forearm transplantation responds to Campath-1H. *Am J Transplant* 2004;**4**:1372.

153 Takemoto SK, Zeevi A, Feng S, *et al.* National conference to assess antibody-mediated rejection in solid organ transplantation. *Am J Transplant* 2004;**4**:1033.

154 Pescovitz MD. The use of rituximab, anti-CD20 monoclonal antibody, in pediatric transplantation. *Pediatr Transplant* 2004;**8**:9.

155 Glotz D, Antoine C, Julia P, *et al.* Intravenous immunoglobulins and transplantation for patients with anti-HLA antibodies. *Transplant Int* 2004;**17**:1.

156 Jordan S, Cunningham-Rundles C, McEwan R. Utility of intravenous immune globulin in kidney transplantation: efficacy, safety, and cost implications. *Am J Transplant* 2003;**3**:653.

157 Jordan SC, Tyan D, Czer L, Toyoda M. Immunomodulatory actions of intravenous immunoglobulin (IVIG): potential applications in solid organ transplant recipients. *Pediatr Transplant* 1998;**2**:92.

158 Wise BV, King KE, Rook AH, Mogayzel PJ Jr. Extracorporeal photopheresis in the treatment of persistent rejection in a pediatric lung transplant recipient. *Prog Transplant* 2003;**13**:61.

159 Dall'Amico R, Murer L. Extracorporeal photochemotherapy: a new therapeutic approach for allograft rejection. *Transfus Apher Sci* 2002;**26**:197.

10 Novel Immunosuppressants

Flavio Vincenti and Ryutaro Hirose

NEW BIOLOGICS

The monoclonal antibodies daclizumab and basiliximab were introduced in the 1990s and marked the emergence of novel biologic agents in renal transplantation. Induction therapy with monoclonal antibodies (anti-IL-2 antibodies) or polyclonal agents (predominantly thymoglobulin) is currently used in approximately 70% of *de novo* renal transplant recipients [1]. Conventional induction therapy has been used to condition the recipient's immune system at the time of transplantation and antigen presentation. The new generation of biologic agents are being developed for chronic therapy with the purpose of displacing maintenance therapy with oral drugs such as the calcineurin inhibitors and corticosteroids [2]. Table 10.1 lists the new biologic agents, their targets and their development status. Currently, only one agent LEA29Y (belatacept) is in phase III trials. However, it is likely that several additional biologic agents will be in advanced clinical development within the next 5 years. While the costimulatory pathway is emerging as an important therapeutic area for immunosuppression therapy, other promising targets include interleukin-15 and adhesion molecules [3].

Table 10.1 Biologic agents in the transplant pipeline.

Antibody	Pharma/Biotech	Status
LEA29Y	Bristol Myers	Phase III trial
Efalizumab*	Xoma-Genetech	Phase II
Alemtuzumab*	Genzyme	IS
Rituximab	Genentech	IS
mIL 5/Fc	Roche	Preclinical
Anti-IL-15	Amgen	Preclinical
Anti-CD40	Bristol Myers	Preclinical
	Chiron	Preclinical
	Novartis	Preclinical

IS, investigator initiated trials.
* US Food and Drug Administration (FDA) approved for other indications.

Alemtuzumab

Alemtuzumab (Campath-1H) is a humanized monoclonal antibody that targets the CD52 antigen expressed on lymphocytes and monocytes. Alemtuzumab is approved for use in chronic lymphocytic leukemia but has recently been used off label for induction therapy in renal transplantation because of its potency as a T-cell depleting agent [4,5]. Alemtuzumab has been administered in one or two doses of 30 mg to induce prolonged lymphocyte depletion and allow drug minimization or safe withdrawal of maintenance immunosuppression. Kirk *et al.* [4] attempted alemtuzumab monotherapy in seven renal transplant recipients, but all seven patients experienced acute rejection, which required the reinstitution of maintenance therapy. Knechtle *et al.* [5] used alemtuzumab induction in combination with sirolimus maintenance therapy in 29 renal transplant recipients. However, 12/29 patients developed acute rejection, several with humoral or vascular features. A recent modification of this regimen that incorporates initial use of calcineurin inhibitors followed by withdrawal has resulted in a lower rejection rate. Potential long-term drawbacks of alemtuzumab include the risk of malignancy and the emergence of a disproportionately large population of memory T cells. Experimentally, severe depletion of lymphocytes results in homeostatic repopulation of T cells with a predominant memory phenotype [6]. This change in T-cell subpopulation could ultimately lead to late episodes of acute rejection and place the allograft at risk of chronic rejection.

Therapies targeting interleukin-15

Interleukin-15 (IL-15) is a cytokine with similar biologic activity to that of IL-2 [7]. While IL-2 results in activation induced cell death, IL-15 promotes antiapoptosis signals. IL-15 is produced by monocyte–macrophage lineage, by epithelial and renal tubule cells but not by T cells. Its role in rejection is suggested by the finding of elevated levels of IL-15 expression in rejecting allografts [8]. Although IL-15 shares the β and common γ class of the IL-2 receptor, it has a distinct high affinity α receptor. Several inhibitors of the IL-15 pathway are likely to be developed for transplantation including direct blockers of IL-15 or the IL-15 α receptor [9,10]. An interesting regimen consisting of a agonist IL-2, a mutant IL-15 Fc and sirolimus induced prolonged graft survival of heart and skin in mice [10]. A potentially attractive use of anti-IL-15 therapy is in conjunction with anti-IL-2 in a calcineurin-free regimen with antiproliferative agents maintenance therapy.

Efalizumab

Efalizumab is a humanized IgG1 monoclonal antibody targeting the CD11a chain of LFA-1 [3]. Efalizumab binds to LFA-1 preventing LFA-1–ICAM interaction. Anti-CD11a has been shown to block T-cell adhesion, trafficking and activation [11]. Pretransplant therapy with anti-CD11a prolonged survival of murine skin and heart allografts and monkey heart allografts. Efalizumab has been approved for use in patients with psoriasis. In a phase I/II open label, dose ranging, multidose, multicenter, renal transplant trial, efalizumab was administered subcutaneously, weekly for 12 weeks following transplantation [12]. Efalizumab was used in two doses (0.5 mg/kg and 2 mg/kg) with a maintenance regimen of full-dose cyclosporine and mycophenolate mofetil (MMF) or half-dose cyclosporine with sirolimus. At 3 months, 7.8% of patients had reversible rejection episodes and at 6 months the cumulative rejection rate was 10.4%. The incidence of acute rejection was similar in all groups. In a subset of 10 patients who received the higher dose efalizumab (2 mg/kg) with full-dose cyclosporine, MMF and steroids, three developed post-transplant lymphoproliferative diseases. While efalizumab appears to provide effective immunosuppression, it should be used in the lower dose (0.5 mg/kg) and with an immunosuppressive regimen that spares calcineurin inhibitors.

Costimulation blockade

Costimulation provides critical signals that activate naïve T cells after they engage alloantigens [13]. The ability of costimulation blockade to induce tolerance or indefinite graft survival in experimental models of transplantation has encouraged the development of several biologic agents against targets in the costimulatory pathway (Fig. 10.1) [14,15]. The CD154–CD40 pathway, originally described in the activation of B cells, also has an important role in T-cell activation. The first clinical effort to block costimulation in renal transplantation was attempted with a monoclonal antibody to CD154 [16,17]. Following the impressive results of Hu5C8 (a humanized anti-CD154) in nonhuman primates, a phase I study was undertaken with chronic intermittent administration of Hu5C8 in combination with a short course of steroids (2 weeks) and MMF in a calcineurin inhibitor free regimen [17]. However, the trial was halted following the occurrence of several thromboembolic events. This complication is not epitope-specific as other antibodies to CD154 were associated with similar thrombotic complications. Thus, direct targeting CD154 will not likely be pursued. However, antibodies against CD40 in preclinical development may prove to be a safer alternative to block the CD40–CD154 pathway.

The second biologic agent to block costimulation is CTL4-Ig, a genetically engineered fusion protein consisting of the extracellular domain of human CTL4 linked to the constant IgG1 Fc region [3]. CTLA4-Ig binds to CD80 and CD86 ligands and sequester them away from CD28, thus preventing costimulatory signals. While CTLA4-Ig has been shown to be effective in autoimmune diseases, CTLA4-Ig had only a modest effect in prolonging graft survival in rhesus monkeys. A second generation CTLA4-Ig, belatacept (LEA29Y), has been re-engineered with two-point mutation in the CTL4 binding sites to increase the avidity to CD80 (twofold) and CD86 (fourfold). Belatacept is 10-fold more effective than CTLA4-Ig *in vitro* on a per dose basis in inhibiting T-cell effective functions.

In a large phase II trial, renal transplant recipients receiving their first or second kidneys were treated with chronic intermittent therapy with belatacept with maintenance therapy

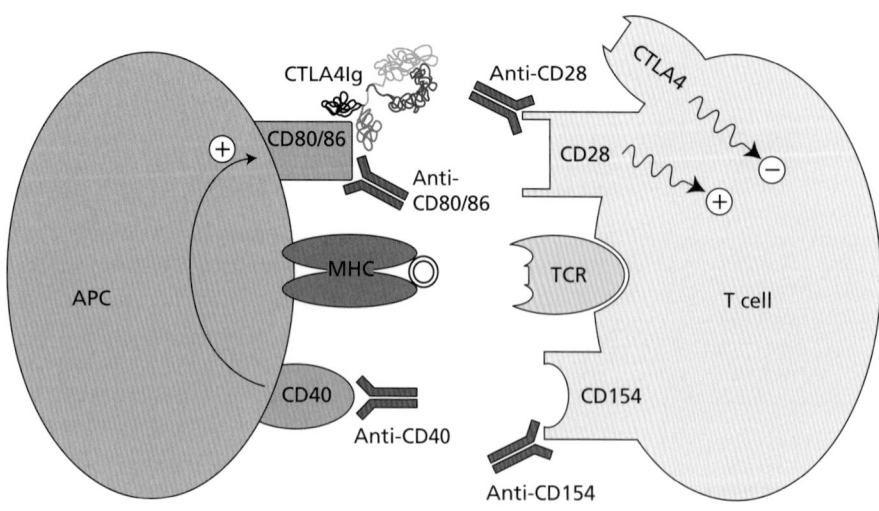

Fig. 10.1 Monoclonal antibodies and fusion receptor proteins against costimulation targets.

consisting of MMF and steroids and were compared with patients treated with a cyclosporine-based regimen with MMF and steroids [18]. All patients had induction therapy with two doses of basiliximab. At 6 months, the acute rejection rate was similar between the belatacept patients and the cyclosporine-treated patients. Patients treated with belatacept had better renal function, lower blood pressure measurements and lower low-density lipoprotein (LDL) values when compared with cyclosporine-treated patients. This study demonstrated that belatacept administered intermittently and chronically can replace calcineurin inhibitors. Belatacept is currently being tested in two phase III trials and additional trials are planned in pediatric patients as well as in a tolerance induction protocol. A particular concern in pediatric patients is their response to primary Epstein–Barr virus (EBV) infection while on therapy with belatacept. However, pediatric patients may greatly benefit from a therapeutic modality that assures compliance and can eliminate calcineurin inhibitors and possibly corticosteroids.

Other biologic agents that block other pathways associated with the costimulation pathway are likely to be tested. Preclinical studies are ongoing with nonagonist anti-CD28 antibodies. Thus, the new biologic agents in preclinical and clinical development hold the promise of improving immunosuppression, minimizing toxicities and enhancing patient compliance.

SMALL MOLECULES

There are several small molecules with immunomodulatory and immunosuppressive properties in clinical development, some of which have novel and interesting mechanisms of action.

FTY720

FTY720 is a novel immunomodulatory drug with a unique mechanism of action. FTY720 is a synthetic structural analog of myriocin, a metabolite of an ascomycete. Initially, it was thought that FTY720 exerted its immunomodulatory effects by causing lymphopenia by inducing lymphocyte apoptosis. Although FTY720 can indeed cause apoptosis of lymphocytes at supraphysiologic concentrations, it has been shown that FTY720 causes a peripheral lymphopenia by affecting lymphocyte trafficking. FTY720 shares structural and functional homology to sphingosine-1-phosphate (S1P), a natural ligand to several G protein coupled receptors. FTY720 displays a novel mechanism of action characterized by the sequestration of lymphocytes in secondary lymphoid tissues. Although first hypothesized to result from a "priming" of lymphocytes to chemokines that attracted lymphocytes to lymph nodes and Peyer patches, it has recently been shown that FTY720 inhibits the egress of lymphocytes from secondary lymphoid organs by acting to internalize S1P1 receptors on lymphocytes without affecting their immunologic function [19]. FTY720-monophosphate (FTY720-P), the active form of the drug, acts as an agonist and signals via the S1P receptor family, binding to S1P1, S1P3 and S1P4, primarily via $S1P_1$ on lymphocytes, the effect of which is to sequester lymphocytes in lymph nodes and Peyer patches by inhibiting their egress from these tissues. This sequestration reduces migration of effector cells to inflammatory tissues and graft sites. These effects have been demonstrated in rodent models and FTY720 seems to also cause apoptosis-independent lymphopenia in humans. In addition, FTY720 may have effects on endothelial cells, promoting their integrity and lessening vascular permeability. FTY720 also seems to ameliorate ischemia-reperfusion injury [20]. Theoretical advantages of such a mechanism of action include the preservation of systemic immune responses to pathogens. The clinical use of FTY720 in the pediatric population, with no antiproliferative effect and lack of chronic nephrotoxicity, may be particularly appealing.

In a recently published study, 20 stable renal transplant recipients on a cyclosporine-based regimen were treated with single oral doses of FTY720 ranging from 0.25 to 3.5 mg [21]. FTY720 was well tolerated with no serious adverse events except for transient asymptomatic bradycardia in 10/24 doses. FTY720-P binds to S1P3 which may mediate the bradycardia effect. The elimination half-life ranged from 89 to 157 hours independent of dose. FTY720 pharmacodynamics were characterized by reversible transient lymphopenia within 6 hours, nadir being 42% of baseline. The lymphocyte count returned to baseline within 72 hours in all dosing cohorts except the highest. A recently published study reported the efficacy and safety results from a phase IIA study that compared four doses of FTY720 with MMF in combination with cyclosporine and steroids in *de novo* renal transplant recipients [22]. There were four groups of patients who received FTY720 ($n = 167$), and this group was compared with a group of 41 patients who received MMF. The 3-month incidence of biopsy-proved rejection rates of the FTY720-treated patients were 23.3%, 34.9%, 17.5% and 9.8%, at daily doses of 0.25, 0.5, 1.0 and 2.5 mg, respectively, versus 17.1% with MMF. As in all clinical trials reported with this drug, some transient bradycardia was noted in the patient groups that were treated with FTY720. The bradycardia was reported as transient, and mostly related to the first dose of FTY720. Based on preliminary results from the phase III trials, Novartis has decided to discontinue the development of FTY720 in transplantation.

FK778

FK778, a new oral immunosuppressive agent under development, is an analog of the active metabolites of leflunomide (Fig. 10.2). FK778 belongs in the class of malononitrilamides. Its mechanism of action is the inhibition of the *de novo*

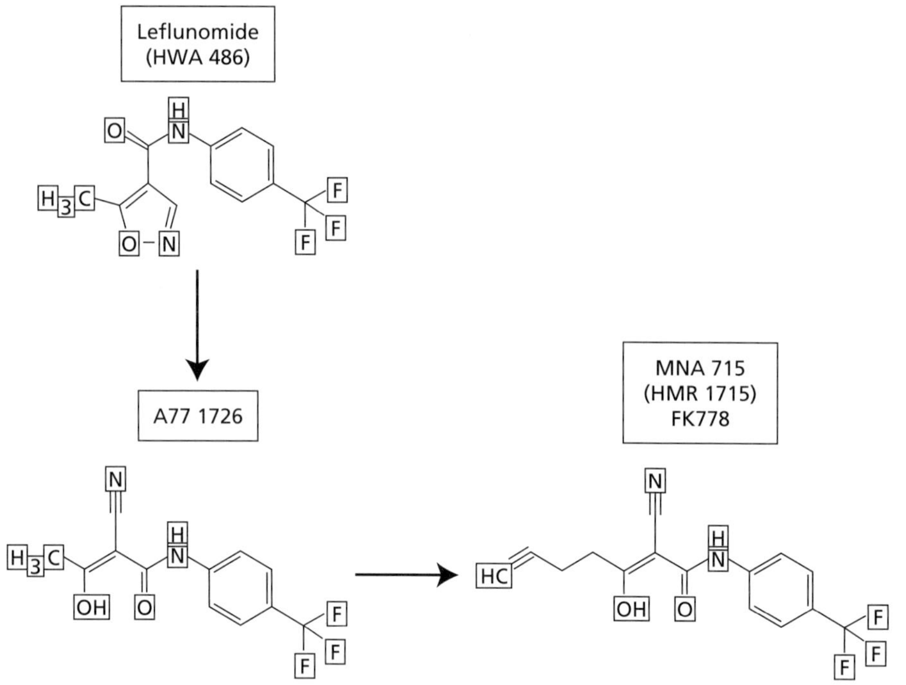

Fig. 10.2 Chemical structure of leflunomide, and its derivatives including FK778.

pathway of pyrimidine synthesis by binding to and inhibiting dihydro-orotate dehydrogenase, thereby blocking T- and B-cell proliferation and strongly suppressing IgM and IgG antibody production. In addition, FK778 appears to have antiviral effects, including the polyomavirus and cytomegalovirus (CMV). Recently, the results of a phase II multicenter trial in renal transplant recipients were published [23]. The trial was conducted in Europe, as a placebo-controlled trial, utilizing two doses of FK778 in combination with tacrolimus and corticosteroids. In this trial, the patients randomized to FK778 were given a loading dose of 600 mg orally and maintained on either 150 or 75 mg/day. In these two groups, the biopsy proven acute rejection rate at 3 months was 28.6% (14/49) and 25.9% (14/54) compared with that of the placebo group of 39% (18/46). The most common adverse event associated with FK778 was anemia, which was reported as reversible upon cessation of FK778. Unfortunately Astellas recently decided not to proceed with the clinical development of FK778 in transplantation.

JAK3 inhibitors

Janus kinase 3 (JAK3) is a tyrosine kinase that is involved in cytokine receptor signaling, such as those for IL-4, IL-7, IL-9 and IL-15 (Fig. 10.3). Because JAK3 is required for the transduction of proliferative signals via the common γ chain of lymphokine receptors, inhibitors of JAK3 can be potentially powerful and useful drugs in transplantation. Other antiproliferatives and inhibitors of signaling often have broad effects on tissues other than lymphocytes; however, with the limited tissue distribution of JAK3, being found primarily on hematopoietic cells, one might predict less systemic side-effects. Individuals with genetically mutant JAK3 exhibit autosomal severe combined immunodeficiency (SCID) and humans mutant in γ chain of the common cytokine receptor have a similar SCID phenotype (X-linked SCID) [24]. This illustrates the importance of the γ chain and JAK3 pathways. There are at least seven JAK3 inhibitors. Several, including PNU156804, NC1153, WHI-P131 and CP-690,550 have shown some efficacy in animal allograft models [25]. CP-690,550 significantly prolonged renal allograft survival in a cynomologous monkey model [26]. Whether JAK3 inhibitors turn out to be prohibitively immunosuppressive remains to be determined.

Overall, there are several small molecules under clinical and preclinical development that may serve to expand further the armamentarium of transplant surgeons and physicians. Some may be particularly suited towards the long-term immunosuppressive management of the pediatric transplant population.

Novartis recently reported preclinical results on a new small molecule (AEB) that inhibits protein kinase C and will initiate clinical trials in renal transplantation [27]. The coming years will prove whether we can continue to improve on the already excellent short-term results of transplantation, as well as improve on the overall clinical outcomes of pediatric transplant patients who to this day are most often subject to lifelong immunosuppression.

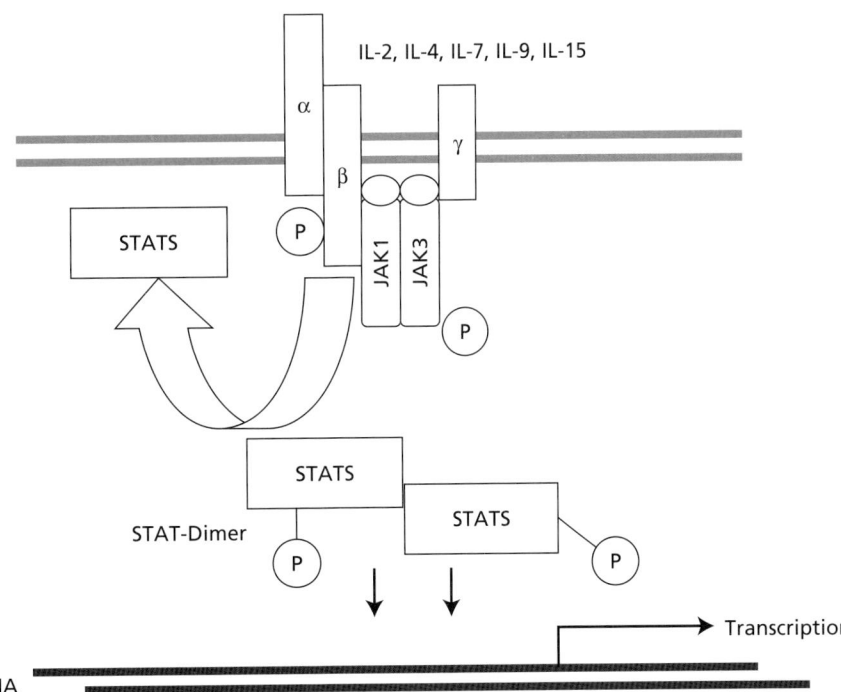

Fig. 10.3 JAK–STAT signaling.

REFERENCES

1 Vincenti F. Induction therapy in kidney transplantation. In: Pereira BJG, Sayegh MH, Blake P., eds. *Chronic Kidney Disease, Dialysis, and Transplantation: Companion to Brenner & Rector's The Kidney.* Philadelphia, PA: Elsevier Saunders, 2005; 647–52.

2 Vincenti F. Chronic induction: What's new in the pipeline? In: Ronco C, Chiaramonte S, Remuzzi G., eds. *Kidney Transplantation: Strategies to Prevent Organ Rejection.* Switzerland: Karger, 2005; 22–9.

3 Vincenti F. What's in the pipeline? New immunosuppressive drugs in transplantation. *Am J Transplant* 2002;**2**:898–903.

4 Kirk AD, Hale DA, Mannon RB, et al. Results from a human renal allograft tolerance trial evaluating the humanized CD52-specific monoclonal antibody alemtuzumab (Campath-1H). *Transplantation* 2003;**76**:120–9.

5 Knechtle SJ, Pirsch JD, Fechner J, et al. Campath-1H induction plus rapamycin monotherapy for renal transplantation: results of a pilot study. *Am J Transplant* 2003;**3**:722–30.

6 Wu Z, Bensinger SJ, Zhang J, et al. Homeostatic proliferation is a barrier to transplantation tolerance. *Nat Med* 2004;**10**:21–3.

7 Waldman T, Tagaya Y, Bamford R. Interleukin-2, interleukin-15, and their receptors. *Int Rev Immunol* 1998;**16**:205.

8 Pavlakis M, Strehlau J, Lipman M, et al. Intragraft IL-15 transcripts are increased in human renal allograft rejection. *Transplantation* 1996;**62**:543–5.

9 Kim SY, Maslinski W, Zheng XX, et al. Targeting the IL-15 receptor with an antagonist IL-15 mutant/Fcg2a protein blocks delayed-type hypersensitivity. *J Immunol* 1998;**160**:5742–8.

10 Zheng XX, Sanchez-Fueyo A, Masayuki S, et al. Favorable tipping the balance between cytopathic and regulatory cells to create transplantation tolerance. *Immunity* 2003;**19**:503–14.

11 Nakakura EK, Shorthouse RA, Zheng B, et al. Long-term survival of solid organ allografts by brief anti-lymphocyte function-associated antigen-1 monoclonal antibody monotherapy. *Transplantation* 1996;**62**:547–52.

12 Vincenti F, Mendez R, Rajagopalan PR, et al. A phase I/II trial of anti-CD11a monoclonal antibody in renal transplantation [Abstract]. *Am J Transplant* 2001;**1**(Suppl 1):276.

13 Sayegh MH, Turka LA. The role of T-cell costimulatory activation pathways in transplant rejection. *N Engl J Med* 1998;**448**:1813–21.

14 Kirk AD, Tadaki DK, Celniker A, et al. Induction therapy with monoclonal antibodies specific for CD80 and CD86 delays the onset of acute renal allograft rejection in non-human primates. *Transplantation* 2001;**72**:377–84.

15 Larsen CP, Elwood ET, Alexander DZ, et al. Long-term acceptance of skin and cardiac allografts after blocking CD40 and CD28 pathways. *Nature* 1996;**381**:434–8.

16 Kirk AD, Knechtle SJ, Sollinger HW, et al. Preliminary results of the use of humanized anti-CD154 in human renal allotransplantation [Abstract]. *Am J Transplant* 2001;**1**(Suppl 1):190.

17 Kirk AD, Burkly LC, Batty DS, et al. Humanized anti-CD154 monoclonal antibody treatment prevents acute renal allograft rejection in non-human primates. *Nat Med* 1999;**5**:686–93.

18 Vincenti F, Larsen C, Durrbach A, et al. Costimulation blockade with belatacept in renal transplantation. *N Engl J Med* 2005;**353**:770–81.

19 Brinkmann V, Cyster JG, Hla T. FTY720: sphingosine 1-phosphate receptor-1 in the control of lymphocyte egress and endothelial barrier function. *Am J Transplant* 2004;**4**:1019–25.

20 Dragun D, Bohler T, Nieminen-Kelha M, et al. FTY720-induced lymphocyte homing modulates post-transplant preservation/reperfusion injury. *Kidney Int* 2004;**65**:1076–83.

21 Budde K, Schmouder RL, Nashan B, *et al*. Pharmacodynamics of single doses of the novel immunosuppressant FTY720 in stable renal transplant patients. *Am J Transplant* 2003;3:846–54.

22 Tedesco-Silva H, Mourad G, Kahan BD, *et al*. FTY720, a novel immunomodulator: efficacy and safety results from the first phase 2A study in *de novo* renal transplantation. *Transplantation* 2004;77:1826–33.

23 Vanrenterghem Y, van Hooff JP, Klinger M, *et al*. The effects of FK778 in combination with tacrolimus and steroids: a phase II multicenter study in renal transplant patients. *Transplantation* 2004;78:9–14.

24 Saemann MD, Zeyda M, Stulnig TM, *et al*. Janus kinase-3 (JAK3) inhibition: a novel immunosuppressive option for allogeneic transplantation. *Transpl Int* 2004;17:481–9.

25 Papageorgiou AC, Wikman LE. Is JAK3 a new drug target for immunomodulation-based therapies? *Trends Pharmacol Sci* 2004;25:558–62.

26 Changelian PS, Flanagan ME, Ball DJ, *et al*. Prevention of organ allograft rejection by a specific Janus kinase 3 inhibitor. *Science* 2003;302:875–8.

27 Wagner J, Evenou J-P, Zenke G, *et al*. The first class oral protein kinase C (PKC) inhibitor NVP-AEBO71 (AEB) prolongs renal allograft survival in non-human primates (NHP) and suppresses lymphocyte proliferation at safe exposures in human proof-of-concept studies. World Transplant Congress Abstract 57. *Amer J Transpl* 2006;(supplement):86.

11 Therapies for the Allosensitized Patient

Alice Peng and Stanley C. Jordan

Despite the well-documented benefits of solid organ transplantation in children, transplant frequency remains lower than desirable because of limited organ availability [1,2]. In patients with high levels of preformed antihuman leukocyte antigen (anti-HLA) antibodies (high PRA; highly-sensitized), transplant rates are even lower because of the additional immunologic barrier with increased rejection risk. Approximately 20–30% of patients on the renal transplant waiting list are classified as sensitized, meaning they have peak PRA levels > 20%, with about half of these having peak PRA levels > 80%. These antibodies result from exposure to non-self HLA antigens, usually from previous transplants, blood transfusions and/or pregnancies [3]. In addition, prior use of homograft material for repair of congenital heart defects is emerging as a key cause of allosensitization in candidates for pediatric heart transplantation. Most data on the prevalence, treatment and outcome of the sensitized transplant candidate come from the study of patients with end-stage renal disease. However, the principles can be broadly applied to other solid organ transplant candidates.

In 2000, only 2.8% of all kidney transplants were performed in patients with PRAs > 80% at the time of transplant (total number of transplants 232) [1,2], despite representing approximately 20% of the waiting list. In the last decade, the transplant rates for these patients has actually decreased by over 50%, in part because of increased sensitivity of antibody detection techniques, but also because the pool of waitlisted patients competing for the scarce donor kidney resources is much greater. If transplanted, these patients experience an increased number of rejection episodes and have poorer graft survivals [2]. The highly sensitized renal transplant candidate is destined to remain waitlisted for extended periods of time on dialysis, an added risk factor for patient and graft survival [1,2]. The financial and emotional costs of maintaining highly sensitized transplant candidates on dialysis for years are enormous. Thus, early transplantation would result in considerable cost savings, reduced morbidity and mortality, and improvement in quality of life, a goal that has been difficult to achieve until recently.

Data by Patel and Terasaki [4] demonstrated the poor outcomes for kidneys transplanted across a positive cross-match (CMX) barrier and established the basis for modern cross-match testing as a means of allocating kidneys. Sensitization is a significant barrier to both access and success in organ transplantation. The risks for transplantation can be assessed using standard assays currently available. Today, the technique(s) used to detect anti-HLA antibody include cytotoxicity (CDC) with or without antihuman globulin (AHG), enzyme-linked immunosorbent assay (ELISA) and flow cytometry (using cells and antigen-coated beads). The development of newer, more sensitive assays has led to an increased ability to define highly sensitized patients and identify donor-specific antibody (DSA). Sensitization can be defined further in terms of risk for allograft loss and antibody-mediated rejection (AMR). Treatments can then be designed to overcome AMR induced by anti-HLA antibodies. However, these treatments may interfere with antibody assessment or monitoring, depending on the protocol used.

The presence of IgG complement fixing antibody specific for donor HLA antigen (class I or II) without the addition of AHG represents an unequivocal contraindication to renal transplantation. Patients transplanted across this barrier are at a very high risk for AMR. The risk is considered moderate to high if antibody detection requires the use of an antiglobulin reagent in the cytotoxicity assay or the use of a binding assay (e.g. ELISA, flow beads). The patient's history of sensitizing events (pregnancies, transplants, transfusions), the duration and thoroughness of the antibody screening history of the patient, the sera used in the CMX (number, timing), antibody titer and potential repeat mismatches are also considered important. Additionally, post-transplant monitoring for antibody should be considered critical to assess acute (and chronic) rejection. This may be even more critical for patients who have undergone treatment to reduce their antibody levels because they are at risk for antibody rebound [5].

Until recently, no therapeutic approaches existed to deal with this problem. Currently, two protocols have emerged. These include the high-dose intravenous immunoglobulin (IVIG) protocol (Cedars-Sinai Protocol) [3,6–8] and the plasmapheresis/ CMVIg protocol (Johns Hopkins Protocol) [9,10]. Some heart transplant groups have also used cyclophosphamide in combination with IVIG.

CEDARS-SINAI PROTOCOL

High-dose IVIG

Intravenous immunoglobulin (IVIG) products were initially developed for use in patients with antibody deficiency. Patients with antibody deficiency often had concomitant autoimmune features. These were noted to improve with IVIG therapy, leading early investigators to the use of IVIG in autoimmune diseases [11]. Our early work showed that IVIG also had inhibitory antibodies to anti-HLA, which led to its use in highly sensitized patients [6,7]. IVIG products are derived from the plasma of thousands of donors. This insures that a wide diversity of antibody repertoire can be administered to patients. We also know that the Fc portion of immunoglobulin G (IgG) is critical for many of the beneficial effects seen in inflammatory and autoimmune disorders [11–15]. The Fc region interacts with Fcγ receptors on immune cells which can either upregulate or dissipate an immune response. The Fc portion of IgG also has the ability to interact with complement components and regulate inflammation by absorption of active complement components and inhibition of C3 convertase activity [11,15]. These attributes are critical to the immunomodulatory and anti-inflammatory effects of IVIG in transplantation. Normal human serum contains natural antibodies of all subclasses that are felt to be important in the maintenance of normal immune homeostasis. These antibodies have immunoregulatory effects and may have ameliorative effects on autoimmunity. They are polyreactive and may have the ability to downregulate deleterious autoantibodies and alloantibodies. IVIG contains high levels of these natural antibodies and appears to have the ability to induce them [6,11]. We first observed this effect on anti-HLA antibodies when we noted that ablation of anti-HLA antibodies by IVIG infusion could be reversed *in vitro* by the addition of dithiothreatol (DTT). Because IVIG products do not contain more than trace amounts of IgM, we hypothesized that IVIG induced IgM natural antibodies that blocked anti-HLA activity [6,8]. These natural autoantibodies may also inhibit the growth of auto- and possibly alloreactive B-cell clones [16]. IVIG inhibits maturation and function of dendritic cells and may affect T-cell activation when present [17]. All of these mechanisms, among many others, suggest that IVIG may have a role in the prevention and treatment of allograft rejection in solid organ transplant recipients.

Data from our group and others have demonstrated that IVIG therapy given to highly sensitized patients results in reduced allosensitization, reduced ischemia-reperfusion injuries, fewer acute rejection episodes and higher successful long-term allograft outcomes for cardiac and renal allograft recipients [3,6–8,18–27]. It has also been confirmed that pretreatment with IVIG results in reductions of anti-HLA antibodies, and is effective in the treatment of allograft rejection episodes [22–25]. These data suggest that pretransplant treatment with IVIG is useful in preventing post-transplant alloimmunizing events, thus reducing or eliminating the risk of antibody-mediated acute rejection episodes.

For the high-dose IVIG protocol (2 g/kg), antibody specificity may be determined by any method; however, it is necessary to identify CDC positive antibody which is often, but not always, directed against HLA. This *in vitro* test is performed using a very sensitive CDC inhibition assay that predicts which patients will benefit from IVIG therapy prior to its administration [3,6]. Currently, none of the binding assays can be used in this inhibition assay because the second step antibodies used in the assay are directed against IgG (i.e. IVIG) itself and not specifically to HLA. In these assays, all results appear positive (no inhibition) when in fact inhibition has clearly occurred by CDC. The FACS CMX test can show the effect of IVIG if the test is performed several days to 1 week after IVIG administration. The kinetics of IVIG interaction with the FACS CMX are still being worked out, but are very promising when analysis of samples is performed 1–5 days after the IVIG infusion. The *in vitro* CDC assay can predict with high reliability the *in vivo* efficacy and eventual down-modulation of antibody among patients awaiting living or deceased donor transplantation. Post-treatment, the patients can continue to be monitored using the CDC assay or after about 3–4 weeks (the half-life of IVIG) by any of the binding methods.

A summary of the Cedars-Sinai high-dose IVIG protocol was recently presented [25]. Briefly, we utilize the *in vitro* IVIG inhibition CMX test to determine if highly sensitized patients are candidates for the IVIG protocol. Patients first undergo a standard T-cell cytotoxicity assay against a random panel of 50 donors to determine PRA. If positive, we then assess the utility of IVIG by incubating IVIG with the positive PRA sera. IVIG is added 1 : 1 and in many cases the cytotoxicity is completely blocked by anti-idiotypic antibodies present in the IVIG. This *in vitro* assay provides an idea of the expected efficacy of IVIG when given *in vivo*. We have also adapted this assay to determine the efficacy of IVIG in single donor/recipient pairs who have a positive CMX. If IVIG is effective in reducing the positive CMX, we then treat the recipient with 2 g/kg IVIG (maximum dose 140 g) monthly until the CMX is negative. We usually do not give more than four doses. We have also adapted this for use in highly sensitized deceased donor transplant candidates who have been on the United Network for Organ Sharing (UNOS) list for > 5 years, have a PRA of > 50% and who receive frequent offers for kidneys from donors with whom they have a positive CMX. These patients have an *in vitro* IVIG PRA, and if suppression or inhibition of the PRA is seen with IVIG, the patients are offered IVIG 2 g/kg monthly for a total of four doses in the hope of achieving desensitization and receiving a CMX compatible kidney or other organ. To date, we have evaluated more than 100 potential recipients for both living donor and cadaver kidneys and have transplanted

70 patients using this protocol (43 living donor and 27 cadaver recipients). The mean PRA for the cadaver recipients was 83%, and nearly all patients had antibodies specific to their donors that were eliminated by IVIG therapy. The incidence of allograft rejection is 28% with a 4-year patient and graft survival of 97.5% and 84.1%, respectively. Five grafts were lost to rejection. The mean serum creatinine at 4 years was 1.4 mg/dL [25].

NIH IGO2 Study

From 1997–2000, the National Institutes of Health (NIH) conducted the IGO2 study, a controlled clinical multicenter double-blinded trial of IVIG vs. placebo in highly sensitized patients awaiting kidney transplantation. The study was designed to determine whether IVIG could reduce PRA levels and improve rates of transplantation without concomitantly increasing the risk of graft loss in this difficult to transplant group. Data from this trial was recently published [8]. Briefly, IVIG was superior to placebo in reducing anti-HLA antibody levels ($P = 0.04$, IVIG vs. placebo) and improving rates of transplantation. The 3-year follow-up shows the predicted mean time to transplantation was 4.8 years in the IVIG group vs. 10.3 years in the placebo group ($P = 0.02$). With a median follow-up of 2 years post-transplant, the viable transplants functioned normally with a mean (+ SE) serum creatinine of 1.68 ± 0.28 (IVIG) vs. 1.28 ± 0.13 mg/dL for placebo ($P = 0.29$). Allograft survival was also superior in the IVIG group at 3 years. From this multicenter double-blinded placebo-controlled trial we concluded that IVIG is superior to placebo in reducing anti-HLA antibody levels and improving transplantation rates in highly sensitized end-stage renal disease (ESRD) patients. Although more acute rejection (AR) episodes were seen in the IVIG treatment group, the 2-year allograft survival and mean serum creatinine values were similar to the placebo group. Transplant rates for highly sensitized ESRD patients awaiting kidney transplants were improved with IVIG therapy.

Thus, it appears that IVIG, alone, offers significant benefits in desensitizing highly HLA sensitized patients and improves the rates of transplantation in this difficult to transplant group without patients experiencing excessive allograft loss.

JOHNS HOPKINS PROTOCOL

In Maryland, a desensitization protocol was developed involving two modalities: plasmapheresis and IVIG or CMV hyperimmune globulin (CMVIg) [9]. Plasmapheresis is known to lower HLA-specific antibody levels in a variety of clinical settings [28–30]. The protocol involves plasmapheresis with one volume exchange every other day with low-dose CMVIg (100 mg/kg) following each plasmapheresis treatment until anti-HLA DSA is eliminated. The strength of reactivity with

the donor is used to estimate the starting titer of DSA and helps to give an indication of how many plamapheresis/CMVIg treatments will be required. This determines the practicality of the Johns Hopkins protocol for desensitization. Tacrolimus and mycophenolate mofetil are begun at standard doses at the same time. The treatment plan is further individualized according to an assessment of the patient's risk. Patients considered low risk (e.g. first transplants with pregnancy as the sensitizing event) will proceed with anti-IL-2 receptor induction antibody and triple drug immunosuppression. Those considered high risk (e.g. third transplants with multiple repeat mismatches) will have splenectomy and/or anti-CD20 antibody added to the treatment plan [10].

In general, the goal is to achieve a negative CMX prior to surgery, but approximately 20% of patients have been transplanted with a low-titer positive cytotoxic CMX with apparently good results. The DSAs are then eliminated after the transplant [10].

With this desensitization protocol, 1- and 3-year patient survival rates have been reported at 94.2% and 87.1%, respectively. The 1- and 3-year death-censored graft survival rates were 87.8% and 83.8%, respectively. The mean serum creatinine was 1.3 mg/dL at a mean follow-up of 23.4 months. No fall off in creatinine was seen with time as the mean serum creatinine at 3 years was 1.4 mg/dL. The incidence of AMR was 40.3%. Most were reported as mild, responding to reinitiation of plasmapheresis and CMVIg and pulse steroids, with creatinine values returning to baseline. Early in the development of their protocol, three graft losses were reported from severe early AMR. All were in high-risk recipients. Since adding splenectomy and/or anti-CD20 antibody to their treatment plan, they report no graft losses from AMR [10].

Post-transplant, antibody screens are performed at regular intervals and are used to trigger biopsies.

NEWER THERAPIES

Rituximab is a genetically engineered chimeric murine/human monoclonal antibody directed against the CD20 antigen found on the surface of normal and malignant pre-B and mature B cells. The antibody is an IgG1 κ immunoglobulin containing murine light- and heavy-chain variable region sequences and human constant region sequences. Rituximab is composed of two heavy chains of 451 amino acids and two light chains of 213 amino acids (based on cDNA analysis) and has an approximate molecular mass of 145 kD. Rituximab has a binding affinity for the CD20 antigen of approximately 8.0 nmol.

Rituximab was developed by IDEC Pharmaceuticals and Genentech, Inc. It was approved by the Food and Drug Administration (FDA) in 1997 for the treatment of relapsed or refractory low-grade or follicular CD20+ B-cell non-Hodgkin's lymphoma (NHL).

Rituximab binds specifically to the CD20 antigen expressed on the surface of both normal and malignant pre-B and mature B cells. The CD20 antigen is not expressed on hematopoietic stem cells, pro-B cells, normal plasma cells or other normal tissues. *In vitro* mechanism of action studies have demonstrated that the Fc portion of rituximab binds human complement and can lead to cell lysis of the targeted cell through complement-dependent cytotoxicity. Additionally, it has been demonstrated that rituximab has significant activity in assays of antibody-dependent cellular cytotoxicity [31]. More recently, rituximab has been shown to induce apoptosis *in vitro* in DHL-4, a human B-cell lymphoma line [32]. The relative extent to which these individual mechanisms account for the observed depletion of normal and malignant B cells *in vivo* is unknown. Treatment of patients with NHL, with either a 4- or 8-week course of rituximab, results in predictable and profound depletion of normal B cells from the circulation [33,34]. Reconstitution of normal B cells typically begins at 6–9 months, with the majority of patients achieving normal circulating B-cell counts by 1 year following therapy. Despite the depth and duration of normal B-cell depletion, normal serum immunoglobulin concentrations do not significantly change [33].

Rituximab has also been studied in a variety of non-malignant autoimmune disorders where B cells and autoantibodies appear to have a role in pathophysiology. Rituximab has been reported to relieve signs and symptoms of rheumatoid arthritis [35,36], lupus [37,38], immune thrombocytopenia [39] and autoimmune anemia [40].

Both our program and Johns Hopkins have begun to explore the use of anti-CD20 in desensitization. Its use is intuitive because reduction or elimination of offending B cells that make anti-HLA antibodies should have a beneficial effect. However, there are problems with this concept. First, anti-CD20 has no effect on plasma cells, which are the primary source of acute antibody production. Second, rituximab has no effect on circulating antibody levels. This might be problematic if this drug were to be used as the sole treatment. It appears that the use of a combination of agents (i.e. plasmapheresis and/or IVIG) might be the best approach for the most optimal management of the allosensitized patient. Because rituximab has little or no effect on antibody levels but has powerful deletional effects on B cells that produce the offending antibodies, it seems prudent to use it with IVIG as synergy would be expected. Our early experience has demonstrated efficacy in highly sensitized patients for whom high-dose IVIG alone has been insufficient to ameliorate a positive cross-match. At Johns Hopkins, anti-CD20 appears to be as effective as splenectomy in the treatment of high-risk patients [10]. However, this agent also poses a significant and prolonged interference with both flow cytometry and cytotoxicity assays, complicating its use in desensitization protocols. Despite this, new approaches to eliminating rituximab from CMX tests have been developed [41].

ANTIBODY-MEDIATED REJECTION

Antibody-mediated rejection (AMR) is emerging as a significant and not uncommon complication of transplantation. The development of anti-HLA antibodies (DSA) in allograft recipients is known to correlate strongly with rejection episodes following transplantation [4]. Indeed, the recognition of AMR has been aided considerably by recent advances in the technology of HLA typing and immunopathology. The ability to distinguish between anti-HLA antibody specific for donor versus third party antibody, which often appears or increases during AMR, has been a significant advancement in this area.

New onset AMR can occur in patients who have apparent negative CMXs with prospective donors prior to transplantation. The reasons for this are unknown, but likely relate to low levels of sensitization that are beyond the ability of current methodologies to recognize. In addition, the presence of antiendothelial cell antibodies may contribute significantly to AMR and are not tested for routinely [42–44]. With the development of desensitizing protocols, an increasing number of patients are being transplanted who are at extremely high risk for AMR. The patient's history of sensitizing events (pregnancies, transplants, transfusions), the duration and thoroughness of the antibody screening history of the patient, the sera used in the CMX (number, timing), antibody titer and potential repeat mismatches are also considered important. If transplanted, these patients experience an increased number of rejection episodes and exhibit poorer long-term allograft survival [4,42–44]. The incidence of AMR has increased in proportion to the use of desensitization protocols used for highly HLA sensitized patients or ABO incompatible transplants [43,44]. The development of anti-HLA antibodies (DSA) in allograft recipients is known to correlate strongly with rejection episodes following transplantation [4,42–45]. Indeed, the recognition of AMR has been aided considerably by recent advances in the technology of HLA typing and immunopathology. Refinements in CMX techniques (antihuman globulin CMX and flow cytometry) and techniques that allow precise identification of antibody specificity (ELISA and flow cytometry solid phase assay using coupled HLA antigens) allow distinction between anti-HLA antibody specific for donor versus third party antibody, which often appears or increases during AMR. This represents a significant advancement both in allocation of organs and in monitoring the success of desensitization protocols. In addition, the diagnosis of AMR has been enhanced in organs undergoing rapid functional deterioration by the emergence of C4d staining of allograft biopsy material as a sensitive indicator of complement activation that occurs in the setting of AMR [45,46].

The evaluation of a patient for AMR should include assessment of the clinical picture, allograft biopsy and testing for DSA. The ability to obtain all this information prior to treating the patient is not always possible, but certain clinical features such as the rapid onset of allograft dysfunction in a high-risk patient should alert the physician to the need for biopsy. In renal transplant biopsies, AMR may be associated with a variety of findings. In the most severe and infrequent form, arteries have fibrinoid necrosis of the walls often with infiltrating neutrophils with or without luminal thrombosis. However, it has recently been recognized that more subtle forms of AMR involve renal allografts. There may be histologic changes consistent with acute tubular necrosis, or there may be scattered neutrophils within peritubular capillary lumina, glomerular capillaries and/or the tubulo-interstitium (see Plate 11.1, facing page 224). In virtually all cases, immunostaining for the C4d complement component, a sensitive marker for AMR, discloses positive staining (> 2/4 +) in the majority of peritubular capillaries (see Plate 11.2, facing page 224). A recent modification of the Banff classification of renal transplant pathology has incorporated these observations, with AMR designated a separate class of rejection. A firm diagnosis of AMR can be made when high-risk patients present with allograft dysfunction, characteristic morphologic findings as detailed above, and the presence of DSA [45,47,48].

We have recently encountered three allosensitized kidney recipients who exhibited the classic findings of thrombotic microangiopathy (TMA) on kidney transplant biopsy with C4d positivity. Both acute vascular rejection and TMA have similar manifestations, including microangiopathic hemolysis, thrombocytopenia and renal failure. In addition, acute vascular rejection is often accompanied by neutrophilic infiltration within the subendothelial layer [49]. Traditionally, TMA has been attributed to the use of calcineurin inhibitors and more recently sirolimus. It can be difficult to differentiate between acute vascular rejection and drug-induced TMA. Mor et al. [50] described five cases of TMA occurring within 2 weeks post-transplant with features of vascular rejection. More recently, Becker et al. [51] described 27 cases of biopsy-confirmed rejection with 14 cases manifesting as TMA or endothelialitis without a cellular infiltrate. Both studies were carried out before the routine use of C4d staining. Thus far there have been no reports of AMR as evidenced by C4d staining presenting as TMA, but we suspect that some of the cases of TMA occurring early post-transplant, especially in highly-sensitized patients, are likely to be a manifestation of AMR, rather than drug effect.

Post-transplant monitoring for antibody is considered critical to assess acute (and chronic) rejection. This may be even more critical for patients who have undergone treatment to reduce their antibody levels because they are at risk for antibody rebound [43,44]. No therapeutic approaches previously existed to deal with this problem. However, three different approaches to the treatment of AMR have recently been advocated [3,6,9,51–53]. All three treatments are designed to overcome AMR induced by anti-HLA antibodies, but may interfere with antibody assessment and monitoring depending on the protocol used; plasmapheresis with low-dose CMVIg or high-dose IVIG. Recent data also suggest that therapy with anti-CD20 may also provide successful reversal of AMR [51,53].

TREATMENT OF AMR WITH HIGH-DOSE IVIG: THE CEDARS-SINAI EXPERIENCE

From our previous experiences with desensitization therapy, we found that IGIV may also have an important role in treating AMR [6,22]. This observation was subsequently confirmed by others [23]. Our early experience showed that patients who developed DSA after transplantation often had evidence of AMR that was resistant to standard immunosuppression. We found that IVIG therapy could inhibit the DSA and result in rapid improvement in AMR. We recently examined outcomes, including incidence and type of AR, patient and graft survival rates, and mean serum creatinine values in 61 highly sensitized patients with positive donor-specific CMX desensitized with IVIG for transplantation. Between January 1999 and January 2004, 61 highly sensitized patients (mean PRA: $69 \pm 23\%$) with positive DSA received kidney transplants at our center (22 deceased donor transplants, 39 living donor transplants). All patients received at least 2 g/kg IGIV (maximum: four 2 g/kg doses) prior to transplantation until a negative or acceptable CMX was obtained. Patients were divided into four groups:

1 Never biopsied ($n = 33$)
2 AR/C4d– ($n = 4$)
3 AR/C4d+ ($n = 20$) and
4 Calcineurin inhibitor (CNI) toxicity/polyoma virus + ($n = 4$).

Patients with AR/C4d– were treated with pulse steroids. Patients with AR/C4d+ were treated with pulse steroids + IVIG (2 g/kg × 1) ± plasmapheresis or thymoglobulin. The mean serum creatinines at 1, 2, 3 and 4 years were examined. At 48 months, the serum creatinines for the first three groups were similar: never biopsied (1.06 ± 0.3 mg/dL); C4d+ (1.4 ± 0.2 mg/dL); and C4d– (1.2 ± 0.3 mg/dL) ($P = $ NS). The patient and graft survival rates at 4 years are 96.5% and 84%, respectively. There were 10 graft losses, seven in the AR/C4d+ group (five from severe unresponsive AMR, two from noncompliance at > 3 years post-transplant). One graft loss was seen in the AR/C4d– group resulting from noncompliance at 2 years. Two grafts were lost in the group who had not undergone biopsy because of nonimmunologic reasons. Excluding those with early graft loss, all AR/C4d+ responded to IVIG + pulse steroid therapy with resolution and no recurrence of AMR.

In summary, AR episodes occurred in 36.5% of patients. Most (32%) were C4d+. AR/C4d+ episodes were responsive to IVIG + pulse steroid therapy in most patients (15/20; 75%); however, a subgroup of patients (AR/C4d+) (5/61; 8.1%) developed severe AMR that was resistant to all forms of therapy, including repeat thymoglobulin, IVIG and plasma exchange. Mean serum creatinine values were similar at 3 years' follow-up. These data suggest that IVIG therapy has great promise for desensitization and treatment of AMR post-transplant [54].

USE OF PLASMAPHERESIS AND IVIG (OR CMVIG) FOR TREATMENT OF AMR

Other approaches to the treatment of AMR include the use of plasmapheresis, usually in combination with low-dose IVIG or CMVIg. This has been accepted as an alternative therapy for C4d+ AMR at many institutions [9,52,55–58]. Rocha et al. [57] treated patients with AMR using plasmapheresis + IVIG. At 1 year, the graft survival rate (81% vs. 84%; $P = NS$) was similar to patients treated for cell-mediated rejection. Despite data showing very poor outcomes in patients with C4d+ AMR episodes [4,42–46], these authors conclude that plasmapheresis + IVIG was efficacious for treatment of AMR. Shah et al. [58] showed that plasmapheresis + thymoglobulin was also very effective in reversing AMR episodes in seven patients. The authors used approximately seven plasmapheresis treatments over the course of 5–10 days. Serum creatinine values returned to baseline in most patients (1.0 ± 1.2 vs. 2 ± 1.4 mg/dL; $P < 0.007$) (post- vs. pretreatment values). One graft loss was seen. These authors conclude that in this small series of patients, thymoglobulin + plasmapheresis is effective in reversing AMR episodes. They theorized that the beneficial effects of thymoglobulin were because of depletion of B cells, although no data were given. Lennertz et al. [55] reported four patients with C4d+ AMR who were treated with plasmapheresis + IVIG. Three of four responded, with one graft loss. Gloor et al. [56] reported 6/6 patients with AMR who responded to plasmapheresis + IVIG. By far the most extensive and meaningful experience with treatment of AMR using plasmapheresis + CMVIg is from the Johns Hopkins University group [9]. With over 3 years of follow-up on 66 patients treated, the patient survival rate is 90.4%, graft survival rate is 78.3% and the mean serum creatinine value is 2.0 ± 1.2 mg/dL. These data suggest that the use of CMVIg + plasmapheresis is beneficial in reversal of AMR episodes.

USE OF ANTI-CD20 MONOCLONAL ANTIBODY IN TREATMENT OF AMR

Rituximab is a relatively new player in the treatment of AMR. Several investigators have begun initial investigations into the use of rituximab for treatment of AMR. The largest series to date is that of Becker et al. [51]. These investigators examined the utility of rituximab in treatment of AMR. The patients were not homogenous, but all had steroid-resistant AR, and 22/27 had been treated with plasmapheresis and

antilymphocyte antibodies. Despite this, the investigators found that the mean serum creatinine values decreased dramatically after rituximab therapy (5.6 ± 1.0 to 0.95 ± 0.7; $P < 0.001$). Five patients lost their grafts (14–688 days post-treatment). After 2 years' follow-up, death censored graft survival was 85%; 22/27 grafts survived. Montgomery et al. [53] reported similar, but not as dramatic, results in a group of 20 patients who had AMR that was resistant to plasmapheresis + CMVIg therapy. Thus, rituximab appears to be a promising new therapy for treatment of AMR. Clearly, more investigations are needed, and the synergistic effects of rituximab used in combination with plasmapheresis and/or IVIG need to be carefully investigated.

NON-HLA ANTIBODY-MEDIATED REJECTION

Recently, Dragun et al. [59] have described a subgroup of kidney transplant recipients with refractory vascular rejection who presented with malignant hypertension and were found to have angiotensin II type 1 receptor antibodies and no evidence of anti-HLA antibodies. Biopsies revealed endarteritis or fibrinoid necrosis with variable staining for C4d but intense staining for tissue factor. Antiendothelial cell antibodies have been previously implicated in the development of acute humoral rejection [60,61]; however, their heterogeneity has made the determination of their relevance difficult. AT1-receptor antibodies may have similarities to antiendothelial cell antibodies because endothelial cells contain AT1 receptors. It is believed that activation of the receptor would activate a signaling cascade mimicking the action of angiotensin II, resulting in damage to the allograft. The authors advocate the use of therapies to remove antibody (such as plasmapheresis and IVIG) and well as blockade of its effects (through blockade of angiotensin receptors with medications such as losartan) [59]. The presence of non-HLA antibodies may explain some of the differences seen in the post-transplant course of allosensitized kidney transplant recipients despite apparent good responses to the desensitization regimens.

CONCLUSIONS

The number of sensitized patients on the kidney transplant waiting list continues to grow. The past few years have seen significant advances in our ability to overcome this immunologic barrier to transplantation. Three novel and effective therapies have evolved: IVIG, plasmapheresis and anti-CD20, for both desensitization of the allosensitized patient and treatment of post-transplant antibody-mediated rejection. Several protocols currently exist, but currently no preferential strategy has emerged. It appears that the optimal treatment, especially for very high-risk allosensitized patients or severe forms of AMR, may involve a combination of the above therapies. This should improve access to transplantation for those patients unable to be transplanted because of their sensitization to HLA antigens and impact the success of transplants of this high immunologic risk population. More work is clearly required in this area, and longer term data regarding patient and graft outcomes are needed, but there is now growing hope for successful transplantation of the very difficult allosensitized patient.

REFERENCES

1 Meier-Kriesche HU, Port FK, Ojo AO, *et al.* Effect of waiting time on renal transplant outcome. *Kidney Int* 2000;**58**:1311–7.

2 Kaplan B, Schold J, Meier-Kriesche HU. Overview of large database analysis in renal transplantation. *Am J Transplant* 2003;**3**:1052–6.

3 Jordan S, Cunningham-Rundles C, McEwan R. Utility of intravenous immune globulin in kidney transplantation: efficacy, safety, and cost implications. *Am J Transplant* 2003;**3**:653–64.

4 Patel R, Terasaki PI. Significance of the positive crossmatch test in kidney transplantation. *N Engl J Med* 1969;**280**:735–9.

5 Lee PC, Terasaki PI, Takemoto SK, *et al.* All chronic rejection failures of kidney transplants were preceded by the development of HLA antibodies. *Transplantation* 2002;**74**:1192–4.

6 Tyan DB, Li VA, Czer L, Trento A, Jordan SC. Intravenous immunoglobulin suppression of HLA alloantibody in highly sensitized transplant candidates and transplantation with a histoincompatible organ. *Transplantation* 1994;**57**:553–62.

7 Jordan SC, Tyan DB. Intravenous gamma globulin (IVIG) inhibits lymphocytotoxic antibody *in vitro* [Abstract]. *J Am Soc Nephrol* 1991;**2**:803.

8 Jordan SC, Tyan D, Stablein D, *et al.* Evaluation of intravenous immunoglobulin as an agent to lower allosensitization and improve transplantation in highly sensitized adult patients with end-stage renal disease: report of the NIH IG02 trial. *J Am Soc Nephrol* 2004;**15**:3256–62.

9 Montgomery RA, Zachary AA, Racusen LC, *et al.* Plasmapheresis and intravenous immune globulin provides effective rescue therapy for refractory humoral rejection and allows kidneys to be successfully transplanted into cross-match-positive recipients. *Transplantation* 2000;**70**:887–95.

10 Montgomery RA, Cooper M, Kraus E, *et al.* Renal transplantation at the Johns Hopkins Comprehensive Transplant Center. *Clin Transpl* 2003:199–213.

11 Kazatchkine MD, Kaveri SV. Immunomodulation of autoimmune and inflammatory diseases with intravenous immune globulin. *N Engl J Med* 2001;**345**:747–55.

12 Samuelsson A, Towers TL, Ravetch JV. Anti-inflammatory activity of IVIG mediated through the inhibitory Fc receptor [see comment]. *Science* 2001;**291**:484–6.

13 Magee JC, Collins BH, Harland RC, *et al.* Immunoglobulin prevents complement-mediated hyperacute rejection in swine-to-primate xenotransplantation. *J Clin Invest* 1995;**96**:2404–12.

14 Toyoda M, Pao A, Petrosian A, Jordan SC. Pooled human gammaglobulin modulates surface molecule expression and induces apoptosis in human B cells. *Am J Transplant* 2003;**3**:156–66.

15 Lutz HU, Stammler P, Bianchi V, *et al.* Intravenously applied IgG stimulates complement attenuation in a complement-dependent autoimmune disease at the amplifying C3 convertase level. *Blood* 2004;**103**:465–72.

16 Hayakawa K, Asano M, Shinton SA, *et al.* Positive selection of natural autoreactive B cells. *Science* 1999;**285**:113–6.

17 Bayry J, Lacroix-Desmazes S, Carbonneil C, *et al.* Inhibition of maturation and function of dendritic cells by intravenous immunoglobulin. *Blood* 2003;**101**:758–65.

18 Glotz D, Haymann JP, Niaudet P, Lang P, Druet P, Bariety J. Successful kidney transplantation of immunized patients after desensitization with normal human polyclonal immunoglobulins. *Transplant Proc* 1995;**27**:1038–9.

19 Glotz D, Antoine C, Julia P, *et al.* Intravenous immunoglobulins and transplantation for patients with anti-HLA antibodies. *Transplant Int* 2004;**17**:1–8.

20 McIntyre JA, Higgins N, Britton R, *et al.* Utilization of intravenous immunoglobulin to ameliorate alloantibodies in a highly sensitized patient with a cardiac assist device awaiting heart transplantation. Fluorescence-activated cell sorter analysis. *Transplantation* 1996;**62**:691–3.

21 De Marco T, Damon LE, Colombe B, Keith F, Chatterjee K, Garovoy MR. Successful immunomodulation with intravenous gamma globulin and cyclophosphamide in an alloimmunized heart transplant recipient. *J Heart Lung Transplant* 1997;**16**:360–5.

22 Jordan SC, Quartel AW, Czer LS, *et al.* Posttransplant therapy using high-dose human immunoglobulin (intravenous gammaglobulin) to control acute humoral rejection in renal and cardiac allograft recipients and potential mechanism of action. *Transplantation* 1998;**66**:800–5.

23 Casadei DH, del C Rial M, Opelz G, *et al.* A randomized and prospective study comparing treatment with high-dose intravenous immunoglobulin with monoclonal antibodies for rescue of kidney grafts with steroid-resistant rejection. *Transplantation* 2001;**71**:53–8.

24 Luke PP, Scantlebury VP, Jordan ML, *et al.* Reversal of steroid- and anti-lymphocyte antibody-resistant rejection using intravenous immunoglobulin (IVIG) in renal transplant recipients. *Transplantation* 2001;**72**:419–22.

25 Jordan SC, Vo A, Bunnapradist S, *et al.* Intravenous immune globulin treatment inhibits crossmatch positivity and allows for successful transplantation of incompatible organs in living-donor and cadaver recipients. *Transplantation* 2003;**76**:631–6.

26 Toyoda M, Zhang X, Petrosian A, Galera OA, Wang SJ, Jordan SC. Modulation of immunoglobulin production and cytokine mRNA expression in peripheral blood mononuclear cells by intravenous immunoglobulin. *J Clin Immunol* 1994;**14**:178–89.

27 Marchalonis JJ, Kaymaz H, Dedeoglu F, Schluter SF, Yocum DE, Edmundson AB. Human autoantibodies reactive with synthetic autoantigens from T-cell receptor beta chain. *Proc Natl Acad Sci USA* 1992;**89**:3325–9.

28 Taube DH, Williams DG, Cameron JS, *et al.* Renal transplantation after removal and prevention of resynthesis of HLA antibodies. *Lancet* 1984;**1**:824–8.

29 Fauchald P, Leivestad T, Albrechtsen D, Willassen Y, Jacobsen A, Flatmark A. Plasma exchange and immunoadsorption prior to renal transplantation in allosensitized patients. *Transplant Proc* 1990;**22**:149–50.

30 Hodge EE, Klingman LL, Koo AP, *et al*. Pretransplant removal of anti-HLA antibodies by plasmapheresis and continued suppression on cyclosporine-based therapy after heart-kidney transplant. *Transplant Proc* 1994;26:2750–1.

31 Reff ME, Carner K, Chambers KS, *et al*. Depletion of B cells *in vivo* by a chimeric mouse human monoclonal antibody to CD20. *Blood* 1994;83:435–45.

32 Piro LD, White CA, Grillo-Lopez AJ, *et al*. Extended rituximab (anti-CD20 monoclonal antibody) therapy for relapsed or refractory low-grade or follicular non-Hodgkin's lymphoma [see comment]. *Ann Oncol* 1999;10:655–61.

33 Maloney DG, Grillo-Lopez AJ, White CA, *et al*. IDEC-C2B8 (rituximab) anti-CD20 monoclonal antibody therapy in patients with relapsed low-grade non-Hodgkin's lymphoma. *Blood* 1997;90:2188–95.

34 McLaughlin P, Grillo-Lopez AJ, Link BK, *et al*. Rituximab chimeric anti-CD20 monoclonal antibody therapy for relapsed indolent lymphoma: half of patients respond to a four-dose treatment program. *J Clin Oncol* 1998;16:2825–33.

35 Edwards JC, Szczepanski L, Szechinski J, *et al*. Efficacy of B-cell-targeted therapy with rituximab in patients with rheumatoid arthritis [see comment]. *N Engl J Med* 2004;350:2572–81.

36 Albert D, Khan K, Stansberry S, Tsai D, Eisenberg R. A phase I trial of rituximab (anti-CD20) for treatment of systemic lupus erythematosus [poster]. American College of Rheumatology Annual Scientific Meeting 2003: LB9. 518.

37 Anolik JH, Campbell D, Felgar RE, *et al*. The relationship of FcγRIIIa genotype to degree of B cell depletion by rituximab in the treatment of systemic lupus erythematosus. *Arthritis Rheum* 2003;48:455–9.

38 Leandro MJ, Edwards JC, Cambridge G. Clinical outcome in 22 patients with rheumatoid arthritis treated with B lymphocyte depletion [see comment]. *Ann Rheum Dis* 2002;61:883–8.

39 Cooper N, Stasi R, Cunningham-Rundles S, *et al*. The efficacy and safety of B-cell depletion with anti-CD20 monoclonal antibody in adults with chronic immune thrombocytopenic purpura. *Br J Haematol* 2004;125:232–9.

40 Gupta N, Kavuru S, Patel D, *et al*. Rituximab-based chemotherapy for steroid-refractory autoimmune hemolytic anemia of chronic lymphocytic leukemia. *Leukemia* 2002;16:2092–5.

41 Bearden CM, Agarwal A, Book BK, *et al*. Pronase treatment facilitates alloantibody flow cytometric and cytotoxic crossmatching in the presence of rituximab. *Hum Immunol* 2004;65:803–9.

42 Fredrich R, Toyoda M, Czer LS, *et al*. The clinical significance of antibodies to human vascular endothelial cells after cardiac transplantation. *Transplantation* 1999;67:385–91.

43 Montgomery RA, Hardy MA, Jordan SC, *et al*. Consensus opinion from the antibody working group on the diagnosis, reporting, and risk assessment for antibody-mediated rejection and desensitization protocols. *Transplantation* 2004;78:181–5.

44 Takemoto SK, Zeevi A, Feng S, *et al*. National conference to assess antibody-mediated rejection in solid organ transplantation. *Am J Transplant* 2004;4:1033–41.

45 Bohmig GA, Exner M, Habicht A, *et al*. Capillary C4d deposition in kidney allografts: a specific marker of alloantibody-dependent graft injury [see comment]. *J Am Soc Nephrol* 2002;13:1091–9.

46 Racusen LC, Colvin RB, Solez K, *et al*. Antibody-mediated rejection criteria – an addition to the Banff 97 classification of renal allograft rejection. *Am J Transplant* 2003;3:708–14.

47 Mauiyyedi S, Pelle PD, Saidman S, *et al*. Chronic humoral rejection: identification of antibody-mediated chronic renal allograft rejection by C4d deposits in peritubular capillaries. *J Am Soc Nephrol* 2001;12:574–82.

48 Onitsuka S, Yamaguchi Y, Tanabe K, Takahashi K, Toma H. Peritubular capillary deposition of C4d complement fragment in ABO-incompatible renal transplantation with humoral rejection. *Clin Transpl* 1999;13(Suppl 1):33–7.

49 Singh N, Gayowski T, Marino IR. Hemolytic uremic syndrome in solid-organ transplant recipients [see comment]. *Transplant Int* 1996;9:68–75.

50 Mor E, Lustig S, Tovar A, *et al*. Thrombotic microangiopathy early after kidney transplantation: hemolytic uremic syndrome or vascular rejection? *Transplant Proc* 2000;32:686–7.

51 Becker YT, Becker BN, Pirsch JD, Sollinger HW. Rituximab as treatment for refractory kidney transplant rejection. *Am J Transplant* 2004;4:996–1001.

52 Schweitzer EJ, Wilson JS, Fernandez-Vina M, *et al*. A high panel-reactive antibody rescue protocol for cross-match-positive live donor kidney transplants. *Transplantation* 2000;70:1531–6.

53 Montgomery R, Simpkins CE, Zachary AA, *et al*. Anti-CD20 rescue therapy for kidneys undergoing antibody-mediated rejection [Abstract]. *Am J Transplant* 2004;4:258.

54 Jordan SC, Vo A, Nast C, *et al*. A four year follow-up of rejection patterns, treatment and outcomes in highly-HLA sensitized crossmatch positive patients transplanted with IVIG desensitization [Abstract]. *Am J Transplant* 2004;4:256.

55 Lennertz A, Fertmann J, Thomae R, *et al*. Plasmapheresis in C4d-positive acute humoral rejection following kidney transplantation: a review of 4 cases. *Therap Apher Dial* 2003;7:529–35.

56 Gloor JM, DeGoey SR, Pineda AA, *et al*. Overcoming a positive crossmatch in living-donor kidney transplantation. *Am J Transplant* 2003;3:1017–23.

57 Rocha PN, Butterly DW, Greenberg A, *et al*. Beneficial effect of plasmapheresis and intravenous immunoglobulin on renal allograft survival of patients with acute humoral rejection. *Transplantation* 2003;75:1490–5.

58 Shah A, Nadasdy T, Arend L, *et al*. Treatment of C4d-positive acute humoral rejection with plasmapheresis and rabbit polyclonal antithymocyte globulin. *Transplantation* 2004;77:1399–405.

59 Dragun D, Muller DN, Brasen JH, *et al*. Angiotensin II type 1-receptor activating antibodies in renal-allograft rejection [see comment]. *N Engl J Med* 2005;352:558–69.

60 Paul LC, Baldwin WM 3rd, van Es LA. Vascular endothelial alloantigens in renal transplantation. *Transplantation* 1985;40:117–23.

61 van der Woude FJ, Deckers JG, Mallat MJ, *et al*. Tissue antigens in tubulointerstitial and vascular rejection. *Kidney Int Suppl* 1995;52:S11–3.

12 Infections Post-Transplantation

Michael Green and Marian G. Michaels

Solid organ transplantation is now accepted therapy for end-stage disease of the kidneys, liver, heart and lungs. Newer procedures, including intestinal and multivisceral transplantation, are also increasingly performed. Accordingly, an expanding number of immunosuppressed children are at risk of developing infection after organ transplantation. This chapter provides an overview of the infectious complications associated with these procedures in children.

PREDISPOSING FACTORS

Factors predisposing to infection after organ transplantation can be divided into those that exist prior to transplant and those secondary to intraoperative and post-transplant activities (Table 12.1).

Table 12.1 Predisposing factors for infection following solid organ transplantation in children.

Pretransplant factors
Underlying disease
Malnutrition
Organ to be transplanted
Age of patient
Previous exposures to infectious agents
Immunization history

Intraoperative factors
Type of surgical reconstruction
Duration of transplant surgery
Exposure to blood products
Technical problems
Exposure to donor-transmitted pathogens

Post-transplant factors
Immunosuppression
Technical problems
Indwelling cannulas
Nosocomial exposures
Community exposures

Pretransplant factors

The organ undergoing transplantation is the most important determinant of the location of infection, especially during the first three postoperative months [1]. For example, the chest, abdomen and urinary tract are the most common sites of infection after thoracic, liver and kidney transplantation, respectively. Explanations for these site-specific infections include local ischemic injury and bleeding, as well as potential soilage with contaminated material.

The underlying illnesses leading to organ failure may also be associated with an increased risk of developing infection after organ transplantation. For example, a history of cystic fibrosis predisposes to pseudomonal and fungal infections after lung transplantation. A history of palliative surgery prior to the transplant increases the technical difficulty of the transplant procedure, enhancing the risk of developing a post-transplant infection [2]. Severity of disease at the time of transplantation is associated with an increased risk of postoperative morbidity and mortality [3]. Similarly, long-standing malnutrition predisposes children to infections before and after transplantation. Attempts to correct nutritional deficits with parenteral alimentation carry attendant risks of catheter-associated infection. Finally, mechanical ventilation while awaiting transplantation increases the risk of colonization and disease with nosocomial pathogens, many of which are resistant to multiple antimicrobial agents.

Age is an important determinant of both susceptibility to certain pathogens and severity of expression of infection after transplantation. Young children undergoing these procedures can experience moderate to severe disease with certain viral (e.g. respiratory syncytial virus [RSV], parainfluenza virus) or bacterial pathogens (coagulase-negative staphylococci) compared with the milder symptoms observed in older children or adult recipients. In contrast, other pathogens, such as *Cryptococcus neoformans*, are rarely found before young adulthood. Age is also associated with severity of infection with cytomegalovirus (CMV) and Epstein–Barr virus (EBV), because primary infections after transplantation (which are more likely to occur in young children) are more severe than those resulting from reactivation [4]. Younger age at the time of transplant has also been associated with a significantly increased rate of infections during the first few years following transplantation [5]. Finally, young children who are not fully immunized remain susceptible to vaccine-preventable infections, or will receive vaccination after transplantation, at a time when their ability to mount an immune response may be hampered [6].

Intraoperative factors

Transplant recipients are at risk of acquiring potential pathogens from their donors that can be active or latent at the time of organ harvesting. Examples of this include CMV [7,8], EBV, *Toxoplasma* and *Histoplasma* spp., hepatitis B and C viruses, and human immunodeficiency virus (HIV). Of these, the use of a donor with either hepatitis B surface antigenemia or HIV seropositivity is contraindicated. The use of hepatitis C-positive donors is controversial, but is usually avoided unless the recipient is also hepatitis C positive. Another donor-related concern is the presence of bacteria or fungi colonizing the respiratory tract of a lung donor; such organisms can cause infection in the postoperative period [9]. Similarly, acute, unrecognized, bacteremia or viremia at the time of organ harvesting may be an additional risk to the recipient.

Operative factors unique to each solid organ transplant procedure can predispose to infectious complications. For example, the type of biliary reconstruction used in liver transplantation has been shown to influence the likelihood of developing an infectious complication after this procedure [10]. Perioperative events can also predispose to infection after transplantation. Injury to the phrenic, vagal or recurrent laryngeal nerves during surgery affect pulmonary toilet and predispose to pneumonia after lung transplantation [11]. Ischemic injury to the allograft during the transplant procedure can reduce its viability and increase the risk of infection. Additional factors, including prolonged operative time, contamination of the operative field and bleeding at or near surgical sites also predispose to postoperative infections.

Post-transplant factors

Immunosuppression is the major risk factor for infection following transplantation. Immunosuppressive regimens continue to evolve in an attempt to achieve more specific control of rejection with the least impairment of immunity. However, all current immunosuppressive regimens interfere with the host's ability to fight infection. Clinical studies of newer immunosuppressive regimens should assess infectious complications so that the full complement of risks can be understood. Treatment of rejection potentially increases the risk for infection. In particular, the use of antilymphocyte preparations, especially OKT3, has been associated with an enhanced risk of infection [12].

Technical problems with the transplant surgery create major risks for infectious complications following transplantation. Examples of technical problems associated with infections include thrombosis of the hepatic artery predisposing to hepatic abscesses and bacteremia following liver transplantation [13], the presence of vesicoureteric reflux predisposing to graft pyelonephritis in renal transplant recipients [11,14], and mediastinal bleeding requiring subsequent re-exploration predisposing to mediastinitis and sepsis in thoracic transplant recipients [7].

The prolonged use of indwelling cannulas is another important risk factor for infection following transplantation. The presence of central venous catheters, uretheral catheters and prolonged endotracheal intubation is associated with the development of bacteremia, urinary tract infections (UTI) and pneumonia, respectively.

Nosocomial exposures constitute the final group of post-transplant risk factors. All transplant recipients are at risk of developing infection with transfusion-associated pathogens. Children undergoing transplantation during the winter months are often nosocomially exposed to common viruses (e.g. RSV, rotavirus). The presence in the hospital of areas that have heavy contamination with pathogenic fungi, such as *Aspergillus* sp., increases the risk of invasive fungal disease in these patients. Finally, nosocomial transmission of multiply resistant bacteria predisposes to infection with these important pathogens.

TIMING OF INFECTIONS

The timing of specific infections is generally predictable, regardless of the type of organ transplanted. Most clinically important infections occur within the first 180 days following transplantation. Risk periods can be divided into three intervals: early (0–30 days after transplantation), intermediate (30–180 days) and late (more than 180 days). In addition, some infections can occur throughout the post-transplant course. While overlap can exist, these divisions provide a useful framework for the approach to a patient with fever after transplantation and serve as a guide to the differential diagnosis.

Early infections (0–30 days)

Early infections are usually associated with the presence of pre-existing conditions or complications of surgery. Bacteria or yeast are the most frequent pathogens recovered in this time period [7,15]. As many as half or more of all bacterial infections developing after transplantation occur during the early post-transplant period [7]. Involvement of superficial or deep surgical wound sites are the most common location of infection during this time period. Technical difficulties, particularly those resulting in anastomotic stenosis, are important risk factors for the development of invasive infection in the first month after most types of organ transplantation.

Intermediate period (31–180 days)

The intermediate period is the typical time of onset of opportunistic infections, including those transmitted from the donor (either organ or blood product) or associated with reactivated viruses. During this period, CMV infection peaks [7,8] and EBV-associated post-transplant lymphoproliferative disorders (PTLD) [16,17], *Pneumocystis jiroveci* pneumonia (PCP) [18,19] and toxoplasmosis may become manifest [20].

Late infections (more than 180 days)

Only limited data on late infectious complications have been published. In general, rates and severity of infection in children more than 6 months after transplantation are similar to those observed in otherwise healthy children [5]. This is most likely explained by the fact that the majority of pediatric transplant recipients are maintained on only low levels of chronic immunosuppression. However, chronic or recurrent infections occur in a subset of transplant recipients who have an uncorrected anatomic or functional abnormality (e.g. vesicoureteric reflux, biliary stricture). In addition, patients with chronic rejection after lung transplantation, manifest as bronchiolitis obliterans, are frequently infected *Pseudomonas* spp., *Stenotrophomonas* and *Aspergillus* [9,21]. Finally, PTLD continues to present in the late time period.

BACTERIAL AND FUNGAL INFECTION

With the exception of infections related to the use of indwelling catheters, sites of bacterial infection tend to occur at or near the transplanted organ; recovery of bacteria with multiple antibiotic resistance is common. Knowledge of surveillance cultures as well as local antimicrobial resistance patterns help guide empiric antibiotic therapy in these patients.

Renal transplantation

Septicemia originating from the urinary tract, the lower respiratory tract or the transplant wound account for most life-threatening infections in the first month after renal transplantation [11]. UTI, especially pyelonephritis, is the most common infectious complication, accounting for up to half of episodes [22]. Gram-negative organisms predominate [22,23]. As many as 40% of children undergoing renal transplantation will develop a UTI; however, severity appears to decrease in association with time from the transplant procedure [5]. Reportedly, one-third of pediatric renal transplant recipients experience recurrent UTI [24]. Of interest, the incidence may be decreased with the use of uteroneocystostomy and prophylactic use of trimethoprim-sulfamethoxazole (TMP-SMZ) [14].

As in immunocompetent children, the development of otitis media and sinusitis as a complication of viral upper respiratory tract infections occurs frequently in children undergoing renal transplantation [5]. However, neither the rate nor the severity of these infections appear to differ from those expected in otherwise healthy children.

Fungal infections are infrequent after renal transplantation. When present, *Candida* spp. predominate, with the urinary tract being the most common site [11]. However, these patients are also at risk of infection with opportunistic fungi such as *Aspergillus* spp. [24].

Liver transplantation

Bacterial and fungal infections are a frequent and early problem following liver transplantation [25,26]. Bacteremia occurs frequently in association with intra-abdominal infection or with use of central venous catheters, but it can occur without an obvious source. Enteric Gram-negative organisms account for more than half of episodes. Bacterial infections involving the abdomen or wound are common in most series and are frequently associated with a technical complication of surgery [27]. Infectious complications of the transplanted liver also occur. Historically, the most important bacterial complication in children undergoing liver transplantation is the development of a hepatic abscess, associated with hepatic artery or portal vein thrombosis, which is often accompanied by persistent bacteremia. Aggressive antimicrobial therapy and percutaneous drainage of the abscess are necessary but retransplantation may be required for survival. Improved surgical technique and aggressive surveillance for the presence of hepatic artery stenosis and thrombosis, potentially allowing for their correction, have virtually eliminated this complication at our center.

Ascending cholangitis is common after liver transplantation and is usually associated with biliary stricture or obstruction [26]. Presentation of infections associated with the biliary tree appeared an average of 7 weeks post-transplant in one recent series [27]. This diagnosis is typically made on clinical grounds in a patient with fever and biochemical evidence of biliary inflammation. Enteric Gram-negative bacteria and enterococcal species are the predominate pathogens. The clinical picture of cholangitis can be identical to that of acute graft rejection. Accordingly, liver biopsy should be performed to differentiate between these processes. A cholangiogram should be undertaken to assess the status of the biliary tract for patients with proven cholangitis.

Candida spp. are the most common fungal pathogens, and infection is usually associated with an intra-abdominal focus or indwelling catheter. Episodes of invasive aspergillosis occur infrequently but can be fatal.

Intestinal transplantation

Only a limited number of children have received intestinal transplants. Many have undergone combined liver-intestinal or multivisceral transplantation. Experience suggests that bacterial infection occurs frequently in these patients [28,29]. Bacteremia, which may be explained in part by disruption of the mucosal barrier associated with harvest injury or rejection, is a frequent finding [28,29]. Coagulase-negative staphylococci, enterococci and Gram-negative enteric bacteria account for most episodes in our series. Intra-abdominal and wound infections occur in more than one-third of patients and are typically diagnosed during the first month after transplantation.

Heart transplantation

Infectious complications, excluding CMV and EBV-associated PTLD, account for 15% of deaths within the first year after cardiac transplantation [30,31]. Bacterial infection of the lower respiratory tract and bloodstream are the most common sites of infection in pediatric heart transplant recipients [7,15,32,33–35]. Mediastinitis is another important infection following thoracic transplantation, particularly if re-exploration of the chest is required. Pathogens associated with mediastinitis include *Staphylococcus aureus* and Gram-negative enteric species. Invasive pneumococcal infection is also noted to occur more frequently after heart transplantation and is not explained by associated asplenia. Risk factors appear to include early age at transplantation, African-American race and idiopathic dilated cardiomyopathy [34].

Fungal infections, while less common than bacterial infections, can be severe after heart transplantation. *Candida* spp. predominate, particularly early after transplantation [36]. However, serious *Aspergillus* infection also occurs [32].

Infants undergoing heart transplantation represent a unique population and appear to be at increased risk for developing serious bacterial or fungal disease. Backer *et al.* [37] reported four serious bacterial infections in 19 infants who underwent heart transplantation. The Pediatric Heart Transplant Study Group also identified infant recipients to be at increased risk for bacterial infections [15].

Heart-lung and lung transplantation

Recipients of lung transplantation are at high risk of developing bacterial infection of the respiratory tract. Pneumonia, the most important infectious complication, may be difficult to diagnose definitively as differentiation between chronic airway colonization and lower respiratory tract infection can be problematic. Gram-negative pathogens and *S. aureus*, often multiply resistant to antimicrobial agents, are frequently recovered in the presence or absence of infection. Radiographic abnormalities are nearly universal with both pneumonia and graft rejection. Accordingly, bronchoalveolar lavage or transbronchial biopsy is often required to help distinguish causes.

Children undergoing lung transplantation because of cystic fibrosis experience a particularly high rate of infectious complications. They usually are colonized with *Pseudomonas* or *Aspergillus* spp. The development of bacteremia resulting from organisms that were present prior to lung transplantation has been frequently reported after transplant in this patient population [21,38,39]. Pre-emptive antibiotic treatment directed against colonizing bacteria and fungi has reduced this complication. However, because of the importance and difficulty in treating some of these bacterial complications, most centers have established protocols for evaluating candidates for the presence of *Burkholderia cepacia* and other multiresistant bacterial organisms prior to transplantation. As the genetics of *B. cepacia* complex becomes more rigorously evaluated, it has been recognized that certain species appear to be more virulent. Colonization with this pathogen is a relative contraindication to transplantation at some centers. Results of synergy testing for multiresistant bacteria from reference laboratories have assisted in the successful transplantation of some patients harboring microbes that would otherwise be considered relative or absolute contraindications to transplantation.

VIRAL INFECTIONS

Viral pathogens, especially herpesviruses, are a major source of morbidity and mortality following organ transplantation. Patterns of disease associated with individual viral pathogens are generally similar among all transplant recipients. However, frequency, mode of presentation and relative severity can differ according to type of organ transplanted and serologic status of the recipient.

Cytomegalovirus

CMV remains one of the most common and important causes of viral infection after solid organ transplantation. Infection can be asymptomatic or symptomatic and may be caused by primary infection, reactivation of latent infection or superinfection with a different strain in a previously seropositive patient. Prior to the use of prophylaxis against CMV, the incidence in children was reported as 22% after kidney [40], 40% after liver [12] and 26% after thoracic [7] organ transplantation. Use of ganciclovir prophylaxis and or pre-emptive treatment has resulted in decreased rate and severity of CMV disease.

Primary CMV infection, typically acquired from an organ donor, is associated with the greatest degree of morbidity and mortality. Reactivation of, or superinfection with, CMV tends to result in milder illness [4]. Patients treated with unusually high doses of immunosuppressants, especially anti-lymphocyte products, experience an increased rate of CMV disease regardless of previous immunity [7,10,40].

In the absence of prophylaxis, symptomatic CMV disease typically manifests 1–3 months after transplantation. The timing of the onset of CMV disease can be affected by the use of preventive strategies; a delay of 1–3 months following discontinuation of prophylaxis has been observed. CMV disease is associated with a characteristic constellation of fever (which may be high grade, prolonged and hectic) and hematologic abnormalities (including leukopenia, atypical lymphocytosis and thrombocytopenia). Disseminated CMV disease is manifest by visceral organ involvement; common sites include the gastrointestinal tract, liver and lungs. The site of involvement can vary according to the type of transplant. Unlike patients with the acquired immunodeficiency syndrome (AIDS), CMV chorioretinitis is rare in organ transplant recipients. Prior to the availability of ganciclovir, fatal disseminated CMV disease occurred in 4%, 14% and 19% of infected children after kidney [40], heart or heart-lung [7], and liver transplantation [12], respectively. Fortunately, mortality resulting from CMV disease has become rare in the ganciclovir era.

Diagnosis of CMV disease is confirmed by a positive viral culture, pp65 antigenemia assay or by detecting the presence of CMV DNA in the blood from a patient with a compatible clinical syndrome. However, the clinician must be aware that results of viral cultures of the urine and even bronchoalveolar lavage specimens are difficult to interpret because patients frequently shed CMV asymptomatically in these secretions. Similarly, the presence of pp65 antigen and CMV DNA in the blood can be misleading, as these assays are often positive in asymptomatic patients. Specificity may be improved by quantitative determination of the pp65 antigen or CMV DNA. Because of this lack of specificity of cultures and these assays, histologic examination of involved organs to confirm the presence of CMV is critical when the diagnosis of invasive CMV disease is being considered.

Antiviral agents with activity against CMV (e.g. ganciclovir and foscarnet) have dramatically improved the survival of transplant recipients with CMV disease. For clinical CMV disease (fever with cytopenia or visceral disease), ganciclovir therapy is given in conjunction with reduction of immunosuppression unless evidence of rejection is present. Clinical response usually occurs 5–7 days after treatment is begun. Recent evidence suggests that patients should be treated until they demonstrate clearance of CMV load as measured by pp65 antigenemia or DNAemia [41]. The role of CMV hyperimmunoglobulin in combination with ganciclovir in the treatment of CMV disease is controversial, although some evidence for improved outcome has been reported in the treatment of CMV pneumonia [42]. Finally, the use of foscarnet or cidofovir should be restricted to patients with apparent or proven resistance to ganciclovir.

Epstein–Barr virus

Recognition of mortality and morbidity of infection resulting from EBV following solid organ transplantation is evolving [8,16,17]. Histologic evaluation is important in differentiating between early lesions (e.g. infectious mononucleosis) and the more ominous PTLD. Variation in severity and extent of disease is related to the degree of immunosuppression and adequacy of the host immune response [17]. Symptomatic EBV infection in general, and PTLD in particular, is more common after primary EBV infection, thus impacting children disproportionately [4]. Onset of clinical symptoms typically occurs within the first year. However, EBV-associated lymphoma tends to occurs later.

The diagnosis of EBV-associated disease is made on the basis of clinical, laboratory and, where appropriate, histopathologic examination. EBV disease is suspected in patients with protracted fever, exudative tonsillitis, lymphadenopathy, organomegaly, leukopenia and/or atypical lymphocytosis [16,17]. Serologic diagnosis is often confounded by the presence of passive antibody acquired at the time of transplantation or during subsequent transfusions. The detection of increased EBV viral load in the peripheral blood identified by quantitative EBV polymerase chain reaction (PCR) has gained wide acceptance as an assay to predict risk for, or presence of, EBV/PTLD [17,43–45]. While extremely sensitive, these assays are limited by their lack of specificity as they are often elevated in asymptomatic patients. Definitive diagnosis of EBV disease (including PTLD) usually requires histologic confirmation. A more complete discussion of the diagnosis and management of PTLD is provided in Chapter 13.

Adenovirus

Adenovirus is the third most important viral infection following liver transplantation, occurring in 10% of 484 pediatric liver transplant recipients in one series [46]. Symptomatic disease (ranging from self-limited fever, gastroenteritis or cystitis to devastating illness with necrotizing hepatitis or pneumonia) occurred in over 60% of infected patients. Infections occurred within the first 3 months after transplantation. The frequency of invasive adenovirus infections after pediatric liver transplantation has decreased markedly with use of tacrolimus-based immunosuppression.

Adenovirus infection in other pediatric organ recipients is less well characterized but can be particularly severe after lung transplantation. Three of 30 pediatric lung transplant recipients developed fatal adenovirus pneumonitis within 1 month of transplantation [47,48]. Adenovirus has also been associated with hemorrhagic cystitis and graft dysfunction in adult renal transplant recipients. As adenovirus, like CMV, can be latent and can reactivate asymptomatically, ascribing a causative role in the pathologic process may be difficult on occasion. This may be particularly true in pediatric intestinal transplant recipients, where adenovirus may be recovered from the gastrointestinal tract in the presence or absence of clinical symptoms in more than half of these children.

Varicella

Many children undergo solid organ transplantation prior to developing immunity against varicella-zoster virus. Accordingly, they are at high risk for developing chickenpox after transplantation while they are maintained on chronic immunosuppressive medications. Infection appears most likely to occur after the transplant recipient enters school [49]. Initial published experience identified high rates of morbidity and even mortality, despite the use of intravenous aciclovir, among pediatric transplant recipients who developed varicella infection [50,51]. Recent experience suggests an improved outcome which may in part be a result of modifications in chronic immunosuppressive regimens that the children are maintained on. Excellent outcomes were observed in pediatric liver transplant recipients treated with intravenous aciclovir and reduction of immunosuppression [52]. Similar results were reported among 28 children developing varicella infection following heart transplantation [49]. Of interest, 14 of these children were managed entirely as outpatients on oral valaciclovir. None of these patients developed any complications of their varicella infection.

Varicella-susceptible transplant recipients should receive VZIG within 72 hours of a varicella exposure. If varicella lesions develop, several options for management now exist. For patients who present with a recent history of exposure to augmented immunosuppression or who appear ill at the time of presentation, it is prudent to hospitalize the patient and administer aciclovir intravenously until fever abates, no new lesions erupt and existent lesions begin to crust. In contrast, children who are maintained on lower levels of immunosuppression who appear reasonably well at the time of diagnosis may be managed on oral valaciclovir as an outpatient [49]. Reduction of immunosuppression should be considered until there is evidence that the varicella infection has resolved clinically. The ability to provide close follow-up of patients managed as outpatients is a necessary requirement for following this therapeutic option.

The use of varicella-zoster virus vaccine is an area of active research for recipients of solid organ transplantation. Based upon promising preliminary experience [53], some centers have begun to provide varicella vaccine to their pediatric transplant recipients. However, most experts feel that additional studies are necessary to confirm the efficacy and safety of this vaccine in children who have received organ transplantation.

BK virus

Recent evidence has identified a potential pathogenic role for BK virus (BKV) among organ transplant recipients. To date, most reports have been limited to recipients of renal transplantation, primarily among adults where rates of infection range between 10 and 60% [54]. However, a recent single-center report documented a rate of 3.5% of BKV in children at least 1 year after a renal transplant [55]. Although experience in adult renal transplant recipients has demonstrated that the majority of BKV infections appear to be associated with reactivation of latent virus in this population, a significant association has been found between the development of BKV disease with a negative serostatus of the recipient in a pediatric series [55].

The major clinical manifestation of BKV infection in renal transplant recipients is tubulointerstitial nephritis. While initial experience with BKV nephropathy (BKVN) was associated with a high incidence of graft loss [56], more recent experience (including the pediatric study) suggests that the presence of BKV infection need not affect mortality rates, severity of renal insufficiency or loss of graft function compared with those without BKV infection [55].

Definitive diagnosis of BKVN requires renal biopsy, although current efforts are focused on evaluating noninvasive diagnostic methods such as screening of urine or blood for the presence of BKV DNA by PCR. At the present time, experience with these approaches are still too limited to endorse either as an acceptable alternative to tissue diagnosis [57]. To date, there is no consensus on the optimal management of BKV disease. Evidence strongly suggests that interventions undertaken late in the course of disease (once the kidney demonstrates interstitial fibrosis and tubular atrophy) are unlikely to be successful. Accordingly, successful management will require early identification of BKVN before progression to irreversible changes occurs. At present, recommended management consists of judicious reduction of immunosuppression combined with active surveillance for rejection [57]. Anecdotal reports suggest that antiviral therapy with cidofovir may be efficacious. However, given its potential nephrotoxic effects and the lack of any prospective comparative data, use of this agent should be undertaken with caution.

Common community-acquired viruses

Although the course of illness has been poorly documented, most children who receive solid organ transplants experience the usual childhood respiratory and gastrointestinal tract illnesses without significant problems. This is especially true when they occur long after transplantation and are not associated with an episode of rejection [5]. Bailey *et al.* [33] noted that most of 43 pediatric heart transplant recipients experienced typical childhood illnesses without resultant fatality. However, infections resulting from RSV, influenza or parainfluenza have led to more severe disease in young children, especially if they develop early after transplant or during periods of maximal immunosuppression [58,59].

OPPORTUNISTIC INFECTIONS

Pneumocystis jiroveci pneumonia

It is well documented that *Pneumocystis jiroveci pneumonia* (PCP) complicates solid organ transplantation. Prior to the widespread use of prophylaxis, the incidence of PCP was 4–35% [18,19]. However, use of prophylaxis has essentially eliminated this problem. PCP typically occurs after the first month following transplantation, reflecting the indolent growth of this pathogen. Whereas most cases occur within the first year, PCP can occur later and should remain in the differential diagnosis for a patient with fever and lower respiratory tract symptoms, particularly if they are not receiving PCP prophylaxis.

Toxoplasmosis

Toxoplasma gondii causes significant infection in immunocompromised hosts [60]. A rare cause of disease in renal and liver transplant recipients [11], it is more often found as an infectious complication after cardiac transplantation [20]. The risk in cardiac recipients may be explained by tropism of the organism for cardiac muscle and subsequent donor transmission. Reactivation of cysts within the graft occurs in the immunosuppressed recipient without previous immunity. This is in contrast to AIDS patients who develop reactivation disease despite the presence of antibody. Four Pittsburgh pediatric cardiac transplant patients developed disease after primary infection [61]. Two had disseminated disease with myocardial involvement; one also developed focal neurologic impairment and severe chorioretinitis. Both patients died despite treatment. Two other patients remain asymptomatic several years after transplantation. Clinical manifestations usually occur 2–24 weeks after transplantation and include fever, pulmonary compromise, chorioretinitis, myocarditis and neurologic disorders. While the optimal prophylactic strategy is unknown, current recommendations include either the use of pyrimethamine or TMP-SMZ given daily for 6 months following transplantation in seronegative recipients of hearts from seropositive donors [57].

Tuberculosis

Tuberculosis is a special concern in immunosuppressed hosts, including recipients of solid organs. While the development of tuberculosis has been rare in our experience, an incidence of 2.4% was reported from a pediatric liver transplant center in the UK [62]. While most cases in this series were felt to represent primary infection acquired after transplantation, transplant recipients with a reactive Mantoux purified protein derivative test (PPD) or who come from areas endemic for tuberculosis are also at increased risk for symptomatic

reactivation after transplantation [63]. Although the risk of reactivation appears greatest in patients who received inadequate therapy for tuberculosis, disease has been reported in patients who received appropriate therapy for tuberculosis prior to transplantation [64]. Accordingly, prior to transplantation a careful history for exposure to tuberculosis is sought, a Mantoux PPD is placed and chest radiographs are reviewed for lesions consistent with healed tuberculosis. Patients with a positive tuberculosis history or a positive PPD receive isoniazid for 6–12 months after transplant [62,65]. Attempts at a more definitive diagnosis are indicated in patients from endemic areas with a negative PPD but suspicious radiograph. Treatment of tuberculosis may be complicated by the potential for drug–drug interactions between isoniazid, rifampin and the patient's immunosuppressive medications. Evidence of side-effects, particularly hepatotoxicity, should be monitored carefully in all pediatric transplant recipients receiving chemotherapy for the treatment of tuberculosis. This may be especially true in pediatric liver transplant recipients who receive allografts from adult donors in whom isoniazid toxicity may be more likely observed than in a child receiving a liver allograft from a pediatric donor.

Other opportunistic infections

Additional opportunistic infections include cryptococcosis, coccidioidomycosis and histoplasmosis. Prior infection with these pathogens is associated with exposure to geographic areas where pathogens are endemic. Because patients often travel to transplant centers distant from their homes, physicians caring for candidates or recipients of solid organ transplantation must be cognizant of the environmental risks for each patient. Experience with coccidioidomycosis in transplant recipients suggests that a minimum of 4 months of antifungal therapy, such as fluconazole, should be given to transplant recipients with this history [66]. Similarities between coccidioidomycosis and other fungal infections suggest that such strategies may be necessary for patients with a positive history of prior fungal infection with pathogens known to recur after resolution of primary infection.

MANAGEMENT AND PREVENTIVE MEASURES

Pretransplant evaluation

Pretransplant evaluation permits preventive interventions and anticipation of post-transplantation complications. An overview of recommended screening for a transplant candidate is provided in Table 12.2. History and physical examination should be performed with particular attention to previous infections, immunizations and drug allergies. Children with cystic fibrosis or those with a prolonged intensive care stay

Table 12.2 Screening protocol for transplant candidate. All tests performed on all candidates except where noted.

Test and pathogen	Comment
*Serologic test**	
HIV-1 and -2	
HTLV-1 and -2	
Hepatitis A virus	Obtain IgG and IgM test
Hepatitis B virus	Hepatitis B surface antigen and anti-core antibody
Hepatitis C virus	
Hepatitis D virus	If hepatitis B serology positive
CMV	Obtain IgG test; obtain urine culture if infant positive
EBV	Obtain viral capsid antigen IgG and EBNA
Herpes simplex virus	
Varicella-zoster virus	
Toxoplasma gondii	Obtain on heart, heart-lung transplant candidates
Measles	Consider immunization if ≥ 3 months anticipated before transplantation
Mumps	Consider immunization if ≥ 3 months anticipated before transplantation
Rubella	Consider immunization if ≥ 3 months anticipated before transplantation
Other tests	
Mycobacterium tuberculosis	Mantoux intermediate PPD skin test with anergy panel
Respiratory tract pathogens	Obtain sputum culture on patients with cystic fibrosis/other heart-lung transplant candidates

CMV, cytomegalovirus; EBNA, Epstein–Barr nuclear antigen; EBV, Epstein–Barr virus; HTLV, human T-cell lymphotrophic virus; Ig, immunoglobulin; PPD, purified protein derivative test.
* IgG antibody measured except where noted.

just prior to transplantation may have colonization with resistant organisms. Pretransplant surveillance cultures in these patients are useful in guiding subsequent antibiotic selection. Evaluation for tuberculosis is performed. Serologic studies (against CMV, EBV, hepatitis B and C, syphilis, HIV, varicella-zoster virus and *Toxoplasma gondii* in the case of heart transplantation) are obtained. Recommended serologic screening for the donor is provided in Table 12.3. Killed-agent vaccines can be safely given. Children expected to have a prolonged wait prior to transplantation may receive live virus vaccination (e.g. varicella and measle-mumps-rubella).

Preventive strategies

Prophylactic regimens for solid organ transplantation vary by center and type of transplant. Perioperative antibiotics are used for the first 48–72 hours to provide prophylaxis against intraoperative soilage, septicemia and wound infection. The choice of antimicrobial agents is dictated by the organ being transplanted, patient characteristics, expected flora and knowledge of the antimicrobial susceptibilities of local pathogens. Surveillance cultures of the donor bronchi or trachea are also useful in heart-lung or lung transplant recipients.

The frequency and severity of CMV infection in transplant recipients prompts consideration of prophylactic strategies.

Potential roles exist for intravenous and oral ganciclovir, as well as valganciclovir [57]. The role of intravenous immunoglobulin (both high-titer anti-CMV and routine intravenous immunoglobulin products) has also been explored [67,68]. Current regimens for the prevention of CMV in pediatric transplant recipients are in flux. Studies are currently underway to determine the appropriate regimen of oral valganciclovir for the prevention of CMV in children. Pending the results of these studies, we typically recommend the use of intravenous ganciclovir alone (for varying durations) for liver, heart and lung transplant recipients; and ganciclovir plus intravenous immunoglobulin containing a high titer of antibody against CMV for high-risk (donor CMV-positive, recipient CMV-negative) intestinal transplant recipients as CMV prophylaxis at our center.

Serial monitoring of the CMV viral load using either the pp65 antigenemia assay or quantitative CMV PCR as an indicator for the use of pre-emptive antiviral therapy has been proposed as an alternative preventative strategy [57,65]. In this approach, only those patients who demonstrate themselves to be at increased risk by the presence of an increased viral load are treated with intravenous or oral ganciclovir. While this strategy has gained acceptance at some centers, experience in pediatric transplant recipients remains limited at this time.

Table 12.3 Serologic screening protcol for organ donor. Immunoglobulin G (IgG) antibody measured except where noted.

Potential pathogen	Comment
HIV-1 and -2	Positive test contraindicates organ use
HTLV-1 and -2	Positive test contraindicates organ use
Hepatitis A virus	Positive IgM result contraindicates organ use
Hepatitis B virus	Obtain complete serologic panel; positive test contraindicates organ use
Hepatitis C virus	Some centers use positive donor only for positive candidate
CMV	Obtain IgG test; obtain urine culture if neonatal donor
EBV	Obtain EBV VCA IgG and anti-EBNA
Toxoplasma gondii	Obtain on heart, heart-lung donor
Treponema pallidum	Obtain reagin test (specific test if positive); positive test contraindicates organ use

CMV, cytomegalovirus; EBNA, Epstein–Barr nuclear antigen; EBV, Epstein–Barr virus; HTLV, human T-cell lymphotrophic virus.

As with CMV, the growing recognition of the importance of EBV infection in pediatric organ transplant recipients has led to an interest in the prevention of EBV infection and PTLD in organ transplant recipients. While a number of strategies are currently being explored (e.g. immunoprophylaxis, monitoring and pre-emptive therapy) [69,70], the efficacies of these approaches have not been established.

Nystatin suspension can be used in pediatric transplant recipients for the first 3 months after transplant in an effort to prevent oropharyngeal candidiasis. TMP-SMZ is used to prevent PCP. This antimicrobial combination has also been shown to decrease the incidence of post-transplant UTIs in renal transplant recipients [22]. In these patients, TMP-SMZ is used twice a day during the initial hospitalization. Renal transplant recipients are usually placed on the single-dose regimen shortly after discharge from hospital. The duration of prophylaxis for PCP is somewhat controversial. Most cases occur during the first year after transplantation. However, because late cases occur, TMP-SMZ is sometimes prescribed indefinitely. The optimal antimicrobial choice for prophylaxis of PCP in children who cannot tolerate sulfa drugs is not known.

REFERENCES

1 Dummer JS, Hardy A, Poorsattar A, Ho M. Early infections in kidney, heart, and liver transplant recipients on cyclosporine. *Transplantation* 1983;**36**:259–67.

2 Cuervas-Mons V, Rimola A, Van Thiel DH, Gavaler JS, Schade RR, Starzl TE. Does previous abdominal surgery alter the outcome of pediatric patients subjected to orthotopic liver transplantation? *Gastroenterology* 1986;**90**:853–7.

3 Hsu J, Griffith BP, Dowling RD, *et al.* Infections in mortally ill cardiac transplant recipients. *J Thorac Cardiovasc Surg* 1989;**98**:506–9.

4 Breinig MK, Zitelli B, Starzl TE, Ho M. Epstein–Barr virus, cytomegalovirus, and other viral infections in children after liver transplantation. *J Infect Dis* 1987;**156**:273–9.

5 Their M, Holmberg C, Lautenschlager I, Hockerstedt K, Jalanko H. Infections in pediatric kidney and liver transplant patients after perioperative hospitalization. *Transplantation* 2000;**69**:1617–23.

6 Burroughs M, Moscona A. Immunization of pediatric solid organ transplant candidates and recipients. *Clin Infect Dis* 2000;**30**:857–69.

7 Green M, Wald ER, Fricker FJ, Griffith BP, Trento A. Infections in pediatric orthotopic heart transplant recipients. *Pediatr Infect Dis J* 1989;**8**:87–93.

8 Dummer JS, White LT, Ho M, Griffith BP, Hardesty RL, Bahnson HT. Morbidity of cytomegalovirus infection in recipients of heart or heart-lung transplants who received cyclosporine. *J Infect Dis* 1985;**152**:1182–91.

9 Dummer JS. Infectious complications. In: Cooper DKC, Novitzky D, eds. *The Transplantation and Replacement of Thoracic Organs*. Norwell, MA: Kluwer Academic Publishers, 1990.

10 Kusne S, Dummer JS, Singh N, *et al.* Infections after liver transplantation: an analysis of 101 consecutive cases. *Medicine (Baltimore)* 1988;**67**:132–43.

11 Zaontz MR, Hatch DA, Firlit CF. Urological complications in pediatric renal transplantation: management and prevention. *J Urol* 1988;**140**:1123–8.

12 Bowman JS, Green M, Scantlebury VP, *et al.* OKT3 and viral disease in pediatric liver transplant recipients. *Clin Transplant* 1991;**5**:294–300.

13 Schroter GP, Hoelscher M, Putnam CW, Porter KA, Hansbrough JF, Starzl TE. Infections complicating orthotopic liver transplantation: a study emphasizing graft-related septicemia. *Arch Surg* 1976;**111**:1337–47.

14 Hanevold CD, Kaiser BA, Palmer J, Polinsky MS, Baluarte HJ. Vesicoureteral reflux and urinary tract infections in renal transplant recipients. *Am J Dis Child* 1987;**141**:982–4.

15 Schowengerdt KO, Naftel DC, Seib PM, *et al.* Infection after pediatric heart transplantation: results of a multiinstitutional study. The Pediatric Heart Transplant Study Group. *J Heart Lung Transplant* 1997;**16**:1207–16.

16 Green M, Michaels MG, Webber SA, Rowe D, Reyes J. The management of Epstein–Barr virus associated post-transplant lymphoproliferative disorders in pediatric solid-organ transplant recipients. *Pediatr Transplant* 1999;**3**:271–81.

17 Paya CV, Fung JJ, Nalesnik MA, *et al.* Epstein–Barr virus-induced posttransplant lymphoproliferative disorders. ASTS/ASTP EBV-PTLD Task Force and The Mayo Clinic Organized International Consensus Development Meeting. *Transplantation* 1999;68:1517–25.

18 Schafers HJ, Cremer J, Wahlers T, *et al. Pneumocystis carinii* pneumonia following heart transplantation. *Eur J Cardiothorac Surg* 1987;1:49–52.

19 Gryzan S, Paradis IL, Zeevi A, *et al.* Unexpectedly high incidence of *Pneumocystis carinii* infection after lung-heart transplantation: implications for lung defense and allograft survival. *Am Rev Respir Dis* 1988;137:1268–74.

20 Luft BJ, Naot Y, Araujo FG, Stinson EB, Remington JS. Primary and reactivated toxoplasma infection in patients with cardiac transplants. Clinical spectrum and problems in diagnosis in a defined population. *Ann Intern Med* 1983;99:27–31.

21 Kaditis AG, Phadke S, Dickman P, Webber S, Kurland G, Michaels MG. Mortality after pediatric lung transplantation: autopsies vs. clinical impression. *Pediatr Pulmonol* 2004;37:413–8.

22 Krieger JN, Brem AS, Kaplan MR. Urinary tract infection in pediatric renal transplantation. *Urology* 1980;15:362–9.

23 Fox BC, Sollinger HW, Belzer FO, Maki DG. A prospective, randomized, double-blind study of trimethoprim-sulfamethoxazole for prophylaxis of infection in renal transplantation: clinical efficacy, absorption of trimethoprim-sulfamethoxazole, effects on the microflora, and the cost–benefit of prophylaxis. *Am J Med* 1990;89:255–74.

24 Peterson PK, Balfour HH Jr, Fryd DS, Ferguson RM, Simmons RL. Fever in renal transplant recipients: causes, prognostic significance and changing patterns at the University of Minnesota Hospital. *Am J Med* 1981;71:345–51.

25 Colonna JO, Winston DJ, Brill JE, *et al.* Infectious complications in liver transplantation. *Arch Surg* 1988;123:360–4.

26 SPLIT Reseach Group. Studies of Pediatric Liver Transplantation (SPLIT): year 2000 outcomes. *Transplantation* 2001;72:463–76.

27 Hollenbeak CS, Alfrey EJ, Sheridan K, Burger TL, Dillon PW. Surgical site infections following pediatric liver transplantation: risks and costs. *Transpl Infect Dis* 2003;5:72–8.

28 Sigurdsson L, Reyes J, Kocoshis SA, Mazariegos G, Abu-Elmagd K, Green M. Bacteremia after intestinal transplantation in children correlates temporally with rejection or gastrointestinal lymphoproliferative disease. *Transplantation* 2000;70:302–5.

29 Green M, Bueno J, Sigurdsson L, Mazareigos G, Abu-Almagd K, Reyes J. Unique aspects of the infectious complications of intestinal transplantation. *Curr Opin Organ Transplant* 1999;4:361–7.

30 Kriett JM, Kaye MP. The Registry of the International Society for Heart Transplantation: seventh official report, 1990. *J Heart Transplant* 1990;9:323–30.

31 Boucek MM, Edwards LB, Keck BM, *et al.* The Registry of the International Society for Heart and Lung Transplantation: Sixth Official Pediatric Report, 2003. *J Heart Lung Transplant* 2003;22:636–52.

32 Baum D, Bernstein D, Starnes VA, *et al.* Pediatric heart transplantation at Stanford: results of a 15-year experience. *Pediatrics* 1991;88:203–14.

33 Bailey LL, Wood M, Razzouk A, Van Arsdell G, Gundry S. Heart transplantation during the first 12 years of life. Loma Linda University Pediatric Heart Transplant Group. *Arch Surg* 1989;124:1221–5.

34 Stovall SH, Ainley KA, Mason EO Jr, *et al.* Invasive pneumococcal infections in pediatric cardiac transplant patients. *Pediatr Infect Dis J* 2001;20:946–50.

35 Gajarski RJ, Smith EO, Denfield SW, *et al.* Long-term results of triple-drug-based immunosuppression in nonneonatal pediatric heart transplant recipients. *Transplantation* 1998;65:1470–6.

36 Doelling NR, Kanter KR, Sullivan KM, Winn KJ, Vincent RN. Medium-term results of pediatric patients undergoing orthotopic heart transplantation. *J Heart Lung Transplant* 1997;16:1225–30.

37 Backer CL, Zales VR, Harrison HL, Idriss FS, Benson DW Jr, Mavroudis C. Intermediate term results of infant orthotopic cardiac transplantation from two centers. *J Thorac Cardiovasc Surg* 1991;101:826–32.

38 Noyes BE, Michaels MG, Kurland G, Armitage JM, Orenstein DM. *Pseudomonas cepacia* empyema necessitatis after lung transplantation in two patients with cystic fibrosis. *Chest* 1994;105:1888–91.

39 Mendeloff EN, Huddleston CB, Mallory GB, *et al.* Pediatric and adult lung transplantation for cystic fibrosis. *J Thorac Cardiovasc Surg* 1998;115:404–13.

40 Palmer SM, Alexander BD, Sanders LL, *et al.* Significance of blood stream infection after lung transplantation: analysis in 176 consecutive patients. *Transplantation* 2000;69:2360–6.

41 Sia IG, Wilson JA, Groettum CM, Espy MJ, Smith TF, Paya CV. Cytomegalovirus (CMV) DNA load predicts relapsing CMV infection after solid organ transplantation. *J Infect Dis* 2000;181:717–20.

42 George MJ, Snydman DR, Werner BG, *et al.* Use of ganciclovir plus cytomegalovirus immune globulin to treat CMV pneumonia in orthotopic liver transplant recipients. The Boston Center for Liver Transplantation CMVIG-Study Group. *Transplant Proc* 1993;25:22–4.

43 Riddler SA, Breinig MC, McKnight JL. Increased levels of circulating Epstein–Barr virus (EBV)-infected lymphocytes and decreased EBV nuclear antigen antibody responses are associated with the development of posttransplant lymphoproliferative disease in solid-organ transplant recipients. *Blood* 1994;84:972–84.

44 Rowe DT, Qu L, Reyes J, *et al.* Use of quantitative competitive PCR to measure Epstein–Barr virus genome load in the peripheral blood of pediatric transplant patients with lymphoproliferative disorders. *J Clin Microbiol* 1997;35:1612–5.

45 Green M, Reyes J, Webber S, Michaels MG, Rowe D. The role of viral load in the diagnosis, management and possible prevention of Epstein–Barr virus associated posttransplant lymphoproliferative disease following solid organ transplantation. *Curr Opin Organ Transplant* 1999;4:292–6.

46 Michaels MG, Green M, Wald ER, Starzl TE. Adenovirus infection in pediatric liver transplant recipients. *J Infect Dis* 1992;165:170–4.

47 Ohori NP, Michaels MG, Jaffe R, Williams P, Yousem SA. Adenovirus pneumonia in lung transplant recipients. *Hum Pathol* 1995;26:1073–9.

48 Bridges ND, Spray TL, Collins MH, Bowles NE, Towbin JA. Adenovirus infection in the lung results in graft failure after lung transplantation. *J Thorac Cardiovasc Surg* 1998;116:617–23.

49 Dodd DA, Burger J, Edwards KM, Dummer JS. Varicella in a pediatric heart transplant population on nonsteroid maintenance immunosuppression. *Pediatrics* 2001;108:E80.

50 Feldhoff CM, Balfour HH Jr, Simmons RL, Najarian JS, Mauer SM. Varicella in children with renal transplants. *J Pediatr* 1981;98:25–31.

51 McGregor RS, Zitelli BJ, Urbach AH, Malatack JJ, Gartner JC Jr. Varicella in pediatric orthotopic liver transplant recipients. *Pediatrics* 1989;**83**:256–61.

52 Pacini-Edelstein SJ, Mehra M, Ament ME, Vargas JH, Martin MG, McDiarmid SV. Varicella in pediatric liver transplant patients: a retrospective analysis of treatment and outcome. *J Pediatr Gastroenterol Nutr* 2003;**37**:183–6.

53 Zamora I, Simon JM, Da Silva ME, Piqueras AI. Attenuated varicella virus vaccine in children with renal transplants. *Pediatr Nephrol* 1994;**8**:190–2.

54 Mylonakis E, Goes N, Rubin RH, Cosimi AB, Colvin RB, Fishman JA. BK virus in solid organ transplant recipients: an emerging syndrome. *Transplantation* 2001;**72**:1587–92.

55 Smith JM, McDonald RA, Finn LS, Healey PJ, Davis CL, Limaye AP. Polyomavirus nephropathy in pediatric kidney transplant recipients. *Am J Transplant* 2004;**4**:2109–17.

56 de Bruyn G, Limaye AP. BK virus-associated nephropathy in kidney transplant recipients. *Rev Med Virol* 2004;**14**:193–205.

57 Green M, Avery R, Preiksaitis J. Guidelines for the prevention and management of infectious complications of solid organ transplantation. *Am J Transplant* 2004;**4**(Suppl 10):5–166.

58 Pohl C, Green M, Wald ER, Ledesma-Medina J. Respiratory syncytial virus infections in pediatric liver transplant recipients. *J Infect Dis* 1992;**165**:166–9.

59 Apalsch AM, Green M, Ledesma-Medina J, Nour B, Wald ER. Parainfluenza and influenza virus infections in pediatric organ transplant recipients. *Clin Infect Dis* 1995;**20**:394–9.

60 Ruskin J, Remington JS. Toxoplasmosis in the compromised host. *Ann Intern Med* 1976;**84**:193–9.

61 Michaels MG, Wald ER, Fricker FJ, del Nido PJ, Armitage J. Toxoplasmosis in pediatric recipients of heart transplants. *Clin Infect Dis* 1992;**14**:847–51.

62 Verma A, Dhawan A, Wade JJ, *et al.* Mycobacterium tuberculosis infection in pediatric liver transplant recipients. *Pediatr Infect Dis J* 2000;**19**:625–30.

63 Singh N, Paterson DL. Mycobacterium tuberculosis infection in solid-organ transplant recipients: impact and implications for management. *Clin Infect Dis* 1998;**27**:1266–77.

64 Lichtenstein IH, MacGregor RR. Mycobacterial infections in renal transplant recipients: report of five cases and review of the literature. *Rev Infect Dis* 1983;**5**:216–26.

65 Higgins R, Kusne S, Reyes J, *et al.* Mycobacterium tuberculosis after liver transplantation: management and guide lines for prevention. *Clin Transplant* 1992;**6**:81–90.

66 Hall KA, Copeland JG, Zukoski CF, Sethi GK, Galgiani JN. Markers of coccidioidomycosis before cardiac or renal transplantation and the risk of recurrent infection. *Transplantation* 1993;**55**:1422–4.

67 Snydman DR, Werner BG, Heinze-Lacey B, *et al.* Use of cytomegalovirus immune globulin to prevent cytomegalovirus disease in renal-transplant recipients. *N Engl J Med* 1987;**317**:1049–54.

68 Snydman DR, Werner BG, Dougherty NN, *et al.* Cytomegalovirus immune globulin prophylaxis in liver transplantation: a randomized, double-blind, placebo-controlled trial. The Boston Center for Liver Transplantation CMVIG Study Group. *Ann Intern Med* 1993;**119**:984–91.

69 Green M, Reyes J, Rowe D. New strategies in the prevention and management of Epstein–Barr virus infections and posttransplant lymphoproliferative disease following solid organ transplantation. *Curr Opin Organ Transplant* 1998;**3**:43–147.

70 McDiarmid SV, Jordan S, Kim GS, *et al.* Prevention and pre-emptive therapy of posttransplant lymphoproliferative disease in pediatric liver recipients. *Transplantation* 1998;**66**:1604–11.

13 Post-Transplant Lymphoproliferative Disorders and Malignancy

Steven A. Webber and Michael Green

Excellent short- and medium-term outcomes are now being achieved in almost all forms of solid organ transplantation in children. This has led to increasing focus on complications and quality of life. Post-transplantation lymphoproliferative disorders (PTLD) represent a major and life-threatening complication of therapeutic immunosuppression and children are disproportionately affected compared to adults. Despite a growing understanding of the pathophysiology of PTLD, its optimal management remains controversial. This chapter provides an overview of the etiology, pathology, clinical manifestations, diagnosis and management of PTLD in pediatric solid-organ transplantation. Nonlymphoid malignancies are extremely rare in pediatric recipients but are a major cause of mortality in adults after solid organ transplantation. The most common forms of nonlymphoid malignancy in pediatric recipients are briefly reviewed.

POST-TRANSPLANTATION LYMPHOPROLIFERATIVE DISORDERS

Etiology and the importance of primary Epstein–Barr virus infection

PTLD are a spectrum of conditions that straddle the borders between infection and malignant neoplasia [1]. It has long been recognized that normal immune surveillance is essential for control of viral infection and for prevention of development of neoplasia. Lymphomas may arise in congenital (e.g. X-linked lymphoproliferative disease) as well as acquired (e.g. acquired immunodeficiency syndrome, AIDS) immunodeficiency syndromes. The association between therapeutic immunosuppression and the development of lymphoid tumors was first recognized in 1968 [2] and an association with Epstein–Barr virus (EBV) infection was soon recognized [3]. Subsequently, a large literature has accrued demonstrating the pivotal role of EBV in most cases of PTLD in pediatric solid organ transplant recipients. Evidence comes both from epidemiologic observations [4] and from demonstration of EBV genome within lesions [5]. We have found that approx-

imately 85–90% of cases in pediatric recipients are EBV driven, including almost all cases arising in the first 3 years after transplantation. EBV negative cases usually arise late after transplantation, generally beyond 5 years, and their etiology remains an enigma. However, the proportion of EBV negative cases does appear to be increasing, particularly in adult transplant recipients [6].

The source of EBV infection is not always clear. What is apparent is that most cases of PTLD occur in children who are seronegative for EBV at the time of transplantation and who subsequently develop primary EBV infection [4,7,8]. Because the vast majority of adults are seropositive at the time of transplantation, it is not surprising that PTLD occurs at a much lower frequency in adult recipients. The strong association between the acquisition of primary EBV infection after transplantation and the risk of PTLD appears to be true for all types of solid organ transplantation with the exception of intestinal transplantation. In the latter setting, EBV seropositive children frequently develop PTLD [9]. For other organs, EBV disease occurs uncommonly in children who are EBV seropositive before transplantation.

Primary EBV infection post-transplantation could come from several sources, including the donor organ(s), perioperative use of blood products or from subsequent community acquisition of the virus. The donor is the most likely source of EBV infection in a seronegative recipient who develops early onset PTLD (e.g. first year). The relatively low incidence of EBV seroconversion and PTLD in the early months after transplantation in seronegative recipients with seronegative donors suggests that perioperative blood transfusion is a less likely source of EBV infection in pediatric solid organ recipients. A small number of studies have now used molecular techniques to demonstrate that EBV was of donor origin [10].

Additional risk factors associated with an increased risk of developing PTLD include the development of cytomegalovirus (CMV) disease and the use of antilymphocyte and/or thymocyte antibodies for prevention or treatment of rejection [11,12]. Caucasian race and male gender have also been found to be risk factors in one review [13]. The relative contribution of specific immunosuppressive regimens to the development of PTLD (e.g. cyclosporine versus tacrolimus as primary immuno-suppressant) remains controversial [12,14–17]. Certainly, the greater the level of T-lymphocyte suppression, the greater will be the risk of developing PTLD. However, the risks of PTLD must then be analyzed in the context of the potential benefits of lower acute rejection rates.

"Incidence" of PTLD

Although the risk of PTLD is highest in the first year after transplantation, the patient remains at indefinite risk. Thus, the "incidence" in any series will depend on postoperative survival and length of follow-up, as well as on case definition. Patients dying soon after transplant are "at risk" for only a very short period. Some reports have therefore quoted the frequency among 30-day survivors. The following range of "incidences" have been reported for pediatric recipients: kidney 1–10% [17,18]; liver 5–14% [12,14,19]; heart 4–10% [8,20,21]; lung/heart-lung 10–20% [21,22]. A more appropriate method of analysis for time-related events is the use of Kaplan–Meier or similar "survival analysis" techniques. In a recent study of 56 cases of PTLD among 1184 primary heart transplant recipients in the Pediatric Heart Transplant Study Group, the probability of freedom from PTLD was 98%, 94% and 92% at 1, 3 and 5 years after transplantation, respectively [23].

A second, and perhaps more important, limitation is the method of case definition of PTLD used within any given center. Most centers do not include infectious mononucleosis and other EBV-associated viral syndromes as cases of PTLD. So-called "early lesions" of normal lymphoid tissues (e.g. lymph nodes, tonsils or adenoids), in which there is architectural preservation (see pathology of PTLD below), form part of the spectrum of lymphoproliferative disorders, but are not generally included as "cases of PTLD" in most studies. Inclusion of these more histologically benign cases will result in a significant increase in incidence of PTLD and will also result in improved overall outcomes, as this group of lesions generally carries a favorable prognosis.

Clinical presentation and diagnostic evaluation of suspected PTLD

EBV infection is increasingly recognized to be associated with a wide range of disease manifestations in pediatric transplant recipients. The spectrum of clinical disease includes a non-specific viral syndrome, mononucleosis and PTLD including EBV-associated malignant lymphoma (e.g. Burkitt lymphoma). This chapter focuses on PTLD. Non-PTLD EBV disease is discussed in Chapter 12.

The diagnosis of EBV disease in pediatric organ transplant recipients is based on clinical history and physical examination (Table 13.1) in combination with laboratory confirma-

Table 13.1 Symptoms and signs of post-transplant lymphoproliferative disorders (PTLD).

Symptoms
Fever
Malaise and lethargy
Weight loss
Sore throat
Abdominal pain, gastrointestinal bleeding, nausea, vomiting and diarrhea
Swollen "glands"
Symptoms of allograft dysfunction, e.g. shortness of breath (lung transplant)
Headache and/or focal neurologic symptoms

Physical signs
Pallor
Lymphadenopathy
Subcutaneous nodules
Tonsillar enlargement
Hepatosplenomegaly
Focal neurologic signs

tion (Table 13.2). The most important factor in making this diagnosis is maintenance of a high index of suspicion at all times. In our experience, earlier diagnosis appears to be correlated with more successful outcomes. Presentation with advanced disease, frequently with comorbid infections, is less common than in previous eras.

In contrast to these severe manifestations, a history of lethargy, malaise, weight loss and fever are now common presentations of PTLD. An additional history of vomiting and/or diarrhea is suggestive of gastrointestinal involvement, which has been increasingly recognized to be a common site of disease in pediatric organ transplant recipients (see Plate 13.1a, facing page 224). This is especially true in intestinal transplant recipients in whom nearly all patients present with involvement of either the transplanted intestinal allograft or their native intestine. Intestinal disease may present with hemorrhage, obstruction or perforation although the highest risk period for the latter may be during therapy when necrosis of transmural lesions may develop.

Additional sites of involvement vary with the type of organ transplant the child received. Pulmonary disease is very common in cardiac recipients and is almost invariably present in lung recipients (see Plate 13.1b, facing page 224). Pulmonary presentation ranges from asymptomatic nodule(s) on routine chest radiograph to life-threatening pulmonary dysfunction in the lung allograft. The latter may resemble lung rejection on chest radiograph with rather diffuse consolidation without clearly defined mass lesions. This may lead to inadvertent augmentation of immunosuppression with severe consequences [22]. Involvement of the liver with EBV disease and PTLD is seen most frequently in liver transplant

115

Routine	Selected patients
Hemoglobin, platelets, white count with differential	Gastrointestinal endoscopy
Serum electrolytes, calcium, renal function	Bone scan
Liver function tests	Bone marrow biopsy
Uric acid	Brain CT/MRI
Lactate dehydrogenase	Lumbar puncture
Quantitative immunoglobulins	Screen for comorbid infections
Serum protein electrophoresis	
EBV serologies (anti-EBNA, VCA and EA)	
EBV viral load by quantitative PCR	
Stools for occult bleeding	
Chest radiograph	
CT scan of chest/abdomen/pelvis	
Core needle or excisional biopsy of lesion(s)	

Table 13.2 Diagnostic evaluation of patient with suspected post-transplant lymphoproliferative disorders (PTLD).

CT, computed tomography; EA, early antigen; EBNA, Epstein–Barr nuclear antigen; EBV, Epstein–Barr virus; MRI, magnetic resonance imaging; NA, nuclear antigen; VCA, viral capsid antigen.

recipients. Interestingly, the heart is the only organ transplant in which there is not a strong tendency for the disease to involve the allograft. In most other solid organ transplants, allograft dysfunction may be a manifestation of PTLD and may mimic acute or chronic rejection.

Other presentations include persistent sore throat, adenopathy and cutaneous nodules, as well as seizures, headaches and focal neurologic lesions with CNS disease (see Plate 13.1c, facing page 224). Multiple sites of disease occur in appproximately 50% of patients (see Plate 13.1d, facing page 224).

Although physical examination may not reveal specific findings, there will frequently be evidence of pallor, weight loss, peripheral adenopathy or hepatosplenomegaly. A full physical examination is essential and should include thorough neurologic examination. Examination of the entire skin and sites of all lymph nodes is warranted. Careful examination of the oropharynx is required.

An overview of the laboratory evaluation for the diagnosis of PTLD is given in Table 13.2. Initial evaluation should include a complete blood count with white cell differential and platelets. Leukopenia, often in association with atypical lymphocytosis, as well as thrombocytopenia is a frequent finding. Anemia is common and may be normocytic and normochromic or may demonstrate findings of iron deficiency when occult gastrointestinal bleeding is present. Rarely, evidence of hemolytic anemia may also be present. Stools should be tested for blood. Organ function (liver, kidney) should be evaluated. Elevations in uric acid and lactate dehydrogenase are common. Serum immunoglobulin levels may be elevated or reduced. Some centers routinely perform serum protein electrophoresis. Although many patients do not demonstrate a monoclonal or oligoclonal gammopathy, if present this provides an additional means of following the patient's response to therapy.

A variety of imaging tests are helpful in the evaluation of the pediatric transplant recipient with suspected PTLD. A chest radiograph often reveals evidence of pulmonary nodular disease and/or evidence of mediastinal lymphadenopathy. The most informative diagnostic study is usually computed tomographic (CT) evaluation of the chest, abdomen and pelvis. Evidence of nodal or extranodal disease will frequently be apparent on CT at one or more sites. In the chest, pulmonary nodules or enlarged mediastinal lymph nodes may be apparent even in the presence of a normal chest radiograph. In the abdomen, disease may be found at normal lymph node sites, within the gastrointestinal tract or at extranodal sites, including the liver, spleen and kidneys. Some centers routinely perform CT or magnetic resonance imaging of the brain. These studies should always be performed if there is any clinical suggestion of CNS disease.

Other studies performed on selected patients as directed by the clinical findings are shown in Table 13.2. Upper and/or lower gastrointestinal endoscopy should be performed when there are gastrointestinal symptoms or evidence of occult gastrointestinal bleeding.

Recently, measurement of EBV viral load in the peripheral blood with polymerase chain reaction (PCR) has been evaluated as a diagnostic tool for patients with symptomatic disease [24,25]. A growing experience suggests elevated EBV viral loads will be present in the vast majority of patients with PTLD. It is important to note that in children the peak of the EBV viral load may be comparable among patients with EBV-associated viral syndromes and those with PTLD. Therefore, marked elevation in viral load is sensitive but not specific for the diagnosis of PTLD. While the measurement of EBV viral load is a promising new diagnostic test, it has several limitations. EBV-PCR assays are not standardized between laboratories and various blood compartments have been utilized including whole blood, plasma and peripheral blood mononuclear cells.

Recent data suggest that whole blood assays correlate well with viral load in peripheral mononuclear cell populations, but correlate poorly with plasma levels [26]. Therefore, either whole blood or peripheral mononuclear cell assays should be utilized. It should also be noted that not every patient with PTLD will have elevated viral loads, even when the lesions are demonstrated to be EBV positive. Conversely, viral loads may be elevated for prolonged periods of time in the absence of evidence of EBV disease or PTLD. Thus, while measurement of the EBV viral load is a useful screening procedure for suspected EBV disease, the test lacks specificity and it cannot replace histologic examination of suspected sites of involvement when the diagnosis of PTLD is contemplated. Finally, clinicians should not rely on serologic tests to make the diagnosis of PTLD as many patients will have positive EBV titers on the basis of passive immunization from blood products (or of maternal origin in infant recipients) and others may seroconvert without manifesting any clinical symptoms. In addition, the immunosuppressive agents used in transplant recipients might result in some patients having falsely negative serologic results even at the time of presentation of EBV disease.

Pathology of PTLD

In general, histologic evaluation is required to confirm the diagnosis of PTLD. Unfortunately, the pathologic description of PTLD has been confusing, with several different classification systems in prior usage. This is regrettable because an understanding of the histology and molecular pathology of these disorders is important for determining therapy and prognosis. More recently, there has been broad agreement that the system of classification of the World Health Organization (WHO) should be routinely employed (Table 13.3) [27]. The pathologic evaluation should be performed by a pathologist with extensive experience in the evaluation of PTLD. Whenever possible, tissue from several involved sites should be obtained because different morphologies may be present at different sites of disease. Fine needle cytology is inadequate for full evaluation.

The most benign end of the histologic spectrum is represented by so-called *early lesions.* The central characteristic

Table 13.3 World Health Organization (WHO) classification of post-transplant lymphoproliferative disorders (PTLD) [27].

Early lesions
   Reactive plasmacytic hyperplasia
   Infectious mononucleosis-like
Polymorphic PTLD
Monomorphic PTLD
   B-cell neoplasms (e.g. diffuse large B-cell lymphoma, Burkitt, myeloma)
   T-cell neoplasms
Hodgkin lymphoma and Hodgkin-like PTLD

of this group of lesions is the diffuse proliferation of mononuclear cells of various sizes, many with plasmacytoid features, but with preservation of normal tissue architecture. These lesions occur in normal lymphoid tissues such as lymph nodes, and in the tonsils and adenoids. *Polymorphic* PTLD also demonstrates lymphoid infiltrates of varying shapes and sizes (see Plate 13.2a, facing page 224). The entire range of lymphocyte differentiation may be seen. However, in these lesions there is effacement and/or destruction of normal tissue architecture. Areas of necrosis are frequently present. These lesions may occur in both nodal tissue and at extranodal sites, and may involve any organ. Large bizarre cells (atypical immunoblasts) may be scanty or abundant. In *monomorphic* ("lymphomatous") PTLD, the destructive lymphoid infiltrate has a much more monotonous appearance, with most cells appearing to be transformed lymphocytes at one stage of differentiation (see Plate 13.2b, facing page 224). These lesions often resemble diffuse large B-cell non-Hodgkin lymphomas seen in the nontransplant population. It is important to recognize that some degree of polymorphism is often seen, although much less pronounced than in polymorphic lesions. Rarely, other specific histologic variants may also be noted including mature plasma cell type predominance, Burkitt lymphoma (see Plate 13.2c, facing page 224) and tumors that strongly resemble Hodgkin lymphoma (see Plate 13.2d, facing page 224) [28].

Further work-up of suspected PTLD includes immunohistochemistry and flow cytometry. These procedures will demonstrate the cell lineage of the lesions. Almost all PTLD are of B-cell origin, although rare cases of T-cell PTLD are seen. It should be noted that variable numbers of T cells (and macrophages) are generally interspersed between the B-cell populations in polymorphic lesions. Molecular studies offer the most definitive assessment of the clonality of the lesions [27,29]. Analysis of host cell clonality is based on the behavior of immunoglobulin genes, which rearrange uniquely in the maturing B cell. Progeny of a B cell that has already arranged its immunoglobulin genes will carry the same rearrangement. Monomorphic lesions are clonal in nature, and analysis of clonality is therefore of little relevance (although is often performed). Polymorphic lesions may be polyclonal, but the majority are also clonal B-cell proliferations. "Early lesions" tend to be polyclonal in nature. Prediction of prognosis based on a search for abnormalities in oncogenes and tumor suppressor genes, or on patterns of gene expression observed in microarray studies, remain research tools at this time. Cytogenetic abnormalities are mostly found in monomorphic disease, especially in Burkitt lymphoma. Few data exist on the presence and significance of cytogenetic abnormalities in polymorphic or other monomorphic PTLD lesions in children.

The pathologist must demonstrate whether PTLD lesions contain evidence of EBV. A number of techniques are available including Southern blot analysis, PCR and *in situ* hybridization. Most programs use *in situ* hybridization with the EBER-1 probe which labels EBV-encoded early RNA transcripts in infected cells. This technique is reliable, rapid and is performed on routinely processed paraffin sections. Overall, approximately 85–90% of pediatric PLTD patients are EBV positive.

Prevention of PTLD

The increased recognition of the importance of PTLD has prompted interest and investigation into disease prevention. The most logical approach would be to immunize all seronegative recipients prior to transplantation. Several vaccine preparations are under evaluation but progress has been slow, despite early optimism from primate work [30]. An alternate strategy would be to avoid transplanting seronegative recipients, especially with a seropositive donor. This approach would effectively exclude many pediatric candidates from receiving organs, and entails tremendous logistical problems because donor EBV serologies are generally not available at the time of acceptance of the donor organ. Various other preventive strategies have been suggested [24,31]. In contrast to CMV, the routine use of antiviral chemoprophylaxis does not appear to be effective in preventing EBV disease or PTLD. Chemoprophylaxis, with short-term intravenous ganciclovir, followed by long-term oral aciclovir therapy was not helpful in preventing PTLD in a randomized trial in pediatric liver transplantation [31]. Several studies have also demonstrated rise in EBV viral load by PCR while patients are receiving therapy with ganciclovir or aciclovir. Despite these observations, many clinicians have considered these agents to be useful and they remain in widespread use in many programs.

Immunoprophylaxis with intravenous immunoglobulin preparations (IVIG) is another potential (but unproven) option for the prevention of EBV-associated complications in solid organ transplantation. Data from a severe combined immunodeficiency (SCID) mouse model [32], as well as anecdotal human experience, support the potential role of IVIG. In a recent multicenter randomized controlled trial in pediatric liver transplantation, CMV hyperimmunoglobulin did not result in statistically significant differences between groups, but there was a trend to disease prevention in the treatment arm (M. Green, unpublished data 2006).

Another appealing preventive strategy is to target patients with evidence of early EBV infection (prior to development of symptoms) for pre-emptive therapy. This targeted approach avoids treatment of all seronegative recipients. Published experience suggests that EBV-PCR levels rise during primary infection, prior to both antibody development and the onset of symptoms. Strategies to prevent progression of early EBV infection to symptomatic disease, including reduction of immunosuppression, addition of antiviral agents, infusion of IVIG or even cellular immunotherapy (see below) could then be instituted. All these strategies require investigation with formal clinical trials.

Management of established PTLD

No randomized trials of any form of therapy for PTLD have been performed. We have recently reviewed the various treatment strategies for PTLD [31,33,34]. Treatment options are also summarized in Table 13.4.

Table 13.4 Treatment strategies for post-transplant lymphoproliferative disorders (PTLD).

Therapy	Comments
First line therapies	
Reduced immunosuppression	Effective in most pediatric recipients, especially in polymorphic PTLD
Antiviral therapy (e.g. ganciclovir)	Widely used but unproven
Chemotherapy	First line for overt malignancy (e.g. Burkitt lymphoma)
Second line therapies	
α-Interferon	May cause severe rejection; rarely used
Intravenous immunoglobulins (containing anti-EBV antibodies)	Unproven (Trial in PTLD prevention inconclusive but with trend to beneficial outcome)
Anti-B cell monoclonal antibodies	Promising results in refractory polymorphic disease Pediatric multicenter trial in progress
Cellular immunotherapy, e.g. autologous (or HLA matched) EBV-specific cytotoxic T-lymphocyte infusions	Promising techniques. Minimal experience in solid organ transplantation. Expensive and labor intensive
Chemotherapy	Established second line therapy for refractory and relapsed PTLD; more often required in adults, monomorphic PTLD and late onset disease
Surgery (± radiation therapy)	Reserved for treatment of local compression of critical structures, bowel obstruction, etc. Also for excisional biopsy of localized, easily accessible lesions at presentation

EBV, Epstein–Barr virus.

Reduction of immunosuppression

In 1984, Starzl et al. [35] reported the reversibility of PTLD by reduction in immunosuppression in cyclosporine-treated patients. This strategy remains the initial mainstay of therapy for most pediatric patients with polymorphic disease. It is also often used as first line therapy in monomorphic disease that is associated with recent primary EBV infection. The goal of this approach is to allow the host to recover natural immune surveillance and subsequently gain control over the proliferation of EBV-infected B cells. In our experience, the majority of polymorphic lesions will respond, although with significant rates of rebound acute cellular rejection. In general, most patients show evidence of clinical response within 2–4 weeks of reduction of immunosuppression, although a belated response has been observed as long as several months in some patients.

The extent to which immunosuppression should be reduced will depend on many factors including the organ transplanted, time from transplantation, prior rejection history and the immunosuppressive regimen used at the time of diagnosis of PTLD. When disease is disseminated or fulminant, complete cessation of all immunosuppression is indicated irrespective of organ transplanted (although corticosteroids should not be completely discontinued because of the potential for adrenal insufficiency). For more localized disease, the optimal method of reduction of immunosuppression is less clear. Discontinuation may improve the chance of achieving remission of PTLD, but will increase the risk of rebound rejection. This dilemma was well illustrated in a large cohort of pediatric heart transplant recipients with PTLD. Death from graft loss from acute and chronic rejection occurred with similar frequency to death from progressive PTLD [23]. Currently, we recommend an aggressive approach to immunosuppression reduction with temporary cessation of calcineurin inhibitor in most cases. This is combined with regular EBV-PCR monitoring and very careful surveillance of graft function (with additional surveillance graft biopsies for heart and lung allografts) to help guide timing of reintroduction of immunosuppressive therapy. If rebound rejection occurs prior to complete resolution of PTLD, second line therapies are indicated (see below). For heart and lung recipients, we generally reintroduce low-dose calcineurin inhibitors for long-term patient management. Liver and kidney recipients are sometimes managed without reintroduction of calcineurin inhibitors, but with adjunctive agents such as mycophenolate mofetil, sirolimus and corticosteroids. Some liver recipients have successfully been maintained long-term off all drug therapy after diagnosis of PTLD.

Responses to reduced immunosuppression in monomorphic PTLD, Hodgkin disease and Hodgkin-like PTLD may be observed, but are much less likely to be complete or durable. In addition, prolonged trials of reduction or cessation of immunosuppression may lead to high rates of rebound acute and chronic rejection leading to graft loss and death. Thus, the role of reduced immunosuppression in these histologies is controversial.

Antiviral chemotherapy

Initial interest in the role of antiviral chemotherapy for treatment of PTLD arose in 1982 when Hanto et al. [36] described a patient whose EBV-associated PTLD lesion appeared to wax and wane in association with starting and stopping aciclovir [36]. Both aciclovir and ganciclovir inhibit lytic EBV DNA replication in vitro and may be of value in treating the lytic phase of EBV infections. Ganciclovir is approximately 10-fold more potent than aciclovir at inhibiting lytic EBV replication in vitro, and has the additional advantage of inhibiting CMV that may be present as a copathogen in some cases of PTLD. Based on Hanto et al.'s report, and the in vitro activity of these agents, use of aciclovir or ganciclovir for the treatment of PTLD has become routine in most centers. However, their efficacy has not been established in prospective comparative clinical trials, and many investigators have questioned their role in the treatment of PTLD. The vast majority of EBV-infected cells within PTLD lesions have been shown to be transformed B cells that are not undergoing lytic infection. Neither aciclovir nor ganciclovir suppress EBV-driven proliferation of B cells in vitro, nor are they active against B cells that are latently infected with EBV. Furthermore, EBV viral loads in the peripheral blood can climb to very high levels, and PTLD may develop, while patients are receiving aciclovir or ganciclovir.

Interferon

The use of interferon has been described in anecdotal reports as a therapeutic option in the management of PTLD [33,37]. Interferon is both a proinflammatory cytokine and a natural antiviral agent and appears capable of controlling proliferation of EBV-infected B cells. Because it is a nonspecific immune stimulant, antidonor responses are often seen and severe rejection can develop during therapy. At the present time, most centers are not routinely using interferon in the management of PTLD.

Intravenous immunoglobulin

A potential role for the use of IVIG for the treatment of PTLD has also been suggested. Several reports have documented an association between loss, or absence, of antibody against at least one of the Epstein–Barr nuclear antigens (EBNA) in EBV infected organ recipients and the subsequent development of PTLD [38]. In addition, a correlation between an increasing level of anti-EBNA antibodies (including those introduced through transfusions) with a decrease in EBV viral load has been demonstrated. Taken together, these reports may provide a rationale for considering the use of antibodies in the prevention and/or treatment of EBV disease and PTLD, even though the primary mechanism for controlling EBV infection appears to be cytotoxic T-cell-mediated immunity. IVIG has been used alone and in combination with α-interferon as treatment for PTLD [37]. Both IVIG and CMV IVIG (CytoGam®, MedImmune, Inc.) have been used in the treatment of some patients with PTLD. As with the use of antiviral agents and interferon, there are no comparative trials evaluating the role of IVIG in general, or CytoGam in particular, in the treatment of PTLD.

Anti-B-cell antibodies

The use of anti-CD21 and anti-CD24 monoclonal antibodies has been reported for the treatment of PTLD in recipients of solid organ and bone marrow transplantation (BMT) [39]. Therapy was most promising for oligoclonal but not monoclonal disease. These two products are no longer available; however, an anti-CD20 human/mouse chimeric monoclonal antibody (rituximab; Genentech Inc. and IDEC pharmaceuticals) is currently commercially available for treatment of certain CD20-positive B-cell non-Hodgkin lymphomas in adult nontransplant recipients. Clinical investigators in France published a retrospective analysis of the use of rituximab in 32 patients with PTLD [40]. The overall response rate was 65% in solid organ transplant recipients, most of whom experienced long-term remission. However, relapse of PTLD developed in approximately 20% of responders a median of 7 months after completing their therapeutic course of rituximab. A pediatric registry has now collected data on 25 children with PTLD refractory to conventional therapy [41]. A complete remission was observed in 17 cases (68%). Overall, the drug was well tolerated. B-cell depletion was typically seen for 6–9 months. Although these results are far from ideal, they are encouraging for a very high-risk group of patients with refractory disease which traditionally has very poor survival.

There are several important questions regarding the use of rituximab. Will the prolonged elimination of B cells by this agent result in additional opportunistic infections or other sequelae? How often will hypogammaglobulinemia develop? If safety is reasonable, should rituximab be used in all patients or only those who fail an initial period of observation on reduced immunosuppression? If relapse occurs after the use of rituximab, how should management proceed? Do newer radio-conjugates of anti-B-cell antibodies offer any advantage over rituximab and are they safe in children? A prospective nonrandomized multicenter trial of rituximab in refractory PTLD in children is currently in progress [41], and a phase III randomized trial as primary therapy is in the planning stages. It is hoped that these studies will answer some of these important questions.

Cellular immunotherapy

Cytotoxic T lymphocytes (CTLs) directed against EBV-specific antigens are thought to be the major source of control over EBV infection in immunocompetent individuals. Withdrawal of immunosuppression reverses the nonspecific suppression of T cells used to prevent rejection and allows the development and expansion of EBV-specific CTLs in patients with symptomatic EBV disease. *Ex vivo* generated bulk cultures of EBV-specific CTLs, or transfusion of unmodified mononuclear cells from matched or closely matched donors, have been used for the management of EBV infection and PTLD in BMT recipients [42] and in a small number of solid organ recipients [43]. Unfortunately, several problems currently limit the applicability of this strategy in solid organ transplantation, where the success has not paralleled that seen after BMT. These techniques remain a research tool limited to a very small number of solid organ transplant centers at this time. Detailed discussion of cellular immunotherapy for treatment of PTLD is outside the scope of this review.

Cytotoxic chemotherapy

In general, the need for chemotherapy appears to be more frequent in adult than in pediatric organ transplant recipients with PTLD. This may, in part, reflect the higher prevalence of monomorphic disease in the adult population. Because of the relatively high toxic mortality rates associated with the use of chemotherapy for PTLD [44], as well as the high likelihood that PTLD in children will respond to more conservative measures, we recommend restricting the use of chemotherapy as primary treatment to patients who have overt malignant disease, such as Burkitt lymphoma. It is unclear whether patients with monomorphic disease with histology of diffuse, large B-cell, non-Hodgkin lymphoma should receive a trial of reduction in immunosuppression or whether they should receive chemotherapy as primary treatment (with or without rituximab). Pediatric patients with refractory polymorphic PTLD have quite high initial response rates to "low dose" chemotherapy with cyclophosphamide and prednisone, although 2-year event-free survival is suboptimal at approximately 58% [44]. The addition of rituximab to a cytoxan-prednisone regimen is currently under investigation [45]. For refractory polymorphic disease, our preference at this time is to give a trial of rituximab before contemplating chemotherapy. Chemotherapy may be particularly useful for treating patients who relapse during reintroduction of immunosuppression necessitated by rejection, or in the rare case of active PTLD with concomitant rejection. For late onset monomorphic disease (not associated with primary EBV infection), most centers use chemotherapy as first line therapy. There have been no comparative trials of different chemotherapy regimens for PTLD and most centers used some form of "CHOP"-based regimen for most cases.

Burkitt-like PTLD is usually treated in comparable fashion to Burkitt lymphoma arising in the nontransplant recipient.

Radiation and surgery

Surgery and radiation are primarily indicated for the management of local complications (e.g. gastrointestinal hemorrhage, perforation, local compression of critical structures). Excisional biopsy may be curative for solitary PTLD lesions, but is usually combined with some reduction in immunosuppression. Thus, almost all patients receive a systemic approach to treatment and EBV-associated PTLD is probably best thought of as a systemic process.

EBV viral load monitoring and the management of PTLD

Although evidence supports measuring EBV viral load in the peripheral blood by quantitative PCR as an adjunct to making the diagnosis of PTLD [24,25], fewer data are available regarding the potential use of serial measurements of the EBV viral load as part of the management of this disease. Based on our experience, we believe that this test provides clinically relevant information regarding a patient's response to therapy [24,34]. Accordingly, we recommend weekly monitoring of the EBV viral load in the peripheral blood for patients diagnosed with EBV-driven PTLD. A decline in viral load suggests that the patient is responding and may identify the time when the patient is at risk for developing rejection. A viral load that remains high for more than 4 weeks, particularly if the patient is not showing evidence of a clinical response, should warrant consideration of a modification in both the child's specific PTLD therapy and immunosuppressive management.

The role of ongoing monitoring after a patient has appeared to respond to treatment is unclear. In our experience, most patients develop rebound elevations in their EBV viral load during serial monitoring after recovery from PTLD. Often this appears to correlate with the reintroduction or augmentation of immunosuppression. To date, viral load rebounds have only rarely been associated with symptoms or evidence of recurrence of PTLD. Because the frequency of rebound in PCR viral load is extremely high, but the rate of recurrent PTLD appears to be less than 10%, the interpretation of elevated EBV viral loads for patients with a past history of PTLD is unclear. Accordingly, we do not routinely recommend following this assay for clinical monitoring of patients who have fully recovered from PTLD. However, monitoring these patients as part of well-designed prospective clinical studies may be important. A significant proportion of patients who have recovered from their PTLD will go on to develop very high EBV viral loads that may persist for months or even years after resolution of their PTLD. An association between this chronic high load state and late malignant transformation has been reported for pediatric thoracic transplant recipients [46].

NON-PTLD MALIGNANCY

In adults, many forms of malignancy occur with increased incidence after solid organ transplantation and death from malignancy with a functioning graft is not rare. This includes an increased risk of recurrence of previously treated (pretransplant) malignant disease, as well as a marked increased risk of many forms of de novo malignancy [47]. Fortunately, non-PTLD malignancy is very rare after pediatric transplantation, and it is estimated that approximately 95% of pediatric post-transplant "tumors" fall into the broad category of lymphoproliferations. Most of the remaining tumors are skin cancers, and reflect the full range of cutaneous malignancy seen in the nontransplant setting. Other forms of cancer have been reported on rare occasions, including a specific association of immunosuppression with smooth muscle ("spindle cell") tumors [48]. These lesions usually demonstrate clonal EBV proliferation and may develop after a prior diagnosis of PTLD. These smooth muscle tumors appear to carry a poor prognosis. It seems likely that an increasing burden of non-PTLD malignancy will be observed as pediatric recipients survive longer and enter adult life.

CONCLUSIONS

Over the last decade, much has been learned about the nature of PTLD. The pivotal role of EBV infection in the majority of cases has been established and the pathologic description of lesions has been simplified in the current WHO classification. It seems likely that further understanding of the molecular pathology may lead to greater ability to define prognosis and optimal treatment regimens. Quantitative PCR techniques for EBV have enhanced the capability for early diagnosis of EBV infection and PTLD, and have proved a useful tool for monitoring response to therapy. A number of exciting new therapies are on the horizon, including use of monoclonal antibodies against B-cell surface antigens and the development of cellular therapies, such as the use of EBV-specific cytotoxic T-cell infusions. The role of chemotherapy, and the optimal regimens, is not yet fully defined. Our understanding of the etiology, behavior and optimal treatment for EBV-negative PTLD remains limited, in part because of the rarity of these lesions in children. Encouragingly, there is an increasing level of interest in PTLD among clinical and basic investigators, as well as recognition of the need for multicenter trials to define optimal prevention and treatment strategies.

REFERENCES

1 Nalesnik MA, Starzl TE. Epstein–Barr virus, infectious mononucleosis, and post-transplant lymphoproliferative disorders. *Transplant Science* 1994;4:61–79.

2 Starzl TE. Discussion of Murry JE, Wilson RE, Tilney NL *et al.* Five years' experience in renal transplantation with immunosuppressive drugs: survival, function, complications and the role of lymphocyte depletion by thoracic duct fistula. *Ann Surg* 1968;**168**:416.

3 Briggs JD, Hamilton DNH, Macsween RNM, *et al.* Infectious mononucleosis, herpes simplex infection and diffuse lymphoma in a renal transplant patient. *Transplantation* 1978;**25**:227.

4 Ho M. Risk factors and pathogenesis of posttransplant lymphoproliferative disorders. *Transplant Proc* 1995;**27**:38–40.

5 Chadburn A, Cesarman E, Knowles DM. Molecular pathology of posttransplant lymphoproliferative disorders. *Semin Diagn Pathol* 1997;**14**:15–26.

6 Nelson BP, Nalesnik MA, Bahler DW, Locker J, Fung JJ, Swerdlow SH. Epstein–Barr virus-negative post-transplant lymphoproliferative disorders: a distinct entity? *Am J Surg Pathol* 2000;**24**:375–85.

7 Webber SA. Post-transplant lymphoproliferative disorders: a preventable complication of solid organ transplantation? [Editorial]. *Pediatr Transplant* 1999;**3**:95–9.

8 Zangwill SD, Hsu DT, Kichuk MR, *et al.* Incidence and outcome of primary Epstein–Barr virus infection and lymphoproliferative disease in pediatric heart transplant recipients. *J Heart Lung Transplant* 1998;**17**:1161–6.

9 Finn L, Reyes J, Bueno J, Yunis E. Epstein–Barr virus infections in children after transplantation of the small intestine. *Am J Surg Pathol* 1998;**22**:299–309.

10 Cen H, Breinig MC, Atchison RW, Ho M, McKnight JLC. Epstein–Barr virus transmission via the donor organ in solid organ transplantation: polymerase chain reaction and restriction fragment length polymorphism analysis of IR2, IR3 and IR4. *J Virol* 1991;**65**:976–80.

11 Swinnen LJ, Costanzo-Nordin MR, Fisher SG, *et al.* Increased incidence of lymphoproliferative disorders after immunosuppression with the monoclonal antibody OKT3 in cardiac transplant recipients. *N Engl J Med* 1990;**323**:1723–8.

12 Newell KA, Alonso EM, Whitington PF, *et al.* Posttransplant lymphoproliferative disease in pediatriac liver transplantation. *Transplantation* 1996;**62**:370–5.

13 Dharnidharka VR, Tejani AH, Ho PL, Harmon WE. Posttransplant lymphoproliferative disorder in the United States: young Caucasian males are at highest risk. *Am J Transplant* 2002;**2**:993–8.

14 Cox KL, Lawrence-Miyasaki LS, Garcia-Kennedy R, *et al.* An increased incidence of Epstein–Barr virus infection and lymphoproliferative disease in young children on FK506 after liver transplantation. *Transplantation* 1995;**59**:524–9.

15 Ciancio G, Siquijor AP, Burke GW, *et al.* Post-transplant lymphoproliferative disease in kidney transplant recipients in the new immunosuppressive era. *Clin Transpl* 1997;**11**:243–9.

16 Webber SA. Fifteen years of pediatric heart transplantation at the University of Pittsburgh: lessons learned and future prospects. *Pediatr Transplant* 1997;**1**:8–21.

17 Dharnidharka VR, Ho PL, Stablein DM, Harmon WE, Tejani AH. Mycophenolate, tacrolimus and post-transplant lymphoproliferative disorder: a report of the North American Pediatric Renal Transplant Cooperative Study. *Pediatr Transplant* 2002; **6**:396–9.

18 Shapiro R, Nalesnik M, McCauley J, *et al.* Posttransplant lymphoproliferative disorders in adult and pediatric renal transplant patients receiving tacrolimus-based immunosuppression. *Transplantation* 1999;**68**:1851–4.

19 Younes BS, McDiarmid SV, Martin MG, *et al.* The effect of immunosuppression on posttransplant lymphoproliferative disease in pediatric liver transplant patients. *Transplantation* 2000;**70**:94–9.

20 Harwood JS, Gould FK, McMaster A, *et al.* Significance of EBV status and post-transplant lymphoproliferative disease in pediatric thoracic transplantation. *Pediatr Transplant* 1999;**3**:100–3.

21 Boyle GJ, Michaels MG, Webber SA, *et al.* Posttransplantation lymphoproliferative disorders in pediatric thoracic organ recipients. *J Pediatr* 1997;**131**:309–13.

22 Sweet SC, Spray TL, Huddleston CB, *et al.* Pediatric lung transplantation at St. Louis Children's Hospital, 1990–1995. *Am J Respir Crit Care Med* 1997;**155**:1027–35.

23 Webber SA, Naftel DC, Fricker FJ, *et al.* and the Pediatric Heart Transplant Study. Lymphoproliferative disorders following pediatric heart transplantation: a multi-institutional study. *Lancet* 2006;**367**:233–9.

24 Green M, Reyes J, Webber S, Michaels MG, Rowe D. The role of the Epstein–Barr viral load in the diagnosis, management and possible prevention of EBV-associated post-transplant lymphoproliferative disease following solid organ transplantation. *Curr Opin Organ Transplant* 1999;**4**:292–6.

25 Rowe DT, Qu L, Reyes J, *et al.* Use of quantitative competitive PCR to measure Epstein–Barr virus genome load in the peripheral blood of pediatric transplant recipients with lymphoproliferative disorders. *J Clin Microbiol* 1997;**35**:1612–5.

26 Wadowsky RM, Laus S, Green M, Webber SA, Rowe D. Comparison of Epstein–Barr virus DNA load measured in whole blood and plasma by TaqMan PCR and in peripheral blood lymphocytes by competitive PCR. *J Clin Microbiol* 2003;**41**:5245–9.

27 Harris NL, Swerdlow SH, Frizzera G, Knowles DM. Post-transplant lymphoproliferative disorders. In: Jaffe ES, Harris NL, Stein H, Vardiman JW, eds. *Pathology and Genetics of Tumours of Haematopoietic and Lymphoid Tissues. World Health Organization Classification of Tumors.* Lyon: IARC Press; 2001: 264–9.

28 Ranganathan S, Webber SA, Ahuja S, Jaffe R. Hodgkin's-like posttransplant lymphoproliferative disorder in children: does it differ from posttransplant Hodgkin's lymphoma? *Pediatr Dev Pathol* 2004;**7**:348–60.

29 Knowles DM, Cesarman E, Chadburn A, *et al.* Correlative morphologic and molecular genetic analysis demonstrates three distinct categories of posttransplant lymphoproliferative disorders. *Blood* 1995;**85**:552–65.

30 Epstein MA, Morgan AJ, Finerty S, *et al.* Protection of cottontop tamarins against Epstein–Barr virus-induced malignant lymphoma by a prototype subunit vaccine. *Nature* 1985;**318**:287–9.

31 Green M, Reyes J, Rowe D. New strategies in the prevention and management of Epstein–Barr virus infection and posttransplant lymphoproliferative disease following solid organ transplantation. *Curr Opin Organ Transplant* 1998;**3**:143–7.

32 Abedi MR, Linde A, Christensson B, Mackett M, Hammarstrom L, Smith C. Preventive effect of IgG from EBV-seropositive donors on the development of human lymphoproliferative disease in SCID mice. *Int J Cancer* 1997;**71**:624–9.

33 Green M, Michaels MG, Webber SA, Rowe D, Reyes J. The management of Epstein–Barr virus associated post-transplant lymphoproliferative disorders in pediatric solid organ transplant recipients. *Pediatr Transplant* 1999;**3**:271–81.

34 Webber SA, Green M. Post-transplant lymphoproliferative disorders: advances in diagnosis, prevention and management in children. *Prog Pediatr Cardiol* 2000;**11**:145–57.

35 Starzl TE, Nalesnik MA, Porter KA, *et al*. Reversibility of lymphomas and lymphoproliferative lesions developing under cyclosporin-steroid therapy. *Lancet* 1984;**1**:583–7.

36 Hanto DW, Frizzera G, Gajl-Peczalska KJ, *et al*. Epstein–Barr virus induced B-cell lymphoma after renal transplantation. *N Engl J Med* 1982;**306**:913–8.

37 Shapiro RS, Chauvenet A, McGuire W, *et al*. Treatment of B-cell lymphoproliferative disorders with interferon alfa and intravenous gamma globulin [Letter]. *N Engl J Med* 1988;**318**:1334.

38 Riddler SA, Breinig MC, McKnight JLC. Increased levels of circulating Epstein–Barr virus-infected lymphocytes and decreased EBV nuclear antigen antibody responses are associated with the development of posttransplant lymphoproliferative disease in solid-organ transplant recipients. *Blood* 1994;**84**:972–84.

39 Fisher A, Blanche S, Le Bidois J, *et al*. Anti-B-cell monoclonal antibodies in the treatment of severe B-cell lymphoproliferative syndrome following bone marrow and organ transplantation. *N Engl J Med* 1991;**324**:1451–6.

40 Milpied N, Vasseur B, Parquet N, *et al*. Humanized anti-CD20 monoclonal antibody (rituximab) in post transplant B-lympho-proliferative disorder: a retrospective analysis on 32 patients. *Ann Oncol* 2000;**11**(Suppl 1):113–6.

41 Webber S, Harmon W, Faro A, *et al*. Anti-CD20 monoclonal antibody (Rituximab) for refractory PTLD after pediatric solid organ transplantation: multicenter experience from a registry and from a prospective clinical trial [Abstract]. *Blood* 2004;**104**:213a.

42 Rooney CM, Smith CA, Ng CYC, *et al*. Use of gene-modified virus-specific T lymphocytes to control Epstein–Barr virus related lymphoproliferation. *Lancet* 1995;**345**:9–13.

43 Gottschalk S, Heslop HE, Rooney CM. Adoptive immunotherapy for EBV-associated malignancies. *Leuk Lymphoma* 2005;**46**:1–10.

44 Gross TG. Low-dose chemotherapy for children with post-transplant lymphoproliferative disease. *Recent Adv Cancer Res* 2002;**159**:96–103.

45 Orjuela M, Gross TG, Cheung YK, Alobeid B, Morris E, Cairo MS. A pilot study of chemoimmunotherapy (cyclophosphamide, prednisone, and rituximab) in patients with post-transplant lymphoproliferative disorder following solid organ transplantation. *Clin Cancer Res* 2003;**9**:3945S–52S.

46 Bingler MA, Miller SA, Boyle GJ, *et al*. Chronic high Epstein–Barr virus load carrier state and risk for late onset PTLD/malignant lymphoma. *J Heart Lung Transplant* 2005;**24**:S113–4.

47 Trofe J, Beebe TM, Buell JF, *et al*. Posttransplant malignancy. *Prog Transplant* 2004;**14**:193–200.

48 Lee ES, Locker J, Nalesnik M, *et al*. The association of Epstein–Barr virus with smooth muscle tumors occurring after organ transplantation. *N Engl J Med* 1995;**332**:19–25.

14 Organ Toxicities

Vikas R. Dharnidharka, Carlos E. Araya and Mark R. Benfield

Solid organ transplant recipients are subjected to multiple organ toxicities as a result of the medications needed to prevent rejection and infection and to treat complications. In most cases, these toxicities are not preventable so transplant physicians attempt to minimize them. This chapter describes the different toxicities that are primarily caused by transplant-related medications. These medications include immunosuppressive agents, antimicrobial agents used in routine prophylaxis and antihypertensive medications. The common organ toxicities of these three classes of agents are listed in Tables 14.1–14.3, respectively. Organ damage from transplant-related infections or post-transplant malignancy is covered elsewhere in this book.

KIDNEY TOXICITY IN NONRENAL TRANSPLANTS

Nephrotoxicity in solid organ transplants other than the kidney (e.g. heart, lung, liver) is most commonly caused by the long-term nephrotoxicity of calcineurin inhibitors (CNIs) such as cyclosporine and tacrolimus. In general, the nephrotoxicity of CNIs can be classified as an acute, functional and dose-dependent decrease in renal blood flow and glomerular filtration rate (GFR) or chronic structural changes and dose-independent interstitial fibrosis [1]. Although the mechanism of nephrotoxicity is not fully understood, several factors have been implicated in the pathogenesis of immunosuppressive-induced nephrotoxicity. Renal and systemic vasoconstriction,

Table 14.1 Common end-organ toxicities of various immunosuppressive agents.

Immunosuppressive agent	End-organ/system	Toxicity
Cyclosporine A	Kidney	Nephrotoxicity
	Cardiovascular	Hypertension
	Nervous system	Seizures, headache
	Gastrointestinal	Hepatotoxicity
Tacrolimus	Metabolic	Diabetes mellitus, hypokalemia, hypomagnesemia
	Nervous system	Neurotoxicity, seizures
	Kidney	Nephrotoxicity
	Gastrointestinal	Diarrhea, abdominal pain
Mycophenolate mofetil	Hematologic	Leukopenia, neutropenia, thrombocytopenia
	Gastrointestinal	Diarrhea, abdominal pain, dyspepsia, bleeding, ulceration
Azathioprine	Hematologic	Leukopenia, neutropenia, thrombocytopenia, anemia
	Gastrointestinal	Nausea, vomiting, diarrhea, pancreatitis, elevated hepatic transaminases
Glucocorticoids	Cardiovascular	Hypertension
	Bone	Growth failure
	Bone	Osteopenia
	Nervous system	Psychosis
	Gastrointestinal	Gastric ulceration
Sirolimus	Metabolic	Hyperlipidemia, hypercholesterolemia
	Hematologic	Leukopenia, thrombocytopenia
	Gastrointestinal	Hepatic artery thrombosis in liver transplants

Table 14.2 Common end-organ toxicities of various antimicrobial agents used for prophylaxis in transplant recipients.

Antimicrobial agent	End-organ/system	Toxicity
Trimethoprim-sulfamethoxazole	Hematologic Gastrointestinal Kidney	Leukopenia Nausea, vomiting, diarrhea Interstitial nephritis, albuminuria
Aciclovir and valaciclovir	Gastrointestinal Hematologic Kidney	Nausea, vomiting, diarrhea, hepatic transaminase elevation Leukopenia, neutropenia, thrombocytopenia Nephrotoxicity
Ganciclovir and valganciclovir	Gastrointestinal Hematologic Kidney	Nausea, vomiting, diarrhea, hepatic transaminase elevation Leukopenia, neutropenia, thrombocytopenia Nephrotoxicity
Clotrimazole	Very few systemic adverse reactions	
Pentamidine	Kidney Hematologic Respiratory Metabolic	Renal failure Leukopenia, thrombocytopenia Dyspnea Hypoglycemia
Dapsone	Hematologic Kidney Gastrointestinal	Hemolytic anemia, methemoglobinemia, aplastic anemia Acute tubular necrosis, albuminuria Nausea, pancreatitis, hepatic transaminase elevation

Table 14.3 Common end-organ toxicities of antihypertensive agents used post-transplantation.

Agent and class	End-organ/system	Toxicity
ACE inhibitors Enalapril, lisinopril	Kidney Metabolic Reproductive Pulmonary	Acute renal failure Hyperkalemia Fetal teratogenicity Chronic cough
Angiotensin receptor blockers Candesartan, telmesartan, irbesartan	Kidney Metabolic Reproductive	Acute renal failure Hyperkalemia Fetal teratogenicity
Beta blockers Propranolol, atenolol, metoprolol	Pulmonary Cardiac Metabolic	Exacerbation of asthma Bradycardia Diabetes mellitus
Calcium-channel blockers Nifedipine, diltiazem	Cardiac Hepatic	Worsened heart failure Liver enzyme elevation
Diuretics Hydrocholorothiazide, furosemide	Metabolic	Hypokalemia Hyperuricemia Hyponatremia
Vasodilators Clonidine, minoxidil	Neurologic Dermatologic	Sedation Hirsutism

ACE, angiotensin-converting enzyme.

increased release of endothelin-1, decreased production of nitric acid and increased expression of transforming growth factor β (TGF-β) are the major adverse pathophysiologic abnormalities of these agents. Over a period of time, these molecular level changes are associated with secondary hyaline vascular changes in the renal parenchyma and accelerate glomerular sclerosis and tubular atrophy [2].

Occasionally, other medications may contribute additive nephrotoxicity (e.g. prolonged use of ganciclovir or acute courses of nephrotoxic antimicrobials such as vancomycin and gentamicin for treatment of infections). Additionally, in heart transplant recipients, it is often difficult to distinguish between the amount of drug-induced nephrotoxicity and the drop in GFR because of poor renal blood flow from a suboptimal pump function of the heart. Recently, sirolimus has been associated with proteinuria in both renal and islet cell transplants [3,4].

Ojo et al. [5] performed a large-scale analysis of United Network for Organ Sharing (UNOS) data on chronic renal failure in nonrenal transplant recipients. In the period 1990–2000, UNOS recorded 69 321 nonrenal transplants within the USA. Of these, 16.5% developed chronic renal insufficiency (CRI) (GFR < 29 mL/min/1.73 m^2). Among these patients with CRI, 28.9% needed maintenance dialysis or transplantation. The occurrence of CRI significantly increased the risk of patient death.

Coopersmith et al. [6] reported their single-center series of 18 renal transplants following previous heart, liver or lung transplantation over an 8-year period. CNI toxicity was a major contributor in 94%. The patient survival rate at 1 and 3 years was no statistically different in these patients compared with those receiving a kidney transplant without previous other solid organ transplant. Other single-center studies have demonstrated a 3–10% incidence of end-stage renal disease (ESRD) with chronic cyclosporine use in cardiac transplants, 7.5% after lung transplantation and 18–73% after liver transplantation [7].

Among 294 orthotopic liver transplants in 221 children between 1984 and 1992 at the University of Wisconsin, the incidence of acute renal failure was 6.2% [8]. The prevalence of abnormal renal function was 33% at any given time period following transplantation. A single-center retrospective review of 125 pediatric lung transplant recipients undergoing first lung transplant and surviving at least 1 year also reveals a high incidence of renal insufficiency among these patients [9]. Serum creatinine nearly doubled from baseline to 1 year, and tripled by 7 years after transplant. The GFR, as estimated by the Schwartz formula, decreased from baseline 163 to 69 mL/min/1.73 m^2 by 10 years (P < 0.01). Seven patients (5.6%) developed ESRD, and by 5 years after transplant 38% of patients reached GFR < 60 mL/min. Older age at transplant and primary diagnosis of cystic fibrosis were both associated with decreased renal survival.

Tables 14.4 and 14.5 depict the most recent registry data available regarding the incidence of various organ system toxicities after pediatric heart or lung transplantation, respectively. Approximately 10% of all pediatric lung or heart transplant recipients will develop abnormal serum creatinine values by 5–7 years post-transplant. Approximately 3% will be on sustained dialysis by that time period and 1% will have received a kidney transplant.

In the immediate postoperative period, preventing hypotension and ensuring adequate renal perfusion can help reduce ischemic injury to the kidney. Close monitoring of CNI levels in peripheral blood and prevention of high CNI drug levels is also helpful and should be standard of care. In particular, levels should be carefully monitored when drugs with known pharmacokinetic interactions (e.g. ketoconazaole, erythromycin) are added. Many centers have now introduced CNI minimization protocols which feature much lower peripheral blood drug levels once the patient is beyond the first few months post-transplant. Industry sponsored drug trials of switch from CNI to sirolimus after the first few months have shown better preservation of renal function at 2–3 years post-transplant [10,11]. Similar prospective data are lacking in a pediatric population, although one retrospective study in a pediatric heart transplant population suggests improvement in renal function [12]. Avoiding drugs with additive nephrotoxicity (such as vancomyin, amphotericin, aminoglycosides) is preferred but not always possible, given the complexities of pediatric transplant patients.

Outcome	Within 1 year	Within 5 years	Within 7 years
Hypertension (%)	45.6	60.4	64.7
Renal dysfunction (%)	5.4	8.4	10.0
Abnormal creatinine < 2.5 mg/dL (%)	3.5	7.0	5.4
Creatinine > 2.5 mg/dL (%)	1.3	0.7	3.1
Long-term dialysis (%)	0.6	0.5	3.1
Renal transplant (%)	0.1	0.2	1.2
Hyperlipidemia (%)	9.9	20.2	23.3
Diabetes (%)	3.2	4.5	4.4
CAV (%)	2.5	11.4	14.3

Table 14.4 Pediatric heart transplant end-organ toxicities (Source: OPTN/SRTR registries of US data up to the year 2003; courtesy of Dr. Richard Fine).

CAV, cardiac allograft vasculopathy.

Table 14.5 Pediatric lung transplant toxicities (Source: OPTN/SRTR registries of US data up to the year 2003; courtesy of Dr. Richard Fine).

Outcome	Within 1 year	Within 5 years
Hypertension (%)	37.8	71.6
Renal dysfunction (%)	6.8	22.1
Abnormal creatinine < 2.5 mg/dL (%)	4.0	10.3
Creatinine > 2.5 mg/dL (%)	1.7	7.4
Long-term dialysis (%)	0.8	2.9
Renal transplant (%)	0.3	1.5
Hyperlipidemia (%)	1.4	2.9
Diabetes (%)	22.5	27.9
Bronchiolitis obliterans (%)	14.6	26.5

CARDIOVASCULAR TOXICITY IN NONHEART TRANSPLANT RECIPIENTS

Cardiovascular disease is the most important risk factor limiting the long-term success of solid organ transplants. It accounts for 40%, 20% and 5% of late mortality after adult renal, liver and lung transplant recipients, respectively [13–15]. Major risk factors for cardiovascular disease in adults include advanced age, male gender, obesity, hypertension, diabetes mellitus, dyslipidemia and tobacco use. Immunosuppressive medications contribute importantly to cardiovascular risk by increasing the likelihood of hypertension, dyslipidemia and diabetes mellitus. CNIs can lead to post-transplant hypertension by renal or peripheral vasoconstriction, impaired nitric oxide-induced vasodilatation and release of the vasoconstrictors endothelin, thromboxane and prostaglandins [16,17]. Glucocorticoids have the potential to cause hypertension by affecting peripheral vascular resistance and circulating volume [18]. There are no data to suggest that mycophenolate mofetil (MMF), azathioprine or sirolimus contribute to the development of post-transplant hypertension.

The prevalence of cardiovascular disease is considerably higher in the kidney transplant patients when compared with the general population up to the age of 80 years [19]. In liver transplant recipients, Johnston et al. [20] evaluated cardiovascular risk scores and demonstrated a relative risk of cardiac death of 2.56 when compared with an age- and gender matched population.

The 5-year results from a study comparing tacrolimus with cyclosporine-based immunosuppression in kidney transplant patients demonstrated that fewer patients treated with tacrolimus required antihypertensive medications [21]. Ligtenberg et al. [22] documented changes in cardiovascular risk factors in stable renal transplant patients converted from cyclosporine to tacrolimus. Using 24-hour ambulatory blood pressure recordings, a significant decline in blood pressure both day

and night was observed and when cyclosporine was resumed the blood pressure returned to preconversion levels. Total and low density lipoprotein cholesterol levels (LDL) decreased and no abnormalities in the fasting glucose levels were noted. A higher prevalence of coronary events were observed by Guckelberger et al. [23] at 10 years' follow-up in liver transplant recipients. However, no difference was seen between the immunosuppressive regimens. Other investigators have found that tacrolimus has a more favorable cardiovascular profile of blood pressure, serum cholesterol level and weight [24]. Silverborn et al. [25] reported the prevalence of new onset cardiovascular risk factors in lung transplant recipients with cyclosporine-based immunosuppression. At 3 years, 90% of patients had at least one risk factor and 40% had developed two or more risk factors. CNI-free immunosuppression protocols have led to significant improvements in blood pressure in patients treated with sirolimus, but the risk of dyslipidemia was higher [26]. Tacrolimus may have direct cardiotoxic potential, but the incidence of hypertrophic cardiomyopathy in adult transplant recipients was only 0.1% [27].

Single-center studies have reported increased cardiovascular disease mortality in pediatric renal transplant patients [28]. However, data on long-term survival in children after solid organ transplantation are lacking. Using ambulatory blood pressure monitoring, post-transplant hypertension has been documented in 62–75% of patients [29,30]. The incidence of hypertension after pediatric kidney, heart, lung and liver transplantation at different time points post-transplant is shown in Table 14.6. A retrospective study of the North American Pediatric Renal Transplant Cooperative Study (NAPRTCS) database demonstrated that patients receiving tacrolimus/MMF/steroids were less likely to require antihypertensive medications at 1 and 2 years post-transplant compared with patients receiving cyclosporine/MMF/steroids [31]. However, in a prospective randomized study of kidney transplants, the prevalence of hypertension was not different in patients

Table 14.6 Incidence of long-term hypertension in pediatric solid organ transplants per registry data (hypertension defined as need for antihypertension medication).

Organ	% Reported			Source
	2 years	5 years	7 years	
Kidney	75	70		NAPRTCS
Liver	14.5/15.7			SPLIT
Heart			64.7	ISHLT
Lung		71.6		ISHLT

Blank cells indicate time periods for which the respective registry has not reported percentages.
ISHLT, International Society for Heart and Lung Transplantation; NAPRTCS, North American Pediatric Renal Transplant Cooperative Study; SPLIT, Special Studies in Pediatric Liver Transplantation.

treated with cyclosporine- or tacrolimus-based immunosuppression after 6 months' follow-up. In this study, the patients treated with tacrolimus had lower total cholesterol levels and the incidence of post-transplant diabetes was similar for both groups [32]. A study by Jain *et al.* [33] analyzed 233 children who received liver transplants. The investigators documented a significant reduction in the incidence and severity of hypertension in the patients treated with tacrolimus when compared with cyclosporine. Direct cardiac toxicity resulting in hypertrophic cardiomyopathy in children undergoing liver and small bowel transplantation has been associated with tacrolimus therapy at higher rates than seen in adults, for reasons that are yet unclear [34–36].

Vascular thrombosis in the early post-transplant period is a relatively greater problem in pediatric solid organ transplant recipients than adult recipients. The reasons for the greater incidence may relate to the smaller size of the blood vessels being anastomosed, lower blood flow rates or greater prothrombotic potential because of underlying diseases such as nephrotic syndrome. In intestinal transplants, thrombosis represents the second most common reason for graft removal at 15.3% (Intestinal Transplant Registry report). The use of very young donors, less than 5 years of age, for pediatric recipients was associated with a very high incidence of thrombosis post-kidney transplant [37]. The incidence of renal vessel thrombosis after kidney transplantation dropped after this practice was stopped [38]. In pediatric liver transplant recipients, the use of sirolimus in the early post-transplant period was associated with higher risk of hepatic artery thrombosis [39].

Lifestyle modifications including dietary changes, weight reduction, exercise and smoking cessation are important in the management of cardiovascular risk factors. Adjustment of the immunosuppressive drug regimens can be a reasonable alternative when risk factor is associated with such therapy. Corticosteroid reduction or withdrawal is associated with a significant decrease in hypertension and post-transplant diabetes [40–42]. The choice of CNI also appears to affect the prevalence of cardiovascular risk factors, because converting patients from cyclosporine to tacrolimus frequently results in a reduction in hypertension and dyslipidemia.

All classes of antihypertensive medications have been used in solid organ transplantation. Calcium-channel blockers reduce the nephrotoxicity of CNI but may interact with the cytochrome P450 system. Beta-blockers have the advantage of providing cardioprotection but may contribute to dyslipidemia and insulin resistance. The angiotensin-converting enzyme (ACE) inhibitors and angiotensin receptor blockers (ARB) are renoprotective agents. However, their use is generally avoided early in renal transplantation because they may decrease renal blood flow. Diuretics are useful in patients with sodium and fluid excess but may contribute to dyslipidemia and insulin resistance. In patients with elevated levels of total cholesterol and LDL cholesterol, the HMG-CoA reductase inhibitors are commonly used. Fibrates are effective in lowering triglyceride levels primarily. These agents may increase the risk of rhabdomyolysis when used in combination or with CNIs and sirolimus. Patients with post-transplant diabetes should maintain adequate glycemic control with lifestyle modifications, insulin, metformin and/or a thiazilidinedione.

METABOLIC TOXICITIES

The three major toxicities related to body metabolism are diabetes mellitus, hyperlipidemia and obesity. Diabetes mellitus is already common in patients needing lung transplants when cystic fibrosis is the predominant cause of end-stage lung disease. Similarly, diabetes mellitus is a common cause or contributor for ESRD in adults, but not in children. New onset diabetes mellitus is a known adverse effect of both glucocorticoids and CNI because these drugs affect insulin secretion and tissue sensitivity and resistance to the effects of insulin. The diabetogenic effect of glucocorticoids is dose dependent. Improvements in appetite, plus the effects of glucocorticoids, lead to develop of obesity, promoting insulin resistance and the development of diabetes mellitus in children.

The CNIs, glucocorticoids and especially the mammalian target of rapamycin (mTOR) inhibitors lead to hyperlipidemia. The increased levels of very low density lipoprotein (VLDL), total cholesterol and triglycerides observed with glucocorticoid therapy are brought about by enhanced activity of acetyl-coenzyme A carboxylase and free fatty acid synthase, as well as inhibition of lipoprotein lipase [43]. Cyclosporine binds to the LDL receptor, increasing serum LDL cholesterol levels. Also, its effects on hepatic lipase and lipoprotein lipase activity impair the clearance of LDL and VLDL [43]. CNI use, especially tacrolimus, is also commonly associated with blood electrolyte abnormalities such as hypomagnesemia, hypophosphatemia and hypokalemia, because of effects upon renal tubular excretion of these electrolytes. After transplantation, most patients experience an improvement in appetite because of absence of organ failure. Glucocorticoids increase the appetite, contributing to obesity after transplantation.

The occurrence of diabetes mellitus in adult renal transplants is quite high at almost 20–30%. Age, family history and ethnicity all impact upon the incidence of diabetes. Kasiske *et al.* [44] determined from a retrospective large-scale analysis of the US Renal Data System (USRDS) database that the risk for diabetes mellitus was higher with greater recipient age, African-American or Hispanic ethnicity, male donor, higher human leukocyte antigen (HLA) mismatch, hepatitis C infection or use of tacrolimus [44]. In long-term liver transplant patients, the prevalence of diabetes was significantly increased compared with the general population [45]. Using the International Society for Heart and Lung Transplantation (ISHLT) registry data, Taylor *et al.* [46] determined that the prevalence of post-transplant diabetes was 33.2% after 5 years and 36.5% after 8 years in heart transplant recipients. In lung transplant recipients, the 5 and 8 year cumulative prevalence was 30.9% and 28.3%, respectively [15]. Furthermore, cystic fibrosis and pretransplant blood glucose level have been identified as independent predictors of post-transplant diabetes in lung transplant recipients [25].

Dyslipidemia is common following solid organ transplantation, particularly after heart and lung transplant. In heart transplant recipients, dyslipidemia has been associated with the development of cardiac allograft vasculopathy [43]. In males with a deceased donor kidney allograft and a history of acute rejection, the rate of graft loss was significantly greater in those with hypercholesterolemia compared with those with normal cholesterol at 5 and 10 years [47]. Of the CNIs, cyclosporine has been associated with a significant greater proportion of hypercholesterolemia and hypertriglyceridemia in renal transplant patients when compared with tacrolimus [48]. Also, a significantly greater proportion of patients receiving cyclosporine-based therapy required lipid lowering medications at 1 and 5 years post-transplant [21]. The same results are observed in patients treated with a combination of tacrolimus and sirolimus when compared with tacrolimus and MMF therapy [49]. In a report by Silverborn et al. [25], lung transplant recipients with hypercholesterolemia had a lower incidence of acute rejection episodes. The authors speculated that the use of statins, which increases systemic concentration of cyclosporine, could have led to a lower cyclosporine dose in those patients.

Data in pediatric transplant recipients

In contrast to adult renal transplant recipients, the incidence of diabetes mellitus in pediatric renal transplant recipients is much lower at 2–4%. The incidence of diabetes mellitus after heart and lung transplantation in children is provided in Tables 14.3 and 14.4. Heart transplant recipients have a similar incidence of diabetes mellitus in comparison with kidney transplant recipients. However, lung transplant recipients have a much higher cumulative diabetes mellitus incidence of 20–30% by 5 years post-transplant, again likely because of the progressive effects of cystic fibrosis in this population. The impact of diabetes mellitus on survival has not been evaluated in the pediatric transplant population. With regards to immunosuppression, the lower corticosteroid doses and target tacrolimus trough levels have also contributed to a decrease in the incidence of diabetes mellitus in pediatric patients. In the recent pediatric multicenter European study there was no difference in the incidence of diabetes mellitus between the tacrolimus and cyclosporine groups [32].

As in adults, the prevalence of dyslipidemia in pediatric transplant recipients is variable. Registry data from the ISHLT reported a cumulative prevalence of hyperlipidemia in heart and lung transplant recipients at 5 years of 21.4% and 4.5%, respectively [50]. In pediatric liver transplant recipients, McDiarmid et al. [51] reported an elevated total cholesterol

level in almost half of the study cohort. In the European study in renal transplant patients, the total cholesterol levels were elevated in the cyclosporine group when compared with the tacrolimus group at 6 months [32].

Obesity is an increasing problem in children who present for transplantation and may have an adverse effect on allograft and patient survival, besides increasing the risk for type II diabetes and hypertension. In pediatric kidney transplants, Hanevold et al. [52] found that obese children aged 6–12 years had higher risk for death than nonobese patients (adjusted relative risk: 3.65 for living donor; 2.94 for deceased donor), and death was more likely as a result of cardiopulmonary disease (27% in obese vs. 17% in nonobese). Overall, graft loss as a result of thrombosis was more common in obese compared with nonobese (19% vs. 10%).

In renal transplant patients, the use of alternate day steroids was associated with lower total cholesterol and triglyceride levels when compared with daily steroid therapy [53]. A reduction in total and LDL cholesterol levels were also observed in patients after corticosteroid withdrawal as early as 3 months post-transplant [41]. Furthermore, early steroid withdrawal reduces the incidence of diabetes mellitus from 30% to 8% at 2 years post-transplant [40].

Several investigators have shown an improvement in blood lipid levels as well as a decreased requirement for lipid-reducing medications after converting patients from cyclosporine to tacrolimus-based immunosuppression [21,22,54]. Earlier studies by Pirsch et al. [48] reported a higher incidence of diabetes mellitus with tacrolimus-based immunosuppression when compared with cyclosporine at 1 year post-transplant (19.9% and 4%, respectively). More recent studies have shown a low incidence of diabetes mellitus in both cyclosporine- and tacrolimus-treated patients [55,56]. However, the initial higher tacrolimus mean daily doses may have contributed to the observed higher incidence of diabetes mellitus.

In patients with elevated levels of total cholesterol and LDL-cholesterol, the HMG-CoA reductase inhibitors are commonly used. Fibrates are effective in lowering triglyceride levels primarily. Patients with post-transplant diabetes should maintain adequate glycemic control with lifestyle modifications, insulin, metformin and/or a thiazilidinedione.

TOXICITIES RELATED TO BONE AND MUSCULOSKELETAL SYSTEM

Several bone and skeletal system adverse effects can be noted after transplantation, including stunted linear growth, osteoporosis/bone loss, higher incidence of fractures and avascular necrosis of the hip joint. These adverse effects are not unexpected, because adult stature and peak bone mass are achieved during childhood growth and development, and organ failure as well as post-transplant medications impact normal bone metabolism. This section briefly outlines some of the bone-related toxicities. A recently published review provides greater detail [57]. Renal and hepatic failure can themselves give rise to an osteodystrophy [58,59]. Post-transplant renal dysfunction, now not uncommon in other solid organ transplants, is probably an additional aggravating factor. Most of the bone-related transplant drug toxicity has been attributed to long-term glucocorticoid use. This class of drugs has many negative effects on bone, including decreased intestinal calcium absorption, increased renal calcium excretion, decreased osteoblastic activity, increased serum parathyroid hormone (PTH) concentrations and increase number of remodeling sites [57]. Many studies have highlighted the higher risk for bone problems with long-term glucocorticoid use, as reviewed by Ward [60]. However, Leonard et al. [61] have questioned this hypothesis based on their studies in patients receiving high-dose intermittent glucocorticoids for nephrotic syndrome. In fact, Julian et al. [62] demonstrated that even in the cyclosporine era, there was widespread osteopenia in transplant recipients. Other factors implicated in bone disease in the post-transplant patient include immobilization and primary disease (such as cystinosis or primary hyperoxaluria).

In adults, most bone-related disease occurs in the form of osteopenia, avascular necrosis of joints and higher incidence of fractures. Thus, young adult kidney transplant recipients under 45 years age have an 87- to 99-fold higher risk of fracture than the general population before transplant, a risk that actually rises transiently post-transplant [63,64]. Avascular necrosis of the hip and other joints is a particular problem in elderly transplant recipients. Abbott et al. [65] reviewed USRDS renal transplant registry data from 1994 to 1998, which revealed that the cumulative incidence of avascular necrosis was 7.1 episodes/1000 person-years from 1994 to 1998. An earlier year of transplant, African-American race, allograft rejection, peritoneal dialysis (vs. hemodialysis) and diabetes were the only factors independently associated with hospitalizations for avascular necrosis. Similarly, the risk for needing hip joint replacement was 5.1 times higher in post-kidney transplant adult patients than the general population. Adult liver transplant recipients also experience higher rates of fracture and avascular necrosis than the general population, with a cumulative incidence of avascular necrosis 33% at 4 years.

In contrast to adults, the predominant osseous effects in children are upon linear growth. Fractures are more common in children with organ transplants than the general population, but the frequency is lower than in adult transplant recipients. Thus, children post-kidney transplant have 2% incidence of fractures and 1% incidence of avascular necrosis within 3–4 years post-transplant. Rates of avascular necrosis were higher in older reports from the 1970s and 1980s, largely because of worse control of renal osteodystrophy and greater dependence on steroids for post-transplant immunosuppression. Children with a liver transplant have a cumulative post-transplant fracture rate of approximately 5%.

Linear body growth is a particularly important issue in pediatric solid organ transplantation [66]. Children with organ failure generally have stunted growth at the time of transplant, even with the use of pretransplant growth hormone therapy. Although organ transplantation leads to catch-up growth in the short term, there is still suboptimal growth in the long term. Younger patients and those with more marked stunting experience the greatest catch-up growth [67]. The reduced final adult height has been attributed to premature closure of the epiphyses because of chronic glucocorticoid administration.

Optimization of growth and minimization of bone disease preorgan transplant is recommended to whatever extent possible. Growth hormone therapy can be used post-transplant to improve linear growth and is effective [68]. No increase in acute rejections or decrease in graft survival was seen, even though growth hormone does possess some immunomodulatory activities. Withdrawal of or reduction in glucocorticoid dosage post-transplant has been associated with some improvements [69]. With the advent of steroid avoidance protocols in pediatric transplantation, linear growth post-transplant can be markedly improved [42,70].

GASTROINTESTINAL TOXICITY IN NONGASTROINTESTINAL ORGAN TRANSPLANTS

Many of the medications used post-transplant can cause gastrointestinal symptoms. In fact, nausea, vomiting and abdominal pain are among the most common side-effects of most of the medications discussed in this chapter. In particular, MMF and azathioprine lead to nausea, vomiting and diarrhea. The exact mechanisms are unknown but include direct cytopathic effects, drug interactions and predisposition to infection [71].

Drug-induced hepatotoxicity, by comparison, is relatively rare in transplant recipients. Issues related to hepatitis C infection or drug interactions resulting from cytochrome C metabolic pathways are much more common. Cyclosporine is associated with mild cholestasis in the early period post-transplant [72]. Azathioprine can lead to damage to endothelial cells within sinusoids, with a variety of clinical manifestations [73]. Glucocorticoids and tacrolimus do not appear to have significant hepatotoxicity. Sirolimus may lead to hepatic artery thrombosis [39]. Right heart failure can lead to hepatic congestion.

Because many transplant medications that are toxic to the gastrointestinal tract are used in combination, it is difficult to ascertain precisely the relative contribution of each medication.

In three large randomized trials of MMF in kidney transplant recipients, the cumulative incidence of gastrointestinal side-effects was 25–40% in placebo or azathioprine groups and 50–55% in the MMF groups [74–76]. The higher 3-g dose of MMF was associated with a higher incidence of gastrointestinal side-effects with no additional benefit in reducing acute rejection rates. In adult lung transplant recipients, 13% experienced gastrointestinal side-effects [77]. Hepatic enzyme elevation with cyclosporine use was reported in as many as 49% of renal transplant recipients in one study [72].

Ettenger and Sarwal recently reviewed the role of MMF in pediatric renal transplantation [78]. The Tricontinental MMF suspension trial showed a higher incidence of gastrointestinal side-effects in the youngest recipients [79,80]. Other European studies have suggested that the adverse effect profile is acceptable [81]. Data in other pediatric organ transplant recipients relate primarily to pharmacokinetics and not to adverse effect profiles.

Acid reflux problems can be minimized by the concomitant use of proton pump inhibitors or H-2 receptor antagonists. The dosage of MMF can be reduced if gastrointestinal symptoms are severe. Monitoring drug levels may be useful. In some cases, the symptoms are so severe that MMF may need to be discontinued. Hepatic enzyme elevation post-transplant because of drug toxicity and not a result of infection is usually reversible or self-limited, but may require cessation of the implicated drug.

HEMATOPOIETIC TOXICITIES

All three major cell lines of the hematopoietic system (i.e. red cells, white cells and platelets) can be affected. Thus, toxicities related to the three cell lines include anemia/erythrocytosis, leukopenia/leukocytosis and thrombocytopenia/thrombocytosis. However, in most cases related to pediatric transplantation, the *decrease* in cell counts are more frequent and of greater clinical importance.

Anemia can be caused by any or a combination of bone marrow suppression, hemolysis or blood loss. Bone marrow suppression can be induced by several of the transplant medications such as mycophenolic acid, azathioprine, the antiviral drugs aciclovir and ganciclovir and their oral analogs valaciclovir and valganciclovir. The sulfur-containing drugs such as trimethoprim-sulfamethoxazole and dapsone can lead to hemolytic anemias. The ACE inhibitors may cause a pure red cell aplasia. Very rarely, the CNIs and OKT3 were associated with hemolytic uremic syndrome [82]. More commonly, poor kidney function from whatever cause can lead to secondary erythropoietin deficiency and anemia. Poor nutritional intake secondary to any organ dysfunction can lead to iron, B vitamin or folic acid deficiencies and nutritional anemia.

The drugs MMF and azathioprine can also cause leukopenia and thrombocytopenia as part of bone marrow suppression by direct nucleic acid synthesis inhibition [83]. Leukopenia and thrombocytopenia may also be seen with pentamidine, sirolimus and trimethoprim-sulfamethoxazole.

Azathioprine caused leukopenia in 3.8% and thrombocytopenia in 2% of 739 inflammatory bowel disease patients [84]. With the use of MMF, severe neutropenia develops (absolute neutrophil count < 500/mm^3) in up to 2% of renal transplant patients, 2.8% of cardiac transplant patients and 3.6% of liver transplant patients. Neutropenia is more common with higher doses of MMF and occurs most commonly 31–180 days post-transplant [74–76]. Other hematologic adverse reactions occurring in renal, cardiac and liver transplant patients, respectively, include anemia (25.6%, 42.9%, 43%), leukopenia (23.2%, 30.4%, 45.8%), thrombocytopenia (10.1%, 23.5%, 38.3%) and leukocytosis (7.1%, 40.5%, 22.4%). Decreases in hemoglobin occurred in 3–19.9%, anemia in 21.6% and leukopenia in 19.2% of patients who received 1440 mg/day mycophenolate sodium (various studies cited previously in the gastrointestinal toxicity section).

The incidence of anemia in pediatric renal transplants has been variable but much higher than in the adult renal transplant population. Previous studies have shown anemia rates of 30–80% at 1 and 5 years post-transplant [85–87]. The incidence of anemia may be increasing in this population with the wider use of MMF in place of azathioprine [86]. In a prospective trial of MMF, anemia and leukopenia were more common after MMF use in renal transplant recipients less than 6 years of age [79].

Anemia should be minimized pretransplant through adequate nutritional intake, therapeutic supplementation and erythropoietin use. Post-transplant, all allograft recipients should have their complete blood counts monitored routinely. Evidence of abnormal counts or levels, especially low levels such as leukopenia, which are deemed to be drug-induced, may require changes in drug doses or even discontinuation. In general, the MMF dosage is reduced when the absolute neutrophil count drops below 1500/mm^3 and the drug is discontinued at absolute neutrophil count (ANC) levels below 1000/mm^3. Paradoxically, studies of steroid avoidance in pediatric renal transplants demonstrated greater leukopenia with MMF use, suggesting a protective effect of steroids in this situation [42,70]. Post-transplant erythrocytosis can, in fact, be treated with ACE inhibitors, a beneficial use of an adverse effect [88].

NEUROTOXICITIES

Neurologic toxicities in solid organ transplant recipients can occur as a result of several mechanisms [89]. Drugs such as CNIs, glucocorticoids, OKT3 and growth hormone can have direct drug toxicities. In most cases, the exact mechanisms by which these drugs lead to neuronal damage is unknown. The CNIs can cause cerebral edema, hypertension or demyelination and lead to encephalopathy [90]. OKT3 can lead to a cytokine release syndrome and acute encephalopathy [91,92]. Chronic steroid use is associated with cerebral atrophy. Both steroids and growth hormone are associated with pseudotumor cerebri development [93]. In addition to drug toxicities, transplant recipients are at risk for vascular ischemic or hemorrhagic events, especially in the postoperative period. Infections and malignancies can also affect the nervous system but are beyond the scope of this chapter.

In general, the incidence of neurologic complications is higher in heart and liver transplant recipients than in kidney transplant recipients. This finding should not be surprising, because heart and liver failure patients tend to have greater hemodynamic compromise and more unstable postoperative periods than kidney transplant recipients. The incidence of neurologic complications following heart transplantation in adults is variable and ranges from 13% to 70% [94,95]. Risk factors associated with a higher incidence of neurologic complications included coexisting diabetes mellitus, renal failure or prior valvular heart disease [94]. In adult liver transplant recipients, the incidence ranges from 13% to 47% [96,97]. Living donor liver transplants who have smaller allograft ischemic times were associated with lower incidence of neurologic complications [97]. The toxicities include encephalopathy, seizures, stroke, focal neurologic deficits and peripheral neuropathies. Approximately 8% of adult kidney transplant recipients experience a stroke post-transplant [89]. Direct drug toxicities such as CNI or OKT3-associated encephalopathy are rare in this population. Because the allograft kidney is transplanted in the iliac fossa, approximately 2% of patients develop an acute femoral neuropathy because of nerve compression after transplant [98].

Wong *et al.* [99] reported that 45% of 135 pediatric lung transplant recipients experienced neurologic complications, including seizures, encephalopathy, headache, depression and focal neurologic deficits. Where the cause was identifiable, cyclosporine toxicity and ischemia were the most frequent etiologies. In 20 children transplanted for fulminant hepatic failure, 20% experienced neurologic complications, a large percentage of which were fatal [100]. The duration of pretransplant coma was strongly associated with the incidence of post-transplant neurotoxicities.

Guarino *et al.* [96] have published guidelines for potential strategies to minimize neurologic complications after liver transplantation, especially in the early postoperative period. In general, these strategies include minimizing the dosage of CNIs, oral administration as soon as possible, strict monitoring of plasma drug and electrolyte levels with prompt corrections, drug withdrawal if necessary and maintenance of hemodynamic stability. These same recommendations are also broadly applicable to other organ transplants.

MISCELLANEOUS TOXICITIES: PULMONARY, SKIN, REPRODUCTIVE/SEXUAL

Various induction antibody agents such as OKT3, daclizumab and basiliximab may rarely cause pulmonary edema post-transplant. Beta-blockade antihypertensive agents may aggravate bronchospasm in patients with coexisting asthma. The ACE inhibitor agents can lead to chronic cough as one of their side-effects, perhaps related to substance P stimulation of C-fiber receptors in the respiratory tract or accumulation of kinins [101]. Right heart dysfunction can lead to pulmonary hypertension.

Skin conditions such as acne vulgaris are often precipitated in teenagers with transplants who receive glucocorticoids or cyclosporine. These two drugs, plus the antihypertensive agent minoxidil, can lead to facial hirsuitism. Cyclosporine use is associated with gingival hyperplasia. There are reports of several types of skin rashes associated with the use of sirolimus [102,103].

Beta-blockers and clonidine (another antihypertensive agent) can potentially lead to sexual dysfunction and impotence, although recent evidence suggest that these effects are overestimated [104]. Pregnancy after transplantation, while often successful, is associated with a 14% spontaneous abortion rate, increased prevalence of pre-eclampsia and greater than 50% prematurity rate [105–108]. Pediatric data are reviewed in greater detail by Armenti *et al.* [106]. ACE inhibitor medications are associated with fetal teratogenicity and should be avoided [109]. CNI, azathioprine or glucocorticoid use does not seem to be associated with increased incidence of fetal teratogenicity [105,110]. A case report of major fetal malformations after MMF use has been published [111].

CONCLUSIONS

There are various organ toxicities associated with the use of medications post-transplant. The large variety of medications often needed precludes elimination of all the toxicities but physicians need to be aware of potential toxicities for early detection and limiting the morbidity. Besides this chapter, several society-sponsored publications also cover specific aspects of transplant management practice and can be helpful guides [108,112–123].

REFERENCES

1 Olyaei AJ, de Mattos AM, Bennett WM. Nephrotoxicity of immunosuppressive drugs: new insight and preventive strategies. *Curr Opin Crit Care* 2001;7:384–9.

2 Myers BD, Ross J, Newton L, Luetscher J, Perlroth M. Cyclosporine-associated chronic nephropathy. *N Engl J Med* 1984;**311**:699–705.

3 Letavernier E, Peraldi MN, Pariente A, Morelon E, Legendre C. Proteinuria following a switch from calcineurin inhibitors to sirolimus. *Transplantation* 2005;80:1198–203.

4 Senior PA, Paty BW, Cockfield SM, Ryan EA, Shapiro AM. Proteinuria developing after clinical islet transplantation resolves with sirolimus withdrawal and increased tacrolimus dosing. *Am J Transplant* 2005;5:2318–23.

5 Ojo AO, Held PJ, Port FK, *et al*. Chronic renal failure after transplantation of a nonrenal organ. *N Engl J Med* 2003;**349**: 931–40.

6 Coopersmith CM, Brennan DC, Miller B, *et al*. Renal transplantation following previous heart, liver, and lung transplantation: an 8-year single-center experience. *Surgery* 2001;**130**:457–62.

7 Wilkinson AH, Cohen DJ. Renal failure in the recipients of nonrenal solid organ transplants. *J Am Soc Nephrol* 1999;**10**: 1136–44.

8 Bartosh SM, Alonso EM, Whitington PF. Renal outcomes in pediatric liver transplantation. *Clin Transplant* 1997;**11**:354–60.

9 Hmiel SP, Beck AM, de la Morena MT, Sweet S. Progressive chronic kidney disease after pediatric lung transplantation. *Am J Transplant* 2005;**5**:1739–47.

10 Russ G, Segoloni G, Oberbauer R, *et al*. Superior outcomes in renal transplantation after early cyclosporine withdrawal and sirolimus maintenance therapy, regardless of baseline renal function. *Transplantation* 2005;**80**:1204–11.

11 Sanchez EQ, Martin AP, Ikegami T, *et al*. Sirolimus conversion after liver transplantation: improvement in measured glomerular filtration rate after 2 years. *Transplant Proc* 2005;**37**:4416–23.

12 Lobach NE, Pollock-Barziv SM, West LJ, Dipchand AI. Sirolimus immunosuppression in pediatric heart transplant recipients: a single-center experience. *J Heart Lung Transplant* 2005;**24**:184–9.

13 Asfar S, Metrakos P, Fryer J, *et al*. An analysis of late deaths after liver transplantation. *Transplantation* 1996;**61**:1377–81.

14 Kasiske BL. Epidemiology of cardiovascular disease after renal transplantation. *Transplantation* 2001;**72**(Suppl):S5–8.

15 Trulock EP, Edwards LB, Taylor DO, *et al*. The Registry of the International Society for Heart and Lung Transplantation: Twentieth Official adult lung and heart-lung transplant report, 2003. *J Heart Lung Transplant* 2003;**22**:625–35.

16 Lucini D, Milani RV, Ventura HO, *et al*. Cyclosporine-induced hypertension: evidence for maintained baroreflex circulatory control. *J Heart Lung Transplant* 1997;**16**:615–20.

17 Miller LW. Cardiovascular toxicities of immunosuppressive agents. *Am J Transplant* 2002;**2**:807–18.

18 Brem AS. Insights into glucocorticoid-associated hypertension. *Am J Kidney Dis* 2001;**37**:1–10.

19 Foley RN, Parfrey PS, Sarnak MJ. Clinical epidemiology of cardiovascular disease in chronic renal disease. *Am J Kidney Dis* 1998;**32**(Suppl 3):S112–9.

20 Johnston SD, Morris JK, Cramb R, Gunson BK, Neuberger J. Cardiovascular morbidity and mortality after orthotopic liver transplantation. *Transplantation* 2002;**73**:901–6.

21 Vincenti F, Jensik SC, Filo RS, Miller J, Pirsch J. A long-term comparison of tacrolimus (FK506) and cyclosporine in kidney transplantation: evidence for improved allograft survival at five years. *Transplantation* 2002;**73**:775–82.

22 Ligtenberg G, Hene RJ, Blankestijn PJ, Koomans HA. Cardiovascular risk factors in renal transplant patients: cyclosporin A versus tacrolimus. *J Am Soc Nephrol* 2001;**12**:368–73.

23 Guckelberger O, Byram A, Klupp J, *et al*. Coronary event rates in liver transplant recipients reflect the increased prevalence of cardiovascular risk-factors. *Transpl Int* 2005;**18**:967–74.

24 Neal DA, Gimson AE, Gibbs P, Alexander GJ. Beneficial effects of converting liver transplant recipients from cyclosporine to tacrolimus on blood pressure, serum lipids, and weight. *Liver Transpl* 2001;**7**:533–9.

25 Silverborn M, Jeppsson A, Martensson G, Nilsson F. New-onset cardiovascular risk factors in lung transplant recipients. *J Heart Lung Transplant* 2005;**24**:1536–43.

26 Gonwa TA, Hricik DE, Brinker K, Grinyo JM, Schena FP. Improved renal function in sirolimus-treated renal transplant patients after early cyclosporine elimination. *Transplantation* 2002;**74**:1560–7.

27 Coley KC, Verrico MM, McNamara DM, Park SC, Cressman MD, Branch RA. Lack of tacrolimus-induced cardiomyopathy. *Ann Pharmacother* 2001;**35**:985–9.

28 Kim MS, Jabs K, Harmon WE. Long-term patient survival in a pediatric renal transplantation program. *Transplantation* 1991;**51**:413–6.

29 Calzolari A, Giordano U, Matteucci MC, *et al*. Hypertension in young patients after renal transplantation: ambulatory blood pressure monitoring versus casual blood pressure. *Am J Hypertens* 1998;**11**:497–501.

30 Giordano U, Matteucci MC, Calzolari A, Turchetta A, Rizzoni G, Alpert BS. Ambulatory blood pressure monitoring in children with aortic coarctation and kidney transplantation. *J Pediatr* 2000;**136**:520–3.

31 Neu AM, Ho PL, Fine RN, Furth SL, Fivush BA. Tacrolimus vs. cyclosporine A as primary immunosuppression in pediatric renal transplantation: a NAPRTCS study. *Pediatr Transplant* 2003;**7**:217–22.

32 Trompeter R, Filler G, Webb NJ, *et al*. Randomized trial of tacrolimus versus cyclosporin microemulsion in renal transplantation. *Pediatr Nephrol* 2002;**17**:141–9.

33 Jain A, Mazariegos G, Kashyap R, *et al*. Comparative long-term evaluation of tacrolimus and cyclosporine in pediatric liver transplantation. *Transplantation* 2000;**70**:617–25.

34 Chang RK, Alzona M, Alejos J, Jue K, McDiarmid SV. Marked left ventricular hypertrophy in children on tacrolimus (FK506) after orthotopic liver transplantation. *Am J Cardiol* 1998;**81**:1277–80.

35 Dhawan A, Mack DR, Langnas AN, Shaw BW Jr, Vanderhoof JA. Immunosuppressive drugs and hypertrophic cardiomyopathy. *Lancet* 1995;**345**:1644–5.

36 Atkison P, Joubert G, Barron A, *et al*. Hypertrophic cardiomyopathy associated with tacrolimus in paediatric transplant patients. *Lancet* 1995;**345**:894–6.

37 Singh A, Stablein D, Tejani A. Risk factors for vascular thrombosis in pediatric renal transplantation: a special report of the North American Pediatric Renal Transplant Cooperative Study. *Transplantation* 1997;**63**:1263–7.

38 Seikaly M, Ho PL, Emmett L, Tejani A. The 12th Annual Report of the North American Pediatric Renal Transplant Cooperative Study: renal transplantation from 1987 through 1998. *Pediatr Transplant* 2001;**5**:215–31.

39 Montalbano M, Neff GW, Yamashiki N, *et al*. A retrospective review of liver transplant patients treated with sirolimus from a single center: an analysis of sirolimus-related complications. *Transplantation* 2004;**78**:264–8.

40 Boots JM, Christiaans MH, Van Duijnhoven EM, Van Suylen RJ, Van Hooff JP. Early steroid withdrawal in renal transplantation with tacrolimus dual therapy: a pilot study. *Transplantation* 2002;**74**:1703–9.

41 Hricik DE, Knauss TC, Bodziak KA, *et al*. Withdrawal of steroid therapy in African American kidney transplant recipients receiving sirolimus and tacrolimus. *Transplantation* 2003; **76**:938–42.

42 Sarwal MM, Yorgin PD, Alexander S, *et al*. Promising early outcomes with a novel, complete steroid avoidance immunosuppression protocol in pediatric renal transplantation. *Transplantation* 2001; **72**:13–21.

43 Kobashigawa JA, Kasiske BL. Hyperlipidemia in solid organ transplantation. *Transplantation* 1997; **63**:331–8.

44 Kasiske BL, Snyder JJ, Gilbertson D, Matas AJ. Diabetes mellitus after kidney transplantation in the United States. *Am J Transplant* 2003; **3**:178–85.

45 Sheiner PA, Magliocca JF, Bodian CA, *et al*. Long-term medical complications in patients surviving > or = 5 years after liver transplant. *Transplantation* 2000; **69**:781–9.

46 Taylor DO, Edwards LB, Boucek MM, *et al*. Registry of the International Society for Heart and Lung Transplantation: twenty-second official adult heart transplant report, 2005. *J Heart Lung Transplant* 2005; **24**:945–55.

47 Wissing KM, Abramowicz D, Broeders N, Vereerstraeten P. Hypercholesterolemia is associated with increased kidney graft loss caused by chronic rejection in male patients with previous acute rejection. *Transplantation* 2000; **70**:464–72.

48 Pirsch JD, Miller J, Deierhoi MH, Vincenti F, Filo RS. A comparison of tacrolimus (FK506) and cyclosporine for immunosuppression after cadaveric renal transplantation. FK506 Kidney Transplant Study Group. *Transplantation* 1997; **63**:977–83.

49 Gonwa T, Mendez R, Yang HC, Weinstein S, Jensik S, Steinberg S. Randomized trial of tacrolimus in combination with sirolimus or mycophenolate mofetil in kidney transplantation: results at 6 months. *Transplantation* 2003; **75**:1213–20.

50 Boucek MM, Edwards LB, Keck BM, Trulock EP, Taylor DO, Hertz MI. Registry of the International Society for Heart and Lung Transplantation: eighth official pediatric report, 2005. *J Heart Lung Transplant* 2005; **24**:968–82.

51 McDiarmid SV, Gornbein JA, Fortunat M, *et al*. Serum lipid abnormalities in pediatric liver transplant patients. *Transplantation* 1992; **53**:109–15.

52 Hanevold CD, Ho PL, Talley L, Mitsnefes MM. Obesity and renal transplant outcome: a report of the North American Pediatric Renal Transplant Cooperative Study. *Pediatrics* 2005; **115**:352–6.

53 Curtis JJ, Galla JH, Woodford SY, Lucas BA, Luke RG. Effect of alternate-day prednisone on plasma lipids in renal transplant recipients. *Kidney Int* 1982; **22**:42–7.

54 McCune TR, Thacker LR II, Peters TG, *et al*. Effects of tacrolimus on hyperlipidemia after successful renal transplantation: a Southeastern Organ Procurement Foundation multicenter clinical study. *Transplantation* 1998; **65**:87–92.

55 First MR, Gerber DA, Hariharan S, Kaufman DB, Shapiro R. Posttransplant diabetes mellitus in kidney allograft recipients: incidence, risk factors, and management. *Transplantation* 2002; **73**:379–86.

56 Johnson C, Ahsan N, Gonwa T, *et al*. Randomized trial of tacrolimus (Prograf) in combination with azathioprine or mycophenolate mofetil versus cyclosporine (Neoral) with mycophenolate mofetil after cadaveric kidney transplantation. *Transplantation* 2000; **69**:834–41.

57 Saland JM. Osseous complications of pediatric transplantation. *Pediatr Transplant* 2004; **8**:400–15.

58 Langman CB. Renal osteodystrophy: a pediatric perspective, 2005. *Growth Horm IGF Res* 2005; **15**(Suppl A):42–7.

59 Ninkovic M, Love SA, Tom B, Alexander GJ, Compston JE. High prevalence of osteoporosis in patients with chronic liver disease prior to liver transplantation. *Calcif Tissue Int* 2001; **69**:321–6.

60 Ward LM. Osteoporosis due to glucocorticoid use in children with chronic illness. *Horm Res* 2005; **64**:209–21.

61 Leonard MB, Feldman HI, Shults J, Zemel BS, Foster BJ, Stallings VA. Long-term, high-dose glucocorticoids and bone mineral content in childhood glucocorticoid-sensitive nephrotic syndrome. *N Engl J Med* 2004; **351**:868–75.

62 Julian BA, Laskow DA, Dubovsky J, Dubovsky EV, Curtis JJ, Quarles LD. Rapid loss of vertebral mineral density after renal transplantation. *N Engl J Med* 1991; **325**:544–50.

63 Stehman-Breen CO, Sherrard DJ, Alem AM, *et al*. Risk factors for hip fracture among patients with end-stage renal disease. *Kidney Int* 2000; **58**:2200–5.

64 Alem AM, Sherrard DJ, Gillen DL, *et al*. Increased risk of hip fracture among patients with end-stage renal disease. *Kidney Int* 2000; **58**:396–9.

65 Abbott KC, Oglesby RJ, Agodoa LY. Hospitalized avascular necrosis after renal transplantation in the United States. *Kidney Int* 2002; **62**:2250–6.

66 Fine RN. Growth following solid-organ transplantation. *Pediatr Transplant* 2002; **6**:47–52.

67 Fine RN. Growth post renal-transplantation in children: lessons from the North American Pediatric Renal Transplant Cooperative Study (NAPRTCS). *Pediatr Transplant* 1997; **1**:85–9.

68 Fine RN, Stablein D, Cohen AH, Tejani A, Kohaut E. Recombinant human growth hormone post-renal transplantation in children: a randomized controlled study of the NAPRTCS. *Kidney Int* 2002; **62**:688–96.

69 Oberholzer J, John E, Lumpaopong A, *et al*. Early discontinuation of steroids is safe and effective in pediatric kidney transplant recipients. *Pediatr Transplant* 2005; **9**:456–63.

70 Sarwal MM, Vidhun JR, Alexander SR, Satterwhite T, Millan M, Salvatierra O Jr. Continued superior outcomes with modification and lengthened follow-up of a steroid-avoidance pilot with extended daclizumab induction in pediatric renal transplantation. *Transplantation* 2003; **76**:1331–9.

71 Behrend M. Adverse gastrointestinal effects of mycophenolate mofetil: aetiology, incidence and management. *Drug Saf* 2001; **24**:645–63.

72 Lorber MI, Van Buren CT, Flechner SM, Williams C, Kahan BD. Hepatobiliary and pancreatic complications of cyclosporine therapy in 466 renal transplant recipients. *Transplantation* 1987; **43**:35–40.

73 Kowdley KV, Keeffe EB. Hepatotoxicity of transplant immunosuppressive agents. *Gastroenterol Clin North Am* 1995; **24**:991–1001.

74 Placebo-controlled study of mycophenolate mofetil combined with cyclosporin and corticosteroids for prevention of acute rejection. European Mycophenolate Mofetil Cooperative Study Group. *Lancet* 1995; **345**:1321–5.

75 A blinded, randomized clinical trial of mycophenolate mofetil for the prevention of acute rejection in cadaveric renal trans-

plantation. Tricontinental Mycophenolate Mofetil Renal Transplantation Study Group. *Transplantation* 1996;**61**:1029–37.

76 Sollinger HW. Mycophenolate mofetil for the prevention of acute rejection in primary cadaveric renal allograft recipients. US Renal Transplant Mycophenolate Mofetil Study Group. *Transplantation* 1995;**60**:225–32.

77 Palmer SM, Baz MA, Sanders L, *et al*. Results of a randomized, prospective, multicenter trial of mycophenolate mofetil versus azathioprine in the prevention of acute lung allograft rejection. *Transplantation* 2001;**71**:1772–6.

78 Ettenger R, Sarwal MM. Mycophenolate mofetil in pediatric renal transplantation. *Transplantation* 2005;**80**(suppl):201–10.

79 Bunchman T, Navarro M, Broyer M, *et al*. The use of mycophenolate mofetil suspension in pediatric renal allograft recipients. *Pediatr Nephrol* 2001;**16**:978–84.

80 Hocker B, Weber LT, Bunchman T, Rashford M, Tonshoff B. Mycophenolate mofetil suspension in pediatric renal transplantation: three-year data from the tricontinental trial. *Pediatr Transplant* 2005;**9**:504–11.

81 Jungraithmayr T, Staskewitz A, Kirste G, *et al*. Pediatric renal transplantation with mycophenolate mofetil-based immunosuppression without induction: results after three years. *Transplantation*. 2003;**75**:454–61.

82 Ducloux D, Rebibou JM, Semhoun-Ducloux S, *et al*. Recurrence of hemolytic-uremic syndrome in renal transplant recipients: a meta-analysis. *Transplantation* 1998;**65**:1405–7.

83 Danesi R, Del Tacca M. Hematologic toxicity of immunosuppressive treatment. *Transplant Proc* 2004;**36**:703–4.

84 Connell WR, Kamm MA, Ritchie JK, Lennard-Jones JE. Bone marrow toxicity caused by azathioprine in inflammatory bowel disease: 27 years of experience. *Gut* 1993;**34**:1081–5.

85 Kausman JY, Powell HR, Jones CL. Anemia in pediatric renal transplant recipients. *Pediatr Nephrol* 2004;**19**:526–30.

86 Mitsnefes MM, Subat-Dezulovic M, Khoury PR, Goebel J, Strife CF. Increasing incidence of post-kidney transplant anemia in children. *Am J Transplant* 2005;**5**:1713–8.

87 Al-Uzri A, Yorgin PD, Kling PJ. Anemia in children after transplantation: etiology and the effect of immunosuppressive therapy on erythropoiesis. *Pediatr Transplant* 2003;**7**:253–64.

88 Montanaro D, Groupuzzo M, Boscutti G, Risaliti A, Bresadola F, Mioni G. Long-term therapy for postrenal transplant erythrocytosis with ACE inhibitors: efficacy, safety and action mechanisms. *Clin Nephrol* 2000;**53**(Suppl):47–51.

89 Ponticelli C, Campise MR. Neurological complications in kidney transplant recipients. *J Nephrol* 2005;**18**:521–8.

90 Torocsik HV, Curless RG, Post J, Tzakis AG, Pearse L. FK506-induced leukoencephalopathy in children with organ transplants. *Neurology* 1999;**52**:1497–500.

91 Min DI, Monaco AP. Complications associated with immunosuppressive therapy and their management. *Pharmacotherapy* 1991;**11**:119S–25S.

92 Parizel PM, Snoeck HW, van den Hauwe L, *et al*. Cerebral complications of murine monoclonal CD3 antibody (OKT3): CT and MR findings. *Am J Neuroradiol* 1997;**18**:1935–8.

93 Zanardi VA, Magna LA, Costallat LT. Cerebral atrophy related to corticotherapy in systemic lupus erythematosus (SLE). *Clin Rheumatol* 2001;**20**:245–50.

94 Perez-Miralles F, Sanchez-Manso JC, Almenar-Bonet L, Sevilla-Mantecon T, Martinez-Dolz L, Vilchez-Padilla JJ. Incidence

of and risk factors for neurologic complications after heart transplantation. *Transplant Proc* 2005;**37**:4067–70.

95 Cemillan CA, Alonso-Pulpon L, Burgos-Lazaro R, Millan-Hernandez I, del Ser T, Liano-Martinez H. [Neurological complications in a series of 205 orthotopic heart transplant patients.] *Rev Neurol* 2004;**38**:906–12.

96 Guarino M, Benito-Leon J, Decruyenaere J, Schmutzhard E, Weissenborn K, Stracciari A. EFNS guidelines on management of neurological problems in liver transplantation. *Eur J Neurol* 2006;**13**:2–9.

97 Saner F, Gu Y, Minouchehr S, *et al*. Neurological complications after cadaveric and living donor liver transplantation. *J Neurol* 2006;**253**:612–7.

98 Sharma KR, Cross J, Santiago F, Ayyar DR, Burke G 3rd. Incidence of acute femoral neuropathy following renal transplantation. *Arch Neurol* 2002;**59**:541–5.

99 Wong M, Mallory GB Jr, Goldstein J, Goyal M, Yamada KA. Neurologic complications of pediatric lung transplantation. *Neurology* 1999;**53**:1542–9.

100 Nachulewicz P, Kaminski A, Kalicinski P, *et al*. Analysis of neurological complications in children transplanted due to fulminant liver failure. *Transplant Proc* 2006;**38**:253–4.

101 Israili ZH, Hall WD. Cough and angioneurotic edema associated with angiotensin-converting enzyme inhibitor therapy: a review of the literature and pathophysiology. *Ann Intern Med* 1992;**117**:234–42.

102 Tracey C, Hawley C, Griffin AD, Strutton G, Lynch S. Generalized, pruritic, ulcerating maculopapular rash necessitating cessation of sirolimus in a liver transplantation patient. *Liver Transpl* 2005;**11**:987–9.

103 Kunzle N, Venetz JP, Pascual M, Panizzon RG, Laffitte E. Sirolimus-induced acneiform eruption. *Dermatology* 2005;**211**:366–9.

104 Barksdale JD, Gardner SF. The impact of first-line antihypertensive drugs on erectile dysfunction. *Pharmacotherapy* 1999;**19**:573–81.

105 Armenti VT, Moritz MJ, Cardonick EH, Davison JM. Immunosuppression in pregnancy: choices for infant and maternal health. *Drugs* 2002;**62**:2361–75.

106 Armenti VT, Moritz MJ, Davison JM. Pregnancy in female pediatric solid organ transplant recipients. *Pediatr Clin North Am* 2003;**50**:1543–60, xi.

107 Davison JM, Bailey DJ. Pregnancy following renal transplantation. *J Obstet Gynaecol Res* 2003;**29**:227–33.

108 McKay DB, Josephson MA, Armenti VT, *et al*. Reproduction and transplantation: report on the AST Consensus Conference on Reproductive Issues and Transplantation. *Am J Transplant* 2005;**5**:1592–9.

109 Tabacova S. Mode of action: angiotensin-converting enzyme inhibition: developmental effects associated with exposure to ACE inhibitors. *Crit Rev Toxicol* 2005;**35**:747–55.

110 Danesi R, Del Tacca M. Teratogenesis and immunosuppressive treatment. *Transplant Proc* 2004;**36**:705–7.

111 Le Ray C, Coulomb A, Elefant E, Frydman R, Audibert F. Mycophenolate mofetil in pregnancy after renal transplantation: a case of major fetal malformations. *Obstet Gynecol* 2004;**103**:1091–4.

112 EBPG Expert Group on Renal Transplantation. European best practice guidelines for renal transplantation. Section IV: Long-term management of the transplant recipient. IV.11.

Paediatrics (specific problems). *Nephrol Dial Transplant* 2002; **17**(Suppl 4):55–8.

113 EBPG Expert Group on Renal Transplantation. European best practice guidelines for renal transplantation. Section IV: Long-term management of the transplant recipient. IV.10. Pregnancy in renal transplant recipients. *Nephrol Dial Transplant* 2002; **17**(Suppl 4):50–5.

114 EBPG Expert Group on Renal Transplantation. European best practice guidelines for renal transplantation. Section IV: Long-term management of the transplant recipient. IV.9.3. Haematological complications. Erythrocytosis. *Nephrol Dial Transplant* 2002;**17**(Suppl 4):49–50.

115 EBPG Expert Group on Renal Transplantation. European best practice guidelines for renal transplantation. Section IV: Long-term management of the transplant recipient. IV.9.2. Haematological complications. Leukopenia. *Nephrol Dial Transplant*2002; **17**(Suppl 4):49.

116 EBPG Expert Group on Renal Transplantation. European best practice guidelines for renal transplantation. Section IV: Long-term management of the transplant recipient. IV.9.1. Haematological complications. Anaemia. *Nephrol Dial Transplant* 2002;**17**(Suppl 4):48–9.

117 EBPG Expert Group on Renal Transplantation. European best practice guidelines for renal transplantation. Section IV: Long-term management of the transplant recipient. IV.8. Bone disease. *Nephrol Dial Transplant* 2002;**17**(Suppl 4):43–8.

118 EBPG Expert Group on Renal Transplantation. European best practice guidelines for renal transplantation. Section IV:

Long-term management of the transplant recipient. IV.5.8. Cardiovascular risks. Immunosuppressive therapy. *Nephrol Dial Transplant* 2002;**17**(Suppl 4):30–1.

119 EBPG Expert Group on Renal Transplantation. European best practice guidelines for renal transplantation. Section IV: Long-term management of the transplant recipient. IV.5.7. Cardiovascular risks. Obesity and weight gain. *Nephrol Dial Transplant* 2002;**17**(Suppl 4):29–30.

120 EBPG Expert Group on Renal Transplantation. European best practice guidelines for renal transplantation. Section IV: Long-term management of the transplant recipient. IV.5.4. Cardiovascular risks. Post-transplant diabetes mellitus. *Nephrol Dial Transplant* 2002;**17**(Suppl 4):28.

121 EBPG Expert Group on Renal Transplantation. European best practice guidelines for renal transplantation. Section IV: Long-term management of the transplant recipient. IV.5.3. Cardiovascular risks. Hyperlipidaemia. *Nephrol Dial Transplant* 2002;**17**(Suppl 4):26–8.

122 EBPG Expert Group on Renal Transplantation. European best practice guidelines for renal transplantation. Section IV: Long-term management of the transplant recipient. IV.5.2. Cardiovascular risks. Arterial hypertension. *Nephrol Dial Transplant* 2002;**17**(Suppl 4):25–6.

123 EBPG Expert Group on Renal Transplantation. European best practice guidelines for renal transplantation. Section IV: Long-term management of the transplant recipient. IV.3.3. Long-term immunosuppression. Toxicity of immunosuppression. *Nephrol Dial Transplant* 2002;**17**(Suppl 4):21–3.

Kidney Transplantation

15 Historical Notes

Vassilios E. Papalois and John S. Najarian

Transplantation is one of the great scientific revolutions of the last 100 years. The amazing achievements in the field during that period resulted from truly inspired, painstaking experimental and clinical work that changed forever the lives of many patients with end-stage organ failure. In particular, pediatric transplantation allowed children to thrive and grow normally; it had a tremendous impact on them and on their families. Pediatric kidney transplantation has developed over the last 50 years thanks to multidisciplinary work by scientists, pediatricians, and surgeons. However, the main driving force for its success was the dedication and determination of the young patients and their families, who kept the hope and dream alive through difficult times and gave the medical teams the courage to continue. We herein review some of the historic hallmarks of this great scientific journey and present the University of Minnesota experience field over the last five decades.

HISTORIC HALLMARKS

The first advance that led to clinical kidney transplantation was the development of vascular anastomosis techniques by Alexis Carrel [1,2]. He described technically successful experimental kidney auto- and allotransplantation in the canine model. In autotransplants, he observed that long-term graft function could be achieved; however, in allotransplants, the graft was soon destroyed. He stated that the major obstacle to allotransplantation was not technical; rather, a biologic phenomenon led to graft destruction. For his achievements, Carrel was awarded the Nobel Prize in 1912.

The phenomenon of graft destruction that Carrel observed was studied in great detail in the 1940s by Gibson and Medawar [3]. By performing skin graft allotransplants in rabbits, they observed that technically successful skin grafts were eventually destroyed. Even more important, they observed that a second skin graft from the same donor was destroyed more rapidly. Histologically, the destroyed grafts showed an inflammatory process. The observation of a vigorous second-set response was the basis for the recognition of graft destruction

as an immune-mediated process. This recognition led to the establishment of our knowledge about allorecognition and rejection, the cornerstones of transplantation immunology. Medawar was awarded the Nobel Prize in 1960.

Medawar's work made it very clear that the future of transplantation depended on the suppression of the immune response. Initially this was carried out by total body recipient irradiation [4], but gradually, less toxic pharmacologic immunosuppression was developed. The use of azathioprine [5], antilymphocyte globulin [6], and cyclosporine [7] were major breakthroughs.

It is important to mention the crucial role of dialysis in saving the lives of patients with end-stage renal failure and in offering a "bridge" until kidney transplantation was possible. In the 1940s, multiple dialysis treatments for renal failure were reported in both adults and children [8–11]. Improvements in dialysis over the years always complemented the advances in transplantation.

The first pediatric kidney transplant was performed by Michon *et al.* [12] in Paris on Christmas Eve 1952. The recipient was a 16-year-old boy who underwent nephrectomy of his right ruptured kidney after a fall, in order to prevent immediate death from hemorrhage. After the nephrectomy, the surgical team discovered that the boy had no left kidney. In view of his constantly rising blood urea level during the postoperative period, portending imminent death, and after weighing the responsibility of removing a healthy organ from a living donor, the team decided to satisfy the (ABO compatible) mother's insistent demand to offer her son his last chance of survival. Her kidney was implanted into her son's iliac region, with anastomosis of the graft ureter to the part of his ureter that remained after the nephrectomy. The ischemia time was limited to 55 minutes. The transplanted kidney excreted urine immediately; the laboratory parameters returned to normal within a few days. The recipient's condition was excellent over the following days. The procedure appeared to be a success. Then, suddenly, on the 21st postoperative day, abrupt onset of anuria indicated rejection and the boy died several days later. This transplant – performed under the most favorable technical and intensive care conditions, using an organ from a living related donor in excellent health with a very short ischemia time – clearly demonstrated that allograft rejection was the major problem.

Two years later, Murray proceeded with kidney transplants between identical twins, thus bypassing the problem of allograft rejection. Murray *et al.* [13] performed the first successful kidney transplant at the Peter Bent Brigham Hospital in Boston on December 23, 1954, between identical twin brothers. The donor kidney was placed retroperitoneally and the renal vessels were anastomosed to the iliac blood vessels. The ureter was implanted into the bladder. This was the first of seven pioneering transplants between identical twins [13]. Of the seven recipients, two were pediatric patients, both 14 years old: a girl with renal failure from subacute glomerulonephritis and a boy with congenital megaloureters and chronic pyelonephritis. Both underwent a transplant in 1957. Unfortunately, the long-term outcome was not successful: the girl's original disease recurred in the graft 7 weeks post-transplant and she died 4 months post-transplant; the boy's graft never functioned and he died 12 days post-transplant.

On October 9, 1959, the first successful transplant between pediatric (12 years old) identical twins was performed by Murray, Goodwin, and Hodges at the University of Oregon in Portland [14]. The recipient had renal failure secondary to chronic glomerulonephritis but enjoyed a full recovery post-transplant. A biopsy of the transplanted kidney obtained 18 years post-transplant showed normal morphology [15]. Murray was awarded the Nobel Prize in 1990 for his achievements.

In the early days of clinical transplantation, total body irradiation was the only immunosuppressive treatment, but it proved to be toxic to the recipient [16,17]. Calne [18] was the first to demonstrate that azathioprine (the imidazole derivative of 6-mercaptopurine synthesized by Elion and Hitchings) prolonged graft survival in dogs. In November 1962, Starzl *et al.* [19] performed the first successful nontwin, living related donor, pediatric kidney transplant in a 12-year-old boy, with a kidney donated by his mother. Immunosuppression consisted of total body irradiation, azathioprine, and prednisone. At the time of Starzl's report, graft survival had been sustained for 3 years.

Soon the interest of transplant pioneers turned to expanding the donor pool by using cadaver donors. In December 1963, Mowbray *et al.* [20] performed the first successful pediatric cadaver kidney transplant in a 17-year-old boy at St. Mary's Hospital in London. Immunosuppression consisted of prednisone and azathioprine; at the time of Mowbray's report, the graft had survived for 586 days.

In the 1960s, pediatric kidney transplantation gained popularity, but skepticism was also expressed [21]. The immediate results of a successful transplant were truly impressive, but long-term results were unknown. Some questioned whether the benefits of the transplant were worth the risks of the operation (which was not a pleasant experience for a child)

and the risks of immunosuppression (especially given the possibly miserable side-effects of long-term corticosteroid therapy). Gradually, more and more clinical series [22–25] demonstrated prolonged patient and graft survival with good quality of life: the balance was in favor of transplantation.

In 1976, Borel [7] in Basel, Switzerland, reported his discovery of a new immunosuppressive agent, cyclosporine, which inhibited cell-mediated cytotoxicity *in vitro*. In 1977, Calne demonstrated that cyclosporine prolonged graft survival in animals more effectively than other available agents [26,27]; in 1978 and 1979, he reported that it improved graft survival in human cadaver kidney transplant recipients [28,29]. The irony was that cyclosporine was potentially nephrotoxic [30,31]. In a way, this was a blessing, in that the fear of nephrotoxicity prevented clinicians from overimmunosuppressing recipients. In 1982, the first use of cyclosporine in pediatric kidney recipients was reported by Starzl *et al.* [32]. It offered excellent long-term results and gradually reduced the need for high-dose steroids, resulting in better growth and more normal sexual maturation of pediatric recipients [33,34].

In the 1980s, the clinical armamentarium against rejection was enriched by the development of OKT3, a murine monoclonal antibody directed against the CD3 complex on mature human T lymphocytes. In pediatric kidney recipients, OKT3 could effectively reverse acute rejection that was resistant to conventional treatment [35,36]. In 1989, the macrolide antibiotic tacrolimus (FK506) (with an immunosuppressive activity similar to cyclosporine) was first used clinically in a pediatric kidney recipient [37] and eventually proved very effective in both adult and pediatric kidney recipients [38,39].

In the 1990s, several new immunosuppressive agents were approved for clinical use, such as mycophenolate mofetil (which inhibits the *de novo* pathway of purine synthesis in T and B lymphocytes) [40] and Neoral® (the microemulsion formulation of cyclosporine), which is superior in both absorption and area-under-the-concentration curve [41]. The 1990s also saw the introduction of two monoclonal antibodies (daclizumab and basiliximab) that block the interleukin-2 receptor expressed on activated T lymphocytes, thereby providing more selective immunosuppression [42,43]. In addition, Thymoglobulin® (a rabbit polyclonal antithymocyte globulin) came into clinical practice as an effective treatment for acute rejection in pediatric kidney recipients [44,45]. These new medications are now used clinically, but randomized trials are needed to determine their effect on long-term graft survival and their long-term side-effects.

A PERSONAL PERSPECTIVE

Patients

The pediatric kidney transplant program at the University of Minnesota started in 1965. Since then, we have performed

Table 15.1 Gender of pediatric kidney recipients, University of Minnesota (January 1, 1967 to December 31, 1999).

Total number of recipients: 730
Male: 428
Female: 302

Primary transplants: 578
Male: 345
Female: 233

Retransplants: 152
Male: 83
Female: 69

Table 15.2 Age of pediatric kidney recipients, University of Minnesota (January 1, 1967 to December 31, 1999).

Age at transplant (years)	Number of recipients
< 1	42
1–5	233
6–12	239
13–17	216

Table 15.3 Donor source for pediatric kidney recipients, University of Minnesota (January 1, 1967 to December 31, 1999).

Donor source	Number of recipients
Cadaver	135
Living related	439
Living unrelated	4

850 kidney transplants in children: 730 such transplants performed between January 1967 and December 31, 1999. Of these 730 recipients, 428 were male; 302, female. In all, 578 underwent primary transplants (345 male, 233 female). A total of 152 underwent secondary transplants (83 male, 69 female) (Table 15.1). With regard to age at transplant, 42 recipients were less than 1 year old; 233, 1–5 years; 239, 6–12 years; and 216, 13–17 years (Table 15.2). The vast majority of donors were living donors (439 related, 4 unrelated) with 135 cadaver donors (Table 15.3). Of the 730 transplants, 75 had no HLA mismatches between the donor and the recipient; 543 had 1–3 and 86 had 4–6 (Table 15.4).

Long-term results

For primary transplant recipients, the 10-year patient survival rate by decade of transplant was 60% in the 1960s, 77% in the 1970s, 87% in the 1980s, and 95% in the 1990s. The rate gradually but significantly increased from one

Table 15.4 A, B, and DR mismatches for pediatric kidney recipients, University of Minnesota (January 1, 1967 to December 31, 1999).

Number of mismatches	Number of recipients
0	75
1–3	543
4–6	86

decade to the next (Fig. 15.1). By donor source (cadaver vs. living), the rate was 67% vs. 58% in the 1960s, 66% vs. 82% in the 1970s, 90% vs. 86% in the 1980s, and 95% vs. 96% in the 1990s. The only significant difference (in favor of living donors) was in the 1970s (Figs 15.2–15.5).

Also, for primary transplant recipients, the 10-year death-censored graft survival rate by decade of transplant was 59% in the 1960s, 51% in the 1970s, 64% in the 1980s, and 78% in the 1990s. The rate gradually but significantly increased in the last three decades (Fig. 15.6). By donor source (cadaver vs. living), the rate was 67% vs. 60% in the 1960s, 51% vs. 52% in the 1970s, 55% vs. 67% in the 1980s, and 55% vs.

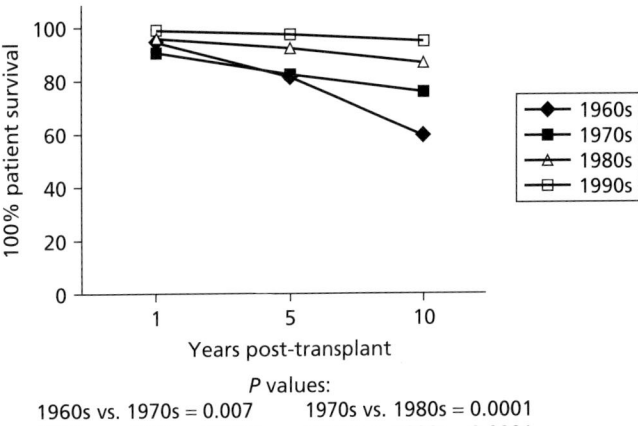

P values:

1960s vs. 1970s = 0.007	1970s vs. 1980s = 0.0001
1960s vs. 1980s = 0.0001	1970s vs. 1990s = 0.0001
1960s vs. 1990s = 0.0001	1980s vs. 1990s = 0.02

Fig. 15.1 Overall patient survival by decade of transplant.

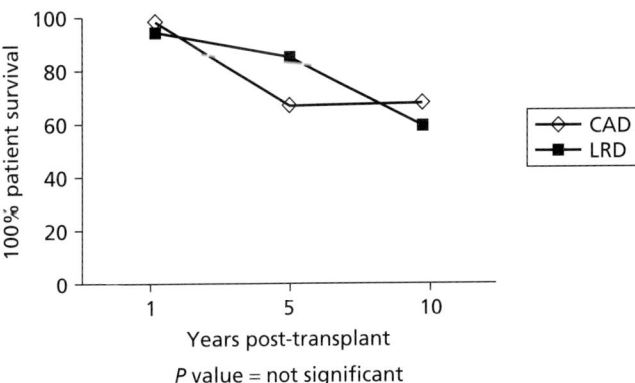

P value = not significant

Fig. 15.2 Patient survival in the 1960s for cadaver (CAD) versus living related donor (LRD) transplants.

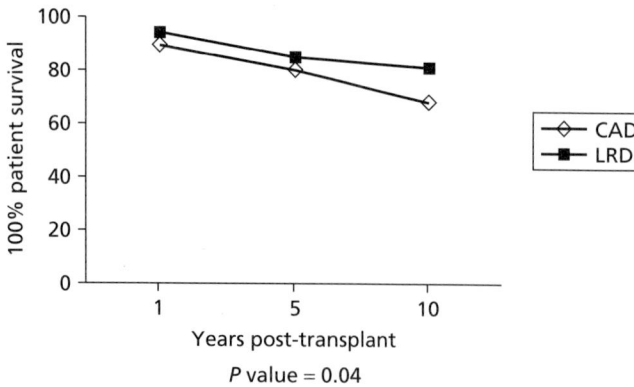

P value = 0.04

Fig. 15.3 Patient survival in the 1970s for cadaver (CAD) versus living related donor (LRD) transplants.

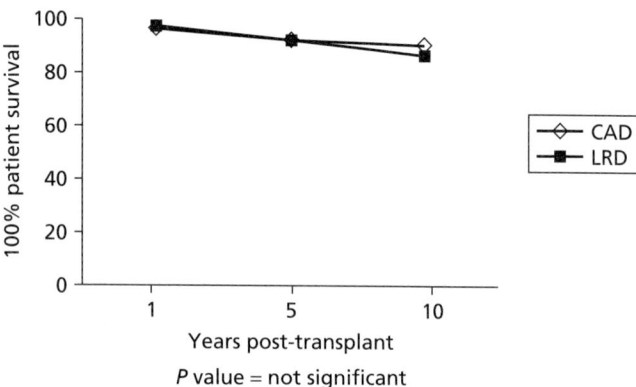

P value = not significant

Fig. 15.4 Patient survival in the 1980s for cadaver (CAD) versus living related donor (LRD) transplants.

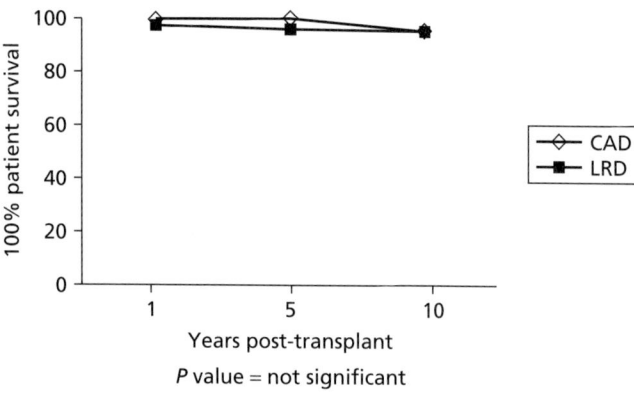

P value = not significant

Fig. 15.5 Patient survival in the 1990s for cadaver (CAD) versus living related donor (LRD) transplants.

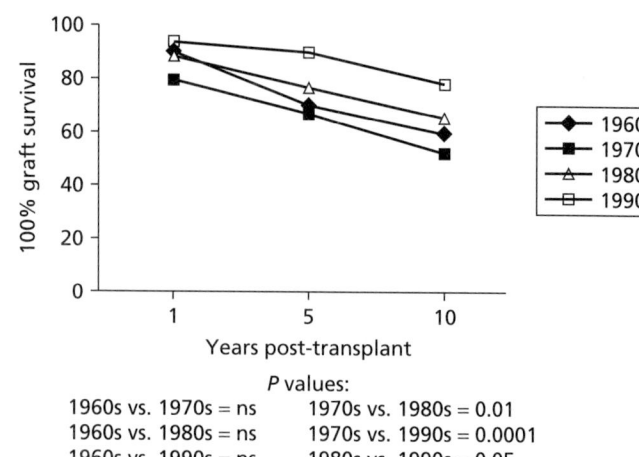

P values:
1960s vs. 1970s = ns   1970s vs. 1980s = 0.01
1960s vs. 1980s = ns   1970s vs. 1990s = 0.0001
1960s vs. 1990s = ns   1980s vs. 1990s = 0.05

Fig. 15.6 Overall death-censored graft survival by decade of transplant.

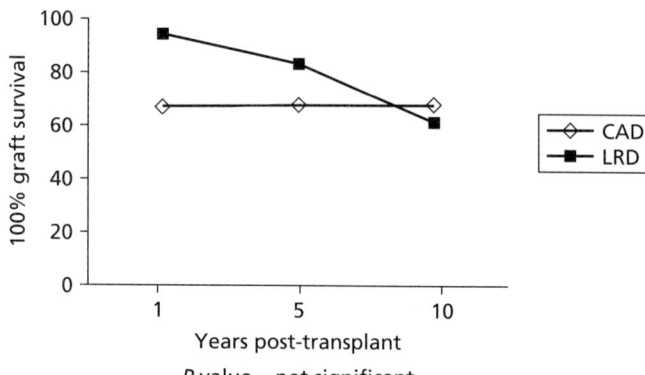

P value = not significant

Fig. 15.7 Death-censored graft survival in the 1960s for transplants performed from cadaver (CAD) versus living related donors (LRD).

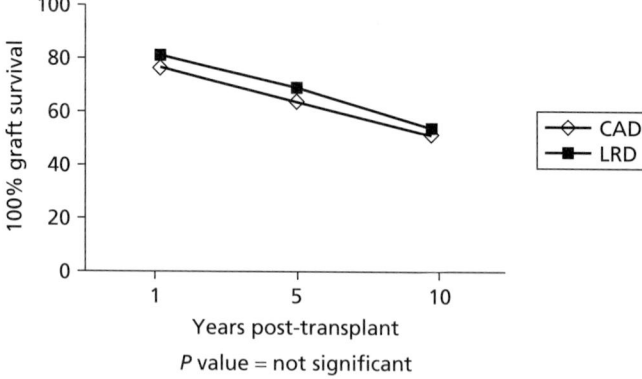

P value = not significant

Fig. 15.8 Death-censored graft survival in the 1970s for cadaver (CAD) versus living related donor (LRD) transplants.

82% in the 1990s. The difference became significant (in favor of living donor) in the last two decades (Figs 15.7–15.10).

The cause of graft loss by decade of transplant is presented in Table 15.5. In the 1960s, death and chronic rejection were the two major causes of graft loss. In the decades to follow, death became a much less important cause of graft loss, while chronic rejection remained the dominant cause.

Insights

Our experience has been progressively presented over the years [22,46–55], but we would like to highlight the following insights.

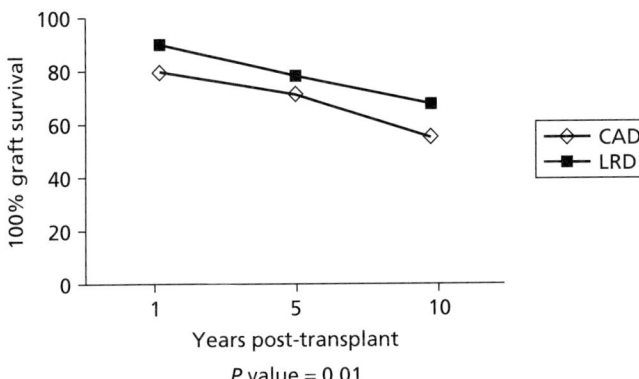

Fig. 15.9 Death-censored graft survival in the 1980s for cadaver (CAD) versus living related donor (LRD) transplants.

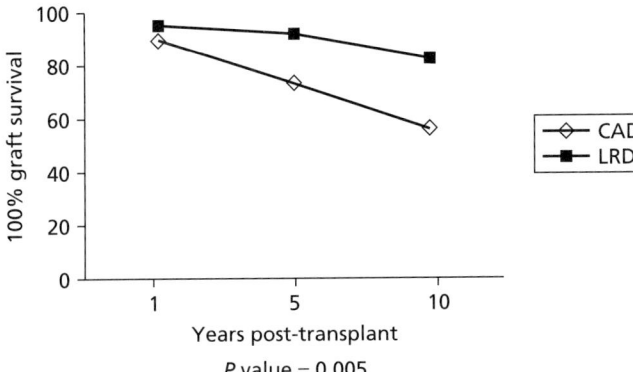

Fig. 15.10 Death-censored graft survival in the 1990s for cadaver (CAD) versus living related donor (LRD) transplants.

Our approach to the timing of the transplant for children is based on two premises:
1 Outcome with living donors is better than with cadaver donors.
2 Infants with chronic renal failure have an increased susceptibility to progressive encephalopathy [56] and infants and children with renal failure have significant growth and developmental delays [57].
Therefore, we always encourage living donor transplants, preferably before dialysis is necessary and before any nutritional and developmental problems are evident.

A highly motivated multidisciplinary team of pediatric nephrologists, neurologists, surgeons, anesthesiologists, psychologists, nutritionists, transplant coordinators, and social workers is vital, in order to evaluate properly each infant and child referred for a possible kidney transplant. Two aspects of the pretransplant evaluation are of special importance for children. First, good nutrition is crucial to limit growth retardation and to prepare these children for the stress of surgery. Second, psychological and social support is extremely important. Many families are unprepared to deal with a chronically ill child. The infant or child with renal failure places a tremendous long-term burden on the entire family. Psychologists, social workers, and transplant coordinators must be very supportive, helping family members to overcome some of this stress and to cope with renal failure, transplantation, and post-transplant treatment.

Finally, a key decision that affects post-transplant outcome but that must be made at the time of the pretransplant evaluation is whether or not to perform a native nephrectomy. A secondary consideration is the timing of the nephrectomy, either pretransplant or at the time of the transplant. Children with recurrent pyelonephritis or with significant nephrotic syndrome require a nephrectomy at least 6 weeks pretransplant, which allows their nutritional status to improve. For infants and small children with reflux nephropathy, polycystic kidneys, or hypoplasia with hypertension, the nephrectomy can be carried out at the time of the transplant [58]. Because we use a midline incision in children weighing less than 16 kg, it is easy to perform a simultaneous bilateral nephrectomy. For older children whose transplant is performed via an extraperitoneal approach, the nephrectomy can be carried out pretransplant.

CONCLUSIONS

Over the last 50 years, a long and fascinating scientific journey has led to the triumph of pediatric kidney transplantation. However, so many challenges must still be faced: maximizing the donor pool, producing more effective immunosuppressants, inducing tolerance (the Holy Grail!), preventing recurrence of the original disease in the transplanted kidney, and improving long-term growth and quality of life. The challenges are

Table 15.5 Cause of graft loss for pediatric kidney recipients, University of Minnesota (January 1, 1967 to December 31, 1999).

Decade of transplant	Number of graft losses: n (%)				
	Technical	Acute rejection	Chronic rejection	Death	Other
1960s	0 (0%)	1 (5%)	10 (48%)	9 (42%)	1 (5%)
1970s	2 (2%)	19 (17%)	64 (57%)	16 (14%)	11 (10%)
1980s	6 (5%)	6 (5%)	65 (56%)	14 (12%)	26 (22%)
1990s	5 (17%)	3 (10%)	12 (40%)	4 (13%)	6 (20%)

formidable. However, the scientific and clinical achievements of the past, fueled by the constant encouragement of our young patients and their families, allow us to face the future with hope and confidence.

ACKNOWLEDGMENT

The authors wish to thank Mary Knatterud for her editorial assistance.

REFERENCES

1 Carrel A. La technique operatoire des anastomoses vasculaires et la transplantation des visceres. *Lyon Med* 1902;**98**:859–64.

2 Carrel A, Guthrie CC. The transplantation of veins and organs. *Am Med* 1905;**10**:1101–2.

3 Gibson T, Medawar PB. The behavior of skin homografts in man. *J Anat* 1943;**77**:299–310.

4 Murray JE, Merrill JP, Dammin GJ, *et al*. Study on transplantation immunity after total body irradiation: clinical and experimental investigation. *Surgery* 1960;**48**:272–84.

5 Schwartz R, Dameshek W. Drug-induced immunological tolerance. *Nature* 1959;**183**:1682–3.

6 Woodruff MFA, Anderson NF. Effect of lymphocyte depletion and thoracic duct fistula and administration of antilymphocytic serum on the survival of skin homografts in rats. *Nature* 1963;**200**:702.

7 Borel JF. Comparative study of *in vitro* and *in vivo* drug effects on cell-mediated cytotoxicity. *Immunology* 1976;**31**:631–41.

8 Fine J, Frank HA, Seligman AM. The treatment of acute renal failure by peritoneal irrigation. *Ann Surg* 1946;**124**:857–78.

9 Murray G, Delorme E, Thomas N. Development of an artificial kidney: experimental and clinical experiences. *Arch Surg* 1947;**55**:505–22.

10 Merrill JP, Thorn GW, Callahan EJ, Smith LH Jr. Use of artificial kidney. I. Technique. *J Clin Invest* 1950;**29**:412–24.

11 Swan H, Gordon HH. Peritoneal lavage in the treatment of anuria in children. *Pediatrics* 1949;**4**:586–95.

12 Michon L, Hamburger J, Oeconomos N, *et al*. Une tentative de transplantation renale chez l'homme: aspects medicaux et biologique. *Presse Med* 1953;**61**:1419–923.

13 Murray JE, Merrill JP, Harrison JH. Kidney transplantation between seven pairs of identical twins. *Ann Surg* 1958;**148**:343–59.

14 Goodwin WE, Mims MM, Kaufman JJ. Human renal transplantation. III. Technical problems encountered in six cases of kidney homotransplantation. *Trans Am Assoc Genitourin Surg* 1962;**54**:116–25.

15 Bohannon LL, Barry JM, Norman DJ, Bennett WM. Renal function 27 years after unilateral nephrectomy for related donor kidney transplantation. *J Urol* 1988;**140**:810–1.

16 Dealy JB Jr, Dammin GJ, Murray JE, Merrill JP. Total body irradiation in man: tissue patterns observed in attempts to increase the receptivity of renal homografts. *Ann N Y Acad Sci* 1960;**87**:572–85.

17 Mathe G, Thomas ED, Ferrebee JW. The restoration of marrow function after lethal irradiation in man: a review. *Transplant Bull* 1959;**6**:407–9.

18 Calne RY. Inhibition of the rejection of renal homografts in dogs by purine analogues. *Transplant Bull* 1961;**28**:445–61.

19 Starzl TE, Marchioro TL, Porter KA, Tanous DF, Carey TA. The role of organ transplantation in pediatrics. *Pediatr Clin North Am* 1966;**13**:381–422.

20 Mowbray JF, Cohen SL, Doak PB, *et al*. Human cadaveric renal transplantation: report of twenty cases. *BMJ* 1965;**2**:1387–94.

21 Riley CM. Thoughts about kidney homotransplantation in children. *J Pediatr* 1964;**65**:797–800.

22 Najarian JS, Simmons RL, Tallent MB, *et al*. Renal transplantation in infants and children. *Ann Surg* 1971;**174**:583–601.

23 Potter DO, Belzer FO, Rames L, *et al*. The treatment of chronic uremia in childhood. I. Transplantation. *Pediatrics* 1970;**45**:432–43.

24 Gonzalez LL, Martin L, West CD, Spitzer R, McEnery P. Renal homotransplantation in children. *Arch Surg* 1970;**101**:232–40.

25 Fine RN, Korsch BM, Edelbrock HH, *et al*. Cadaveric renal transplantation in children. *Lancet* 1971;**1**:1087–91.

26 Kostakis AJ, White DJG, Calne RY. Prolongation of rat heart allograft survival by cyclosporin A. *Int Res Commun Syst Med Sci* 1977;**5**:280.

27 Calne RY, White DJG. Cyclosporin A: a powerful immunosuppressant in dogs with renal allografts. *Int Res Commun Syst Med Sci* 1977;**5**:595–6.

28 Calne RY, White DJG, Thiru S, *et al*. Cyclosporin A in patients receiving renal allografts from cadaver donors. *Lancet* 1978;**2**:1323–7.

29 Calne RY, Rolles K, White DJG, *et al*. Cyclosporin A initially as the only immunosuppressant in 34 recipients of cadaveric organs: 32 kidneys, 2 pancreases, and 2 livers. *Lancet* 1979;**2**:1033–6.

30 Canadian Multicenter Transplant Group. A randomized clinical trial of cyclosporine in cadaveric renal transplantation. *N Engl J Med* 1983;**309**:809–15.

31 Merion RM, White DJG, Thiru S, Evans DB, Calne RY. Cyclosporine: five years' experience in cadaveric renal transplantation. *N Engl J Med* 1984;**310**:148–54.

32 Starzl TE, Iwatsuki S, Malatack JJ, *et al*. Liver and kidney transplantation in children receiving cyclosporin A and steroids. *J Pediatr* 1982;**100**:681–6.

33 Tejani A, Butt KMH, Khawar MR, *et al*. Cyclosporine experience in renal transplantation in children. *Kidney Int* 1986;**30**:35–43.

34 Brodehl J, Bokenkamp A, Hoyer PF, Offner G. Long-term results of cyclosporin A therapy in children. *J Am Soc Nephrol* 1992;**2**:S246–54.

35 Goldstein G, Barnes L, Hirsch RL. OKT3 monoclonal antibody reversal of renal and hepatic rejection in pediatric patients. *J Pediatr* 1987;**111**:1046–50.

36 Leone MR, Alexander SR, Barry JM, *et al*. OKT3 monoclonal antibody in pediatric kidney recipients with recurrent and resistant allograft rejection. *J Pediatr* 1987;**111**:45–50.

37 Jensen CWB, Jordan ML, Schneck FX, *et al*. Pediatric renal transplantation under FK 506 immunosuppression. *Transplant Proc* 1991;**23**:3075–7.

38 Starzl TE, Fung J, Jordan M, *et al*. Kidney transplantation under FK 506. *JAMA* 1990;**264**:63–7.

39 Schneck FX, Jordan ML, Jensen CWB, *et al*. Pediatric renal transplantation under FK 506 immunosuppression. *J Urol* 1992;**147**:1585–7.

40 Ransom JT. Mechanism of action of mycophenolate mofetil. *Ther Drug Monit* 1995;**17**:681–4.

41 Wahlberg J, Wilczek HE, Fauchald P, *et al.* Consistent absorption of cyclosporine from a microemulsion formulation assessed in stable renal transplant recipients over a one-year study period. *Transplantation* 1995;**60**:648–52.

42 Vincenti F, Kirkman R, Light S, *et al.* Interleukin-2 receptor blockade with daclizumab to prevent acute rejection in renal transplantation. Daclizumab Triple Therapy Study Group. *N Engl J Med* 1998;**338**:161–5.

43 Nashan B, Moore R, Amlot P, *et al.* Randomized trial of basiliximab versus placebo for control of acute cellular rejection in renal allograft recipients. CHIB 201 International Study Group. *Lancet* 1997;**350**:1193–8.

44 Broyer M, Gagnadoux MF, Guest G, Niaudet P. Triple therapy including cyclosporine A versus conventional regimen: a randomized prospective study in pediatric kidney transplantation. *Transplant Proc* 1987;**19**:3582–5.

45 Bell L, Giardin C, Sharma A, Goodyer P, Mazer B. Lymphocyte subsets during and after rabbit antithymocyte globulin induction in pediatric renal transplantation: sustained T cell depletion. *Transplant Proc* 1997;**29**:6S–9S.

46 DeShazo CV, Simmons RL, Bernstein DM, *et al.* Results of renal transplantation in 100 children. *Surgery* 1974;**76**:461–8.

47 Miller LC, Bock GH, Lum CT, Najarian JS, Mauer SM. Transplantation of the adult kidney into the very small child: long-term outcome. *J Pediatr* 1982;**100**:675–80.

48 Nevins TE, Knaak M, So SKS, *et al.* Preliminary results of low-dose cyclosporin A in pediatric renal transplantation. *Int J Pediatr Nephrol* 1986;**7**:91–3.

49 Nevins TE. Transplantation in infants less than 1 year of age. *Pediatr Nephrol* 1987;**1**:154–6.

50 Chavers BM, Matas AJ, Nevins TE, *et al.* Results of pediatric kidney transplantation at the University of Minnesota. In: Terasaki PI, ed. *Clinical Transplants 1989*. Los Angeles, CA: UCLA Tissue Typing Laboratory, 1990: 253–66.

51 Najarian JS, Frey DJ, Matas AJ, *et al.* Renal transplantation in infants. *Ann Surg* 1990;**212**:353–67.

52 Najarian JS, Almond PS, Mauer SM. Renal transplantation in the first year of life: the treatment of choice for infants with end-stage renal disease. *J Am Soc Nephrol* 1992;**2**:S228–33.

53 Chavers BM, Matas AJ, Gillingham KJ, Schmidt WJ, Najarian JS. Pediatric renal transplantation at the University of Minnesota: the cyclosporine years. In: Terasaki PI, Cecka JM, eds. *Clinical Transplants 1994*. Los Angeles, CA: UCLA Tissue Typing Laboratory, 1995: 203–12.

54 Matas AJ, Najarian JS. Kidney transplantation. In: O'Neil JA, Rowe MI, Grosfeld JL, Foncalsrud EW, Coran AG, eds. *Pediatric Surgery*. St. Louis, MO: Mosby, 1998: 563–80.

55 Papalois VE, Najarian JS. Surgical technique and management of pediatric kidney transplantation. In: Tejani AH, Harmon WE, Fine RN, eds. *Textbook of Pediatric Transplantation*. Copenhagen: Munskgaard, 2000: 176–85.

56 Rotundo A, Nevins TE, Lipton M, *et al.* Progressive encephalopathy in children with chronic renal insufficiency in infancy. *Kidney Int* 1982;**21**:486–91.

57 Rizzoni T, Basso T, Setari M. Growth in children with chronic renal failure on conservative treatment. *Kidney Int* 1984;**26**:52–8.

58 Khwaja K, Humar A, Najarian JS. Kidney transplants for children under 1 year of age: a single-center experience. *Pediatr Transplant* 2003;**7**:163–7.

16 Recipient Characteristics

Sharon M. Bartosh

The number of children who develop renal failure and require renal replacement therapy is relatively low in comparison with adult populations and represents 1.3% of the total reported renal failure cases in the USA [1]. According to the 2004 US Renal Data System (USRDS) report, new cases of end-stage renal disease (ESRD) for children 0–19 years in 2002 was 1200 for an incident rate of 15 per million population per year [1]. The incidence of ESRD in children has increased slightly in the past decade (Fig. 16.1) [1].

INDICATIONS FOR RENAL REPLACEMENT THERAPY AND TREATMENT OF ESRD

Renal replacement therapy is indicated when significant complications from chronic renal insufficiency are present. These complications include but are not strictly limited to: symptoms of uremia not responsive to standard medical therapies; failure to thrive because of limitations in total caloric intake; delayed psychomotor development; hypervolemia; hyperkalemia; and metabolic bone disease resulting from renal osteodystrophy [2]. Most if not all pediatric nephrologists caring for infants, children and adolescents with ESRD would advocate renal transplantation as the optimal renal replace-

ment therapy. Children are transplanted at such a high rate that 86% of those alive 4 years after beginning therapy for ESRD have a functioning transplant [3].

In addition to improved rehabilitation, pediatric renal transplantation provides superior survival compared with dialysis. In 1993–97, approximately 92% of children beginning therapy with a transplant survived 5 years, compared with 81% of those on hemodialysis and 83% of those receiving peritoneal dialysis [1]. Annual death rates among children awaiting deceased donor renal transplants has remained relatively unchanged since 1992. Children 6–10 years of age have significantly lower death rate (17 per 1000 patient-years at risk) than other ages, while children 1–5 years of age have significantly higher mortality rates (61 per 1000 patient-years at risk), approaching that observed for adults [4]. The mortality of children 1–5 years of age on dialysis is three times higher than for those children who receive a transplant [5,6].

Choice of modality for treatment of pediatric ESRD varies with patient age, gender and race. Compared with adults, there is greater use of peritoneal dialysis or transplantation as primary therapy. When considering children younger than 4 years of age who begin dialysis as their primary mode of renal replacement therapy, 72% are treated with peritoneal dialysis [1]. However, the initial use of hemodialysis has grown steadily since the early 1990s [1]. Of those children who are on dialysis immediately prior to transplantation, 62% are receiving hemodialysis and 38% are receiving peritoneal dialysis [1]. By the 18th month of ESRD treatment, transplant is the dominant modality present in the prevalent population [1]. Increased willingness or ability to transplant pediatric ESRD patients is also reflected in data showing that 2 years following the onset of treatment of ESRD, 44.5% of children under 19 years of age had a functioning graft in comparison to only 15% of adults in the 20–44 age group [1].

White children are more likely to receive a transplant than children from other racial groups. (Fig. 16.2) [1]. Nonwhite children are twice as likely to be treated with hemodialysis [7]. Transplantation rates corrected for dialysis patient years by recipient's race and gender for both deceased donor and living-related donors in 1999–2002 is found in Figure 16.2

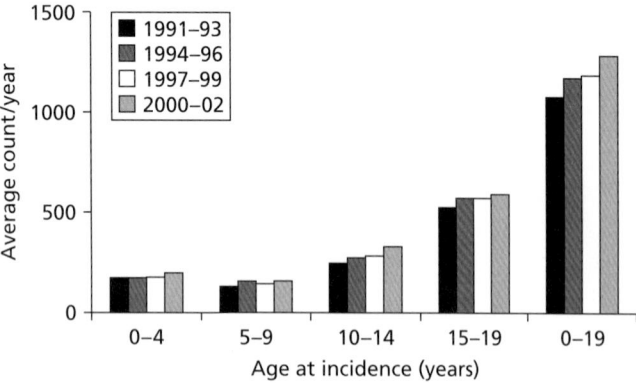

Fig. 16.1 Count of pediatric end-stage renal disease (ESRD) patients.

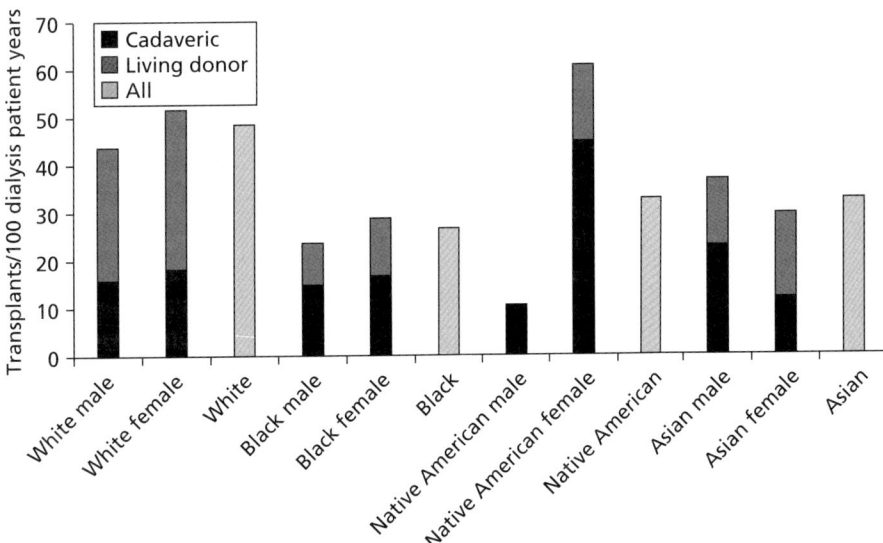

Fig. 16.2 Pediatric transplant rates, 1999–2002.

[1]. African-American children have lower overall transplant rates and lower living donor rates than white children.

There are few if any reasons to withhold transplantation from children with ESRD. Absolute contraindications to transplantation are:
1 Active or untreated malignancy.
2 Chronic active infection with hepatitis B.
3 Severe multiorgan failure that precludes a combined transplant with a kidney.
4 Positive current direct cross-match.
5 Debilitating, irreversible brain injury.
  Relative contraindications to transplantation are:
1 ABO incompatibility with the donor.
2 Positive direct cross-match within previous 3–12 months (with multiple desensitization protocols currently being utilized, this must be analyzed on a case-by-case basis).
3 Active autoimmune disease such as systemic lupus erythematosus or antiglomerular basement membrane (anti-GBM) disease with high levels of anti-GBM antibodies.
4 HIV infection (with current availability of antiretroviral therapy, some centers are re-evaluating this policy on a case-by-case basis) [8].
5 Psychomotor retardation or psychiatric illness of such severity that custodial care is required.
6 Chronic infection with hepatitis C virus.
7 Serious long-standing noncompliance with medical management.
8 Lack of adequate home supervision or family support of a transplant patient [2,9].

CHARACTERISTICS OF PEDIATRIC KIDNEY TRANSPLANTS

The annual number of kidney transplants received by chil-

dren under the age of 18 years has been 674–767 over the past 5 years, which represents approximately 4% of the total number of kidney transplants performed in the USA [1].

Type of transplant

Overall, 17% of children reported as newly incident ESRD will undergo pre-emptive transplantation [1]. In specialized pediatric renal transplant centers, the percentage of pre-emptive transplants is higher at 25% for primary transplants [10]. Pre-emptive transplantation in children demonstrates no deleterious effects in living donor or deceased donor recipients and presents an opportunity to limit the period of uremia as well as avoid procedures that may permanently compromise blood vessels or result in injury to the peritoneal membrane [11]. Although pre-emptive transplantation has clear advantages, many children require a course of dialysis – particularly when nephrectomies are necessary in preparation for transplantation – to correct metabolic, nutritional or orthopedic problems prior to transplant; until a suitable donor is found; or particularly in conditions such as congenital nephrotic syndrome [2,12]. The rate of pre-emptive transplantation differs significantly between recipients of living (33%) and deceased donor (13%) source organs; between males (28%) and females (20%); between age groups, with rates of 20%, 24%, 28%, 23% and 20% for recipients 0–1, 2–5, 6–12, 13–17 and 18–20 years old; and across races with whites, African-Americans and Hispanics having pre-emptive transplantation rates of 30%, 15% and 16%, respectively [10].

Since 1995, living donors have become the dominant source of organs for children receiving their first transplants, accounting for 57% of all pediatric renal transplants in 2002 compared with 41% in adults [4]. Parents comprise 82% of living donors, with mothers contributing 56% of kidneys [10].

The percentage of children receiving deceased donor transplants increases from zero in children less than 12 months, to 35% in children 1–5 years, to 40% in those 6–10 years and to 46% in the 11–17 year age group [4]. At the end of 2002, 708 children under the age of 18 years accounted for 1.4% of the deceased donor kidney waiting list in the USA [4]. Of the pediatric patients on the deceased donor waiting list at the end of 2002, 70% were in the 11–17 year age range [4]. For children awaiting transplantation, the median time to transplant has decreased for children less than 10 years of age and is significantly shorter than for adults [4]. In 2002, the median waiting times were 195, 373 and 471 days for children 1–5, 6–10 and 11–17 years old, respectively [13]. The use of deceased donors less than 10 years of age has declined over the past 10 years [10]. Among deceased donor transplants, only 2% have come from donors less than 24 months of age, and 24% from donors between 2 and 10 years of age [10]. There is essentially no use of "extended criteria donor" kidneys in pediatric recipients [4]. Thirteen percent of deceased donor allografts received by children are machine perfused and 68% have cold ischemia times of 24 hours or less, with 0.3% having cold ischemia times exceeding 48 hours [10].

Patient characteristics

The mean age of children starting ESRD treatment is 12.3 years and this has not changed over time [1]. Renal failure is more common in older children, with the average incidence rate in adolescents 15–19 years old being 26 per million compared with 15 per million in children aged 10–14 years, 8 per million in children aged 5–9 years, and 9 per million in the youngest cohort aged 0–4 years. Subsequently, the vast majority of children receiving kidney transplants are adolescents (Fig. 16.3) [1].

Within the pediatric ESRD population there are large variations in incidence rates of ESRD by race, with the highest rates seen in African-American children followed by Native Americans [1]. The higher overall incidence of ESRD for African-American children is primarily the result of an almost threefold excess of ESRD among African-Americans

Table 16.1 Age at index transplant by race and diagnosis. Numbers in table are percentages.

	Age at index transplant (years)				
	0–1	2–5	6–12	13–17	> 17
Race					
White	77	64	62	59	55
Black	7	14	14	19	25
Hispanic	10	16	17	16	13
Other	6	6	6	6	7
Diagnosis					
Renal plasias*	29	25	17	11	9
Obstructive uropathy	19	23	16	14	10
FSGS†	1	9	13	12	15
Other	51	44	54	62	65

* Aplastic, hypoplastic or dysplastic kidneys.
† Focal segmental glomerulosclerosis.

compared with whites in the 15–19-year-old cohort (60 per million vs. 20 per million) [1]. In a cohort of 8713 pediatric renal transplants, registered over a 17-year period in the North American Pediatric Renal Transplant Cooperative Study, white patients comprised 62% of the cohort, African-American patients 16% and Hispanic patients 16% [10]. The percentage of white patients in a given year has decreased from as high as 72% in 1987 to less than 57% in 2001 [10]. Coincident with the increasing prevalence of focal segmental glomerulosclerosis as an etiologic diagnosis for ESRD in the older pediatric age groups, the racial makeup of children undergoing transplantation also changes with age, with 64% of children under the age of 5 years and 58% of children over 13 years of age being white (Table 16.1) [10]. There are clear disparities across both age and racial groups. Black and Native American children are less likely to receive a transplant than children of other races. The most prevalent diagnoses leading to ESRD vary between African-American patients and white children, with glomerulonephritis accounting for ESRD in a larger percentage of African-American than white children [14].

Gender disparity is quite striking in pediatric renal transplantation. The reasons become obvious when the etiologies of ESRD in children are examined. The unbalanced distribution is most evident in children under 5 years of age, where 68% of all transplanted children are male [10]. This is largely because males comprise the majority of aplasia, hypoplasia or dysplasia and obstructive uropathy diagnoses and the fact that the relative incidence of these diagnoses decreases with age. Forty percent of male patients carry one of these diagnoses compared with 21% of females [10]. Male predominance continues throughout adolescence and adulthood.

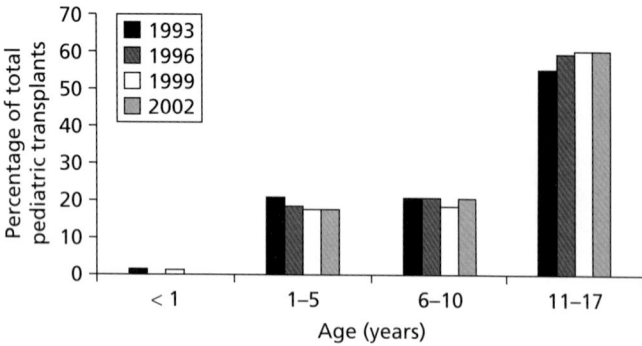

Fig. 16.3 Age distribution of children receiving kidney transplants.

Etiology of ESRD

The etiology of ESRD in children is substantially different from causes of ESRD in adults. The largest single disease group causing ESRD in children is primary glomerulonephritis, accounting for approximately 25% of all reported causes, followed by cystic, hereditary or congenital diseases, accounting for 50% [10]. Etiologies of ESRD in transplanted children in the USA are found in Table 16.2 [10]. While younger patients are more likely to carry a primary diagnosis of cystic, hereditary or congenital disease, in older children ESRD is more often caused by primary or secondary glomerulonephritis (see Table 16.1) [10]. Another distinguishing feature between pediatric and adult ESRD populations is that many of the causes of childhood ESRD are associated with various inherited and sporadic syndromes, and metabolic disorders with multi-system organ dysfunction such as congenital heart disease, central nervous system disorders, skeletal malformations and gastrointestinal disorders. Several diseases leading to ESRD are unique to the child such as congenital and infantile nephrotic syndrome, primary hyperoxaluria, autosomal recessive polycystic kidney disease, nephropathic cystinosis and hemolytic

Table 16.2 Etiology of end-stage renal disease (ESRD) in transplanted children.

	Transplanted patients (%)
Obstructive uropathy	16
Aplasia, dysplasia or hypoplasia	16
Focal segmental glomerulonephritis	11
Reflux nephropathy	5
Unspecified glomerulonephritis	3.5
Prune belly syndrome	3
Hemolytic uremic syndrome	3
Membranoproliferative glomerulonephritis	3
Polycystic kidney disease	3
Medullary cystic disease	3
Congenital nephrotic syndrome	2.5
Alport nephritis	2
Cystinosis	2
Pyelonephritis or interstitial nephritis	2
Systemic lupus erythematosus	2
IgA nephropathy	1
Henoch–Schönlein purpura	1
Membranous nephropathy	< 1
Wegener glomerulonephritis	< 1
Oxalosis	< 1
Tumor	< 1
Diabetes	< 1
Sickle cell	< 1
Drash syndrome	< 1
Goodpasture glomerulonephritis	NA*

* Not available.

uremic syndrome. Unlike in adults, diabetes and hypertension as a cause of ESRD account for a very small number of children undergoing renal transplantation in the USA [10].

Blood type and transfusions

Forty-eight percent of pediatric recipients are blood group O, 36% are blood group A, 12% are blood group B and 4% are blood group AB (unpublished analysis of NAPRTCS database). This is not dissimilar to the distribution of blood types in adult kidney transplant recipients [15]. Overall, 88% of donor and recipient blood types in pediatric kidney transplants are identical (82% in living donor and 94% in deceased donor) [10].

The percentage of pediatric living donor transplant recipients receiving donor-specific transfusions has decreased from 40% in 1987 to 17% in 1990, 4% in 1993 and 0.9% since January 2000 (unpublished analysis of NAPRTCS database) in association with a diminished positive transfusion effect in the cyclosporine era [16]. If donor-specific transfusions are given they are usually administered under the immunologic cover of concomitant immunosuppression to decrease the development of cytotoxic antibodies to donor lymphocytes [17].

Nondonor-specific transfusion rates have also declined over the past decade. Prior to the widespread utilization of cyclosporine, large studies established that blood transfusions powerfully enhanced renal allograft outcome [18]. More recent reports confirm a favorable effect of limited blood transfusions [1–5] on the risk of acute rejection [19,20] and graft survival [20]. Multiple (more than five) pretransplant blood transfusions have been shown to be a risk factor for graft failure [19]. The total number of random transfusions given to pediatric renal transplant recipients differs by donor type. Currently, 47% of living donor graft recipients and 31% of deceased donor graft recipients enter transplantation having had no previous transfusions, while 14% and 30%, respectively, have had more than five transfusions [10]. This represents a sizable decrease in the use of transfusions pretransplantation over the past decade.

The majority (68%) of children receiving a first transplant have a panel reactive antibody (PRA) of zero. Twenty-five percent have a PRA of 1–19 and 3% have a PRA above 80. Adult statistics are similar, with 80% of adult renal transplant recipients having a PRA of 0–9, 12% with PRA of 10–79 and 4% having a PRA above 80 at the time of transplant [13].

HLA matching

Children receiving living donor transplants achieve matching at least three alleles in 51% of patients, and matching at four alleles in 18%. Six antigen mismatch is found in 12% of pediatric living donor transplants [10]. In contrast, adults receiving living donor transplants achieve matching at least three alleles in 30%, at four alleles in 18% and at no alleles

Table 16.3 Percentage of HLA mismatches in children and adults.

HLA-A, -B and -DR	Living donor		Cadaveric donor	
	Pediatric	Adult	Pediatric	Adult
0	3	9	2	15
1	5	6	2	2
2	18	19	6	6
3	51	28	14	14
4	8	13	25	24
5	3	15	25	26
6	12	8	25	12

in 7% [15]. Pediatric patients receive more poorly matched deceased donor kidneys than adults [21]. Approximately 5% of pediatric patients receive nationally shared, HLA-matched kidneys, compared with 14% of adults [15]. In deceased donor pediatric transplants, 50% of transplants are four or five HLA mismatches and 25% are six antigen mismatches [10]. Adult deceased donor transplants have 40% three or four antigen mismatches, 21% five antigen mismatches and 12% six antigen mismatches (Table 16.3) [10,15].

Nephrectomy and splenectomy

The indications for nephrectomy prior to transplantation are severe hypertension resistant to medical treatment, persistent nephrotic syndrome, recurrent infections related to urinary tract anomalies and respiratory compromise or feeding problems directly related to enlarged polycystic kidneys [2]. Twenty-three percent of children undergoing renal transplantation undergo native kidney nephrectomies [10].

Previously splenectomy was routinely performed in some centers in an effort to decrease acute rejection. A prospective trial performed at the University of Minnesota demonstrated only slightly improved graft survival and a higher incidence of deaths secondary to sepsis [22]. Currently, splenectomy is performed in less than 1% of pediatric renal transplants (unpublished analysis of NAPRTCS database).

Growth, bone health and development

Achieving adequate growth in children with chronic renal insufficiency has been challenging because diminished growth rates may develop once glomerular filtration rate (GFR) falls below 75 mL/min/1.73 m^2 body surface area [23]. This growth failure is age-dependent in that young infants and adolescents with chronic renal insufficiency are most susceptible [24,25]. Growth failure correlates with the presence of renal osteodystrophy, particularly when the GFR decreases below 30 ml/min/1.73 m^2 body surface area [23] and usually persists on dialysis, particularly for children older than 6 years [10]. For children undergoing renal transplantation, the mean height

deficit calculated as a height standard deviation score (Height Z score) and corrected for age and gender is –1.45 [10]. This represents an improvement from a mean of –2.2 in 1987. This improvement can be attributed to improved management of renal osteodystrophy and metabolic acidosis, aggressive nutritional supplementation and the use of recombinant human growth hormone. The degree of growth retardation at the time of transplantation is most severe in younger children with a diagnosis of aplastic or hypoplastic kidneys or obstructive uropathy, in males versus females, and in those who have received a prior transplant [10,26,27]. Twelve percent of transplant recipients received growth hormone prior to their transplant in 1997, compared with 7% in 1995 [10].

Although no reports detailing the presence of renal osteodystrophy at the time of transplantation are available, 32–45% of children with chronic renal insufficiency have hyperparathyroidism, indirect evidence of renal bone disease [10]. Eighty-four percent of children receiving peritoneal dialysis have abnormal bone histology consisting of osteitis fibrosa, adynamic bone lesions or osteomalacia [28].

Delayed puberty is a common finding in ESRD [29]. Onset of puberty is delayed by an average of 2.5 years once the GFR decreases below 25 mL/min/1.73 m^2 body surface area [30]. Information regarding baseline pubertal status of children who are undergoing renal transplantation is not readily available.

Seventy-six percent of children with ESRD on peritoneal dialysis and 52% of those on hemodialysis are attending school full-time [10]. While these numbers are encouraging, particularly for children on peritoneal dialysis, children with ESRD are clearly at risk for impaired school performance and academic achievement [31–33]. In addition, neurodevelopmental delay and small head circumference is commonly seen in infants and young children with chronic renal insufficiency and ESRD [34,35]. Deficits in performance IQ and visual motor skills have also been documented in children undergoing renal transplantation [36]. The degree of cognitive performance impairment is positively correlated with earlier onset and increased duration of ESRD [37].

Anemia

The correction of anemia with the introduction recombinant human erythropoietin is probably the most important factor that has improved the quality of life in patients with renal failure in the last 15 years. The current Dialysis Outcomes Quality Initiative Guidelines (DOQI) recommend a target range for hematocrit of 33–36% and for hemoglobin of 11–12 g/dL [38]. Although baseline data at the time of transplantation are not available, inferences can be made from the pediatric dialysis population. Hemoglobin levels in children on dialysis tend to be lower than those in adult patients [1]. Levels differ little by gender but more so by race [1]. At the end of 2002, more than 70% of pediatric dialysis patients had a hemoglobin value meeting K/DOQI target of 11 g/dL or higher [1].

Infection risks

Fifty-three to 82% of pediatric renal transplants are cytomegalovirus (CMV) negative at the time of transplantation [39–41]. This is in keeping with epidemiologic studies which show that beyond the neonatal period, the prevalence of CMV seropositivity increases with age. Fifty-seven percent of pediatric renal transplant recipients are Epstein–Barr virus negative at the time of transplant [42].

Morbidity and mortality from vaccine preventable diseases remain a significant concern for immunocompromised patients. Given the variable serologic conversion rate of a number of vaccines when given in the post-transplant period and concern regarding a risk for heightened immunoresponsiveness and acute rejection in the renal allograft, every effort should be made to immunize the child with chronic renal failure prior to transplantation [43]. Little has been documented regarding pediatric immunization status at the time of transplantation. One of the most potentially devastating post-transplant infections in the immunologically naïve child is varicella. We know that prior to availability of the varicella vaccine, 7% of children undergoing renal transplantation were varicella antibody negative [44].

Retransplantation

The pediatric retransplantation rate in the USA is approximately 15% [45]. Of those children who are receiving first repeat transplants, there is a lower rate of living donor grafts performed compared with primary transplants (52% vs. 23%) and a smaller percentage of recipients under 6 years of age (15% vs. 24%). More than half of all children receiving non-primary transplants are older than 12 years. When comparing primary with retransplants, no differences in patient demographics are seen with regard to gender, race, donor age or cold storage time [45]. The incidence of 2-DR mismatches are significantly increased for second compared with primary transplants (40% vs. 27%) [45].

REFERENCES

1 US Renal Data System. *USRDS 2004 Annual Data Report.* Bethesda, MD: National Institutes of Health, National Institute of Diabetes and Digestive and Kidney Diseases, 2004 (available at www.usrds.org).

2 Davis ID, Bunchman TE, Grimm PC, *et al*. Pediatric renal transplantation: indications and special considerations: a position paper from the pediatric committee of the American Society of Transplant Physicians. *Pediatr Transplant* 1998;2:117–29.

3 US Renal Data System. *USRDS 2003 Annual Data Report.* Bethesda, MD: National Institutes of Health, National Institute of Diabetes and Digestive and Kidney Diseases, 2003 (available at www.usrds.org).

4 Magee JC, Bucavalas JC, Farmer DG, *et al*. Pediatric transplantation. *Am J Transplant* 2004:4:54–71.

5 Wood EJ, Hand M, Briscoe DM, *et al*. Risk factors for mortality in infants and young children on dialysis. *Am J Kidney Dis* 2001;37:573–9.

6 Seihalz M, Ho PL, Emmett L, Tejani A. The 12th annual report of the North American Pediatric Renal Transplant Cooperative Study: renal transplantation from 1987 through 1998. *Pediatr Transplant* 2001;5:215–31.

7 US Renal Data System. *USRDS 2002 Annual Data Report.* Bethesda, MD: National Institutes of Health, National Institute of Diabetes and Digestive and Kidney Diseases, 2002 (available at www.usrds.org).

8 Anonymous. Solid organ transplantation in the HIV-infected patient. *Am J Transplant* 2004:4:83–8.

9 Yaden O, Grimm P, Ettenger R. Renal transplantation in children. In: Holliday M, Barratt T, Avner E, eds. *Pediatric Nephrology*, 3rd edn. Williams and Wilkins, 1994: 1390–418.

10 *2004 Annual Report of the North American Pediatric Renal Transplant Co-Operative Study* (available at spitfire.emmes.com/study/ped/).

11 Fine RN, Tejani A, Sullivan EK. Pre-emptive renal transplantation in children: report of the North American Pediatric Renal Transplant Co-Operative Study. *Clin Transplant* 1994:8:474–8.

12 Holmberg C, Laine J, Ronnholm K, Ala-Houhala M, Jalanho H. Congenital nephrotic syndrome. *Kidney Int* 1996;49(Suppl 53): S51–6.

13 *2004 Annual Report of the US Scientific Registry for Transplant Recipients and the Organ Procurement and Transplantion Network.* Rockville, MD: US Department of Health and Human Services Administration, Office of Special Programs, Division of Transplantation; Richmond, VA: UNOS (available at www.ustransplant.org).

14 Benfield MR, McDonald RA, Bartosh S, Ho PL, Harmon W. Changing trends in pediatric transplantation: 2001 Annual Report of the North American Pediatric Renal Transplant Cooperative Study. *Pediatr Transplant* 2003;7:321–35.

15 *2003 Annual Report of the US Scientific Registry for Transplant Recipients and the Organ Procurement and Transplantation Network.* Rockville MD: US Department of Heath and Human Services Administration, Office of Special Programs, Division of Transplantation; Richmond, VA: UNOS (available at www.ustransplant.org).

16 Lundgren G, Groth CG, Albrechtsen D, *et al*. HLA-matching in cyclosporine treated renal transplant recipients: a prospective Swedish-Norwegian multicenter study. *Clin Transplant* 1986: 79–85.

17 Potter D, Feduska N, Melzer J, *et al*. Twenty years of renal transplantation in children. *Pediatrics* 1986;77:465–70.

18 Opelz G, Graver B, Terasaki PI. Induction of high kidney graft survival rate by multiple transfusion. *Lancet* 1981;i:223–5.

19 Chavers BM, Sullivan EK, Tejani A, Harmon WE. Pre-transplant blood transfusion and renal allograft outcome: a report of the North American Pediatric Renal Transplant Cooperative Study. *Pediatr Transplant* 1997;i:22–8.

20 Niaudet P, Dudley J, Charbit M, *et al*. Pretransplant blood transfusions with cyclosporine in pediatric renal transplantation. *Pediatr Nephrol* 2000;14:451–6.

21 Cecka JM, Gjertson DW, Terasaki PI. Pediatric renal transplantation: a review of the UNOS data. United Network For Organ Sharing. *Pediatr Transplant* 1997;1:55–64.

22 Sutherland DER, Fryd DS, So SKS, *et al.* Long-term effects of splenectomy versus no splenectomy in renal transplant patients: reanalysis of a randomized prospective study. *Transplantation* 1984;38:619–24.

23 Hodson EM, Shaw PF, Evans RA, *et al.* Growth retardation and renal osteodystrophy in children with chronic renal failure. *J Pediatr* 1983;103:35–40.

24 Karlberg J, Schaefer F, Hennicke M. Early age-dependent growth impairment in chronic renal failure. *Pediatr Nephrol* 1996;10:283–7.

25 Schaefer F, Seidel C, Bending A. Pubertal growth in chronic renal failure. *Pediatr Res* 1990;28:5–10.

26 Tejani A, Sullivan K. Long-term follow-up of growth in children post-transplantation. *Kidney Int* 1993;44(Suppl 43):S56–8.

27 Tejani A, Fine R, Alexander S, Harmon W, Stablein D. Factors predictive of sustained growth in children after renal transplantation. North American Pediatric Renal Transplant Cooperative Study. *J Pediatr* 1993;22:397–402.

28 Salusky IB, Coburn JW, Brill J, *et al.* Bone disease in pediatric patients undergoing dialysis with CAPD or CCPD. *Kidney Int* 1988;33:975–82.

29 Wuhl E, Schaefer F. Puberty in chronic renal failure. *Adv Ren Replace Ther* 1999;6:335–43.

30 Scharer K. Study group on pubertal development in chronic renal failure: growth and development of children with chronic renal failure. *Acta Paediatr Scand* 1990;Suppl 336:90–2.

31 Groothoff JW, Grootthenhuis M, Domerholt A, *et al.* Impaired cognition and schooling in adults with end stage renal disease since childhood. *Arch Dis Child* 2002;87:380–5.

32 Broyer M, LeBihan C, Charbit M, *et al.* Long term social outcome of children after kidney transplantation. *Transplantation* 2004;77:1033–7.

33 Brouhard BH, Donaldson LA, Lawry KW, *et al.* Cognitive functioning in children on dialysis and post-transplantation. *Pediatr Transplant* 2000;4:261–7.

34 Davis ID, Chang P, Nevins TE. Successful renal transplantation accelerates development in young uremic children. *Pediatrics* 1990;86:594–600.

35 Bawden HN, Acott P, Carter J, *et al.* Neuropsychological functioning in end-stage renal disease. *Arch Dis Child* 2004;89:644–7.

36 Fennell RS, Fennell EB, Carter RL, *et al.* A longitudinal study of the cognitive function of children with renal failure. *Pediatr Nephrol* 1990;4:1–15.

37 Fennell RS, Rasbury WC, Fennell EB, Morris M. Effects of kidney transplantation on cognitive performance in a pediatric population. *Pediatrics* 1984;74:273–8.

38 Anonymous. NKF-DOQI Clinical Practice Guidelines for the treatment of anemia of chronic renal disease: Update 2000. *Am J Kidney Dis* 2001;37:S182–238.

39 Iragorri S, Pillay D, Scrine M, *et al.* Prospective cytomegalovirus surveillance in paediatric renal transplant patients. *Pediatr Nephrol* 1993;7:55–60.

40 Niaudet P, Raguin G, Lefevre J, *et al.* Serological status of cytomegalovirus and outcome of renal transplantation. *Kidney Int* 1983;23(Suppl 14):S50–3.

41 Robinson LG, Hilinski J, Graham F, *et al.* Predictors of cytomegalovirus disease among pediatric transplant recipients within one year of renal transplantation. *Pediatr Transplant* 2002:6:111–8.

42 Ellis D, Jaffe R, Green M, *et al.* Epstein–Barr virus-related disorders in children undergoing renal transplantation with tacrolimus-based immunosuppression. *Transplantation* 1999;68:997–1003.

43 Anonymous. Guidelines for vaccination of solid organ transplant candidates and recipients. *Am J Transplant* 2004;4(Suppl 10):160–3.

44 Gershon AA. Immunizations for pediatric transplant patients. *Kidney Int* 1993;44(Suppl 43):S87–90.

45 Tejani A, Sullivan EK. Factors that impact on the outcome of second renal transplants in children. *Transplantation* 1996;62:606–11.

17 Evaluation of the Candidate

Uptal D. Patel and Susan E. Thomas

The goal of organ transplantation is to restore the health and improve the quality of life of the recipient [1]. Kidney transplantation dramatically improves patient survival when compared with maintenance dialysis and is therefore the treatment of choice for end-stage renal disease (ESRD) [2–4]. In children and adolescents, additional benefits include improved growth, school attendance and cognitive functioning [1,5]. While the primary diagnoses leading to ESRD have remained stable over the past decade [6], many of these diseases may cause continued problems after transplantation if not adequately addressed. Thus, in order to optimize the chances for successful renal transplantation, a thorough evaluation of the patient with advanced chronic kidney disease (CKD) or ESRD is necessary. Table 17.1 outlines essential components of the evaluation of the candidate for kidney transplantation.

Table 17.1 Evaluation of the candidate for kidney transplantation.

Assessment	Pediatric transplantation nephrologist, surgeon, coordinator, urologist, nurse, social worker, child psychologist, dietitian, pharmacist, anesthesiologist
Histocompatability testing	ABO/Rh; HLA typing [Class I (A, B), Class II (DR)]; panel reactive antibody level (PRA); initial and final cross-matches (complement-dependent cytotoxicity or flow cytometry)
History	Etiology of renal disease, renal biopsy results, previous transplants (ABO, HLA, PRA, induction therapy, rejection therapy, CAD or LRD), dialysis method (access, frequency, duration), urologic abnormalities, native urine output, previous procedures and surgeries, other organ disease, transfusion history (number, dates, type), allergies, erythropoietin therapy, family history of kidney disease
Physical examination	Height, weight, OFC if < 10 years, BP, complete physical examination including vessels, pelvic exam (age appropriate), dental exam
Laboratory studies	Na, K, Cl, CO_2, BUN, Cr, Ca, Mg, Phos, CBC/diff/plt, PT, PTT, Glu, Chol, Trig, Alb, Alk Phos, Bili, AST, ALT, GGT, pregnancy test, monthly PRA
Serology studies	CMV (IgG, IgM), EBV (IgG, IgM), toxoplasmosis (IgG, IgM), HIV (ELISA, Western blot), Hep B (sAg, antibody), Hep C (IgG, IgM, PCR), VZV (IgG, IgM), HSV (IgG, IgM), MMR (if indicated)
Vaccinations	Hep B, DTaP/Td, HIB, IPV, MMR, Varicella, Pneumococcal conjugate vaccine (< 2 years), Pneumococcal polysaccharide vaccine (> 2 years), influenza, Hep A (for children living in or traveling to high-risk areas), influenza
Other studies	PPD with controls, urinalysis, urine culture, spot urine protein/creatinine ratio, CXR, cardiac ECHO, EKG, pap smear (within 1 year if age appropriate), VCUG or urodynamics, MRV (for assessment of IVC patency if indicated), US (kidneys, ureters, post-void bladder, abdomen, pelvis)
Updates every 6–12 months pretransplant	Physical examination, brief evaluation with pediatric transplant team (nephrologist, surgeon, nurse, dietitian and social worker); Na, K, Cl, CO_2, BUN, Cr, Ca, Mg, Phos, Alb, Alk Phos, Bili, AST, ALT, GGT, CBC/diff/plt, CMV (IgG, IgM), EBV (IgG, IgM), HIV (ELISA, Western blot), Hep B (sAg, antibody), Hep C (IgG, IgM, PCR), VZV (IgG, IgM)

TIMING

The transplant evaluation should begin once the patient's course towards ESRD is inevitable. Receiving a transplant before initiating dialysis (pre-emptive transplantation) may occur if a living donor is available. Patients who do not have a living donor must be placed on the deceased donor transplantation list. For adults, US federal guidelines require that waiting time can only accumulate after the transplant evaluation is complete and the measured or estimated creatinine clearance is less than 20 mL/min. All children, however, may be placed on the deceased donor list upon completion of the transplant evaluation even while awaiting live donor evaluation. For live donation, children may be transplanted at any level of renal function, but typically transplantation occurs when the creatinine clearance is less than 20 mL/min, and the risks of morbidity from impending ESRD outweigh the risks associated with transplantation. Indications for transplantation in pediatrics have been well addressed and include growth impairment, electrolyte disturbances, uremia, persistent anemia, metabolic acidosis and metabolic bone disease [7,8]. With advances in the medical management of CKD over the last decade, however, individual indications have become less relevant. Treatments for CKD now include the use of growth hormone for growth impairment, erythropoietin with oral or intravenous iron for anemia, bicarbonate supplementation for metabolic acidosis, vitamin D and phosphorus binders for metabolic bone disease, and use of aggressive nutrition and fluid management [9–11]. Therefore, determining the best time for a pre-emptive transplant in children with CKD can be a more difficult decision and is often dependent on the presence of a combination of abnormalities and overall level of kidney function.

CONTRAINDICATIONS

There are a few generally accepted contraindications to transplantation in adults [12]. No absolute contraindications exist for children because in general the benefits greatly outweigh the risks of remaining on dialysis. However, a few relative contraindications must be considered. Active infections require careful evaluation and may require therapy prior to transplantation. Although uncommon in children, infection with the hepatitis C virus (HCV) is associated with significant morbidity and mortality in the immunosuppressed transplant recipient [13].

Until recently, patients with human immunodeficiency virus (HIV) were excluded from transplantation under the premise that the required immunosuppression would exacerbate an already immunocompromised state [14]. However, recent advances with highly active antiretroviral therapy have dramatically improved the prognosis of individuals living with HIV. Many HIV-infected adult patients have tolerated immunosuppression and have allograft survival rates comparable to that of HIV-negative transplant recipients [15]. Until the results of ongoing multicenter trials evaluating transplantation in HIV-infected patients are available, HIV infection should no longer be an absolute contraindication for transplantation and cases should be considered individually.

Active malignancy precludes transplantation until treatment with chemotherapy is completed and life expectancy is established. However, pre-existing malignancy is a relative contraindication. Observation during an appropriate disease-free interval before transplantation is a reasonable approach. In children with Wilms tumor, kidney transplantation has been successful without disease recurrence [16]. Registry data support general recommendations that advocate a 2-year disease-free interval for most invasive tumors (e.g. renal tumors, Wilms tumor, lymphoma), but no waiting period for *in situ* cancers of the cervix and skin or incidental renal tumors [17].

While the primary etiology of kidney disease is not a contraindication to transplantation, many diseases can recur in the allograft [18]. In some cases, recurrence may lead to graft failure. Special approaches to management may be required for diseases that may recur such as focal glomerulosclerosis, antiglomerular basement membrane (anti-GBM) disease, immunoglobulin A (IgA) nephropathy, membranoproliferative glomerulonephritis, hemolytic uremic syndrome–thrombotic thrombocytopenic purpura, systemic lupus erythematosus, Henoch–Schönlein purpura and primary hyperoxaluria [18–21]. However, recurrence in the transplant is not inevitable for these diseases. Thus, once the appropriate precautions have been taken, the possibility of disease recurrence itself should not preclude transplantation.

Several other conditions mandate carefully reconsidering transplantation. Immunological conditions include elevated levels of circulating anti-GBM antibodies, ABO incompatibility and the presence of cytotoxic antilymphocyte antibody against the donor. Finally, patients with severe permanent brain injury or multiorgan failure are also unlikely to realize the benefit of transplantation.

RETRANSPLANTATION

While most centers perform repeat transplantations in suitable candidates, subsequent transplants may be associated with higher rates of graft failure [22]. Prior graft loss is one of the major causes of high sensitization, particularly with early graft failure [23]. Because up to 10% of transplants in children are repeat transplants, sensitization may be a significant barrier to timely receipt of subsequent allografts [24]. In those patients who do undergo retransplantation, the role of primary allograft nephrectomy is not clear [25,26] and should be individualized.

DIALYSIS VERSUS PRE-EMPTIVE TRANSPLANT

Most patients, family members and transplant programs prefer that children avoid dialysis and proceed directly with a pre-emptive transplant for management of impending ESRD. The benefit of a pre-emptive transplant is to maximize survival by avoiding vascular complications related to hemodialysis, peritoneal complications related to peritoneal dialysis, and other morbidity and mortality associated with dialysis [27,28]. Overall, recipients of pre-emptive transplantation have improved patient and allograft survival [28,29].

A critical component to the success of pre-emptive transplantation is timely referral for transplant evaluation. Sufficient time to evaluate the candidate appropriately and plan for transplantation is necessary and should occur when the estimated glomerular filtration rate (GFR) is approximately 30 mL/min/1.73 m^2 [30]. Because obstructive uropathy is the most common etiology of renal failure in children, many children with advanced CKD will have polyuria which prevents volume-related complications that may otherwise prompt earlier initiation of dialysis. However, the etiology of renal disease in adolescents includes more immunologic renal diseases (e.g. focal segmental glomerulosclerosis). Complications such as hypertension, nephrotic syndrome and hyperkalemia may necessitate interim dialysis and potentially even nephrectomy, subsequently decreasing the chance of pre-emptive transplantion in this group [31].

Some programs may be concerned that avoiding dialysis prior to transplantation may impact medical nonadherence after transplantation. They presume that children who have never had to comply with a medical routine may then find it difficult to make the transition to the strict medical adherence required after transplantation [32]. In response, some programs only utilize pre-emptive transplant in highly motivated families and in small children. Conversely, adolescents at high risk for nonadherence may be placed on dialysis for a period of time to be "educated" regarding adherence. While nonadherence is a legitimate concern that impacts long-term graft survival, no data support this practice.

NATIVE NEPHRECTOMY

In certain instances, pretransplantation bilateral native nephrectomy with short-term dialysis may minimize problems after transplantation. Nephrotic syndrome is a common feature of many causes of ESRD in children, such as focal segmental glomerulosclerosis, congenital nephrotic syndrome, membranoproliferative glomerulonephritis, systemic lupus erythematosus, nephritis and membranous nephropathy. In addition to the adverse consequences of massive proteinuria such as edema, nutritional deficits and hyperlipidemia, a hypercoaguable state increases the risk of graft thrombosis [33].

In order to minimize these complications, pretransplantation native nephrectomy has been performed and found to be beneficial in some cases [34,35].

Other conditions that require consideration of nephrectomy include severe polyuria, severe electrolyte wasting, recurrent pyelonephritis and severe hypertension [36]. One-third of children who require renal transplantation have congenital malformations of the urinary tract (obstructive uropathy) or kidneys (renal aplasia, hypoplasia or dysplasia) resulting in severe polyuria. Maintenance of euvolemia can be challenging post-transplant, and chronic dehydration may exacerbate the nephrotoxic effects of many required medications. Recurrent pyelonephritis with vesicoureteral reflux has been managed with pretransplant nephrectomy; however, whether this lowers the incidence of infection post-transplant is not clear [37]. Chronic hypertension, a common complication of ESRD resulting from the glomerulonephritides, is associated with decreased patient and allograft survival. In those with refractory hypertension before transplantation, native nephrectomy may improve blood pressure control, reduce the number of antihypertensive medications required and improve surgical outcomes [38]. Finally, children with XY gonadal dysgenesis and renal failure (Drash syndrome) may benefit from native nephrectomy because the frequency of Wilms tumor is high [39].

While most nephrectomies are performed surgically, medical nephrectomy may be performed in some cases. In the past, metallic salts have been used [40], while more recently high-dose nonsteroidal anti-inflammatory drugs (NSAIDs) [41] and bilateral renal artery embolization [42] have been successful. If NSAIDs are used, discontinuation prior to transplantation is imperative in order to avoid NSAID toxicity to the allograft. One successful approach to delay the need for bilateral nephrectomy in young children with congenital nephrotic syndrome includes unilateral nephrectomy with use of an angiotensin-converting enzyme inhibitor and an NSAID [43].

BLADDER EVALUATION

Many children develop ESRD from urinary tract abnormalities and bladder dysfunction (e.g. posterior urethral valves, neurogenic bladder, vesicoureteral reflux, outflow obstruction, prune belly syndrome or bladder extrophy). An abnormal lower urinary tract, if not corrected prior to transplantation, may adversely impact recipient and graft survival [44]. Thus, a coordinated urologic evaluation with pediatric urologist and nephrologist is vital. For successful transplantation, the bladder should have adequate volume and drainage in order to support the urine output from the transplant and native kidneys. Inadequate bladder capacity or elevated end-filling pressures may require bladder augmentation or substitution prior to transplantation. Inadequate drainage prior to or following transplantation may require intermittent self-catheterization or creation of a continent urinary diversion [45]. In those patients with questionable bladder function, pretransplant cystometrogram helps to determine how the bladder is behaving during filling. In addition, a voiding cystoureterogram allows the physician to observe the bladder and ureters during voiding in order to determine if there is inadequate drainage or vesicoureteral reflux. In those patients with reflux and recurrent urinary tract infections, either correction of the reflux by an antireflux procedure or a nephroureterectomy prior to or at the time of transplant may be necessary in order to avoid complications such as recurrent infections or sepsis.

VASCULAR EVALUATION

The vasculature must be adequately assessed prior to transplantation. The arterial anastomosis is performed to the aorta in small children (end-to-side) and to the common iliac artery (end-to-side) in older children. The venous anastomosis is performed to the inferior vena cava (IVC) in small children and to the external iliac or common iliac vein (end-to-side) in older children. Therefore, children who have had prior femoral catheters for dialysis or other medical care need to be evaluated for adequate vascular patency. Patients with prolonged femoral catheters or recurrent scarring processes of the abdomen such as peritonitis or multiple surgeries may also be predisposed to thromboses of the IVC and should be screened with magnetic resonance venogram [46]. Alternatively, computed tomography (CT) or ultrasound may also be used to confirm IVC patency.

EXTRARENAL DISEASE

Evaluation of the candidate for extrarenal disease is imperative in order to ensure that there are no other factors that may adversely affect their health with kidney transplantation. While several important conditions that impact morbidity and mortality in adults require careful evaluation (e.g. coronary heart, cerebrovascular and peripheral arterial diseases), fewer exist in children. Nonetheless, an important component of the transplantation evaluation is to detect and treat reversible medical conditions that increase the risks of transplantation.

Cardiovascular disease

Hypertension is common in children before and after transplantation. Poorly controlled hypertension may lead to left ventricular hypertrophy (LVH), which can be ascertained by echocardiography. The presence of LVH should prompt intensified hypertension management prior to and following

transplantation. Echocardiography also provides an assessment of cardiac function; diminished cardiac output may impair renal allograft perfusion and thus influence blood pressure treatment goals or trigger additional therapies.

Pulmonary disease

Several pulmonary disorders may influence management and impact outcomes in the transplant recipient. Many children with renal hypoplasia or dysplasia have pulmonary hypoplasia, which has been associated with increased mortality [47]. Pulmonary hypertension may develop in some patients, especially in those with prolonged dialysis through an arteriovenous fistula [48]. While pulmonary hypertension is associated with decreased survival, it may resolve in some patients following transplantation [48]. All patients should discontinue smoking because it is associated with an increased risk of patient and allograft loss [49].

Infection

In order to prevent infectious complications following transplantation, the candidate should be free of all active infection and given prophylaxis for certain indicated infections. Sites of potential subclinical infection that should be excluded prior to transplantation include the skin, teeth, sinuses, urinary tract and dialysis access sites (hemodialysis and peritoneal dialysis catheters). Evidence for tuberculosis should be sought with history, physical examination, chest X-ray and purified protein derivative (PPD) skin testing. Transplant candidates should also be tested for HIV.

Two important pathogens that should be evaluated prior to transplantation are cytomegalovirus (CMV) and Epstein–Barr virus (EBV). Recipients who are CMV-negative and receive a CMV-positive kidney are at risk for developing CMV infection or disease. Given the frequent morbidity and mortality associated with CMV disease after renal transplantation, many programs administer anti-CMV agents during the peri- and postoperative periods. Preferred agents include ganciclovir, valganciclovir or CMV-specific immunoglobulin (CytoGam®) [50,51]. An additional benefit for patients at-risk for CMV who receive pooled human immunoglobulin may be improved graft survival [52]. Recipients who are EBV-negative and receive an EBV-positive kidney are at a much higher risk for developing post-transplant lymphoproliferative disease (PTLD). Measures to manage this risk following transplantation include limiting patient exposure to aggressive immunosuppression and, perhaps, more frequent serologic surveillance [53].

If possible, routine childhood immunizations should be completed prior to immunosuppression [54]. In particular, attenuated live virus vaccines such as varicella and measles should be administered at least 2 months prior to transplantation because administration of live virus vaccines following transplantation is contraindicated. Other childhood vaccines (i.e. influenza, pneumococcus, hepatitis A and B, and others excluding live virus vaccines) should also be administered prior to transplantation because immunosuppression following transplantation may impair an adequate immunologic response. However, they may be given 12 months following transplantation provided that allograft function is stable and there have been no rejection episodes [54].

Gastrointestinal disease

Viral hepatitis can cause progressive liver disease and death; however, its presence is not an absolute contraindication to transplantation. While hepatitis B virus infection in ESRD patients has decreased, HCV infection has become more common in adults. The incidence and impact in younger transplant recipients is not well known; however, HCV infection is prevalent in children with ESRD and duration of dialysis appears to be a significant risk factor [55].

Malignancy

Growth of malignant cells favored by immunosuppression following transplantation accounts for the increased incidence of most tumors in renal transplant recipients when compared with age-matched controls. Screening for malignancies that may be present in the candidate requires a targeted evaluation in adults. In children, however, only a prior history of malignancy warrants further evaluation. Excluding recurrence and ensuring observation for an appropriate disease-free interval has been completed is a reasonable approach.

TRANSPLANTATION IN SPECIAL PATIENT GROUPS

In the past, patient and allograft survival in young children was poor compared with that of older children and adults [56]. While outcomes were especially poor in infants younger than 1 year, infants with allograft function at 1 year now have excellent long-term allograft survival [57,58].

Transplantation in mentally impaired children raises ethical dilemmas for many centers [59]. One reasonable course of action is to pursue the family's wishes following intensive discussions between the physicians, family, psychologist and social worker. It may then be reasonable to proceed if the patient is found to be cooperative, have a long life expectancy and be able to take medications under supervision by a reliable long-term caregiver. While the decision of whether or not to transplant a patient with mental retardation requires careful individual consideration, excellent patient and graft survival rates have been achieved [60]. In addition, patient quality of life and health judged by their support person can improve significantly after transplantation [60].

As in adults, the incidence of multiorgan transplantation in children is increasing in incidence. Transplantation of non-renal organs is often complicated by chronic renal disease, and treatment of ESRD with kidney transplantation in these patients is associated with a significantly lower risk of death when compared with dialysis [61]. Not surprisingly, many centers now perform combined transplantations including heart and kidney, liver and kidney, and pancreas and kidney. For bone marrow transplant recipients who develop ESRD, use of the kidney from the donor source of the bone marrow transplant should be considered [62,63]. Thus, in specific cases, potential candidates for kidney transplants must also be considered as candidates for other organ transplantation concurrently or in the future. While there is no well-defined approach to these difficult cases, open communication between the transplant surgery and various medical transplant teams may facilitate optimal care and planning.

PSYCHOSOCIAL ISSUES

While the psychosocial evaluation may be difficult given patients from diverse cultures and backgrounds, the primary goal is to identify if there are any potential risk factors that may result in an increased risk of postoperative nonadherence and subsequent morbidity or mortality [64]. Nonadherence with immunosuppressive medications is a major cause of allograft failure, accounting for up to 30–70% of long-term graft loss among children and adolescents [65,66]. The presence of substance abuse, nonadherence with dialysis or serious psychopathology mandates further evaluation and treatment. Although uncommon in children, patients with a history of alcohol and/or substance abuse are more likely to have difficulties with adherence [67] and documentation of a drug-free interval or rehabilitation prior to transplantation may be necessary. In addition, patients who are nonadherent with therapies prior to transplantation (e.g. dialysis and medication prescriptions, clinic visits) are also more likely to be nonadherent after transplantation. However, a variety of factors may be related to nonadherence among children with ESRD, including psychological distress and depression [68], which makes predicting future nonadherence with immunosuppression difficult. In general, pediatric patients should not be denied transplantation for previous nonadherent behaviors. Finally, patients with cognitive or personality disorders should be evaluated by a pediatric social worker, psychologist and/or psychiatrist. Psychiatric diagnoses are associated with nonadherence and graft loss [69]. In addition, patients and providers should be aware that the high doses of corticosteroids used after transplantation may exacerbate psychiatric symptoms.

The relationship between family functioning, social support and medication adherence has been long established [70]; however, these factors are not routinely evaluated prior to transplantation. Parental and family functioning variables that may be beneficial to understand include assessments of parent stress [66], problematic parent–child interactions [65,66,68], child behavior problems [66,68], lack of parental supervision [68] and parental psychiatric illness [68].

REFERRAL BIAS

Given that renal transplantation is the treatment of choice for pediatric patients with ESRD, efforts to allocate kidneys equitably must be addressed. A series of steps must be traversed during the transplant process, including being medically suitable, being interested in transplantation, completing the pretransplant workup, and movement up a waiting list to eventual transplantation [71]. Barriers at several steps are responsible for differences observed by race, gender and income in access to deceased donor renal transplantation in adults [71]. Even among children with ESRD, there are racial disparities in access to the deceased donor waiting list [72], as well as for successful completion of pre-emptive transplantation [28]. While reasons for these disparities are poorly characterized, a variety of social and contextual factors may be responsible for limiting living-related kidney donation to children in certain settings [73]. Gender disparities also exist among both children and adults. Female patients with ESRD face barriers to receiving a pre-emptive transplantation [28] and to being activated for deceased donor transplantation [74]. Decreased rates of placement on the deceased donor waiting list are also associated with treatment at a for-profit dialysis facility, as compared with not-for-profit facility [75]; however, the strength of this association in the pediatric dialysis population has not been established.

In conclusion, physicians treating patients with ESRD should be aware that disparities by race, gender and economic status exist; however, they should not permit personal or cultural bias to limit access to transplantation.

EVALUATION UPDATES

Pediatric candidates, expressed as the percentage of all candidates on the waiting list, have remained stable at approximately 3% for the last 4 years, although the continued disproportionate growth of adult candidates has led to, and will continue to lead to, a gradual decline in the percentage of the waiting list represented by pediatric candidates [58]. Nonetheless, conditions that may change the chances for successful renal transplantation may develop over relatively short periods of time. Thus, candidates for kidney transplantation should be re-evaluated at regular intervals of 6–12 months. Evaluation updates should include a simplified version of the initial evaluation visit (see Table 17.1).

CONCLUSIONS

Significant advancements in pediatric transplantation over the past several decades have clearly established this remarkable therapy as the optimal treatment for ESRD, especially among children. Transplantation not only reverses the metabolic and growth derangements associated with CKD and ESRD, but it also improves the psychological well-being and development of the child [1,7]. Careful evaluation of the candidate is crucial to the success of kidney transplantation.

REFERENCES

1 Davis ID, Chang PN, Nevis TE. Successful renal transplantation accelerates development in young ureic children. *Pediatrics* 1990;86:594–600.
2 Suthanthiran M, Strom TB. Renal transplantation. *N Engl J Med* 1994;331:365–76.
3 Wolfe RA, Ashby VB, Milford EL, *et al*. Comparison of mortality in all patients on dialysis, patients on dialysis awaiting transplantation, and recipients of a first cadaveric transplant. *N Engl J Med* 1999;341:1725–30.
4 McDonald SP, Craig JC, for the Australian and New Zealand Paediatric Nephrology Association. Long-term survival of children with end-stage renal disease. *N Engl J Med* 2004;350:2654–62.
5 Fennell RS III, Rasbury WC, Fennell EB, Morris MK. Effects of kidney transplantation on cognitive performance in a pediatric population. *Pediatrics* 1984;74:273–8.
6 Benfield MR, McDonald RA, Bartosh SM, Ho PL, Harmon WE. Changing trends in pediatric transplantation: 2001 annual report of the North American Pediatric Renal Transplant Cooperative Study. *Pediatr Transplant* 2003;7:321–35.
7 Davis ID, Bunchman TE, Grimm PC, *et al*. Pediatric renal transplantation: indications and special considerations. A position paper from the Pediatric Committee of the American Society of Transplant Physicians. *Pediatr Transplant* 1998;2:117–29.
8 Matas AJ, Chavers BM, Nevins TE, *et al*. Recipient evaluation, preparation, and care in pediatric transplantation: the University of Minnesota protocols. *Kidney Int* 1996;53:S99–102.
9 Fine RN, Kohaut EC, Brown D, Perlman AJ. Growth after recombinant human growth hormone treatment in children with chronic renal failure: report of a multicenter randomized double-blind placebo-controlled study. Genentech Cooperative Study Group. *J Pediatr* 1994;124:374–82.
10 Brungger M, Hulter HN, Krapf R. Effect of chronic metabolic acidosis on the growth hormone/IGF-1 endocrine axis: new cause of growth hormone insensitivity in humans. *Kidney Int* 1997;51:216–21.
11 Sanchez CP, Goodman WG, Salusky IB. Prevention of renal osteodystrophy in predialysis patients. *Am J Med Sci* 1999;317:398–404.
12 McKay DB, Milford EL, Sayegh MH. Clinical aspects of renal transplantation. In: Brenner BM, Rector FC, eds. *The Kidney*, 5th edn, Philadelphia: Saunders, 1995.
13 Fabrizi F, Martin P, Ponticelli C. Hepatitis C virus infection and renal transplantation. *Am J Kidney Dis* 2001;38:919–34.

14 Spital A. Should all human immunodeficiency virus-infected patients with end-stage renal disease be excluded from transplantation? The views of US transplant centers. *Transplantation* 1998;**65**:1187–91.

15 Abbott KC, Swanson SJ, Agodoa LY, Kimmel PL. Human immunodeficiency virus infection and kidney transplantation in the era of highly active antiretroviral therapy and modern immunosuppression. *J Am Soc Nephrol* 2004;**15**:1633–9.

16 Pais E, Pirson Y, Squifflet JP, *et al*. Kidney transplantation in patients with Wilms' tumor. *Transplantation* 1992;**53**:782–5.

17 Kasiske BL. Evaluation and management of prospective kidney recipients. In: Norman DJ, Turka LA, eds. *Primer on Transplantation*, 2nd edn. Mt Laurel, NJ: American Society of Transplantation; Malden, MA: Blackwell Science, 2001.

18 Seikaly MG. Recurrence of primary disease in children after renal transplantation: an evidence-based update. *Pediatr Transplant* 2004;**8**:113–9.

19 Ramos EL, Tisher CC. Recurrent diseases in the kidney transplant. *Am J Kidney Dis* 1994;**24**:142–54.

20 Hariharan S, Adams MB, Brennan DC, *et al*. Recurrent and *de novo* glomerular disease after renal transplantation: a report from Renal Allograft Disease Registry (RADR). *Transplantation* 1999;**68**:635–41.

21 Briggs JD, Jones E. Recurrence of glomerulonephritis following renal transplantation. Scientific Advisory Board of the ERA-EDTA Registry. European Renal Association–European Dialysis and Transplant Association. *Nephrol Dial Transplant* 1999;**14**:564.

22 Tejani A, Sullivan EK. Factors that impact on the outcome of second renal transplants in children. *Transplantation* 1996;**62**:606–11.

23 Sautner T, Gnant M, Banhegyi C, *et al*. Risk factors for development of panel reactive antibodies and their impact on kidney transplantation outcome. *Transplant Int* 1992;**5**:S116–20.

24 Vella JP, O'Neill D, Atkins N, Donohoe JF, Walshe JJ. Sensitization to human leukocyte antigen before and after the introduction of erythropoietin. *Nephrol Dial Transplant* 1998;**13**:2027–32.

25 Douzdjian V, Rice JC, Carson RW, Gugliuzza KK, Fish JC. Renal retransplants: effect of primary allograft nephrectomy on early function, acute rejection and outcome. *Clin Transplant* 1996;**10**:203–8.

26 Abouljoud MS, Deierhoi MH, Hudson SL, Diethelm AG. Risk factors affecting second renal transplant outcome, with special reference to primary allograft nephrectomy. *Transplantation* 1995;**60**:138–44.

27 Fine RN, Tejani A, Sullivan EK. Pre-emptive renal transplantation in children: report of the North American Pediatric Renal Transplant Cooperative Study (NAPRTCS). *Clin Transplant* 1994;**8**:474–8.

28 Kasiske BL, Snyder JJ, Matas AJ, *et al*. Pre-emptive kidney transplantation: the advantage and the advantaged. *J Am Soc Nephrol* 2002;**13**:1358–64.

29 Mange KC, Joffe MM, Feldman HI. Effect of the use or nonuse of long-term dialysis on the subsequent survival of renal transplants from living donors. *N Engl J Med* 2001;**344**:726–31.

30 National Kidney Foundation. K/DOQI clinical practice guidelines for chronic kidney disease: evaluation, classification, and stratification. *Am J Kidney Dis* 2002;**39**:S1–266.

31 Warady BA, Hebert D, Sullivan EK, Alexander SR, Tejani A. Renal transplantation, chronic dialysis, and chronic renal insufficiency in children and adolescents. 1995 Annual Report of the North American Pediatric Renal Transplant Cooperative Study. *Pediatr Nephrol* 1997;**11**:49–64.

32 Blowey DL, Hebert D, Arbus GS, *et al*. Compliance with cyclosporine in adolescent renal transplant recipients. *Pediatr Nephrol* 1997;**11**:547–51.

33 Harmon WE, Stablein D, Alexander SR, Tejani A. Graft thrombosis in pediatric renal transplant recipients: a report of the North American Pediatric Renal Transplant Cooperative Study. *Transplantation* 1991;**51**:406–12.

34 Kim MS, Primack W, Harmon WE. Congenital nephrotic syndrome: pre-emptive bilateral nephrectomy and dialysis before renal transplantation. *J Am Soc Nephrol* 1992;**3**:260–3.

35 Fujisawa M, Iijima K, Ishimura T, *et al*. Long-term outcome of focal segmental glomerulosclerosis after Japanese pediatric renal transplantation. *Pediatr Nephrol* 2002;**17**:165–8.

36 Benfield MR. Current status of kidney transplant: update 2003. *Pediatr Clin North Am* 2003;**50**:1301–34.

37 Erturk E, Burzon DT, Orloff M, Rabinowitz R. Outcome of patients with vesicoureteral reflux after renal transplantation: the effect of pretransplantation surgery on post-transplant urinary tract infections. *Urology* 1998;**51**:27–30.

38 Power RE, Calleary JG, Hickey DP. Pre-transplant bilateral native nephrectomy for medically refractory hypertension. *Ir Med J* 2001;**94**:214–6.

39 Hu M, Zhang GY, Arbuckle S, *et al*. Prophylactic bilateral nephrectomies in two paediatric patients with missense mutations in the WT1 gene. *Nephrol Dial Transplant* 2004;**19**:223–6.

40 Avram MM, Lipner HI. Medical nephrectomy: use of metallic salts as an alternative to bilateral renal infarction. *N Engl J Med* 1976;**295**:1080.

41 Baumelou A, LeGrain M. Medical nephrectomy with anti-inflammatory non-steroidal drugs. *BMJ* 1982;**284**:234.

42 Olivero JJ, Frommer JP, Gonzalez JM. Medical nephrectomy: the last resort for intractable complications of the nephrotic syndrome. *Am J Kidney Dis* 1993;**21**:260–3.

43 Kovacevic L, Reid CJ, Rigden SP. Management of congenital nephrotic syndrome. *Pediatr Nephrol* 2003;**18**:426–30.

44 Churchill BM, Jayanthi RV, McLorie GA, Khoury AE. Pediatric renal transplantation into the abnormal urinary tract. *Pediatr Nephrol* 1996;**10**:113–20.

45 Koo HP, Bunchman TE, Flynn IT, *et al*. Renal transplantation in children with severe lower urinary tract dysfunction. *J Urol* 1999;**161**:240–5.

46 Thomas SE, Hickman RO, Tapper D, *et al*. Asymptomatic inferior vena cava abnormalities in three children with end-stage renal disease: risk factors and screening guidelines for pretransplant diagnosis. *Pediatr Transplant* 2000;**4**:28–34.

47 Wood EG, Hand M, Briscoe DM, *et al*. North American Pediatric Renal Transplant Cooperative Study. Risk factors for mortality in infants and young children on dialysis. *Am J Kidney Dis* 2001;**37**:573–9.

48 Yigla M, Nakhoul F, Sabag A, *et al*. Pulmonary hypertension in patients with end-stage renal disease. *Chest* 2003;**123**:1577–82.

49 Kasiske BL, Klinger D. Cigarette smoking in renal transplant recipients. *J Am Soc Nephrol* 2000;**11**:753–9.

50 Boudreaux JP, Hayes DH, Mizrahi S, *et al.* Decreasing incidence of serious cytomegalovirus infection using gancyclovir prophylaxis in pediatric liver transplant patients. *Transplant Proc* 1993;**25**:1872.

51 Ham JM, Bunchman TE, Campbell DA Jr, *et al.* Cytomegalovirus and Epstein–Barr virus-acquired immunity after Sandoglobulin prophylaxis in the pediatric renal transplant population. *Transplant Proc* 1994;**26**:20–1.

52 Bunchman TE, Parekh RS, Kershaw DB, *et al.* Beneficial effect of Sandoglobulin upon allograft survival in the pediatric renal transplant recipient. *Clin Transplant* 1997;**11**:604–7.

53 Axelrod DA, Holmes R, Thomas SE, Magee JC. Limitations of EBV-PCR monitoring to detect EBV associated post-transplant lymphoproliferative disorder. *Pediatr Transplant* 2003;**7**:223–7.

54 Lopez MJ, Thomas S. Immunization of children after solid organ transplantation. *Pediatr Clin North Am* 2003;**50**:1435–49.

55 Molle ZL, Baqi N, Gretch D, *et al.* Hepatitis C infection in children and adolescents with end-stage renal disease. *Pediatr Nephrol* 2002;**17**:444–9.

56 Najarian JS, Simmons RL, Tallent MB, *et al.* Renal transplantation in infants and children. *Ann Surg* 1971;**174**:583–601.

57 Laine J, Holmberg C, Salmela K, *et al.* Renal transplantation in children with emphasis on young patients. *Pediatr Nephrol* 1994;**8**:313–9.

58 Magee JC, Bucuvalas JC, Farmer DG, *et al.* Pediatric transplantation. *Am J Transplant* 2004;**4**:54–71.

59 Baqi N, Tejani A, Sullivan EK. Renal transplantation in Down syndrome: a report of the North American Pediatric Renal Transplant Cooperative Study. *Pediatr Transplant* 1998;**2**:211–5.

60 Benedetti E, Asolati M, Dunn T, *et al.* Kidney transplantation in recipients with mental retardation: clinical results in a single-center experience. *Am J Kidney Dis* 1998;**31**:509–12.

61 Ojo AO, Held PJ, Port FK, *et al.* Chronic renal failure after transplantation of a nonrenal organ. *N Engl J Med* 2003;**349**:931–40.

62 Butcher JA, Hariharan S, Adams MB, *et al.* Renal transplantation for end-stage renal disease following bone marrow transplantation: a report of six cases, with and without immunosuppression. *Clin Transplant* 1999;**13**:330–5.

63 Thomas SE, Hutchinson RJ, DebRoy M, Magee JC. Successful renal transplantation following prior bone marrow transplantation in pediatric patients. *Pediatr Transplant* 2004;**8**:507–12.

64 Olbrisch ME, Benedict SM, Ashe K, Levenson JL. Psychological assessment and care of organ transplant patients. *J Consult Clin Psychol* 2002;**70**:771–83.

65 Wolff G, Strecker K, Vester U, Latta K, Ehrich JH. Non-compliance following renal transplantation in children and adolescents. *Pediatr Nephrol* 1998;**12**:703–8.

66 Gerson AC, Furth SL, Neu AM, Fivush BA. Assessing associations between medication adherence and potentially modifiable psychosocial variables in pediatric kidney transplant recipients and their families. *Pediatr Transplant* 2004;**8**:543–50.

67 Lurie S, Shemesh E, Sheiner PA, *et al.* Non-adherence in pediatric liver transplant recipients: an assessment of risk factors and natural history. *Pediatr Transplant* 2000;**4**:200–6.

68 Simoni JM, Asarnow JR, Munford PR, *et al.* Psychological distress and treatment adherence among children on dialysis. *Pediatr Nephrol* 1997;**11**:604–6.

69 Shaw RJ, Palmer L, Blasey C, Sarwal M. A typology of non-adherence in pediatric renal transplant recipients. *Pediatr Transplant* 2003;**7**:489–93.

70 Rapoff MA. *Adherence to Pediatric Medical Regimens.* New York, NY: Kluwer Academic/Plenum Publishers, 1999.

71 Alexander GC, Sehgal AR. Barriers to cadaveric renal transplantation among blacks, women, and the poor. *JAMA* 1998;**280**:1148–52.

72 Furth SL, Garg PP, Neu AM, *et al.* Racial differences in access to the kidney transplant waiting list for children and adolescents with end-stage renal disease. *Pediatrics* 2000;**106**:756–61.

73 Hidalgo G, Tejani C, Clayton R, *et al.* Factors limiting the rate of living-related kidney donation to children in an inner city setting. *Pediatr Transplant* 2001;**5**:419–24.

74 Garg PP, Furth SL, Fivush BA, Powe NR. Impact of gender on access to the renal transplant waiting list for pediatric and adult patients. *J Am Soc Nephrol* 2000;**11**:958–64.

75 Garg PP, Frick KD, Diener-West M, Powe NR. Effect of the ownership of dialysis facilities on patients' survival and referral for transplantation. *N Engl J Med* 1999;**341**:1653–60.

18 Donor Evaluation, Surgical Technique and Perioperative Management

Zoran Vukcevic, Demetrius Ellis, Mark Bellinger and Ron Shapiro

Kidney transplantation has become a highly successful treatment for end-stage renal disease in pediatric recipients [1]. This chapter focuses on donor selection and evaluation, technical aspects of implantation and perioperative management. There are important differences between adults and children regarding these three areas, and successful transplantation in pediatric recipients is dependent on understanding these differences.

DONOR SELECTION AND EVALUATION
(Tables 18.1 & 18.2)

In the USA, there were 769 pediatric kidney transplantations in 2002, compared with 661 in 1993. In 2002, deceased donor renal transplants accounted for 327 (43%) cases, while 442 (57%) cases were with living donors. The proportion of living donor renal transplants was inversely related to recipient age. By comparison, 41% of adult kidney transplantations were with living donors in 2002 [2,3].

Deceased donor kidneys for pediatric recipients tend to come from young and middle-aged adult donors with normal renal function and no significant pathology, and are transplanted with a short cold ischemia time. In the past, children were preferentially allocated kidneys from young deceased donors under 10 years of age. Unfortunately, these donors were associated with poor outcomes, because of a high rate of technical complications; young recipients seemed particularly susceptible to graft failure, often related to graft thrombosis. There are, however, individual centers reporting good outcomes with very young donors.

Table 18.1 Contraindications to deceased kidney donation.

Absolute	Relative
Chronic renal disease	Hypertension
Malignant tumor (except primary brain tumor)	Bacterial sepsis
Positive HBsAg test	Anti-HCV Ab positive
Positive HIV test	Prolonged cold ischemia time
Untreated systemic bacterial, fungal or viral infections	Donor ATN
Prolonged warm ischemia time	

ATN, acute tubular necrosis; HbsAg, hepatitis B surface antigen; HCV Ab, hepatitis C virus antibody; HIV, human immunodeficiency virus.

Table 18.2 Exclusion criteria for living renal donation.

Absolute	Relative
Age < 18 years	Anatomical abnormalities of the donor kidney (urologic, vascular)
Diabetes	
Proteinuria (> 300 mg/24 hours)	Obesity (> 30% over ideal weight)
Abnormal glomerular filtration rate (creatinine clearance < 75 mL/min)	Psychiatric disorders
History of thrombosis or thromboembolism	Hypertension
Medically significant illness (cardiovascular disease, recent malignancy, lung disease)	Hematuria (including microscopic)
History of bilateral kidney stones	

Older deceased donors over the age of 50 years are also less likely to be utilized for children. Donation after cardiac death (DCD) donors are similarly much less likely to be used in pediatric recipients. There is essentially no use of extended criteria donor (ECD) kidneys in pediatric recipients. In 1998, 17 children received ECD deceased donor kidneys, but the number fell to just one in 2002.

Interestingly, even though living donor renal transplant is undoubtedly the preferred treatment modality when dealing with renal failure in children, recent reports support the finding that the difference in short-term graft survival between deceased donor kidneys and living donor kidneys appears to be decreasing [4]: 1-year age-unadjusted graft survival in children older than 1 year ranged from 93% to 95% for deceased donor kidney transplants and 94% to 96% for living donor kidney transplants. These similar outcomes probably reflect, at least in part, the greater selectivity in the utilization of deceased donors in pediatric recipients.

The use of living donors for renal transplantation was historically an early development in the field, and preceded the use of deceased donors. The first successful kidney transplant was a living donor case between two identical twins in Peter Bent Brigham Hospital in Boston on December 23, 1954.

Living donors are evaluated according to generally accepted criteria. Evaluation of the donor represents a medical and moral responsibility [5,6]. Living donors must be in excellent physical and psychological health, must not be coerced to donate, and must not be paid to donate. As long as donor and recipient have a negative T-cell cross-match, the transplant operation can be carried out. This is true for both related and nonrelated donors who are ABO compatible (Rh factor compatibility is unnecessary).

The Organ Procurement and Transplantation Network (OPTN) and United Network of Organ Sharing (UNOS) have formed the Ad Hoc Living Donor Committee [7], which has proposed guidelines for potential kidney transplant living donor evaluation, including provisions for an independent donor team, psychiatric and social screening, and appropriate medical, radiologic, and anesthesia evaluation. An attending physician and surgeon should screen all potential donors.

Donor kidney function should be tested to determine serum creatinine, calculated creatinine clearance, and urine protein excretion. Donors should undergo imaging studies to determine:

1 the presence of two kidneys of normal size and appearance; and

2 the renal vascular and urinary drainage anatomy.

Donors are judged unsuitable for kidney donations for a variety of reasons. In general, anyone at risk of developing acquired renal disease should be excluded.

SURGICAL TECHNIQUE AND PERIOPERATIVE CARE

The surgical plan must be established before transplantation, so that necessary urologic procedures, including cystoscopy with fulguration of residual posterior urethral valve leaflets, vesicostomy closure, or nephrectomy with or without ureterectomy may be performed either prior to or at the time of transplantation.

Attention to the technical details of renal transplantation in children and infants is critical [8]. These issues are almost entirely a function of the recipient's size. Pediatric patients with a body weight over 30 kg can be treated surgically as small adults, and the procedure can be performed using the standard pelvic extraperitoneal approach. Smaller children and infants need an individualized approach. The key issue is appropriate matching of blood vessel size and anticipation of circulatory volume requirements.

For infants and children with a body weight of less than 10 kg, the transplant incision is a midline laparotomy, with mobilization of the right colon and terminal ileum to the left side of peritoneal cavity. The distal aorta and inferior vena cava and their respective iliac branches are mobilized (Fig. 18.1). Lumbar branches are divided only as necessary. An adult donor kidney is often used, usually from a parent, and anastomoses at the level of infrarenal inferior vena cava and aorta are performed.

For toddlers and older children, with a body weight between

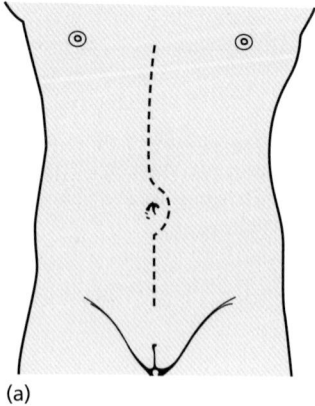

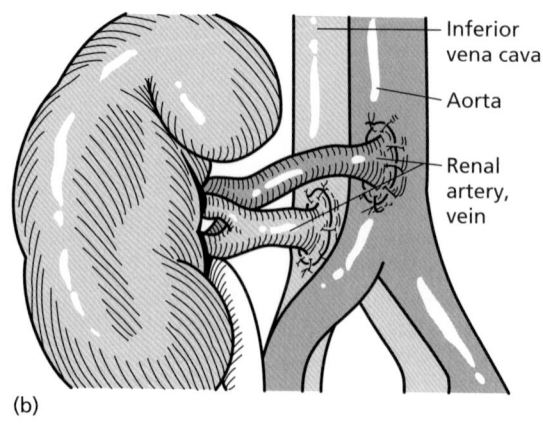

(a)   (b)

Inferior vena cava

Aorta

Renal artery, vein

Fig. 18.1 Midline approach to the very small pediatric kidney recipient, with vascular anastomosis at the level of the inferior vena cava and aorta.

10 and 30 kg, there is some variability regarding the incision and placement of the allograft. Our preference is to anastomose to the largest appropriate recipient vessel, as the external iliac vessels are frequently too small, until the body weight exceeds 30 kg. In children with a body weight of less than 20 kg, we almost always make a midline incision and perform the vascular anastomoses at the level of the inferior vena cava and the infrarenal aorta or the right common iliac artery. In children weighing between 20 and 30 kg, the inferior vena cava or right common iliac vein and the right common iliac artery can be used (the left side can be used in a retransplant setting), with either a midline transperitoneal approach or a retroperitoneal exposure. This view is not universally accepted; some surgeons prefer to use and can achieve excellent results with the standard retroperitoneal external iliac approach for patients who weigh more than 20 kg. A few even use this approach for children who weigh 10–20 kg.

In contrast to the variability surrounding the selection of vessels and site for vascular anastomosis, ureteral reimplantation is not particularly different from the standard approach used in adults. With intraperitoneally placed kidneys, it is not necessary to make a retroperitoneal tunnel for the ureter, although some surgeons may prefer to do so.

In small children and infants, an adult sized kidney may occupy the entire right side of the abdomen, displacing the large and small intestine toward the left side of the abdominal cavity. In this circumstance, although abdominal wound closure is generally not a problem, prolonged ileus occasionally may result, and therefore removal of the nasogastric tube and institution of enteral feeding may be delayed. When biopsy of the intraperitoneal allograft is required, the lateral edge of the allograft is almost always easily accessible to an ultrasound-guided percutaneous approach.

Vascular anastomosis

There are many slightly different techniques of vascular anastomosis for the renal transplant procedure. The simplest approach is to place two sutures, one at each corner of the vessel, and then anastomose two sides successively. A popular variation is to place two sutures in the middle to provide traction and minimize inadvertent suture of the back wall. Some surgeons perform one side of the vessel anastomosis from within, borrowing from techniques used in liver transplantation. Others use a single-stitch technique, particularly for the arterial anastomosis. As it may be necessary to use different techniques in different situations, familiarity with these technical variations is useful.

The vein is customarily anastomosed first, in an end-to-side fashion. Suture material of 6-0 or 7-0 polypropylene is commonly used. The artery is also sutured end-to-side, with either 6-0 or 7-0 polypropylene. End-to-end anastomosis to the internal iliac artery is generally not utilized in small children.

There are different adjunctive measures performed while the vessels are being sutured. A popular local maneuver is to wrap the deceased donor kidney in an *ice blanket* during the actual performance of the anastomosis (crushed ice is within the laparotomy pad and not in direct contact with the kidney). The kidney remains cold until reperfusion. With living donor kidneys, the donor vessels are too short to allow an ice blanket, and continual topical cooling during the performance of the vascular anastomoses will minimize ischemic damage.

Ureteral reimplantation

The most common technique of ureteroneocystostomy is extravesical. It involves incision of the bladder wall musculature at the bladder dome for a distance of 2–3 cm to expose the bladder wall mucosa. A small incision is made in the distal mucosa. The ureter is trimmed to an appropriate length, and cut usually at an angle. The anastomosis of full-thickness ureter to the bladder mucosa is performed with running or interrupted sutures. Absorbable surgical material (e.g. 6-0 polyglyconate) is almost always used. The bladder muscle layer may then be reapproximated for a short distance, enough to create a submucosal tunnel, but not so long as to constrict the ureter. This concept of the submucosal tunnel was adopted from a technique described by Lich et al. [9], originally proposed to correct reflux in children.

Variations of the extravesical technique range from not reapproximating bladder wall musculature, to using only a single suture to telescope the ureter into the bladder before reapproximating the muscle layer (the ureter is not actually sutured to the bladder mucosa).

In the case of a double ureter there are two options. The ureters can be implanted separately into the bladder, or they can be partially anastomosed on the "back table" and then implanted as a single unit. With either variation, it is important to dissect minimally the ends of the ureters so as not to disturb the blood supply.

The original open technique, attributed to Politano and Leadbetter [10], involves producing a large opening in the bladder, fashioning a submucosal tunnel, and performing a ureteroneocystostomy from within.

Possible ureteropelvic junction obstruction in the transplanted ureter may be of no functional importance. On the other hand, it may result in significant obstruction. It is not always possible to predict the outcome at the time of transplantation. Ureteropelvic junction obstruction may not even be noticed because the ureter has not been dissected proximally enough to uncover it. Options for correcting obstruction include simple stenting at the time of transplant, performance of a pyelovesicostomy or pyeloureterostomy end-to-side or end-to-end to the native ureter, or performance of an endopyelotomy through a nephrostomy.

There are techniques that avoid the bladder altogether, useful if the donor ureter has been stripped and is ischemic. The native ureter is used for end-to-end or side-to-end anastomosis to the proximal transplant ureter or pelvis (with or without native nephrectomy). Ureteroureterostomies and pyeloureterostomies are generally always stented for 6 weeks.

The goal of these techniques is to perform a watertight, technically perfect anastomosis, and use a healthy nonischemic donor ureter.

PERIOPERATIVE CARE

Prior to transplantation, many children are maintained on either hemodialysis or peritoneal dialysis for months while awaiting a suitable kidney. Optimizing the child's general health, nutrition and growth, to avoid the complications of renal failure, such as poor growth, decline in neurologic and mental function, renal osteodystrophy, anemia, cardiomegaly and hypertension, is certainly necessary [11]. Potential sources of infection must be eradicated, and urinary tract abnormalities that may hinder allograft function should be corrected at the time of transplantation. Severe uncontrollable hypertension, or proteinuria, in spite of adequate renal replacement therapy, may be an indication for bilateral native nephrectomy. In children already on dialysis, a treatment immediately before transplantation may be necessary to optimize serum electrolytes, correct acid–base disturbances and improve hemostasis. Removal of excessive amounts of fluid should be avoided, to maintain intravascular volume and allograft perfusion.

Intraoperative management of the recipient is focused on prevention of complications from underlying systemic disease and maintenance of optimal perfusion of the transplanted kidney. In pediatric renal transplant recipients, the most important intraoperative issue is to expand the circulatory volume to allow for adequate perfusion of the adult donor allograft. An adult graft may sequester up to 250 mL of blood, and in infants almost 50% of the cardiac output may be directed toward perfusion of the transplanted kidney. Although low intravascular volume caused by dialysis is routinely corrected by administration of intravenous fluids (usually crystalloids) before reperfusion of the grafted kidney, the anesthesiologist actually needs to *volume overload* the child to ensure adequate perfusion of the allograft. Before cross-clamp release, central venous pressure (CVP) should be maintained at 8–12 cm H_2O, and mean arterial pressure (MAP) above 70 mmHg. If the MAP is inadequate to achieve good renal perfusion of an adult kidney, dopamine infusion of up to 5 µg/kg/min may be started, and is the pressor of choice because of beneficial splanchnic (and renal) vasodilatation. During completion of the vascular anastomoses, 20% mannitol (1 g/kg) and intravenous furosemide (frusemide) (1 mg/kg), are given before the cross-clamps are released. Intraoperative blood gasses may need to be monitored frequently, because clamping of the aorta or iliac artery, and

accumulation of lactic acid, can result in metabolic acidosis and vasoconstriction.

The critical issue is to obtain optimal perfusion of the allograft and its immediate function. Hypotension after cross-clamp release in an infant or child with inadequate circulatory volume and an underperfused allograft is a potential catastrophe. Intravenous 25% albumin (0.5 g/kg/dose), furosemide (1–2 mg/kg/dose), sodium bicarbonate (1 mEq/kg) and 20% mannitol (0.3–0.5 g/kg/dose) or 0.9% normal saline solution (10–20 mL/kg/bolus) may be used to promote urine output in the immediate post unclamping or immediate postoperative period.

Various hemodynamic and acid–base disturbances may be seen on reperfusion of the transplanted kidney. Hyperkalemia following removal of the cross-clamp is possible, and is often treated with infusions of sodium bicarbonate, and occasionally insulin and glucose. Hypertension, reflecting the large intravenous volume infusions administered, is also common. Mild to moderate acidosis may be seen with the release of acidic substances from the kidney and the lower extremity. These changes should be closely monitored, and appropriate treatment promptly instituted.

Attention to the intravascular volume and electrolyte and acid–base stability is essential to ensure good renal function during the first 48 postoperative hours. Urine output is replaced milliliter for milliliter, usually with 0.45% or 0.9% saline solution. During the first 24–48 postoperative hours, urine output frequently exceeds 5 mL/kg/hour. For these patients, we reduce the concentration of dextrose in maintenance fluid to 1%, to prevent hyperglycemia and excessive osmotic diuresis (the standard urinary replacement solution at our center is 1% glucose, 0.5 normal saline and one ampule of $NaHCO_3$/L). Additional fluid boluses of normal saline or 5% albumin may be given if there is a reduction in urine output below 1.5 mL/kg/hour. In conjunction with these fluid boluses, administration of intravenous furosemide (1 mg/kg) may improve urine output. In infants and young children, close monitoring of fluid balance and repeated physical examination are essential to prevent electrolyte imbalance and fluid overload, which may result in severe hypertension and pulmonary edema. On the other hand, reduction of intravascular volume and acute tubular necrosis should be also avoided. A bladder catheter inserted intraoperatively is kept *in situ* postoperatively, and is usually removed after 3–5 days, to diminish the risk of urinary tract infection.

Postoperative oliguria is an alarming sign, and immediate measures must be undertaken to improve urine output. Besides the easily correctable problems, such as hypovolemia or a malfunctioning catheter, other possible causes include early rejection, vascular occlusion, acute tubular necrosis (ATN), urinary extravasation, or obstruction. A child with delayed graft function, congestive heart failure, or marked electrolyte abnormalities may need hemodialysis or peritoneal dialysis postoperatively.

Urologic disorders and pediatric renal transplantation

It is generally accepted that renal transplantation into a poorly functioning bladder or anomalous lower urinary tract reduces allograft function and survival after transplantation [11]. Approximately 15–25% of children with end-stage renal disease have associated urologic abnormalities that may lead to lower urinary tract dysfunction. Children at risk for bladder dysfunction include those with posterior urethral valves, myelodysplasia, urogenital sinus anomalies, and the prune belly syndrome. A study evaluating 300 pediatric cadaveric renal transplant recipients was performed, looking specifically at the etiology of end-stage renal disease [12]. The 5-year graft survival was approximately 70% in the group of patients with cystic or acquired renal disease, but only 30% in patients with obstructive uropathy. Other studies have confirmed lower allograft survival rates or worse renal function following transplantation in children with posterior urethral valves. These data have led to the conclusion that uncorrected abnormalities of the lower urinary tract may both cause renal failure and contribute to allograft dysfunction and failure. Such patients are at increased risk for urinary tract infection, surgical complications and graft loss [13,14].

Because satisfactory urinary drainage is necessary for a successful renal transplantation, it is very important to establish a stable urinary reservoir and storage system before transplantation. The connection between upper urinary tract dysfunction and reservoir (bladder) storage pressure has been widely accepted. Acceptable intravesical pressure of well below 30 cm H_2O should be maintained within the range of working bladder volumes. McGuire et al. [15] demonstrated that the presence of bladder leak point pressures (terminal bladder pressures) above 40 cm H_2O are associated with upper tract deterioration. Previously, others have suggested that normal bladder filling pressures are below 20 cm H_2O. Adequate urinary drainage is necessary for successful renal transplantation. Establishing a stable urinary reservoir and storage system before transplantation appears to be the best approach.

Pretransplant investigation must be tailored to the cause of end-stage renal disease and a history or suspicion of lower urinary tract dysfunction. Each pediatric patient with renal failure who is considered for transplantation should be screened for bladder dysfunction. Screening includes elimination interview, complete history and physical examination, with evaluation of external genitalia, lower spine, perineum, neurologic examination, and inspection of stomas and surgical scars. Urinalysis and urine cultures should be performed in all patients who are not anuric, and urinary tract infection should be treated before any instrumentation of urethra is conducted. A voiding diary may be helpful in the assessment of incontinence. Postvoid renal ultrasound provides a noninvasive assessment of anatomic details and residual urine

volumes. All children with a history of urinary tract infection, lower urinary tract abnormality or an abnormal renal ultrasound should undergo further evaluation. Essential study for all children with suspected urologic disorder is a voiding cystourethrogram (VCUG), which defines urethral and bladder anatomy, confirms the presence or absence of vesicoureteral reflux and provides information about bladder emptying. A formal urodynamic evaluation (cystometrogram) should be performed if neurovesical dysfunction is suspected. Cystoscopy and retrograde contrast studies may be performed if further anatomic details are required.

The role of the pediatric urologist is to define the presence or nature of lower tract dysfunction, to correct or compensate for the dysfunction (improving or stabilizing renal function when possible), and to provide the plan for satisfactory management and long-term monitoring. An individualized urologic evaluation is especially important for infants and young children, because their inability to cooperate with procedures or verbalize concepts such as sensation of bladder filling may influence the results of testing. Urologic evaluation must address both structure and function of the lower urinary tract.

MANAGEMENT

In patients with a dysfunctional lower urinary tract, the goal of therapy is to provide a sterile, compliant, nonrefluxing, low pressure reservoir that is continent and easily emptied. The approach to peritransplantation urologic management or reconstruction is highly individualized. It requires understanding of the disease involved, the natural history of end-stage renal disease, the resources and the ability of both children and caretakers to comply with specific interventions, and the proposed timing of the transplantation.

Initial approach to the hostile bladder before transplantation usually involves pharmacologic agents. In some individuals, clean intermittent catheterization may be required to maintain safe pressure and periodic emptying. If intermittent catheterization is necessary, patient and/or family cooperation must be demonstrated before transplantation. Vesicoureteral reflux resulting from urethral obstruction, neurovesical dysfunction or prune belly syndrome may cause renal dysplasia and renal failure. Low-grade primary reflux (grades 1 and 2), without a history of urinary tract infection, may require no treatment. However, if recurrent urinary tract infection or high-grade reflux is documented, a surgical approach may be necessary. Grade 3 and 4 reflux without marked ureteral tortuosity or upper tract stasis may best be managed with ureteroneocystostomy before transplantation. Correction of reflux by transurethral subureteric injection of polytetra-fluoro ethylene (PTFE) or collagen may be applicable in certain patients. Nephrectomy or nephroureterectomy may be appropriate for patients with huge refluxing megaureters and poorly functioning kidneys, if the ureter is not needed for

165

bladder augmentation. Management of the lower ureter varies. Leaving the ureteral stump *in situ* avoids perivesical scarring, which may increase the difficulty of the subsequent transplantation procedures.

Many of these children have a combination of several of the following: diminished compliance, elevated postvoid residual volume, diminished bladder volume, vesicoureteral reflux and incontinence. Consideration for management include first intermittent catheterization and/or anticholinergic medications. Bladder augmentation with detubularized bowel, native ureteral augmentation (ureterocystoplasty) or "autoaugmentation" (detrusorrhaphy) is advocated for many of these children to help reduce intravesical pressure and hyperreflexic contractions, especially in children with neurogenic bladders. Children with augmentation cystoplasty often require intermittent catheterization. This procedure is not recommended for children younger than 5 years. Patients with prior cutaneous urinary diversion need complete radiologic and urodynamic evaluation. If rehabilitation of the defunctionalized bladder (undiversion) is possible, it should be performed with the goal of establishing a bladder reservoir, with adequate compliance, capacity and emptying. If the date of transplantation is known, urinary undiversion to refunctionalize the bladder, or augmentation cystoplasty may best be performed 3–6 months prior to transplantation.

Post-transplant urologic monitoring is necessary to ensure that reconstructive and bladder management strategies are adequate to maintain upper tract stability. If urinary infection, secondary reflux, hydronephrosis or other dysfunction develops, prompt re-evaluation and change in the management plan must be considered.

CONCLUSIONS

Kidney transplantation in pediatric recipients is a highly successful therapy. Key elements of donor selection involve utilizing essentially ideal deceased donors from young or middle-aged adults, or appropriate living donors. Details of implantation vary with the size of the recipient, but emphasize the utilization of the largest possible recipient vessels for anastomosis, and appropriate intraoperative fluid management (the latter may require frank overhydration). Postoperative fluid management is generally guided by the urine output. Urologic issues should be evaluated prior to transplantation, and should be corrected either prior to or at the time of transplantation, depending on the individual needs of the patient.

REFERENCES

1 Colombani PM, Dunn SP, Harmon WE, *et al*. Pediatric transplantation. *Am J Transplant* 2003;3(Suppl 4):53–63.

2 Seikaly M, Ho PL, Emmett L, Tejani A. The 12th annual report of the North American Pediatric Renal Transplant Cooperative Study: renal transplantation from 1987 through 1998 (updated at www.naprtcs.org). *Pediatr Transplant* 2001;5:215–31.

3 Harmon WE, Hulbert-Shearon TE, Magee JC, *et al*. Improvements in outcomes in pediatric renal transplantation: children less than 10 years of age now have the best graft survival rates. *Am J Transplant* 2003;3(Suppl 5):285.

4 Benfield MR, McDonald RA, Bartosh S, Ho PL, Harmon W. Changing trends in pediatric transplantation: 2001 annual report of the North American Pediatric Renal Transplant Cooperative Study. *Pediatr Transplant* 2003;7:321–35.

5 Lennerling A, Forsberg A, Meyer K, Nyberg G. Motives for becoming a living kidney donor. *Nephrol Dial Transplant* 2004;**19**:1600–5.

6 Koller H, Mayer G. Evaluation of the living kidney donor. *Nephrol Dial Transplant* 2004;**19**(Suppl 4):41–4.

7 Abecassis M, Adams M, Adams P, *et al*. Consensus statement on the live organ donor. *JAMA* 2000;**284**:2919–26.

8 Shapiro R. The transplant procedure. In: Shapiro R, Simmons R, Starzl T, eds. *Renal Transplantation*. Stamford, CT: Appleton & Lange: 103–43.

9 Lich R, Howerton LW, Davis LA. Recurrent urosepsis in children. *J Urol* 1961;**86**:554–8.

10 Politano VA, Leadbetter. An operative technique for the correction of vesicoureteral reflux. *J Urol* 1958;**79**:932–41.

11 Ellis D, Gilboa N, Bellinger M, Shapiro R. Renal transplantation in infants and children. In: Shapiro R, Simmons R, Starzl T, eds. *Renal Transplantation*. Stamford, CT: Appleton & Lange: 427–69.

12 Churchill BM, Sheldon CA, McLorie GA, Arbus GS. Factors influencing patient and graft survival in 300 cadaveric pediatric renal transplants. *J Urol* 1988;**140**:1129–33.

13 Koo H, Bunchman T, Flynn J, *et al*. Renal transplantation in children with severe lower urinary tract dysfunction. *J Urol* 1999;**161**:240–5.

14 Luke P, Herz D, Bellinger M, *et al*. Long-term results of pediatric renal transplantation into a dysfunctional lower urinary tract. *Transplantation* 2003;**76**:1578–82.

15 McGuire EJ, Woodside JR, Borden TA, *et al*. Prognostic value of urodynamic testing in myelodysplastic patients. *J Urol* 1981;**126**:205–9.

19 Pathology of the Kidney Allograft

Arthur H. Cohen

Structural and immunopathologic abnormalities in the transplanted kidney vary in pathogenic mechanisms, structures involved, clinical correlations and diagnostic specificity. It is appropriate to divide them into pathologies of rejection and nonrejection lesions [1]. The gold standard for diagnosing the varied lesions in the allograft is the core biopsy; fine needle aspiration may be very useful in the early post-transplant setting.

TRANSPLANT BIOPSY

Because of the distribution of certain rejection-related lesions, especially of arterial inflammation, the concept of "more is better" has attraction; as documented by Sorof *et al.* [2], two cores increase the sensitivity of diagnosing acute rejection by approximately 10% over one core as often obtained in many centers. Because morphologic changes of acute rejection as well as some other lesions are patchy, the larger the amount of kidney sampled, the greater the likelihood for relevant and complete diagnoses. Processing of the biopsy depends upon the clinical setting. If a glomerular lesion is suspected, then the biopsy should be divided into three parts and evaluated by light microscopy, immunofluorescence and electron microscopy, as for a native kidney. If no glomerulopathy is suspected, then the tissue should be fixed and processed for light microscopy and immunofluorescence. In all instances, immunostain for C4d either on frozen sections with immunofluorescence or on paraffin embedded or frozen sections with immunoperoxidase must be performed (see below) [1,3,4]. The standard stains for light microscopy, which, in our practice, include periodic acid–Schiff, periodic acid–methenamine silver (Jones) and Masson trichrome in addition to hematoxylin and eosin, are a necessity [5]. Although I do not recommend completely sectioning the entire block, a sufficient number of sections must be available for evaluation to meet minimum requirements for adequacy; this includes at least two arterial cross-sections, minimum of seven glomeruli and not entirely subcapsular cortex, which is not representative [1,6]. Although a biopsy may not meet adequacy, it may still be diagnostic; for example, if only a single artery is present but is involved with intimal infiltration by lymphocytes, this is diagnostic of cell-mediated arterial rejection. Alternatively, a sufficient amount of cortex without acute inflammation of the interstitium does not completely exclude rejection because of the patchy nature of this process.

REJECTION-RELATED INJURY

Although the traditional manner of considering rejection is to divide the lesions into three distinct processes based upon temporal and pathologic information, perhaps a more logical way is to approach rejection with the prime consideration of pathogenic mechanisms. Thus, the following descriptions are based upon immunopathologic mechanisms of rejection [1]. The two mechanisms of injury are caused by T cells (cell-mediated rejection) and by antibody (humoral rejection), alone or together.

Cell-mediated rejection

Acute cellular rejection typically appears 1–6 weeks following engraftment although it may occur at any time, including after many years. T cells may infiltrate the tubulo-interstitium, glomeruli and arteries; these sites may be affected separately or together. It is convenient to describe the different anatomic locations of this form of rejection separately; indeed, these are classified as distinctive morphologic and clinical forms.

Tubulo-interstitial rejection

This is the most common location for, and form of cell-mediated rejection. T lymphocytes accumulate in the peritubular capillaries and extend into the interstitium.

The interstitial infiltrate, of activated T cells with variable numbers of monocytes/macrophages and occasional eosinophils and plasma cells, is associated with edema; furthermore, infiltration of tubule walls (tubulitis) by activated T cells is integral to and necessary for diagnosis of this form of rejection

167

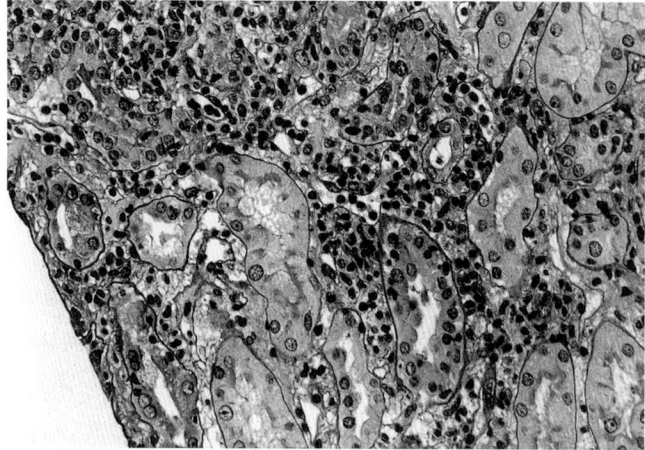

Fig. 19.1 Acute cell-mediated tubulo-interstitial rejection. The interstitium is edematous and infiltrated by numerous lymphocytes which are also in peritubular capillaries and in the walls of tubules (periodic acid–Schiff).

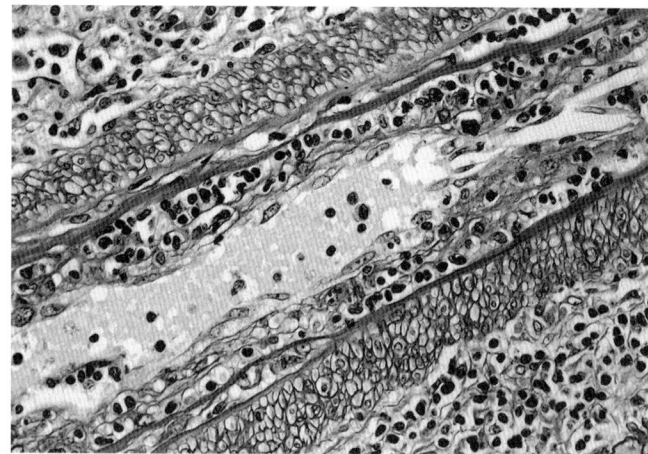

Fig. 19.2 Acute cell-mediated arterial rejection. Lymphocytes are beneath swollen endothelial cells (periodic acid–Schiff).

(Fig. 19.1). This results in epithelial cell damage and often in disruption to the tubular walls. Interstitial foci of Tamm–Horsfall protein are commonly identified; approximately 60% of acutely rejecting transplants may be so affected [7]. The clinicopathologic entity known as subclinical rejection, a process detected by protocol transplant biopsies, is characterized by cell-mediated acute tubulo-interstitial rejection.

Arterial rejection

As this is a type of cell-mediated rejection, it should be pointed out here that the term "arterial rejection" can signify either this cell-mediated process or an antibody-mediated one; thus, "arterial/vascular rejection" should not be used without further modification, as the common assumption is that arterial rejection indicates the antibody-mediated process, largely because of its historic use. This form of rejection is characterized by the accumulation of mononuclear leukocytes, including mostly lymphocytes, with accompanying lymphoblasts and monocytes in arterial walls. They undermine endothelial cells of arteries and arterioles (Fig. 19.2). This is termed endarteritis or endothelialitis. It does not affect all arteries; larger ones are more typically involved. Leukocytes adherent to the luminal aspect of endothelial cells do not have diagnostic significance, although that finding should spur a careful search for the diagnostic feature either in deeper sections of the same or another vessel [8]. There is little or no necrosis; leukocytes only infrequently extend into the muscularis, although lymphocytes may surround affected arteries. Arterial cell-mediated rejection has been reported in approximately 50% of kidneys with tubulo-interstitial rejection. It confers a more ominous prognosis, as this lesion is less responsive to corticosteroids [8].

Glomerular rejection

Lymphocyte and monocyte infiltration of glomeruli is not common in the course of acute tubulo-interstitial rejection; few leukocytes may accumulate in some glomerular capillaries associated with swelling of endothelium (transplant glomerulitis) with little clinical significance. However, more severe glomerular inflammation and cellular damage may infrequently occur (Fig. 19.3); this is termed acute transplant or allograft glomerulopathy and may be the dominant morphologic feature [9,10]. It may be found in the absence of tubulo-interstitial rejection, although arterial endarteritis may coexist. In the past, this lesion was thought to be induced by cytomegalovirus (CMV) infection; currently it is considered a severe form of cell-mediated rejection. It is present in a minority of biopsies performed for acute rejection.

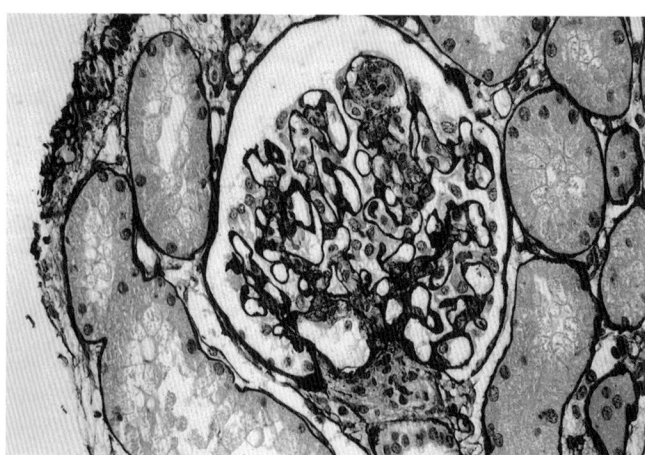

Fig. 19.3 Acute cell-mediated glomerular rejection. Numerous lymphocytes and fewer monocytes are in capillary lumina (periodic acid–methenamine silver).

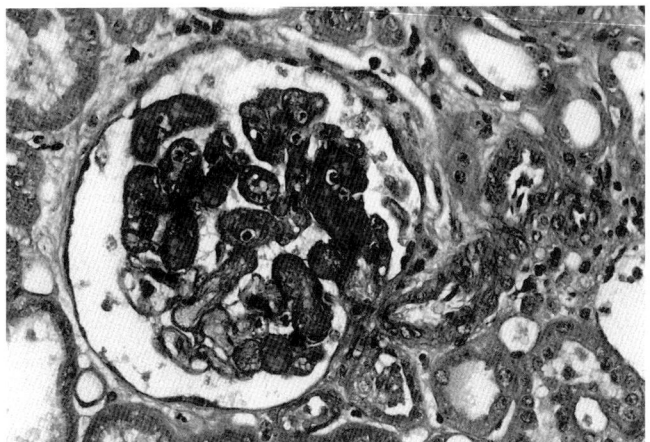

Fig. 19.4 Hyperacute rejection. The glomerular capillary lumina contain fresh thrombi, some of which incorporate neutrophils (Masson trichrome).

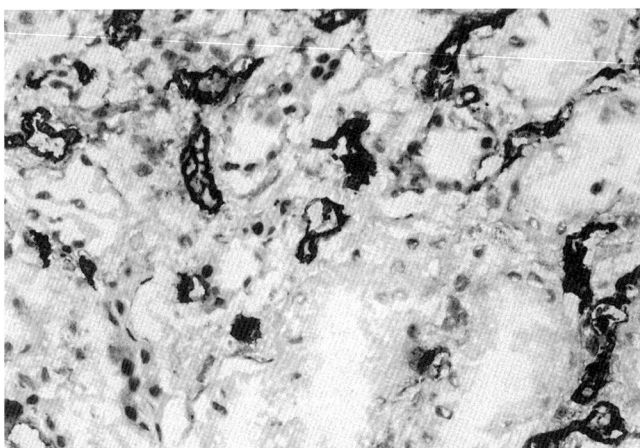

Fig. 19.5 Acute antibody-mediated rejection. Immunoperoxidase stain for C4d on frozen section. Peritubular capillary walls are positive.

Antibody-mediated rejection

This immunopathologic form of rejection is the result of donor-specific antibodies directed against endothelial antigens. This results in three distinctive forms of rejection: hyperacute rejection, acute humoral rejection and chronic rejection [1,11]. The pathologies are different and may require different microscopic methods to identify.

Hyperacute rejection

This lesion, the result of preformed circulating antibodies at the time of rejection binding to and damaging endothelial cells, causes prompt intravascular thrombosis and cortical necrosis [1,12]. There is accumulation of neutrophils in the thrombi; these cells may be first observed in peritubular and glomerular capillaries in biopsies performed upon establishment of circulation and followed by coagulation within a short period of time (Fig. 19.4).

Acute rejection

Acute rejection has been recently subclassified into two reasonably distinctive types affecting different vascular beds: arterial and peritubular capillary [4,13]. In both instances, antibodies are directed against endothelial cells. A third type (acute tubular injury) is also occasionally described. The diagnosis of antibody-mediated (humoral) rejection often requires the identification of C4d, a stable breakdown product of the complement component C4. Following C4 fixation consequent to antibody binding to antigen, C4 is cleaved into C4a and C4b by activated C1; C4b binds covalently to nearby molecules such as proteins and carbohydrates. Bound C4b is inactivated to C4d which remains covalently bound at the same site. Thus, C4d is a long-lasting marker of complement activation at an anatomic site and its presence can be used as a surrogate of immune complex formation at that site, as is the case with antibody-mediated rejection. C4d positivity has been associated with donor-specific anti-HLA antibodies in the vast majority of patients. It is the form of humoral rejection affecting peritubular capillaries and/or characterized by acute tubular cell injury which is identified by finding C4d in the walls of peritubular capillaries (Fig. 19.5). The identification of C4d in tissue sections requires immunohistochemistry; methods for both indirect immunofluorescence on frozen tissue sections and immunoperoxidase on frozen or on paraffin-embedded sections are available, although most laboratories prefer immunofluorescence [11,12,14].

In acute arterial antibody-mediated rejection, there is fibrin in and "fibrinoid" necrosis of the muscularis with variable leukocytic infiltration and not infrequently with luminal thrombosis (Fig. 19.6). Mononuclear leukocytes are sparse;

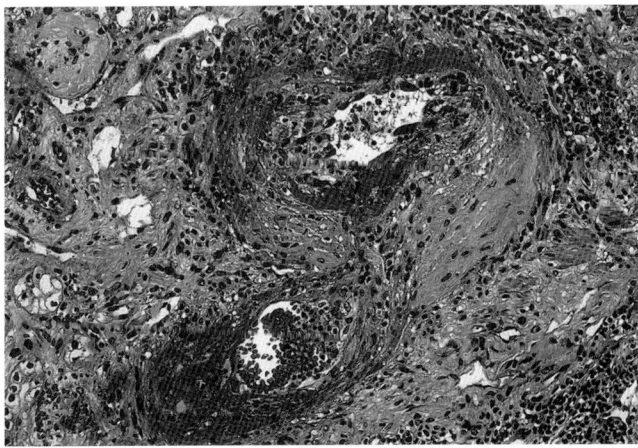

Fig. 19.6 Acute antibody-mediated rejection. There is fibrin with accompanying inflammation in the artery wall (periodic acid–Schiff).

neutrophils and eosinophils are slightly more common. Parenchymal infarction or hemorrhage usually ensues. Immunofluorescence discloses immunoglobulin G (IgG), IgM, C3 and fibrin in the walls of affected arteries. This classic arterial rejection is decidedly uncommon currently and is associated with poor graft prognosis.

The peritubular capillary form has inconstant light microscopic abnormalities, ranging from peritubular capillary and sometimes glomerular capillary inflammation to acute tubular cell injury and/or necrosis to no abnormalities. Acute cell-mediated rejection may coexist. Consequently, it is clear that relying only on light microscopic examination of the allograft biopsy can very well result in incomplete and incorrect diagnoses. It is strongly recommended that all transplant biopsies be examined routinely for the presence of C4d regardless of the morphologic features [13].

Studies by Colvin *et al*. have documented C4d-associated humoral rejection to coexist with acute cell-mediated rejection in approximately 35% of the biopsies and be not uncommonly documented in approximately 61% of biopsies with chronic rejection (see below) [15].

CHRONIC TRANSPLANT REJECTION

The changes in kidneys of patients with gradual loss of renal function over months to years, with onset as early as 3 months post-transplant, are often those that have been designated as chronic rejection. The morphologic abnormalities affect all tissue components to varying degrees, with prominent arterial lesions, sometimes characteristic glomerular lesions, and significant tubular atrophy with interstitial fibrosis [1,16].

Arteries display marked intimal thickening with fibrosis, accumulation of variable numbers of monocytes/macrophages, some with abundant cytoplasmic lipid (foam cells), sometimes circumferential arrangement of myointimal cells beneath endothelium replicating a neo-media, and with calcification, all resulting in luminal narrowing, sometimes to a considerable degree (Fig. 19.7). The internal elastic lamina is often segmentally disrupted and/or duplicated. Arteries of all sizes may be involved, although larger arteries are preferentially affected so that it may not be possible to diagnose this important lesion on a kidney biopsy. Arterioles are relatively spared, exhibiting muscular hypertrophy and insudative lesions; however, these changes are generally mild in comparison to other chronic disorders affecting renal transplants.

The glomerular changes are quite heterogeneous but are characterized primarily by variable increase in mesangial matrix and cellularity and double-contoured capillary walls [10]. There may be lobular accentuation of the architecture. Mesangiolysis and microaneurysm formation, while morphologically impressive, are infrequent components of the glomerular damage. Segmental sclerosis is a common complicating lesion (Fig. 19.8). Immunofluorescence is inconstant,

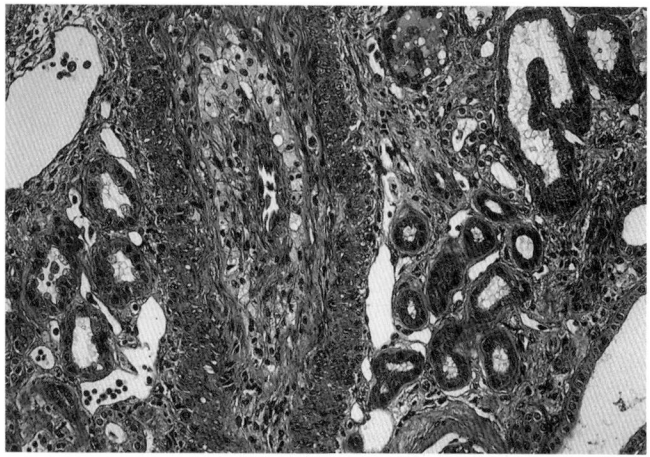

Fig. 19.7 Chronic rejection. The artery wall is thick, primarily resulting from infiltration of foam cells and lymphocytes in the intima. The lumen is considerably narrowed (Masson trichrome).

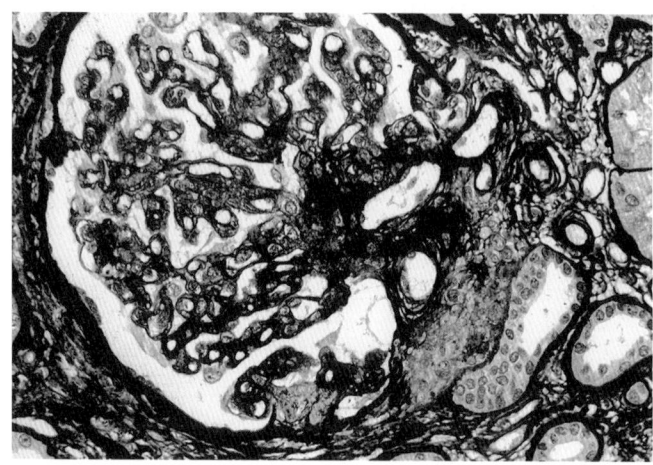

Fig. 19.8 Chronic transplant glomerulopathy. There is slight accentuation of lobular architecture with widening of mesangial regions. Many capillary walls are double-contoured (periodic acid–methenamine silver).

with segmental granular deposits of IgM, lesser IgG and C3 in mesangial regions and/or capillary walls, usually in intermediate degrees of intensity. Ultrastructural examination discloses the double-contoured capillary walls to be the result of new basement membrane formation beneath endothelial cells, and less commonly a consequence of peripheral migration and interposition of mesangium. Electron-dense deposits are not common. The foot processes of podocytes are largely effaced. These changes together constitute the entity known as chronic transplant glomerulopathy which is morphologically specific for chronic rejection but, because this lesion is present in no more than approximately 30% of kidneys with chronic rejection, it does have limited diagnostic significance. The differential diagnosis of chronic transplant glomerulopathy needs to be considered. The major entities from which it must be distinguished, especially at the light microscopic

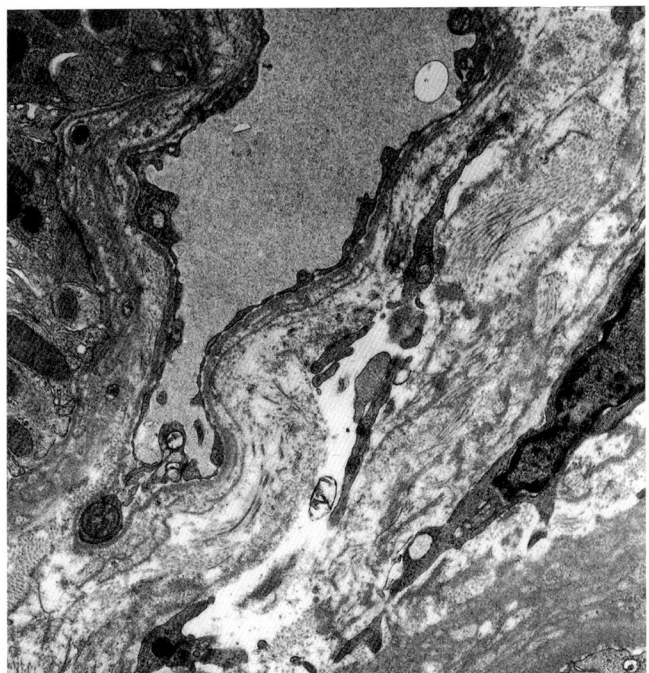

Fig. 19.9 Electron micrograph of peritubular capillary with multilayered basement membrane.

level, include membranoproliferative glomerulonephritis, type I (*de novo* or recurrent primary or secondary forms), chronic thrombotic microangiopathies, and focal and segmental glomerulosclerosis. It should be clear, however, that use of electron microscopy and immunofluorescence easily allow for distinction in most instances [5].

The tubulo-interstitial changes have no specificity and are those accompanying any chronic damage to kidneys. However, in contrast to other lesions, the chronically rejected kidney may have considerable tubular drop-out in addition to marked atrophy. Calcifications in the fibrotic interstitium are common; ossification may rarely occur.

The peritubular capillaries are abnormal [11,17]. C4d deposition has been detected in more than 50% of kidneys with chronic rejection. This suggests that this form of antibody-mediated rejection contributes to chronic rejection. Ultrastructural abnormalities of these vessels include multiple layers of basement membranes, suggesting repetitive damage and repair of endothelial cells with production of new basement membrane material during the healing phases (Fig. 19.9). Some investigators have correlated the multilayered basement membranes with C4d positivity and chronic transplant glomerulopathy.

CALCINEURIN INHIBITOR TOXICITY

The structural abnormalities typically encountered in transplant biopsies are virtually identical for cyclosporine and tacrolimus; thus, the changes described are for both agents [18,19].

Acute toxicity

Acute decline in renal function may be associated with structural lesions of tubules or arterioles or may have no anatomic findings. The tubular abnormalities are most often of cellular injury characteristically within the spectrum of acute tubular necrosis, with irregular flattening of cells and, for proximal tubular cells, reduction in or loss of brush border staining. In addition or as the sole abnormality, the cytoplasm of cells in relatively few tubular profiles contain uniform small vacuoles (isometric vacuoles). These are clear by electron microscopy, similar to those induced by osmotic agents but are usually less widely distributed and of smaller size. Although these vacuolar changes were at one time considered virtually pathognomonic of calcineurin inhibitor toxicity, they are relatively infrequently encountered at present, probably because of lower doses of these drugs.

Arteriolar abnormalities include initial necrosis of smooth muscle cells including cells of the juxtaglomerular apparatus with resultant decreased production of renin; insudative lesions (hyalinosis) replace the vacuoles created by individual cell necrosis. These hyaline "deposits" are typically nodular and are in the media or in subadventitial sites with a beaded appearance (Fig. 19.10). Some reports have documented these changes to be reversible with modification of therapy, although this is not a widely shared view [20].

Thrombotic microangiopathy, a more common lesion in the early days of cyclosporine use, has declined in prevalence although it has not disappeared. It is uncertain whether this represents a manifestation of toxicity or is an idiosyncratic reaction. It is of interest that switching from one calcineurin inhibitor to the other because of a thrombotic microangiopathy

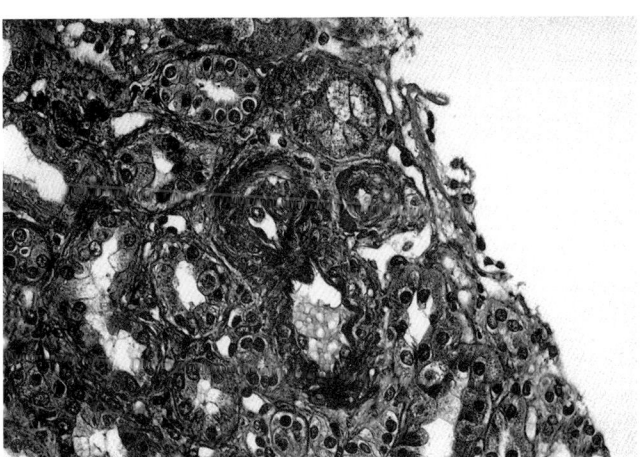

Fig. 19.10 Cyclosporine arteriolopathy. The wall of the small arteriole has several subadventitial nodular areas of hyalinosis (Masson trichrome).

171

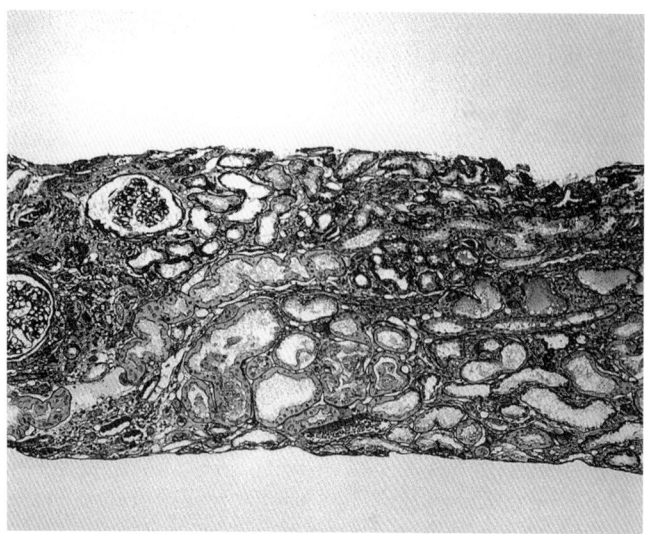

Fig. 19.11 Chronic calcineurin inhibitor toxicity. Tubular atrophy with interstitial fibrosis is arranged in elongated zones ("stripes") (periodic acid–Schiff).

is not associated with recurrence, although both have been implicated in the development of this lesion. The changes in the kidney are those of thrombotic microangiopathies occurring in the nontransplant setting. However, the only abnormality may be few fresh thrombi in few capillaries in few glomeruli. In the absence of acute rejection, especially antibody mediated, this should alert the pathologist to a calcineurin inhibitor-induced lesion.

Chronic toxicity is characterized by patchy tubular atrophy with interstitial fibrosis (termed "striped fibrosis") (Fig. 19.11). It is important to distinguish these changes from those of chronic rejection, hypertension or nephrosclerosis, chronic

interstitial nephritis, chronic glomerulopathies (recurrent or *de novo*) and all other forms of chronic damage. In its most "pure" state, chronic calcineurin inhibitor toxicity does not include arterial intimal fibrosis, thereby differentiating it from chronic rejection and nephrosclerosis. Furthermore, there are no glomerular changes intrinsic to calcineurin inhibitor toxicity; the presence of chronic transplant glomerulopathy precludes chronic toxicity, although focal and segmental glomerulosclerosis may arise as a complication to long-standing toxicity [18,19]. The presence of interstitial lymphocytes is not particularly helpful as a point of differentiation. It should be noted that calcineurin inhibitor toxicity may coexist with rejection and other chronic changes but that morphologic confirmation of toxicity would be obscured by the other lesions.

Chronic allograft nephropathy is a term that was coined to indicate that there were times at which the pathologic processes responsible for chronic structural damage in the transplant could not be specifically identified or distinguished from one another. For example, at times it is not possible to distinguish chronic rejection from chronic calcineurin inhibitor toxicity from nephrosclerosis. However, each of these entities may clearly have specific pathologic lesions and, when present, the term chronic allograft nephropathy is not appropriate. Unfortunately, currently this term is used indiscriminately to indicate chronic damage of any type in the transplant, thus mixing many pathologic processes together and possibly obscuring treatment and prognostic data. Several methods for distinguishing chronic rejection from calcineurin inhibitor toxicity have been advocated. These include analysis of interstitial collagen type [21] and assessment of tissue mRNA for laminin β2 and transforming growth factor β (TGF-β), both of which are more elevated in cyclosporine toxicity [22].

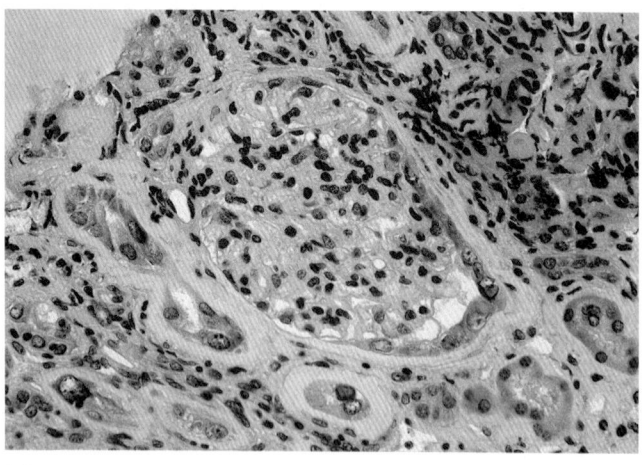

(a)

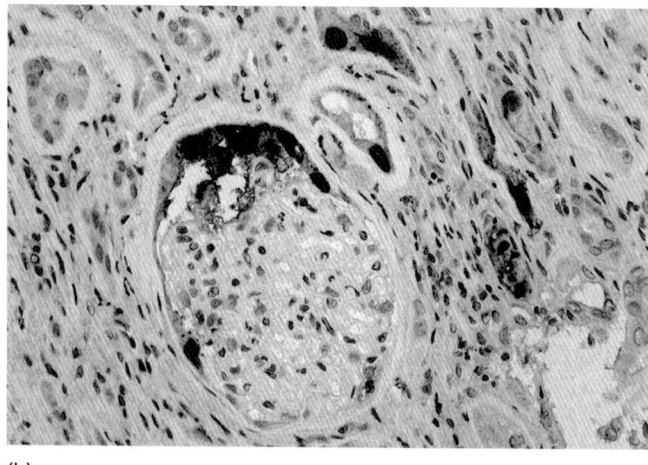

(b)

Fig. 19.12 Polyoma virus infection. (a) Nuclei of some tubular cells and parietal epithelial cells are enlarged, hyperchromatic or vesicular. One contains an inclusion (hematoxylin and eosin). (b) Immunostain (anti-SV40) indicating nuclear positivity.

INFECTIONS

While many microorganisms have been described in transplanted kidneys resulting from immunosuppression, currently the most common and clinically and pathologically important is polyoma virus, in particular the BK strain. Its incidence has greatly increased since the more frequent use of tacrolimus and mycophenolate; with these agents, it is estimated that 3–5% of patients develop this infection in the graft. BK is related to JC virus and the animal strain SV40 [23,24]. The human viruses reside in tubular epithelium and becomes reactivated in the immunosuppressed state. The major changes affect tubular epithelium, particularly of collecting ducts of outer cortex and medulla; nuclei are enlarged, typically hyperchromatic, although some may have a prominent vesicular appearance and some have intranuclear inclusions (Fig. 19.12a). The cells display degenerative features. An acute interstitial nephritis, with plasma cells and fewer lymphocytes and monocytes, often accompanies the infection. Tubulitis may also be present, simulating acute cellular rejection. The identification of the virus requires immunostaining with monoclonal antibodies (Fig. 19.12b). These are commercially available to all three strains and can easily be used on paraffin-embedded material. Some laboratories use anti-BK and others prefer anti-SV40. By electron microscopy, the viruses are 40–45 nm in diameter and are usually aggregated in a paracrystalline array. Urothelium may also be infected and be responsible for ureteral stenosis. Reduction of immunosuppression often results in disappearance of the virus, although it may also cause acute rejection.

REFERENCES

1 Colvin RB. Renal transplant pathology. In: Jennette JC, Olson JL, Schwartz MM, Silva FG, eds. *Heptinstall's Pathology of the Kidney*, 5th edn. Philadelphia: Lippincott-Raven, 1998: 1409–540.

2 Sorof JM, Vartanian RK, Olson JL, *et al.* Histopathological concordance of paired renal allograft biopsy cores: effect on the diagnosis and management of acute rejection. *Transplantation* 1995;**60**:1215–9.

3 Nickeleit V, Zeiler M, Gudat F, Thiel G, Mihatsch MJ. Detection of the complement degradation product C4d in renal allografts: diagnostic and therapeutic implications. *J Am Soc Nephrol* 2002;**13**:242–51.

4 Mauiyyedi S, Crespo M, Collins AB, *et al.* Acute humoral rejection in kidney transplantation. II. Morphology, immunopathology, and pathologic classification. *J Am Soc Nephrol* 2002;**13**:779–87.

5 Cohen AH, Nast CC. Kidney: non-neoplastic conditions. In: Damjanov I, Linder J, eds. *Anderson's Pathology*, 10th edn. St. Louis: Mosby, 1996: 2073–137.

6 Colvin RB, Cohen AH, Saiontz C, *et al.* Evaluation of pathologic criteria for acute renal allograft rejection: reproducibility, sensitivity, and clinical correlation. *J Am Soc Nephrol* 1997;**8**:1930–41.

7 Cohen AH, Border WA, Rajfer J, Dumke A, Glassock RJ. Interstitial Tamm–Horsfall protein in rejecting renal allografts: identification and morphologic pattern of injury. *Lab Invest* 1984;**50**:519–25.

8 Nickeleit V, Vamvakas EC, Pascual M, Poletti BJ, Colvin RB. The prognostic significance of specific arterial lesions in acute renal allograft rejection. *J Am Soc Nephrol* 1998;**9**:1301–8.

9 Hiki Y, Leong AS, Mathew TH, *et al.* Typing of intraglomerular mononuclear cells associated with transplant glomerular rejection. *Clin Nephrol* 1986;**26**:244–9.

10 Maryniak RK, First MR, Weiss MA. Transplant glomerulopathy: evolution of morphologically distinct changes. *Kidney Int* 1985;**27**:799–806.

11 Mauiyyedi S, Colvin RB. Humoral rejection in kidney transplantation: new concepts in diagnosis and treatment. *Curr Opin Nephrol Hypertens* 2002;**11**:609–18.

12 Collins AB, Schneeberger EE, Pascual MA, *et al.* Complement activation in acute humoral renal allograft rejection: diagnostic significance of C4d deposits in peritubular capillaries. *J Am Soc Nephrol* 1999;**10**:2208–14.

13 Racusen LC, Colvin RB, Solez K, *et al.* Antibody-mediated rejection criteria: an addition to the Banff 97 classification of renal allograft rejection. *Am J Transplant* 2003;**3**:708–14.

14 Regele H, Bohmig GA, Habicht A, *et al.* Capillary deposition of complement split product C4d in renal allografts is associated with basement membrane injury in peritubular and glomerular capillaries: a contribution of humoral immunity to chronic allograft rejection. *J Am Soc Nephrol* 2002;**13**:2371–80.

15 Mauiyyedi S, Pelle PD, Saidman S, *et al.* Chronic humoral rejection: identification of antibody-mediated chronic renal allograft rejection by C4d deposits in peritubular capillaries. *J Am Soc Nephrol* 2001;**12**:574–82.

16 Sibley RK. Morphologic features of chronic rejection in kidney and less commonly transplanted organs. *Clin Transplant* 1994; **8**:293–8.

17 Gough J, Yilmaz A, Mishkulin D, *et al.* Peritubular capillary basement membrane reduplication in allografts and native kidney disease: a clinicopathologic study of 278 consecutive renal specimens. *Transplantation* 2001;**71**:1390–3.

18 Mihatsch MJ, Thiel G, Basler V, *et al.* Morphological patterns in cyclosporine-treated renal transplant recipients. *Transplant Proc* 1985;**17**:101–6.

19 Mihatsch MJ, Thiel G, Ryffel B. Morphological diagnosis of cyclosporine nephrotoxicity. *Semin Diagn Pathol* 1998;**5**:104–21.

20 Hamahira K, Iijima K, Tanaka R, Nakamura H, Yoshikawa N. Recovery from cyclosporine-associated arteriolopathy in childhood nephrotic syndrome. *Pediatr Nephrol* 2001;**16**:723–7.

21 Abrass CK, Berfield AK, Stehman-Breen C, Alpers CE, Davis CL. Unique changes in interstitial extracellular matrix composition are associated with rejection and cyclosporine toxicity in human renal allograft biopsies. *Am J Kidney Dis* 1999;**33**:11–20.

22 Koop K, Bakker RC, Eikmans M, *et al.* Differentiation between chronic rejection and chronic cyclosporine toxicity by analysis of renal cortical mRNA. *Kidney Int* 2004;**66**:2038–46.

23 Nickeleit V. Nephropathy due to polyomavirus type BK. *N Engl J Med* 2000;**342**:1361–3.

24 Drachenberg CB, Beskow CO, Cangro CB, *et al.* Human polyoma virus in renal allograft biopsies: morphological findings and correlation with urine cytology. *Hum Pathol* 1999;**30**:970–7.

20 Post-Transplant Management

Jodi M. Smith and Ruth A. McDonald

Pediatric kidney transplantation differs in some aspects of perioperative and post-transplant care from adult transplantation because of differences in primary renal disease, patient size, immunologic responsiveness, medication pharmacokinetics, as well as growth and development issues. Improvements in transplantation technology and immunosuppression over the last decade have resulted in improved renal allograft survival rates in the pediatric patient. Complications including infection, rejection, post-transplant lymphoproliferative disease (PTLD) and growth failure continue to be especially problematic in the pediatric patient. Close monitoring, prevention, early detection and prompt management of complications help to minimize the risks of post-operative morbidity and mortality.

INPATIENT MANAGEMENT

Small children may require massive volume expansion in order to maintain adequate perfusion of the adult sized kidney. It may be prudent to keep the small child intubated in the early postoperative phase if there is evidence of pulmonary edema. Routinely, the patient is placed on continuous electrocardiographic monitoring, cutaneous pulse oximeter and central venous pressure monitoring. Ongoing assessment of the patient's respiratory status by examination, oximetry and chest X-ray (CXR) is important because of the fluid challenge. This is especially important if the child is receiving medications that trigger cytokine release (e.g. OKT3, anti-thymocyte globulin). A set of baseline laboratory tests is obtained, including creatinine (Cr), blood urea nitrogen (BUN), calcium, phosphorus, magnesium, electrolytes, urine analysis and complete blood count, as well as arterial blood gases and coagulation tests, if clinically indicated. Laboratory studies should be reassessed daily with more frequent follow-up of critical values or a concerning trend. Vital signs are monitored frequently, daily weights are obtained and meticulous attention is given to recording all of the patient's inputs and outputs. The use of perioperative intravenous antibiotics is program specific, but many centers use a first generation cephalosporin for the first 24–48 hours in the nonallergic patient. Gastritis prophylaxis is important for patients on high-dose steroids and may also be beneficial for patients on mycophenolate mofetil (MMF). Combination therapy using antacids and a histamine-2 antagonist is often the most efficacious. In the patient who has delayed graft function, avoid magnesium-containing antacids to prevent the development of hypermagnesemia.

Radiology

In the immediate postoperative period, it is important to get a baseline study of renal perfusion and excretion. Renal transplant recipients are often taken from the recovery room directly to nuclear medicine for a ^{99m}Tc-MAG3 radionuclide renal scan, especially if the patient is oligoanuric. The results help the clinician to evaluate for renal artery thrombosis, obstruction and urinary leak. A renal ultrasound with Doppler should also be obtained, particularly in the anuric patient, to assess for renal vascular thrombosis. After these initial studies, the patient should be reimaged as necessary (e.g. decrease in urine output) to evaluate renal blood flow, rule out obstruction and assess for suspected urinary leak or lymphocele.

Fluid and electrolyte management

Meticulous fluid and electrolyte management is critical for pediatric patients because they often require additional intravascular volume repletion in the perioperative period to establish diuresis and avoid delayed graft function. This is especially critical in the situation where a small child needs to perfuse an adult donor kidney. Frequent vital signs, physical examinations, daily weights and close attention to monitoring input and output are essential to determine the safety of volume administration, particularly in the patient with cardiac disease or smaller patients who risk pulmonary edema with fluid challenge. Central venous pressure monitoring may be used to help assess intravascular volume status but needs to be evaluated in the context of the child's size.

Supplemental loop diuretics or osmotic agents (mannitol) may be needed to facilitate diuresis in the oliguric patient. Some centers use "renal dose dopamine" to enhance renal vasculature dilatation but this is controversial [1–3]. Medications associated with cytokine release such as polyclonal and monoclonal T-cell antibodies need to be administered carefully in the volume-expanded patient. In addition, excessive volume administration may complicate blood pressure management. Output is replaced with intravenous (IV) fluid, usually 1/2 normal saline with dextrose and water. In some cases, the postoperative diuresis is so large that hyperglycemia can result when 5% dextrose is used for urine replacement. Therefore, at our center, we administer 5% dextrose in water at 500 mL/m^2/24 hours to cover insensible losses and use 2.5% dextrose 1/2 normal saline for urine replacement, only adding potassium when the serum potassium falls below 4 mEq/L. Urine output is usually replaced cc/cc throughout the first 24 hours with a gradual tapering off of IV urine replacement as the patient's oral intake increases. Most patients start oral intake on their first postoperative day.

High volume diuresis may deplete electrolytes, depending on the type of fluid replacement administered. Postoperative evaluation of electrolytes should include close monitoring of serum sodium, potassium, chloride, bicarbonate, calcium, phosphorus and magnesium. Supplementation should be tailored to electrolyte levels.

At the time of transplantation, most patients have normal or elevated serum phosphorus levels. With delayed graft function, phosphate binders may be necessary to control hyperphosphatemia. With improved urine output, phosphaturia occurs as a result of hyperparathyroidism and/or the effect of calcineurin inhibitors. The goal phosphate level depends on the patient's age, with higher levels acceptable in the young growing child. Oral phosphate supplements include preparations that contain potassium phosphate or a combination of sodium and potassium phosphate in either tablet or powder form. The choice of supplement depends on the patient's serum potassium and palatability.

Many patients have an elevated serum magnesium pre-transplant. Once good allograft function is established, hypomagnesemia may occur because of calcineurin inhibitor-induced renal magnesium wasting [4,5]. A complication often seen with oral magnesium-containing preparations is diarrhea. Supplementation with magnesium protein complex (133 mg elemental magnesium/tablet) may result in less stool output.

Patients with chronic renal failure often have metabolic acidosis and this may be exacerbated because of increased acid production associated with surgery. Supplemental sodium bicarbonate may be needed in the postoperative period, especially in those with delayed graft function. Patients who are undergoing a substantial diuresis and receiving high volume IV fluid may also need addition of bicarbonate-containing solution to avoid metabolic acidosis.

Glucose management can be problematic, especially in the pediatric patient with type 1 diabetes mellitus or those receiving tacrolimus. In some cases, an insulin drip may be required to maintain glycemic control. Once on a stable diet, patients can be switched to subcutaneous administration of long-acting insulin with a sliding scale of a short-acting preparation. Corticosteroids complicate glycemic control and increased doses of insulin may be needed, especially when the patient is on higher doses of steroids in the first few months after transplant.

Wound and catheter care

Wound care is per standard surgical routine with close attention to the amount and quality of wound drainage. Attention should also be paid to central line and dialysis access care. Occasionally, patients on peritoneal dialysis may have impressive peritoneal fluid accumulation, presumably as a result of peritoneal irritation from long-standing exposure to dextrose-containing dialysate. Intermittent drainage of the abdomen via the peritoneal catheter may be warranted.

Urologic care

Serious urologic anomalies are present in approximately 20% of children who undergo renal transplantation. The most common etiologies include posterior urethral valves, vesicoureteral reflux (VUR) and prune belly syndrome. Some of these children have undergone urinary diversion or bladder augmentation as a consequence of these malformations. Salvatierra et al. [6] have reported success with ureteral implantation in the small capacity, defunctionalized, non-neurogenic bladder. All children should have urologic evaluation, including a voiding cystourethrogram (VCUG), prior to transplantation. Those with abnormalities should be evaluated by a pediatric urologist and considered for cystometrics prior to transplantation [7,8]. In children with significant bladder abnormalities, a urologist should be included as part of the transplant team. In general, a catheter (Foley) is usually kept in the bladder for the first 5 postoperative days to avoid stressing the ureterocystostomy.

Blood pressure management

It is important to avoid severe hypertension and hypotension in the immediate postoperative period. Hypertension secondary to high fluid intake, corticosteroids and calcineurin inhibitors is problematic because of the risk of seizure, as well as the stress placed on the renal arterial anastomosis. Hypotension and underperfusion of the adult-sized kidney in the pediatric patient is equally problematic. The agents of choice for treatment of hypertension in the immediate postoperative period are calcium-channel blockers, especially because they may offer protection against calcineurin inhibitor induced graft dysfunction [9]. Both nifedipine and amlodipine have been used in the pediatric transplant patient [10]. In general, angiotensin-converting enzyme (ACE) inhibitors and angiotensin II receptor antagonists are avoided in the first few weeks after transplant as they may induce renal insufficiency in the setting of diminished effective arterial blood volume. Hydralazine as well as β- and α-adrenergic receptor blockers can usually be used safely in moderation. Diuretics may be helpful if hypervolemia is contributing to hypertension. The treatment of choice for hypotension post-transplant is volume expansion with crystalloid and/or colloid. If possible, avoid vasopressors because of the risk of renal vasoconstriction.

Infection surveillance and prevention

In the child, both elevation and depression of core body temperature can indicate infection. Close daily attention to the patient's vital signs and physical examination is critical, including evaluation of wounds, indwelling catheters and drains. Lines, drains and urinary catheters should be discontinued as soon as medically indicated to avoid risk of infection. Urine should be cultured and the sediment examined routinely as part of post-transplant management. Evaluation for suspected infection in the pediatric patient should include physical examination; culture of urine, blood, as well as drains, spinal and peritoneal fluid if indicated; CXR; evaluation of the blood for active cytomegalovirus (CMV) infection by antigenemia assay, rapid viral isolation or polymerase chain reaction (PCR) [11] and for Epstein–Barr virus (EBV) activity by PCR [12]. Results of the above and the patient's clinical condition should guide therapy and further testing.

Some centers provide prophylaxis against urinary tract infection as well as against *Pneumocystis carinii* (PCP) by instituting daily co-trimoxazole. Other centers use co-trimoxazole PCP prophylaxis three times weekly during the first 3 months post-transplant. Alternatively, dapsone or pentamidine inhalation can be used if the patient is allergic to co-trimoxazole. Oral antifungal treatment is often given for the first 3–6 months post-transplant, usually in the form of nystatin or clotrimazole troches. Viral prophylaxis is almost routinely used by all centers and must be adjusted for estimated glomerular filtration rate (GFR) in the post-transplant period. The Schwartz formula (C_{SCH}) for estimated GFR:

$$C_{SCH} \text{ (mL/min per 1.73 m}^2) = \text{height (centimeters)} \times k \div \text{serum Cr (mg/dL)},$$

where k = 0.55 in children and pubertal girls, 0.7 in pubertal boys [13]. Strategies to prevent CMV disease include high-dose oral aciclovir (ACV), intravenous immunoglobulin (IVIG) (standard or high-titer anti-CMV) and IV or oral ganciclovir (GCV) or valganciclovir. Patients with a history of oral or genital herpes simplex should receive ACV prophylaxis if they are not receiving GCV. Many programs have EBV prophylaxis

strategies in the high-risk pediatric patient. Some centers use either ACV or GCV in addition to IVIG in the EBV seronegative patient receiving a kidney from an EBV seropositive donor. EBV detection can be monitored and quantified by PCR and some transplant programs adjust the level of the patient's immunosuppression based on the degree of EBV activity [14,15].

IMMUNOSUPPRESSION

There are a variety of factors that influence the choice and use of immunosuppressive therapies. With the dramatic improvements in short-term graft survival in the past decade, the transplant community has started to focus on improving long-term graft survival. The goal remains to find the best combination that will optimize graft survival while limiting the side-effects. As such, many centers now consider patient-specific factors in choosing which medication regimen the transplant recipient will receive. A discussion of the medications used for induction and maintenance of immunosuppression is found in Chapter 9.

COMPLICATIONS

Acute transplant dysfunction

Immediate oliguria or anuria can have several etiologies including hypovolemia, acute tubular necrosis (ATN) resulting from ischemia, thrombosis of the renal artery or vein, urinary extravasation, urinary obstruction, hyperacute rejection and external compression resulting from hematoma, seroma or lymphocele. Initial evaluation should confirm patency and correct position of the Foley catheter, vital signs and examination to assess volume status, as well as the patient's hematocrit. In the immediate postoperative period, it is essential to evaluate perfusion and function by radionuclide renal scan and renal ultrasound with Doppler studies of the renal vessels. After the initial studies, re-evaluate as necessary to assess renal blood flow, resistive indices, rule out obstruction and fluid collection. Doppler interrogation can demonstrate alterations in local renal hemodynamics such as reduction, absence or reversal of diastolic flow, in addition to arterial or venous thrombosis. Reductions in diastolic flow results from increased renal resistance to blood flow. This can be caused by parenchymal edema, external compression of vascular structures, venous kinking or thrombosis. If recovery of graft function is delayed or if graft function deteriorates, a biopsy may be necessary to determine the etiology. A North American Pediatric Renal Transplant Cooperative Study (NAPRTCS) analysis confirms that percutaneous renal transplant biopsies can be safely performed in the pediatric population [16].

The most common cause of delayed graft function (DGF) is ischemic renal injury or ATN. The 2004 NAPRTCS annual report shows that DGF, defined as the need for dialysis in first week after transplant, is observed in 5.2% of living donor (LD) and 17.4% deceased donor (DD) transplants [16]. LD recipients with significantly higher rates of DGF include those with a history of more than five blood transfusions, prior transplant and African-American race. Risk factors for DGF in DD recipients include African-American race, cold ischemia time longer than 24 hours, absence of T-cell induction antibody therapy, more than five random blood transfusions, repeat transplant, absence of HLA-DR matching, and donor age less than 2 years [17]. Renal dysfunction caused by ATN usually recovers but may take days to weeks or months. Management of patients with ATN includes dialysis as well as other renal failure support.

Hyperacute rejection (immediate) and accelerated acute rejection (within the first week of transplant) must always be considered in the differential diagnosis of early renal dysfunction. Hyperacute rejection is caused by a response with antidonor antibodies against HLA, ABO or other antigens [18], resulting in rapid destruction of the graft. The only treatment for hyperacute rejection is removal of the kidney. Patients with a history of or at risk for hyperacute rejection may benefit from plasmapheresis pre- and post-transplant [19].

If there are signs of thrombosis, a thorough workup for hypercoagulability is indicated (see the section on Vascular and hematological complications below) and hyperacute rejection should be ruled out. If such abnormalities are found to be the cause of graft loss, precautions need to be considered with future transplantation such as peritransplant high-dose IVIG, plasmapheresis, antilymphocyte antibody therapy and anticoagulation, depending on the etiology of thrombosis. If peritransplant IVIG is used, careful selection of the preparation with less sucrose and monitored administration are necessary to avoid the complication of acute renal failure [20].

The most common cause of renal dysfunction after the initial week remains acute and chronic allograft nephropathy. Other causes include obstruction resulting from ureteral stenosis, lymphocele, infection (bacterial, fungal and viral), drug toxicity, vascular stenosis, PTLD and dehydration. Imaging studies, laboratory data, cultures and renal biopsy may be needed to confirm diagnosis.

Cyclosporine (CSA) and tacrolimus are nephrotoxins and can cause allograft dysfunction. Both CSA and tacrolimus are substrates for a member of the P450 cytochrome system, CYP3A4. This results in potential interactions between CSA and tacrolimus metabolism and other medications and substances that use or affect that metabolic pathway. Some medications increase drug levels, such as macrolide antibiotics, whereas others decrease levels, including antiseizure medications and rifampin. In addition, some foods such as grapefruit juice can change absorption of calcineurin inhibitors. CSA and tacrolimus nephrotoxicity can occur concomitantly with acute cellular rejection and ATN. If the biopsy lacks histologic evidence of rejection or ATN, then a trial reduction of CSA or tacrolimus may be indicated.

Obstruction and urine leak

If a renal ultrasound demonstrates peritransplant fluid collection, aspiration may be indicated to rule out bleeding, urinoma, seroma or lymph. In the case of increasing abdominal girth resulting from peritoneal fluid accumulation, aspiration or drainage of fluid through an existing peritoneal catheter should be performed and the fluid should be analyzed for BUN and Cr, as a urine leak may extravasate into the peritoneal space. Obstruction may be caused by kinking of the ureter, blockage at the implantation site of the ureter, or the development of a lymphocele, urinoma or blood clot. Rarely, disintegration of the distal ureter or rupture of the bladder can cause the urine leak. If obstruction or urinary leak is suspected, a radionuclide scan with furosemide washout may be helpful with examination for tracer accumulation in the peritoneal cavity, scrotal, vulval or inguinal area. If urinary extravasation is diagnosed, urgent exploration and correction of the underlying problem with possible repeat ueterocystostomy or pyelo-ureterouererostostomy using the host ureter is indicated [21–23]. In some circumstances, nephrostomy placement or ureteral stenting may be needed to ensure adequate drainage of the kidney.

Lymphoceles can be problematic and occasionally cause obstruction of urine or vascular perfusion. If the lymphocele is not obstructive, it should be closely followed but no intervention is indicated. When conservative treatment fails, drainage may be warranted. Nonsurgical treatment with repeated percutaneous drainage, with or without instillation of sclerosing agents such as povidone-iodine [24] or alcohol [25] can be attempted. High recurrence rates and long-term catheterization with increased risk of infection are potential drawbacks [25]. In some cases, surgical drainage may be needed by open or laparoscopic fenestration of the lymphocele [26].

Late ureteral complications can present as obstruction or extravasation of urine and can be the result of fibrosis following ischemia resulting from compromised ureteral blood flow or acute rejection. Acute management includes placement of a percutaneous nephrostomy or ureteral stent. Operative management includes ureterocystostomy and uretero- or pyeloureterocystostomy using the native ureter [21–23]. Techniques for evaluation include a radionuclide renal scan and renal ultrasound, but further studies such as arteriography and cystoscopy with retrograde studies may be needed to confirm the diagnosis.

Vascular and hematologic complications

Postoperative bleeding may require exploration to control hemorrhage and evacuation of any hematoma that is causing renal compression. Prompt diagnosis with expeditious restoration of renal hemodynamics can result in a good outcome. Delayed diagnosis and intervention can increase the incidence of infection, graft failure and patient death.

Vascular thrombosis is the third leading cause of graft failure in pediatric renal transplant recipients, with an incidence varying from 0.7% to 5.0% [27]. Thrombosis can be seen as late as 2 weeks post-transplant following initial engraftment and function. Risk factors include recipient under 2 years of age, deceased donor age less than 5 years, cold ischemia time longer than 24 hours, ATN and history of a previous renal transplant. The use of antibody induction therapy, deceased donors older than 5 years of age and increasing recipient age were factors that decreased the risk for thrombosis [27]. In addition, underlying thrombophilic disorders have been identified as increasing the risk of allograft loss resulting from thrombosis. Protein C and S deficiencies [28], factor V Leiden mutation [29], prothrombin gene abnormalities [30] and antiphospholipid antibodies [31] have been recognized as risk factors for arterial or venous thrombosis of renal allografts. More recently, the presence of antiendothelial antibodies detected by immunoflorescence has been associated with graft thrombosis [32]. In addition, NAPRTCS recently reported a significantly higher rate of graft thrombosis in pediatric patients on peritoneal dialysis [33]. Thrombosis should be suspected in the case where immediate function is followed by oliguria. Doppler studies of the renal vessels and radionuclide renal scanning using ^{99m}Tc-diethylenetriamine pentaacetic acid (DTPA) or ^{99m}Tc-MAG3 can establish the diagnosis. If thrombosis is suspected, surgical exploration, thrombectomy and anticoagulation with heparin, streptokinase [34] or urokinase [35,36] may salvage the kidney. Transplant nephrectomy is indicated if thrombosis is irreversible. Certain patients with a thrombotic history may require antithrombotic therapy, which should be started as soon as it is felt to be clinically safe in the immediate postoperative period. Heparin, low-molecular weight heparin, warfarin and aspirin should be considered, depending on the clinical case.

Renal arteriostenosis should be suspected in the patient with severe or escalating hypertension with or without graft dysfunction. Initial evaluation can include Doppler studies of the renal artery but the gold standard is arteriography. Stenosis is managed using either balloon angioplasty, stenting or operative repair. The specific approach varies with the clinical situation and requires collaboration between members of the transplant and interventional radiology teams.

Neurologic and psychiatric complications

In the immediate postoperative period, psychiatric disturbances can arise and may represent a reaction to steroids or hospitalization. The most common psychiatric manifestations seen in pediatric patients are behavioral disorders such as angry outbursts, mood swings and uncooperative behavior.

Depression and anxiety may also occur. Family support and psychotherapy are important to provide a calm reassuring environment and may alleviate many fears and anxieties.

Neurologic complications include altered mental status, seizure, central nervous system (CNS) infection, cerebral vascular accident and malignancy. The differential diagnosis should include metabolic disturbance, drug reaction, infection, thrombotic disorder, hypertension and hypotension. Neurologic workup should include collection of blood for chemistries, culture, viral studies, drug levels and coagulation studies if indicated; imaging by computed tomography or magnetic resonance; and lumbar puncture for cultures and tests for bacterial, fungal and viral pathogens, including EBV PCR.

Infection

The risk of infection is a serious threat in the immunosuppressed renal transplant patient [37]. Urinary tract infections are common after transplantation. Pyuria, fever and allograft tenderness may not always be present because of the immunosuppression. Antibiotic therapy should be started with cultures pending, and subsequently adjusted depending on sensitivity. A VCUG should be performed to rule out reflux but, if present, prophylactic daily antibiotics should be instituted once treatment therapy is complete. Contamination during urine collection is not uncommon in children who have a catheterizable stoma. We have found success in obtaining uncontaminated urine by passing a large sterile catheter that maintains contact with the stoma walls, followed by the passage of a smaller sterile catheter through the larger catheter channel.

Discussion of the viral complications of transplantation is found in Chapter 12.

Recurrence of original disease in allograft

Before the introduction of CSA, acute rejection and chronic allograft nephropathy were the leading causes of graft loss. However, with improvements in antirejection therapy, recurrence of the primary disease has a more prominent role in graft dysfunction [38]. Recurrence rates in focal segmental glomerulosclerosis (FSGS), the most common glomerular disease causing end-stage renal disease (ESRD) in children, can be as high as 50% [39]. Factors that may be predictive of recurrence include onset of original disease before age 6 years, rapid progression to ESRD from onset of proteinuria and mesangial proliferation in the native biopsy specimen [40]. Recurrent FSGS usually presents as persistent proteinuria. The risk of graft loss is high, up to 50%, especially in those who develop nephrotic range proteinuria within 2 weeks of transplant [41]. Therapy such as high-dose CSA, methylprednisolone and plasma exchange has been successful in some cases [39,42].

The Finnish type of congenital nephrotic syndrome (CNS) is caused by autosomal recessive inheritance of defects in the *NPHS1* gene on chromosome 19, which codes for the glomerular protein nephrin [43]. Although no recurrence of the basic disease has been reported [44–46], nine CNS patients have developed post-transplant nephrotic syndrome [47–50]. The episodes were usually preceded by a viral infection. Some patients responded to prednisone and/or cyclophosphamide, but five patients lost their grafts. Analysis of the NAPRTCS data demonstrates an increased risk of graft loss in patients with CNS resulting from thrombosis, most likely because of their hypercoaguable state [46]. However, Holmberg *et al.* [44] reported no graft loss resulting from thrombosis in patients who had bilateral nephrectomy and received peritoneal dialysis at least 3 months prior to transplantation. Care should be taken to eliminate all risk factors for hypercoaguability in these vulnerable patients. In addition, NAPRTCS data reveal these patients were at higher risk for death with a functioning graft, which was primarily because of increased incidence of infection. Patients with CNS have lower immunoglobulin levels resulting from nephrosis, which may increase susceptibility for infection. Attention should be paid to eliminate risk factors for infection, which may improve patient and graft survival [51]. Future studies should involve screening patients with other types of nephrotic syndrome for abnormalities in nephrin [52] and the recently reported CD2-associated protein, which interacts with nephrin in maintaining integrity of the podocyte slit diaphram [53]. It is to be hoped that knowledge of the molecular pathophysiology will lead to treatments for the primary disease and recurrence in the allograft.

Hemolytic uremic syndrome (HUS) has been reported to recur in up to 50% of children following renal transplantation. HUS has also been seen in response to CSA, tacrolimus and antilymphocyte therapy in patients with other primary nephropathies [39]. It is controversial whether CSA or antilymphocyte therapy should be used in the immunosuppressive management of the patient whose primary disease was HUS [54]. Recurrence of HUS in the allograft has been shown to occur more frequently in patients with a history of atypical HUS (20%) as compared with those who had diarrhea-positive HUS (less than 1%) [55]. Among patients with atypical HUS, patients with factor H deficiency have been shown to have a higher risk of recurrence [55].

Primary oxalosis, most often resulting from the absent or dysfunctional liver enzyme alanine-glyoxylate aminotransferase, is associated with renal failure caused by the deposition of calcium oxalate crystals. The high rate of recurrence in the allograft has led to the development of aggressive pre- and post-transplant fluid and electrolyte management [56], which has improved graft survival. More recently, liver transplantation to replace the abnormal enzyme has been successful in either preventing primary renal failure or prolonging renal allograft survival [57].

Membranoproliferative glomerulonephritis (MPGN) types I and II both recur with high frequency in allograft biopsies, but only rarely are associated with graft loss [58]. Cystinosis, an inherited metabolic disorder that results in renal failure, does not cause kidney dysfunction in the allograft [59].

DISCHARGE PLANNING

Discharge planning and patient and caregiver education should be started as soon as possible. Special attention should be given to the home support system, especially in the case where a parent is the donor. Medication boxes and notebook/checkbox systems are often helpful to organize a complicated medication regimen. Although we recommend that the patient be involved in their care, we do stress that the parent, not the patient, is responsible. Outpatient management with schedules for laboratory assessment and clinic visits should be outlined and it must be stressed that they are mandatory. Families should be counseled on the high risk of rejection and infection in the post-transplant period. It should be emphasized that a kidney transplant is not a cure; it is an alternative renal replacement therapy, requiring close adherence to medication schedules.

OUTPATIENT MANAGEMENT

The length of the hospitalization post-transplant has decreased over the past decade to a mean of 7 days. Frequent laboratory assessment and clinic follow-up is warranted. It is not uncommon for the patient to be evaluated by either laboratory tests or clinic visits daily during the first few weeks after transplant. The frequency of clinic visits and laboratory assessment tapers off during the first year depending on the patient's clinical status. Laboratory assessment include electrolytes, BUN, Cr, calcium, phosphorus, albumin, magnesium, urine analysis, urine culture and complete blood count with quarterly assessment of liver function and lipid profile, as well as iron studies in the patient with anemia. Viral surveillance for EBV, BK virus and CMV is becoming increasingly common practice. Estimates of GFR should be performed once the serum Cr has reached its nadir. C_{SCH} [13] can be used as an estimate but should be confirmed by a formal study such as iothalamate clearance [60]. Cr clearance studies should be repeated as clinically indicated. Renal ultrasound is followed on a yearly basis and more frequently in the patient who develops complications.

The cause and pathogenesis of post-transplant hypertension is multifactorial including side-effects of steroid and calcineurin inhibitor therapy, rejection, transplant renal artery stenosis, high renin output from native kidneys, as well as pre-existing disease, *de novo* or recurrent disease in the allograft. If the patient is on antihypertensive therapy, an

179

electrocardiogram and/or cardiac echocardiogram should be obtained annually. Consideration should be made to switch patients to an ACE inhibitor after the first several months post-transplant. Close monitoring for complications of ACE therapy such as acute deterioration of renal function and hyperkalemia is important. Acute deterioration or progressive worsening of hypertension may indicate functionally significant renal artery stenosis. Doppler studies of the renal artery may be suggestive but arteriography remains the gold standard. Balloon dilatation, stenting and corrective surgery of the stenosed artery are potential treatment options.

Post-transplant bone disease is problematic, especially in the growing child. Parathyroid hormone (PTH) is measured yearly in the patient with normal renal function and every 6 months in patients with chronic renal insufficiency. Vitamin D supplements are initiated, if clinically indicated. A high index of suspicion for avascular necrosis and fracture should be maintained. Studies are needed to define interventional measures, such as treatments with bisphosphonates, to reduce the risks of bone disease in the pediatric transplant patient.

Currently, there are no clear treatment guidelines for the management of post-transplant hyperlipidemia in the pediatric patient. There are compliance issues with dietary intervention and lipid-lowering agents. The use of 3-hydroxy-3-methylglutaryl (HMG) coenzyme A (CoA) reductase inhibitors has not been studied in the pediatric renal transplant population.

Dental examination is required every 6 months with antibiotic prophylaxis. Ophthalmology evaluation is recommended yearly. Gynecological follow-up is recommended yearly if the patient is over 18 years, sexually active or has irregular menstrual bleeding.

Medication adherence

Poor adherence with immunosuppressive medications is a major factor in the late loss of renal allografts. In adult renal transplant recipients, rates of noncompliance range from 2% to 18% [61]. Among pediatric renal transplant recipients, the range of noncompliance is reported between 5% and 50% [62–65]. Among adolescents, Ettenger et al. [64] reported rates of noncompliance as high as 64%. The exact incidence of noncompliance is difficult to monitor because of underdetection and under-reporting. In addition, there is the potential mislabeling of the etiology of graft loss as chronic rejection rather than noncompliance [66]. Identified risk factors for noncompliance include female gender, adolescent age, race, distance from transplant center, low socioeconomic status, lack of social supports, complexity and duration of medical regimen, and cosmetic side-effects of medication [67–70]. A recent longitudinal study of adherence demonstrated that adolescents with excessive anger were at higher risk for missing medications [71].

There are several recommendations for facilitating treatment adherence [61,67,69,71,72]. Special attention should be given to the home support system, especially in the case where a parent is the donor. Although we recommend that the patient be involved in their care, we do stress that the parent, not the patient, is responsible. Close post-transplant monitoring is mandatory. This follow-up has to be sustained over the long term despite years of stable graft function because of the late manifestations of noncompliance. The complexity of the medical regimen demands excellent pre- and post-transplant patient and family education. Efforts to simplify the regimen should be made on an ongoing basis. Establishment of a primary health-care provider has been found to improve patient compliance. More personal and individualized approaches to follow-up may be necessary in certain cases. The health-care provider can contribute by simplifying medication regimens when possible, following up on missed visits, acknowledging patients' efforts and providing ongoing encouragement. The availability of long-term support through counseling may improve adherence.

Many factors come into play in determining the optimal time for transplant, including primary disease, family dynamics, psychosocial support, growth and development, dialysis success, availability of donors and optimal immunosuppressive therapy. Another important factor to address when considering when to transplant the adolescent is peer dynamics. The physical changes that accompany transplant may dramatically impact compliance in an atmosphere of peer pressure. Delaying the transplant until after graduation from high school should be considered if this is a viable option.

Immunizations

Currently, there are no guidelines for the immunization of solid organ transplant recipients. In general, immunizations are withheld until 1 year post-transplant and the resumption should be according to the American Academy of Pediatrics recommendations with "catch-up" immunizations given as necessary [73]. Supplemental immunization with pneumococcal and influenza vaccine is recommended [73]. As yet, there are no formal recommendations for the general use of hepatitis A vaccine for the pediatric solid organ transplant recipient. The decision on whether this should be administered should be made on a case-by-case basis. Regarding the immunization of house-hold contacts, they are able to receive measles–mumps–rubella (MMR) and the varicella zoster virus (VZV) vaccines but they should be counseled to receive the inactivated polio vaccine (IPV) [73].

Nutrition

There is a paucity of data regarding dietary recommendations for children following renal transplantation. Much of what is recommended is in response to clinical and biochemical factors observed in individual patients. Energy and protein needs are significantly increased immediately after transplant. Protein needs are probably 150–200% of recommended daily allowance (RDA) for age and weight. It is important to meet these needs to achieve wound healing and to help prevent muscle wasting associated with high-dose steroids. Supplemental enteral or parenteral nutrition is indicated in patients who cannot meet their requirements by oral intake in the first few days post-transplant.

Young children, who have been exclusively tube fed while on dialysis, are not generally ready to wean from tube feeding in the immediate post-transplant period. However, many of these patients are interested in oral feeding after transplant, because of the resolution of uremia and prednisone-induced appetite enhancement. These children are given a regimen of a standard pediatric tube feeding formula plus water to meet 100% of their nutritional and fluid needs after transplant. Ad lib intake of oral foods is encouraged and daily food intake records are kept. Tube feeding formula is tapered slowly as oral intake increases; the amount of formula decrease is based on weight gain and reported oral intake. Children who were eating even a few bites of food on a regular basis prior to transplant wean off tube feeding much faster than those who were receiving no oral intake.

The child also needs to have adequate fluid intake. The quantity ranges from 1.5 to 4 L/day depending on the size of the child, their activity and the ambient temperature. Achieving these fluid goals can be a challenge especially in the dialysis patient who was previously fluid restricted. Water and milk, rather than sugar-containing beverages, are encouraged. If the child has a gastrostomy (g-tube), it can be used for some portion of the fluid intake. Parents can keep track of fluid intake during the day and give the remainder of the child's requirement with boluses throughout the day or by nocturnal drip tube feedings.

Sugars and/or simple carbohydrates are generally limited during the early post-transplant period (first 4–6 weeks) because of hyperglycemia associated with high doses of prednisone and calcineurin inhibitors, especially tacrolimus [74]. A low sodium diet (less than 2–3 g/day) has traditionally been prescribed for transplant patients because of sodium retention associated with high doses of prednisone and calcineurin inhibitor-induced hypertension. There are no data demonstrating the long-term efficacy of low sodium diet in transplant patients, but patients with hypertension may benefit from a moderate restriction [74]. Serum potassium levels often rise with the administration of calcineurin inhibitors and can be especially problematic with tacrolimus. In these cases, a low potassium diet is prescribed, and in some cases the use of an exchange resin (Kayexalate®) is necessary. As serum phosphorus levels fall after transplant, a high phosphorus diet is encouraged. This can be achieved by increasing dairy intake, as long as serum potassium is not elevated. In most cases, a child cannot take in enough dietary phosphorus to maintain normal serum levels, and a supplement is necessary. Patients may require up to 2–3 g/day phosphorus. Magnesium levels also fall in most patients after transplant and, in these cases, a supplement is necessary, as transplant patients cannot take in enough dietary magnesium to achieve normal serum levels. Calcium and vitamin D needs are increased in the post-transplant patient. It is thought that the RDA (800 mg/day of calcium for children and adults, 1300 mg/day for adolescents) is probably insufficient. A recommendation of 1.5 g/day of calcium for adults has been made, which is 188% of the RDA [74]. If the same recommendation were made for adolescents, this would extrapolate to 2.4 g/day calcium. Calcium supplements are given in the form of calcium gluconate or calcium glubionate, rather than calcium carbonate, to avoid phosphorus binding. If a child is eating well and taking in high amounts of dairy products, we do not generally supplement calcium. Vitamin D is supplemented if the PTH is elevated.

A major concern in the transplant patient is long-term excess energy and fat intake, with subsequent excessive weight gain leading to obesity, hyperlipidemia and increased risk of cardiovascular disease. It is important to monitor weight gain and to make aggressive efforts to decrease high fat foods for children who are gaining weight excessively. A diet low in saturated fat plus regular aerobic and weight-bearing exercise have been shown to have a major role in keeping weight gain down and lowering lipid levels in both adults and children post-transplant [75–79].

Growth and development

Growth retardation continues to be a significant concern for both patients and their families post-transplant. NAPRTCS data found that at the time of transplantation, the mean height deficit for all pediatric transplant recipients exceeded 2.0 SD [80]. Recipients who were 1 year of age or younger had accelerated growth during the first year after transplant. In contrast, adolescent recipients had a deceleration in growth after transplantation. This suggests that delaying transplantation beyond the 12th year is disadvantageous in terms of height improvement and greater attempts should be made to facilitate transplantation prior to adolescence. The use of corticosteroids as part of the immunosuppressive therapy post-transplant contributes to poor growth. An NAPRTCS analysis found that patients receiving alternate-day steroids had better growth with no adverse effect on graft survival or function [81]. NAPRTCS, in conjunction with the National Cooperative Growth Study, evaluated the outcome of renal transplant patients who received growth hormone for a minimum of 1 year post-transplant [82]. Growth velocity was increased for up to 3 years post-transplant. No significant decrease in 5-year graft survival rates or renal function was observed [83].

Quality of life

Improved patient and graft survival rates have led clinicians to take a closer look at quality of life issues in this young population. Back to school issues and academic performance post-transplant have been specifically addressed. School re-entry can be limited by numerous factors. Alteration of physical appearance with heightened self-awareness may cause children, especially adolescents, to be reluctant to return to the classroom. Anxiety on the part of parents and school personnel can be significant. It is the role of the health-care team to educate both parents and school personnel about the importance of returning to school [84]. An NAPRTCS analysis evaluated school performance in 40 renal transplant recipients at a mean age of 13 years and a mean of 3 years post-transplant [85]. A significantly greater number of transplant recipients were enrolled in combined regular and special classrooms when compared with controls (30% vs. 9%). The incidence of hearing loss, motor delay, language/speech delay and visual impairment was similar between the two groups. School achievement scores for math, reading and written language were similar in transplant recipients and controls [86,87]. Frequent absenteeism with numerous physician visits can also contribute to academic difficulties.

CONCLUSIONS

Renal transplantation remains the goal for the pediatric patient with ESRD. Recent advances in technology and immunosuppression have greatly enhanced patient and graft survival, while reducing significant complications. Future research must be directed at improved operative techniques, induction of allograft tolerance, reduction of rejection episodes, prevention of serious infectious and neoplastic complications as well as enhanced growth and development of the child.

REFERENCES

1 Flancbaum L, Dick M, Choban PS, Dasta JP. Effects of low-dose dopamine on urine in oliguric, critically ill, renal transplant patients. *Clin Transplant* 1998;**12**:256–9.

2 Bund M, Seitz W, Kirchner E. Is preventative perioperative dopamine administration of value? *Anaesthesiol Reanim* 1995; **20**:76–81.

3 Kadieva VS, Friedman L, Margolius LP, Jackson SA, Morrell DF. The effect of dopamine on graft function in patients undergoing renal transplantation. *Anesth Analg* 1993;**76**:362–5.

4 Barton CH, Vaziri ND, Martin DC, Choi S, Alikhani S. Hypomagnesemia and renal magnesium wasting in renal transplant recipients receiving cyclosporine. *Am J Med* 1987;**83**: 693–9.

5 Niederstadt C, Steinhoff J, Erbsloh-Moller B, *et al.* Effect of FK506 on magnesium homeostasis after renal transplantion. *Transplant Proc* 1997;**29**:3161–2.

6 Salvatierra O Jr, Sarwal M, Alexander S, *et al.* A new, unique and simple method for ureteral implantation in kidney recipients with small, defunctionalized bladders. *Transplantation* 1999;**68**:731–8.

7 Gonzalez R, Reinberg Y, Nguyen DH. Urologic evaluation in renal transplantation. *Dial Pediatr Urol* 1989;**12**:2–4.

8 Burns MW, Watkins SL, Mitchell ME, Tapper D. Treatment of bladder dysfunction in children with end-stage renal disease. *J Pediatr Surg* 1992;**27**:170–4.

9 Kiberd BA. Cyclosporine-induced renal dysfunction in human renal allograft recipients. *Transplantation* 1989;**48**:965–9.

10 Silverstein DM, Palmer J, Baluarte HJ, *et al.* Use of calcium-channel blockers in pediatric renal transplant recipients. *Pediatr Transplant* 1999;**3**:288–92.

11 The TH, van den Bern AP, van Son WJ, *et al.* Monitoring for cytomegalovirus after organ transplantation: a clinical perspective. *Transplant Proc* 1993;**25**:5–9.

12 Nadasdy T, Park C-S, Peiper SC, *et al.* Epstein–Barr virus infection-associated renal disease: diagnostic use of molecular hybridization technology in patients with negative serology. *J Am Soc Nephrol* 1992;**2**:1734–42.

13 Schwartz GJ, Haycock GB, Edelmann CM Jr, Spitzer A. A simple estimate of glomerular filtration rate in children derived from body length and plasma creatinine. *Pediatrics* 1976;**58**:259–63.

14 Green M, Michaels MG, Webber SA, Rowe D, Reyes J. The management of Epstein–Barr virus associated post-transplant lymphoproliferative disorders in pediatric solid-organ transplant recipients. *Pediatr Transplant* 1999;**3**:271–81.

15 McDiarmid SV, Jordan S, Lee GS, *et al.* Prevention and pre-emptive therapy of post-transplant lymphoproliferative disease in pediatric liver recipients. *Transplantation* 1998;**66**:1604–11.

16 Benfield MR, Herrin J, Feld L, *et al.* Safety of kidney biopsy in pediatric transplantation: a report of the Controlled Clinical Trials in Pediatric Transplantation Trial of Induction Therapy Study Group. *Transplantation* 1999;**67**:544–7.

17 Tejani AH, Sullivan EK, Alexander SR, *et al.* Predictive factors for delayed graft function (DGF) and its impact on renal graft survival in children: a report of the North American Pediatric Renal Transplant Cooperative Study (NAPRTCS). *Pediatr Transplant* 1999;**3**:293–300.

18 Tilney NL. Early course of a patient. In: Morris P, ed. *Kidney Transplantation.* Philadelphia: WB Saunders, 1988: 278–83.

19 Alkhunaizi AM, de Mattos AM, Barry JM, Bennett WM, Norman DJ. Renal transplantation across the ABO barrier usin A2 kidneys. *Transplantation* 1999;**67**:1319–24.

20 Haskin JA, Warner DJ, Blank DU. Acute renal failure after large doses of intravenous immune globulin. *Ann Pharmacother* 1999;**33**:800–3.

21 Salomon L, Saporta F, Amsellem D, *et al.* Results of pyelou-reterostomy after ureterovesical anastomosis complications in renal transplantation. *Urology* 1999;**53**:908–12.

22 Ghasemian SM, Guleria AS, Khawand NY, Light JA. Diagnosis and management of the urologic complications of renal transplantation. *Clin Transplant* 1996;**10**:218–23.

23 Rosenthal JT. Surgical management of urological complications after kidney transplantation. *Semin Urol* 1994;**12**:114–22.

24 Rivera M, Marcen R, Burgos J, *et al.* Treatment of posttransplant lymphocele with povidone-iodine sclerosis: long-term follow-up. *Nephron* 1996;**74**:324–7.

25 Sawhney R, Dágostino HB, Zinck S, *et al.* Treatment of post-operative lymphoceles with percutaneous drainage and alcohol sclerotherapy. *J Vasc Interv Radiol* 1996;7:241–5.

26 Bischof G, Rockenschaub S, Berlakovich G, *et al.* Management of lymphoceles after kidney transplantation. *Transpl Int* 1998;11:277–80.

27 Singh A, Stablein D, Tejani A. Risk factors for vascular thrombosis in pediatric renal transplantation. *Transplantation* 1997; 63:1263–7.

28 Fischereder M, Göhring P, Schneeberger H, *et al.* Early loss of renal transplants in patients with thrombophilia. *Transplantation* 1998;65:936–9.

29 Irish AB, Green F, Gray DWR, Morris PJ. The factor V Leiden (R506Q) mutation and risk of thrombosis in renal transplant recipients. *Transplantation* 1997;64:604–7.

30 Oh J, Schaefer F, Veldmann A, *et al.* Heterozygous porthrombin gene mutation: a new risk factor for early renal allograft thrombosis. *Transplantation* 1999;68:575–8.

31 Wagenknecht DR, Becker DG, LeFor WM, McIntyre JA. Antiphospholipid antibodies are a risk factor for early renal allograft failure. *Transplantation* 1999;68:241–6.

32 Kooijmans-Coutinho MF, Hermans J, Schrama E, *et al.* Interstitial rejection, vascular rejection, and diffuse thrombosis of renal allografts: predisposing factors, histology, immunohistochemistry, and relation to outcome. *Transplatation* 1996;61: 1338–44.

33 Vats AN, Donaldson L, Fine RN, Chavers BM. Pretransplant dialysis status and outcome of renal transplantation in North American children: a NAPRTCS study. *Transplantation* 2000; 69:1414–9.

34 Ismail H, Kalicinski P, Drewniak T, *et al.* Primary vascular thrombosis after renal transplantation in children. *Pediatr Transplant* 1997;1:43–7.

35 Bedani PL, Galeotti R, Mugnani G, *et al.* Successful local arterial urokinase infusion to reverse late postoperative venous thrombosis of a renal graft. *Nephrol Dial Transplant* 1999;14:2225–7.

36 Lee G, Watson CW, Mammen KJ, Phillips-Hughes J, Morris PJ. Successful selective thrombilysis of a spontaneous transplant renal vain thrombosis. *BJU Int* 1999;83:869–70.

37 Dharnidharka VR, Stablein DM, Harmon WE. Post-transplant infections now exceed acute rejection as cause for hospitalization: a report of the NAPRTCS. *Am J Transplant* 2004;4:384–9.

38 Mathew TH. Recurrence of disease following transplantation. *Am J Kidney Dis* 1988;12:85–96.

39 Fine RN, Ettenger RB. Renal transplantation in children. In: Morris P, ed. *Kidney Transplantation Principles and Practice.* Philadelphia: WB Saunders, 1988: 635–91.

40 Ettenger RB. Renal transplantation. In: Barakat A, ed. *Renal Disease in Children.* New York: Springer-Verlag, 1990: 371–84.

41 Seuggutuvan P, Cameron JS, Hartley RB, *et al.* Recurrence of focal segmental glomerulosclerosis in transplanted kidneys: analysis of incidence and risk factors in 59 allografts. *Pediatr Nephrol* 1990;4:21–8.

42 Ingulli E, Tejani A, Butt K, *et al.* High-dose cyclosporine therapy in recurrent nephrotic syndrome following renal transplantation. *Transplantation* 1990;49:219–21.

43 Holthofer H, Ahola H, Solin M, *et al.* Nephrin localizes at the podocyte filtration slit area and is characteristically spliced in the human kidney. *Am J Pathol* 1999;155:1681–7.

44 Holmberg C, Antikainen M, Rönnholm K, Ala-Houhala M, Jalanko H. Management of congenital nephrotic syndrome of the Finnish type. *Pediatr Nephrol* 1995;9:87–93.

45 Mahan JD, Mauer M, Sibley RK, Vernier RL. Congenital nephrotic syndrome: evolution of medical management and results of renal transplantation. *J Pediatr* 1984;105:549–57.

46 Kim M, Stablein D, Harmon W. Renal transplantation in children with congenital nephrotic syndrome: a report of the North American Pediatric Renal Transplant Cooperative Study (NAPRTCS). *Pediatr Tranplant* 1998;2:305–8.

47 Laine J, Jalanko H, Holthofer H, *et al.* Post-transplantation nephrosis in congenital nephrotic syndrome of the Finnish type. *Kidney Int* 1993;44:867–74.

48 Sigström L, Hansson S, Jodal U. Long-term survival of a girl with congenital nephrotic syndrome and recurrence of proteinuria after transplantation. *Pediatr Nephrol* 1989;3:C169.

49 Lane PH, Schnapper HW, Vernier RL, Bunchman TE. Steroid-dependent nephrotic syndrome following renal transplantation for congenital nephrotic syndrome. *Pediatr Nephrol* 1991;5: 300–3.

50 Flynn JT, Schulman SL, deChadarevian JP, *et al.* Treatment of steroid-resistant post-transplant nephrotic syndrome with cyclophosphamide in a child with congenital nephrotic syndrome. *Pediatr Nephrol* 1992;6:553–5.

51 Kim MS, Primack W, Harmon WE. Congenital nephrotic syndrome: pre-emptive bilateral nephrectomy and dialysis before renal transplantation. *J Am Soc Nephrol* 1992;3:260–3.

52 Furness PN, Hall LL, Shaw JA, Pringle JH. Glomerular expression of nephrin is decreased in acquired human nephrotic syndrome. *Nephrol Dial Transplant* 1999;14:1234–7.

53 Shih N, Li J, Karpitskii V, *et al.* Congenital nephrotic syndrome in mice lacking CD2-associated protein. *Science* 1999;286:312–5.

54 Herbert D, Sibley RK, Mauer SM. Recurrence of hemolytic uremic syndrome in renal transplant recipients. *Kidney Int* 1986;30:551–8.

55 Loirat C, Niaudet P. The risk of recurrence of hemolytic uremic syndrome after renal transplantation in children. *Pediatr Nephrol* 2003;18:1095–101.

56 Scheinman JI. Primary hyperoxaluria: therapeutic strategies for the 90s. *Kidney Int* 1991;40:389–99.

57 Watts RW. Treatment of renal failure in the primary hyperoxalurias. *Nephron* 1990;56:1–5.

58 Alexander SR. Controversies in pediatric renal transplantation. *AKF Nephrol Lett* 1990;7:5–21.

59 Broyer M, Gagnadoux MF, Guest G. In: Hamberger J, Crossnier J, Grunfeld JP, eds. *Advances in Nephrology.* Chicago: Year Book Medical, 1987: 307–34.

60 Seikaly MG, Browne R, Bajaj G, Arant BS Jr. Limitations to body length/serum creatinine ratio as an estimate of glomerular filtration in children. *Pediatr Nephrol* 1996;10:709–11.

61 Schweizer RT, Rovelli M, Palmeri D, *et al.* Noncompliance in organ transplant recipients. *Transplantation* 1990;49:374–7.

62 Morgenstern BZ, Murphy M, Dayton J, *et al.* Noncompliance in a pediatric renal transplant population. *Transplant Proc* 1994;26:129.

63 Meyers KE, Weiland H, Thomson PD. Pediatric renal transplantation noncompliance. *Pediatr Nephrol* 1995;9:189.

64 Ettenger RB, Rosenthal JT, Marik JL, *et al.* Improved cadaveric renal transplant outcome in children. *Pediatr Nephrol* 1991;5:137.

65 Beck DE, Fennell RS, Yost RL, *et al.* Evaluations of an educational program on compliance with medication regimens in pediatric patients with renal transplants. *J Pediatr* 1980;**96**:1094–7.

66 Ishitani M, Isaacs R, Norwood V, Nock S, Lobo P. Predictors of graft survival in pediatric living-related kidney transplant recipients. *Transplantation* 2000;**70**:288–92.

67 Meyers KE, Thomson PD, Weiland H. Noncompliance in children and adolescents after renal transplantation. *Transplantation* 1996;**62**:186–9.

68 Cole BR. Noncompliance to medical regimens. In: Tejani AH, Fine RN, eds. *Pediatric Renal Transplantation.* New York: Wiley-Liss, 1994: 397.

69 Bunchman TE. Compliance in pediatric transplant. *Pediatr Transplant* 2000;**4**:165–9.

70 Foulkes LM, Boggs SR, Fennell RS, Skibinski K. Social support, family variables, and compliance in renal transplant children. *Pediatr Nephrol* 1993;**7**:185.

71 Penkower L, Dew MA, Ellis D, *et al.* Psychological distress and adherence to the medical regimen among adolescent renal transplant recipients. *Am J Transplant* 2003;**3**:1418–25.

72 Siegel EG, Mahan JD, Johnson RS. Solid organ transplantation in adolescents: the blessing and the curse. *Adolesc Med* 1994;**5**:293–310.

73 American Academy of Pediatrics. *2003 Red Book Report on the Committee of Infectious Diseases.*

74 Warady BA, Hebert D, Sullivan EK, Alexander SR, Tejani A. Renal transplantation, chronic dialysis, and chronic renal insufficiency in children and adolescents. The 1995 Annual Report of the North American Pediatric Renal Transplant Cooperative Study. *Pediatr Nephrol* 1997;**11**:49–64.

75 Fennell EB, Fennell RS, Mings E, Morris MK. The effects of various modes of therapy for end-stage renal disease on cognitive performance in a pediatric population: a preliminary report. *Int J Pediatr Nephrol* 1986;**7**:107–12.

76 Fine RN. Renal transplantation for children: the only realistic choice. *Kidney Int Suppl* 1985;**17**:S15–7.

77 United States Renal Data System (USRDS). *The 1997 Annual Report.* Bethesda: National Institutes of Health, National Institute of Diabetes and Digestive and Kidney Diseases, 1997.

78 Kohaut EC, Tejani A. The 1994 annual report of the North American Pediatric Renal Transplant Cooperative Study. *Pediatr Nephrol* 1996;**10**:422–34.

79 Cecka JM, Gjerston DW, Terasaki PI. Pediatric renal transplantation: a review of the UNOS data. *Pediatr Transplant* 1997;**1**:55–64.

80 McEnery PT, Stablein DM, Arbus G, Tejani A. Renal transplantation in children: a report of the North American Pediatric Renal Transplant Cooperative Study. *N Engl J Med* 1992;**326**:1727–32.

81 Jabs K, Sullivan K, Avner ED, Harmon WE. Alternate day steroid dosing improves growth without adversely affecting graft survival or long-term graft function. *Transplantation* 1996;**61**:31–6.

82 Mentser M, Breen TJ, Sullivan, Fine RN. Growth hormone treatment of renal transplant recipients: the National Cooperative Growth Study experience: a report of the National Cooperative Growth Study and the North American Pediatric Renal Transplant Cooperative Study. *J Pediatr* 1997;**131**:S20–4.

83 Tejani A, Cortes L, Stablein DM. Clinical correlates of chronic rejection in pediatric renal transplantation: a report of the North American Pediatric Renal Transplant Study Group. *Transplantation* 1996;**61**:1054–8.

84 Davis ID. Pediatric renal transplantation: back to school issues. *Transplant Proc* 1999;**31**:61S–2S.

85 Brouhard B, Donaldson K, Lawry K, *et al.* Quality of life of children post transplantation compared to children on dialysis. For the North American Pediatric Renal Transplant Cooperative Study. *Pediatr Transplant* 1998;**2**(Suppl 1):80.

86 Fennell RS, Fennell EB, Carter RL, *et al.* A longitudinal study of the cognitive function of children with renal failure. *Pediatr Nephrol* 1990;**4**:11–5.

87 Lawry KW, Brouhard BH, Cunningham RJ. Cognitive functioning and school performance in children with renal failure. *Pediatr Nephrol* 1994;**8**:326–9.

21 Outcomes and Risk Factors

Alicia M. Neu and Barbara A. Fivush

Because the number of pediatric kidney transplants performed at any one institution is relatively small, in the past reports of outcomes in pediatric kidney transplantation were often anecdotal and descriptive, and could not critically consider the multiple variables that may affect transplant graft and patient survival. For this reason, in 1987, the North American Pediatric Renal Transplant Cooperative Study (NAPRTCS) was created to collect data and define standard clinical practices and outcomes for this population. This organization has grown considerably, and at the time of the 2001 NAPRTCS Annual Report there were 150 participating centers located throughout the USA, Canada, Mexico and Costa Rica [1]. These centers voluntarily contribute data on their transplant recipients and, as a result, this database provides comprehensive and accurate information of outcomes for pediatric kidney transplant recipients. The 2001 NAPRTCS Annual Report contained data on 7545 kidney transplants in 6878 patients transplanted since 1987 [1]. Data from previously published NAPRTCS annual reports will largely serve as the basis for this chapter. Pediatric data from the Organ Procurement and Transplantation Network (OPTN)/Scientific Registry of Transplant Recipients (SRTR) Annual Report, which gathers data on adult and pediatric transplant patients, will also be presented. Finally, data from pediatric kidney transplant and end-stage renal disease databases maintained in Europe will be presented as available.

REJECTION

Acute rejection

Although acute rejection remains a significant problem post-transplantation, recent data reveal a substantial decline in the frequency of acute rejection in pediatric kidney transplant recipients. The 2001 NAPRTCS Annual Report reveals that the probabilities of acute rejection have decreased from 57% and 70% in living donor (LD) and deceased donor (DD) transplants performed in 1987–88 to 32% in LD and 36% in DD transplants performed in 1999–2000 [1,2]. It should

be noted that rejection in NAPRTCS is defined as treatment with antirejection medication and biopsy verification is not required [2]. Table 21.1 details risk factors associated with first rejection episode for both LD and DD grafts [3]. Risk factors for rejection in both LD and DD grafts include black race, the presence of at least one DR mismatch and the absence of anti-T-cell antibody prophylaxis [1–3]. Although a previous report of the NAPRTCS suggested that deceased donor age less than 5 years was associated with an increased risk for rejection, more recent analysis of this database no longer identifies this as a risk factor, presumably because of the decreased use of kidneys from very young donors for pediatric recipients [3,4].

Late acute rejection

Late acute rejection is defined as a first acute rejection occurring beyond the first year post-transplant. A review of NAPRTCS data in 1998 examined 1471 patients who were rejection free at the end of 1 year, 327 (22%) of whom subsequently developed a rejection episode [4]. Risk factors for late acute rejection include age over 6 years at transplantation (relative risk [RR] 1.7; $P < 0.001$) and black race (RR 1.5; $P < 0.002$) [4].

Reversibility of acute rejection

NAPRTCS data reveal that the ability to completely reverse an acute rejection episode, defined as return of serum creatinine to pre-rejection baseline, has improved with the introduction of newer treatments for rejection [1,2]. In the early years of the NAPRTCS database, only 52% of rejection episodes in LD recipients were completely reversed, compared with 65% in more recent cohorts [1,2]. In NAPRTCS, complete reversal was less likely with increasing number of rejections, increased recipient age and late acute rejection, while use of polyclonal or monoclonal induction therapy had no effect [1,5].

Chronic allograft nephropathy

Chronic allograft nephropathy is an incompletely understood clinicopathologic entity also known as chronic rejection,

Table 21.1 Relative risk (RR) of first rejection in pediatric renal transplant recipients. Reprinted from Seikaly *et al.* [3] with permission.

Characteristic	Living donor		Deceased donor	
	RR	P value	RR	P value
Recipient race (black vs. nonblack)	1.29	0.001	1.18	0.005
Recipient age (< 24 months)	0.77	0.018	1.15	0.317
HLA-DR mismatch				
One mismatch vs. zero	1.57	< 0.001	1.18	0.041
Two mismatch vs. zero	1.13	0.208	1.32	0.001
No induction therapy	1.31	< 0.001	1.26	< 0.001
Prior random transfusions				
1–5 vs. none	0.97	0.576	1.05	0.391
> 5 vs. none	1.18	0.028	1.26	< 0.001
1–5 vs. > 5	0.72	< 0.001	0.84	0.002
Donor-specific transfusions	1.12	0.169	–	–
Preoperative immunotherapy	0.99	0.804	–	–
Cold storage time	–	–	1.14	0.010

transplant glomerulopathy or transplant nephropathy [6]. Recent NAPRTCS data reveal that chronic allograft nephropathy is the cause of allograft loss in over one-third of cases [1]. Various studies in pediatric kidney transplant patients have identified acute rejection, increasing number of rejections, late acute rejection, repeat transplant, deceased donor source, deceased donor age under 5 years, black race, low cyclosporine dose of less than 5 mg/kg/day at 30 days post-transplant, lower calculated creatinine clearance at 1 year post-transplant and high panel reactive antibody (PRA) pretransplant as significant risk factors for chronic allograft nephropathy [7–11]. Acute rejection is one of the important risk factors for chronic allograft nephropathy and an early study using NAPRTCS data revealed that a single acute rejection was associated with a relative risk for chronic allograft nephropathy of 3.1, while multiple acute rejection episodes increased that relative risk to 4.3 [8]. More recent data from NAPRTCS suggest that with reduction in acute rejection rates, the incidence of chronic allograft nephropathy has decreased and the relative risk of graft failure from chronic

allograft nephropathy in patients transplanted between 1995 and 2000 compared with those transplanted between 1987 and 1994 was 0.66 ($P = 0.005$) [12].

GRAFT SURVIVAL

Causes of graft loss

NAPRTCS data reveal that with the reduction in acute rejection rates, the most common cause of graft loss in pediatric kidney transplant patients is now chronic allograft nephropathy. Causes of both index and subsequent graft failure from the most recent published NAPRTCS annual report are listed in Table 21.2 [1]. In addition to chronic and acute rejection, common causes of graft failure include thrombosis (12.0%) and recurrence of original disease (6.3%) [1]. Recently, the Late Effects of Renal Insufficiency in Children (LERIC) study, a national Dutch long-term follow-up study, reported outcomes in 397 kidney transplants performed in 231 patients who

Table 21.2 Causes of graft failure. Reprinted from Benfield *et al.* [1] with permission.

Cause	Index graft failures		Subsequent graft failures		Total graft failures	
	(*n* = 1605)	%	(*n* = 237)	%	(*n* = 1842)	%
Chronic rejection	520	32.4	78	32.9	598	32.5
Acute rejection	244	15.2	31	13.1	275	15.0
Vascular thrombosis	186	11.6	35	14.8	221	12.0
Death	162	10.1	17	7.2	179	9.7
Recurrence of original disease	95	5.9	21	8.9	116	6.3

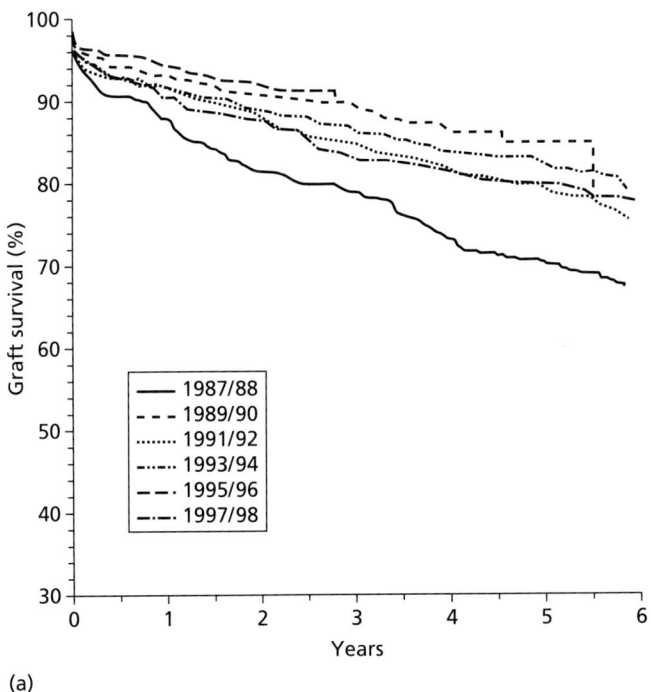
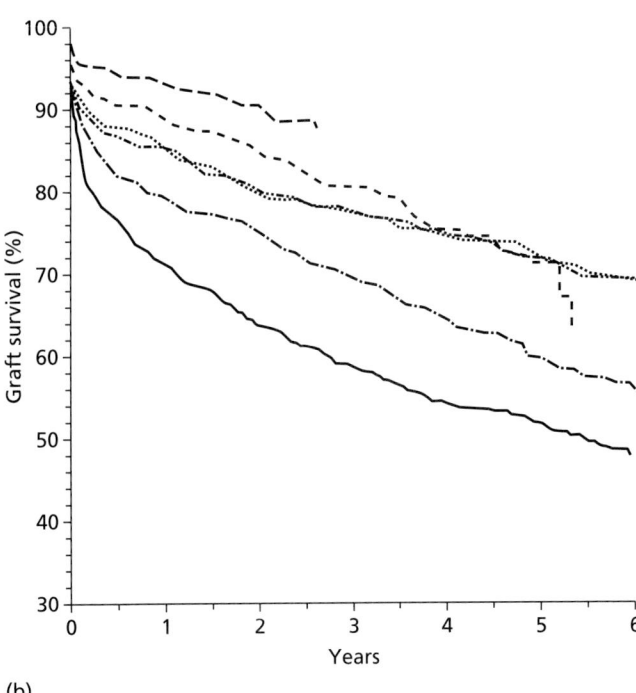

(a)

(b)

Fig. 21.1 Percentage of living donor (a) and deceased donor (b) graft survival among pediatric kidney transplants in North American Pediatric Renal Transplant. Pediatric Renal Transplant Cooperative Study (NAPRTCS) by cohort year. Reprinted from Benfield *et al.* [1] with permission.

reached end-stage between 1972 and 1992 at age 0–15 years [13]. This analysis revealed that 29.7% of graft failures in this cohort of patients were caused by acute rejection, 52.2% to chronic graft nephropathy and 9.1% to thrombosis [13].

Graft survival rates

Graft survival rates in pediatric kidney transplant recipients have improved significantly over the last decade. Figure 21.1 demonstrates that among NAPRTCS patients, the cumulative

distribution of graft survival has improved significantly with each cohort year, and 1-year graft survival in LD and DD recipients, respectively, has increased from 91% and 81% in transplants performed between 1987 and 1994, to 94% and 93% for transplants performed between 1995 and 2000 (*P* < 0.001) [1]. The improvement has been especially dramatic in the youngest patients, and data from the SRTR reveal that graft survival rates in young pediatric patients are among the best of all transplants [14,15]. As shown in Figure 21.2, recipients under the age of 10 years who received a LD

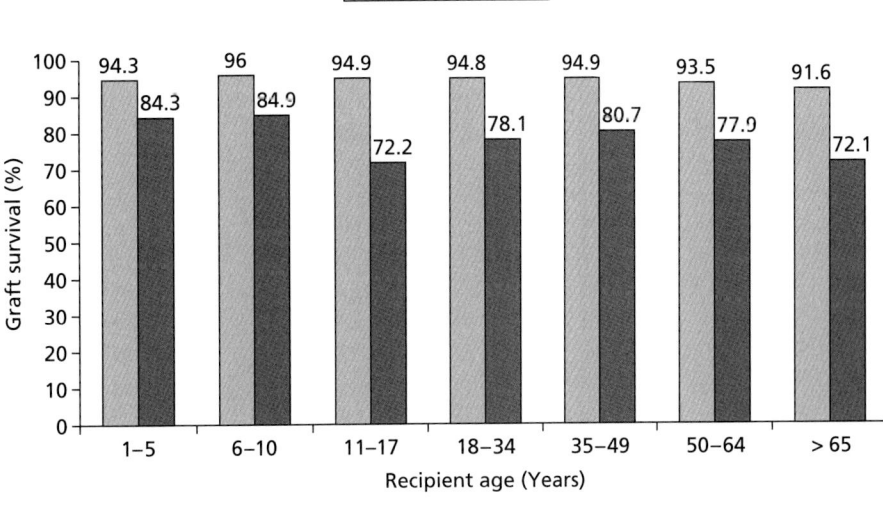

Fig. 21.2 Adjusted 1- and 5-year graft survivals among living donor kidney transplants by recipient age from the 2003 Organ Procurement and Transplantation Network (OPTN)/ Scientific Registry of Transplant Recipients (SRTR) Annual Report [15]. Reprinted from Magee *et al.* [14] with permission.

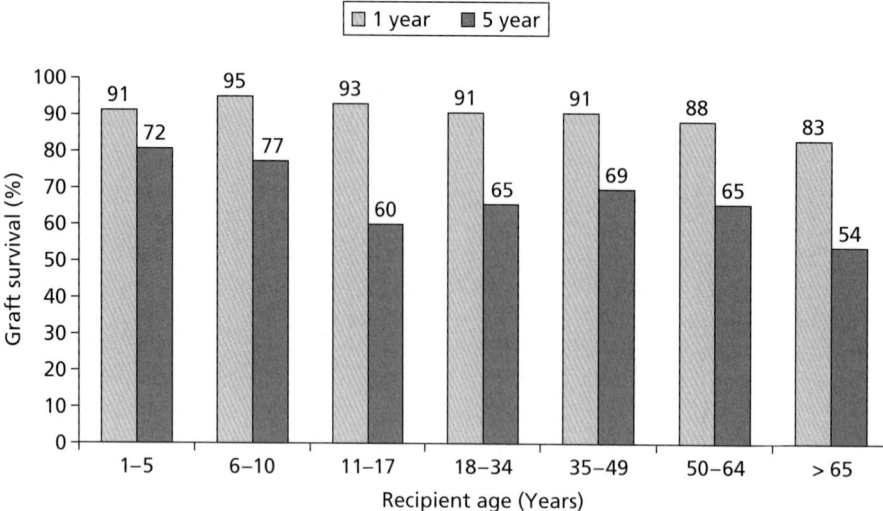

Fig. 21.3 Adjusted 1- and 5-year graft survival among deceased donor kidney transplants by recipient age, from the 2003 Organ Procurement and Transplantation Network (OPTN)/ Scientific Registry of Transplant Recipients (SRTR) Annual Report [15]. Reprinted from Magee *et al.* [14] with permission.

transplant have 5-year adjusted graft survival rates better than all age groups of adults [14,15]. Similar results for recipients of DD grafts are shown in Figure 21.3 [14,15]. These figures also reveal that although the youngest patients have the best long-term survival, adolescent kidney transplant recipients do not enjoy the same outcome [14,15]. For recipients of LD grafts aged 11–17 years, the 5-year adjusted graft survival is only 72%, while 5-year adjusted graft survival in adolescent recipients of DD grafts is only 60% [14,15]. The reason for these poor outcomes is not known, and although there has been speculation about the role of nonadherence, an unexplained high frequency of graft thrombosis and the high incidence of focal and segmental glomerulosclerosis (FSGS) recurrence in this age group, thus far there have been no studies to define clearly the role of these or other factors in the poor graft survival seen in adolescent patients [14–19].

Risks for graft failure

Using NAPRTCS data, relative risks for graft failure have been derived using Cox proportional hazards regression models. For recipients of LD grafts, risk factors for graft failure include black race (RR 2.0; $P < 0.001$), more than five random blood transfusions pretransplant (RR 1.6; $P < 0.001$) and absence of HLA-B locus match (RR 1.6; $P < 0.002$) [3]. Risk factors for graft failure in recipients of DD grafts include donor age less than 6 years (RR 1.22; $P = 0.025$), recipient age < 24 months (RR 1.95; $P < 0.001$), prior transplant (RR 1.32; $P = 0.003$), no induction therapy (RR 1.26; $P = 0.001$), more than five random blood transfusions pretransplant (RR 1.29; $P = 0.001$), absence of HLA-B locus match (RR 1.21; $P = 0.009$), absence of HLA-DR match (RR 1.25; $P = 0.002$), black race (RR 1.41; $P < 0.001$), prior dialysis (RR 1.37; $P = 0.012$) and cold ischemia time longer than 24 hours (RR 1.18; $P = 0.023$) [3]. It should be noted that this analysis was performed on NAPRTCS data through

1998 and, consistent with the data from SRTR, more recent data from NAPRTCS reveal that 1-year graft survival rates in recipients under the age of 24 months have improved from 88% and 78% in LD and DD transplants performed between 1987 and 1994 to 96% and 94% in LD and DD transplants performed between 1995 and 2000 [1]. These data suggest that multivariate analyses performed on this more recent cohort may not demonstrate the risk of graft failure associated with young recipient age seen in analyses performed on earlier cohorts.

PATIENT SURVIVAL

As seen in Figure 21.4, data from SRTR demonstrate that patient survival is generally better for pediatric than adult kidney transplant recipients [14]. In addition, data from the re-established European Renal Association-European Dialysis and Transplant Association (ERA-EDTA) demonstrate significant improvement in patient survival in recent years and the relative risk of death among pediatric recipients of a first kidney transplant between 1995 and 2000 was reduced by 42% (adjusted hazards ratio [AHR] 0.58; 95% confidence interval [CI], 0.34–1.00) compared with pediatric patients transplanted between 1980 and 1984 [20]. These data are shown in Figure 21.5 [20].

Among transplant patients in NAPRTCS, the most common causes of death are infection (34%), cardiopulmonary causes (15%) and malignancy (12%) [1]. Data from the ERA-EDTA also identifies infection as a leading cause of death in children transplanted in Europe, where it was responsible for over 20% of deaths [20]. There is some concern that infection rates in pediatric renal transplantation may be increasing, perhaps as a result of more potent immunosuppressive medications, and a recent analysis of NAPRTCS data revealed that risk for hospitalization resulting from

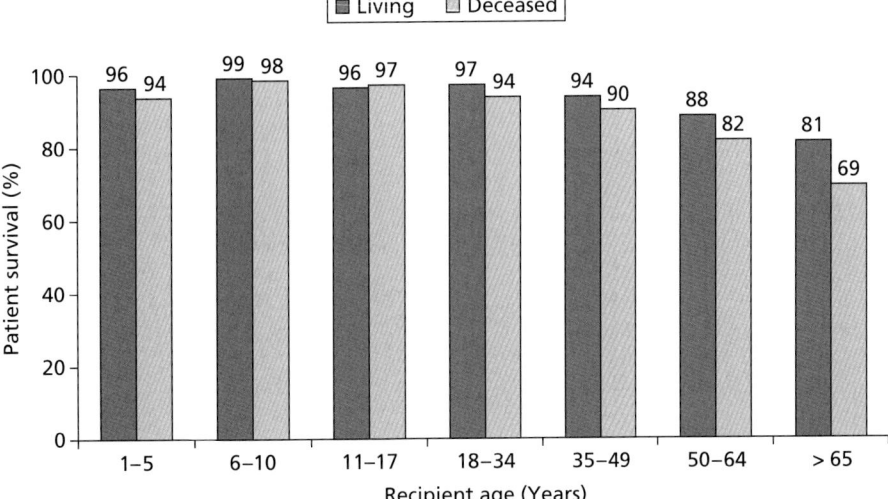

Fig. 21.4 Adjusted 5-year patient survival of living and deceased donor kidney transplants by recipient age from the 2003 Organ Procurement and Transplantation Network (OPTN)/ Scientific Registry of Transplant Recipients (SRTR) Annual Report [15]. Reprinted from Magee *et al.* [14] with permission.

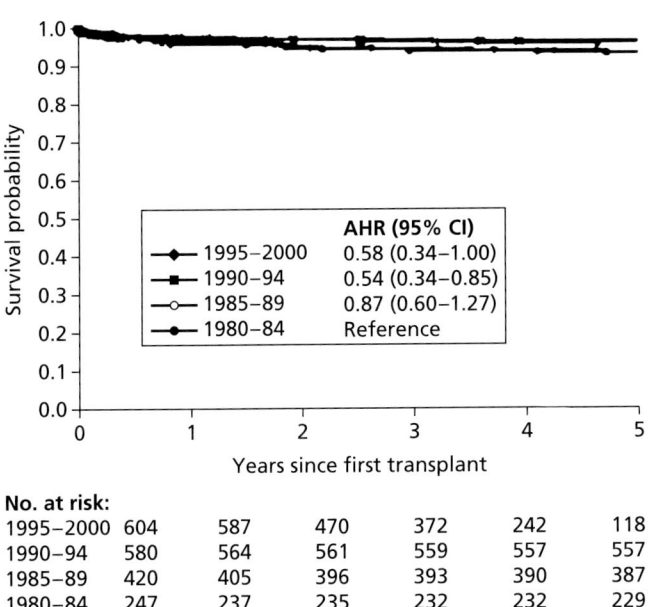

No. at risk:

1995–2000	604	587	470	372	242	118
1990–94	580	564	561	559	557	557
1985–89	420	405	396	393	390	387
1980–84	247	237	235	232	232	229

Fig. 21.5 Probability of patient survival in recipients of a first renal transplant aged 0–19 years by cohort (adjusted for age, gender and donor type). The relative risk of death was expressed as adjusted hazards ratio (AHR). Reprinted from van der Hiejden *et al.* [20] with permission.

infection now exceeds the risk resulting from acute rejection in the first 24 months post-transplant [21].

CONCLUSIONS

Outcomes in pediatric kidney transplantation, including acute rejection rates, graft and patient survival have improved dramatically in the last decade. These improvements are in part related to the development of newer immunosuppressive medications and advances in transplantation immunobiology, but the use of pediatric kidney transplantation databases has also allowed the identification of risk factors specific for pediatric patients which, in turn, has allowed changes in clinical practice and more focused research that have likely contributed greatly to the recent improvements. Areas of concern include the poorer outcomes seen in black and adolescent patients, and further study is needed to identify the factors associated with the poorer outcomes in these patients.

REFERENCES

1 Benfield MR, McDonald RA, Bartosh S, Ho PL, Harmon W. Changing trends in pediatric transplantation: 2001 Annual Report of the North American Pediatric Renal Transplant Cooperative Study. *Pediatr Transplant* 2003;7:321–35.

2 Benfield MR. Current status of kidney transplant: update 2003. *Pediatr Clin North Am* 2003;50:1301–34.

3 Seikaly M, Ho PL, Emmett L, Tejani A. The 12th Annual Report of the North American Pediatric Renal Transplant Cooperative: Renal transplantation from 1987 through 1998. *Pediatr Transplant* 2001;5:215–31.

4 Tejani AH, Stablein DM, Sullivan EK, *et al.* The impact of donor source, recipient age, pre-operative immunotherapy and induction therapy on early and late acute rejections in children: a report of the North American Pediatric Renal Transplant Cooperative Study (NAPRTCS). *Pediatr Transplant* 1998;23:318–24.

5 McDonald R, Ho PL, Stablein DM, Tejani A, North American Pediatric Renal Transplant Cooperative Study (NAPRTCS). Rejection profile of recent pediatric renal transplant recipients compared with historical controls: a report of the North American Pediatric Renal Transplant Cooperative Study (NAPRTCS). *Am J Transplant* 2001;1:55–60.

6 Womer KL, Vella JP, Sayegh MH. Chronic allograft dysfunction: mechanisms and new approached to therapy. *Semin Nephrol* 2000;20:126–47.

7 Tejani A, Sullivan EK. The impact of acute rejection on chronic rejection: a report of the North American Pediatric Renal Transplant Cooperative Study. *Pediatr Transplant* 2000;**4**:107–11.

8 Tejani A, Cortes L, Stablein D. Clinical correlates of chronic rejection in pediatric renal transplantation: a report of the North American Pediatric Renal Transplant Cooperative Study. *Transplantation* 1996;**61**:1054–8.

9 Guyot C, Nguyen JM, Cochat P, *et al*. Risk factors for chronic rejection in pediatric renal allograft recipients. *Pediatr Nephrol* 1996;**10**:723–7.

10 Birk PE, Matas AJ, Gillingham KJ, *et al*. Risk factors for chronic rejection in pediatric renal transplant recipients: a single center experience. *Pediatr Nephrol* 1997;**11**:395–8.

11 Broyer M, Charbit M, Lebihan M, *et al*. Loss of graft by chronic rejection in a series of pediatric kidney transplantation: predictive value of biopsy. *Transplant Proc* 1998;**30**:2815.

12 Tejani A, Ho PL, Emmett L, Stablein DM. Reduction in acute rejections decreases chronic rejection graft failure in children: a report of the North American Pediatric Renal Transplant Cooperative Study (NAPRTCS). *Am J Transplant* 2002;**2**:142–7.

13 Groothoff JW, Cransberg K, Offringa M, *et al*. Long-term follow-up of renal transplantation in children: a Dutch Cohort Study. *Transplantation* 2004;**78**:453–60.

14 Magee JC, Bucuvalas JC, Farmer DG, *et al*. Pediatric transplantation. *Am J Transplant* 2004;**4**(Suppl 9):54–71.

15 2003 OPTN/SRTR Annual Report: Transplant Data 1993–2002. HHS/HRSA/SPB/DOT;UNOS; URREA. www.ustransplant.org

16 Shaw RJ, Palmer L, Blasey C, Sarwal M. A typology of non-adherence in pediatric renal transplant recipients. *Pediatr Transplant* 2003;**7**:489–93.

17 Smith JM, Ho PL, McDonald RA, North American Pediatric Renal Transplant Cooperative Study. Renal transplant outcomes in adolescents: a report of the North American Pediatric Renal Transplant Cooperative Study. *Pediatr Transplant* 2002;**6**:493–9.

18 Singh A, Stablein D, Tejani A. Risk factors for vascular thrombosis in pediatric renal transplantation: a special report of the North American Pediatric Renal Transplant Cooperative Study. *Transplantation* 1997;**63**:1263–7.

19 Baum MA, Ho M, Stablein D, Alexander SR, North American Pediatric Renal Transplant Cooperative Study. Outcome of renal transplantation in adolescents with focal segmental glomerulosclerosis. *Pediatr Transplant* 2002;**6**:488–92.

20 van der Hiejden BJ, van Dijk PCW, Verrier-Jones K, Jager KJ, Briggs JD. Renal replacement therapy in children: data from 12 registries in Europe. *Pediatr Nephrol* 2004;**19**:213–21.

21 Dharnidharka VR, Stablein DM, Harmon WE. Post-transplant infections now exceed acute rejection as cause for hospitalization: a report of the NAPRTCS. *Am J Transplant* 2004;**3**:384–9.

Liver Transplantation

22 Historical Notes

Silvio Nadalin, Massimo Malagó and Christoph E. Broelsch

The history of pediatric liver transplantation (LT) has spanned more than 50 years. Experimental work in the laboratory has been critical to each major step in the evolution of liver surgery and LT. Evidence obtained through animal models has been transferred to the clinic and, conversely, problems encountered in patients have been brought back to the animal laboratory for clarification. This flux has been continuous for almost 50 years and resulted in enormous technical developments, improved immunosuppression and clarification of previously enigmatic physiologic principles. Essential components of the success in this field have included advances in surgical techniques, organ preservation and transplant immunology as well as perioperative care of the transplant patient.

LT is the culmination of a long history of innovations made by liver surgeons based on hemorrhage control, appreciating the occurrence of regeneration and understanding the anatomy of the liver [1]. Resective and transplant liver surgery influenced each other reciprocally during their historic evolutions: advances in liver transplantation surgery were based on the evolution of the surgical technique of liver resection, and innovative concepts in oncologic liver surgery were developed in the light of new technical features used for liver transplantation.

The first evocation of the concept of liver transplantation was in 1951 by Lortat-Jakob during his studies of right hepatectomy [2,3]. He understood that the ability of the surgeon to remove a large volume of liver tissue safely depended not only on a detailed knowledge of the anatomy, but also on the extraordinary capacity of the liver to regenerate after resection. In this way he anticipated what would become some of the basic principles of segmental LT.

Almost 30 years later, the well-established technique of full-size LT led Pichlmayr to extend the limits of standard resective liver surgery accepted at the time. By combining the techniques of LT and major liver surgery, he advanced the now well-know techniques of *in situ* and *ex situ* major liver resections [4–7].

Contemporaneously, expertise in standard oncologic liver resection based on the segmental anatomy of the liver became regarded as an unequivocal prerequisite for the performance of segmental LT at the beginning of the 1980s. Conversely, the growing experiences in segmental liver transplantation improved the anatomic and hemodynamic knowledge of the liver, permitting the performance of extended liver resections starting in the late 1990s [8–10].

EXPERIMENTAL BACKGROUND AND EVOLUTION OF LIVER TRANSPLANTATION

Lortat-Jakob first alluded to the concept of liver transplantation during his 1951 studies on right hepatectomy [2,3].

Heterotopic liver transplantation

Transplantation of the whole liver was first reported in 1955 by Welch, who described the heterotopic insertion of an auxiliary hepatic allograft into the right pelvis of non-immunosuppressed dogs [11]. The clinical significance of auxiliary heterotopic LT lies in its use as a method of temporary hepatic support in potentially reversible liver failure or as the first step of eventual staged and easier method of liver transplantation. Because of the lack of immunosuppression and the exclusion of the graft from splanchnic circulation (the vascular anastomoses were performed by connecting the graft to iliac vessels only), shrinkage of the transplanted liver was observed within a short time, probably secondary to lack of hepatotrophic substances.

Physiologic and hemodynamic studies followed, proposing various models of auxiliary heterotopic LT aimed at avoiding the atrophy of the graft observed by Welch *et al.* [12–16]. Slapak *et al.* [17,18] finally demonstrated that the atrophy of the graft (i.e. Welch's model) was not secondary to a lack of trophic portal substances but mainly secondary to a low vascular flow situation. According to this observation, Wexler *et al.* [19] later developed an auxiliary LT model *without* portal blood flow or portocaval shunt with the expectation that the host liver function would not be impaired as a result of portal diversion, and potential recovery and regeneration of the host liver would be possible.

Orthotopic liver transplantation

In 1958, Moore et al. [20] described the standard technique of canine orthotopic liver transplantation.

The early 1960s began the era of orthotopic liver replacement based on the importance of portal revascularization of the graft. The field was soon divided into two major schools, each with a different focus. The first school, guided by Moore in Boston (fellow, Sir Roy Calne), was most concentrated on the technical feasibility of the transplantation in animals without any adjuvant treatment. The second school, guided by Starzl (in Miami first and then in Chicago) studied the consequences of substraction of portal flow on liver growth ("Eck fistula model"). After the meeting of the two schools in White Sulphur Spring (April 1960), Starzl moved to Denver (Colorado University) with an international team of experts to investigate various areas of liver transplantation: technical aspects, graft conservation (Bretschneider), hemodynamic tolerance (Putnam), coagulation (Groth) and immunosuppression (Starzl and Terasaki).

Segmental liver transplantation

At the beginning of the 1960s, Dagradi et al. [21] began studies of liver anatomy, identifying the liver as an assemblement of different sectors, each with anatomic and functional independence based upon its own pedicle of inflow and outflow. From this, he developed the preliminary anatomic studies of segmental ("sectorial") LT with the objective being to use different sectors of the same liver to reach an optimal graft–recipient size match and eventually to obtain segmental grafts from living donors. Based on some principles of auxiliary liver transplantation, Dagradi et al. [22] developed two models of heterotopic segmental LT (i.e. left lateral segments): one in the left hypocondrium and the other in the right iliac fossa. In both situations, they performed different kind of vascular connections – physiologic and nonphysiologic ones – in order to study the hemodynamics of the graft and the competitive system between graft and host liver.

A few years later, Smith [23] discussed the applicability of partial LT from living donor in humans, based on her experimental experience in partial LT in dogs, cats and monkeys. By describing a precise technique of dissection of the donor liver that yielded a left lateral segment, Smith et al. presented for the first time a possible technique of partial left lateral orthotopic LT in the human from a living donor.

In 1982, Bax et al. [24] were the first to report the orthotopic nonauxiliary homotransplantation of a part of the liver in dogs with good long-term survival.

CLINICAL EVOLUTION OF PEDIATRIC LIVER TRANSPLANTATION

Full-size liver transplantation

The first clinical attempt at liver replacement was made by Starzl [25] on March 1, 1963 in a 3-year-old child who had developed end-stage liver disease from biliary atresia, but "he bled to death as we worked desperately to stop the hemorrhage. The operation could not be completed."

This attempt was followed in 1963 by transplantation of four adult patients who all died, after an otherwise successful transplant, from pulmonary embolism emanating from clots formed in the veno-venous bypass tubing. It was the beginning of a self-imposed moratorium of more than 3 years, which they used in the surgical laboratory for refining preservation techniques and immunosuppressive therapy.

The trials were resumed in 1967. Kempe, Chairman of Pediatrics at the University of Colorado, supported the trials. Starzl et al. [26] performed the next eight transplantations in infants and children. All survived surgery; four died after 2–6 months from the development of gangrene in a portion of the transplanted liver with infection and lethal sepsis. This series of fatal complications was attributed to inadequate immunosuppression, followed by rejection. The other four children had a remarkably long survival time. Two of them who had been transplanted for liver cancer died of recurrence more than 1 year post-transplant; the third one, whose original disease was biliary atresia, survived 2.5 years before dying from chronic rejection. The last patient was transplanted on January 20, 1970; she became the longest surviving recipient of a liver, being currently 32.5 years post-transplant, off medication for about 8 years (T.E. Starzl, personal communication, 2002). Her original disease was biliary atresia with an incidental hepatocellular cancer which never recurred.

Between March 1963 and July 1976, 111 LTs were performed but with 1-year survival of only 28%. Causes of such poor results were technical and medical problems (80%) (i.e. thrombosis, hemorrhage, air embolism and biliary complication) and acute rejection (20%) [27].

From July 1976 to December 1977, after technical and diagnostic improvements the pediatric and adult 1-year survival rate doubled from 34% to 62% and from 20% to 41%, respectively.

Based on these improved results, the development of other liver transplant centers was undertaken. In Europe, the first attempt at liver transplantation in a 10-month-old child with biliary atresia was performed on June 6, 1968 in Cambridge, UK, by Sir Roy Calne (who made many research contributions in transplantation immunology and pioneered the development of kidney and liver transplantation in Europe). Like Starzl's first attempt, the child died during surgery. The first successful liver transplantation in Europe was performed by Otte [28] on March 17, 1971 in a 17-month-old child with biliary atresia. The child recovered uneventfully until he developed acute rejection, which was reversed by steroids; sadly he died 7 weeks after transplantation from massive intrathoracic bleeding caused by a liver biopsy. A long-term moratorium followed this case until the LT program was finally resumed in 1984. The four children transplanted that year are currently alive, including the first patient to receive a reduced liver graft who is currently, worldwide, the longest survivor with her original cut-down liver [29].

All the earliest LT patients were treated with a drug regimen that had been developed for kidney grafts: azathioprine and steroids, with sometimes the addition of antilymphocyte globulins. Because of inadequate immunosuppression, long-term survival was observed in less than one-third of patients. At the beginning of the 1980s, the introduction of cyclosporine led to a significant increase of graft and patient survival rates. By March 1980, liver trials with cyclosporine A immunosuppression began in Denver. Twelve patients entered the study between March and September 1980; 11 patients lived for 1 year or longer [30].

In October 1986, the eight centers of Europe and the USA that had experience with at least 20 pediatric liver transplants (Boston, Brussels, Cambridge, Dallas, Hannover, Minneapolis, Pittsburgh and Los Angeles) met for an update on the actual status of pediatric LT. Long-term (> 1 year) patient survival reached 57–83%; all centers used cyclosporine-based primary immunosuppression; the major indications – biliary atresia being the most frequent one – were already clearly delineated.

Since the implementation of LT for end-stage liver disease, there has been a strong disparity between organ demand and the cadaveric donor supply for children. This initially resulted in a pretransplant mortality for children listed for LT of approximately 25% and was disproportionally high compared with adult patients [31]. The problem of size mismatch and the different epidemiology of pediatric donorship and terminally diseased children were responsible for the disparity [32]. This stimulated the development of technical innovations, based on the segmental anatomy of the liver, which facilitated transplanting parts of a large cadaveric donor liver into smaller recipients (i.e. reduced-size LT, split LT and living donor LT).

Reduced size liver transplantation

The first step to solve the size mismatch problem was the introduction of reduced-size liver transplantation (RSLT). With this approach, after explantation from a cadaver donor, a liver resection is performed on the back table to tailor the size of the graft to that of a single recipient. The remaining resected liver tissue is discarded. In pediatric RSLT, either the left lateral segment (Couinaud's segments II–III) or the full left lobe (Couinaud's segments II–IV) is usually retained.

The technique was originally described by Bismuth and Houssin [33], was validated in the late 1980s and later became standard practice worldwide, with 1-year survival rates of approximately 80% [34–38].

Although RSLT increases the number of pediatric donor organs, it does not increase the total number of organs available for transplantation; indeed, it actually disadvantages the adult recipient pool, which is continuously growing [39].

Split liver transplantation

The disadvantage of RSLT (a discarded liver segment) was solved by the introduction of split liver techniques. Split liver transplantation (SLT) evolved from the RSLT and was first described by Pichlmayr et al. [40]. This technique allowed the preparation of two split grafts by dividing all vascular and biliary structures and parenchyma for the benefit of two recipients: one recipient receiving a right lobe graft, the other receiving a left lobe (segments 2–4) or left lateral one (segments 2–3) (usually the right lobe is transplanted into an adult and the left lobe or the left lateral segment into a child).

In 1989, Pichlmayr et al. [41,42] were the first to report a case of transplanting one donor liver into two recipients. The first series was reported by Broelsch et al. [43] at the University of Chicago and the technique was further validated in the early 1990s [44–46].

Technically, SLT is a complex procedure that can be performed in two ways, both of which require precise knowledge of the liver anatomy and extensive experience with liver resection techniques and all technical modalities of liver graft implantation. In the ex situ technique [43,45], the splitting is performed on the (ex vivo) back table, similar to the RSLT technique. The technique for procuring a left lateral segment from a live donor, which has been shown to be safe and reproducible, led the Hamburg team to adopt an in situ split in heart-beating cadaveric donors [47]; they were soon followed by the UCLA group [48]. Major advantages of this technique are the perfect hemostasis of the cut surface, less biliary complications and shorter back table surgery with the inherent risk of rewarming of the graft.

Today, morbidity and mortality have been shown to be comparable between the two procurement methods [49]. Unfortunately, the wider application of the split technique is still hindered by the lack of experience and unwillingness of some centers to split every suitable donor liver [50]. Altogether, SLT significantly increases the donor pool and has had an important impact on the waiting list and on the outcome of pediatric liver transplantation [50–54].

Recent comprehensive studies confirm that SLTs generally lead to less favorable results for individual recipients, but also lead to more individuals getting the benefit of a liver transplant. While initially holding great promise and being adopted as standard policy by many pediatric transplant centers, early experience demonstrated a higher incidence of technical complications and decreased graft and patient survival rate in recipients of right lobe grafts. Unfortunately, detailed extensive data are not yet available.

Living donor liver transplantation

Pediatric living donor liver transplantation (LDLT) originated as a response to the disparity in adult and pediatric waiting list times, which accounted for pediatric waiting list mortality rates exceeding 25% in major pediatric liver transplant centers [36]. The development of LDLT in USA and Europe has been driven by the shortage of donor organs despite the innovative techniques for cadaveric liver transplantation such as RSLT and SLT [55]. Additionally, LDLT was the only option in Japan where organ procurement from brain-dead donors was not legal until recently.

From a technical point of view, LDLT was first proposed by Dagradi *et al.* [21,22] as heterotopic transplantation and successively by Smith [23] in 1969. LDLT was first reported in two patients by Raia *et al.* [56] in 1989. Both recipients died shortly after the procedure of medical complications but lived long enough to establish the technical feasibility of the procedure. This was soon followed by a report from Strong *et al.* [57] in Australia, where the first successful transplant of a child using the mother's left lobe was performed in July 1989. Before the initial reports by Raia and Strong, an extensive ethical appraisal of the concept of LDLT was in progress at the University of Chicago, where clinical ethicists and transplant physicians convened a year-long series of seminars and discussions open to the entire university community [58]. The introduction of LDLT required a balance between the presumed benefits of an elective transplant for the recipient and the risk of morbidity or even mortality of LDLT. At the beginning, the principles of equipoise and coercion were the main ethical problems the Chicago group had to deal with for the introduction of pediatric LDLT [58,59]. From these meetings, a proposal was submitted to the institutional review board and a successful LDLT was performed by Broelsch in November 1989. He subsequently initiated the systematic use of LDLT in children with end-stage liver disease [60]. Between November 1989 and July 1996, 100 LDLTs were performed, with 1-year patient and graft survival rates of 88% and 72%, respectively. Similar results were reproduced worldwide, confirming the effectiveness of the procedure [61,62].

LDLT has several advantages for the child and the transplant population as a whole. First, it increases the number of organs directly available for the pediatric population. Second, most recipients receive their transplant on an elective basis and thus should incur lower morbidity and mortality rates and decrease overall cost. Third, the minimal cold ischemia time and the use of healthy donors may contribute to the absence of primary nonfunction.

The application of LDLT for children with end-stage liver disease profoundly impacted organ waiting list times and markedly decreased waiting list mortality [63]. Pediatric LDLT is now accepted therapy for children throughout the world and frequently accounts for 50% or more of all pediatric liver transplantations performed at regional referral centers [28,63].

Despite the impressive results of LDLT, considerable debate persists concerning donor safety. Risks to the donor include those associated with invasive presurgical testing and the surgical procedure. These risks are accepted by the potential donors in exchange for the knowledge that a child's life may be saved without the uncertainty of the cadaveric waiting list. Up-to-date donor outcomes from multiple centers have been excellent [64,65].

The development of segmental hepatic grafts has expanded the supply of size-appropriate organs, allowing children who otherwise would have died on the waiting list the opportunity to undergo LT. Recently, the association between graft type, recipient age and graft survival was better defined. Among children < 3 years of age, LDLT graft provides superior graft survival compared with RLT and SLT. In older children, it appears that cadaveric organs may offer better outcome [66,67]. While reduced and split grafts produce overall inferior outcomes in the national experience, they remain an important and necessary tool in the pediatric center's armamentarium. They provide appropriately sized grafts in children without a suitable living donor and for those for whom no cadaveric pediatric donor is available, and they can yield an excellent outcome in experienced centers. It is apparent that the technical complexities and perioperative events surrounding these procedures have significant impact on outcome. This emphasizes the importance of experience, attention to continued technical refinement, and judicious selection of appropriate donors for specific recipients.

Until artificial organs or xenotransplantation becomes a reality, thus rendering operating on a healthy subject part of medical history, LDLT will remain essential, in conjunction with cadaveric transplantation, in the cure of patients affected by end-stage liver disease [68,69].

REFERENCES

1 Hardy KJ. Liver surgery: the past 2000 years. *Aust N Z J Surg* 1990;**60**:811–7.

2 Lortat-Jacob JL, Robert HG. Well defined technic for right hepatectomy. *Presse Med* 1952;**60**:549–51.

3 Belghiti J. The first anatomical right resection announcing liver donation. *J Hepatol* 2003;**39**:475–9.

4 Pichlmayr R, Weimann A, Oldhafer KJ, *et al*. Role of liver transplantation in the treatment of unresectable liver cancer. *World J Surg* 1995;**19**:807–13.

5 Oldhafer KJ, Lang H, Schlitt HJ, *et al*. Long-term experience after *ex situ* liver surgery. *Surgery* 2000;**127**:520–7.

6 Pichlmayr R, Grosse H, Hauss J, *et al*. Technique and preliminary results of extracorporeal liver surgery (bench procedure) and of surgery on the *in situ* perfused liver. *Br J Surg* 1990;**77**:21–6.

7 Pichlmayr R, Gubernatis G, Lamesch P, Raygrotzki S, Hauss J. The European liver surgery topic: recent developments in liver surgery (*in situ* protection and *ex situ* operation). *Langenbecks Arch Chir Suppl II Verh Dtsch Ges Chir* 1989:257–61.

8 Lang H, Radtke A, Liu C, et al. Extended left hepatectomy: modified operation planning based on three-dimensional visualization of liver anatomy. *Langenbecks Arch Surg* 2004;389:306–10.

9 Lang H, Sotiropoulos GC, Malago M, Broelsch CE. Mesohepatectomy, caudate lobectomy and resection of hilar bifurcation with biliary reconstruction by 6 hepaticojejunostomies for Klatskin tumor. *Hepatogastroenterology* 2003;50:1327–9.

10 Lang H, Sotiropoulos GC, Fruhauf NR, et al. Extended hepatectomy for intrahepatic cholangiocellular carcinoma (ICC): when is it worthwhile? Single center experience with 27 resections in 50 patients over a 5-year period. *Ann Surg* 2005;241:134–43.

11 Goodrich EO Jr, Welch HF, Nelson JA, Beecher TS, Welch CS. Homotransplantation of the canine liver. *Surgery* 1956;39:244–51.

12 Gliedman ML, Pangan J, Minkowitz S, Popowitz L, Karlson KE. Heterotopic liver transplantation after liver damage. *Trans Am Soc Artif Intern Organs* 1965;11:205–12.

13 van der Heyde MN, Vink M, Stol H, Dicke HW, Schalm SW. Heterotopic auxiliary liver transplantation. 3. Functional competition: cause of atrophy of the auxiliary liver transplant. *Arch Chir Neerl* 1966;18:293–8.

14 Hagihara P, Absolon KB. Experimental studies on homologous heterotopic liver transplantation. *Surg Gynecol Obstet* 1964;119:1297–304.

15 Marchioro TL, Porter KA, Dickinson TC, Faris TD, Starzl TE. Physiologic requirements for auxiliary liver homotransplantation. *Surg Gynecol Obstet* 1965;121:17–31.

16 Slapak M, Beaudoin JG, Lee HM, Hume DM. Auxiliary liver homotransplantation: a new technique and an evaluation of current techniques. *Arch Surg* 1970;100:31–41.

17 Slapak M, Wexler M, Mizumoto R, et al. The role of arterial portal and systemic venous blood on regeneration of the canine liver. *Br J Surg* 1970;57:392.

18 Tretbar LL, Beven EG, Hermann RE. The effects of portacaval shunt and portal flow occlusion on canine auxiliary liver homotransplants. *Surgery* 1967;61:733–8.

19 Wexler MJ, Farkouh EF, Farrer PA, Slapak M, MacLean LD. Auxiliary liver transplantation: a successful model without portal blood or portacaval shunt. *Ann Surg* 1972;175:357–74.

20 Moore FD, Wheele HB, Demissianos HV, et al. Experimental whole-organ transplantation of the liver and of the spleen. *Ann Surg* 1960;152:374–87.

21 Dagradi A, Marzoli GP, Radin S, et al. Possibilities of sectional liver transplantation in man. *Langenbecks Arch Chir* 1968;322:533–7.

22 Dagradi A, Marzoli GP, Gamba A, et al. Experimental auxiliary liver transplantations: sectorial, total and in plurivisceral association. *Helv Chir Acta* 1968;35:309–20.

23 Smith B. Segmental liver transplantation from a living donor. *J Pediatr Surg* 1969;4:126–32.

24 Bax NM, Vermeire BM, Dubois N, et al. Orthotopic nonauxiliary homotransplantation of part of the liver in dogs. *J Pediatr Surg* 1982;17:906–13.

25 Starzl TE. *Memoirs of a Transplant Surgeon. The Puzzle People.* Pittsburgh; 1992.

26 Starzl TE, Groth CG, Brettschneider L, et al. Orthotopic homotransplantation of the human liver. *Ann Surg* 1968;168:392–415.

27 Starzl TE, Koep LJ, Halgrimson CG, et al. Fifteen years of clinical liver transplantation. *Gastroenterology* 1979;77:375–88.

28 Otte JB. History of pediatric liver transplantation. Where are we coming from? Where do we stand? *Pediatr Transplant* 2002;6:378–87.

29 Otte JB, de Ville de Goyet J, Sokal E, et al. Size reduction of the donor liver is a safe way to alleviate the shortage of size-matched organs in pediatric liver transplantation. *Ann Surg* 1990;211:146–57.

30 Starzl TE, Klintmalm GB, Porter KA, Iwatsuki S, Schroter GP. Liver transplantation with use of cyclosporin A and prednisone. *N Engl J Med* 1981;305:266–9.

31 Malago M, Rogiers X, Broelsch CE. Reduced-size hepatic allografts. *Annu Rev Med* 1995;46:507–12.

32 Emond JC, Whitington PF, Thistlethwaite JR, Alonso EM, Broelsch CE. Reduced-size orthotopic liver transplantation: use in the management of children with chronic liver disease. *Hepatology* 1989;10:867–72.

33 Bismuth H, Houssin D. Reduced-sized orthotopic liver graft in hepatic transplantation in children. *Surgery* 1984;95:367–70.

34 Strong R, Ong TH, Pillay P, et al. A new method of segmental orthotopic liver transplantation in children. *Surgery* 1988;104:104–7.

35 Broelsch CE, Emond JC, Thistlethwaite JR, et al. Liver transplantation, including the concept of reduced-size liver transplants in children. *Ann Surg* 1988;208:410–20.

36 Broelsch CE, Emond JC, Thistlethwaite JR, et al. Liver transplantation with reduced-size donor organs. *Transplantation* 1988;45:519–24.

37 Ringe B, Pichlmayr R, Burdelski M. A new technique of hepatic vein reconstruction in partial liver transplantation. *Transpl Int* 1988;1:30–5.

38 Ong TH, Lynch SV, Pillay SP, et al. Reduced-size orthotopic liver transplantation in children: an experience with seven cases. *Transplant Proc* 1989;21:2443–4.

39 Busuttil RW, Goss JA. Split liver transplantation. *Ann Surg* 1999;229:313–21.

40 Pichlmayr R, Ringe B, Gubernatis G, Hauss J, Bunzendhal H. Transplantation of a donor liver to two recipients (splitting transplantation): a new method in the further development of segmental liver transplantation. *Langenbecks Arch Chir* 1988;373:127–30.

41 Pichlmayr R, Ringe B, Gubernatis G, Hauss J, Bunzendahl H. Transplantation of a donor liver to 2 recipients (splitting transplantation): a new method in the further development of segmental liver transplantation. *Langenbecks Arch Chir* 1988;373:127–30.

42 Pichlmayr R, Bretschneider HJ, Kirchner E, et al. Ex situ operation on the liver: a new possibility in liver surgery. *Langenbecks Arch Chir* 1988;373:122–6.

43 Broelsch CE, Emond JC, Whitington PF, et al. Application of reduced-size liver transplants as split grafts, auxiliary orthotopic grafts, and living related segmental transplants. *Ann Surg* 1990;212:368–75; discussion 375–7.

44 Bismuth H, Morino M, Castaing D, et al. Emergency orthotopic liver transplantation in two patients using one donor liver. *Br J Surg* 1989;76:722–4.

45 Otte JB, de Ville de Goyet J, Alberti D, Balladur P, de Hemptinne B. The concept and technique of the split liver in clinical transplantation. *Surgery* 1990;**107**:605–12.

46 Otte JB, de Ville de Goyet J, Reding R, *et al*. Pediatric liver transplantation: from the full-size liver graft to reduced, split, and living related liver transplantation. *Pediatr Surg Int* 1998;**13**:308–18.

47 Rogiers X, Malago M, Gawad K, *et al*. *In situ* splitting of cadaveric livers: the ultimate expansion of a limited donor pool. *Ann Surg* 1996;**224**:331–9; discussion 339–41.

48 Goss JA, Yersiz H, Shackleton CR, *et al*. *In situ* splitting of the cadaveric liver for transplantation. *Transplantation* 1997;**64**:871–7.

49 Azoulay D, Astarcioglu I, Bismuth H, *et al*. Split-liver transplantation. The Paul Brousse policy. *Ann Surg* 1996;**224**:737–46; discussion 746–8.

50 Colledan M, Segalin A, Spada M, *et al*. Liberal policy of split liver for pediatric liver transplantation: a single centre experience. *Transpl Int* 2000;**13**(Suppl 1):S131–3.

51 Broering DC, Mueller L, Ganschow R, *et al*. Is there still a need for living-related liver transplantation in children? *Ann Surg* 2001;**234**:713–21; discussion 721–2.

52 Broering DC, Kim JS, Mueller T, *et al*. One hundred thirty-two consecutive pediatric liver transplants without hospital mortality: lessons learned and outlook for the future. *Ann Surg* 2004;**240**:1002–12.

53 Spada M, Gridelli B, Colledan M, *et al*. Extensive use of split liver for pediatric liver transplantation: a single-center experience. *Liver Transpl* 2000;**6**:415–28.

54 Gridelli B, Spada M, Petz W, *et al*. Split-liver transplantation eliminates the need for living-donor liver transplantation in children with end-stage cholestatic liver disease. *Transplantation* 2003;**75**:1197–203.

55 Trotter JF, Wachs M, Everson GT, Kam I. Adult-to-adult transplantation of the right hepatic lobe from a living donor. *N Engl J Med* 2002;**346**:1074–82.

56 Raia S, Nery JR, Mies S. Liver transplantation from live donors. *Lancet* 1989;**2**:497.

57 Strong RW, Lynch SV, Ong TH, *et al*. Successful liver transplantation from a living donor to her son. *N Engl J Med* 1990;**322**:1505–7.

58 Singer PA, Siegler M, Whitington PF, *et al*. Ethics of liver transplantation with living donors. *N Engl J Med* 1989;**321**:620–2.

59 Singer PA, Lantos JD, Whitington PF, Broelsch CE, Siegler M. Equipoise and the ethics of segmental liver transplantation. *Clin Res* 1988;**36**:539–45.

60 Broelsch CE, Whitington PF, Emond JC, *et al*. Liver transplantation in children from living related donors: surgical techniques and results. *Ann Surg* 1991;**214**:428–37; discussion 437–9.

61 Reding R, de Goyet Jde V, Delbeke I, *et al*. Pediatric liver transplantation with cadaveric or living related donors: comparative results in 90 elective recipients of primary grafts. *J Pediatr* 1999;**134**:280–6.

62 Inomata Y, Tanaka K, Uemoto S, *et al*. Living donor liver transplantation: an 8-year experience with 379 consecutive cases. *Transplant Proc* 1999;**31**:381.

63 Emond JC, Heffron TG, Kortz EO, *et al*. Improved results of living-related liver transplantation with routine application in a pediatric program. *Transplantation* 1993;**55**:835–40.

64 Renz JF, Roberts JP. Long-term complications of living donor liver transplantation. *Liver Transpl* 2000;**6**(Suppl 2):S73–6.

65 Lo CM. Complications and long-term outcome of living liver donors: a survey of 1508 cases in five Asian centers. *Transplantation* 2003;**75**(Suppl):S12–5.

66 Emond JC. Living donor liver transplantation in children: what to recommend? *Am J Transplant* 2004;**4**:293–4.

67 Abt PL, Rapaport-Kelz R, Desai NM, *et al*. Survival among pediatric liver transplant recipients: impact of segmental grafts. *Liver Transpl* 2004;**10**:1287–93.

68 Broelsch CE, Testa G, Alexandrou A, Malago M. Living related liver transplantation: medical and social aspects of a controversial therapy. *Gut* 2002;**50**:143–5.

69 Surman OS. The ethics of partial-liver donation. *N Engl J Med* 2002;**346**:1038.

23 Recipient Characteristics

Udeme D. Ekong, Estella M. Alonso and Peter F. Whitington

In making the decision to proceed with transplantation, the benefits must be carefully weighed against the potential morbidity and mortality associated with the procedure and ongoing care. This chapter provides an overview of the indications for pediatric liver transplantation and discusses specific aspects of some of the more common diseases leading to liver transplantation in children.

GENERAL INDICATIONS FOR LIVER TRANSPLANTATION IN CHILDREN

Diseases that progress to liver failure account for over 90% of pediatric liver transplants performed. Table 23.1 shows data from Studies of Pediatric Liver Transplantation (SPLIT) where primary liver disease diagnosis is summarized. Cholestatic disease comprises 54.4% of the total population and is the most common disease among both registered and transplanted patients; with 39.6% of patients specifically diagnosed with biliary atresia. Of the 613 children transplanted with biliary atresia as the primary liver disease diagnosis, 84.2% were less than 5 years of age. Metabolic disease was the primary diagnosis in 12.5% of patients, fulminant liver failure in 11.8% and cirrhosis in 9.7%.

Biliary atresia is by far the most frequent single indication in all series. Parenchymal liver diseases, including chronic hepatitis and certain metabolic diseases, and fulminant hepatic failure are also common indications. Cirrhosis is neither a specific disease entity nor a general indication for transplantation. It is an anatomic diagnosis with functional implications. Determining when a transplant should be performed involves estimating the functional reserve of the cirrhotic liver and its potential for supporting life of reasonable quality. Cirrhosis is an indication for immediate liver transplantation when there is evidence of functional hepatic decompensation. Evidence of decompensation includes coagulopathy, ascites, frequent or massive gastrointestinal hemorrhage, malnutrition and growth failure, and frequent severe bacterial infections.

Growth failure is a transplant indication that warrants further discussion. Growth is a sensitive measure of liver function in childhood. The integrated metabolic functions of the liver permit growth to proceed, and failure of metabolic function is often first manifest as growth failure. The infant with biliary atresia and cirrhosis may continue to grow reasonably normally, perhaps with some nutritional support, until the liver begins to decompensate. At that time, growth will cease and no effort at nutritional support will cause it to resume. The infant cannot improve as a candidate for transplantation beyond that time, even though growth arrest may precede other evidence of decompensation by several months. The point of growth arrest is, therefore, the ideal time to transplant an infant with biliary atresia and cirrhosis. Caution is required when making this assessment. If growth failure is observed in an infant with biliary atresia and otherwise normal liver function (e.g. a normal bilirubin), the patient may have a correctable cause of growth failure, such as postsurgical bowel disease or bile diversion leading to malabsorption.

Patients known to have cirrhosis should be followed at regular intervals to monitor growth, progression of their disease and to determine the optimal time for transplantation. If a child will receive living donor liver transplantation then the procedure should be performed for the previously mentioned indications. Patients without this option are dependent on allocation through the United Network of Organ Sharing (UNOS). Prior to 2002, priority for deceased donor liver allocation in the UNOS system was primarily based on waiting time. Various ranking systems were used to establish broad categories of medical urgency and patients within these categories were distinguished only by waiting time. Under those circumstances, physicians frequently listed their patients for transplantation weeks to months before the procedure was essential to ensure that the candidate would have accumulated adequate waiting time when the need became more urgent. In February 2002, UNOS adopted the Model for End-Stage Liver Disease (MELD) and Pediatric End-Stage Liver Disease (PELD) allocation system, which was designed to prioritize patients by acuity of illness rather than waiting time [1–3].

Table 23.1 Primary diagnosis by transplant status. Studies of Pediatric Liver Transplantation (SPLIT) 2003.

Primary diagnosis	Regd/no Tx ($n = 648$) n	First Tx on registry ($n = 1491$) n
Cholestatic	*343*	*821*
Biliary atresia	235	613
Alagille syndrome	16	45
Byler disease	6	22
Idiopathic cholestasis	15	17
TPN-induced cholestasis	19	28
PSC	25	45
Biliary strictures	1	2
Neonatal hepatitis	14	14
Other	12	35
Fulminant liver failure	*61*	*192*
Acute hepatitis A	0	2
Subacute hepatitis B	0	1
Subacute hepatitis C	2	2
Unknown	40	164
Autoimmune hepatitis	8	7
Subacute	8	4
Other	5	12
Metabolic disease	*84*	*185*
α_1-Antitrypsin deficiency	21	48
Wilson disease	4	15
Tyrosinemia	6	20
Primary hyperoxaluria	7	10
Cystic fibrosis	15	21
Urea cycle defects	7	26
Crigler–Najjar	0	8
Glycogen storage disease	3	8
Neonatal hemochromatosis	10	10
Other	11	19
Tumor	*20*	*76*
Hepatocellular cancer	3	8
Hepatoblastoma	11	53
Hemangioendothelioma	5	10
Other	1	5
Toxicity	*9*	*10*
Accidental OD	0	5
Attempted suicide	5	0
Drug induced	4	5
Cirrhosis	*88*	*123*
Neonatal hepatitis	6	11
Hepatitis B	0	1
Hepatitis C	6	12
Autoimmune hepatitis	34	48
Unknown	28	30
Other	14	21
Other	*43*	*84*
Budd–Chiari syndrome	0	8
Congenital hepatic fibrosis	14	14
Other	29	61

OD, overdose; PSC, primary sclerosing cholangitis; TPN, total parenteral nutrition; Tx, transplant.

MANAGEMENT OF SPECIFIC DISEASES

Cholestatic liver disease

Overall, 1 in 2500 live births is affected with a neonatal cholestatic disorder [4]. *Biliary atresia* is by far the most common cholestatic disease in children, accounting for 50–75% of liver transplants performed [5]. Early diagnosis with an attempt to provide biliary drainage with a Kasai procedure is still recommended. Even when the Kasai procedure is performed before 3 months of age, approximately 75% of children will eventually require transplantation [6,7]. Without a Kasai procedure, children with biliary atresia progress to chronic liver failure with cirrhosis, portal hypertension and malnutrition. With its increasing effectiveness, an argument has been raised as to whether liver transplantation should be the primary therapy, or should only be used after other management efforts fail. Survival statistics following Kasai procedure show that this approach is as good as early transplantation [8–11]. Ten-year survival following a successful portoenterostomy performed before 60–90 days of age at North American and European centers with the most experience is approximately 30–40% [12–14], while 10-year survival following portoenterostomy performed before 60 days of age in Japan approximates 60% [15]. The age at referral of the patient for evaluation is therefore one of the most important factors determining surgical outcome, together with the experience of the center performing the portoenterostomy [16].

Following a Kasai procedure there are three possible outcomes:

1 Good biliary drainage and marked improvement in liver enzymes accompanied by a period of normal growth. Some of these children will present with recurrent cholangitis as infants.

2 No improvement in biliary drainage and progression to end-stage liver disease before 2 years of age.

3 Improvement in biliary flow with reduction of the serum bilirubin but progression to cirrhosis with growth failure, portal hypertension and synthetic function failure as young children [17].

There is no standardized protocol for postoperative treatment of patients with biliary atresia in the USA. Therapeutic options include antibiotic prophylaxis of cholangitis [18]; short courses of corticosteroid pulse therapy for refractory cholangitis [19]; empiric use of ursodeoxycholic acid to stimulate bile flow and as a cytoprotective agent [20]; optimization of nutrition through the use of a medium-chain triglyceride containing infant formula; and prevention of fat-soluble vitamin deficiencies [21].

Some chronic cholestatic disorders of childhood, notably *Alagille syndrome*, produce severe symptoms, but do not progress to end-stage liver disease [22]. When estimating the value of liver transplantation, the morbidity of the liver disease should be weighed carefully against the potential morbidity and mortality of transplantation. Complications such as pruritus, growth failure, bone disease, hypercholesterolemia and xanthomatosis, neuropathy and malnutrition must not only be severe and have a major effect on the patient, they must also be refractory to all other treatment in order to qualify as indications for transplantation. However, it is important to note that while hypercholesterolemia in patients with Alagille syndrome is often refractory to treatment, it does not pose any significant risk for cardiovascular disease, as such it is not a reason for transplantation. We have used partial external biliary diversion (PEBD) for the relief of intractable pruritus and disfiguring xanthomas in Alagille syndrome patients (AGS) who failed conventional medical therapy [23]. PEBD was introduced as a therapy for children with intrahepatic cholestatic diseases 17 years ago by Whitington and Whitington [24]. It is designed to divert a portion of total biliary output via a surgically constructed conduit connecting the dome of the gallbladder to the abdominal skin via an interposed jejunal segment with formation of a stoma. The stoma is created in the right lower quadrant of the abdomen and drains bile directly into a stoma bag to allow for daily disposal (usually 30–150 mL/day) [25]. PEBD alters the enterohepatic recirculation of bile salts in such a way that hepatic excretory function improves. This has proved to be very effective therapy of progressive familial intrahepatic cholestasis (PFIC). However, the pathophysiology of cholestasis in Alagille syndrome is different from that in PFIC, and it is thought that PEBD in Alagille syndrome lowers serum bile salt concentration by causing the bile acid pool to be continuously depleted, and lowers serum cholesterol probably by shunting away bile salts and biliary cholesterol [23]. Given the demonstrated effectiveness of PEBD in a select group of Alagille syndrome patients who had failed medical therapy, and the fact that results of liver transplantation can be unpredictable in Alagille syndrome (45–100%) [26–29], it is reasonable to proceed with PEBD in Alagille syndrome patients who have morbid complications of cholestasis in the absence of progressive liver disease, and who are unresponsive to medical therapy.

Familial cholestatic syndromes are often recessively inherited, with a highly variable natural history, even within the same family [30]. The disease may be present with mild cholestasis and controllable pruritus, or early clinical deterioration with cirrhosis. These children can be managed medically or sometimes with biliary diversion to improve cholestasis and diminish progressive fibrosis [25]. Some children may slowly improve or stabilize as they grow older and never require liver transplantation, while others have their development, sleep patterns and activities of daily life severely impacted by severe pruritus, or severe cholestasis inducing malabsorption with growth failure resulting in the need for liver transplantation [30].

Metabolic diseases

The question of expected quality of life following liver transplantation is paramount in evaluating whether a child with a metabolic disease is a suitable candidate for transplantation. *Urea cycle defects* can be managed with diet and medications, but unexpected hyperammonemic episodes are common and cause brain injury. Liver transplantation can correct hyperammonemia related to metabolic errors involving the urea cycle, but not central nervous system injury. Early diagnosis, aggressive support and early liver transplantation before neurological damage occurs is therefore essential [31].

Tyrosinemia can present as acute liver failure in infancy or with a more insidious onset in childhood. Current approach to treating these patients includes the use of the agent NTBC, [2-(2-nitro-4-trifluoromethylbezoyl)-1-3-cyclohexanedione], which inhibits tyrosine catabolism and reduces formation of succinyl acetone and other toxic intermediates [32,33]. Therapy is usually started as soon as the diagnosis is confirmed, with a positive response being seen in 90% of treated patients. Although NTBC may diminish the risk for hepatocellular carcinoma, treated patients should still be monitored frequently with α-fetoprotein and imaging. Those patients with decompensated cirrhosis and/or signs of hepatocellular carcinoma should be transplanted.

Patients with *Crigler–Najjar* syndrome can be effectively treated for a time with phototherapy and the enteric administration of bilirubin-binding agents. However, the risk for developing kernicterus is great [34], As a result, liver transplantation should be considered before brain damage occurs. Unfortunately, there is no good way to predict when this complication will occur. As a result, these patients are usually managed medically until age 10–12 years, at which time liver transplantation is performed [35–39].

With improvement in the survival of *cystic fibrosis* (CF) patients, advanced liver disease is now considered the third leading cause of death in these patients [40,41]. In a longitudinal study of the epidemiology of liver disease in CF, liver disease was found to occur mainly in the first decade with a prevalence of 18% at 2 years, 29% at 5 years and 41% at 12 years, remaining stable thereafter. Pancreatic insufficiency and history of meconium ileus were the main predictive factors for cystic fibrosis-related liver disease (CF-LD) in that series. Factors such as male gender, cystic fibrosis transmembrane conductance regulator (CFTR) mutation, chronic colonization with *Pseudomonas aeruginosa* and severity of pulmonary disease do not seem to influence the prevalence of liver disease [42]. The primary consequence of liver disease in CF is portal hypertension with massive splenomegaly, hypersplenism, varices and ascites. Although individual complications of CF-LD can be managed temporarily without transplantation, liver transplantation remains the only curative treatment for liver failure [43]. Although there are published reports of liver transplantation and immunosuppression not affecting pulmonary function or infection status [43–47], the experience is not uniform [48].

α$_1$-*Antitrypsin deficiency* is the metabolic disease for which liver transplantation is most frequently performed [49,50].

Most individuals with the genetic defect will have no liver disease and progression to end-stage liver disease in children with PIZZ phenotype occurs only in a minority [51]. Approximately 10% will have neonatal cholestasis which usually resolves after a few months. A small proportion develops macronodular cirrhosis, characteristically before 20 years of age [52]. Liver transplantation has a role only in the patient with hepatic insufficiency or early malignancy. Patients with neonatal cholestasis that resolves should be observed for the onset of cirrhosis with yearly physical and biochemical evaluations.

Wilson disease, if diagnosed early, can be managed medically for long periods with chelating agents. However, should the child present with fulminant liver failure or established cirrhosis, liver transplantation would be indicated [17].

Defects of mitochondrial function, which include defects of fatty acid β-oxidation and oxidative phosphorylation, have variable clinical presentations ranging from mild to severe liver dysfunction and mild to severe central nervous system impairment. The consideration for liver transplantation must be made on an individual basis, depending on the extrahepatic manifestations.

Hepatic tumors

Hepatoblastoma is the most common primary hepatic tumor in childhood accounting for 0.8–2.0% of all pediatric cancers [53]. Unfortunately, more than 50% of patients are unsuitable for radical surgery at diagnosis because of huge intrahepatic extension of the tumor and/or the presence of extrahepatic disease [53]. Data obtained from the Children's Cancer Study Group [54–56] suggested that preoperative chemotherapy could be the best strategy to treat all children with hepatoblastoma, irrespective of the extent of tumor at diagnosis. An international multicenter study, SIOPEL-1, was launched between January 1990 and February 1994 to study the efficacy of preoperative chemotherapy with a cisplatin-based regimen (cisplatin and doxorubicin) [57]. The results showed that complete resection was possible in 77% of patients with a 5-year event-free survival of 66% and a 5-year overall survival of 75% [57]. Some tumors that cannot be primarily resected should be re-evaluated after aggressive chemotherapy. Extensive resection of even 85% of the liver parenchyma can be accomplished with recovery of liver function. In cases where resection is truly not possible, liver transplantation is performed when it is judged that the maximum benefit of chemotherapy has been obtained. Exploratory laparotomy may be useful to evaluate for extrahepatic extension before proceeding with the transplant procedure. This avoids the risk of finding unexpected metastasis at the time of transplantation. Outcomes following liver transplantation for this indication are comparable to transplantation for other diagnoses [58]. Ideal transplant candidates include children with tumors that are completely confined to the liver, but which

are unresectable, despite a definite response to chemotherapy. Furthermore, recent data suggest that children presenting with metastatic hepatoblastoma with lung metastases that clear with chemotherapy [58,59] may have reasonable outcomes as well. The place of post liver transplant chemotherapy in the treatment plan is still uncertain [58].

The outcome of liver transplantation in children with *hepatocellular carcinoma* has been suboptimal. Patients with multifocal disease or singular lesions larger than 5 cm have a high rate of recurrence after liver transplantation, even when treated with adjuvant chemotherapy [60,61]. The prognosis is far better for patients with chronic liver disease or metabolic disease who have tumors just above the limits of detection by ultrasound or computed tomography (CT) scan (0.5–1.0 cm) or small foci of tumor in their explanted liver [61]. *Cholangiocarcinomas* and *sarcomas* involving the liver are not considered indications for transplantation because of the high probability of recurrence. Large benign *hemangiomas* and *hemangioendotheliomas* that cannot otherwise be treated are rare indications for transplantation. Transplantation therapy should never be considered in the treatment of metastatic disease to the liver.

Acute hepatic failure

The Pediatric Acute Liver Failure Study Group (PALFSG), a multicenter collaborative network sponsored by the National Institutes of Health (NIH), has improved our understanding of acute liver failure by collecting detailed clinical and epidemiologic data on children with this disorder. An interim analysis of 139 patients (Squires, personal communication) revealed a two-peak curve of incidence with the largest number of cases observed in infants (less than 1 year of age), and the second peak observed between 13 and 16 years of age. An etiology could not be determined in 50% of cases in this series, with half of these indeterminant cases being less than 1 year of age. The next largest patient group was children with acetaminophen toxicity who constituted 15% of the cohort.

Making the decision to proceed with liver transplantation in a child with fulminant hepatic failure is difficult. Although most children with this diagnosis will require transplantation, some may recover with medical support [62,63]. Furthermore, the outcome after liver transplantation is not as good as with chronic liver disease, with survival in most series averaging approximately 60%. Therapeutic decisions made for children with acute liver failure are made primarily based on experience and clinical research in adult patients. This is problematic because the etiologies and clinical progression of acute liver failure in children is distinct from that of adults. O'Grady *et al.* [64] were the first to develop a prognostic classification, which has gained wide acceptance as the "King's College Criteria." This system emphasizes etiology, age, time course of disease and coagulation as the most important predictors. Although this system provides some guidance for selection of liver transplant candidates, it does not identify all candidates who will require transplantation. An alternative classification, the Clichy criteria, relies on level of encephalopathy, age and factor V activity levels to predict the need for liver transplantation [65]. In this schema, transplantation is recommended if, in the presence of coma or confusion (i.e. grade 3 or 4 encephalopathy), a patient under 30 years of age has a factor V level less than 20% or a patient over 30 years of age has a factor V level of less than 30%. In a head-to-head comparison, both systems have high positive predictive values but unacceptably low negative predictive values to be used as sole determinants [66]. Both systems are most accurate 48 hours before death compared with at the time of admission.

Our work in children and adults with fulminant failure has led to an aggressive empiric approach to management [62]. All patients are listed for transplant at presentation, with transplantation being performed as soon as a donor becomes available. A patient showing signs of stabilization or evidence of recovering function while awaiting graft availability has an outlook for spontaneous recovery as good as with liver transplantation, so the decision to transplant is reversed. Patients with nonicteric fulminant failure represent a special group that has a better prognosis, with more than 50% recovering spontaneously [67]. In contrast, fulminant Wilson disease is associated with a particularly poor prognosis [68].

The development of aplastic anemia has been observed in patients treated with transplantation for acute liver failure secondary to indeterminate hepatitis (sporadic non-A-G hepatitis) [69]. Marrow aplasia or hypoplasia can present either before or after transplantation. The mechanism is unknown, but presumably represents involvement of the bone marrow with the same virus that caused the liver disease. It is a disheartening complication, as these patients are cured of their liver disease only to die of aplastic anemia.

Specific management strategies differ among major centers. There is no specific therapy for fulminant hepatic failure except hepatic replacement [63]. Management, therefore, is directed at life support and prevention and treatment of complications to allow recovery to occur if possible or to provide a suitable candidate for liver transplantation. Management should be in an intensive care unit setting. It is logical to assume that improved life support, monitoring for the detection of complications and the management of life-threatening complications, as are provided in an intensive care setting, will improve the overall survival. In addition to routine monitoring, daily or more frequent evaluation of neurologic function is essential to follow the progress of hepatic encephalopathy. Encephalopathy should be aggressively treated and every effort made to prevent the onset of cerebral edema [70]. In our opinion, exchange transfusions or plasmapheresis may be indicated in the patient awaiting transplantation. Although it is true that these therapies do not improve the outcome of fulminant hepatic failure in the patient managed without transplantation, they can improve the general clin-

ical condition of the patient and perhaps delay central nervous system injury until transplantation can be performed. If evidence of advanced and irreversible cerebral edema is detected, transplantation should not be performed. If the cerebral perfusion pressure falls consistently below 50 mmHg and/or the intracranial pressure is consistently higher than 20 mmHg, liver transplantation is unlikely to restore normal brain function [70,71].

Another important aspect of supportive care is management of coagulopathy. The risk for spontaneous bleeding increases sharply as the prothrombin activity drops below 10% of normal. At our center we institute pre-emptive therapy with transfusion of fresh frozen plasma (FFP) when the prothrombin activity drops below 10% to prevent spontaneous bleeding. Platelet infusion for secondary thrombocytopenia and cryoprecipitate to replenish the fibrinolytic system may also be required. Plasmapheresis can be performed to temporarily improve hemostasis [14]. However, the indications for initiating these therapies are not standardized across centers. Most clinicians agree that coagulation needs to be corrected prior to an invasive procedure. In addition to FFP infusions, we have used recombinant factor VIIa (rFVIIa) in children with liver failure to treat hemorrhagic complications and as pre-emptive therapy to reduce the risk of spontaneous and procedure-related bleeding [72]. This treatment option has increased our institution's use of diagnostic liver biopsy and intracranial pressure monitoring in patients with acute liver failure awaiting transplantation. We have not observed thrombotic complications attributed to this therapy, although we avoid use of rFVIIa in the setting of disseminated intravascular coagulation. Prospective studies are necessary to further demonstrate the cost–benefit relationship of this expensive new therapy.

Survival after liver transplantation performed for this indication is somewhat reduced compared with general survival rates [62,73–76]. In the pediatric acute liver failure (ALF) study, overall short-term survival was 79%. The best survival was for children with acetaminophen poisoning (95%), with only one child requiring transplantation. Survival for indeterminate cases was somewhat less (82%).

Referral to a transplant center

The best time for referral is as soon as the patient is identified as having a condition that will require transplantation. Examples of patients with chronic liver disease who should be referred are infants with biliary atresia who remain jaundiced post Kasai procedure, patients with metabolic disease poorly controlled by medication and patients with cirrhosis for any reason. Early referral allows the transplant center to have maximum input into the pretransplant management strategy. Transplant centers have extensive experience in children with advanced liver disease and can be of help to the primary physician in the management of complications before transplantation, improve diagnosis and suggest alternative therapies. The primary physician can facilitate the referral by communicating the indications for referral to the patient's insurance provider and providing some preliminary orientation of the family to the transplant evaluation process. The mutual goal should be to develop a close working relationship between the family, the primary physician and the transplant center. This type of partnership is essential for the optimal coordination of postoperative care.

In the setting of acute liver disease, all patients with non-A, non-B hepatitis or Wilson disease and encephalopathy should be transferred immediately and directly to a transplant referral center. However, the need to initiate a transplant referral for a patient with acute hepatitis and coagulopathy but normal mental status is less obvious. The best approach is to contact the transplant center as soon as the patient develops coagulopathy. The transplant physicians and the primary physician should then communicate daily to monitor the patient's progress. We generally recommend transfer when the prothrombin time is ≥ 19 s (mean factor VII activity is 20% of normal). Patients with acute liver failure can deteriorate quickly and the transplant center is better equipped to manage a bleeding complication or sudden and rapidly advancing encephalopathy.

REFERENCES

1 Wiesner RH, McDiarmid SV, Kamath PS, *et al.* MELD and PELD: application of survival models to liver allocation. *Liver Transpl* 2001;7:567–80.

2 Freeman RB Jr, Wiesner RH, Harper A, *et al.* The new liver allocation system: moving toward evidence-based transplantation policy. *Liver Transpl* 2002;8:851–8.

3 McDiarmid SV, Merion RM, Dykstra DM, Harper AM. Selection of pediatric candidates under the PELD system. *Liver Transpl* 2004;10(Suppl 2):S23–30.

4 Balistreri WF, Grand R, Hoofnagle JH, *et al.* Biliary atresia: current concepts and research directions: summary of a symposium. *Hepatology* 1996;23:1682–92.

5 Busuttil RW, Seu P, Millis JM, *et al.* Liver transplantation in children. *Ann Surg* 1991;213:48–57.

6 Otte JB, de Ville de Goyet J, Reding R, *et al.* Sequential treatment of biliary atresia with Kasai portoenterostomy and liver transplantation: a review. *Hepatology* 1994;20(Part 2):41S–8S.

7 Goss JA, Shackleton CR, Swenson K, *et al.* Orthotopic liver transplantation for congenital biliary atresia: an 11-year, single-center experience. *Ann Surg* 1996;224:276–84; discussion 284–7.

8 Grosfeld JL, Fitzgerald JF, Predaina R, *et al.* The efficacy of hepatoportoenterostomy in biliary atresia. *Surgery* 1989;106:692–700; discussion 700–1.

9 Lilly JR, Karrer FM, Hall RJ, *et al.* The surgery of biliary atresia. *Ann Surg* 1989;210:289–94; discussion 294–6.

10 Hasegawa T, Fukui Y, Tanano H, *et al.* Factors influencing the outcome of liver transplantation for biliary atresia. *J Pediatr Surg* 1997;32:1548–51.

11 Kobayashi A, Itabashi F, Ohbe Y. Long-term prognosis in biliary atresia after hepatic portoenterostomy: analysis of 35 patients who survived beyond 5 years of age. *J Pediatr* 1984;105:243–6.

12 Karrer FM, Price MR, Bensard DD, *et al.* Long-term results with the Kasai operation for biliary atresia. *Arch Surg* 1996;131:493–6.

13 Laurent J, Gaultier F, Bernard O, *et al.* Long-term outcome after surgery for biliary atresia: study of 40 patients surviving for more than 10 years. *Gastroenterology* 1990;99:1793–7.

14 Howard ER, MacLean G, Nio M, *et al.* Survival patterns in biliary atresia and comparison of quality of life of long-term survivors in Japan and England. *J Pediatr Surg* 2001;36:892–7.

15 Ohi R. Biliary atresia: a surgical perspective. *Clin Liver Dis* 2000;4:779–804.

16 McKiernan PJ, Baker AJ, Kelly DA. The frequency and outcome of biliary atresia in the UK and Ireland. *Lancet* 2000;355:25–9.

17 McDiarmid SV, Millis MJ, Olthoff KM, So SK. Indications for pediatric liver transplantation. *Pediatr Transplant* 1998;2:106–16.

18 Mones RL, DeFelice AR, Preud'Homme D. Use of neomycin as the prophylaxis against recurrent cholangitis after Kasai portoenterostomy. *J Pediatr Surg* 1994;29:422–4.

19 Karrer FM, Lilly JR. Corticosteroid therapy in biliary atresia. *J Pediatr Surg* 1985;20:693–5.

20 Balistreri WF. Bile acid therapy in pediatric hepatobiliary disease: the role of ursodeoxycholic acid. *J Pediatr Gastroenterol Nutr* 1997;24:573–89.

21 Chin SE, Shepherd RW, Cleghorn GJ, *et al.* Pre-operative nutritional support in children with end-stage liver disease accepted for liver transplantation: an approach to management. *J Gastroenterol Hepatol* 1990;5:566–72.

22 Whitington PF. Chronic cholestasis of infancy. *Pediatr Clin North Am* 1996;43:1–26.

23 Emerick KM, Whitington PF. Partial external biliary diversion for intractable pruritus and xanthomas in Alagille syndrome. *Hepatology* 2002;35:1501–6.

24 Whitington PF, Whitington GL. Partial external diversion of bile for the treatment of intractable pruritus associated with intrahepatic cholestasis. *Gastroenterology* 1988;95:130–6.

25 Emond JC, Whitington PF. Selective surgical management of progressive familial intrahepatic cholestasis (Byler's disease). *J Pediatr Surg* 1995;30:1635–41.

26 Cardona J, Houssin D, Gaultier F, *et al.* Liver transplantation in children with Alagille syndrome: a study of twelve cases. *Transplantation* 1995;60:339–42.

27 Hoffenberg EJ, Narkewicz MR, Sondheimer LM, *et al.* Outcome of syndromic paucity of interlobular bile ducts (Alagille syndrome) with onset of cholestasis in infancy. *J Pediatr* 1995;127:220–4.

28 Quiros-Tejeira RE, Ament ME, Heyman MB, *et al.* Variable morbidity in alagille syndrome: a review of 43 cases. *J Pediatr Gastroenterol Nutr* 1999;29:431–7.

29 Quiros-Tejeira RE, Ament ME, Heyman MB, *et al.* Does liver transplantation affect growth pattern in Alagille syndrome? *Liver Transpl* 2000;6:582–7.

30 Alagille D. Liver transplantation in children: indications in cholestatic states. *Transplant Proc* 1987;19:3242–8.

31 Msall M, Batshaw ML, Suss R, *et al*. Neurologic outcome in children with inborn errors of urea synthesis: outcome of urea-cycle enzymopathies. *N Engl J Med* 1984;**310**:1500–5.

32 Ros J, Vilaseca MA, Lambruschini N, *et al*. NTBC as palliative treatment in chronic tyrosinaemia type I. *J Inherit Metab Dis* 1999;**22**:665–6.

33 Holme E, Lindstedt S. Tyrosinaemia type I and NTBC (2-(2-nitro-4-trifluoromethylbenzoyl)-1,3-cyclohexanedione). *J Inherit Metab Dis* 1998;**21**:507–17.

34 Jansen PL. Diagnosis and management of Crigler–Najjar syndrome. *Eur J Pediatr* 1999;**158**(Suppl 2):S89–94.

35 Fox IJ, Chowdhury JR, Kaufman SS, *et al*. Treatment of the Crigler–Najjar syndrome type I with hepatocyte transplantation. *N Engl J Med* 1998;**338**:1422–6.

36 Green RM, Gollan JL. Crigler–Najjar disease type I: therapeutic approaches to genetic liver diseases into the next century. *Gastroenterology* 1997;**112**:649–51.

37 Gridelli B, Lucianetti A, Gatti S, *et al*. Orthotopic liver transplantation for Crigler–Najjar type I syndrome. *Transplant Proc* 1997;**29**:440–1.

38 Rela M, Muiesan P, Vilca-Melendez H, *et al*. Auxiliary partial orthotopic liver transplantation for Crigler–Najjar syndrome type I. *Ann Surg* 1999;**229**:565–9.

39 Shevell MI, Majnemer A, Schiff D. Neurologic perspectives of Crigler–Najjar syndrome type I. *J Child Neurol* 1998;**13**:265–9.

40 FitzSimmons SC. The changing epidemiology of cystic fibrosis. *J Pediatr* 1993;**122**:1–9.

41 Scott-Jupp R, Lama M, Tanner MS. Prevalence of liver disease in cystic fibrosis. *Arch Dis Child* 1991;**66**:698–701.

42 Lamireau T, Monnereau S, Martin S, *et al*. Epidemiology of liver disease in cystic fibrosis: a longitudinal study. *J Hepatol* 2004;**41**:920–5.

43 Fridell JA, Bond GJ, Mazariegos GV, *et al*. Liver transplantation in children with cystic fibrosis: a long-term longitudinal review of a single center's experience. *J Pediatr Surg* 2003;**38**:1152–6.

44 Mack DR, Traystman MD, Colombo JL, *et al*. Clinical denouement and mutation analysis of patients with cystic fibrosis undergoing liver transplantation for biliary cirrhosis. *J Pediatr* 1995;**127**:881–7.

45 Noble-Jamieson G, Valente J, Barnes ND, *et al*. Liver transplantation for hepatic cirrhosis in cystic fibrosis. *Arch Dis Child* 1994;**71**:349–52.

46 Couetil JP, Soubrane O, Houssin DP, *et al*. Combined heart-lung-liver, double lung-liver, and isolated liver transplantation for cystic fibrosis in children. *Transpl Int* 1997;**10**:33–9

47 Della Rocca G, Pompei L, Pugliese F, *et al*. Anaesthesia for liver transplantation in cystic fibrosis patients. *Eur J Pediatr Surg* 1998;**8**:278–81.

48 Molmenti EP, Squires RH, Nagata D, *et al*. Liver transplantation for cholestasis associated with cystic fibrosis in the pediatric population. *Pediatr Transplant* 2003;**7**:93–7.

49 Whitington PF, Balistreri WF. Liver transplantation in pediatrics: indications, contraindications, and pretransplant management. *J Pediatr* 1991;**118**:169–77.

50 Alagille D. α$_1$-Antitrypsin deficiency. *Hepatology* 1984;**4**(Suppl):11S–14S.

51 Sveger T. The natural history of liver disease in α$_1$-antitrypsin deficient children. *Acta Paediatr Scand* 1988;**77**:847–51.

52 Sveger T. α$_1$-Antitrypsin deficiency in early childhood. *Pediatrics* 1978;**62**:22–5.

53 Exelby PR, Filler RM, Grosfeld JL. Liver tumors in children in the particular reference to hepatoblastoma and hepatocellular carcinoma: American Academy of Pediatrics Surgical Section Survey, 1974. *J Pediatr Surg* 1975;**10**:329–37.

54 Evans AE, Land VJ, Newton WA, *et al*. Combination chemotherapy (vincristine, adriamycin, cyclophosphamide, and 5-fluorouracil) in the treatment of children with malignant hepatoma. *Cancer* 1982;**50**:821–6.

55 Douglass EC, Green AA, Wrenn E, *et al*. Effective cisplatin (DDP) based chemotherapy in the treatment of hepatoblastoma. *Med Pediatr Oncol* 1985;**13**:187–90.

56 Quinn JJ, Altman JJ, Robinson HT, *et al*. Adriamycin and cisplatin for hepatoblastoma. *Cancer* 1985;**56**:1926–9.

57 Pritchard J, Brown J, Shafford E, *et al*. Cisplatin, doxorubicin, and delayed surgery for childhood hepatoblastoma: a successful approach – results of the first prospective study of the International Society of Pediatric Oncology. *J Clin Oncol* 2000;**18**:3819–28.

58 Otte JB, Pritchard J, Aronson DC, *et al*. Liver transplantation for hepatoblastoma: results from the International Society of Pediatric Oncology (SIOP) study SIOPEL-1 and review of the world experience. *Pediatr Blood Cancer* 2004;**42**:74–83.

59 Perilongo G, Brown J, Shafford E, *et al*. Hepatoblastoma presenting with lung metastases: treatment results of the first cooperative, prospective study of the International Society of Paediatric Oncology on childhood liver tumors. *Cancer* 2000;**89**:1845–53.

60 Olthoff KM, Millis JM, Rosove MH, *et al*. Is liver transplantation justified for the treatment of hepatic malignancies? *Arch Surg* 1990;**125**:1261–6; discussion 1266–8.

61 Klintmalm GB. Liver transplantation for hepatocellular carcinoma: a registry report of the impact of tumor characteristics on outcome. *Ann Surg* 1998;**228**:479–90.

62 Emond JC, Aron PP, Whitington PF, *et al*. Liver transplantation in the management of fulminant hepatic failure. *Gastroenterology* 1989;**96**:1583–8.

63 Whitington PF. Fulminant hepatic failure in children. In: Suchy FJ, Sokol RJ, Balistreri WF, eds. *Liver Disease in Children*, 2nd edn. Philadelphia: Lippincott Williams & Wilkins, 2001: 63–88.

64 O'Grady JG, Alexander GJ, Hayllar KM, Williams R. Early indicators of prognosis in fulminant hepatic failure. *Gastroenterology* 1989;**97**:439–45.

65 Bismuth H, Samuel D, Castaing D, *et al*. Orthotopic liver transplantation in fulminant and subfulminant hepatitis: the Paul Brousse experience. *Ann Surg* 1995;**222**:109–19.

66 Pauwels A, Mostefa-Kara N, Florent C, Levy VG. Emergency liver transplantation for acute liver failure: evaluation of London and Clichy criteria. *J Hepatol* 1993;**17**:124–7.

67 Alonso EM, Sokol RJ, Hart J, *et al*. Fulminant hepatitis associated with centrilobular hepatic necrosis in young children. *J Pediatr* 1995;**127**:888–94.

68 Sternlieb I. Wilson's disease: indications for liver transplants. *Hepatology* 1984;**4**:15–7S.

69 Tzakis AG, Arditi M, Whitington PF, *et al*. Aplastic anemia complicating orthotopic liver transplantation for non-A, non-B hepatitis. *N Engl J Med* 1988;**319**:393–6.

70 Lidofsky SD, Bass NM, Prager MC, *et al.* Intracranial pressure monitoring and liver transplantation for fulminant hepatic failure. *Hepatology* 1992;**16**:1–7.

71 Lidofsky SD. Liver transplantation for fulminant hepatic failure. *Gastroenterol Clin North Am* 1993;**22**:257–69.

72 Brown JB, Emerick KM, Brown DL, *et al.* Recombinant factor VIIa improves coagulopathy caused by liver failure. *J Pediatr Gastroenterol Nutr* 2003;**37**:268–72.

73 Bismuth H, Samuel D, Castaing D, Williams R, Pereira SP. Liver transplantation in Europe for patients with acute liver failure. *Semin Liver Dis* 1996;**16**:415–25.

74 Chenard-Neu MP, Boudjema K, Bernuau J, *et al.* Auxiliary liver transplantation: regeneration of the native liver and outcome in 30 patients with fulminant hepatic failure: a multicenter European study. *Hepatology* 1996;**23**:1119–27.

75 Nicolette L, Billmire D, Faulkenstein K, *et al.* Transplantation for acute hepatic failure in children. *J Pediatr Surg* 1998;**33**:998–1002; discussion 1002–3.

76 Superina RA, Pearl RH, Roberts EA, *et al.* Liver transplantation in children: the initial Toronto experience. *J Pediatr Surg* 1989;**24**:1013–9.

24 Evaluation of the Candidate

Binita M. Kamath and Elizabeth B. Rand

Pediatric liver transplantation is one of the most successful solid organ transplants with the United Network for Organ Sharing (UNOS), reporting 1- and 3-year patient survival approaching and exceeding 90% and 80%, respectively (varying with age) [1]. Liver transplant recipients can expect to enjoy essentially normal quality of life and successfully attain goals such as returning to school, completing pregnancy and even engaging in Olympic level athletic competition [2]. One of the key factors in achieving this level of transplant success is the appropriate selection and evaluation of candidates for liver transplantation. In this chapter, the stages of evaluation of the recipient are outlined, beginning with the goals of evaluation, the indications for and contraindications to transplant, the medical evaluation of the candidate and then the process of listing itself. Clearly, the care of children with end-stage liver disease does not end with listing for transplantation and therefore the management of children awaiting liver transplantation is also discussed.

GOALS OF EVALUATION

The primary purpose of evaluation of a candidate for liver transplantation is to determine if a particular child can be expected to benefit from transplantation. It is important to ensure that other relevant medical and surgical treatments have been considered and that liver transplantation remains overall the best option. Other goals of a complete evaluation are to optimize nutritional and medical therapy for the child awaiting liver transplantation, to provide education to the patient and family, and to predict the optimal timing of transplantation.

INDICATIONS FOR LIVER TRANSPLANTATION

The primary indication for liver transplantation is the existence of life-threatening liver disease secondary to acute liver failure, chronic end-stage liver disease or, more rarely, metabolic diseases corrected by liver replacement. In addition,

liver transplantation is also offered prior to the development of life-threatening complications for severe progressive liver disease refractory to maximal medical management. The determination of the severity of liver disease requires an assessment of the life-sustaining functions of the liver and how they can be sustained without the need for transplantation. The major functions of the liver can be grouped into five general categories which can be assessed individually: protein synthesis, bile formation and excretion, metabolic functions (including glucose homeostasis), immunologic function and hemodynamic function. Any patient with chronic liver disease who has clinically significant abnormalities in two or more areas will likely greatly benefit from liver transplantation. Children with only one area of significant dysfunction may well be equally well sustained with other therapies, although a severe abnormality in one area may indicate a need for evaluation for transplantation. If possible, a delay in liver transplantation allows the child to grow, complete immunizations, receive fewer total years of immunosuppression and potentially benefit from medical and surgical advances.

In addition to transplantation for acute liver failure and end-stage chronic liver disease, a smaller number of children undergo liver transplantation because of metabolic diseases with primarily extrahepatic manifestations [3]. For example, the urea cycle defects interrupt conversion of ammonia into urea causing hyperammonemia and brain toxicity. Liver transplantation is curative as the liver is the major site of ammonia metabolism despite an otherwise structurally and functionally normal liver [4]. Similarly, in primary hyperoxaluria, systemic oxalate crystal deposition results in renal failure and cardiac arrhythmia but liver transplantation restores normal oxalate metabolism.

CONTRAINDICATIONS TO PEDIATRIC LIVER TRANSPLANTATION

It is important to identify contraindications to liver transplantation at the earliest stage of the evaluation process. As surgical techniques and medical management have improved,

Absolute contraindications	Relative contraindications
Extrahepatic malignancy	Malignancy that is considered cured or curable by standard oncologic criteria

Infection
  Uncontrolled systemic or local invasive infection
  AIDS
	Infection
	  Treatable infection
	
	  HIV infection

Extrahepatic disease
  Irreversible massive brain injury
  Uncorrectable congenital anomalies affecting major organs
  Multisystem organ failure
	Extrahepatic disease
	  Progressive extrahepatic disease (i.e. renal insufficiency)
	  Substance abuse

Table 24.1 Contraindications to pediatric liver transplantation.

AIDS, acquired immunodeficiency syndrome; HIV, human immunodeficiency virus.

the list of contraindications has shortened dramatically (Table 24.1). Absolute contraindications are conditions in which liver transplantation is futile and will not improve overall survival or quality of life, and can be grouped into categories including extrahepatic malignancy, overwhelming sepsis and terminal or irreversible extrahepatic disease, and even these may not be absolute if specific interventions can be made. Relative contraindications to liver transplantation include a recent history of malignancy and incompletely treated systemic infection. An active alcohol or substance abuse problem in the candidate or a primary caregiver may also constitute a relative contraindication. All relative contraindications require careful evaluation by the transplant center, and institution of treatment that may make the child an appropriate candidate. Past contraindications, such as human immunodeficiency virus (HIV) infection and intestinal failure, no longer eliminate a child from receiving transplantation, as HIV can be well controlled with current therapies, and combined liver and intestinal transplants have improving survival rates.

MEDICAL EVALUATION OF THE CANDIDATE

The medical evaluation of the candidate begins with recognition of the patient's original diagnosis and an assessment of complications arising from liver failure, enabling the team to determine the indication for and urgency of liver transplantation. The process requires specific blood cultures, radiologic studies and consultations with specialists (Table 24.2).

Potential contraindications are identified. Comorbidities and/or anatomic variations that could alter perioperative or postoperative management and surveillance for viral and other infections are documented. An assessment of the nutritional status of the candidate is an essential part of the evaluation process. Malnutrition should be treated if necessary, as optimal nutritional status at the time of surgery improves outcome considerably. The evaluation also addresses psycho-

logic factors in terms of the child's understanding of his or her illness and the parents' understanding of the transplant process and their child's prognosis.

Assessment for extrahepatic disease that might impact on perioperative or postoperative management is an important part of the evaluation for transplantation and will vary with the underlying liver disease. Children with Alagille syndrome, for example, will require careful cardiac and renal consultation given the known involvement of those organs in this syndrome. With appropriate pretransplant evaluation and candidate selection, the outcome of liver transplantation in Alagille syndrome is comparable to other nonsyndromic patients [4,5]. Another important group of patients who require careful evaluation are those with syndromic biliary atresia. Approximately 20% of infants with biliary atresia have syndromic features such as portal vein anomalies, situs inversus, malrotation and cardiac anomalies, all of which may impact liver transplant surgery and outcome.

Evaluation at the time of listing for liver transplantation includes testing required by UNOS for all organ recipients as well as screening for exposure to viral infections that will impact care following liver transplantation. Radiologic evaluation will also vary based on underlying disease, but at a minimum should include duplex Doppler ultrasound of the hepatic vessels at the time of listing and chest X-ray. Table 24.2 lists the laboratory, radiologic and other testing performed at the time of listing for liver transplantation. In general, Doppler ultrasound is an adequate modality for screening for vascular anomalies; however, in certain cases, such as syndromic biliary atresia or if abnormalities are detected on ultrasound, additional imaging with magnetic resonance angiography may be indicated [6].

The concept of living related donation should be introduced during the evaluation process. Often, parents will raise this possibility even before the transplant team. It is important to provide an objective presentation of living donation with a clear outline of the risks. Living donor transplantation

Table 24.2 Evaluation of the candidate for pediatric transplantation.

Blood work

Hematology

Complete blood count, prothrombin time/INR*, partial thromboplastin time, fibrinogen, blood type with antibody screen

Chemistry

Electrolytes (sodium*, potassium), blood urea nitrogen, creatinine*, albumin*, total bilirubin*, conjugated bilirubin, hepatic enzymes (alkaline phosphatase, alanine aminotransferase, aspartate aminotransferase, gammaglutamyl transferase), ammonia, α-fetoprotein, ferritin, iron, cholesterol, triglycerides, thyroid function tests, amylase, lipase, vitamin A, D and E levels

Serology

Hepatitis B (surface antigen, surface antibody, core antibody, e antigen, e antibody), hepatitis C (HCV antibody, PCR if antibody positive), hepatitis A IgG, EBV IgG and PCR, CMV IgG and antigenemia, HIV, HSV IgG, measles, IgG, varicella IgG, rubella IgG

Radiology/other

Doppler ultrasound of hepatic vessels

Chest radiograph

Electrocardiogram (and echocardiogram, if indicated)

Consultations

Transplant surgeon

Pediatric hepatologist

Transplant coordinator

Nutritionist

Anesthesiologist

Social worker

Psychologist

Medical consults as needed: cardiology, neurology, nephrology

* Required by UNOS at time of listing.

CMV, cytomegalovirus; EBV, Epstein–Barr virus; HCV, hepatitis C virus; HIV, human immunodeficiency virus; HSV, herpes simplex virus; IgG, immunoglobulin G; INR, international normalized ratio; PCR, polymerase chain reaction; UNOS, United Network for Organ Sharing.

clearly offers the advantage of surgery at an earlier stage in the course of the disease and moreover offers the opportunity to time the transplantation optimally in an elective fashion. However, this process also exposes the living donor to risks of morbidity and mortality, which may have particular impact when a parent or caregiver is involved. Review of the data suggests that there is a clear advantage in living donor liver transplantation in the youngest and smallest patients, less than 2 years of age, with improved graft survival and reduced mortality over deceased donor organs [7,8]. Most likely this finding is the result of reduced waiting time for infants with available live donors. In contrast, for older children, liver donor transplantation does not seem to offer any benefits over deceased donor grafts and is actually associated with a higher risk of graft loss and a trend towards higher mortality (possibly because a left lateral segment may be too small in a larger child).

Discussions surrounding living related transplantation predominantly involve evaluation of the donor; however, an assessment of the candidate's suitability is also important. For instance, in a child with short gut syndrome, a size-matched graft with duct-to-duct anastomosis at surgery is optimal (to prevent the further loss of intestine to construction of a Roux-en-Y anastomosis) and therefore living related donation is made more complex. Special live donor considerations also exist for specific pediatric diseases; for example, potential related donors for a child with Alagille syndrome must be evaluated carefully as affected individuals may appear clinically healthy. A liver biopsy and/or cholangiogram is indicated as part of the donor assessment for potential related donors in Alagille syndrome.

Every attempt is made to include the child in age-appropriate discussion of liver transplantation throughout the evaluation process. An older child may sign an assent form and is encouraged to ask as many questions as possible of the liver transplant team. It may also be appropriate for the candidate to meet post-transplant patients during this time. It is important for the older child to be made aware of the need for medication compliance and alcohol avoidance.

LISTING FOR TRANSPLANTATION

Once the need for liver transplantation is established and no contraindications exist, patients are listed for a deceased donor graft, regardless of whether a potential living donor exists. In 2002, the pediatric end-stage liver disease (PELD) score was implemented to allocate deceased donor livers based on the severity of liver disease [9,10]. At the same time, the model for end-stage liver disease (MELD) was implemented for adults. In this system the PELD and MELD scores rank children and adults on a continuous numeric scale related to the 3-month probability of death (or need for intensive care for children). MELD and PELD scoring were based on similar underlying principles and each relies solely on objective and measurable parameters. The Studies of Pediatric Liver Transplantation (SPLIT) provided a pediatric data set required to develop and validate the current PELD equation [11]. Based on the children enrolled in this population, the factors that predicted death or transfer to the intensive care unit (ICU) within 3 months of listing were international normalized ratio (INR), total bilirubin, serum albumin, age < 1 year, and height < 2 standard deviations from the mean for age and gender (Table 24.3). The PELD score seeks to accurately predict death or transfer to ICU within 3 months of listing and this model was validated in a separate population of children at a large single center prior to implementation [12].

The Status 1 assignation has been retained outside the MELD/PELD calculations for children and adults meeting specific criteria. Patients assigned Status 1 must be located in the ICU. There are five allowable diagnostic groups, as listed in Table 24.4. Fulminant hepatic failure is defined as hepatic

Table 24.3 Pediatric end-stage liver disease (PELD) scoring system.

Factors
Total bilirubin
INR
Serum albumin
Age < 1 year
Height < 2 standard deviations from mean

PELD score = $10 \times [0.480 \times \log_e$ (total bilirubin mg/dL)
$+ 1.857 \times \log_e$ (INR)
$- 0.687 \times \log_e$ (albumin g/dL)
$+ 0.436$ (if patient is < 1 year of age)
$+ 0.667$ (if patient has growth failure)]

INR, international normalized ratio.

Table 24.4 Status 1 classification and exceptions for metabolic disease.

Requirements for Status 1 classification for children
Acute liver failure
Primary nonfunction of a transplanted liver
Hepatic artery thrombosis in postoperative period
Acute decompensated Wilson disease
Chronic liver disease (with a PELD score > 25 and meeting other criteria)

Patients listed as Status 1 must be hospitalized in an intensive care unit

Metabolic disease
Urea cycle disorder
Organic acidemia

Patients with these conditions are assigned a PELD score of 30.
If the candidate is not transplanted within 30 days, they may be listed as Status 1

encephalopathy within 8 weeks of the onset of liver disease and, in addition, ventilator dependence or hemodialysis. Primary nonfunction of a transplanted liver must be diagnosed within 7 days of implantation and hepatic artery thrombosis within 14 days of transplantation. Children (but not adults) with chronic liver disease may also be designated Status 1 if they have a PELD score > 25 and in addition are mechanically ventilated, require dialysis for renal failure, have neurologic failure or have had a recent significant gastrointestinal bleed. Children with diagnoses outside these five categories may also be assigned Status 1 by special exception after a formal request from the transplant team to the UNOS regional review board.

Although PELD (currently used for children up to 12 years old) and MELD scores rank both children and adults on the same scale, certain provisions exist to benefit children. Pediatric candidates (< 12 years) have priority to receive livers from pediatric donors (< 18 years) over adults with the same score. Only children with chronic liver disease may be assigned Status 1. Children with certain metabolic diseases may receive additional PELD points (see Table 24.4). The numeric value of the PELD is used for scoring purposes, without adjustment, even though children have a lower probability of death at any given score. Finally, the PELD score is not capped at a value of 40 as is the MELD score, so children can achieve a score above all adults, except those who are Status 1.

At the time of implementation of the new policy of liver donor allocation based on PELD and MELD scores, there was a concern that children would have reduced access to available donor livers. The developers and implementers of the MELD/PELD system knew that there would need to be continuous revision and improvement as more prospective data showed the impact of the system on liver transplantation. Since the implementation of the PELD/MELD system, the percentage of deceased donor liver transplants has actually increased by 4% in the pediatric population (compared with a 2% increase in adults) [12]. Furthermore, fewer patients are now dying on the waiting list for liver transplantation, including those children < 2 years of age who previously had a high death rate on the liver waiting list. Initial data also suggest that transplant outcomes, in terms of patient and graft survival, are similar after introduction of the new scoring system. Therefore, it appears that implementation of the PELD scoring system has not adversely affected children's access to liver transplantation and subsequent outcomes. This assessment is undermined, however, by the observation that since implementation of the PELD system, a large proportion of children are transplanted with PELD scores (or Status 1 assignment) by exception. The allocation of donor livers in the pediatric population reveals two extremes, with almost half of all children currently being transplanted at Status 1 and half of the remainder being transplanted at a PELD score < 10. The significant number of children being transplanted with low PELD scores may suggest that some children are being transplanted too early. A minority of children listed as Status 1 have diagnoses of acute liver failure, primary nonfunction or hepatic artery thrombosis. Many children are being granted Status 1 by exception, thereby undermining the original intent of the MELD/PELD system in allocation. It has been suggested that the assignation of Status 1 be modified by prioritizing children with acute liver failure (including primary nonfunction and hepatic artery thrombosis) above any other Status 1 child, defining the Status 1 chronic liver disease criteria more strictly and eliminating the Status 1 by exception category altogether.

Further assessment is needed to determine if PELD score is an accurate predictor of disease severity in children. The PELD/MELD scoring system was instituted as a mechanism to determine that the sickest individuals receive organs first and therefore the system is continuously undergoing critical assessment and modification in order to retain this discrimination.

MANAGEMENT OF THE CHILD AWAITING LIVER TRANSPLANTATION

Once a child has been placed on the waiting list for liver transplantation it remains important to optimize all aspects of the patient's care prior to surgery. Management of complications of chronic liver disease such as esophageal varices should continue as per the standard of care. Particular attention should be placed on enhancing a child's nutrition as it is the only intervention at this time that may improve the outcome after surgery.

Patients on the waiting list for liver transplantation also require periodic reassessment of their clinical status, based on clinical information and laboratory data. The PELD score may thus be reassigned, if appropriate. The frequency of reassessment is determined by the current PELD score and ranges from patients at Status 1 requiring recertification every 7 days and those with a PELD score ≥ 25 requiring recertification every 14 days, to children with a score < 10 requiring recertification only annually [1].

Nutritional support

Malnutrition is common in patients with end-stage liver disease [13]. The delivery of adequate nutritional support to a patient with hepatic insufficiency is complicated by increased energy expenditure, malabsorption secondary to gut edema, cholestasis and poor intake. Regardless of the indication for liver transplantation, the importance of nutritional support at every stage of the management of liver disease cannot be underestimated [14]. Not only does good nutrition counteract some of the problems of liver disease specifically (i.e. the poor digestion and absorption of fat calories and fat-soluble vitamins in cholestasis), but it also provides overall improved health by enhancing immune function, wound healing, motor development and cognitive skills. Nutritional assessment in infants with liver disease may be difficult as an increase in weight may reflect worsening organomegaly or ascites rather than true growth. Anthropometric measurements can be very helpful in tracking body composition and should be used whenever possible. Infants with chronic cholestasis benefit from concentrated high-caloric density formula, especially protein hydrolysate products such as Pregestimil® (Mead Johnson Nutritionals), which is favored for its high content of medium chain triglycerides (MCT) and supplementation with essential fatty acids. High-density protein hydrolysate formulas with increased MCT are also available for children over 1 year of age. The caloric density of spoon and table foods can be enhanced by the addition of MCT oil or other supplements for the cholestatic infant or child; butter and/or household oils can also be used and will work well, especially in the noncholestatic patient.

Well-child care

Standard well-child care is vitally important for children with chronic liver disease and particularly those awaiting liver transplantation. Minor infections and intercurrent illnesses can further compromise nutrition and general health in these vulnerable children who require close monitoring and early intervention for these problems. General pediatric follow-up can also help in evaluation of nutritional management, general development, hearing and vision screening, and infection surveillance. Complete immunization including all standard immunizations is of the utmost importance for transplant candidates, as immunization may be less effective in children on immunosuppressive medications. In addition to the standard vaccinations, many centers suggest that children awaiting liver transplantation receive immunization against influenza, pneumococcus and hepatitis A, where age appropriate. Some centers use passive immunization against respiratory syncytial virus (RSV) for young infants awaiting transplantation.

CONCLUSIONS

Evaluation of the candidate for pediatric liver transplantation is a vital step in ensuring a successful outcome from surgery. The process requires a multidisciplinary approach and involves an assessment of the candidate's underlying illness and indication for transplant, the severity of liver disease and timing of transplant, and then a medical and psychosocial evaluation. The process of listing an individual for liver transplantation has changed dramatically in the last few years with the advent of the PELD scoring system, and preliminary data indicate that fewer children are now dying on the waiting list. Continued careful evaluation of candidates, combined with a listing mechanism that allocates organs to the sickest individuals first, will ensure that pediatric liver transplantation remains one of the most successful solid organ transplants.

REFERENCES

1 United Network for Organ Sharing. Available at www.unos.org (accessed August 2005).

2 Bucuvalas JC, Ryckman FC. Long-term outcome after liver transplantation in children. *Pediatr Transplant* 2002;**6**:30–6.

3 Florman S, Shneider B. Living-related liver transplantation in inherited metabolic liver disease: feasibility and cautions. *J Pediatr Gastroenterol Nutr* 2001;**33**:520–1.

4 Kasahara M, Kiuchi T, Inomata Y, *et al.* Living-related liver transplantation for Alagille syndrome. *Transplantation* 2003; **75**:2147–50.

5 Maldini G, Torri E, Lucianetti A, *et al.* Orthotopic liver transplantation for alagille syndrome. *Transplant Proc* 2005;**37**: 1174–6.

6 Ravindra KV, Guthrie JA, Woodley H, *et al.* Preoperative vascular imaging in pediatric liver transplantation. *J Pediatr Surg* 2005;**40**:643–7.

7 Abt PL, Rapaport-Kelz R, Desai NM, *et al.* Survival among pediatric liver transplant recipients: impact of segmental grafts. *Liver Transpl* 2004;**10**:1287–93.

8 Roberts JP, Hulbert-Shearon TE, Merion RM, Wolfe RA, Port FK. Influence of graft type on outcomes after pediatric liver transplantation. *Am J Transplant* 2004;**4**:373–7.

9 Wiesner RH, McDiarmid SV, Kamath PS, *et al.* MELD and PELD: application of survival models to liver allocation. *Liver Transpl* 2001;**7**:567–80.

10 Freeman RB Jr, Wiesner RH, Harper A, *et al.* The new liver allocation system: moving toward evidence-based transplantation policy. *Liver Transpl* 2002;**8**:851–8.

11 McDiarmid SV, Anand R, Lindblad AS. Development of a pediatric end-stage liver disease score to predict poor outcome in children awaiting liver transplantation. *Transplantation* 2002; **74**:173–81.

12 McDiarmid SV, Merion RM, Dykstra DM, Harper AM. Selection of pediatric candidates under the PELD system. *Liver Transpl* 2004;**10**(Suppl 2):S23–30.

13 Protheroe SM, Kelly DA. Cholestasis and end-stage liver disease. *Baillieres Clin Gastroenterol* 1998;**12**:823–41.

14 Ramaccioni V, Soriano HE, Arumugam R, Klish WJ. Nutritional aspects of chronic liver disease and liver transplantation in children. *J Pediatr Gastroenterol Nutr* 2000;**30**:361–7.

25 Donor Evaluation, Surgical Technique and Perioperative Management

Jean C. Emond, Steven J. Lobritto and Dominique Jan

Transplantation for children with liver disease has become well-established therapy with excellent outcomes as the norm. As in all transplantation, access to a donor liver has become the limiting step in the procedure. Aspects of the waiting list, including regional variations in organ supply, the practice of split liver transplantation (SLT) and living donor liver transplantation (LDLT), are all part of the educational issues the parents face in adjusting to the reality of transplantation in their newly diagnosed child. In this light, although LDLT has demonstrated superior results in small children [1], and is considered a standard option in pediatric liver transplantation, its use has remained limited to approximately 10–15% of the transplants in children for the past 5 years (Fig. 25.1). In this chapter, we review elements of donor selection, provide a brief overview of the surgical technique and present a detailed approach to perioperative care for children undergoing liver transplantation.

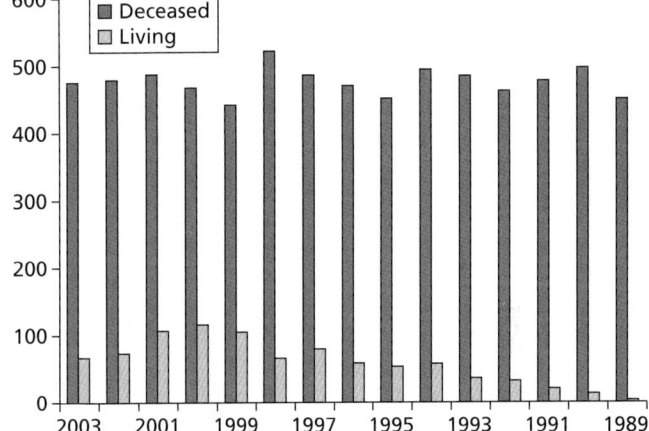

Fig. 25.1 Pediatric living and deceased donor transplantation in the USA (United Network of Organ Sharing [UNOS]).

DONOR SELECTION

Living donors

The evaluation and selection of living donors for liver transplantation in children has been widely studied over the past decade and has become largely standardized [2]. The standard algorithm that we have used is reproduced in Table 25.1.

The issue of informed consent, which we first studied in the original trials of LDLT in Chicago [3] has been of primal importance and has been revived comprehensively in the recent extension to adult–adult LDLT. The risk of donor death may be as high as 0.5% for adult–adult LDLT, which is 10-fold the risk faced by renal donors [4]. In contrast, left lateral segment donation, the standard procedure in pediatric LDLT, seems to have a much lower risk, approaching that faced by renal donors [5]. In our opinion, recent data suggesting that LDLT offers the best outcomes in very small children simplify the initial conversations with the parents regarding the feasibility and safety of living donation.

Living donor evaluation process (Table 25.1)

The evaluation has not changed in the past decade and is based on three steps: initial screening, medical assessment of the health risks for the donor and assessment of the suitability of the potential graft. An independent donor advocate team, which takes medical responsibility in terms of care of the donor, ideally performs the medical and psychologic assessment of donor suitability. This step confirms that the donor is healthy, truly committed to the donation and not coerced [6]. This is obviously relatively simple in parent–child transplantation in which, unlike adult LDLT, donor–recipient relationships are straightforward and benefits are aligned. Centers generally follow State guidelines for selection of the living donor including age restrictions and assessments to exclude chronic medical illness. Blood testing is used to rule out important infectious diseases, underlying liver disease and disorders of hemostasis. The details and extent of this testing remains the subject of some debate and is beyond the scope of this chapter. Blood type compatibility has been required,

Table 25.1 Living donor evaluation criteria.

Phase I Age	I Relation	II Psychosocial support	II Medical evaluation	II Laboratory evaluation	III Graft assessment
18–60 years	Emotionally related to recipient ABO compatible Negative serology for hepatitis and HIV	Psychosocial support systems adequate as determined by pediatric transplant team, psychiatry and social services	Comprehensive history and physical examination negative for acute or chronic illness affecting operative risk	Hematologic, serum chemistry, liver, and kidney function normal Normal ECG and CXR Negative serology for hepatitis and HIV	Volumetric MRI scan excludes occult mass lesions, documents adequate liver volume Graft represents ≥ 50% of expected recipient liver mass Arteriography documents arterial supply for the anticipated graft (for adult LDLT only)

ECG, electrocardiogram; CXR, chest X-ray; HIV, human immunodeficiency virus infection; LDLT, living donor liver transplantation; MRI, magnetic resonance imaging.

although recent data would suggest that ABO-incompatible liver transplants do rather well, modeling after the techniques practiced in renal transplantation in this setting [7].

Graft assessment is the final aspect of donor selection. Size matching is the most obvious constraint, and organs from living donors can either be too large, too small or just right. The liver has a tremendous ability to accommodate disparities in graft size with either regeneration or apoptotic reductions in hepatocyte mass [8]. Large livers have been managed utilizing temporary enlargement of the peritoneal cavity with prosthetic closure, with attention to position of the graft and alignment of the vessels [9]. This leads to selection of the donor based on body size and may affect the extent of the resection in the donor. Babies under 5 kg may not be able to receive a graft from a large adult male; however, surprising accommodations have been observed in clinical practice. Figure 25.2 depicts the standard resections available to generate partial liver grafts from either living or deceased donors [5]. In general, small children have been served with resection of the adult anatomic left lateral lobe (Couinaud segments 2 and 3), which produces a graft of approximately 250 g which is adequate for a recipient up to 20 kg or so. The intermediate

graft (the full left lobe) is usually between 250 and 500 g and has been used for medium-sized children and even adults, although in our hands these grafts have been plagued by technical problems, consistent with the poor results seen in older children with LDLT observed in the Scientific Registry of Transplant Recipients (SRTR) database [1]. Finally, adult-sized teenagers are served with right lobe grafts, bringing all the donor selection issues faced in adult–adult LDLT, although preserving the emotional alignment of the parent and child.

Assessment of the health of the donor's liver can be performed by laboratory tests, imaging and liver biopsy. The use of liver biopsy remains an issue of some contention, with current practice ranging from selective biopsy (our own practice) in the face of abnormal laboratory tests or imaging (steatosis), to routine biopsy of all donors. This was a subject of vigorous discussion at a recent international meeting and is not likely to be readily resolved (International Consensus Conference on the Living Liver Donor, Vancouver BC, September 2005). Assessment of the vessels and the biliary tree is now often performed without the use of invasive tests such as angiography and cholangiography, which have been supplanted by cross-sectional imaging obtained

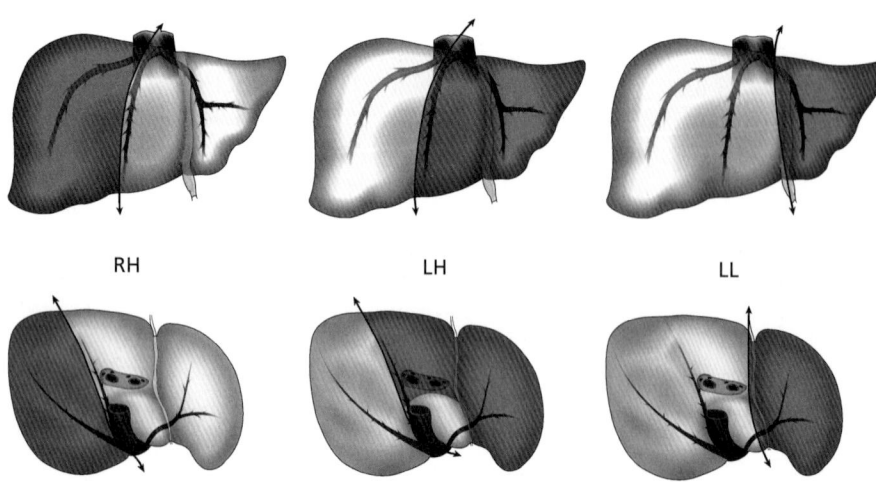

RH   LH   LL

Fig. 25.2 Potential transections for the preparation of partial liver grafts: LL, left lateral lobe (Couinaud II and III); LH, full left lobe (segments II, III and IV); and RH, right lobe (segments V–VIII). Adapted from Salame *et al.* [5].

Table 25.2 Demographics of the organ supply in the USA (United Network of Organ Sharing [UNOS]).

	2004	2003	2002	2001	2000	1999	1998	1997	1996
All ages	4959	5997	5649	5612	5382	5200	4935	4684	4522
< 1 year	88	65	66	61	74	61	60	52	61
1–5 years	178	142	152	171	169	163	196	193	168
6–10 years	120	98	125	148	133	150	149	135	142
11–17 years	510	495	472	468	501	479	535	560	576
18–34 years	1668	1691	1704	1659	1525	1432	1420	1376	1323
35–49 years	1632	1601	1489	1516	1440	1404	1224	1139	1128
50–64 years	1505	1379	1165	1131	1126	1050	945	907	854
65+ years	619	519	467	447	398	452	405	321	270
Unknown	0	4	3	11	16	9	1	1	0

either by magnetic resonance imaging (MRI) or computed tomography (CT). High-quality cholangiograms have been obtained using CT and are extremely intriguing [10]. Detailed three-dimensional reconstructions of biliary and vascular anatomy by CT imaging has been developed by Peitgen and others [11]. These studies produce detailed anatomic information that is used for planning the resection and estimating the functional capacity of both the graft and the remnant remaining in the donor.

Deceased donor selection

Table 25.2 depicts the available supply of deceased donors (DD) available for the transplantation of children over the past decade. The United Network of Organ Sharing (UNOS) data indicate that in 2003 there were 65 donors less than 1 year of age, 142 between 1 and 5 years, 98 from 6 to 10 years and 495 from 11 to 17 years. These 800 pediatric donors compare favorably with the number of children who need liver transplantation each year, some 600 or so. That same year, 478 children received DD transplants and 68 LDLT. There is general agreement that the rate of mortality on the waiting list for children has declined as a result of many factors including the success of split liver transplantation as well as LDLT. A major outcome study of pediatric liver transplantation, the Studies of Pediatric Liver Transplantation (SPLIT) database, (a multicenter observational study consisting of pediatric liver transplant candidates enrolled between 1995 and 2005) reported 106 deaths on the waiting list in their cohort of 2578 listed children, a rate of 4.1% (SPLIT Annual Report 2005, Tables 1–5). UNOS data suggest that waiting list mortality varies substantially by age cohort. For example, in 2004, 28 children under 1 year of age died on the waiting list from the 295 added to the list that year (9.5%). This ratio was lower for children between 1 and 5 years (18/214; 8.4%), and lowest for children between 6 and 10 years (2/105; 1.8%). Children between 11 and 17 years had a death to new candidate listed ratio of 5.9% (data from UNOS: http://www.optn.org/). The lower rate of waiting list mortality observed in the SPLIT data may reflect center effect. In general, while there seems to be enough size-matched pediatric liver donors to serve much of the candidate pool, the mortality of children on the waiting list remains an issue of concern, especially because it seems to vary between centers and regions.

As in the selection of grafts for adults, the immediate concern in selecting DD is prevention of the transmission of infectious diseases or cancer. This is titrated against the urgency of the medical condition of the recipient. In contrast to adult donors, who are often older, carry evidence of past viral exposure and are in an age demographic in which cancer may occur, pediatric donors tend to be young and healthy and are usually suffering from trauma or another sudden cause of death so the risk of occult liver disease is exceedingly low. The use of expanded criteria organ donors, whose use is associated with an increased risk of graft failure has not been well studied in children [12]. We have been very aggressive in using nearly all pediatric donors offered to our center because many of the clinical parameters used to decline organs in the past have not affected our graft outcomes. It is our clinical impression that livers in children seem to be very tolerant of shock and regenerate with normal architecture. Despite using organs from donors with long "down time," high doses of vasopressors, large blood loss and markedly elevated aminotransferases, we have not seen a case of primary non-function of a pediatric donor liver in more than a decade. Another group of potential donor organs long considered inappropriate for liver transplantation, newborn livers, have been used successfully in recent years because of improvements in surgical technique, particularly with the introduction of microsurgical techniques for arterial and biliary reconstruction [13].

With respect to size matching of whole livers for children, we use livers from donors up to twice the weight of the recipients with little hesitation. We are careful to avoid abdominal compression by the use of temporary prosthetic closure in some 20% of cases. If the livers are too large, they are either reduced (small donors) or split, in which the larger lobe goes to a large child or small adult recipient and the left lateral segment is retained for use in the small baby. It is easy to misjudge the abdominal pressure and all efforts must be made to avoid tight closure in a baby that may lead to hepatic compression, arterial thrombosis, renal dysfunction, respiratory complications and other potentially catastrophic events.

Split livers

Since our initial report in 1990, split livers, in which two patients are transplanted with lobes of a single donor liver, have been proposed as a solution to the pediatric organ shortage [14]. Since then, excellent results have been reported by many centers dividing livers between an adult (usually a right trisegment) and a child (left lateral segment) [15]. In the 2005 SPLIT annual report, 217/1626 DD transplants (13.3%) in children were from split liver donors (SPLIT annual report 2005, Tables 3–4). The actual percentage of split graft volume is lower because centers contributing to the SPLIT database disproportionately represent centers performing this procedure. The real challenge has been the effective allocation of the split donor between two competing recipients and often two competing centers. The allocation of split livers must take into consideration that the most severe crisis in organ access is faced by adults, who account for some 95% of the waiting list. In our practice, we have performed split liver transplantation in children when the adult liver is allocated to the pediatric recipient, requiring us to reduce the liver to fit the child and reallocating the right lobe to the adult pool. In this instance, an adult who would not otherwise receive a transplant is able to use the right lobe, albeit with a slightly increased risk of graft failure than if they had received the whole liver. We prefer, when possible, to offer living donation to pediatric patients, because the results are superior to both split and even size-matched whole organs, especially for the smallest patients [16]. Others strongly disagree with this approach and have promoted split livers in children as a way to avoid living donation [17].

In summary, the use of a broad range of methods, including aggressive use of pediatric DD grafts, splitting and LDLT have greatly reduced the risk of dying on the waiting list for children in the past decade.

SURGICAL PROCEDURES FOR DONOR AND RECIPIENT

Detailed surgical techniques are beyond the scope of this chapter and have been well described in previous publications [18]. A few technical details of interest are highlighted with speculation about potential future developments.

Procurement of the deceased donor

The procedure for cadaveric procurement has been extensively described and is little modified for children [19]. Very careful handling of the vessels is important and, when pos-

sible, procurement of the splenic or carotid arteries should be considered to provide optimal visceral conduits for arterial reconstruction.

Living donor operation (left lateral segment donation)

Following standard preoperative preparation, the donor is anesthetized and a generous abdominal incision is made. Recently, Cherqui [20] has describe a technique for full laparoscopic procurement of the left lateral lobe of a living donor with extraction of the graft though a pelvic transverse incision. This group has performed at least 17 laparoscopic procurements with excellent results in the recipients (D. Cherqui, personal communication). The left triangular ligament and gastrohepatic ligaments are incised, and the left hepatic artery exposed near its origin from the proper hepatic artery. The left portal vein is exposed posteriorly near the caudate lobe, and the small vessels to this lobe are then divided. The left bile duct is then divided, ideally distal to the insertion of the duct of segment 4, although the entire left duct can be used without morbidity. The liver parenchyma is then divided just to the right of the round ligament for left lateral hepatectomy and in the plane of the gallbladder fossa for total left hepatectomy, depending upon the amount of parenchyma to be transplanted. Following parenchyma transection, which is perfomed without hepatic ischemia, the liver graft is free on its hepatic artery, portal vein and left hepatic vein. These are then clamped and divided, and the liver graft is rapidly flushed with heparinized preservation solution via the portal vein and the hepatic artery is carefully flushed. The portal vein can be extended by using DD iliac vein segments. In most instances, a single bile duct is available for anastomosis.

Recipient operation

Intraoperative monitoring and vascular access in pediatric liver transplant is usually achieved with a peripheral arterial catheter, a percutaneously inserted silastic central venous line, and supplemental peripheral venous access for blood and fluid infusions. These, combined with non-invasive monitoring of P_{O_2} and end-tidal CO_2, are sufficient in nearly all cases.

The recipient operation in the baby or small child is performed with a bilateral subcostal incision. The liver is carefully mobilized with exposure of the vena cava. The hilar dissection is performed with meticulous care, preserving the bile duct in patients with native anatomy and the Roux limb from the Kasai procedure in biliary atresia cases. With careful dissection it is possible to reuse the Roux in nearly all cases. The arteries are divided high in the hilum to preserve all the options for reimplantation. We try to mobilize the proper hepatic artery proximal to the gastroduodenal artery, preserving that branch intact if length will allow. The portal vein is carefully skeletonized by removing the collar of lymph nodes back to the common hepatic artery for optimal flexibility. If the portal vein is atretic, it is best to plan to extend it, either with iliac vein from a deceased donor or else with internal jugular vein from the host in the case of a living donor. If a whole liver is used, the vena cava need not be liberated from the liver, but in the case of a partial graft in which the hepatic vein of the graft will be anastomosed to the host vena cava, the small hepatic veins from the vena cava to the liver are individually ligated and oversewn, as much as possible prior to cross-clamp. After the donor liver has been prepared, the vena cava is clamped and the recipient liver is excised. Children tolerate clamping of the vena cava and the portal vein with few hemodynamic effects. However, we are careful to limit the cross-clamp time to avoid prolonged stasis in the mesenteric and caval circulations, thereby avoiding the accumulation of products of anaerobic metabolism and proximal thrombosis. We frequently flush the vena cava and the portal vein to ensure patency during the creation of the anastomoses. Ideally, the clamp time can be limited to not much over 30 minutes. For a left lobe or left lateral segment graft we use a triangulated anastomosis which rotates the liver into the right upper quadrant [21] while a whole liver is implanted with a standard caval reconstruction. The reduced graft is then retracted gently to the right allowing the portal vein of the graft to meet the portal vein of the host for end-to-end reconstruction with little redundancy. The clamps are then removed, allowing portal refilling with careful attention to metabolic restoration. After reperfusion, the artery is reconstructed in all tranquility, using precise microvascular technique [22]. Roux-en-Y hepaticojejunostomy is used to reconstitute the bile ducts [23]. In selected cases, however, we have used primary anastomoses of donor and recipient bile ducts with good success. This approach is especially important in children with short gut, in whom creation of a Roux would result in further shortening of the available digestive surface. We have not used biliary stents or external drainage in children.

POSTOPERATIVE CARE

Donors

The care of donors following LDLT has been relatively straightforward, comparable with that required for routine cases of hepatic resection. Care of the living donors in New York State has recently been standardized in State health regulations following the highly publicized death of a living donor in 2001 (New York State Department of Health). Patients are usually awake and extubated following the procedure and are observed in the intensive care unit (ICU) overnight. They are transferred to a transplantation inpatient unit where nursing care is available at a ratio of no less than one nurse to four patients. A brief course of antibiotics is administered with parenteral fluid therapy. Peristalsis usually appears within 72 hours and donors are ambulatory by this time. The median hospital stay has been 6 days in our series. No donor since the second case has required readmission to the hospital. Biliary leaks, which occur in up to 5% of right lobe donors for adults, are uncommon in our experience with an incidence of 1% in our series of nearly 100 living donors for pediatric recipients.

Recipients

Improvements in surgical technique and anesthesia over the past decade have simplified the postoperative care of the pediatric liver transplant recipient, with rapid transition out of the ICU and early discharge home becoming the rule [24–27]. As with all major operations, the postoperative care of the potential pediatric liver transplant recipient begins with judicious management in the preoperative period. Preoperative care to address the complications of liver insufficiency, management of portal hypertension, optimization of nutritional state, suppression of infectious complications and correction of metabolic derangements has been shown to decrease both the morbidity and mortality associated with the transplant operation [28–35]. With the widespread use of LDLT, it is possible to choose the optimal time for operative intervention and minimize pretransplant morbidity [16]. The preoperative care challenges are predictive of the needs and postoperative issues of the liver recipient. The medicosurgical team model of preoperative and postoperative management affords the patient the best result, combining the skills and expertise of both disciplines [36].

Preoperative factors affecting post-transplant care

Chronic cholestatic liver disease

All liver transplant recipients are not equal. The majority of pediatric liver transplants are still performed to address liver insufficiency from disorders of chronic cholestasis [37]. Patients with biliary cirrhosis have special nutritional requirements, with particular detail to fat malabsorption and overall calorie delivery [38]. In addition, cirrhotic patients may enter a liver transplant with profound synthetic dysfunction and hypersplenism putting them at greater risk of intraoperative blood loss resulting from coagulation defects and thrombocytopenia. Patients with advanced portal hypertension may decompensate in the preoperative period, having their liver transplant performed in the setting of uncontrolled ascites, relative hypoxia, renal insufficiency, electrolyte disarray or recent gastrointestinal hemorrhage. In addition, these patients are immunosuppressed by their underlying disorders and are at risk of infectious complications postoperatively.

Beside the problems common to any chronic cholestatic cirrhosis there are special considerations with implications for postoperative management depending on the specific underlying disorder. For example, the pediatric patient with biliary atresia has usually had prior abdominal surgery, increasing the risk of operative blood loss and inadvertent enterotomies during the surgical dissection at the time of liver transplantation. In addition, patients with biliary atresia may have other associated anomalies such as cardiac disease and gastrointestinal malrotation [39,40]. Some syndromic cholestatic disorders are associated with pulmonary hypertension. Patients with progressive familial intrahepatic cholestasis have defects in intestinal function leading to difficulties with severe diarrhea in the postoperative period, compromising the delivery of nutritional support and medications [41,42]. Similarly, patients with primary sclerosing cholangitis may have underlying bowel disease, infectious complications and chronic dependency on pain medications, each with implications for management after transplantation [43]. One final example would be the patient with chronic cholestasis in the setting of long-term dependency on parenteral nutrition who may have significant underlying pulmonary disease and marginal gastrointestinal absorptive capacity [44,45]. It is only with this thorough knowledge of the preoperative condition of the patient that the optimum postoperative care can be rendered.

Fulminant liver failure

Patients with fulminant hepatic failure pose unique issues in the perioperative period [46,47]. The cause of liver failure varies in this group and may be associated with other major organ injury too. This heterogeneous group of patients will differ by their prior medical comorbid disorders which may have specific implications for postoperative management. Patients in this group are at specific risk of severe encephalopathy and life-threatening cerebral edema. The pre- and postoperative management of fluids, electrolytes, blood pressure and cerebral perfusion pressure must be judicious to permit patient survival with or without liver transplantation [46]. The perioperative management of these patients often necessitates the placement of an intracranial pressure monitoring device for optimal delivery of care [48]. Volume control with hypertonic saline and rapid correction of coagulopathy with activated factor VII have been introduced. Factor VII correction seems to have reduced the risk of bleeding from the device placement. Insertion risks and infection are balanced by the improved ability to monitor and manage cerebral hypertension to insure the best possible transplant outcome [49]. Unfortunately, the risk of cerebral hypertension does not end immediately after successful liver transplantation and can persist into the second and third postoperative day [50]. These patients often have severe coagulation anomalies placing them at increased risk of intraoperative bleeding. In addition, these patients have an increased risk of sepsis and

should be monitored closely in the postoperative period with empiric antibiotic coverage to improve outcomes [32].

Metabolic liver disease

Patients with metabolic liver disease include those with disorders such as urea cycle defects, glycogen storage disease, neonatal hemochromatosis, tyrosinemia, Crigler–Najjar type 1, α_1-antitrypsin deficiency and Wilson disease [26,51–57]. Patients in this category may have specific medication and dietary restrictions entering liver transplant which need to be adjusted in the postoperative period. Some of these patients require urgent neonatal liver transplant that further complicates the postoperative care because of technical complications and immature physiology [58]. Some of the metabolic patients have associated organ injuries, such as brain and lung involvement, that will affect postoperative tolerance to medications and other care issues. Portal hypertension can be absent in these patients and some are at risk for postoperative hepatocellular carcinoma [59].

Retransplantation

The last general group of patients with specific considerations in the postoperative period includes those undergoing repeat liver transplantation. The patient in need of a second liver transplant is at increased risk of perioperative issues including increased blood loss, inadvertent bowel injury, poor wound healing and severe acute cellular rejection [60]. These patients may have significant altered renal function from prior medication exposure affecting their postoperative management. The outcomes in such patients will also depend on the degree of liver insufficiency entering retransplant, the nutritional status of the patient and the presence of associated biliary or vascular injuries. The choice of medications to prevent rejection will often need to be more aggressive than that utilized during the first transplant. The presence of infections such as cytomegalovirus (CMV) and post-transplant lymphoproliferative disease should be monitored with vigilance.

OPERATIVE FACTORS AFFECTING POST-TRANSPLANT CARE

It is crucial that information regarding intraoperative events is passed from the anesthesia and surgical team to the ICU personnel and the hepatology team. We advocate an integrated multidisciplinary postoperative care team because the surgical team may be involved in other operations or else be physically taxed after operating through the night. Parameters such as blood loss, plasma infused, hourly urine output, endotracheal tube size and position, medications infused, intraoperative vitals, intraoperative laboratory results, warm and cold ischemia times, types of vascular access and monitoring modalities are

Table 25.3 Postoperative management.

Intravenous fluids: lactated Ringer's at 1.5–2 times weight-based maintenance rate
Acid suppression with IV histamine blockers followed by an enteral proton pump inhibitor
Antibacterial agents: enterics, *Staphylococcal* species and enterococcus
    CMV prophylaxis: IV ganciclovir for 7 days followed by high-dose aciclovir
    Fungal prophylaxis: oral nystatin aspirin – vascular thrombosis prophylaxis
Immunosuppressive agents
    Steroids
    Antimetabolites (azathioprine or MMF)
    Calcineurin blocker (cyclosporine or tacrolimus)
    Monoclonal IL-2 receptor antagonists (daclizumab or basiliximab)
    Antilymphocyte globulin (antithymocyte globulin or muromonab/CD3)
Narcotic pain medication (fentanyl or morphine) and sedation (short-acting anxiolytics)
Laboratory monitoring parameters
Mechanical ventilation and weaning parameters
Renal dose dopamine and diuretics

CMV, cytomegalovirus; IL-2, interleukin 2; MMF, mycophenolate mofetil.

presented by the anesthesia team. The surgical team needs to report the type of graft, donor attributes, color and texture of the graft following reperfusion, details regarding biliary and vascular anastomoses, any bowel injuries or spillage, number and type of drains and type of wound closure. This communication will permit the postoperative management team to predict likely needs and expected complications from intraoperative findings and events.

The type of graft used has important implications for postoperative management. Up to 50% of children receive technical variant grafts such as split right or left lobes, or living donor liver grafts [13,15,16,61–63]. These partial liver transplants can have complicated vascular and biliary anastomoses, creating postoperative problems with graft perfusion and biliary outflow [21,23,64,65]. In addition, partial liver grafts with a cut edge can predispose to biliary leaks and postoperative infection [23]. The outcomes of these types of transplants seem to correlate with the experience of the operative team and use of these grafts should be confined to centers of excellence.

Initial postoperative ICU care

After the operative team has communicated the course and findings to both the intensivist and the hepatology team, the continuity of the patient's care is insured. We favor the use of standard protocol postoperative orders and care algorithms. The initial management of the patient will include transferring portable monitoring devices to those of the ICU, re-establishing lines and infusions and re-establishing mechanical ventilation. A rapid yet thorough assessment is made to evaluate adequacy of ventilation, hemodynamic stability, vascular access and monitoring modalities. The patient's fluid status is assessed by vitals, central venous pressure (CVP) monitoring, capillary refill and weight comparison with preoperative values. A set of metabolic and hematologic admission laboratory tests are

obtained to assess the need for electrolyte and fluid adjustments, further blood products, acid–base balance, adequacy of oxygenation and ventilation and overall liver function. Chest and abdominal radiographs are obtained to check line, drain and endotracheal tube placement. We favor a single abdominal sonogram with Doppler within 12 hours to assess vascular patency and to exclude large intra-abdominal collections. Others have reported more frequent sonographic surveillance [66].

Postoperative management

Transplant teams commonly use standardized order sets with weight-based dosing to minimize medication errors and omissions [26,67,68]. The typical postoperative orders include the general categories listed in Table 25.3. Intravenous (IV) fluids are administered to provide the necessary intravascular volume to ensure adequate graft and vital organ perfusion. Typically, a buffered resuscitation fluid such as lactated Ringer's is delivered at 1.5–2 times the calculated weight-based maintenance rate. The fluid rate is adjusted to optimize organ perfusion as estimated by a CVP of 4–10 mm water, and urine output is monitored closely. The acid–base balance and serum electrolytes are used to make adjustments in fluid constituents. Particular attention is given to the presence of hyperkalemia and metabolic acidosis, two early clues to graft vascular insufficiency or major dysfunction. In patients at risk for cerebral edema, the delivery of fluid requires a balance between maintaining adequate intravascular volume and avoiding increasing intracranial pressures. Diuretics such as furosemide and renal-dose dopamine are often administered to stimulate renal function after caval cross-clamping. Cirrhotic patients are sodium avid and commonly retain fluids for weeks following liver transplantation [69]. Such patients often require diuretics during this period of adaption.

219

Acid suppression with IV histamine blockers followed by an enteral proton pump inhibitor are administered to decrease the risk of superficial gastric ulceration and gastrointestinal bleeding. If mycophenolate mofetil (MMF) is included in the immunosuppression regimen then proton pump inhibitors are maintained to prevent drug-induced intestinal injury. Perioperative standard antibacterial agents are administered to provide coverage for both Gram-negative and Gram-positive organisms with particular attention to *Staphylococcal* species and enterococcus [70]. Patients with prior bacterial infection, delayed wound closure, intraoperative gut injury or spillage are continued on antibacterials for longer periods as appropriate. These patients are at risk for antibiotic-resistant infections. Prophylactic antibiotic exposure should be limited to prevent the emergence of resistant organisms such as methicillin-resistant *Staphylococcus* aureus and vancomycin-resistant enterococcal species. Other prophylactic antimicrobials are administered to prevent opportunistic infections. We provide CMV prophylaxis to all recipients with a combination of IV ganciclovir for 7 days followed by either oral ganciclovir or high-dose aciclovir delivered for the first 3 months following liver transplantation. Recipients at particular risk of CMV include those who are CMV-naïve who have a donor with prior CMV exposure [71]. The peak incidence of CMV infection that affects the graft or the gut is about 6 weeks. *Pneumocystis* prophylaxis is achieved with co-trimoxazole administered three times per week for the first post-transplant year. Fungal prophylaxis is usually achieved with oral nystatin administered during the period of steroid administration. Patients on long-term preoperative antibiotics, those with fulminant hepatic failure, biliary leaks or documented invasive fungal infection are treated with long-term fluconazole with careful attention to calcineurin drug levels.

Aspirin is administered for the first postoperative month for vascular thrombosis prophylaxis, although this practice has never been studied rigorously [72]. This is not universally accepted at all centers nor is the administration of heparin, dextrans or prostacyclin [70,73].

Immunosuppressive agents are administered to prevent acute cellular rejection. Most centers use some combination of steroids, antimetabolites (azathioprine or MMF) and a calcineurin blocker (cyclosporine or tacrolimus) [74]. Some centers are attempting steroid-free or steroid-less protocols which involve some combination of one of the monoclonal interleukin 2 (IL-2) receptor antagonists (daclizumab or basiliximab) or antilymphocyte globulin (antithymocyte globulin or muromonab/CD3) with conventional agents [75,76]. For patients with renal insufficiency, calcineurin inhibitors may be delayed by intention and these globulin-mediated immunosuppressant agents may provide a bridge until improved renal function permits conventional agents. Sirolimus has also been used in renal protective protocols but has limited use in the immediate postoperative period as it has been associated with hepatic artery thrombosis and impedes wound healing

[77]. Because of their inherent neurotoxicity, it is our center practice not to use either calcineurin-blocking agent until the recipient shows signs of neurologic recovery post liver transplant. This neurotoxicity, characterized by demyelinization of both gray and white matter, may lead to seizures that are exacerbated by concurrent hypomagnesemia [78,79].

Although occasional patients may be extubated in the operating room, most patients remain on mechanical ventilation during the operative day. Patients without prior lung disease with a well-functioning graft are usually extubated on the first postoperative day as sedation is withdrawn. Patients with delayed graft function should remain mechanically ventilated until signs of improved graft function and mentation. Patients with pre-existing lung disease, preoperative sedation or prolonged preoperative ventilator dependency are weaned and extubated as tolerated. Common factors delaying timely extubation include poorly positioned endotracheal tubes, atelectasis, transient diaphragmatic dysmotility, right reactive pleural effusion, fluid overload and excess sedation. Infants are particularly susceptible to gastric dilatation and well positioned gastric decompression tubes are essential during positive pressure ventilation.

Narcotic pain medication (fentanyl or morphine) and sedation (short-acting anxiolytics) are essential to the management of the pediatric liver transplant recipient. Most sedation can be removed permitting extubation as above. Narcotics are usually required for the first 3–4 postoperative days with conversion to non-narcotic analgesics thereafter. Prolonged narcotic use has been associated with delayed return of gut function and ineffective ventilation and should be avoided.

Laboratory monitoring parameters are used to assess graft function, metabolic balance and adequacy of ventilatory support. Drug levels are monitored after the first 2 postoperative days.

Postoperative indicators of graft function

Upon transport to the ICU, the patient is monitored for indicators of graft function. The earliest predictor of graft function is the appearance and consistency of the liver after reperfusion in the operative suite [80]. Bile production is commonly observed during the operation as well. Hemodynamic stability with diuresis, good acid–base balance and signs of neurologic recovery are all clinical indicators of good graft function. In patients with elevated intracranial pressure at the time of transplant, return of neurologic function my lag behind other signs of stable graft function. Intracranial pressure monitoring is essential in comatose patients [50]. Abnormalities in coagulation are common in the first 24–48 hours after transplantation. We expect to see progressive improvement in coagulation times without the use of plasma infusions. We do not routinely correct abnormalities in coagulation in the absence of bleeding, although supplemental vitamin K should be considered in recipients with chronic cholestatic disease as the indication for liver transplantation. Serum bilirubin levels are a poor initial indicator as these values are diluted by volume shifts intraoperatively and may actually rise postoperatively despite excellent graft function. Unexpected rises in serum bilirubin may indicate graft congestion, a bile leak, sepsis, drug toxicity, hemolysis, intraperitoneal bleeding or small-for-size syndrome with reperfusion injury.

Primary non-function of the implanted liver has become a rare event in recent years. The surgical team may report a liver with poor color and firm texture at the time of reperfusion. Hemodynamic instability, oliguria, acidosis, persistent coagulopathy and failure to recover neurologic function are signs of graft non-function. The grafts at greatest risk are those with advanced steatosis, those from elderly donors and those with prolonged ischemic insult, which are rarely used in children [81,82]. Damaged or ischemic livers release aminotransferases so laboratory tests demonstrating rising hepatic enzymes necessitate emergent liver imaging to detect acute arterial thrombosis, which is correctable. Our group advocates angiography with thrombolysis and stent placement over open revision. Image-guided therapy is more precise for rescuing the hepatic artery because most early thromboses are caused by intimal flaps rather than anastomotic problems [66,72]. Immediate relisting for urgent retransplantation is indicated.

Hemodynamic indicators

The postoperative hemodynamics of the recipient are monitored in a number of ways: routine vitals by intra-arterial catheterization, CVP monitoring, urine output, skin perfusion and acid–base balance. Pulmonary arterial catheters are rarely used in children. Postoperative hypertension is commonly observed and is likely the result of volume shifts, medications and discomfort. The preoperative cirrhotic physiology is often indistinguishable from sepsis; it is characterized by low system vascular resistance, wide pulse pressure, relative hypotension and super-normal cardiac output. Asymptomatic bradycardia is a common observation in the early postoperative period and rarely requires intervention. Possible etiologies include excessive intravascular volume, normalization of preoperative vasodilatory tone, vagal stimulation or injury during transplantation, medications, venous access position or mechanical ventilation [83]. Antihypertensive agents that do not lower heart rate may therefore be needed in the perioperative period.

Postoperative indicators of surgical complications

Surgical complications can usually be recognized early in the postoperative course while still in the ICU setting. Early reoperation for bleeding is no longer common, but is required in the setting of ongoing blood loss. Postoperative bleeding may be a function of diffuse coagulopathy or a focal bleeding vessel. Management of this postoperative complication is similar in approach to that practiced in non-transplant abdominal surgery. Initial management consists of correction of clotting anomalies and appropriate volume and blood product resuscitation with surgery reserved for severe or persistent bleeding.

Early bile leaks are readily detected by bile drainage from abdominal drains. Because bile leaks may resolve spontaneously, we do not recommend routine immediate surgical exploration. An abdominal sonogram should be performed to exclude an undrained intra-abdominal collection or vascular thrombosis [84,85]. Anastomotic biliary leaks may have a delayed presentation as edema may initially mask this event. Perforation of the bowel may also present after the first few days as steroids and narcotics mask symptoms. If an intestinal perforation is suspected, reoperation is essential [86]. Chylous ascites may represent transient disruption of lymphatics, but may be an indication of a bowel perforation [87]. Early analysis of ascites for cell count, bilirubin, amylase and triglycerides will often suggest an etiology for the finding and will help guide medical and/or surgical intervention. Appropriate drainage of collections and empiric antibacterial and antifungal agents appear prudent.

Postoperative laboratory indicators

Elevated aminotransferases after pediatric liver transplant is a common event (Table 25.4). The differential diagnosis for this observation is reperfusion injury, infection, vascular thrombosis, pressure necrosis, medications and thermal surface injury. Acute cellular rejection in the first few days after liver transplantation is unusual with the peak incidence around 1 week to 10 days [26,74]. Abdominal sonogram with vascular Doppler analysis is essential to evaluate the

Table 25.4 Differential diagnoses of postoperative laboratory abnormalities.

Elevated aminotransferases
Reperfusion injury
Infection
Vascular thrombosis
Pressure necrosis
Medication reaction
Thermal surface injury
Rejection

Elevated cholestatic enzymes and bilirubin
Reperfusion injury
Biliary leaks
Medication reaction
Infection
Graft congestion
Biliary obstruction
Rejection

patency of all hepatic vessels. If the sonogram is inconclusive, then more invasive studies including hepatic angiography or surgical exploration is indicated. Early vascular thrombosis after liver transplantation is a medical emergency that may result in graft loss or severe necrosis. Some patients have been reported to have severe acidosis and hyperkalemia leading to cardiac arrhythmias [88,89]. Unfortunately, even if the graft can be salvaged after correction of a vascular obstruction, focal or diffuse biliary injury may occur requiring eventual graft replacement.

Abnormal elevations in cholestatic enzymes, alkaline phosphatase and gamma-glutamyltranspeptidase, and bilirubin are commonly observed in the post-transplant period (Table 25.4). These elevations may indicate reperfusion injury, biliary leaks, drug reactions, infection, graft congestion, biliary obstruction or rejection. In patients with chronic preoperative cholestasis, the serum bilirubin drops dramatically after transplant compared with preoperative values as a result of volume shifts and serum dilution. These values rise in the first few postoperative days as tissue bilirubin is mobilized and intravascular volume normalizes. Imaging is of limited value to assess rises in cholestatic enzymes and liver biopsy is often required to determine the cause in persistent cases [68,69].

Postoperative ascites

Ascites after liver transplant surgery is quite common. High drainage output is a direct function of mismatch in overall intake and output of fluids. Cirrhotic renal physiology favors salt and water retention and persists for weeks following liver replacement therapy predisposing to ascites formation [21,69]. Patients receiving small-for-size grafts have relative congestion from hyperperfusion and are prone to ascites formation. Relative mismatch of donor and recipient vascular size may also contribute to ascites in the post-transplant period [21]. Chylous ascites may be related to lymphatic disruption, and can be confirmed by lipid measurements and responds rapidly to fat-restricted diets [87]. Bilious ascites always merits investigation to exclude leaks, collections and bowel disruptions [90,91]. The management of ascites in the postoperative period depends on the underlying etiology. The general approach would be to limit fluid intake, mobilize fluids with diuretics and to replace protein loses with salt-poor albumin products. Although uncommon, hepatic outflow obstruction can occur, particularly in partial grafts. Hepatic venography with pressure measurements may be indicated for persistent transudative ascites.

Postoperative fever

Fever in the postoperative period is common. The cause of fever varies with the time from transplantation and is a quite non-specific finding. Early fevers are usually the result of pulmonary atelectasis, responding to chest physical therapy,

incentive spirometry and early mobilization from bed. A careful search must be made to exclude bacterial infections, especially in patients with multiple intravenous catheters and drains. The blood, sputum and urine should be cultured to pinpoint infection. The wound should be carefully examined to exclude cellulitis or infected collections. The volume and nature of ascites drainage should be assessed with careful analysis to exclude peritonitis, bile leaks and bowel perforations. Extremities should be examined to exclude underlying thrombosis in patients with indwelling catheters and in those chronically immobilized. Liver tests should be reviewed to exclude acute cellular rejection and vascular insufficiency. A liver biopsy may need to be performed after sonographic imaging proves negative to clarify the etiology of fevers in patients with liver test anomalies. The skin should be examined for rashes, and the patient's medication list should be reviewed and minimized to exclude drug-induced fevers. The febrile patient with diarrhea should have full stool studies performed including analysis for CMV infection and *Clostridium difficile*. Empiric therapy with metronidazole should be considered in patients at greatest risk especially if diarrhea is bloody. Patients with delayed wound closure and a Gore-tex® skin patch should be continued on antibiotics until wound closure. Common post-transplant infections involve *Staphylococcal* species, enterococcus, candidal species, rotavirus, CMV and respiratory syncytial virus [29,30,92–94].

Postoperative nutritional management

Nutrition support is often an important issue in the pretransplantation period. Although the need for special formulas may no longer be necessary after successful liver transplantation, outcomes are certainly affected by continued efforts at nutritional repletion [34,95,96]. Luckily, steroids stimulate excessive oral intake, and the hypermetabolic state improves post-transplant to permit assimilation of calories. In fact, after a period of catch-up growth parents should be warned to avoid excess calories, as obesity is not uncommon after successful liver transplantation, affecting overall health in a negative way. Dietary counseling by the nutritional support staff is crucial to ensure proper care during this transition period.

The typical postoperative course

The general course for an uncomplicated pediatric liver transplantation is an ICU stay of 24–48 hours with termination of mechanical ventilation within 12–24 hours of transplantation. Patients are weaned off dopamine after successfully extubation and IV fluids are reduced to maintenance rates after 24 hours. Enteral medications are generally started immediately after transplant as tolerated. Oral feeds are started usually around 6–12 hours after extubation and advanced as tolerated to regular within 24–48 hours. Most medications are delivered enterally with the exception of antibiotics, initial steroids and ganciclovir. Patients receive physical, feeding and pulmonary therapies to stimulate early ambulation and mobilization from bed to avoid unnecessary postoperative complications. Patients remain in private rooms without isolation during their initial hospitalization. Recipients and their families are taught medication administration and side-effects. After stable liver tests and medication levels are achieved, when the patient can enterally nourish and hydrate themselves, and when the patient is comfortable and mobile enough to function, they are discharged to home with weekly outpatient follow-up. Median length of stay should be approximately 7–10 days for uncomplicated transplants. After discharge, patients are seen weekly and more frequently if indicated. Sutures are removed 3 weeks after transplantation although most children are closed with subcuticular sutures to avoid the need for painful staple removals.

Pearls and pitfalls regarding the postoperative care of the pediatric liver recipient

1 Know your patient's pretransplant state to anticipate post-operative needs.
2 Keep communication between members of the care team open.
3 Acidosis is an ominous perioperative sign.
4 Unexplained liver test elevations should prompt a search for a vascular occlusion.
5 Avoid unnecessary renal toxic medications including aminoglycosides and nonsteroidal anti-inflammatory agents.
6 Post-transplant patients can have acetaminophen if needed.
7 Avoid fluid overload after liver transplantation.
8 Approximately 10% of pediatric liver transplant patients will require early operative exploration.
9 Just because some immunosuppression is good does not mean that more is better.
10 Know your drug interactions.
11 Late bile duct obstructions can present insidiously and are frequently missed by noninvasive studies.
12 Patients do not always do what you tell them to do.
13 Liver transplant is not an experiment, but it does remain a high-risk sport.

REFERENCES

1 Roberts JP, Hulbert-Shearon TE, Merion RM, Wolfe RA, Port FK. Influence of graft type on outcomes after pediatric liver transplantation. *Am J Transplant* 2004;**4**:373–7.
2 Renz JF, Mudge CL, Heyman MB, *et al.* Donor selection limits use of living-related liver transplantation. *Hepatology* 1995;**22**:1122–6.
3 Singer PA, Siegler M, Whitington PF, *et al.* Ethics of liver transplantation with living donors. *N Engl J Med* 1989;**321**:620–2.
4 Malago M, Testa G, Marcos A, *et al.* Ethical considerations and rationale of adult-to-adult living donor liver transplantation. *Liver Transpl* 2001;**7**:921–7.
5 Salame E, Goldstein MJ, Kinkhabwala M, *et al.* Analysis of donor risk in living-donor hepatectomy: the impact of resection type on clinical outcome. *Am J Transplant* 2002;**2**:780–8.
6 Abecassis M, Adams M, Adams P, *et al.* Live Organ Donor Consensus Group. Consensus statement on the live organ donor. *JAMA* 2000;**284**:2919–26.
7 Kozaki K, Egawa H, Kasahara M, *et al.* Therapeutic strategy and the role of apheresis therapy for ABO incompatible living donor liver transplantation. *Ther Apher Dial* 2005;**9**:285–91.
8 Samstein B, Emond J. Liver transplants from living related donors. *Annu Rev Med* 2001;**52**:147–60.
9 Emond JC. Liver transplantation in children: advances in patient selection, technique and immunosuppression. *Zhonghua Min Guo Xiao Er Ke Yi Xue Hui Za Zhi* 1997;**38**:249–54.
10 Yeh BM, Breiman RS, Taoli B, *et al.* Biliary tract depiction in living potential liver donors: comparison of conventional MR, mangafodipir trisodium-enhanced excretory MR, and multi-detector row CT cholangiography – initial experience. *Radiology* 2004;**230**:645–51.
11 Harms J, Bartels M, Bourquain H, *et al.* Computerized CT-based 3D visualization technique in living related liver transplantation. *Transplant Proc* 2005;**37**:1059–62.
12 Amin MG, Wolf MP, TenBrook JA Jr, *et al.* Expanded criteria donor grafts for deceased donor liver transplantation under the MELD system: a decision analysis. *Liver Transpl* 2004;**10**:1468–75.
13 Guarrera JV, Emond JC. Advances in segmental liver transplantation: can we solve the donor shortage? *Transplant Proc* 2001;**33**:3451–5.
14 Emond JC, Whitington PF, Thistlethwaite JR, *et al.* Transplantation of two patients with one liver: analysis of a preliminary experience with 'split-liver' grafting. *Ann Surg* 1990;**212**:14–22.
15 Renz JF, Yersiz H, Reichert PR, *et al.* Split-liver transplantation: a review. *Am J Transplant* 2003;**3**:1323–35.
16 Emond JC. Living donor liver transplantation in children: what to recommend? *Am J Transplant* 2004;**4**:293–4.
17 Washburn K, Halff G, Mieles L, Goldstein R, Goss JA. Split-liver transplantation: results of statewide usage of the right trisegmental graft. *Am J Transplant* 2005;**5**:1652–9.
18 Abu-Elmagd K, Fung J, Bueno J, *et al.* Logistics and technique for procurement of intestinal, pancreatic, and hepatic grafts from the same donor. *Ann Surg* 2000;**232**:680–7.
19 Jan D, Renz J. Donor selection and procurement of multivisceral and isolated intestinal allografts. *Curr Opin Transplant* 2005; **10**:137–41.
20 Cherqui D. Laparoscopic liver resection. *Br J Surg* 2003;**90**: 644–6.
21 Emond JC, Heffron TG, Whitington PF, Broelsch CE. Reconstruction of the hepatic vein in reduced size hepatic transplantation. *Surg Gynecol Obstet* 1993;**176**:11–7.
22 Guarrera JV, Sinha P, Lobritto SJ, *et al.* Microvascular hepatic artery anastomosis in pediatric segmental liver transplantation: microscope vs loupe. *Transpl Int* 2004;**17**:585–8.
23 Reichert PR, Renz JF, Rosentha P, *et al.* Biliary complications of reduced-organ liver transplantation. *Liver Transpl Surg* 1998; **4**:343–9.

24 Emond JC. What's new in transplantation. *J Am Coll Surg* 2002; **194**:636–41.

25 Emre S. Living-donor liver transplantation in children. *Pediatr Transplant* 2002;**6**:43–6.

26 Rand EB, Olthoff KM. Overview of pediatric liver transplantation. *Gastroenterol Clin North Am* 2003;**32**:913–29.

27 McDiarmid SV. Management of the pediatric liver transplant patient. *Liver Transpl* 2001;**7**(Suppl 1):S77–86.

28 Lichtor JL, Emond J, Chung MR, Thistlethwaite JR, Broelsch CE. Pediatric orthotopic liver transplantation: multifactorial predictions of blood loss. *Anesthesiology* 1988;**68**:607–11.

29 Their M, Holmberg C, Lautenschlager I, Hockerstedt K, Jalanko H. Infections in pediatric kidney and liver transplant patients after perioperative hospitalization. *Transplantation* 2000; **69**:1617–23.

30 Bouchut JC, Stamm D, Boillot O, Lepape A, Floret D. Postoperative infectious complications in paediatric liver transplantation: a study of 48 transplants. *Paediatr Anaesth* 2001;**11**:93–8.

31 Balistreri WF. Transplantation for childhood liver disease: an overview. *Liver Transpl Surg* 1998;**4**(Suppl 1):S18–23.

32 Alonso MH, Ryckman FC. Current concepts in pediatric liver transplant. *Semin Liver Dis* 1998;**18**:295–307.

33 Hasegawa T, Fukui Y, Tanano H, *et al.* Factors influencing the outcome of liver transplantation for biliary atresia. *J Pediatr Surg* 1997;**32**:1548–51.

34 McDiarmid SV. Risk factors and outcomes after pediatric liver transplantation. *Liver Transpl Surg* 1996;**2**(Suppl 1):44–56.

35 Quak SH. Pre-liver transplantation management of children. *Ann Acad Med Singapore* 1991;**20**:534–9.

36 Ganschow R, Nolkemper D, Helmke K, *et al.* Intensive care management after pediatric liver transplantation: a single-center experience. *Pediatr Transplant* 2000;**4**:273–9.

37 Whitington PF, Emond JC, Black DD, *et al.* Indications for liver transplantation in pediatric patients. *Clin Transplant* 1991; **5**:155–60.

38 Cohran VC, Heubi JE. Treatment of pediatric cholestatic liver disease. *Curr Treat Options Gastroenterol* 2003;**6**:403–15.

39 Carmi R, Magee CA, Neill CA, Karrer FM. Extrahepatic biliary atresia and associated anomalies: etiologic heterogeneity suggested by distinctive patterns of associations. *Am J Med Genet* 1993; **45**:683–93.

40 Kataria R, Kataria A, Gupta DK. Spectrum of congenital anomalies associated with biliary atresia. *Indian J Pediatr* 1996;**63**: 651–4.

41 Chen F, Ananthanarayanan M, Emre S, *et al.* Progressive familial intrahepatic cholestasis, type 1, is associated with decreased farnesoid X receptor activity. *Gastroenterology* 2004;**126**:756–64.

42 van Mil SW, Klomp LW, Bull LN, Houwen RH. FIC1 disease: a spectrum of intrahepatic cholestatic disorders. *Semin Liver Dis* 2001;**21**:535–44.

43 Narumi S, Roberts JP, Emond JC, Lake J, Ascher NL. Liver transplantation for sclerosing cholangitis. *Hepatology* 1995;**22**: 451–7.

44 Garcia S, Ruza F, Gonzalez M, *et al.* Evolution and complications in the immediate postoperative period after pediatric liver transplantation: our experience with 176 transplantations. *Transplant Proc* 1999;**31**:1691–5.

45 Kelly DA. Nutritional factors affecting growth before and after liver transplantation. *Pediatr Transplant* 1997;**1**:80–4.

46 Ascher NL, Lake JR, Emond JC, Roberts JP. Liver transplantation for fulminant hepatic failure. *Arch Surg* 1993;**128**:677–82.

47 Daas M, Plevak DJ, Wijdicks EF, *et al.* Acute liver failure: results of a 5-year clinical protocol. *Liver Transpl Surg* 1995;**1**:210–9.

48 Jalan R. Intracranial hypertension in acute liver failure: pathophysiological basis of rational management. *Semin Liver Dis* 2003;**23**:271–82.

49 Blei AT, Olafsson S, Webster S, Levy R. Complications of intracranial pressure monitoring in fulminant hepatic failure. *Lancet* 1993;**341**:157–8.

50 Keays R, Potter D, O'Grady J, *et al.* Intracranial and cerebral perfusion pressure changes before, during and immediately after orthotopic liver transplantation for fulminant hepatic failure. *Q J Med* 1991;**79**:425–33.

51 Matern D, Starzl TE, Arnaout W, *et al.* Liver transplantation for glycogen storage disease types I, III, and IV. *Eur J Pediatr* 1999;**158**(Suppl 2):S43–8.

52 Whitington PF, Alonso EM, Boyle JT, *et al.* Liver transplantation for the treatment of urea cycle disorders. *J Inherit Metab Dis* 1998;**21**(Suppl 1):112–8.

53 Peeters PM, Sieders E, De Jong KP, *et al.* Comparison of outcome after pediatric liver transplantation for metabolic diseases and biliary atresia. *Eur J Pediatr Surg* 2001;**11**:28–35.

54 Ghishan FK, Greene HL. Liver disease in children with PiZZ alpha 1-antitrypsin deficiency. *Hepatology* 1988;**8**:307–10.

55 Bertolani MF, Pellegrino AM, Summa C, Scalera E. [Tyrosinosis. A difficult diagnosis of late infancy]. *Minerva Pediatr* 1990;**42**: 1–7.

56 Hasegawa T, Tzakis AG, Todo S, *et al.* Orthotopic liver transplantation for ornithine transcarbamylase deficiency with hyperammonemic encephalopathy. *J Pediatr Surg* 1995;**30**:863–5.

57 Muiesan P, Rela M, Kane P, *et al.* Liver transplantation for neonatal haemochromatosis. *Arch Dis Child Fetal Neonatal Ed* 1995;**73**:F178–80.

58 Durand P, Debray D, Mandel R, *et al.* Acute liver failure in infancy: a 14-year experience of a pediatric liver transplantation center. *J Pediatr* 2001;**139**:871–6.

59 Kim SZ, Kupke KG, Ierardi-Curto L, *et al.* Hepatocellular carcinoma despite long-term survival in chronic tyrosinaemia I. *J Inherit Metab Dis* 2000;**23**:791–804.

60 Deshpande RR, Rela M, Girlanda R, *et al.* Long-term outcome of liver retransplantation in children. *Transplantation* 2002;**74**: 1124–30.

61 Broelsch CE, Emond JC, Whitington PF, *et al.* Application of reduced-size liver transplants as split grafts, auxiliary orthotopic grafts, and living related segmental transplants. *Ann Surg* 1990; **212**:368–75; discussion 375–7.

62 Emond JC. Clinical application of liver-related liver transplantation. *Gastroenterol Clin North Am* 1993;**22**:301–15.

63 Renz JF, Emond JC, Yersiz H, Ascher NL, Busuttil RW. Split-liver transplantation in the United States: outcomes of a national survey. *Ann Surg* 2004;**239**:172–81.

64 Renz JF, Reichert PR, Emond JC. Biliary anatomy as applied to pediatric living donor and split-liver transplantation. *Liver Transpl* 2000;**6**:801–4.

65 Stevens LH, Emond JC, Piper JB, *et al.* Hepatic artery thrombosis in infants: a comparison of whole livers, reduced-size grafts, and grafts from living-related donors. *Transplantation* 1992;**53**: 396–9.

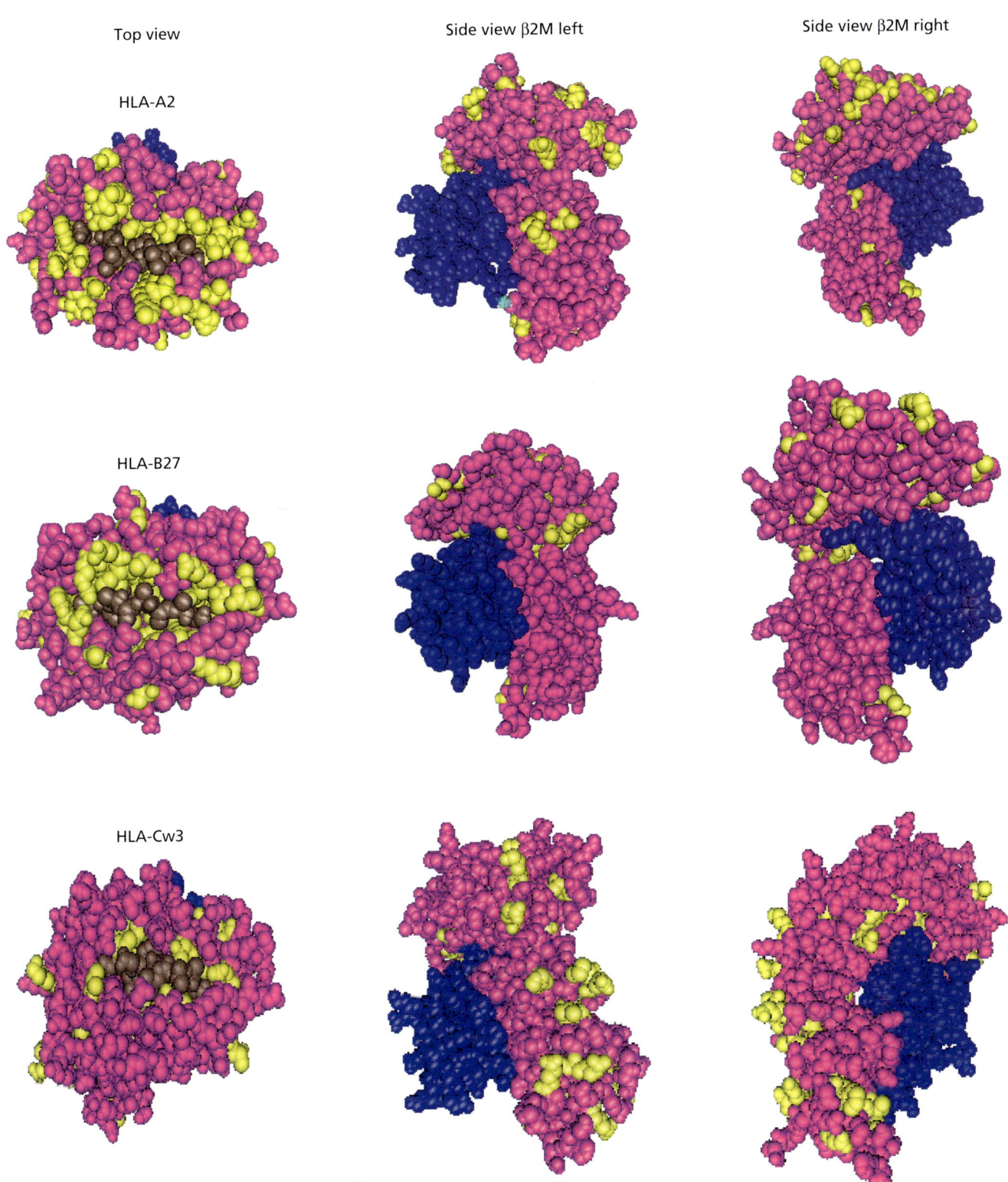

Top view

Side view β2M left

Side view β2M right

HLA-A2

HLA-B27

HLA-Cw3

Plate 4.1 Polymorphic residues on class I molecules controlled by HLA-A, HLA-B and HLA-C loci.

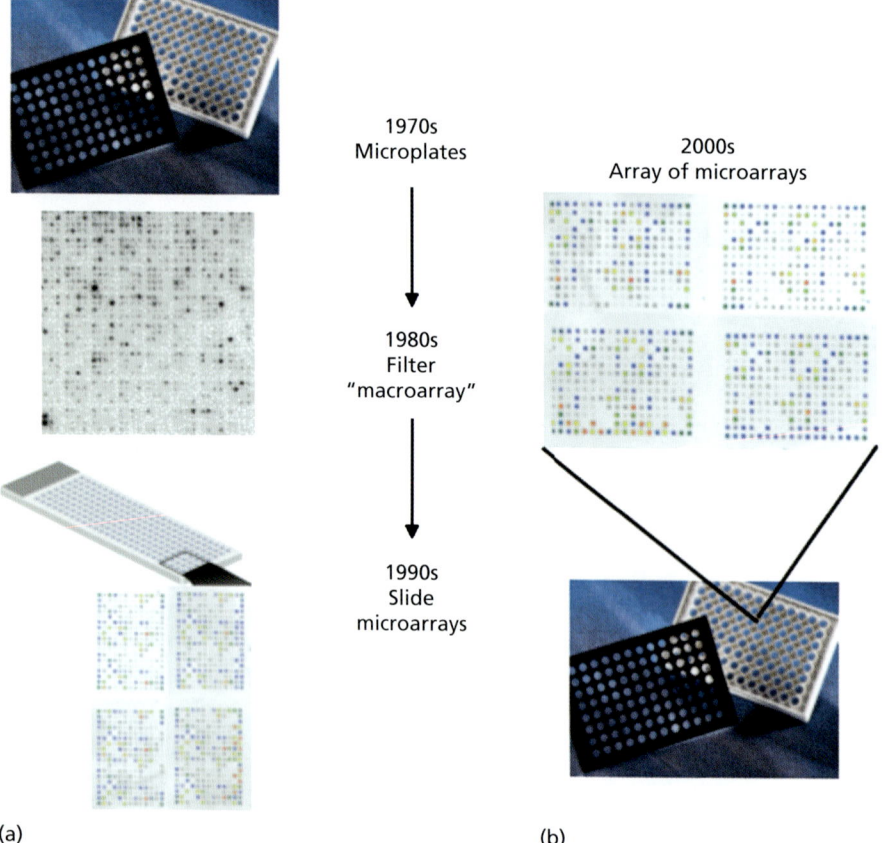

1970s
Microplates

1980s
Filter
"macroarray"

1990s
Slide
microarrays

2000s
Array of microarrays

(a)

(b)

Plate 6.1 Evolution of array-based expression assays over the past 30 years. (a) The advent of multiple-well plates revolutionized how enzymatic assays were run in the 1970s. Their use provided both cost savings and improved assay reproducibility precision because robotic liquid handling could be used for reagent dispensing. A similar format of using parallel analysis was replicated in the 1980s in hybridization-based assays using membrane filter "macroarrays." Spots of gene-specific cDNA clones were used as hybridization probes. Radioactively labeled mRNA pools hybridized to these membranes then permitted the levels of several different genes to be assayed together in parallel. The technology migrated toward further miniaturization on to glass slides at much higher probe density with the advent of "microarray" technology in the 1990s. The use of fluorescent dyes (Cy3 and Cy5) and laser-based scanning in the process reduced dependence on radioactive detection without sacrificing sensitivity. (b) An emerging advance in microarray profiling is the development of plate-based "array of microarrays" where approximately 1000 probes can be spotted on to the grid of a standard 96-well microplate.

Plate 6.2 Clustering of 67 renal biopsies by global mRNA profiling and a minimum gene set that classifies acute rejection into three AR classes. (a) Expression data from 1340 differentially expressed genes were used to cluster 67 pediatric renal biopsy samples. Acute rejection samples cluster into three of four branches of this tree. Prediction analysis of microarrays (PAM) class prediction was used to identify the minimum gene set that differentiates acute rejection biopsies. Genes are ranked by degree of differential expression across user selected sample groups. In this analysis, the 1340 differentially expressed genes from twelve AR-I, nine AR-II and five AR-III biopsies were used as the learning set and a fivefold expression cut-off identified 97 informative genes. (b) Functional clusters of the informative genes are illustrated and the acute rejection (AR) samples group consistently with the comprehensive expression profiles. (c) Based on this small subset of genes, the phenotype and PAM classification scores are in 96% concordance with our previous report (Sarwal M, Chua MS, Kambham N, *et al.* Molecular heterogeneity in acute renal allograft rejection identified by DNA microarray profiling. *N Engl J Med* 2003;**349**:125–38). One AR-I sample, while loosely clustering with other AR-I biopsies, has an intermediate PAM score and phenotypes as AR-II in this analysis. Like many of the AR-II patients, this patient also had urinary tract infection at the time of biopsy. Figure published in modified form in Mansfield ES & Sarwal MM. Arraying the orchestration of allograft pathology. *Am J Transplant* 2004;**4**:853–62, and reproduced with the permission of the *American Journal of Transplantation*.

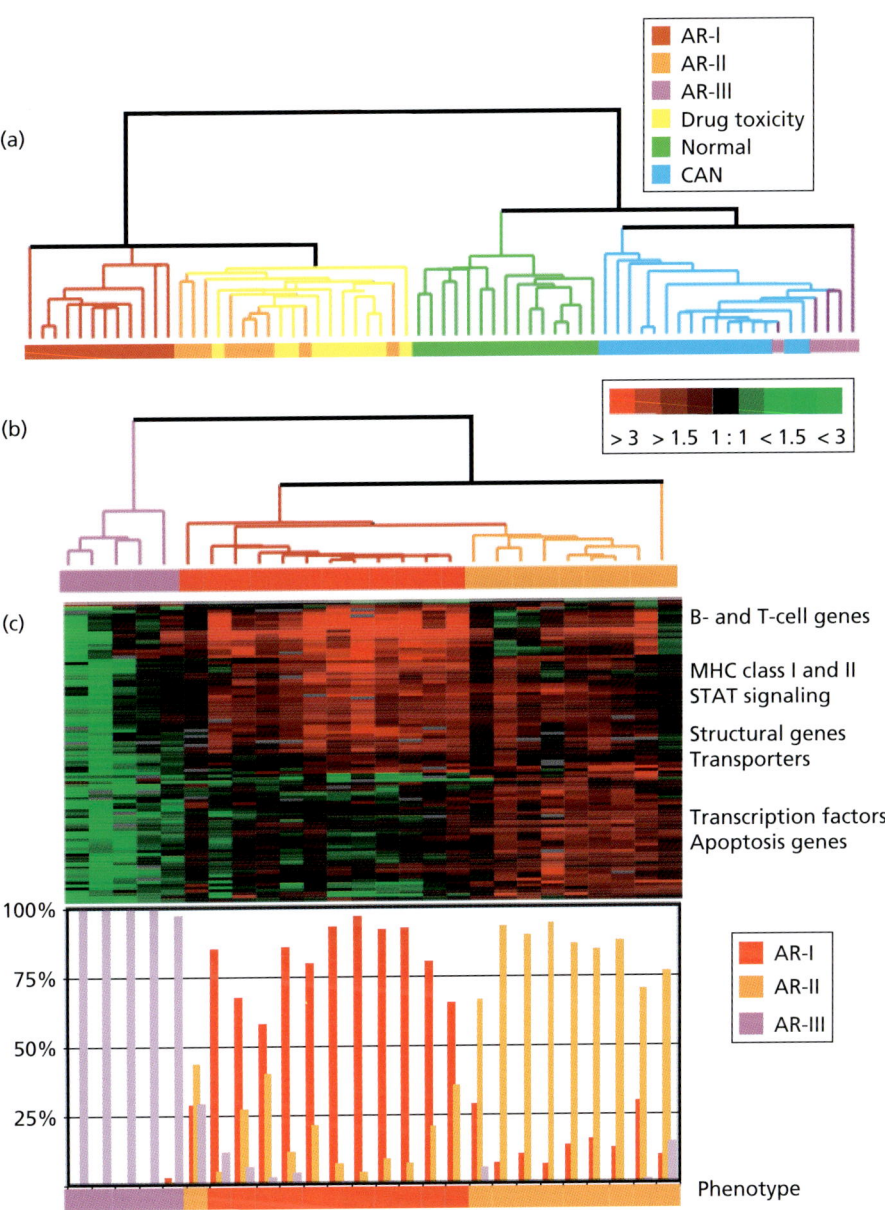

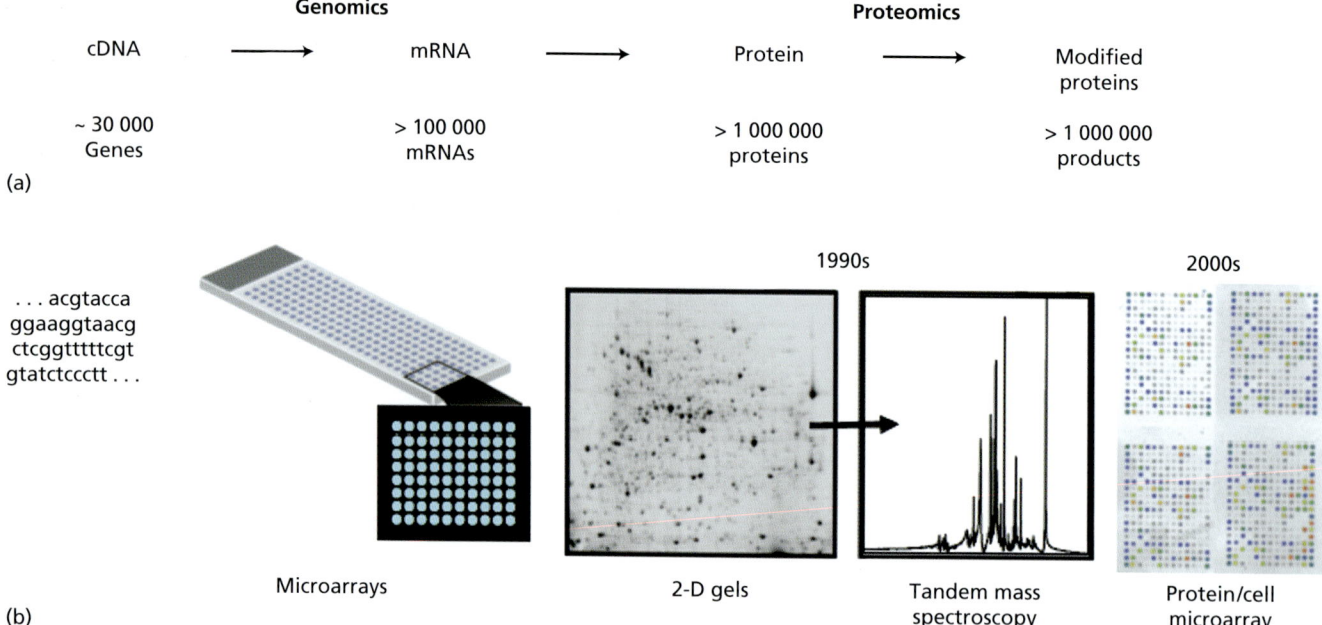

Genomics

cDNA $\longrightarrow$ mRNA $\longrightarrow$ **Proteomics** Protein $\longrightarrow$ Modified proteins

~ 30 000 Genes   > 100 000 mRNAs   > 1 000 000 proteins   > 1 000 000 products

(a)

. . . acgtacca ggaaggtaacg ctcggtttttcgt gtatctccctt . . .

1990s   2000s

Microarrays   2-D gels   Tandem mass spectroscopy   Protein/cell microarray

(b)

Plate 6.3 Evolution of proteomics parallels genomics. The emerging field of proteomics builds on the advances from genomic technology and parallels the complexity of molecular biology. (a) High-density cDNA microarrays have revolutionized the understanding of biology and opened the field of genomics, the study of the mRNA expression at the genome scale. (b) The 30–50 000 genes stored in genomic DNA are selectively transcribed to over 100 000 different mRNA molecules which result from alternatively spliced variants in different tissues. The relative abundance of all mRNA species can be measured simultaneously using microarrays. Similarly, post-translational modification of translated proteins results in an even higher abundance of different proteins in the living organism. High-resolution two-dimensional gels (2D-gel) and tandem mass-spectroscopy can be used to structurally identify gene products at the protein level, a process that is both labor intensive and costly to implement. Consequently, the field of proteomics is increasing using array-based approaches developed in genomics laboratories to identify the spectrum of proteins within cells or on their surface in cell-based microarray technology (Soen Y, Chen DS, Kraft DL, Davis MM, Brown PO. Detection and characterization of cellular immune responses using peptide-MHC microarrays. *PLoS Biol* 2003;**1**:E65.).

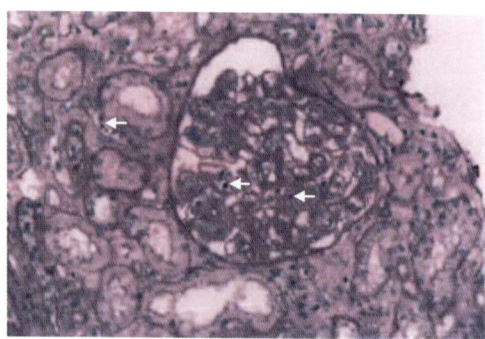

Plate 11.1 Renal biopsy from a patient with antibody-mediated acute rejection. The glomerular and peritubular capillaries contain scattered neutrophils (arrows). The interstitium is mildly edematous and tubular cells show focal degenerative change. (Periodic acid–Schiff × 80)

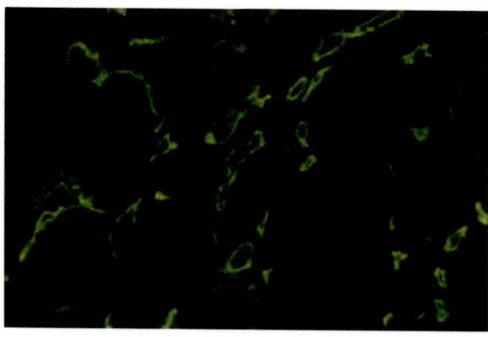

Plate 11.2 Renal biopsy from a patient with AMR stained with fluoresceinated antiserum to C4d. There is bright linear staining of peritubular capillaries (× 80).

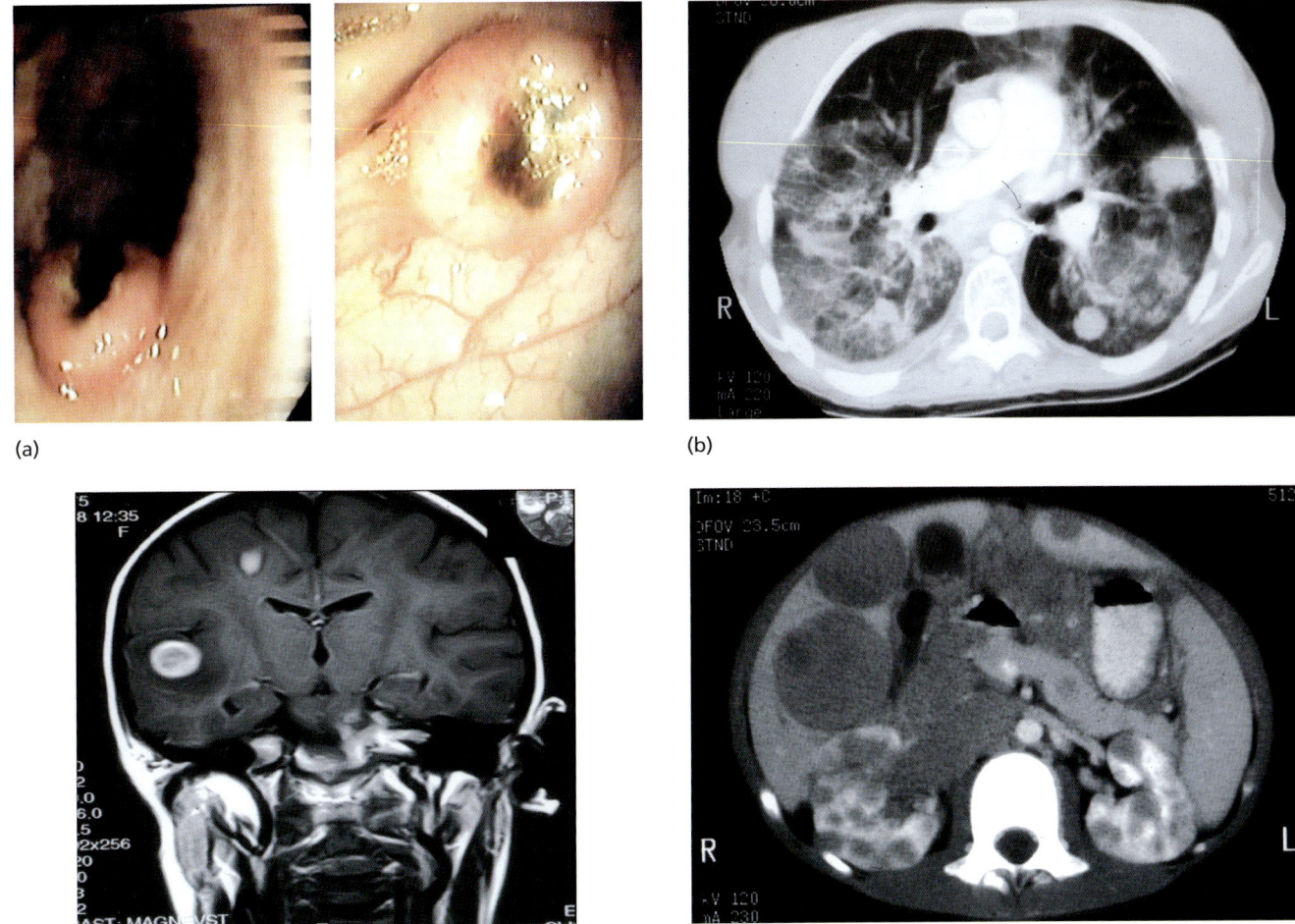

(a)

(b)

(c)

(d)

Plate 13.1 Clinical spectrum of post-transplant lymphoproliferative disorders (PTLD). (a) Characteristic umbilicated nodules of intestinal PTLD. (b) Chest involvement is relatively common, particularly in cardiac and lung recipients. Patchy infiltrates, discrete nodules and mediastinal adenopathy may all be seen. (c) Central nervous system disease is rare but frequently fatal. (d) Multiorgan involvement is seen in this case of Burkitt lymphoma.

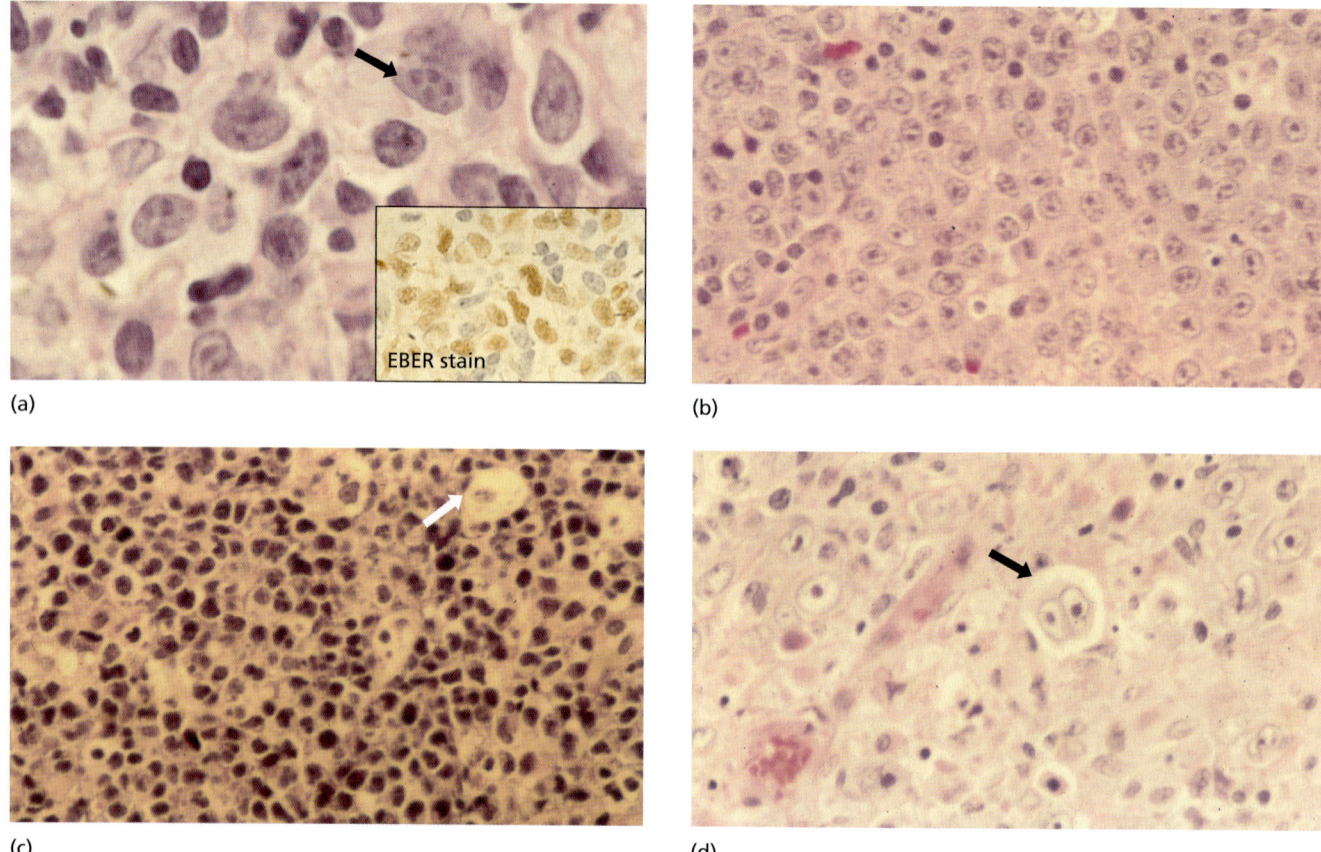

(a)

(b)

(c)

(d)

Plate 13.2 Pathologic spectrum of disease. (a) Polymorphic lesions demonstrate significant pleomorphism with variable numbers of large abnormal cells (arrow) that represent transformed B cells. These usually stain positive for Epstein–Barr virus (EBV) (inset). (b) In monomorphic disease there is much more cellular monotony. Most resemble diffuse large B-cell non-Hodgkin lymphomas.

(c) One specific form of monomorphic disease seen in children is Burkitt or Burkitt-like lymphoma. The so-called starry sky appearance (arrow) represents areas of macrophage ingestion of dying cells. (d) Hodgkin disease and Hodgkin-like PTLD are rare forms of PTLD that are often EBV positive in this population. Typical Reed–Sternberg cell is seen (arrow).

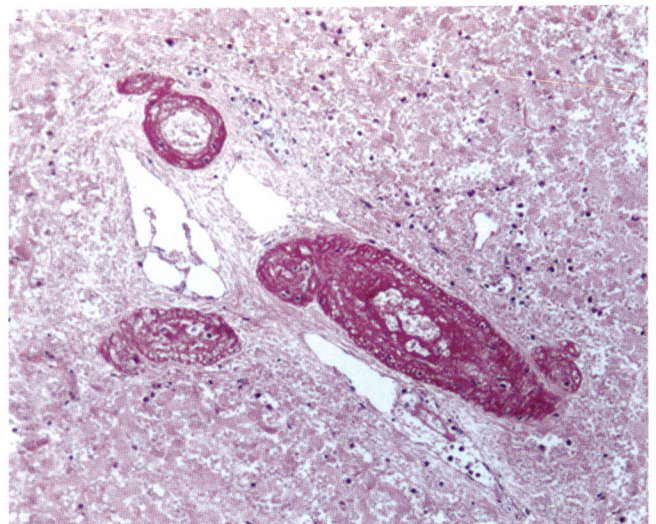

Plate 26.1 Acute humoral rejection. ABO mismatch, an AB liver was used in an A patient with resulting infarction and hepatic failure over the next few days (see Brantley SG, Jaffe R, Esquivel CO, Ramsey G. Acute humoral rejection of an ABO-unmatched liver allograft in a pediatric recipient. *Pediatr Pathol* 1988;8:467–75). Periodic acid–Schiff (PAS) stain highlights the arteries in which there was very extensive immunoglobulin M (IgM) deposition and anti-B was eluted.

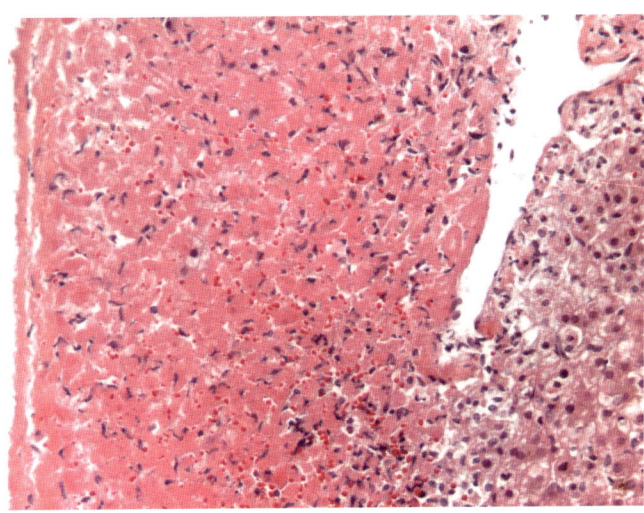

Plate 26.2 Early ischemia. Portion of the needle biopsy shows necrosis. Evaluation of the significance of this finding on biopsy requires careful correlation with hepatocellular enzymes. In this instance, an intraoperative and incidental biopsy, the hepatocellular enzymes had already normalized.

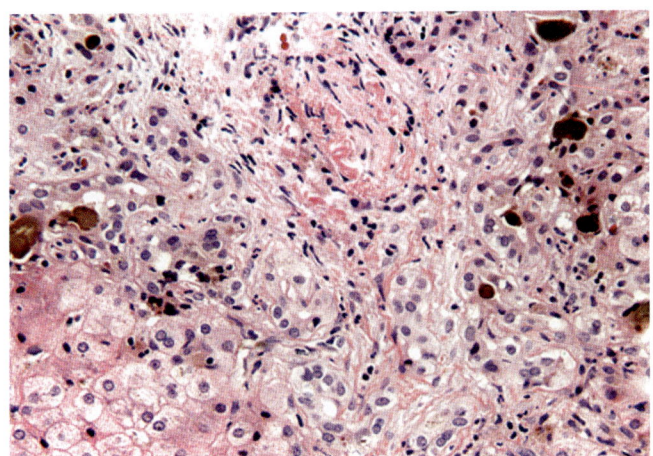

Plate 26.3 Biliary changes. A corona of inspissated Hering ducts surround a portal area that shows little cellular infiltrate but bile ductular proliferation. The liver was eventually removed for obstruction resulting from refractory inspissation of the bile ducts.

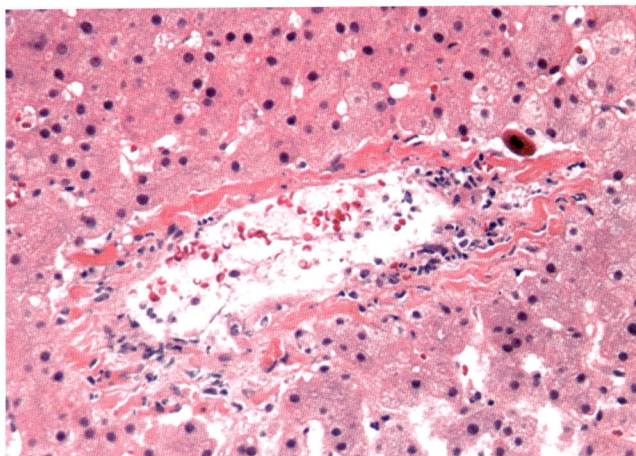

Plate 26.4 Central venulitis. The accumulation of mononuclear cells in and around the central vein has a wide differential. This represents an otherwise normal allograft in the first week.

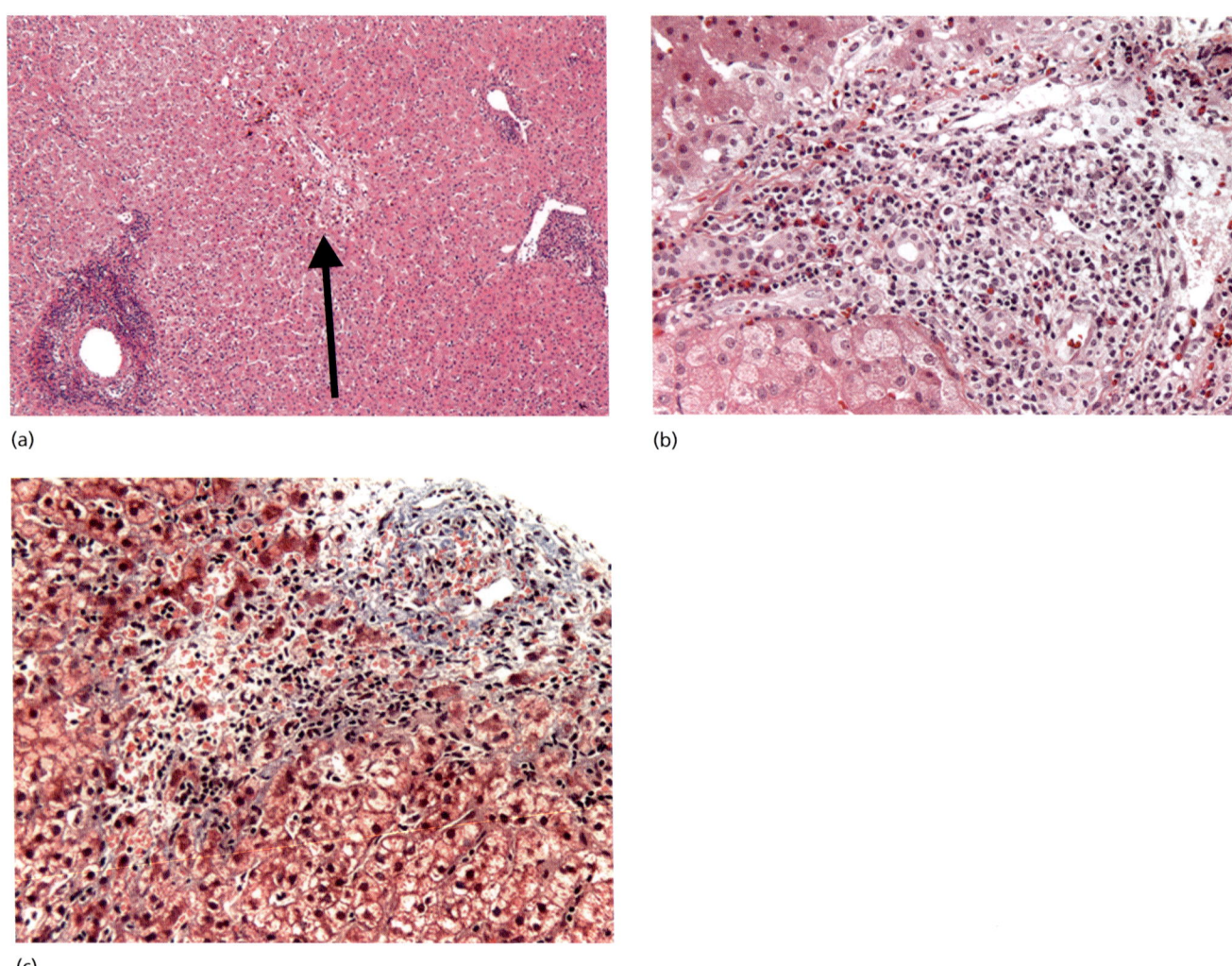

(a)

(b)

(c)

Plate 26.5 (a) Acute cellular rejection. Low power view shows the infiltration that expands portal areas and highlights the central hepatocellular dropout (arrow). (b) Acute cellular rejection. The cellular infiltrate is mixed in nature and the portal venulitis is prominent. (c) Acute cellular rejection. There is damage to pericentral hepatocytes with red cell extravasation and a notable mononuclear presence (Trichrome). Recovery is slow, often weeks. Other causes of centrilobular damage such as venous occlusion and hepatitis should be excluded.

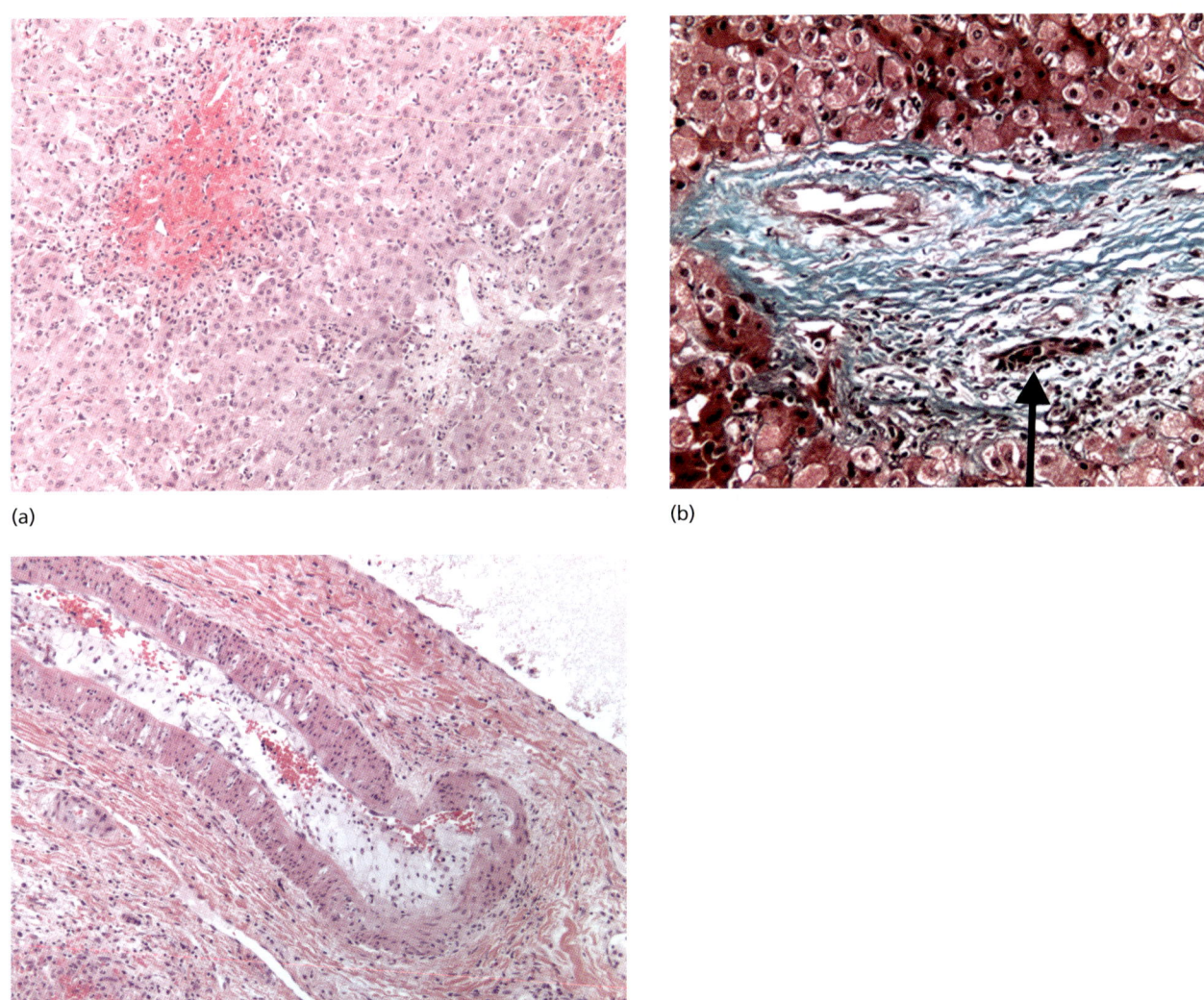

(a)

(b)

(c)

Plate 26.6 (a) Chronic rejection. Portal areas are barely recognizable because of loss of structures, primarily biliary elements. The central damage with red cell extravasation is seen. (b) Chronic rejection. Biopsy prior to the hepatectomy (a) shows a scarred portal area almost devoid of cellular infiltrate and a badly damaged syncytial biliary epithelial remnant (arrow) (Trichrome). (c) Chronic rejection. The hilar vessels display the expected arterial changes of an allograft obliterative vasculopathy.

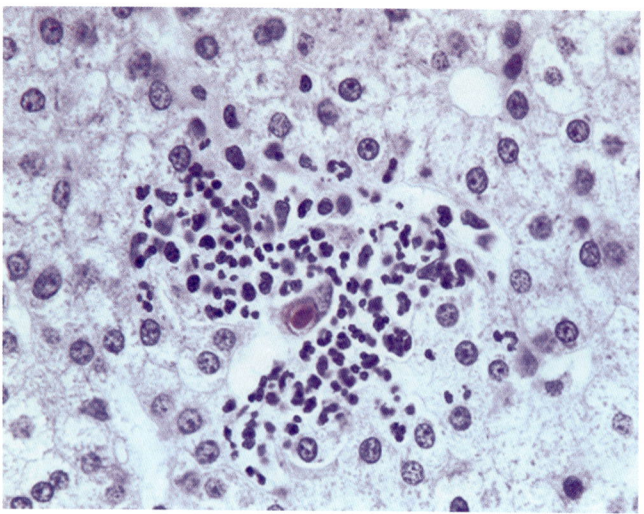

Plate 26.7 Cytomegalovirus. An infected cell is surrounded by neutrophils and the reaction is confined.

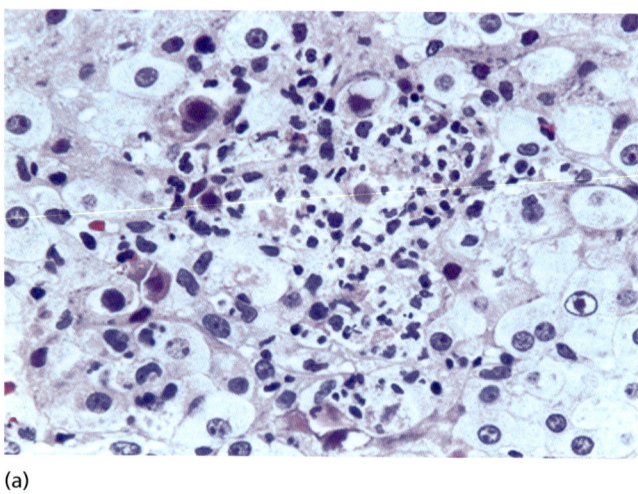

(a)

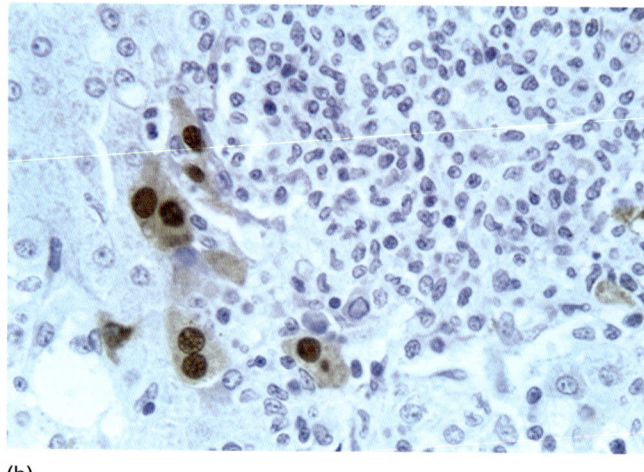

(b)

Plate 26.8 (a) Adenovirus. A circumscribed zone of hepatocyte dropout is filled with monocytes and few neutrophils. Enlarged nuclei contain viral inclusions. (b) Adenovirus. Antibody to adenovirus confirms the identity of the inclusions.

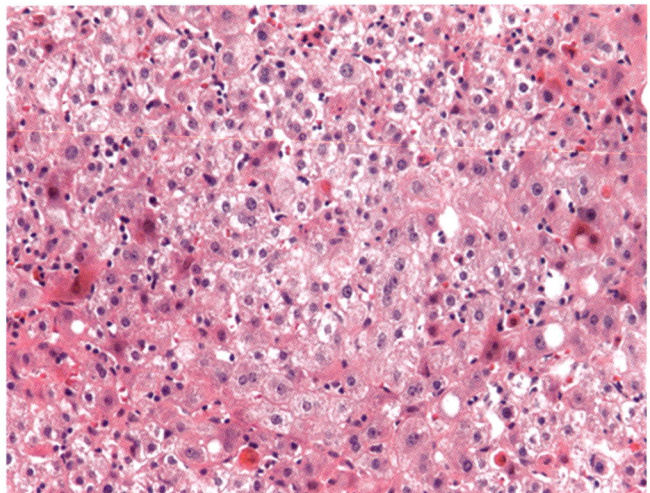

Plate 26.9 Hepatitis C. Recurrent hepatitis C within 1 month of transplantation. The differential diagnosis from acute rejection requires correlation with viral load though the lobular effects are unlike those of rejection.

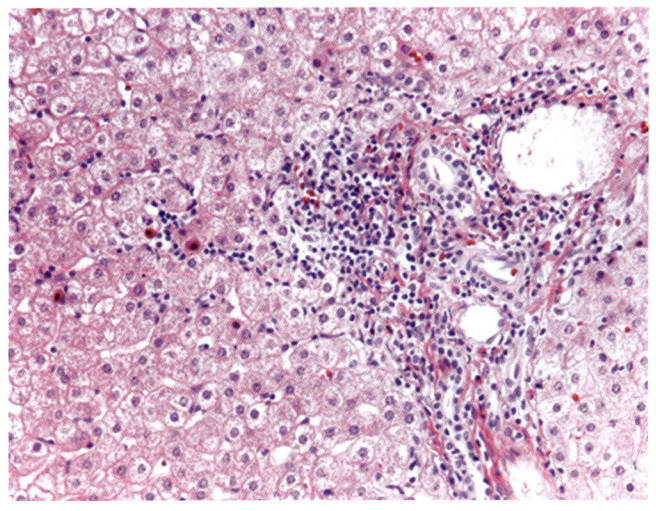

(a)

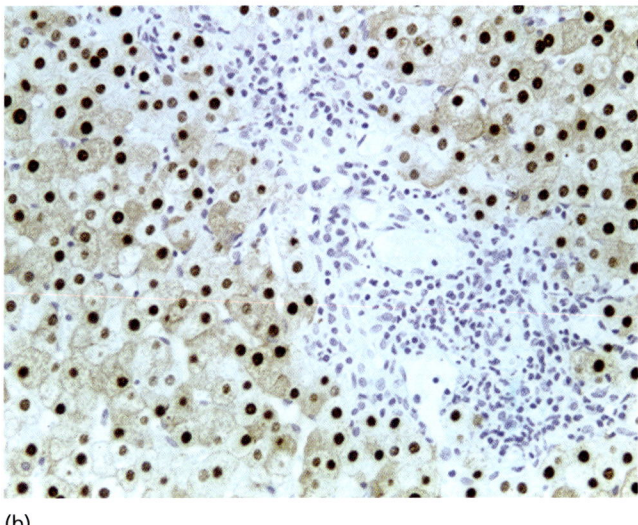

(b)

Plate 26.10 (a) Hepatitis B. The portal infiltrate is not distinguishable from acute rejection although venulitis is not prominent. (b) Hepatitis B. Immunostain for hepatitis B core antigen reveals extensive nuclear staining, some membrane and cytoplasmic staining. The presence of acute rejection and hepatitis B can be difficult to discern.

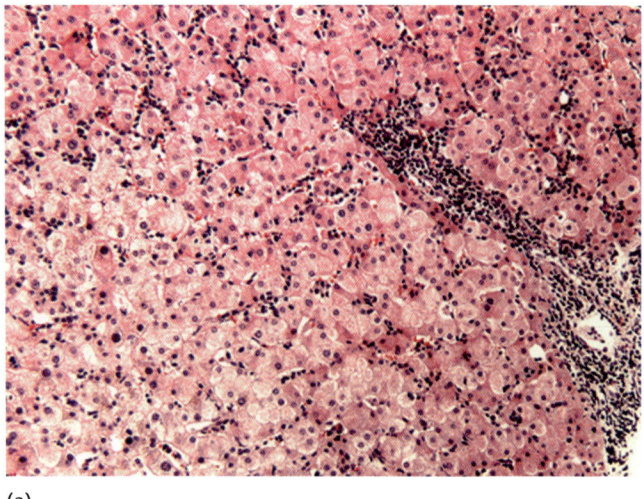

(a)

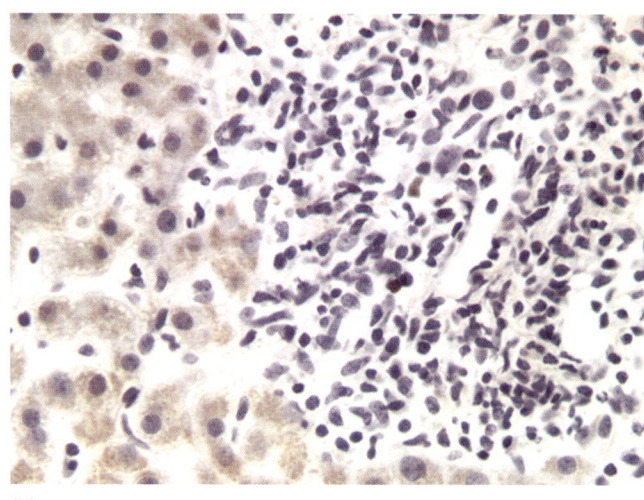

(b)

Plate 26.11 (a) EBV hepatitis. The hepatitis was associated with high EBV-PCR and mildly deranged hepatocellular enzymes.

(b) EBV hepatitis. EBER-1 probe. The number of EBER-1 reactive cells in EBV hepatitis is generally low.

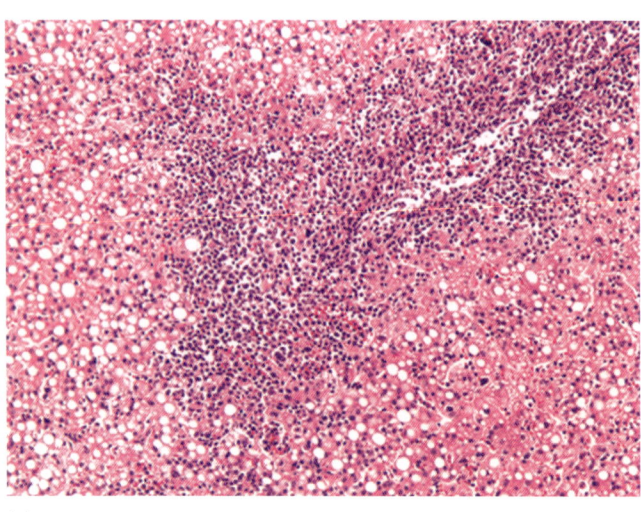

(a)

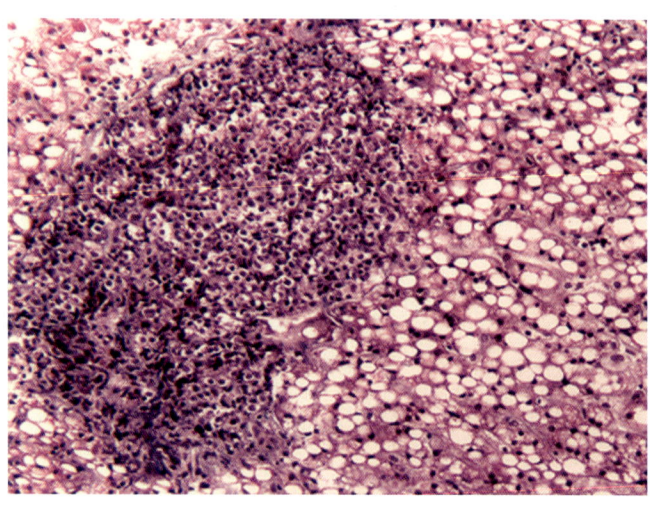

(b)

Plate 26.12 (a) Post-transplant lymphoproliferative disease, polymorphous. A dense portal heterogeneous lymphoid infiltrate was associated with prominent venulitis. EBER-1 probe showed many reactive nuclei, but the majority of cells were CD3⁺.

(b) Post-transplant lymphoproliferative disease, monomorphous. The cells were uniformly CD20⁺/EBER-1⁺. The infiltrate is monotonous, without a population of reactive inflammatory cells.

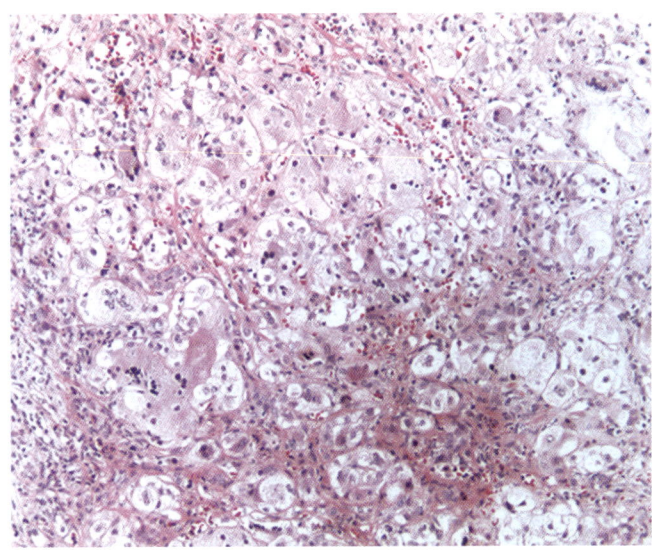

Plate 26.13 Recurrent giant cell hepatitis. Giant cell hepatitis with autoimmune hemolytic anemia recurred within weeks of transplantation.

66 Dalgic A, Dalgic B, Demirogullari B, et al. Clinical approach to graft hepatic artery thrombosis following living related liver transplantation. *Pediatr Transplant* 2003;7:149–52.

67 Emond JC, Rosenthal P, Roberts JP, et al. Living related donor liver transplantation: the UCSF experience. *Transplant Proc* 1996;28:2375–7.

68 Jain A, Mazariengos G, Kashyap R, et al. Pediatric liver transplantation in 808 consecutive children: 20-years experience from a single center. *Transplant Proc* 2002;34:1955–7.

69 McCormick PA, McIntyre N. Pathogenesis and management of ascites in chronic liver disease. *Br J Hosp Med* 1992;47:738–44.

70 Wolf DC, Freni MA, Boccagni P, et al. Low-dose aspirin therapy is associated with few side effects but does not prevent hepatic artery thrombosis in liver transplant recipients. *Liver Transpl Surg* 1997;3:598–603.

71 Couchoud C, Cucherat M, Haugh M, Pouteil-Noble C. Cytomegalovirus prophylaxis with antiviral agents in solid organ transplantation: a meta-analysis. *Transplantation* 1998;65:641–7.

72 Heffron TG, Pillen T, Welch D, et al. Hepatic artery thrombosis in pediatric liver transplantation. *Transplant Proc* 2003;35:1447–8.

73 Mazzaferro V, Esquivel CO, Makowka L, et al. Hepatic artery thrombosis after pediatric liver transplantation: a medical or surgical event? *Transplantation* 1989;47:971–7.

74 Renz JF, Lightdale J, Mudge C, et al. Mycophenolate mofetil, microemulsion cyclosporine, and prednisone as primary immunosuppression for pediatric liver transplant recipients. *Liver Transpl Surg* 1999;5:136–43.

75 Reding R, Gras J, Sokal E, Otte JB, Davies HF. Steroid-free liver transplantation in children. *Lancet* 2003;362:2068–70.

76 Eason JD, Nair S, Cohen AJ, Blazek JL, Loss GE Jr. Steroid-free liver transplantation using rabbit antithymocyte globulin and early tacrolimus monotherapy. *Transplantation* 2003;75:1396–9.

77 Trotter JF. Sirolimus in liver transplantation. *Transplant Proc* 2003;35(Suppl):193S–200S.

78 McDiarmid SV. Liver transplantation: the pediatric challenge. *Clin Liver Dis* 2000;4:879–927.

79 Ghaus N, Bohlega S, Rezeig M. Neurological complications in liver transplantation. *J Neurol* 2001;248:1042–8.

80 Sano K, Makuuchi M, Takayama T, et al. Technical dilemma in living-donor or split-liver transplant. *Hepatogastroenterology* 2000;47:1208–9.

81 Maring JK, Klompmaker IJ, Zwaveling JH, et al. Poor initial graft function after orthotopic liver transplantation: can it be predicted and does it affect outcome? An analysis of 125 adult primary transplantations. *Clin Transplant* 1997;11:373–9.

82 Hwang S, Lee SG, Lee YJ, et al. A case of primary non-function following adult-to-adult living donor liver transplantation. *Hepatogastroenterology* 2002;49:1412–4.

83 McDonnell N, Ames WA, Potter D. Bradycardia in children less than two years of age during liver transplantation. *Transpl Int* 1998;11:237–8.

84 Peh WC, Olliff SP. The role of the radiologist in liver transplantation. *Ann Acad Med Singapore* 1993;22:688–95.

85 Griffith JF, John PR. Imaging of biliary complications following paediatric liver transplantation. *Pediatr Radiol* 1996;26:388–94.

86 Renz JF, Rosenthal P, Roberts JP, Ascher NL, Emond JC. Planned exploration of pediatric liver transplant recipients reduces posttransplant morbidity and lowers length of hospitalization. *Arch Surg* 1997;132:950–5; discussion 955–6.

87 Gaglio PJ, Leevy CB, Koneru B. Peri-operative chylous ascites. *J Med* 1996;27:369–76.

88 Kaku R, Matsumi M, Fujii H, et al. [A case of severe acute hyperkalemia during pre-anhepatic stage in living-related liver transplantation]. *Masui* 2002;51:1003–6.

89 Acosta F, Sansano T, Contreras RF, et al. Changes in serum potassium during reperfusion in liver transplantation. *Transplant Proc* 1999;31:2382–3.

90 Egawa H, Uemoto S, Inomata Y, et al. Biliary complications in pediatric living related liver transplantation. *Surgery* 1998;124:901–10.

91 Egawa H, Inomata Y, Uemoto S, et al. Biliary anastomotic complications in 400 living related liver transplantations. *World J Surg* 2001;25:1300–7.

92 George DL, Arnow PM, Fox A, et al. Patterns of infection after pediatric liver transplantation. *Am J Dis Child* 1992;146:924–9.

93 George DL, Arnow PM, Fox AS, et al. Bacterial infection as a complication of liver transplantation: epidemiology and risk factors. *Rev Infect Dis* 1991;13:387–96.

94 Gladdy RA, Richardson SE, Davies HD, Superina RA. *Candida* infection in pediatric liver transplant recipients. *Liver Transpl Surg* 1999;5:16–24.

95 Amii LA, Moss RL. Nutritional support of the pediatric surgical patient. *Curr Opin Pediatr* 1999;11:237–40.

96 Hade AM, Shine AM, Kennedy NP, McCormick PA. Both under-nutrition and obesity increase morbidity following liver transplantation. *Ir Med J* 2003;96:140–2.

26 Pathology of the Liver Allograft

Maria Parizhskaya and Ronald Jaffe

The interpretation of liver transplant histopathology is a prime example of the close interrelationship between clinical monitoring, laboratory values and the features of the tissue on the slide. Without the clinical context, and in the absence of serum enzyme and bilirubin levels, serology, viral polymerase chain reaction (PCR) and therapeutic drug monitoring, allograft histopathology is likely to be misleading. Allograft diagnosis is not an example of "the answer is on the slide"; quite the contrary, the answer is in the synthesis and histopathology adds an important dimension to the evaluation of the post-transplanted organ. That is not to say that patterns of tissue response have no intrinsic information, clearly they do in the aggregate, but for the individual patient, decisions about changes in treatment should be made on the basis of an integrated interpretation. Ideally, a new program will embark on a system of patient monitoring that allows for informed surveillance monitoring in order to get a baseline for the expected liver features at various time points after transplantation. It is naïve to assume that the features in the tissues will not be affected by advances and changes in immune modulation regimens. For that reason alone, the features described in this review should be treated with some reserve by programs whose therapeutic practice differs from ours. The in-house experience within the transplant team is critical.

DONOR EVALUATION

Pediatric liver transplantation in our institution and others carries a negligible risk for "primary graft non-function," and there does not appear to be any firm clinical rationale for the histopathologic examination of the donor organ for damage, fat or granulomas, and most of the large programs do not use it. Obviously, in the infant donor, the risk of an undiagnosed metabolic condition should be acknowledged, but frozen needle biopsy is not likely to be contributory.

HANDLING OF ALLOGRAFT LIVER TISSUES

Needle biopsies are widely used to diagnose the various conditions involving the hepatic allograft. Triage of unfixed liver tissue is determined by clinical information. Clinical suspicion of cholangitis warrants cultures; a differential diagnosis of viral infection, including recurrent hepatitis B and C, indicates viral PCR or cultures, appropriate serology, or immunohistochemical staining, depending on the virus.

In the routine diagnostic service, 6–10 levels of each needle core are stained with hematoxylin and eosin (H&E), and one each with periodic acid–Schiff (PAS) diastase and trichrome in order to demonstrate the portal features and fibrosis. Immunostains for cytomegalovirus (CMV) early antigen, adenovirus, herpes simplex and varicella-zoster viruses are performed only if indicated by H&E morphology [1], and *in situ* hybridization for Epstein–Barr virus (EBV) early RNA (EBER-1 probe) is carried out on clinical suspicion in the correct histopathologic context.

In the examination of allograft hepatectomies, particular attention must be paid to the hilar area [2]. After the extrahepatic stumps of the arteries, veins and bile ducts have been dissected and examined, a rectangular hilar block, sliced at 3-mm intervals, should be obtained. Leaks, fistulas, vascular thromboses and infiltrates can be identified. At least one of the slices should be snap-frozen for immunohistochemistry or documentation of immune deposits by immunofluorescence if indicated.

PRIMARY ALLOGRAFT FAILURE

Hyperacute rejection is virtually unknown in the liver, and early humoral rejection is very unusual but can occur in the first weeks after transplantation. The morphology of early humoral rejection may not be diagnostic on percutaneous needle biopsy, because complement and immunoglobulin deposition affects larger hilar arteries that are not represented. There are damaged central veins with fibrin accumulation, erythrocyte extravasation and sinusoidal distention leading to centrizonal thrombosis and hemorrhagic coagulative necrosis (see Plate 26.1, facing page 224) [3].

HARVESTING-RELATED INJURY

Harvesting-related damage manifests early and is characterized by hepatocellular ballooning, primarily centrilobular, but it can occupy the entire lobule if severe. There may be hepatocellular necrosis – both centrizonal and spotty – canalicular cholestasis and portal changes such as edema and bile ductular proliferation. Hyperalimentation effect may compound the cholestasis. Portal cellularity can vary significantly, some of the cellularity being donor in origin, and neutrophils accompany the bile ductular proliferation. Damage may be more severe in the subcapsular area; therefore extensive necrosis and hemorrhage in a biopsy specimen (particularly a wedge biopsy) may not represent the entire liver (see Plate 26.2, facing page 224) [4]. Close correlation with the trajectory of the hepatocellular enzyme profile is absolutely essential in order to avoid errors in this period.

VASCULAR DISORDERS

Hepatic arterial thrombosis alone, or in combination with portal vein thrombosis, remains a major problem in very small recipients [1,5]. Biopsy may be of little value in the diagnosis of hepatic artery thrombosis because of paucity of changes, but in some the findings are similar to those of harvesting-related ischemia with centrizonal hepatocellular ballooning, canalicular cholestasis, centrizonal collapse and coagulative necrosis.

As is true for many other situations, the differential diagnosis of early allograft damage can best be elucidated with the full knowledge of the hepatocellular and biliary enzymes. A liver that does not rapidly return to baseline enzyme and synthetic levels is likely to be caused by donor organ damage prior to death or in the retrieval, transport or implantation phase. A liver that works well but fails after an interval is more likely to have acquired vascular compromise.

In hepatic venous outflow obstruction there may be ascites. The liver is enlarged and the biopsy reveals prominent centrilobular sinusoidal dilatation, congestion and hemorrhage together with progressive atrophy and loss of hepatocytes.

BILIARY DISORDERS

In the early postoperative period there is a possibility of a false-positive diagnosis of a biliary problem. The damage caused by harvesting and ischemia, in addition to cholestasis and hepatocellular ballooning, can induce neutrophilic cholangitis and pericholangitis, as well as bile ductular proliferation. Sepsis

and parenteral nutrition can induce portal bile plugs, thus simulating extrahepatic biliary obstruction. All of these findings are compounded in partial (split or reduced and living-related) liver allografts. In some instances, ultrasonography or cholangiography may be needed, because the morphologic features of biliary obstruction can be simulated by other processes [6]. Neutrophils in and around the bile ducts can also signify bacterial cholangitis or intra-abdominal abscess.

Features of biliary fistulas can be encountered on the biopsy [1]. In biliary–portal fistula, the portal venous system contains clumps of bile with a surrounding giant cell reaction. In a vascular–biliary fistula, the portal bile ducts are filled with erythrocytes.

Biliary complications are now the single most common finding after 5 years in the pediatric population who present with hyperbilirubinemia and elevated gamma-glutamyltransferase (GGT) levels [7]. Chronic biliary disease can be accompanied by extensive portal chronic inflammation, mimicking acute rejection. The two features that are of diagnostic importance in the differential diagnosis are the presence of bile ductular proliferation, not seen in acute rejection alone, and concentric edema and fibrosis around larger bile ducts when these are represented in the biopsy (see Plate 26.3, facing page 224). Centrilobular canalicular cholestasis accompanied by hepatocellular ballooning will be common to biliary obstruction, bile duct loss in chronic rejection, arterial ischemia and parenteral nutrition. While biliary obstruction is often caused by stenosis of an anastomosis and is reparable, biliary strictures can also be a manifestation of ischemia resulting from allograft vascular disease.

ACUTE CELLULAR REJECTION

Acute cellular rejection can occur as early as day 3 following transplantation and is most common during the first 2 months, but can occur months or even years later if there are changes in immunosuppression. In acute cellular rejection, the portal areas are expanded by a mixed cellular infiltrate that is composed predominantly of T lymphocytes but also contains eosinophils, macrophages, few plasma cells and neutrophils. The infiltrate is centered on the biliary epithelial cells that show a spectrum of histologic alterations, including cytoplasmic vacuolation or eosinophilia, enlarged nuclei with anisonucleosis, nuclear crowding and overlap, prominent nucleoli and, in more severe cases, syncytial transformation of epithelial cells and eventual loss of interlobular bile ducts. Endotheliitis is feature of acute rejection and is seen in portal veins but perhaps more consistently in or around central veins (see Plate 26.4, facing page 224) [8,9]. Initially, lymphocytes accumulate along the luminal surface of the veins and adhere to enlarged endothelial cells. With advancing degree of involvement, the endothelium is lifted from its underlying connective tissue and lymphocytes accumulate

Table 26.1 Rejection Activity Index (RAI) after Banff Schema [10].

Category	Criteria	Score
Portal inflammation	Mostly lymphocytic inflammation involving a minority of the triads	1
	Expansion of most or all of the triads by a mixed infiltrate	2
	Marked expansion of most or all of the triads by a mixed infiltrate with inflammatory spillover into the periportal parenchyma	3
Bile duct inflammation, damage	A minority of the ducts are infiltrated by inflammatory cells and show mild reactive changes	1
	Most or all of the ducts are infiltrated by inflammatory cells. Some ducts show degenerative changes	2
	As above for 2, with most or all of the ducts showing degenerative changes or focal lumenal disruption	3
Venous endothelial inflammation	Subendothelial lymphocytic infiltration involving some portal and/or hepatic venules	1
	Subendothelial infiltration involving most or all of the portal and/or hepatic venules	2
	As above for 2, with moderate to severe perivenular inflammation and associated perivenular hepatocyte necrosis	3

Note: Total score = sum of components (RAI 1–3 mild rejection, RAI 4–6 moderate rejection, RAI 7–9 severe rejection).

in the subendothelial zone. Mononuclear infiltrates including monocytes are commonly seen in otherwise normal allografts in the first week. Pericentral hepatocellular dropout with erythrocyte extravasation in the presence of lymphocytes signifies more extensive damage. The hepatic lobules, however, are relatively spared in acute rejection. An uncommon pattern of acute rejection has hepatocellular damage with Councilman bodies at the limiting plate.

The "severity" of acute rejection is graded by using the Banff schema which utilizes the three classic criteria of a mixed cellular portal infiltrate, portal and/or pericentral venulitis, and biliary epithelial damage (see Plate 26.5a,b, facing page 224) [10]. While the grading system (Table 26.1) has proven clinical utility, it is not absolutely predictive and is not validated for the pediatric patient population. Some "severe" acute rejection episodes respond rapidly to adjustments in immunosuppression while others, ostensibly "mild" or "moderate," may be corticosteroid-resistant and require more potent immunosuppressants. Some patients manifest their rejection by virtue of the pericentral activity (i.e. mononuclear cell infiltrate around the central veins, red cell extravasation and eventual centrizonal hepatocyte necrosis) in the virtual absence of portal signs. This centrizonal pattern of acute rejection is recapitulated consistently in the same individual over time, responds slowly to enhanced immunosuppression and must be distinguished from venous outflow obstruction which usually lacks the lymphocytic component (see Plate 26.5c, facing page 224). The differential diagnosis of central venulitis, however, is not limited to acute rejection and should include conditions such as autoimmune and viral hepatitis, especially EBV infection, drug or toxin reactions, and sometimes vascular compromise [11,12].

An unusual pattern of acute rejection is the "hepatitic" pattern. Teenagers who become noncompliant and present with elevated liver enzymes and low or undetectable drug levels may show this pattern. Biopsy from some of these children has shown disproportionate lobular inflammatory activity with mild to moderate portal changes simulating hepatitis. Restoring drug levels to the therapeutic range was associated with resolution, although in some children this was a slow process. In this situation, in which the clinical diagnosis is so compelling and the serologic studies are negative, a diagnosis of rejection with a lobular or "hepatitic" pattern is made.

To add to the complexity, a partially treated acute rejection can be difficult to recognize without a clinical history of change in the immunosuppressive treatment prior to the biopsy. A partially treated rejection is characterized by disparity between persisting biliary epithelial damage and partial resolution of the cellular infiltrate [1].

CHRONIC REJECTION

A working recommendation for the histopathologic staging and reporting of chronic rejection by an international panel has been published as the International Banff Schema [13]. Progressive bile duct loss, arterial loss and obliterative arteriopathy are features of chronic rejection, although the latter is not well represented in biopsies. The principal diagnostic feature on biopsy is therefore bile duct loss (subject to sampling variation and regeneration) and cholestasis, so that biliary disease is the prime differential diagnosis (see Plate 26.6a–c, facing page 224). In contrast to the previously mentioned biliary complications, however, bile ductular proliferation at the interface zone is unusual even for chronic rejection with loss of bile ducts. Chronic ductopenic rejection has become very rare in our population on current immunosuppression unless therapy has been reduced for life-threatening infection or the patient is noncompliant [14,15]. Features of acute rejection that accompany those of chronic rejection should be recognized as such because there is evidence that some features of chronic rejection are reversible [16].

INFECTIONS

Because of changes in monitoring for antigenemia and prophylaxis, CMV hepatitis has become more unusual in our transplant population. CMV hepatitis is characterized by haphazardly scattered microabscesses, sometimes with a mixture of mononuclear cells, surrounding damaged hepatocytes. Nuclear and cytoplasmic CMV inclusions are noted in the vast majority cases if a number of sections are carefully examined (see Plate 26.7, facing page 224). Immunostaining for early intermediate CMV antigen (which can be seen in the nucleus of still untransformed cells) yields very rare additional cases but does give some indication of the degree of active viral replication. Because damage is local, confined to the infected hepatocytes, portal inflammation tends to be sparse, with a few lymphocytes and plasma cells unless there is CMV infection in a portal area, biliary or endothelial, in which case the local reaction is more exuberant.

Infection with herpes simplex or varicella-zoster viruses leads to foci of necrosis varying in size and randomly distributed across the liver. The nuclear inclusions should be sought and confirmed by immunohistochemistry.

The histopathology of adenovirus hepatitis is characteristic. Circumscribed granulomas, filled with monocytes, entrap or are surrounded by enlarged hepatocytes that have nuclear inclusions, which can be confirmed by immunohistochemistry, *in situ* hybridization or, if required, by electron microscopy (see Plate 26.8a,b, facing page 224) [1].

Patients infected with hepatitis B or C are at high risk of recurrence in the allograft. *De novo* cases are rare in the allograft because of current immunization and transfusion practices. Liver biopsy must be read in the context of knowing the DNA/RNA and serologic status of the patient. The histopathologic features of hepatitis B and C in the allograft are similar to that in the host – lobular activity with Kupffer cell activation and spotty hepatocellular necrosis is accompanied by a portal infiltrate (less heterogeneous than in acute rejection) that concentrates on the area of the limiting plate and is associated with piecemeal necrosis (see Plate 26.9, facing page 224). Recurrent hepatitis C infection differs histopathologically from hepatitis B in that nodular lymphoid aggregates are common in the portal areas, and bile duct damage can be seen that mimics acute rejection. A predominantly lymphocytic portal infiltrate that is disproportionate to the usually small amount of biliary epithelial damage is in favor of hepatitis C infection rather than rejection. Foci of central venulitis can appear in recurrent viral hepatitis either as part of the underlying disease or as a manifestation

of coexistent rejection [12]. Distinction between these two processes may be difficult and subjective and correlation with quantitative PCR levels is needed. Unfortunately, there is a tendency to overlook the features of acute rejection in patients who have known viral hepatitis, and this can lead to organ loss (see Plate 26.10a,b, facing page 224).

A subgroup of patients with cholestatic variant of recurrent hepatitis C infection has been described [17,18]. These patients present with jaundice, hyperbilirubinemia, high hepatitis C virus RNA levels and frequent allograft failure. Besides the usual morphologic features of hepatitis C virus infection, their biopsies show areas of confluent necrosis, bridging fibrosis, hepatocellular ballooning and prominent bile ductular proliferation.

Seroconversion in previously EBV-negative pediatric recipients is high within the first few months after liver transplantation [19,20]. As with other hepatitides, biopsies are best interpreted when the serology and EBV-DNA status are known, but this is not always possible because in children EBV hepatitis in the allograft may be the first manifestation of the infection. EBV hepatitis can have lobular and portal components (see Plate 26.11a,b, facing page 224). The lobules show small lymphocytes in sinusoids, Kupffer cell hyperplasia and lobular disarray with hepatocellular damage depending on the severity. Central venulitis with mononuclear cells can be present in EBV hepatitis. Portal infiltrates tend to be more lymphocytic, less heterogeneous than in acute rejection but can be quite extensive. The portal infiltrate is generally disproportionate to the mild biliary epithelial damage. Phenotyping of the infiltrating cells is of little help because the lymphocytes in both EBV hepatitis and rejection are T cells. Large, transformed immunoblasts are sparse and may be difficult to recognize. EBER-1 probe is of some but limited help because only few of the lymphoid cells in EBV hepatitis are expected to be positive, but the presence of more than a single infected cell in a child is significant in our experience. The most difficult differential diagnosis is that between EBV hepatitis and acute rejection when the immunosuppression has been lowered for some time, and rising liver enzymes lead to a clinical suspicion of rejection. Strict adherence to the morphologic criteria for rejection and an absence of nuclear EBER-1 staining may make this distinction easier, and correlation with quantitative EBV-PCR levels can be helpful, especially in the face of chronic and persistent active EBV hepatitis.

POST-TRANSPLANT LYMPHOPROLIFERATIVE DISEASE

Post-transplant lymphoproliferative disease (PTLD) is closely associated with immunosuppression and EBV infection [19–21]. In polymorphous PTLD there is a diffuse heterogeneous proliferation of lymphoid cells, including small and large cleaved and noncleaved lymphocytes, immunoblasts, plasmacytoid and plasma cells (see Plate 26.12a, facing page 224). The lesions of monomorphous PTLD are composed of sheets of large, transformed immunoblasts. They are often "malignant" appearing with areas of necrosis and difficult to distinguish from large cell or Burkitt lymphoma (see Plate 26.12b, facing page 224). The PTLD infiltrate obscures the normal hepatic landmarks and is usually associated with a nodule or a mass that is visible on computed tomography (CT) scan. EBER-1 probe will, in most pediatric cases, demonstrate nuclear positivity in the majority of infiltrating B lymphoid cells. The diagnosis of PTLD is usually not difficult, but it is the diagnosis of rejection following the decrease in immunosuppression that presents the same dilemma as that described above.

EBV-RELATED SMOOTH MUSCLE TUMOR

Smooth muscle tumors containing EBV may involve the allograft, as well as extrahepatic sites [22]. These tumors typically occur in a setting of prior or ensuing diagnosis of PTLD. They are composed of fascicles of spindled smooth muscle cells showing nuclear staining with EBER-1 probe.

DRUG REACTIONS

According to Sherlock [23], "hepatic drug reactions can mimic almost all patterns of liver injury seen in man." The other processes going on simultaneously in transplanted livers, new drugs and the combinations of drugs and active biologic therapeutic agents make this area even more confounding. To this complexity must be added the hepatic effects of parenteral nutrition.

RECURRENCE OF PRIMARY DISEASE IN THE ALLOGRAFT

Autoimmune hepatitis recurs or can appear *de novo* [24,25]. The histologic features recapitulate those in the native liver (i.e. plasma cell rich infiltrate concentrating on the area of the limiting plate). These histologic features are accompanied by positive serum autoantibodies on which the diagnosis is based. Giant cell hepatitis with autoimmune hemolytic anemia has a high incidence of recurrence in the allograft (see Plate 26.13, facing page 224). Occasional examples of recurrent metabolic disease are recorded [26]. It is important to be aware of the original disease when confronted with an allograft liver biopsy.

The Transplant Pathology Internet Service (TPIS) offers a useful resource for all aspects of transplant pathology at http://tpis.upmc.edu.

REFERENCES

1 Jaffe R, Yunis EJ. Pediatric liver transplantation: diagnostic pathology. *Perspect Pediatr Pathol* 1989;**13**:44–81.

2 Demetris AJ, Jaffe R, Starzl TE. A review of adult and pediatric post-transplant liver pathology. *Pathol Annu* 1987;**22**:347–86.

3 Demetris AJ, Jaffe R, Tzakis A, *et al*. Antibody-mediated rejection of human orthotopic liver allografts: a study of liver transplantation across ABO blood group barriers. *Am J Pathol* 1988;**132**:489–502.

4 Russo PA, Yunis EJ. Subcapsular hepatic necrosis in orthotopic liver allografts. *Hepatology* 1986;**6**:708–13.

5 Sieders E, Peeters PM, TenVergert EM, *et al*. Early vascular complications after pediatric liver transplantation. *Liver Transpl* 2000;**6**:326–32.

6 Lerut J, Gordon RD, Iwatsuki S, *et al*. Biliary tract complications in human orthotopic liver transplantation. *Transplantation* 1987;**43**:47–51.

7 Lopez-Santamaria M, Martinez L, Hierro L, *et al*. Late biliary complications in pediatric liver transplantation. *J Pediatr Surg* 1999;**34**:316–20.

8 Porter KA. Pathology of liver transplantation. *Transplant Rev* 1969;**2**:129–70.

9 Ludwig J, Batts KP, Ploch M, *et al*. Endotheliitis in hepatic allografts. *Mayo Clin Proc* 1989;**64**:545–54.

10 Banff schema for grading liver allograft rejection: an international consensus document. An International Panel. *Hepatology* 1997;**25**:658–63.

11 Krasinskas AM, Ruchelli ED, Rand EB, *et al*. Central venulitis in pediatric liver allografts. *Hepatology* 2001;**33**:1141–7.

12 Demetris AJ. Central venulitis in liver allografts: considerations of differential diagnosis. *Hepatology* 2001;**33**:1329–30.

13 Update of the international Banff schema for liver allograft rejection: working recommendations for the histopathologic staging and reporting of chronic rejection. An International Panel. *Hepatology* 2000;**31**:792–9.

14 Cao S, Cox KL, Berquist W, *et al*. Long-term outcomes in pediatric liver recipients: comparison between cyclosporine A and tacrolimus. *Pediatr Transplant* 1999;**3**:22–6.

15 Cacciarelli TV, Dvorchik I, Mazariegos GV, *et al*. An analysis of pretransplantation variables associated with long-term allograft outcome in pediatric liver transplant recipients receiving primary tacrolimus (FK506) therapy. *Transplantation* 1999;**68**:650–5.

16 Blakolmer K, Seaberg EC, Batts K, *et al*. Analysis of the reversibility of chronic liver allograft rejection implications for a staging schema. *Am J Surg Pathol* 1999;**23**:1328–39.

17 Taga SA, Washington MK, Terrault N, *et al*. Cholestatic hepatitis C in liver allografts. *Liver Transpl Surg* 1998;**4**:304–10.

18 Demetris AJ, Eghtesad B, Marcos A, *et al*. Recurrent hepatitis C in liver allografts: prospective assessment of diagnostic accuracy, identification of pitfalls, and observations about pathogenesis. *Am J Surg Pathol* 2004;**28**:658–69.

19 Ho M, Miller G, Atchison RW, *et al*. Epstein–Barr virus infections and DNA hybridization studies in post-transplantation lymphoma and lymphoproliferative lesions: the role of primary infection. *J Infect Dis* 1985;**152**:876–86.

20 Ho M, Jaffe R, Miller G, *et al.* The frequency of Epstein–Barr virus infection and associated lymphoproliferative syndrome after transplantation and its manifestations in children. *Transplantation* 1988;**45**:719–27.

21 Cacciarelli TV, Reyes J, Jaffe R, *et al.* Primary tacrolimus (FK506) therapy and the long-term risk of post-transplant lymphoproliferative disease in pediatric liver transplant recipients. *Pediatr Transplant* 2001;**5**:359–64.

22 Lee ES, Locker J, Nalesnik M, *et al.* The association of Epstein–Barr virus with smooth-muscle tumors occurring after organ transplantation. *N Engl J Med* 1995;**332**:19–25.

23 Sherlock S. The spectrum of hepatotoxicity due to drugs. *Lancet* 1986;**2**:440–4.

24 Birnbaum AH, Benkov KJ, Pittman NS, *et al.* Recurrence of autoimmune hepatitis in children after liver transplantation. *J Pediatr Gastroenterol Nutr* 1997;**25**:20–5.

25 Gupta P, Hart J, Millis JM, *et al. De novo* hepatitis with autoimmune antibodies and atypical histology: a rare cause of late graft dysfunction after pediatric liver transplantation. *Transplantation* 2001;**71**:664–8.

26 Jaffe R. Liver transplant pathology in pediatric metabolic disorders. *Pediatr Dev Pathol* 1998;**1**:102–17.

27 Brantley SG, Jaffe R, Esquivel CO, Ramsey G. Acute humoral rejection of an ABO-unmatched liver allograft in a pediatric recipient. *Pediatr Pathol* 1988;**8**:467–75.

27 Post-Transplant Management

Kyle Soltys, Robert Squires, Rakesh Sindhi and George V. Mazariegos

After the first successful transplant in a child with liver cancer, pediatric liver transplantation has successfully evolved into a life-saving option for children with end-stage liver disease and a host of derangements of hepatic metabolism. The current success of liver transplantation in children can best be appreciated in the historical context of the developments that have allowed it to occur. Once the initially overwhelming technical challenges of liver transplantation in children were overcome, survival outcome was equally impacted by the difficult immunosuppressive, infectious disease and nutritional management in these children. The introduction of cyclosporine in 1980 and tacrolimus in 1989, with or without induction immunosuppression, have allowed for adequate immunosuppression to be realized. Since that time, pediatric transplantation has continued to evolve, with clear improvements in perioperative mortality despite the increasingly complex techniques associated with living-related and technical variant cadaveric allografts. Preventing late graft loss in children remains a significant challenge to the transplant community. This chapter focuses on the postoperative management of children who have undergone liver transplant. For simplicity, the chapter has been divided into sections that highlight the important aspects of management of children during the various chronologic stages after transplant: from the perioperative patient to the long-term survivor.

MANAGEMENT IN EARLY POSTOPERATIVE PERIOD

The advances in the technical aspects of liver transplantation have paralleled improvements in intraoperative monitoring and management of these challenging patients. As operative times and blood loss have decreased and perioperative invasive monitoring has improved, children have become increasingly stable in the perioperative period. Nonetheless, liver transplantation remains a complex procedure that is performed in children who often have multiple comorbidities. Several important postoperative factors must be taken into consideration. Graft loss in the early period is usually multifactorial, with

donor, recipient and technical factors having important roles. Multivariate analysis of the SPLIT registry revealed cadaveric technical variant grafts, transplant for fulminant hepatic failure, recipients with increased height deficits (> 2 standard deviations [SD] from the mean) and those with continuous hospitalization pretransplant as significant risk factors for death [1,2].

Surgical complications

Liver dysfunction should always prompt a thorough evaluation for surgical complications, which complicate interpretation of biopsy results. An early and prompt diagnosis of the common surgical complications in pediatric transplant is essential for successful outcome.

Hepatic artery complications

Hepatic arterial complications are more common after pediatric liver transplantation than in adults. Hepatic artery stenosis (HAS) occurs in approximately 5% of cases [3,4]. Although HAS can be accompanied by graft dysfunction, a significant percentage have little impact on routine liver function tests. If discovered prior to progression to thrombosis, good long-term patency can be achieved with both operative and percutaneous techniques. Because of the relative insensitivity of routine liver injury tests (aspartate aminotransferase [AST], alanine aminotransferase [ALT]) in diagnosing HAS, surveillance allograft ultrasound evaluation of the hepatic artery is important [5,6]. A resistive index less than 0.5, systolic acceleration and foci of peaking velocities are suggestive of HAS and should be further evaluated by angiography. Newer techniques, including computed tomography (CT) angiography are currently evolving; however, angiography remains the gold standard for diagnosis of HAS and hepatic artery thrombosis (HAT) [7]. Angiographic diagnosis of HAS is defined as a 50% reduction in normal luminal caliber, and if diagnosed in the perioperative period should be operatively repaired. If discovered later in the postoperative period, balloon angioplasty has emerged as a promising nonoperative technique [8].

HAT occurs in 4–6% of pediatric liver transplants in experienced centers [4]. Some studies suggest that recipients under 10 kg, under 3 years of age and with hepatic arterial diameters of less than 2 mm have an increased risk of HAT [4]. Other factors associated with HAT include prolonged cold ischemia times, use of blood products and postoperative cytomegalovirus (CMV) infection. Medical therapies aimed at reduction in thrombotic complications, including dextran, heparin, prostaglandins and aspirin, have had little evidence-based support.

The presentation of HAT is extremely variable and differs in its timing in relation to transplantation. A severe fulminant course with coagulopathy, fever, transaminasemia, biliary sepsis and biliary anastamotic breakdown may be seen with early thrombosis. As the biliary system is dependent on arterial flow, it is the most affected in cases of HAT. Once hepatic synthetic function becomes severely altered and ischemic type biliary damage occurs (e.g. strictures, leaks), operative thrombectomy is contraindicated and emergent re-transplant after control of biliary leakage and sepsis becomes the treatment of choice. If HAT is diagnosed early, often with protocol Doppler studies, before significant graft dysfunction or biliary necrosis occurs, operative exploration and thrombectomy with intraoperative intrahepatic tissue plasminogen activator (TPA) administration should be undertaken. Reconstruction with aortic conduit grafts is preferred if arterial inflow is questionable on exploration. Long-term sequelae of HAT such as biliary strictures may still develop. A high index of suspicion can help facilitate prompt diagnosis and treatment.

Use of hyperbaric oxygen in unrepairable or recurrent HAT has been shown to lengthen time to retransplantation, possibly by hastening the development of collaterals [9]. Late HAT is often asymptomatic because of the development of a rich collateral network of vessels from surrounding organs and the diaphragm. Attempts at operative repair should not be undertaken in this situation as a large proportion of these patients survive with normal allograft function. Any operative exploration in these patients should be carefully considered, as disruption of graft-sustaining collateral arterial circulation will likely occur. In a review of 29 children with HAT, Stringer et al. [10] demonstrated 83% survival with 40% surviving without retransplantation. Of those managed conservatively, 85% had normal or mildly abnormal liver function with a median follow-up of 4 years.

Patients experiencing significant late allograft dysfunction resulting from HAT should be carefully monitored for septic complications, intrahepatic bilomas, abscesses and strictures. Most of these problems can be managed percutaneously, thus controlling life-threatening complications during evaluation for retransplantation [11]. Attempts at graft salvage in this situation are almost uniformly unsuccessful, often leading to significant delays in retransplantation, increased patient morbidity and eventual mortality.

Anticoagulation

Although the majority of centers employ postoperative prophylactic anticoagulation, little research has been carried out to verify the practice. Early studies demonstrated that a close balance between pro- and anticoagulant factors must be maintained in the post-transplant setting and the intra-operative use of plasma should be limited. The perioperative use of dextran and heparin was found to be effective in the prevention of HAT by multivariate analysis ($P < 0.02$) [12].

Portal vein complications

Portal vein thrombosis (PVT) occurs less frequently than HAT, complicating approximately 1–5% of pediatric liver transplants and may present with ascites, or liver dysfunction or recurrent varices [3,13,14]. Liver ultrasound should be immediately performed in any child with upper gastro-intestinal bleeding after transplant. PVT is more common in patients requiring venous reconstructions or interposition grafts, portosystemic shunts (operative or spontaneous) and those who have undergone splenectomy. Portal vein stenosis (PVS) is a more common entity, with an overall incidence of 1–10% in one large series [13]. In this series, PVS became symptomatic at a mean of 50.8 months after transplant and presented with bleeding, ascites, increased liver functions tests (LFTs) or splenomegaly and thrombocytopenia. Diagnosis was confirmed with venogram and all were initially managed percutaneously with an initial 66% success rate. One-quarter of those successfully managed percutaneously required repeat venoplasty and stenting after recurrent stenosis; however, none required operative intervention. Of the eight patients found to have PVT on venogram, two were successfully managed with urokinase thrombolysis. The remaining patients were medically managed or underwent surgical decompression. Those patients successfully treated percutaneously had an improved survival compared with those who failed such interventions. Early PVT or significant stenosis in the initial postoperative period is usually best managed by surgical repair.

Hepatic venous outflow complications

The venous outflow of the allograft can be impaired by hepatic venous stenosis or thrombosis and complicates approximately 2% of pediatric liver transplants. Technical variant and living-related allografts were found to have a higher rate of hepatic venous complications (4% and 2%, respectively) when compared with whole grafts (1%) and younger patients were also found to have a higher incidence of this complication. Retransplantation also carries an increased risk of hepatic venous complications, with an incidence of up to 5% in patients receiving their third allograft. Outflow obstruction presents after the second postoperative month with ascites, elevated LFTs or splenomegaly. Percutaneous approaches to the initial management of outflow complications have become more successful with a combination of balloon venoplasty and stenting successful in up to 75% of cases [13]. Anticoagulation in this group is an important adjunct to radiologic procedures and failures can often be managed medically with good long-term results. Retransplantation is rarely needed in this setting.

Biliary complications

Biliary complications continue to cause significant morbidity after pediatric liver transplant. Large single-center and multi-center studies have found the overall incidence of biliary complications to be 15–30% [15,16]. Although considerable controversy exists, some studies suggest an increased rate of biliary morbidity associated with the use of technical variant and living-related allografts [17].

Biliary complications in the early postoperative period usually consist of leaks which, if left untreated, lead to significant sepsis. The presentation is generally within 1–4 weeks and is associated with abdominal pain, bilous drain output, ileus, fever and enteric bacteremia. In split liver allografts, the cut surface is a potential source of leak. These are generally benign and, if adequately drained, will often resolve with conservative treatment. Persistent leak from the cut surface should prompt investigation into hepatic arterial supply and the biliary drainage of that segment. As the majority of pediatric grafts are drained by hepaticojejunostomy, endoscopic methods of diagnosis and therapy are not technically possible and percutaneous approaches are generally required [18]. Non-invasive diagnosis of biliary leak with ultrasound, CT scan and biliary scintography is possible; however, once discovered, only cholangiography allows adequate mapping of the biliary tree for operative and interventional planning. Anastamotic leaks are a more significant cause of morbidity because of the direct connection with the bowel and operative drainage of the resultant biloma is usually necessary, with open revision of the biliary anastomosis or conversion to enteric-drained anastamoses. When anastamotic leaks are managed with percutaneous stenting, late postoperative strictures may result.

Biliary strictures (Fig. 27.1) tend to present several months into the postoperative course, with cholangitis or graft dysfunction [16]. Diagnosis relies on ultrasound, biopsy and subsequent cholangiography. Ultrasound diagnosis is based on the presence of ductal dilatation (defined as bile ducts with diameters greater than adjacent portal venous tributaries); however, marked dilatation may not always be present in allografts despite significant ductal obstruction. Biopsies usually reveal significant cholangitis and ductal proliferation, often prompting a more focused investigation of the biliary system. The use of noninvasive magnetic resonance cholangiopancreatography (MRCP) has begun to be used in the pediatric population; however, relatively few publications have examined its utility [19]. Once again, percutaneous transhepatic

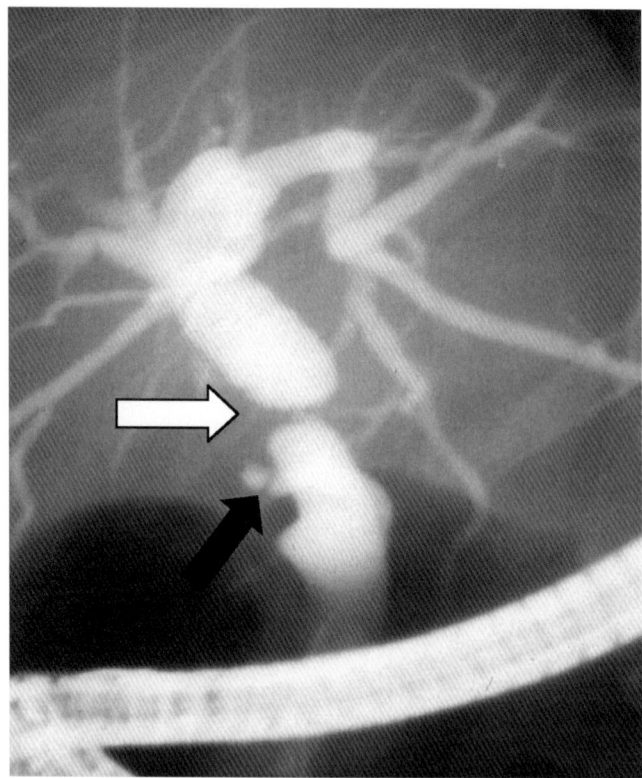

Fig. 27.1 Endoscopic retrograde cholangiographic appearance of an anastomotic biliary stricture (white arrow). Note the ligated cystic duct stump of the recipient (black arrow).

cholangiography remains the gold standard for initial diagnosis and treatment of biliary strictures [18]. Initial catheter drainage of the obstructed system allows for control of biliary sepsis. Balloon dilatation of isolated strictures with or without stent placement is successful in treating a large majority of strictures (up to 90% of cases) with a relatively low incidence of complications [20]. It should be again stressed that any postoperative biliary complication should prompt an immediate investigation of hepatic arterial patency.

Nonsurgical complications of the allograft

Primary nonfunction

Primary nonfunction (PNF) is defined as a graft failure within 90 days of transplant without evidence of technical complication or acute rejection. PNF is characterized by encephalopathy, coagulopathy and progressive renal and multisystem organ failure. Although several donor-related factors such as macrovesicular steatosis, donors at extremes of age, prolonged cold ischemia times, prolonged intensive care unit (ICU) stays and elevated creatinine have been shown to increase the risk of PNF, each liver offer should be individualized according to the potential recipient. The overall risk–benefit ratio should be evaluated carefully and decisions based on the available data should be reviewed by a number of physicians prior to proceeding with transplantation.

Acute cellular rejection

Diagnosis of acute cellular rejection (ACR) begins with clinical suspicion. The majority of episodes are discovered prior to the development of significant allograft dysfunction by screening periodic LFTs and are generally characterized by elevated transaminases. A detailed work-up of possible technical complications should promptly ensue, with Doppler ultrasound evaluation of the allograft for arterial or venous insufficiency and biliary ductal dilatation. Although excellent sensitivity for ACR is reported using LFTs, ACR can occur in the face of normal LFTs and usually presents with acute ascites, peripheral edema, fever or right upper quadrant tenderness. The gold standard for diagnosing ACR remains the liver biopsy. Percutaneous liver biopsy can be performed at the bedside with little associated morbidity. Small patients and those with segmental allografts should be biopsied under ultrasound guidance. Careful evaluation and correction of the coagulation profile should be performed prior to performing an allograft liver biopsy. A post-procedure chest X-ray and hematocrit should also be checked and close monitoring of vital signs should also be employed. The timing of ACR in pediatric liver transplant varies by the type of immunosuppression employed in the perioperative period. A review of the 2002 Studies of Pediatric Liver Transplantation (SPLIT) data revealed an overall 60% risk of rejection after 36 months, with 73% of these rejections occurring in the first 3 months. Initial immunosuppression with tacrolimus resulted in a statistically significant decrease in the probability of rejection [1].

Treatment of ACR should begin with a steroid bolus with or without a steroid recycle. Baseline immunosuppression should also be augmented with close follow-up of LFTs and levels. With prompt normalization, a rapid conversion to oral steroids and a weekly taper should be adequate. If LFTs remain persistently elevated, or in the case of ACR without LFT elevation, repeat allograft biopsy should be performed to follow the histologic response to treatment. Empiric therapy of ACR, especially persistent ACR, should be avoided. Biopsy-proven steroid-resistant ACR should be promptly treated with antibody preparations. The 2002 SPLIT data revealed a 11% rate of steroid-resistant ACR [1].

Extrahepatic complications and post-transplant issues

Infectious complications

Early infections in the pediatric transplant patient should be divided into those related to the procedure, such as biliary leaks and bowel perforations, and those not directly related to the operation, such as pneumonia and catheter-related sepsis [21]. A detailed review of infections complications is found in Chapter 12; however, some pertinent points are presented here. In the early postoperative period, nontechnical infectious complications substantially contribute to morbidity. Analysis of the SPLIT database revealed respiratory complications and pneumonias in 18% of patients, with 39% experiencing culture-positive bacterial infections [2]. Intra-abdominal sepsis and catheter-related bloodstream infections were the most common sources of bacterial infections.

Overall, surgical complications, including enteric and biliary leaks and vascular thromboses, dramatically increase the risk of bacterial and fungal sepsis. Invasive fungal infections are associated with decreased patient and graft survival, and prompt diagnosis and aggressive treatment are essential to rescue the patient. Bowel perforation remains a feared complication of transplant, and breakdown of enteroenteric anastamoses may lead to overwhelming sepsis. Technical aspects of enteric anastamoses such as two-layered anastamosis and avoidance of tension on the suture line should be stressed. Careful closure of mesenteric defects should also be employed to avoid internal herniation and volvulus. Bowel perforation can also result from inadvertent enterotomies while dissecting in hostile, often reoperative abdominal cavities. This is especially true in cases of biliary atresia with previous hepatic portoenterostomy.

Surgical site infections following pediatric orthotopic liver transplantation are increased by prolonged operative and cold ischemia times, large volume intraoperative transfusions, preoperative ascites and hypoalbuminemia [22]. Use of OKT3 and rejection have also been associated with increased surgical site infections.

Fungal infections can be particularly devastating in the post-transplant patient, with a peak incidence in the first 2 months. The SPLIT database defined a 9.8% fungal infection rate. Risk factors included transplantation for fulminant hepatic failure, retransplantations, prolonged operative times and the use of high-dose steroids and broad-spectrum antibiotics. Aggressive drainage of fluid collections, débridement of devitalized tissue and use of potent antifungal therapy can reduce the morbidity and mortality of invasive fungal infections. Prophylaxis in high-risk patients should also be considered, although use of perioperative fluconazole can interfere with tacrolimus metabolism. Although over 80% of fungal infections are caused by *Candida* species, an increasing awareness should be lent to *Aspergillus* species, as antemortem diagnosis is achieved in only 50% of patients. The availability of voriconazole and high-dose liposomal amphotericin has afforded a viable treatment option to patients infected with *Aspergillus*.

Viral infections can have a devastating effect in the immunosuppressed child in the early postoperative period. Common pathogens include CMV, Epstein–Barr virus (EBV), herpes simplex virus (HSV), adenovirus and influenza viruses. In the pediatric age group, many patients have no prior protective exposure to these viruses and primary infection is thus encountered during immunosuppression [23]. Recent advances in prophylaxis and pre-emptive therapy have been successful in decreasing the early morbidity associated with EBV, CMV and HSV to an incidence of < 5%. Because of the lack of effective treatments, disseminated viremia, necrotizing pneumonitis and bacterial superinfection can result from common respiratory viruses such as influenza and adenovirus in the early postoperative period [23].

Post-transplant nutrition

The nutritional goal in the immediate postoperative period is to provide adequate nutrition to facilitate replenishment of the pretransplant nutritional deficit associated with chronic liver disease and to allow for the additional recovery from the stress of major abdominal surgery. Although limited studies have been performed in this area, aggressive nutritional therapy facilitates wound healing, decreases infectious complications and hastens successful weaning from the ventilator. Rapid use of enteral tube feeding should be considered in malnourished patients with intraoperative placement of postpyloric enteral feeding tubes. This strategy has been shown to increase total early postoperative caloric and protein intakes and to decrease postoperative infectious complications. Parenteral nutrition is sparingly used at some centers and is indicated if prolonged postoperative ileus or gastrointestinal complications of surgery limit the possibility of enteral feeding [24–29].

LONG-TERM MANAGEMENT

Etiology of late graft loss

Several large single-center studies have begun to define the etiology of graft failure and death in children who have undergone liver transplantation [30–37]. Although the short-term survival of liver transplant recipients has dramatically improved over the past two decades, similar improvements in late graft survival still need to be realized. In older studies, a significant proportion of pediatric patients had significant graft dysfunction contributing to their death. An early study demonstrated significant mortality associated with acute or chronic rejection, accounting for 17% of late deaths [30].

In a later study from the Pittsburgh group, 1- and 10-year survival rates of 85.5% and 82.9% were reported with extremely low rates of mortality after the 1-year mark (0.32% per year). Despite using a tacrolimus-based steroid-sparing immunosuppresive protocol, the primary etiology of late mortality was found to be infectious in nature, accounting for 60% of the deaths in this group with post-transplant lymphoproliferative disease (PTLD) accounting for an additional 20% of late deaths, although PTLD mortality has decreased

significantly with current EBV monitoring. Noncompliance accounted for 10% of late deaths with recurrent hepatic malignancy, complications of cystic fibrosis and complications after retransplant for hepatitis completing the group. This study was the first to examine the changing etiology in late mortality after pediatric liver transplant under newer immunosuppresive protocols because acute or chronic rejection were not causes of late graft loss [31]. This most likely reflects a chronologic change in immunosuppresion from cyclosporine to tacrolimus. Other centers may note similarly improved results with modern cyclosporine preparations such as Neoral®.

Overall, the most common causes of late (> 1 year posttransplant) patient and graft loss include infection, PTLD, malignancy and noncompliance. Significant post-transplant morbidities associated with chronic immunosuppression include renal insufficiency, hypertension, hyperglycemia and hyperlipidemia. Technical complications have also been found to contribute to a significant number of late graft loss and must be sought for in cases of late graft dysfunction.

Complications of chronic immunosuppression

Post-transplant lymphoproliferative disease

Although most studies examining late graft loss in pediatric transplantation are relatively small, PTLD has been a significant cause of late mortality. Post-transplant infection with EBV results in a spectrum of diseases, from mononucleosis syndromes and plasma cell hyperplasia (reactive hyperplasias) to neoplastic PTLD. Histologic examination of neoplastic PTLD demonstrates disruption of normal underlying architecture by proliferating monoclonal or polyclonal lymphocytes. Although a small subpopulation of PTLD (5–10%) is not associated with EBV, in situ hybridization of most histologic specimens in these patients reveals the presence of EBV-encoded RNA. Early studies found that primary tacrolimus use in pediatric patients was associated with a 15% long-term risk of PTLD, with almost 80% of these cases occurring in the first 2 years after transplant. Infants and toddlers comprise the majority of transplant waiting list patients and are usually EBV-naïve, thus increasing their risk of developing a primary infection while immunosuppressed and accordingly increasing their risk of developing clinical disease [38,39]. In contrast, clinical disease rarely occurs in children who are seropositive prior to transplant. The diagnosis of EBV disease in children after liver transplantation hinges on the clinical history and physical examination coupled with confirmatory laboratory and radiologic studies. A high index of suspicion in these high-risk patients is warranted and leads to early diagnosis and institution of therapy. Patients often complain of sporadic fever, lethargy and malaise. Weight loss, diarrhea and gastrointestinal complaints are often common, as are symptoms of allograft dysfunction. Persistent sore throat, adenopathy, headaches, seizures and cutaneous lesions may also been seen. Physical examination may reveal adenopathy, tonsillar changes and hepatosplenomegaly. Standard laboratory evaluation may show leukopenia amd atypical lymphocytosis, anemia and thrombocytopenia. Hemoccult-positive stool specimens suggest gastrointestinal involvement and LFTs may also be elevated. The current availability of well-validated tests to measure EBV viral load in the peripheral blood allows clinicians to monitor the replication of EBV in the recipient and follow the response to treatment. Further evaluation of PTLD is guided by initial findings and contrast-enhanced CT scanning of the head, neck, chest, abdomen and pelvis, and endoscopy should be performed if indicated by initial studies. Histologic examination of tissue is optimal and surgical and/or endoscopic specimens should be promptly submitted for fresh staining with the EBER-1 probe by experienced pathologists. An evaluation for CD20 staining should also be performed [40].

The well-described permissive role of immunosuppression in the replication of EBV has vastly improved the outcome of recipients experiencing EBV-associated disease. Clearly, PTLD prevention by optimization of immunosuppression is the ideal to strive for; however, the balance between this and rejection is often difficult to achieve. Rapid tapering of steroids or their complete avoidance is an initial measure. Reliable polymerase chain reaction (PCR) monitoring of EBV loads in the peripheral blood has led to the era of pre-emptive therapy of EBV viremia prior to its evolution to PTLD. For prospective monitoring to be efficient, the frequency of monitoring needs to be sufficient to catch relevant rises in EBV load. As the highest risk for EBV infection in seronegative patients after liver transplant is in the first 3 months post-transplant, we monitor EBV PCR every 2 weeks for this time period. After 3 months, monitoring periods increase and EBV PCR is checked every 3–4 months for 1–2 years. Response to elevated EBV PCR is graded according to the degree of elevation. Mild increases prompt reduction in immunosuppression to tacrolimus levels of 3–5 ng/mL until EBV PCR levels are normal or biopsy-proven rejection occurs. With more significant PCR elevations, immunosuppression is similarly decreased and investigation for clinical disease begins with an enhanced screening CT scan of the head, neck, chest, abdomen and pelvis. The presence of any suspicious nodes or masses will prompt biopsy and treatment with ganciclovir (5 mg/kg i.v. b.i.d.) and Cytogam® (100 mg/kg q.o.d. × 3) as a biweekly dosage until levels have normalized [39].

In children with documented PTLD, immunosuppression should be stopped completely; successful reduction in size or disappearance of lesions is usually seen [39–41]. A prompt fall in EBV PCR levels predicts a good clinical response in this situation, often before lesions shrink. PTLD that is unresponsive to this treatment plan should be treated with the anti-CD20 human/mouse chimeric monoclonal antibody, rituximab, if shown to be CD20 positive by biopsy. Complete

remission rates of 60–70% have been documented in children; the drug is well tolerated and although up to 20% recur, most can be cured with retreatment. B-cell depletion persists for up to 9 months after rituximab and children should thus be carefully monitored for infectious complications and immunoglobulins supplemented with intravenous immunoglobulin (IVIG) in cases of documented hypogammaglobulinemia. For PTLD refractory to rituximab, low-dose cytotoxic chemotherapy and prednisone has been effective. Cytotoxic chemotherapy is also, by nature, immunosuppressive and allows complete elimination of calcineurin inhibitors around the time of its administration.

Renal insufficiency

Nephrotoxicity is a frequent side-effect of calcineurin inhibitors (CNI) used after liver transplant. Pre-existing renal disease clearly increases these side-effects; however, the overall incidence of renal dysfunction in children after liver transplant has not been elucidated. Renal function seems to sharply decline in the first months after transplant and then stabilize over the ensuing postoperative year; however, post-transplant renal function does not reach pretransplant levels when measured by calculated glomerular filtration rate (GFR) or by inulin and para-amino-hippurate (PAH) clearance. If followed for 5 years, GFR remains stable, suggesting that duration of CNI exposure does not affect renal function, as long as the overall cumulative dose remains low. Initial losses in GFR are likely the results of perioperative stress and high initial CNI levels [41–43]. Careful avoidance of dehydration and the chronic use of nephrotoxic agents such as nonsteroidal anti inflammatory agents and aminoglycosides are important, as is avoidance of drugs that rapid increase CNI levels (Table 27.1). Follow-up of renal function should rely on actual measurement of 24-hour creatinine clearance, rather than calculation, as calculated values and serum creatinine have been shown to be inaccurate in this population. Furthermore, it seems that dose reduction of CNIs will benefit patients with nephrotoxicity if done prior to development of permanent renal insufficiency [15,42].

Other complications of immunosuppression

Cardiovascular complications

Although there is growing concern in the adult transplant population regarding CNI-induced hypertension, diabetes and hyperlipidemia, relatively little work has been carried out to quantitate the deleterious cardiovascular effects of chronic CNI use in children. In one study of 10-year survivors of pediatric liver transplant using ciclosporin-based immunosuppression, 38% of patients developed hypertension and 25% required chronic use of antihypertensives. Hyperlipidemia was also found in 45% of these patients; however, none had levels elevated enough to warrant therapy. Diabetes developed in 10% of the population; however, the majority of cases

Table 27.1 Medications that effect calcineurin inhibitor (CNI) levels and renal toxicity.

Medications that decrease CNI levels
Anticonvulsants
  Barbiturates
  Phenytoin
  Carbamazepine
Rifampin
St. John's wort

Medications that increase CNI levels
Calcium-channel blockers
  Verapamil
  Diltiazem
  Nicardipine
  Amlodipine
Azole antifungals
  Fluconazole
  Ketoconazole
  Itraconazole

Macrolide antibiotics
  Erythromcycin
  NOT azithromycin
Corticosteroids
Somatostatin
Amiodarone
Grapefruit juice

Medications that increase renal toxicity
Vancomycin
Aminoglycosides
Bactrim
Aciclovir
Ganciclovir
Amphotericin

were steroid dependent [44]. The overall impact these risk factors will have in the long-term survivor of a pediatric liver transplant is not known.

Neurologic complications
The acute neurologic complications of liver transplant and immunosuppression are well-known entities and include cerebral edema, seizures and permanent sequelae of hepatic encephalopathy [45]. No long-term effects of chronic CNI use have been described; however, some studies have suggested impaired cognitive abilities in children after liver transplant. Fortunately, similar cognitive studies demonstrate normal neurodevelopmental outcome 4 years after transplant, suggesting that a "catch-up" period is required [46].

Hematologic complications
Anemia remains a significant problem after orthotopic liver transplantation in children, with an incidence of approximately

25% 5 years after transplant. A large majority of these are multifactorial and not responsive to iron therapy [47]. Although most immunosuppressive and drug-related etiologies are secondary to myelosuppressive effects, studies have shown that a decrease in CNI levels and use of different agents can improve anemia. Cases of tacrolimus-induced hemolytic anemia are prevalent in the literature and should be treated by initially decreasing the dosage. If not effective, a change to cyclosporine or sirolimus is indicated. Aplastic anemia is a dreaded complication of liver transplant and is more common in patients transplanted for fulminant hepatitis. The cause of aplastic anemia remains elusive, however, and mortality rates from pancytopenia can reach 70% in pediatric cases and 100% in elderly patients [48]. Graft-versus-host disease (GVHD) is another rare etiology of anemia; however, diagnosis is critical in maintaining survival. The clinical picture of pancytopenia, unexplained fever and classic rash should prompt bone marrow biopsy, donor-derived chimerism studies and corticosteroid administration with lowered CNI levels. Mortality rates in untreated severe GVHD can reach 90% with gastrointestinal, pulmonary and neurologic involvement [49].

Endocrine complications
Post-transplant diabetes mellitus (PTDM) is a relatively common complication in the post-transplant setting and can occur in up to 7% of the pediatric population following renal transplantation [50]. Several factors increase the risk of PTDM, including a positive family history of type 2 diabetes mellitus, use of tacrolimus and hyperglycemia in the first 2 weeks after transplant [51,52]. The effects of the increasing incidence of type 2 diabetes mellitus in the general pediatric population on the incidence of PTDM have not been elucidated. Also, the long-term consequences of PTDM in this population are unknown, although PTDM has been shown to significantly increase the morbidity associated with adult orthotopic liver transplantation.

Growth and development
Growth retardation and malnutrition are common complications of chronic liver disease because of decreased intake, malabsorption and relative growth hormone resistance. In patients receiving transplants for biliary atresia at less than 1 year of age, average height increases to normal levels in the third postoperative year [24]. An improvement in growth in post-transplant patients has also been demonstrated when corticosteroids are stopped. Factors associated with continued poor growth include severe pretransplant malnutrition, surgical complications of the transplant and allograft dysfunction. Development of adequate support systems and teaching of developmental feeding skills and food intake are important, although up to 30% of children may require continued enteral nutritional support after transplant. Many factors affect growth post-transplant; however, one factor that can be influenced by the physician is avoidance of excessive

corticosteroid use. Considerable data demonstrate the growth suppressive effects of corticosteroids and improved growth after reduction or withdrawal of steroids [24–29].

Psychosocial development after transplant is a complex process involving an initial decline in social skills and overall learning skills. This is likely secondary to prolonged hospitalization, surgical and psychological stress associated with the procedure and chronic illness prior to the transplant. Despite this, with successful liver transplant and improvement in nutrition, there is a great improvement in development and at 3 years, 82% of children attend school and live "normal" lives. Ten-year survivors enjoy a 100% rate of school attendance, with only one-third requiring special education. Despite these excellent results, it is important to realize that up to 25% of pediatric liver transplant survivors have learning problems and early assistance can greatly benefit them. Long-term studies have clearly demonstrated that the majority of children achieve normal psychosocial milestones within 5 years after liver transplant and that early intervention with those patients that lag behind can improve overall outcomes and adherence. Studies have demonstrated that inferior psychosocial development is associated with decreased graft survival; however, it is unclear if pre-existing graft dysfunction confounds this finding [44,46,53].

Long-term immunosuppresive management

Avoidance of late acute cellular rejection and chronic rejection

Although the majority of acute cellular rejection occurs in the early postoperative period, late ACR can present with more atypical features such as centrilobular changes and be more difficult to treat [54]. Although the incidence of graft loss resulting from chronic rejection has been found to be diminished with use of primary tacrolimus-based immunosuppression, it remains an important cause of late graft loss in pediatric liver transplants [55]. Several single-center studies have found chronic rejection to account for 5–30% of late graft loss, with variation in timing and frequency likely caused by differing immunosuppressive protocols. Loss of bile ducts in more than 50% of portal tracts and obliterative foam cell arteriopathy leading to fibrosis are characteristic pathologic markers of chronic rejection as described by the recent international Banff panel [56]. Although several risk factors have been found in single-center studies to increase the risk of chronic rejection in pediatric liver transplant, a great deal of variability was seen in these studies and few were solely performed in the pediatric population. Multivariate analysis of one large pediatric center found a higher risk of chronic rejection in African-American recipients, those receiving cadaveric grafts and those with autoimmune diseases such as primary sclerosing cholangitis (PSC) and autoimmune hepatitis (AIH) [57]. Other factors suggested to be associated with chronic rejection

include: frequent episodes of ACR, positive lymphocytotoxic cross-matching, use of cyclosporine, late ACR episodes, CMV disease, gender mismatch and young recipient age [57–59]. Although approximately 30% cases of chronic rejection respond to conventional immunosuppression, the remainder have progressive deterioration in graft function with development of cholestasis and portal hypertension ultimately requiring retransplantation [58].

Noncompliance

Nonadherence remains a significant source of morbidity and late graft loss after pediatric liver transplantation. In the study by Sudan et al. [30], noncompliance led to 17% of late deaths after liver transplant. This was the third most common etiology of graft loss 1 year after transplant and was found to affect predominantly older children 5–8 years after transplant. Nonadherence in the pediatric population is complex, as the primary responsibility for medication administration begins with the primary caregiver and is then transferred to the patient at a varying age. This transition occurs at a relatively early age (approximately 12 years) and counseling about adherence issues should similarly shift at this time. The ability to predict and demonstrate noncompliance in this population has only recently been investigated [60–62]. A recent study revealed that comparing standard deviations of tacrolimus trough levels in pediatric liver transplant recipients was consistent with a panel assessment of compliance in these patients. The standard deviation of levels was found to predict biopsy-proven rejection episodes, while patient, caregiver and clinician scaled questionnaire reports were unable to do so. In further examination of the reasons for noncompliance, forgetfulness was the most frequently cited, while drug side-effects were a rare rationale for nonadherence. It is also important to realize that pediatric transplant recipients may have certain degrees of post-traumatic stress, fostered by years of chronic illness and surgical procedures [62,63]. Children who had positive scores on the PTSD reaction index were found to be significantly more noncompliant when compared with those without positive scores, and those patients treated for symptoms of PTSD became compliant [62,63].

Immunosuppression minimization and withdrawal

Achieving optimal long-term immunosuppression in children is clearly important if we are to minimize late acute cellular rejection and chronic rejection while reducing patient morbidity and mortality from infection or extrahepatic complications.

Close clinical follow-up is crucial to any management plan. Data suggests that monotherapy with tacrolimus can be achieved and that specific levels need not be maintained late after transplant if rejection history is benign and liver function is normal [64]. Most children will not require steroids after the first year [65]. Some children can be withdrawn from immunosuppression completely [66] and emerging data on immunologic assays that may assist in the prediction of the tolerant state will greatly impact the prospective withdrawal or minimization of immunosuppression [67–69].

REFERENCES

1 Martin SR, Atkison P, Anand R, Lindblad AS and the SPLIT Research Group. Studies of Pediatric Liver Transplantation 2002. Patient and graft survival and rejection in pediatric recipients of a first liver transplant in the United States and Canada. *Pediatr Transplant* 2004;**8**:273–83.

2 The SPLIT Research Group. Studies of Pediatric Liver Transplantation (SPLIT): Year 2000 outcomes. *Transplantation* 2001; **72**:463–76.

3 Zanotelli ML, Vieira S, Alencastro R, *et al.* Management of vascular complications after pediatric liver transplantation. *Transplant Proc* 2004;**36**:945–6.

4 Heffron TG, Pillen T, Welch D, *et al.* Hepatic artery thrombosis in pediatric liver transplantation. *Transplant Proc* 2003;**35**: 1447–8.

5 Nishida S, Kato T, Levi D, *et al.* Effect of protocol Doppler ultrasonography and urgent revascularization on early hepatic artery thrombosis after pediatric liver transplantation. *Arch Surg* 2002;**137**:1279–83.

6 Kaneko J, Sugawara Y, Akamatsu N, *et al.* Prediction of hepatic artery thrombosis by protocol Doppler ultrasonography in pediatric living donor liver transplantation. *Abdom Imaging* 2004;**29**:603–5.

7 Cheng YF, Chen CL, Huang TL, *et al.* 3 DCT angiography for detection of vascular complications in pediatric liver transplantation. *Liver Transpl* 2004;**10**:248–52.

8 Hasegawa T, Sasaki T, Kimura T, *et al.* Successful percutaneous transluminal angioplasty for hepatic artery stenosis in a an infant undergoing living-related liver transplantation. *Pediatr Transplant* 2002;**6**:244–8.

9 Mazariegos GV, O'Toole K, Mieles LA, *et al.* Hyperbaric oxygen therapy for hepatic artery thrombosis after liver transplantation in children. *Liver Transpl Surg* 1999;**5**:429–36.

10 Stringer MD, Marshall MM, Muiesan P, *et al.* Survival and outcome after hepatic artery thrombosis complicating pediatric liver transplantation. *J Pediatr Surg* 2001;**36**:888–91.

11 Dalgic A, Dalgic B, Demirogullari B, *et al.* Clinical approach to graft hepatic artery thrombosis following living related liver transplantation. *Pediatr Transplant* 2003;**7**:149–52.

12 Mazzaferro V, Esquivel CO, Makowka L, *et al.* Hepatic artery thrombosis after pediatric liver transplantation: medical or surgical event? *Transplantation* 1989;**47**:971–7.

13 Buell JF, Funaki B, Cronin DC, *et al.* Long-term venous complications after full-size and segmental pediatric liver transplantation. *Ann Surg* 2002;**236**:658–66.

14 Cheng YF, Vhen CL, Huang TL, *et al.* Risk factors for intraoperative portal vein thrombosis in pediatric living donor liver transplantation. *Clin Transplant* 2004;**18**:390–4.

15 McDiarmid SV. Current status of liver transplantation in children. *Pediatr Clin North Am* 2003;**50**:1335–74.

16 Kling K, Lau H, Colombani P. Biliary complications of living related pediatric liver transplant patients. *Pediatr Transplant* 2004;**8**:178–84.

17 Sieders E, Peeters PMJG, TenVergert EM, *et al.* Analysis of survival and morbidity after pediatric liver transplantation with full-size and technical-variant grafts. *Transplantation* 1999;**68**: 540–5.

18 Lorenz JM, Funaki B, Leef JA, Rosenblum JD, Van Ha T. Percutaneous transhepaticcholangiography and biliary drainage in pediatric liver transplant patients. *Am J Roentgenol* 2001; **176**:761–5.

19 Pilleul F, Guibaud L, Dugougeat F, Lachaud A, Pracros JP. MR cholangiography in pediatric population with biliary complications after liver transplantation. *J Radiol E* 2000;**81**:793–8.

20 Lorenz JM, Denisin G, Funaki B, *et al.* Balloon dilatation of biliary-enteric strictures in children. *Am J Roentgenol* 2005;**184**: 151–5.

21 Bouchut JC, Stamm D, Boillot O, Lepape A, Floret D. Postoperative infectious complication in paediatric liver transplantation: a study of 48 transplants. *Pediatr Anaesth* 2001;**11**:93–8.

22 Hollenbeak CS, Alfrey EJ, Sheridan K, Burger TL, Dillon PW. Surgical site infections following pediatric liver transplantation: risks and costs. *Transpl Infect Dis* 2003;**5**:72–8.

23 Green M. Viral infections and pediatric liver transplantation. *Pediatr Transplant* 2002;**6**:20–4.

24 Alonso G, Duca P, Pasqualini T, D'Agostino D. Evaluation of catch-up growth after liver transplantation in children with biliary atresia. *Pediatr Transplant* 2004;**8**:255–9.

25 Holt RI, Broide E, Buchanan CR, *et al.* Orthotopic liver transplantation reverses the adverse nutritional changes of end-stage liver disease in children. *Am J Clin Nutr* 1997;**65**:534–42.

26 Cabre E, Gassull, M. Nutritional aspects of liver disease and transplantation. *Curr Opin Clin Nutr Metab Care* 2001;**4**:581–9.

27 Campos ACL, Matias JEF, Coelho JCU. Nutritional aspects of liver transplantation. *Curr Opin Clin Nutr Metab Care* 2002;**5**: 297–307.

28 Ramaccioni V, Soriano HE, Arumugam R, Klish WJ. Nutritional aspects of chronic liver disease and liver transplantation in children. *J Pediatr Gastroenterol Nutr* 2000;**30**:361–7.

29 Heubi JE, Heyman MB, Shulman RJ. The impact of liver disease on growth and nutrition. *J Pediatr Gastroenterol Nutr* 2002;**35**(Suppl 1):S55–9.

30 Sudan DL, Shaw BW, Langnas AN. Causes of late mortality in pediatric liver transplant recipients. *Ann Surg* 1998;**227**:289–95.

31 Fridell JA, Jain A, Reyes J, *et al.* Causes of mortlity beyond 1 year after primary pediatric liver transplant under tacrolimus. *Transplantation* 2002;**74**:1721–4.

32 Jain A, Mazariegos G, Kashyap R, *et al.* Pediatric liver transplantation: a single center experience spanning 20 years. *Transplantation* 2002;**73**:941–7.

33 Wallot MA, Mathot M, Janssen M, *et al.* Long-term survival and late graft loss in pediatric liver transplant recipients: a 15-year single-center experience. *Liver Transpl* 2002;**8**:615–22.

34 Langham MR, Tzakis AG, Gonzalez-Peralta R, *et al.* Graft survival in pediatric liver transplantation. *J Pediatr Surg* 2001;**36**: 1205–9.

35 Sieders E, Peeters PMJG, TenVergert EM, *et al.* Graft loss after pediatric liver transplantation. *Ann Surg* 2002;**235**:125–32.

36 Goss JA, Shackleton CR, McDiarmid SV, *et al.* Long-term results of pediatric liver transplantation: an analysis of 569 transplants. *Ann Surg* 1998;**228**:411–20.

37 Vo Thi Diem H, Evrard V, Tran Vinh H, *et al.* Pediatric liver transplantation for biliary atresia: results of primary grafts in 328 recipients. *Transplantation* 2003;**75**:1692–97.

38 Cacciarelli TV, Reyes J, Jaffe R, *et al.* Primary tacrolimus (FK506) therapy and the long-term risk of post-transplant lymphoproliferative disease in pediatric liver transplant recipients. *Pediatr Transplant* 2001;**5**:359–64.

39 Green M, Webber S. Posttransplantation lymphoproliferative disorders. *Pediatr Clin North Am* 2003;**50**:1471–91.

40 Green M. Management of Epstein–Barr virus induced post-transplant lymphoproliferative disease in recipients of solid organ transplantation. *Am J Transplant* 2001;**1**:103–8.

41 Smets F, Sokal EM. Lymphoproliferation in children after liver transplantation. *J Pediatr Gastroenterol Nutr* 2002;**34**:499–505.

42 Arora-Gupta N, Davies P, McKiernan P, Kelly DA. The effect of long-term calcineurin inhibitor therapy on renal function in children after liver transplantation. *Pediatr Transplant* 2004;**8**:145–50.

43 Bartosh SM, Alonso EM, Whitington PF. Renal outcomes in pediatric liver transplantation. *Clin Transplant* 1997;**11**:354–60.

44 Avitzur Y, De Luca E, Cantos M, *et al.* Health status 10 years after pediatric liver transplantation: looking beyond the graft. *Transplantation* 2004;**78**:566–73.

45 Mueller AR, Platz KP, Beechstein WO, *et al.* Neurotoxicity after orthotopic liver transplantation: a comparison between cyclosporine and FK506. *Transplantation* 1994;**58**:155–70.

46 Baum M, Freier C, Chinnock RE. Neurodevelopmental outcome of solid organ transplantation in children. *Pediatr Clin North Am* 2003;**50**:1493–503.

47 Maheshwari A, Mishra R, Thuluvath PJ. Post-liver-transplant anemia: etiology and management. *Liver Transpl* 2004;**10**:165–73.

48 Iglesias-Berengue J, Lopez-Espinosa JA, Ortega-Lopez J, *et al.* Hematologic abnormalities in liver-transplanted children during medium- to long-term follow-up. *Transplant Proc* 2003;**35**:1904–6.

49 Taylor AL, Gibbs P, Bradley JA. Acute graft versus host disease following liver transplantation: the enemy within. *Am J Transplant* 2004;**4**:466–74.

50 Greenspan LC, Gitelman SE, Leung MA, Glidden DV, Mathias RS. Increased incidence in post-transplant diabetes mellitus in children: a case–control analysis. *Pediatr Nephrol* 2002;**17**:1–5.

51 Al-Uzri A, Stablein DM, Cohn RA. Post-transplant diabetes mellitus in pediatric renal transplant recipients: a report of the North American Pediatric Renal Transplant Cooperative Study (NAPRTCS). *Transplantation* 2001;**72**:1020–24.

52 Preeti JR, Thuluvath PJ. Outcome of patients with new-onset diabetes mellitus after liver transplantation compared with those without diabetes mellitus. *Liver Transpl* 2002;**8**:708–13.

53 Qvist E, Jalanko H, Holmberg C. Psychosocial adaptation after solid organ transplantation in children. *Pediatr Clin North Am* 2003;**50**:1505–19.

54 Sellers M, Singer A, Maller E, *et al.* Incidence of late acute rejection and progression to chronic rejection in pediatric liver recipients. *Transplant Proc* 1997;**29**:428–9.

55 Cao S, Cox KL, Berquist W, *et al.* Long-term outcomes in pediatric liver recipients: comparison between cyclosporine and tacrolimus. *Pediatr Transplant* 1999;**3**:22–6.

56 Demetris A, Adams D, Bellamy C. Update of the International Banff Schema for liver allograft rejection: working recommendations for the histopathologic staging and reporting of chronic rejection. *Hepatology* 2000;**31**:792.

57 Gupta P, Hart J, Cronin D, *et al.* Risk factors for chronic rejection after pediatric liver transplantation. *Transplantation* 2001;**72**:1098–102.

58 Wiesner RH, Batts KP, Krom RAF. Evolvong concepts in the diagnosis, pathogenesis and treatment of chronic hepatic allograft rejection. *Liver Transpl Surg* 1999;**5**:388–400.

59 Milkiewicz P, Gonson B, Saksena S, *et al.* Increased incidence of chronic rejection in adult patients transplanted for autoimmune hepatitis: assessment of risk factors. *Transplantation* 2000;**70**:477–80.

60 Rianthavorn P, Ettenger RB, Malekzadeh M, Marik JL, Struber M. Noncompliance with immunosuppressive medications in pediatric and adolescent patients receiving solid-organ transplants. *Transplantation* 2004;**77**:778–82.

61 Falkenstein K, Flynn L, Kirkpatrick B, Casa-Melley, Dunn S. Non-compliance in children post-liver transplant. Who are the culprits? *Pediatr Transplant* 2004;**8**:233–6.

62 Shemesh E, Shneider BL, Savitsky JK, *et al.* Medication adherence in pediatric and adolescent liver transplant recipients. *Pediatrics* 2004;**113**:825–32.

63 Lurie S, Shemesh E, Sheiner PA, *et al.* Non-adherence in pediatric liver transplant recipients: an assessment of risk factors and natural history. *Pediatr Transplant* 2000;**4**:200–6.

64 Varela-Fascinetto G, Treacy SJ, Vacanti JP. Approaching operational tolerance in long-term pediatric liver transplant recipients receiving minimal immunosuppression. *Transplant Proc* 1997;**29**:449–51.

65 Jain A, Mazariegos G, Kashyap R, *et al.* Reasons why some children receiving tacrolimus therapy require steroids more than 5 years post liver transplantation. *Pediatr Transplant* 2001;**5**:93–8.

66 Mazariegos GV. Withdrawal of immunosuppression in liver transplantation: lessons learned from PTLD. *Pediatr Transplant* 2004;**8**:210–3.

67 Mazariegos GV, Zahorchak AF, Reyes J, *et al.* Dendritic cell subset ratio in tolerant, weaning and non-tolerant liver recipients is not affected by extent of immunosuppression. *Am J Transplant* 2005;**5**:314–22.

68 Thomson AW, Mazariegos GV, Reyes J, *et al.* Monitoring the patient off immunosuppression: conceptual framework for a proposed tolerance assay study in liver transplant recipients. *Transplantation* 2001;**72**:S13–22.

69 Mazariegos GV, Reyes J, Webber SA, *et al.* Cytokine gene polymorphisms in children successfully withdrawn from immunosuppression after liver transplantation. *Transplantation* 2002;**73**:1342–5.

28 Outcomes and Risk Factors

Marc L. Melcher and John P. Roberts

Although pediatric liver transplantation has been effective for many forms of irreversible acute and chronic liver disease, the availability of liver grafts is limited, and the necessary financial and human resources are substantial. Advances are continually being made in patient selection, operative technique and immunosuppressant therapy. Optimization of these advances and the limited resources to maximize the benefits to patients requires continual reassessment of the outcomes and risk factors associated with pediatric liver transplantation. In addition, patients and families benefit from clear articulation of the most up-to-date and comprehensive assessment of the risks and outcomes of liver transplantation.

The number of pediatric liver transplants performed annually is significantly lower than the number of adult liver transplants. Therefore, this continual assessment of risk factors and outcomes had been based on single institutions reviewing their own data, and is hindered by small patient numbers that reduce the statistical power necessary to find differences in populations. In recognition of this problem, national and international databases have been created.

The Studies of Pediatric Liver Transplantation (SPLIT) database has collected data since 1995 from a consortium of 38 pediatric liver transplant centers in North America [1]. The US Scientific Registry of Transplant Recipients (SRTR) database consists of data collected since 1987 by the Organ Procurement and Transplantation Network (OPTN) on organ donors and recipients in the USA [2]. It includes data from all transplant centers in North America and allows for comparison of center outcomes with national outcomes. Further information can be drawn from the small number of randomized studies in the pediatric population.

Studies from single institutions and multicenter databases have identified risk factors associated with the recipients, the donor organs and the techniques used that adversely affect mortality and morbidity. Although liver recipient mortality and graft survival continue to be the most commonly followed outcomes, the success of the liver transplant field has made it possible to study long-term and often more subtle outcomes that only become evident years after a transplant. These include renal function, psychosocial development, catching up on growth, and intelligence.

MORTALITY AND GRAFT SURVIVAL

The most recently reported multicenter survival results available for children come from the SPLIT database for transplant recipients between 1995 and 2002 [1]. One-year, 2-year and 3-year patient survival rates were 86.3%, 84.3% and 83.8%, respectively (Fig. 28.1). One-year, 2-year and 3-year graft survival rates were 80.2%, 76% and 75.3%, respectively. There is a trend towards better outcomes in later years.

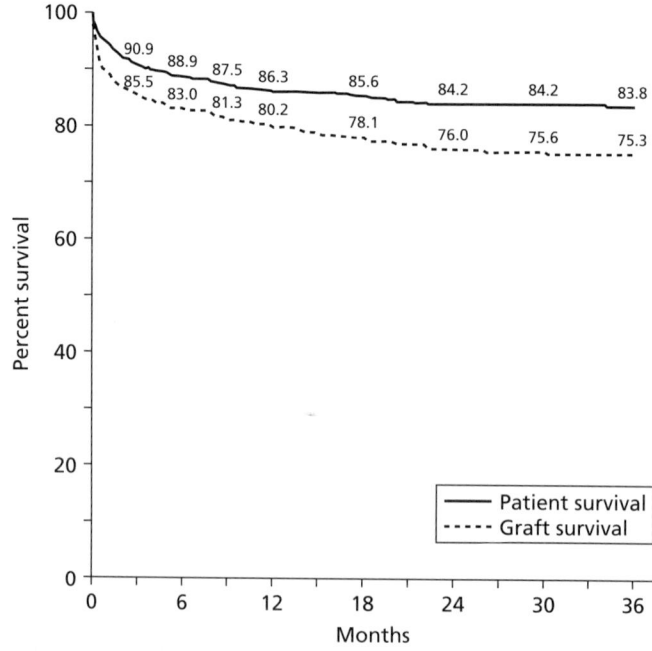

Fig. 28.1 Kaplan–Meier probability of pediatric liver recipient and graft survival in the SPLIT database through 2002. From Martin *et al.* [1] with permission.

Earlier but somewhat overlapping data on pediatric liver transplants come primarily from single institutions. Three of the largest series are from Los Angeles, CA, Pittsburgh, PA, and Brussels, Belgium. Data from the University of California, Los Angeles (UCLA) experience of 256 patients reveal 1-year, 3-year and 5-year patient survival rates of 78%, 77% and 75%, respectively, for the time period 1984–92 and 1-year, 3-year and 5-year patient survival rates of 88%, 85% and 85%, respectively, for the 184 children who received transplants 1993–97 [3]. The improvement in survival rates was most pronounced in children under 1 year old. At Pittsburgh Children's Hospital between October 1989 and October 1996, the actuarial patient survival rate of the 278 patients studied was 87% at 1 year, 85% at 3 years and 85% at 5 years; graft survival was 80% at 1 year, 78% at 3 years and 78% at 5 years [4]. All these Pittsburgh children received tacrolimus after surgery for immunosuppression. Patient and graft survival rates were lower before 1989 when cyclosporine A was part of the standard immunosuppressive regimen. A review of 376 children who received transplants in Brussels, Belgium between March 1984 and July 2000 similarly showed improving survival trends. Overall, the 1-year, 5-year and 10-year survival rates were 95.7%, 91.4% and 90.4%, respectively [5]. In a multivariate analysis, those patients who received transplants after 1991 had significantly higher survival rates and improved graft survival. Finally, the University of Hamburg, Germany, recently published a series of 132 consecutive pediatric liver transplants in which there was 100% survival at 6 months [6]. The authors of these studies attribute the improvements to better patient selection, improved ICU care, optimized use of immunosuppressants and protocol standardizations.

RECIPIENT RISK FACTORS

To optimize placement of the limited supply of liver grafts, the waiting list prioritization algorithm the PELD (pediatric end-stage liver disease) score, and the patient's disease, age, size and nutritional status have all been studied. The findings from these studies have influenced treatment strategies in the preoperative setting, the timing of transplant and the indications for transplant.

PELD score

To assure that liver grafts are going to the patients with the greatest need, the PELD score was instituted in 2002 to establish the patient's priority on the donor organ list. Variables used to calculate the PELD score include age, serum albumin, serum bilirubin, the International Normalization Ratio for the prothrombin time, and growth failure. The specific goal of developing the PELD score was to create an objective and verifiable point system that would predict survival time for patients on the waiting list. While it appears that progress towards this goal has been made [7], use of the PELD score poses the question of whether patients with higher scores do worse after receiving a transplant. Studies from the SPLIT research group identified higher PELD scores as predictive of increased length of postoperative hospital stay [8] and poor graft survival [1]. However, possibly because they have only been used since 2002, higher PELD scores have not yet been correlated with poorer patient survival. The increased hospital stay associated with increasing degree of illness of the patient suggests that earlier transplantation may result in better outcomes.

Age

The effect of recipient age on graft rejection, graft survival and patient survival has been studied using both the multicenter SPLIT database and several single institutional series. Analysis of the SPLIT database shows that the incidence of graft rejection is lower in patients aged 6 months or less at the time of transplant [1]. This lower rejection rate does not translate to lower risk of graft loss or patient death.

However, a separate multivariate analysis of data from this database found that when the patients who specifically had fulminant hepatic failure were analyzed, the risk of death was greater in children less than 1 year old than in those older than 1 year [9]. Moreover, a single institution study from UCLA suggests that all patients less than 1 year had a greater risk of death after surgery [3].

Patient size and nutritional status

Inherent in end-stage liver disease is the presence of protein-energy malnutrition and a reduction in the body cell mass, both of which are secondary to alterations in glucose, lipid and protein metabolism [10,11]. In addition, the nutrient intake of pediatric patients has been measured to be only 63% of the daily recommended intake [12]. As a result, children on the transplant list are underweight and short for their age. Moreover, the degree of malnutrition, based on weight scores and lean body mass, experienced by children on the transplant list correlates with the degree of hepatic dysfunction [13].

Several studies have correlated one or more variables linked to malnutrition with postoperative outcomes of liver recipients. A study of the UCLA experience in the 1980s showed that children whose height was greater than 1 standard deviation (SD) below the mean had significantly more infections and complications, and a higher mortality than children whose height was within 1 SD of the mean [14].

These findings were confirmed by a review of the SPLIT database patients from 1995 through 2002 [1]. In this study, patients whose weight, height, or both, were more than 2 SD less than the mean for their age had significantly worse graft survival and increased risk of postoperative death.

Despite the above findings, data proving that aggressive enteral or parenteral nutritional support decrease pediatric liver transplantation mortality or morbidity are lacking.

Previous grafts

Eleven to twenty-six percent of pediatric liver recipients require retransplantation [1,3,15]. The only data on the risk that having a previous graft has on outcome come from single institutions. Studies from UCLA and from Stanford University suggest that patients receiving more than one graft have an increased mortality risk [3,15]. The greater technical difficulty of reoperation and increased stress of a second operation probably contribute to these worse outcomes.

DISEASE-DEPENDENT FACTORS

Indications for liver transplantation in the pediatric population include biliary atresia, fulminant liver failure, malignancy and metabolic diseases.

Biliary atresia

Although biliary atresia is the most common indication for liver transplantation in children, a successful Kasai hepatoportoenterostomy can also treat the cholestasis of biliary atresia and delay or obviate the need for a transplant. However, long-term results of hepatoportoenterostomy are poor, and the patients who undergo this procedure for biliary drainage often require a transplant later in the course of their disease. Therefore, some have advocated transplantation as the primary treatment. However, because liver transplant outcomes in very young patients appear to be less successful than in older patients, a hepatoportoenterostomy may be beneficial as a bridge to transplant.

Results from Belgium support the strategy to delay transplant until the patient is older [16]. In a retrospective study of 328 patients with biliary atresia treated in Brussels between 1984 and 2000, patients had actuarial survival rates of 87%, 83% and 81% at 1, 5 and 10 years, respectively. When the results were broken down by patient age, the 1-year survival rates were 85%, 86%, 83% and 100% for children under the age of 1 year, 1–3 years, 3–6 years and over 6 years, respectively. Therefore, the 26 patients who received a transplant after age 6 appear to have tolerated the transplant better than the younger patients.

These findings suggest that performing a Kasai hepatoportoenterostomy first may improve outcome by enabling patients to go through their transplant after reaching the age of 6. A review of 42 pediatric liver transplants for biliary atresia at the University of California, San Francisco (UCSF), 1988–2002, suggests that patients who receive transplants after a biliary drainage procedure, do not have an increased risk of perioperative complications despite the technical challenge of a second operation [17]. The above findings would suggest that patients with a substantial expectation of a successful Kasai operation should have this operation performed [18].

Fulminant hepatic failure

Fulminant hepatic failure, defined as severe liver dysfunction and encephalopathy within 8 weeks of initial symptoms, is rare in children, but the mortality rate approaches 90% for those who are not treated for this disease.

According to the SPLIT database, approximately 12.9% of pediatric liver transplants are performed for fulminant hepatic failure [9]. Not only were pediatric patients with fulminant hepatic failure more likely to die while on the transplant list, they also did worse postoperatively when compared with patients with biliary atresia [1,9]. Preoperative factors associated with significantly poorer outcomes in patients with fulminant hepatic failure consisted of severe encephalopathy and the need for preoperative dialysis. Both of these factors are probably indicative of the severity of disease. Moreover, of those who receive a transplant, children with fulminant hepatic failure do worse if they are less than 1 year old [9].

Malignancy

Hepatoblastoma is the most common primary tumor in children that leads to the need for a liver transplant [1,19]. A multi-institutional, international study run by the International Society of Pediatric Oncologists, SIOPEL 1, prospectively followed 138 children with hepatoblastoma who were treated preoperatively with cisplatin and doxorubicin. Children with tumors deemed unresectable by partial hepatectomy as well as children requiring rescue after partial hepatectomy were recommended to have a transplant. Twelve children received a liver graft. The Kaplan–Meier survival rates for these 12 children were 75% at 5 years and 66% at 10 years. Two patients died from uncontrolled tumor relapse; both had vena caval and portal vein invasion. Other studies confirm that the survival rate is worse for patients receiving transplants for liver tumors than for patients with biliary atresia [20].

Other diseases

Several metabolic and genetic diseases that result in liver failure also have broad extrahepatic consequences. Cystic fibrosis, tyrosinemia type I, Crigler–Najjar type I, mitochondrial diseases and bile acid biosynthesis disorders have been indications for liver transplantation in children. However, the extrahepatic disease negatively influences long-term outcome [21]. For example, approximately 3.5% of pediatric transplants are performed for cholestatic disease associated with cystic fibrosis [22]. In this group of recipients, most postoperative deaths are associated with pulmonary and septic episodes rather than dysfunction of the liver graft.

DONOR ORGAN FACTORS

The percentage of patients between the ages of 1 and 5 who die while on the waiting list has been higher than the percentage of patients who die on the waiting list from any other age group under 50 years old [23]. This problem has been partially attributed to the shortage of age- and size-matched organs, especially for infants. Therefore, in addition to optimizing the waiting list algorithm, there has been pressure to extend the criteria of acceptable donor organs by increasing the donor age range – by using surgically reduced livers, splitting cadaver grafts and using living donors.

Donor age

There appears to be a bimodal effect of donor age and size on graft survival. Experience from 278 patients from the Children's Hospital of Pittsburgh suggests that the graft survival from donors less than 1 year old or less than 10 kg in weight is shorter than grafts from other types of donors [4]. This may be a result of the 50% graft loss attributed specifically to vascular thrombosis of the smaller donor's vessels. Grafts from donors older than 18 years do not survive as long as grafts from younger donors in pediatric patients [1]. Donor age has not been shown to affect recipient survival.

Technical variants

The shortage of size-matched livers from deceased donors that are suitable for pediatric patients has led to the development of partial liver grafts from living and deceased donors. The hope is to reduce mortality while on the pediatric liver waiting list, which contained 584 patients in November 2004 [24].

These donor grafts include reduced size grafts, the left lateral segment or the right or left lobe of the liver. Deceased donor livers can be split into usable grafts *in situ* or *ex vivo*. Usually, the left lateral lobe is offered to a child and the remaining liver is offered to an adult. However, this complicates the liver allocation system because the split livers are generally considered to be of lower quality than whole livers in adults [25]. Therefore, an adult patient for whom the primary liver offer is made has little incentive to allow the graft to be split and the lateral segment to be used in a child. Additionally, controversy exists as to whether pediatric patients receiving split livers from deceased donors do worse than patients receiving living donor livers or whole organs [26].

Two separate analyses of first-time pediatric liver transplant recipients from 1989 to 2000 in the US SRTR suggest that living donor partial grafts placed in patients less than 2 years old have a significantly lower risk of graft failure than split deceased donor grafts (Fig. 28.2) [26,27]. Moreover, the findings published from the SPLIT database suggest patients do better when receiving whole cadaveric grafts than when they receive split cadaveric grafts [1]. Finally, none of the above studies found an advantage for older children receiving living donor partial grafts.

There does not appear to be a clear association between graft type or whether the graft is from a living or cadaveric donor and rejection early after transplantation, although there is evidence for decreased rejection in the long term [28].

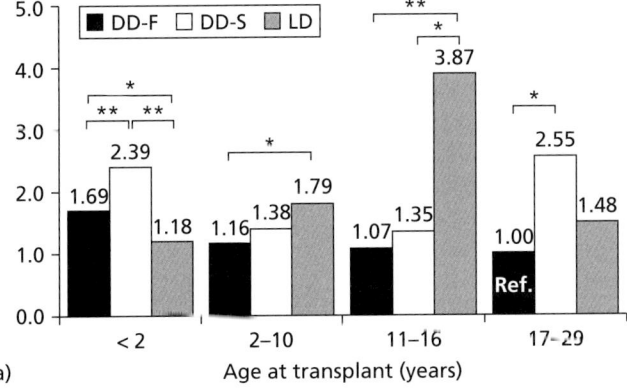

(a)

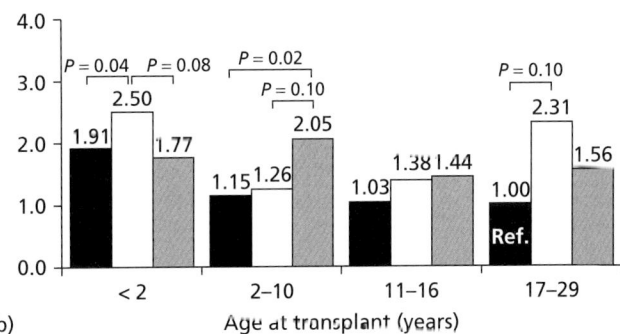

(b)

Fig. 28.2 Relative risk of (a) graft failure and (b) patient mortality 1 year after transplant by age group and graft type. DD-F, full-sized deceased donor grafts; DD-S, split or reduced sized deceased donor grafts; LD, living donor grafts. Adjustments include recipient race, ethnicity, sex, diagnosis, life support, medical urgency status at

transplant, ABO compatibility, year of transplant and transplant center. Within each age group, all statistically significant differences in outcomes between graft types are indicated with brackets. *$P < 0.05$ for the comparison indicated; **$P < 0.001$ for the comparison indicated. From Roberts *et al.* [26] with permission.

ABO incompatibilities

The use of ABO incompatible donor livers in children less than 2 years of age has yielded interesting results. Several series have found that these very young children have good survival outcomes after transplantation with ABO incompatible organs [29]. This contrasts with the outcome in older children and adults, in which the outcome of ABO incompatible transplantation is markedly worse than for transplantation with a compatible organ. The reason why this immunologic privilege exists at the younger age is unclear [29].

RISK FACTORS ASSOCIATED WITH TECHNICAL COMPLICATIONS

Vascular complications

Vascular complications including hepatic artery thrombosis, portal vein thrombosis and postoperative hemorrhage are credited as the most common causes of graft failure that require retransplant in children [1]. In patients tracked in the SPLIT database through 2002, hepatic artery thromboses were reported in 8.3% of patients within the first 90 days after transplant and were cited as the cause of graft failure in 36% of 121 cases. Although the use of split and reduced sized livers has reduced the waiting time on the pediatric liver transplantation list, it has contributed to the technical difficulty of the operation but not significantly to the rate of hepatic artery thrombosis.

Early diagnosis with abdominal ultrasound and early operative repair of hepatic artery thrombosis may prevent graft loss, but the long-term outcome of these salvaged grafts with respect to biliary complications needs further study [30]. Minimizing the use of cryopreserved venous extensions appears to have markedly decreased the portal thrombosis rate, thereby increasing graft survival [31].

Bile duct strictures and leaks

The anastomosis between small recipient ducts and the small ducts of pediatric livers provides for a high rate of biliary duct anastomotic leaks and strictures. Approximately one-third of recipients require intervention – either reoperation or dilatation using an interventional radiology approach – to address leaks and strictures [32].

POST-TRANSPLANT RISK FACTORS

Immunosuppressants

In the last 15 years, four important changes that have improved graft and patient survival while minimizing side-effects have been the introduction of new calcineurin inhibitors, the optimization of their dosing, attempts to withdraw steroids sooner after transplantation and the use of prophylactic antibacterial and antiviral agents to increase the therapeutic index of immunosuppressive drugs.

In adults, prospectively collected results reported by the US Multicenter FK506 Liver Study Group suggest that adult liver transplant recipients have significantly fewer episodes of rejection when treated with tacrolimus (a.k.a. FK506) than with cyclosporine A (CSA) [33]. The retrospective data from the multicenter SPLIT database showed that patients who received tacrolimus had significantly fewer episodes of rejection than those who received cyclosporine. This confirms studies of data from retrospective, single institutional series that showed significantly fewer episodes of rejection [34] or a trend towards to lower rejection rates with tacrolimus [15,35].

Both regimens have significant side-effect profiles, including renal insufficiency and neurologic sequelae; however, because systemic CSA causes hirsuitism and gingival overgrowth, tacrolimus has been used increasingly in the pediatric population.

Steroids have long been a mainstay of immunosuppressant therapy in adults and children. However, several centers have developed protocols to withdraw steroids earlier after transplant because of frequently observed side-effects, including growth retardation, in children. When long-term growth after transplant is measured, the growth of patients who have had steroids withdrawn within 1 or 2 years of receiving a transplant is more likely to approach normal than is the growth of patients who continued to take steroids more than 2 years after transplant [36,37].

CAUSES OF DEATH AND GRAFT LOSS

Infections

The use of strong immunosuppressants in children who require liver transplants has led to a high infection rate after transplantation. In fact, approximately 80% of pediatric liver recipients require hospitalization for an infection during the first decade after transplantation [38]. Although viral infections are the most frequent cause of subsequent hospitalizations, bacterial infections are the most common cause of death postoperatively and remain a significant cause of death for many years after transplantation [1,5]. Fungal and viral (cytomegalovirus [CMV], Epstein–Barr virus [EBV]) infections can also cause death. The use of prophylactic agents has minimized the severity of infections seen in the post-transplant period; in particular, CMV infections.

Graft failure, including primary nonfunction, acute artery thrombosis, recurrent disease and rejection can all contribute to patient death [1].

Rejection

In spite of the risks posed by calcineurin inhibitor therapy, it continues to be used because of its efficacy in preventing graft rejection. While 44% of pediatric recipients experience some rejection within the first 6 months of transplant, acute rejection causes fewer than 1% of deaths in the era of tacrolimus [1]. This is a remarkable change from the era in which cyclosporine A was primarily used and the graft loss caused by acute or chronic rejection was 11% [34]. Currently, most primary episodes of rejection are successfully treated with corticosteroids with or without other drugs.

Chronic rejection can be as high as 25% within 10 years of receiving a transplant [38]. Poor compliance with immunosuppressant therapy, especially a problem in adolescents, was most predictive of development of chronic rejection [38].

OTHER OUTCOMES

Lymphoma

Post-transplant lymphoproliferative disease (PTLD), caused by EBV, occurs in approximately 10% of pediatric liver transplant patients [39]. In this disorder, B lymphocytes and occasionally T lymphocytes undergo uncontrolled proliferation. Cytotoxic T lymphocytes usually are capable of eliminating cells containing rapidly dividing virus. However, typical post-transplant immunosuppressive therapy suppresses these cells, allowing for the development of PTLD.

Risk factors associated with developing PTLD include placement of EBV-positive grafts in EBV-negative recipients, having a newly acquired EBV infection within 3–6 months after transplant, coinfection with CMV, young recipient age and intensive use of immunosuppressants such as cyclosporine A, tacrolimus and OKT3 [39,40].

Withdrawal or minimization of immunosuppression, antiviral therapy, immunotherapy and chemotherapy are part of the multifaceted strategy to treat PTLD. When left untreated, the mortality for transplant patients with PTLD is approximately 50% [39,41]. Therefore, some argue for the complete withdrawal of immunosuppressants despite the increased risk of rejection [42]. Intravenous gangciclovir may effectively prevent the production of new viral particles and subsequent infection of additional lymphocytes. Anti-B-cell antibodies against the cell surface protein CD20 have been used successfully to treat disseminated disease and bulky tumors in children [39].

A controversial area is the monitoring of children in the postoperative period for the presence of EBV viral genomes in the peripheral blood by polymerase chain reaction (PCR). The presence of these genomes is addressed with modification of immunosuppression and antiviral therapy. The efficacy of this approach has not been rigorously tested [43,44].

Chronic renal failure

Intensive use of calcineurin inhibitors, immunosuppressants, tacrolimus and CSA is also associated with nephrotoxiticity. The glomerular filtration rate has been calculated to be on average 35% lower than pretransplant levels just 3 months after transplant and initiation of calcineurin inhibitors [45]. Ten years after transplant and calcineurin inhibitor therapy, 77% of pediatric patients are reported to have mild to severe renal failure [38]. Replacement or minimization of the calcineurin inhibitor with other agents such as sirolimus (aka rapamycin) can improve creatinine clearance [46].

Growth and development

Before their transplants, children with chronic liver disease fail to achieve many of their growth milestones. This is not surprising considering the malnutrition, anorexia and malabsorption associated with chronic liver failure. In addition, the liver produces important growth factors such as insulin-like growth factor-I [47]. A liver transplant offers these patients the possibility of catching up on their growth. The benefits of a functional graft may offset the negative growth effects of the immunosuppressants, including steroids.

In fact, multiple studies have shown that many pediatric patients who exhibit pretransplantation growth failure catch up on their growth after receiving a transplant. The degree of "catch up" growth depends on the age at transplantation. On average, children at UCSF who received a transplant between February 1988 and June 1999 for nontumor indications and survived 1 year, exhibited significant catch-up growth approaching the 50th percentile if their transplant occurred before age 2; however, growth increases were often erased at ages when healthy peers underwent their prepubertal growth acceleration (Fig. 28.3) [48]. A similar review of the children receiving a liver transplant at UCLA between 1984 and 1996 found that the z-score for height deficit was −1.72 SD before surgery and rose to −1.37 SD 2 years after surgery [49]. However, there was no continuing improvement after 2 years. Factors associated with a worse ability to catch-up on growth include receiving a transplant at an older age, fulminant hepatic failure and tumor. A review of children receiving a liver transplant specifically for biliary atresia also found that those who received a transplant before they were 1 year old were more likely to catch-up to their healthy peers than were children receiving transplants later in life [50].

In contrast to these studies, a study on patients with Alagille syndrome, an autosomal dominant syndrome with many manifestations including growth retardation and cholestasis, showed that these patients do not receive much growth benefit from liver transplantation [51]. The growth retardation in Alagille syndrome is thought to be secondary to several factors other than chronic liver failure. Growth

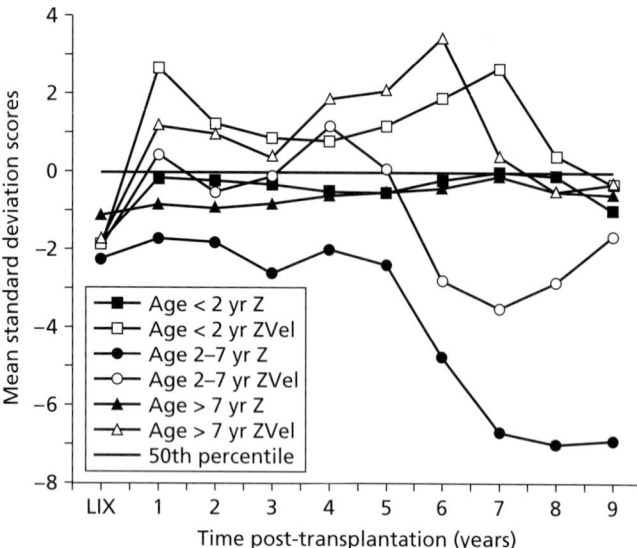

Fig. 28.3 Plot of post-transplantation height (solid shapes) and growth (open shapes) mean standard deviation scores by age. The solid line (0 SD score) represents the 50th percentile for height and growth velocity. Children transplant at an age less than 2 years catch up to the 50th percentile within 1 year (solid squares). From Renz *et al.* [48] with permission.

factor hormone supplementation has not been helpful in children with Alagille syndrome [51].

Psychosocial development

Although recipients of liver transplants tend to score their quality of life as "good" years after receiving their transplant, comprehensive neurocognitive testing shows that up to 50% of these patients have subtle cognitive, emotional and intelligence disturbances [52–54].

When a group of 15 children with liver transplants was compared with other patients with chronic diseases such as cystic fibrosis, the liver transplant recipients did worse on language skill and memory function testing [53]. The presence of deficits in language performance correlated with the number of days in hospital during the first year of life and with younger age at transplant. Malnutrition, drug toxicities and metabolic derangements may all contribute to these outcomes.

CONCLUSIONS

The dramatic success of liver transplantation in children has raised the importance of long-term outcomes other than mortality and graft loss and has highlighted the long waiting list of patients whom this operation benefits. Refinement in techniques and operative care have raised the 1-year survival

rate to above 90%, and the current immunosuppressant regimens have successfully reduced graft loss secondary to rejection to a few percentage points. However, malignancies, chronic renal failure, psychosocial development and growth failure have become increasingly relevant as the number of long-term survivors rapidly increases. As in adults, the powerful immunosuppressants come with a price. Ten percent of patients will develop PTLD and, in the long term, a significant percentage will develop chronic renal failure. The development of new drugs and techniques that reduce these unwanted consequences will require carefully structured studies to differentiate subtle differences in these long-term outcomes. While clear advances have been made based on single center series and multicenter databases, randomized controlled trials will become increasingly important.

REFERENCES

1 Martin SR, Atkison P, Anand R, Lindblad AS. Studies of Pediatric Liver Transplantation 2002: patient and graft survival and rejection in pediatric recipients of a first liver transplant in the United States and Canada. *Pediatr Transplant* 2004;8:273–83.

2 US Transplant, Scientific Registry of Transplant Recipients. 2004.

3 Goss JA, Shackleton CR, McDiarmid SV, *et al*. Long-term results of pediatric liver transplantation: an analysis of 569 transplants. *Ann Surg* 1998;228:411–20.

4 Cacciarelli TV, Dvorchik I, Mazariegos GV, *et al*. An analysis of pretransplantation variables associated with long-term allograft outcome in pediatric liver transplant recipients receiving primary tacrolimus (FK506) therapy. *Transplantation* 1999;68:650–5.

5 Wallot MA, Mathot M, Janssen M, *et al*. Long-term survival and late graft loss in pediatric liver transplant recipients: a 15-year single-center experience. *Liver Transpl* 2002;8:615–22.

6 Broering DC, Kim JS, Mueller T, *et al*. One hundred thirty-two consecutive pediatric liver transplants without hospital mortality: lessons learned and outlook for the future. *Ann Surg* 2004;240:1002–12; discussion 1012.

7 McDiarmid SV, Merion RM, Dykstra DM, Harper AM. Selection of pediatric candidates under the PELD system. *Liver Transpl* 2004;10(Suppl 2):S23–30.

8 Bucuvalas JC, Zeng L, Anand R. Predictors of length of stay for pediatric liver transplant recipients. *Liver Transpl* 2004;10:1011–7.

9 Baliga P, Alvarez S, Lindblad A, Zeng L. Posttransplant survival in pediatric fulminant hepatic failure: the SPLIT experience. *Liver Transpl* 2004;10:1364–71.

10 Cabre E, Gassull MA. Nutritional aspects of liver disease and transplantation. *Curr Opin Clin Nutr Metab Care* 2001;4:581–9.

11 Campos AC, Matias JE, Coelho JC. Nutritional aspects of liver transplantation. *Curr Opin Clin Nutr Metab Care* 2002;5:297–307.

12 Sheperd RW, Chin SE, Cleghorn GJ, *et al*. Malnutrition in children with chronic liver disease accepted for liver transplantation: clinical profile and effect on outcome. *J Paediatr Child Health* 1991;27:295–299.

13 Roggero P, Cataliotti E, Ulla L, *et al*. Factors influencing malnutrition in children waiting for liver transplants. *Am J Clin Nutr* 1997;**65**:1852–7.

14 Moukarzei AA, Napim I, Vargas J, *et al*. Effect of nutritional status on outcome of orthotopic liver transplantation in pediatric patients. *Transplant Proc* 1990;**22**:1560–3.

15 Zajicek A, Esquivel C, Millan M, *et al*. Thirteen years' experience in pediatric liver transplantation: differences between tacrolimus and cyclosporine. *Transplant Proc* 2002;**34**:1976–8.

16 Diem HV, Evrard V, Vinh HT, *et al*. Pediatric liver transplantation for biliary atresia: results of primary grafts in 328 recipients. *Transplantation* 2003;**75**:1692–7.

17 Visser BC, Suh I, Hirose S, *et al*. The influence of portoenterostomy on transplantation for biliary atresia. *Liver Transpl* 2004;**10**:1279–86.

18 Dolgin SE. Answered and unanswered controversies in the surgical management of extrahepatic biliary atresia. *Pediatr Transplant* 2004;**8**:628–31.

19 Otte JB, Pritchard J, Aronson DC, *et al*. Liver transplantation for hepatoblastoma: results from the International Society of Pediatric Oncology (SIOP) study SIOPEL-1 and review of the world experience. *Pediatr Blood Cancer* 2004;**42**:74–83.

20 Abt PL, Desai NM, Crawford MD, *et al*. Survival following liver transplantation from non-heart-beating donors. *Ann Surg* 2004;**239**:87–92.

21 Shneider BL. Pediatric liver transplantation in metabolic disease: clinical decision making. *Pediatr Transplant* 2002;**6**:25–9.

22 Molmenti EP, Squires RH, Nagata D, *et al*. Liver transplantation for cholestasis associated with cystic fibrosis in the pediatric population. *Pediatr Transplant* 2003;**7**:93–7.

23 OPTN/SRTR 2003 Annual Report Transplant Data 1993–2002. Chapter V: Pediatric Transplantation 2003 [cited; available from: www.ustransplant.org].

24 Organ Procurement and Transplant Network. 2004.

25 Merion RM, Rush SH, Dykstra DM, *et al*. Predicted lifetimes for adult and pediatric split liver versus adult whole liver transplant recipients. *Am J Transplant* 2004;**4**:1792–7.

26 Roberts JP, Hulbert-Shearon TE, Merion RM, Wolfe RA, Port FK. Influence of graft type on outcomes after pediatric liver transplantation. *Am J Transplant* 2004;**4**:373–7.

27 Abt PL, Rapaport-Kelz R, Desai NM, *et al*. Survival among pediatric liver transplant recipients: impact of segmental grafts. *Liver Transpl* 2004;**10**:1287–93.

28 Toyoki Y, Renz JF, Mudge C, *et al*. Allograft rejection in pediatric liver transplantation: comparison between cadaveric and living related donors. *Pediatr Transplant* 2002;**6**:301–7.

29 Egawa H, Oike F, Buhler L, *et al*. Impact of recipient age on outcome of ABO-incompatible living-donor liver transplantation. *Transplantation* 2004;**77**:403–11.

30 Dalgic A, Dalgic B, Demirogullari B, *et al*. Clinical approach to graft hepatic artery thrombosis following living related liver transplantation. *Pediatr Transplant* 2003;**7**:149–52.

31 Buell JF, Funaki B, Cronin DC, *et al*. Long-term venous complications after full-size and segmental pediatric liver transplantation. *Ann Surg* 2002;**236**:658–66.

32 Kling K, Lau H, Colombani P. Biliary complications of living related pediatric liver transplant patients. *Pediatr Transplant* 2004;**8**:178–84.

33 A comparison of tacrolimus (FK506) and cyclosporine for immunosuppression in liver transplantation. The US Multicenter FK506 Liver Study Group. *N Engl J Med* 1994;**331**:1110–5.

34 Jain A, Mazariegos G, Kashyap R, *et al*. Pediatric liver transplantation in 808 consecutive children: 20-years experience from a single center. *Transplant Proc* 2002;**34**:1955–7.

35 McDiarmid SV, Busuttil RW, Ascher NL, *et al*. FK506 (tacrolimus) compared with cyclosporine for primary immunosuppression after pediatric liver transplantation: results from the US Multicenter Trial. *Transplantation* 1995;**59**:530–6.

36 Diem HV, Sokal EM, Janssen M, Otte JB, Reding R. Steroid withdrawal after pediatric liver transplantation: a long-term follow-up study in 109 recipients. *Transplantation* 2003;**75**:1664–70.

37 Lopez-Espinosa J, Yeste D, Iglesias J, *et al*. Analysis of growth during prepubertal years in long-term survivors after pediatric orthotopic liver transplantation. *J Pediatr Endocrinol Metab* 2004;**17**:1221–9.

38 Avitzur Y, De Luca E, Cantos M, *et al*. Health status ten years after pediatric liver transplantation: looking beyond the graft. *Transplantation* 2004;**78**:566–73.

39 Holmes RD, Sokol RJ. Epstein–Barr virus and post-transplant lymphoproliferative disease. *Pediatr Transplant* 2002;**6**:456–64.

40 Heo JS, Park JW, Lee KW, *et al*. Posttransplantation lymphoproliferative disorder in pediatric liver transplantation. *Transplant Proc* 2004;**36**:2307–8.

41 Collins MH, Montone KT, Leahey AM, *et al*. Post-transplant lymphoproliferative disease in children. *Pediatr Transplant* 2001;**5**:250–7.

42 Hurwitz M, Desai DM, Cox KL, *et al*. Complete immunosuppressive withdrawal as a uniform approach to post-transplant lymphoproliferative disease in pediatric liver transplantation. *Pediatr Transplant* 2004;**8**:267–72.

43 Kogan-Liberman D, Burroughs M, Emre S, Moscona A, Shneider BL. The role of quantitative Epstein–Barr virus polymerase chain reaction and preemptive immunosuppression reduction in pediatric liver transplantation: a preliminary experience. *J Pediatr Gastroenterol Nutr* 2001;**33**:445–9.

44 McDiarmid SV. Management of the pediatric liver transplant patient. *Liver Transpl* 2001;**7**(Suppl. 1):S77–86.

45 Arora-Gupta N, Davies P, McKiernan P, Kelly DA. The effect of long-term calcineurin inhibitor therapy on renal function in children after liver transplantation. *Pediatr Transplant* 2004;**8**:145–50.

46 Casas-Melley AT, Falkenstein KP, Flynn LM, Ziegler VL, Dunn SP. Improvement in renal function and rejection control in pediatric liver transplant recipients with the introduction of sirolimus. *Pediatr Transplant* 2004;**8**:362–6.

47 Maes M, Sokal E, Otte J. Growth factors in children with end-stage liver disease before and after liver transplantation: a review. *Pediatr Transplant* 1997;**1**:171–5.

48 Renz JF, de Roos M, Rosenthal P, *et al*. Posttransplantation growth in pediatric liver recipients. *Liver Transpl* 2001;**7**:1040–55.

49 McDiarmid SV, Gornbein JA, DeSilva PJ, *et al*. Factors affecting growth after pediatric liver transplantation. *Transplantation* 1999;**67**:404–11.

50 Alonso G, Duca P, Pasqualini T, D'Agostino D. Evaluation of catch-up growth after liver transplantation in children with biliary atresia. *Pediatr Transplant* 2004;**8**:255–9.

51 Quiros-Tejeira RE, Ament ME, Heyman MB, *et al.* Variable morbidity in alagille syndrome: a review of 43 cases. *J Pediatr Gastroenterol Nutr* 1999;**29**:431–7.

52 Adeback P, Nemeth A, Fischler B. Cognitive and emotional outcome after pediatric liver transplantation. *Pediatr Transplant* 2003;**7**:385–9.

53 Krull K, Fuchs C, Yurk H, Boone P, Alonso E. Neurocognitive outcome in pediatric liver transplant recipients. *Pediatr Transplant* 2003;**7**:111–8.

54 Wayman KI, Cox KL, Esquivel CO. Neurodevelopmental outcome of young children with extrahepatic biliary atresia 1 year after liver transplantation. *J Pediatr* 1997;**131**:894–8.

Heart Transplantation

29 Historical Notes

Steven A. Webber and William H. Neches

Historically, credit for the first pediatric heart transplant is given to Kantrowitz *et al.* [1] who, in 1967, transplanted the heart of an anencephalic infant into a 3-week-old with tricuspid atresia. The following year, Cooley *et al.* [2] transplanted the heart and lungs of another anencephalic newborn into a 3-month-old infant with atrioventricular septal defect and pulmonary hypertension. While both of these infants only survived a few hours after surgery, these pioneering procedures emphasized the technical feasibility of thoracic organ transplantation in childhood. These transplants were performed following many years of laboratory experimentation with heterotopic and orthotopic transplantation in small and large animals. The race to "be the first" may well have been part of the driving force behind the timing of these first pediatric transplants, although there is also evidence to suggest that these pioneering surgeons believed that successful thoracic transplantation was feasible in both children and adults by the end of the 1960s.

EXPERIMENTAL HEART TRANSPLANTATION: 1905–67

The earliest attempts to transplant the heart date back to 1905, when Carrel and Guthrie [3] transplanted the heart of a small dog into the neck of a larger one. The heart beat for approximately 2 hours. Mann *et al.* [4] recorded further attempts at heterotopic transplantation in 1933. Graft survival for as long as 8 days was recorded. Importantly, the first observations of cardiac allograft rejection were made during these experiments: "*Histologically the heart was completely infiltrated with lymphocytes, large mononuclears and polymorphonuclears.*" Several other groups experimented with heterotopic transplantation during the 1940s and 1950s. These early experiments are well reviewed by Lansman *et al.* [5].

The key barriers to orthotopic transplantation were preservation of the graft and maintenance of the recipient circulation. In 1953, Neptune *et al.* [6] reported experimental orthotopic transplantation of the heart-lung block with both animals "placed in an ordinary beverage cooler for the production of hypothermia." Three dogs underwent such a procedure with survival for up to 6 hours. In 1957, Webb and Howard [7] reported on "Restoration of function of the refrigerated heart." Canine hearts, heparinized and flushed with potassium citrate, were cooled to 4°C and were shown to function adequately when subsequently transplanted heterotopically. The same authors reported (also in 1957) technically successful orthotopic heart-lung transplants in six dogs, although with maximal survival of only 22 hours [8]. The following year, 1958, Goldberg *et al.* [9] at the University of Maryland, reported the first experimental orthotopic cardiac transplants. This was an important advance because the authors described a technique for leaving a cuff of recipient left atrium incorporating the pulmonary veins. Tedious anastomosis of individual pulmonary veins was therefore avoided. However, the allograft only supported the circulation for approximately 20 minutes. Slightly greater success was achieved by Webb *et al.* [10] who performed orthotopic heart transplants in 12 dogs using their previously described technique of "refrigeration" to preserve the donor heart and a pump oxygenator to maintain the recipient animal. Ten of the 12 animals survived from 30 to 450 minutes.

In 1960, Lower and Shumway [11], at Stanford, published a milestone report of a refined technique for orthotopic heart transplantation. Implantation was by suture anastomosis and combining the pulmonary vein and caval anastomoses into two "atrial cuffs" reduced ischemic time. The recipient was protected by moderate hypothermia (30°C) induced by surface cooling and by cardiopulmonary bypass and the graft was preserved by immersion of the excised heart in iced saline (4°C). This technique formed the basis for subsequent clinical heart transplantation. Survival up to 21 days was achieved, with several animals returning to normal activities after surgery. The animals received no immunosuppression and soon died of acute cellular rejection. Similar results were obtained by Kondo *et al.* [12] who reported (1965) on their results of applying the Lower and Shumway technique to puppies. In these studies, the animals were cooled to 16°C and the transplant was performed under circulatory arrest. Although no immunosuppression was used, one animal survived for 213 days.

Another crucial milestone in experimental heart transplantation during the 1960s was the use of intermittent or continuous immunosuppression. The Stanford group showed that reduced voltage on the electrocardiogram was an indicator of rejection and that treatment with methylprednisone and azathioprine could restore normal voltage [13]. At around the same time there was increasing interest in the use of a number of immunosuppressive therapies, mainly in experimental kidney transplantation [14]. These therapies included azathioprine, 6-mercaptopurine, actinomycin-C, as well as usage of anti-lymphocyte serum and globulin, and whole body irradiation. By 1967, the improved surgical results of experimental cardiac transplantation, and the benefits of various immunosuppressive therapies, led several groups to believe that the time was right for the first attempts at human cardiac transplantation.

THE FIRST HUMAN HEART TRANSPLANTS: DECEMBER 1967

It was clear in the mid-1960s that one of the major barriers to successful human heart transplantation was the lack of a widely accepted definition of brain death. This meant that cardiac function of the donor had to cease before donor procurement could proceed, resulting in a hypoxic-ischemic insult to the donor heart. Hardy *et al.* [15], at the University of Mississippi, made plans for the first allotransplant of the heart in January 1964. A potential recipient was already on cardiopulmonary bypass but "the prospective human donor lingered on in the recovery ward" [15]. A decision was made to proceed with a xenotransplant using a chimpanzee as the donor. This was the first recorded heart transplant in a human. The donor was able to sustain the recipient circulation for only approximately 2 hours. This was the first of eight attempts at xenotransplantation of the heart in humans, with the longest surviving graft beating for only 20 days [16].

On December 3, 1967 the first cardiac allotransplanta-tion procedure was performed by Christian Barnard at the Groote Schuur Hospital in Cape Town, South Africa [17]. The recipient was a 54-year-old man with end-stage ischemic heart disease. The donor was a young man with severe brain injury, who was declared dead only after all electrocardiographic activity ceased. The heart was then resuscitated by placing the donor on cardiopulmonary bypass. The patient recovered after the operation but died 18 days later of *Pseudomonas* pneumonia. The first pediatric heart transplant followed only 3 days later, in the early morning hours of December 6, 1967. The procedure was performed by Kantrowitz *et al.* at the Maimonides Medical Center in Brooklyn, New York. A previous attempt at an infant heart transplantation had been abandoned by the same team the prior summer (June 1966). The donor was an anencephalic infant who had been transferred to the transplant center from another hospital. After cessation of the donor heart beat, the heart could not be successfully perfused and resuscitated and the transplant was aborted. On December 4, 1967, a second anencephalic infant was transferred to Maimonides Medical Center. The recipient was felt to have tricuspid atresia, although in fact was later found to have severe Ebstein malformation with functional pulmonary atresia. A systemic-to-pulmonary shunt had been performed on the third day of life, but the infant developed severe heart failure and pulmonary edema. On November 24, it was decided to offer the family the option of orthotopic heart transplantation. A consent form for the operation was signed by the parents over a week before Barnard's first transplant in South Africa. Both donor and recipient were blood group A, and the "irradiated hamster test disclosed no evidence of major incompatibility." In the early hours of December 6, the donor heart rhythm became irregular and both infants were brought to the operating room where external cooling was begun by immersion in iced water (Fig. 29.1). Donor cardiac activity

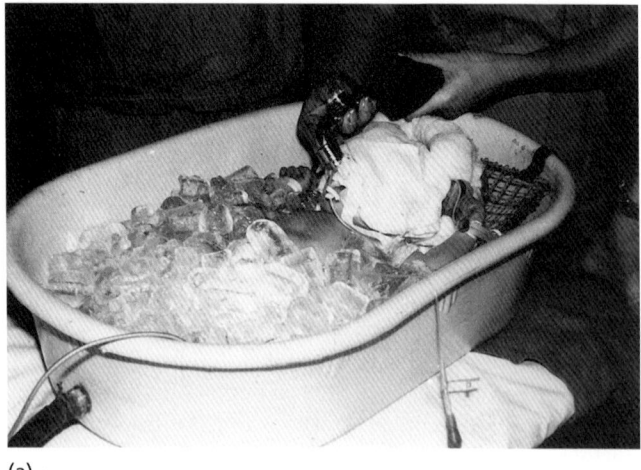

(a)

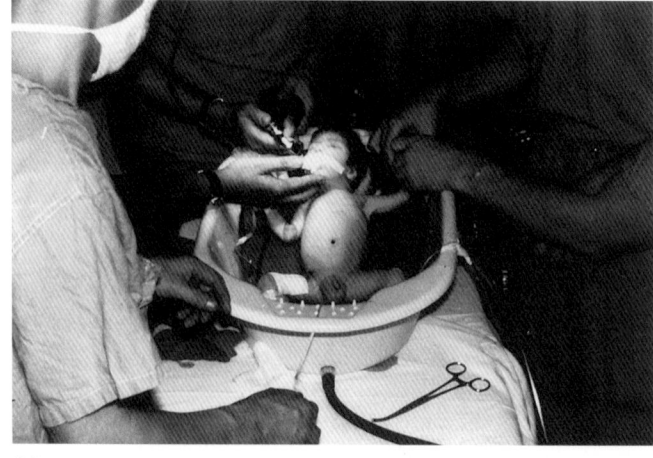

(b)

Fig. 29.1 The first pediatric heart transplant was performed on December 6, 1967. Hypothermia was induced by placing both the donor (a) and the recipient (b) in baths of iced water.

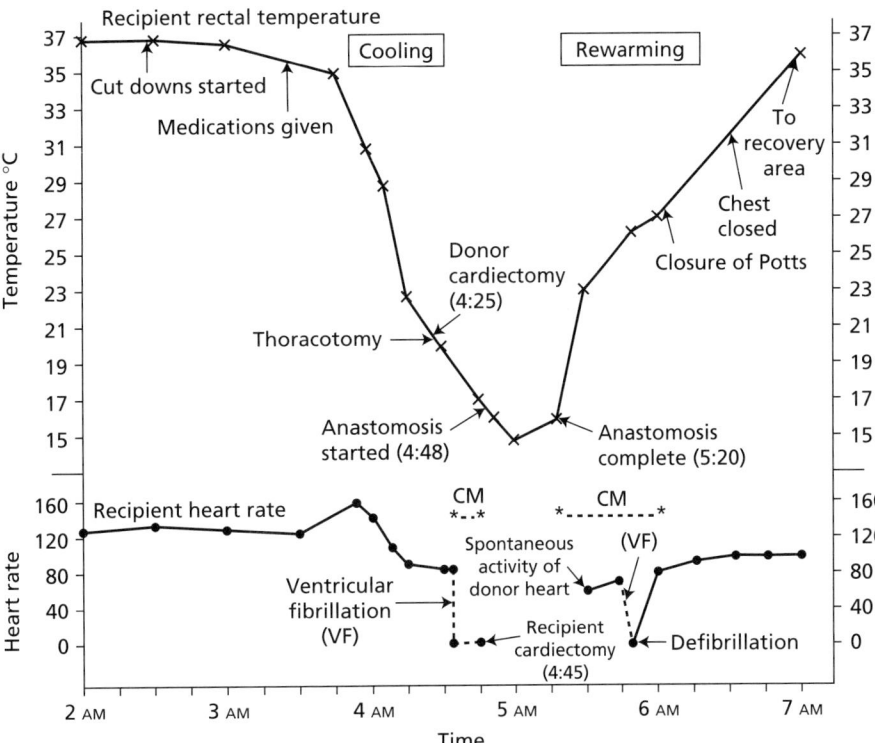

Fig. 29.2 Operative details of the first pediatric heart transplant procedure.

ceased at a temperature of 27°C and the chest was opened bilaterally through the fourth intercostal space. The excised heart was immersed in normal saline at 5°C. The recipient heart developed ventricular fibrillation as the chest was opened

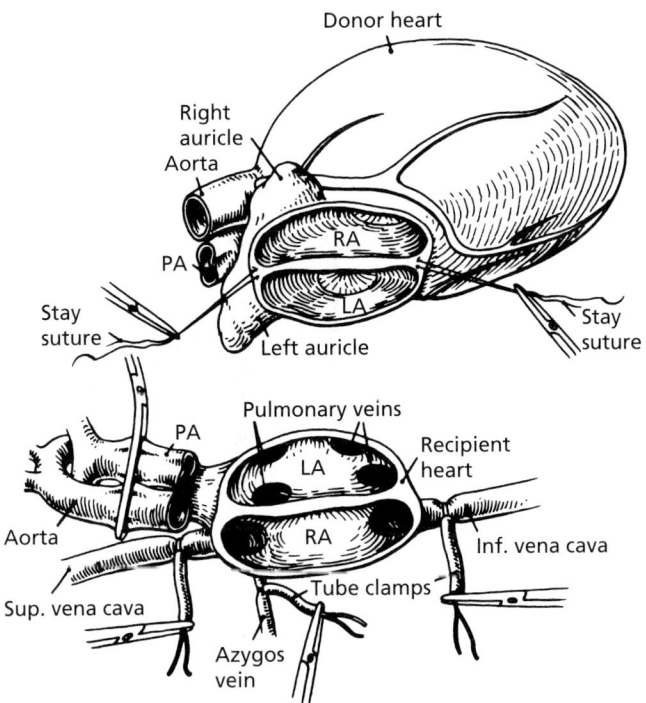

Fig. 29.3 Surgical technique of the first pediatric heart transplant. The drawing was made shortly after the procedure.

through bilateral anterior thoracotomies (Fig. 29.2). Internal cardiac massage was then performed ("manual systole") as the recipient was cooled to 17°C. The implantation essentially used the technique of Lower and Shumway (Fig. 29.3), although the procedure was performed under circulatory arrest. After implantation (achieved in 32 minutes), internal massage was again performed while the infant was rewarmed with the use of warmed normal saline placed in the tub and within the chest cavity. Sinus rhythm resumed after 10 minutes, and an episode of ventricular fibrillation responded to a single internal defibrillation. Initially the infant appeared to do well and was moving all limbs spontaneously. However, after several hours metabolic and respiratory acidosis ensued and after approximately 6 hours cardiac arrest occurred. Attempts at resuscitation failed. Autopsy revealed a good surgical result with appropriate hemostasis from the suture lines. However, the aortopulmonary shunt had been incompletely closed. The same surgeons continued their efforts at orthotopic heart transplantation, with a second procedure in a 57-year-old man 1 month later. This patient survived only 10.5 hours after transplantation [1].

INITIAL ENTHUSIASM FOLLOWED BY A PERIOD OF DESPONDENCY: 1968–80

Following Barnard and Kantrowitz, a large number of surgeons attempted heart transplants in 1968. By the end of that year, some 102 procedures were recorded from 17 countries.

Mean survival for these early transplants was only 29 days [2]. Over the next decade, enthusiasm for human heart transplantation declined worldwide, as it became apparent that the therapeutic armamentarium for controlling allograft rejection was inadequate for achieving allograft and patient survival [18]. Surgeons at a small number of centers, most notably Stanford University, persevered with attempts at heart transplantation in selected adults. The Stanford group also started to transplant a few adolescents, performing seven procedures between 1974 and 1980. Although only corticosteroids and azathioprine were used for immunosuppression, four of these patients survived longer than 10 years from transplantation [19]. Experience in a larger cohort of adult recipients transplanted in the 1970s at the same institution emphasized that such long-term survival was the exception rather than the rule [20]. Despite these disappointing results, significant improvements in survival were achieved prior to the introduction of cyclosporine. These improvements reflected a number of developments including improved preservation of the donor heart (enabling distant procurement) [21], improved selection of donor and recipients, and the development of the transvenous cardiac bioptome by Dr. Phillip Caves along with the development of a grading system for the diagnosis of acute rejection by Dr. Margaret Billingham [22]. The treatment of severe acute rejection was also greatly enhanced by the development of rabbit antithymocyte globulin preparations [23]. In addition, donor organ availability improved as the concept of brain death became accepted [24,25].

THE MODERN ERA OF PEDIATRIC HEART TRANSPLANTATION: 1980–2007

Cyclosporine was first discovered in 1976, during a screening program of fungal extracts at the Sandoz laboratories in Basle, Switzerland. The potent immunosuppressive efficacy was soon apparent and human trials developed rapidly. The favorable impact on survival of adult heart transplant recipients was immediately apparent [26,27] and led to renewed interest in pediatric heart transplantation in Stanford, at the University of Pittsburgh (1982), and subsequently at a number of other centers around the world. The earliest recipients were older children and adolescents, but it was not long before infants and younger children were also considered to be suitable recipients. Bailey *et al.* [28,29], as a result of extensive work in the animal laboratory, suggested that the neonate might make an excellent solid organ recipient. Their first attempt at neonatal transplantation was a baboon-to-human xenotransplant in a 2.2-kg 12-day-old infant with aortic and mitral atresia [30]. The infant only survived for 20 days but the surgical feasibility of newborn transplantation for hypoplastic left heart syndrome had been demonstrated.

Orthotopic newborn heart transplantation was introduced at Loma Linda, in November 1985 [31]. The first recipient was a 4-day-old infant with hypoplastic left heart syndrome, a condition generally considered to be lethal at that time, despite the recent introduction of a palliative operation by Norwood *et al.* [32]. During the 1990s, transplantation for hypoplastic left heart syndrome became the fastest growing area of pediatric heart transplantation [33]. More recently, improved results of staged surgical palliation for hypoplastic left heart syndrome and the long wait times for donor organs for neonatal candidates have led many centers to abandon transplantation as the primary procedure of choice for infants with this condition.

Many other challenges have been overcome, and milestones achieved, in the field of pediatric heart transplantation over the last 15 years. Early results with transplantation for previously palliated complex congenital heart disease were disappointing [34]. However, with improved patient selection and increased surgical experience, results comparable to transplantation for cardiomyopathy can now be achieved [35]. Immunosuppressive regimens have been refined and introduction of new drugs, such as tacrolimus, mycophenolate mofetil and sirolimus, has enhanced the armamentarium of immunosuppressive agents for use in children. Fetal echocardiography has evolved since the late 1980s and "lethal" congenital heart disease can now be reliably diagnosed *in utero*. This has raised new ethical issues about the place of fetal listing for transplantation [36]. The development of ventricular assist devices for pediatric usage, and increasing experience with extracorporeal membrane oxygenation, has enabled the most critically sick children to be successfully bridged to transplantation [37]. Work on further miniaturization of ventricular assist devices is in progress in several centers. Recognition that pediatric recipients, including neonates, are not immune from the development of chronic graft vasculopathy raises ethical issues about the justification for pediatric transplantation, including the ethics of retransplantation [38]. The major challenge at the turn of the millennium is the prevention of acute and chronic rejection through improved drug therapy and, ideally, through induction of donor-specific tolerance. The first attempts to induce donor-specific tolerance in pediatric heart transplantation commenced in 1997 at the University of Pittsburgh, with the introduction of a clinical trial of intrathymic inoculation of donor bone marrow concomitant with pediatric thoracic transplantation [39]. Further trials of tolerance induction should follow, with neonatal recipients being the obvious candidates. The shortage of donor organs remains a critical issue, and death on the waiting list remains high, especially for children receiving mechanical circulatory support with extracorporeal membrane oxygenation (ECMO). The use of ABO-incompatible transplants has recently been advocated by the Toronto group for neonatal and infant candidates, because antibodies to the major blood group antigens are not produced until later in infancy [40]. Such a strategy may improve survival for select infants with high wait-list mortality. No comprehensive solution to the donor shortage will occur unless xenotransplantation can be shown to be safe, efficacious and socially acceptable.

Enormous progress has been made in the field of pediatric heart transplantation over the last two decades. It is now accepted therapy for end-stage heart disease in all pediatric age groups. Much remains to be done, however, and pediatric heart transplantation continues to be a palliative, rather than a curative therapy.

REFERENCES

1 Kantrowitz A, Haller JD, Joos H, Cerruti MM, Carstensen HE. Transplantation of the heart in an infant and an adult. *Am J Cardiol* 1968;**22**:782–90.

2 Cooley DA, Bloodwell RD, Hallman GL, *et al*. Organ transplantation for advanced cardiopulmonary disease. *Ann Thorac Surg* 1969;**8**:30–46.

3 Carrel A, Guthrie CC. The transplantation of veins and organs. *Am J Med* 1905;**11**:1101–2.

4 Mann FC, Priestley JT, Markowitz J, Yates YM. Transplantation of the intact mammalian heart. *Arch Surg* 1933;**26**:219–24.

5 Lansman SL, Ergin MA, Griepp RB. The history of heart and heart-lung transplantation. In: Thompson ME, ed. *Cardiac Transplantation: Cardiovascular Clinics*, F.A. Davis, 1990: 1–19.

6 Neptune WB, Cookson BA, Bailey CP, *et al*. Complete homologous heart transplantation. *Arch Surg* 1953;**66**:174.

7 Webb WR, Howard HS. Restoration of function of the refrigerated heart. *Surg Forum* 1957;**8**:302.

8 Webb WR, Howard HS. Cardiopulmonary transplantation. *Surg Forum* 1957;**8**:313.

9 Goldberg M, Berman EF, Akman LC. Homologous transplantation of the canine heart. *J Intern Coll Cardiol* 1958;**30**:575.

10 Webb WR, Howard HS, Neely WA. Practical methods of homologous cardiac transplantation. *J Thorac Surg* 1959;**37**:361.

11 Lower RR, Shumway NE. Studies on orthotopic homotransplantation of the canine heart. *Surg Forum* 1960;**11**:18–25.

12 Kondo Y, Gradel F, Kantrowiyz A. Homotransplantation of the heart in puppies under profound hypothermia· long survival without immunosuppressive treatment. *Ann Surg* 1965; **162**: 837.

13 Lower RR, Dong E Jr, Shumway ME. Long-term survival of cardiac homografts. *Surgery* 1965;**58**:110.

14 Brent L. *A History of Transplantation Immunology*. Academic Press, 1997: 306–24.

15 Hardy JD, Chavez CM, Kurrus FD, *et al*. Heart transplantation in man: developmental studies and report of a case. *JAMA* 1964;**188**:1132–40.

16 Michler RE, Chen JM. Cardiac xenotransplantation: experimental advances, ethical issues, and clinical potential. In: Emery RW, Miller LW, eds. *Handbook of Cardiac Transplantation*. Mosby, 1996: 231–46.

17 Bernard CN. The operation. A human cardiac transplant: an interim report of a successful operation performed at Groote Schuur Hospital, Cape Town. *S Afr Med J* 1967;**41**:1271–4.

18 Griepp RB. A decade of human heart transplantation. *Transplant Proc* 1979;**11**:285.

19 Baum D, Kaye MP, Miller WW. Pediatric heart, heart-lung, and lung transplantation: historical perspective. *Prog Pediatr Cardiol* 1993;**2**:1–3.

20 Shumway N. The development of heart and heart-lung transplantation at Stanford. *Eur J Cardiothorac Surg* 1993;**7**:5–7.

21 Watson DC, Reitz BA, Baumgartner WA, *et al*. Distant heart procurement for transplantation. *Surgery* 1979;**86**:56.

22 Caves PK, Stinson EB, Billingham ME, Rider AK, Shumway NE. Diagnosis of human cardiac allograft rejection by serial cardiac biopsy. *J Thorac Cardiovasc Surg* 1973;**66**:461–6.

23 Bieber CP, Griepp RB, Oyer PE, *et al*. Use of rabbit antithymocyte globulin in cardiac transplantation. *Transplantation* 1976;**22**:478.

24 Report of the Ad Hoc Committee of the Harvard Medical School to examine the definition of brain death: a definition of irreversible coma. *JAMA* 1968;**205**:337–40.

25 Black PM. Brain death. *N Engl J Med* 1978;**299**:338.

26 Oyer PE, Stinson EB, Jamieson SW, *et al*. Cyclosporine in cardiac transplantation: A 2 1/2 year follow up. *Transplant Proc* 1983; **15**:2546–52.

27 Grattan MT, Moreno-Cobral CE, Starnes VA, *et al*. Eight-year results of cyclosporine-treated patients with cardiac transplants. *J Thorac Cardiovasc Surg* 1990;**90**:500–9.

28 Bailey LL, Li Z, Lacour-Gayet F, *et al*. Orthotopic cardiac xenotransplantation in the cyclosporine-treated neonate. *Transplant Proc* 1983;**15**(Suppl 1):2956–9.

29 Bailey LL, Jang J, Johnson W, Jolley WB. Orthotopic cardiac xenografting in the newborn goat. *J Thoracic Cardiovasc Surg* 1985;**89**:242–7.

30 Bailey LL, Nehlsen-Cannarella SL, Conception W, Jolley WB. Baboon to human cardiac xenotransplantation in a neonate. *JAMA* 1985;**254**:3321–9.

31 Bailey LL, Nehlsen-Cannarella SL, Doroshow RW, *et al*. Cardiac allotransplantation in newborns as therapy for hypoplastic left heart syndrome. *N Engl J Med* 1986;**315**:949–51.

32 Norwood WI, Lang P, Hansen D. Physiologic repair of aortic atresia-hypoplastic left heart syndrome. *N Engl J Med* 1983;**308**:23–6.

33 Boucek M, Novick R, Bennett L, *et al*. The Registry of the International Society of Heart and Lung Transplantation: second official pediatric report, 1998. *J Heart Lung Transplant* 1998;**17**:1141–60.

34 Trento A, Griffith BP, Fricker FJ, *et al*. Lessons learned in pediatric heart transplantation. *Ann Thorac Surg* 1989;**48**:617–23.

35 Webber SA, Fricker FJ, Michael M, *et al*. Orthotopic heart transplantation in children with congenital heart disease. *Ann Thorac Surg* 1994;**58**:1664–9.

36 Michaels MG, Frader J, Armitage J. Ethical considerations in listing fetuses as candidates for neonatal heart transplantation. *JAMA* 1993;**269**:401–3.

37 Del Nido PJ Armitage JM, Fricker FJ, *et al*. Extracorporeal membrane oxygenation support as a bridge to pediatric heart transplantion. *Circulation* 1994,**90**(Part 2):66–9.

38 Ubel PA, Arnold RM, Caplan AL. Rationing failure: the ethical lessons of the retransplantation of scarce vital organs. *JAMA* 1993;**270**:2469–74.

39 Webber SA, Pham Si, Zeevi A, *et al.* A clinical trial of intrathymic inoculation of donor bone marrow cells with concomitant pediatric heart transplantation: preliminary observations (Abstract). *Transplantation* 1999;**67**:S33.

40 West LJ, Pollock-Barziv SM, Dipchand AI, *et al.* ABO-incompatible heart transplantation in infants. *N Engl J Med* 2001;**344**:793–800.

30 Recipient Characteristics

Charles E. Canter and David C. Naftel

The Registry of the International Society for Heart and Lung Transplantation (ISHLT) [1] has recorded a steady range of 347–386 annual pediatric (ages newborn to 18 years) heart transplantations performed around the world over the past decade. This volume is approximately 10% of the total cardiac transplants recorded in the database over this time period [2]. Pediatric cardiac transplant recipients come to transplantation for intractable symptoms associated with cardiomyopathies or structural congenital heart anomalies. Previous consensus reports [3–5] have published criteria that are acceptable reasons to pursue cardiac transplantation in children. These guidelines can be summarized as follows:

• Progressive heart failure, deterioration of ventricular function or functional status despite optimal medical care with digitalis, diuretics and angiotensin-converting enzyme (ACE) inhibitors. Experience with beta-blocker therapy for heart failure with systolic dysfunction in children is accumulating, with reports of favorable efficacy [6–8]. Its use has been associated with sufficient palliation to remove patients from listing for transplantation [8]. Resynchronization therapy in children with biventricular or multisite pacing remains a promising investigational therapy [9,10].
• Need for ongoing intravenous inotropic or mechanical circulatory support.

• Complex congenital heart disease unamenable to conventional surgical repair or palliation or where the surgical procedure carries a higher risk of mortality than transplantation.
• Malignant arrhythmia unresponsive to medical treatment, catheter ablation or an automatic implantable defibrillator.
• Progressive pulmonary hypertension that could preclude cardiac transplantation at a later date.
• Growth failure secondary to cardiac disease.

This chapter focuses on the demographics, cardiac disease etiology and severity of illness in pediatric recipients using data from the registry of the ISHLT and from the Pediatric Heart Transplant Study Group (PHTSG) database, focusing on the changes in recipient characteristics that have occurred over the decade. The PHTSG is a North American multi-institutional group, which has collected data since 1993. In that time its database includes 40% of the pediatric heart transplant recipients within the ISHLT database and currently includes 1645 subjects who have undergone heart transplantation.

DEMOGRAPHICS

Figure 30.1 illustrates the age distribution of pediatric heart transplant recipients within the ISHLT database [1]. In the

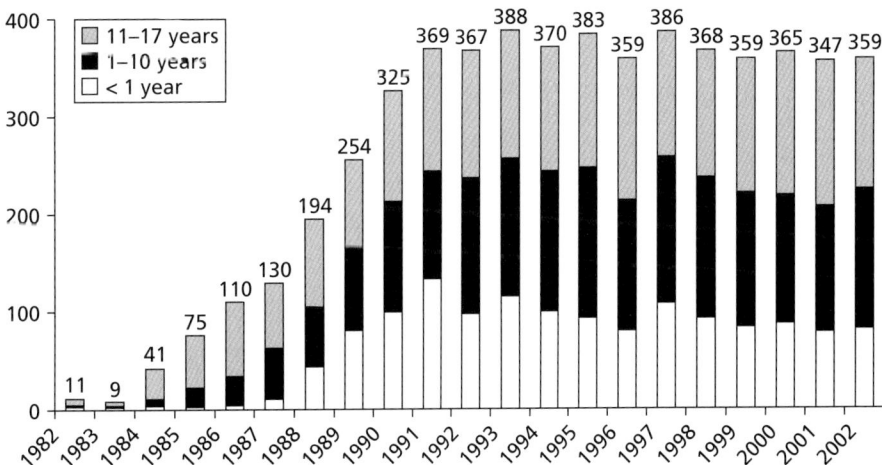

Fig. 30.1 Age distribution of pediatric heart recipients by year of transplant in the International Society for Heart and Lung Transplantation (ISHLT) database [1].

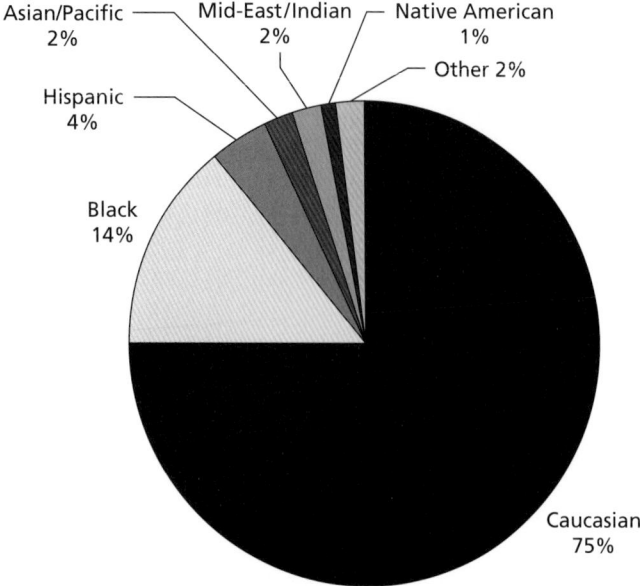

Fig. 30.2 Distribution of ethnicity within the Pediatric Heart Transplant Study Group database 1993–2003.

past 10 years, infants (newborn to 12 months of age) have comprised approximately 20–25% of the transplants performed each year. The remaining transplants have generally been split between older children (1–10 years of age) and adolescents (11–17 years of age). Within the PHTSG database, infant recipients compose approximately 39%, with children aged 1–12 years making up 35% of the total and adolescents (over 12 years) composing 24% of the group. These percentages have remained substantially unchanged over the course of the entire 11 years (1993–2003) that the PHTSG has collected data.

Within the PHTSG, 58% of the recipients have been male and 42% have been female. Figure 30.2 gives the ethnicity breakdown of pediatric heart transplant recipients within the PHTSG. Caucasians make up 75% of the total; followed by blacks at 14%; Hispanics at 4%; Asian/Pacific at 3%; Middle-Eastern/Indian at 1.8%; and Native American at 0.6%.

ETIOLOGY OF CARDIAC DISEASE

Cardiomyopathies and structural congenital heart disease comprise the two primary diagnostic groups of pediatric heart transplant recipients. ISHLT registry data [1] have demonstrated that the diagnosis of cardiomyopathy is responsible for approximately 75% of adolescent pediatric heart transplant recipients (Fig. 30.3); 50% of the diagnoses between 1 and 10 years of age (Fig. 30.4); and only 25% of infant recipients (Fig. 30.5). Recently, ISHLT data have suggested that the proportion of infants transplanted for cardiomyopathies in the last 4 years has substantially increased from over 25% to 35–40%.

Cardiomyopathies account for 42% of the diagnoses of the pediatric heart transplant recipients in the PHTSG. Figure 30.6 illustrates that dilated cardiomyopathies comprised 76% of the cardiomyopathy diagnoses within the PHTSG; restrictive cardiomyopathy 12%; myocarditis 8%; and hypertrophic cardiomyopathies 5%. The etiology of the dilated cardiomyopathy was anthracycline toxicity in 18 patients, indicating that selected pediatric patients with a past history of neoplasm have undergone heart transplantation. The diagnosis of restrictive cardiomyopathy is disproportionately represented in these transplant recipients compared to general prevalence of pediatric restrictive cardiomyopathy [11,12]. This discrepancy likely reflects the lack of efficacy of conventional medical management for this condition and the progressive rise in pulmonary vascular resistance that is frequently observed [13–15].

Figures 30.3 and 30.4 also illustrate the increasing number of cardiac retransplantations that have been performed in the pediatric age group. The percentage of patients aged 1–17 years who underwent cardiac retransplantation in the ISHLT database doubled in the era 1996–2003 compared to the 1988–95 era.

Congenital heart disease, mainly hypoplastic left heart syndrome, has been the predominant diagnosis in infants undergoing cardiac transplantation. Transplantation for congenital

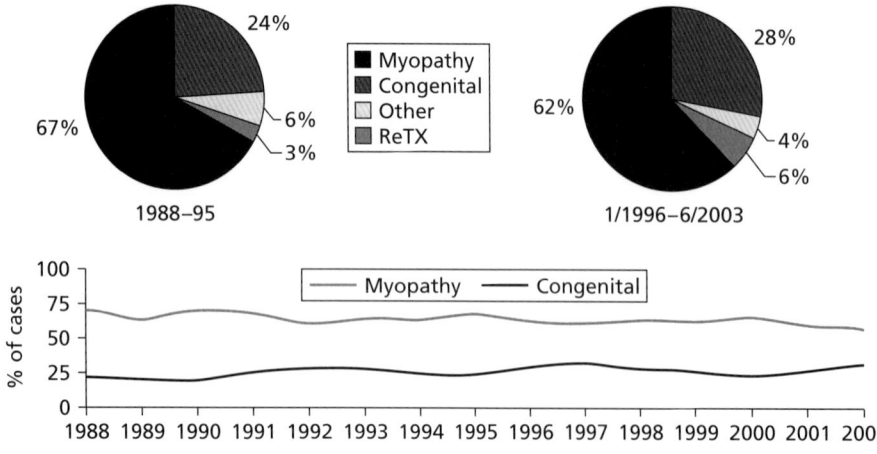

Fig. 30.3 Diagnoses for pediatric heart transplant recipients 11–17 years of age in the International Society for Heart and Lung Transplantation (ISHLT) database [1]. ReTX, retransplants.

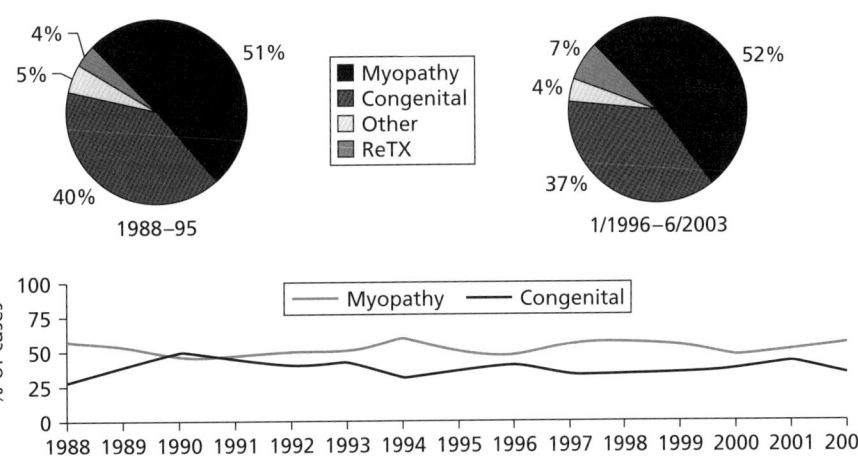

Fig. 30.4 Diagnoses for pediatric heart transplant recipients 1–10 years of age from the International Society for Heart and Lung Transplantation (ISHLT) database [1]. ReTX, retransplants.

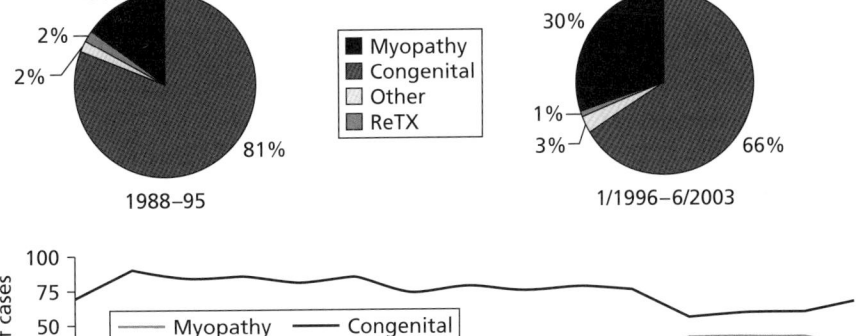

Fig. 30.5 Diagnoses for pediatric heart transplant recipients less than 1 year of age in the International Society for Heart and Lung Transplantation (ISHLT) database [1]. ReTX, retransplants.

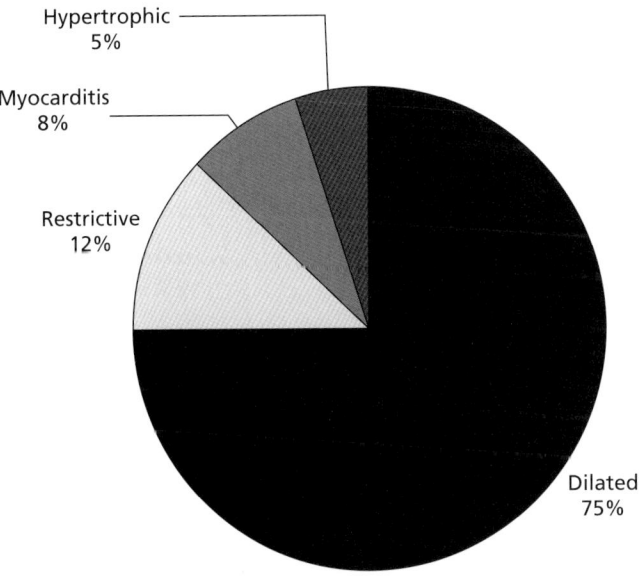

Fig. 30.6 Distribution of cardiomyopathy subtypes within the Pediatric Heart Transplant Study Group (PHTSG) recipients transplanted with a diagnosis of cardiomyopathy.

heart disease in infants is generally utilized as primary therapy, whereas in older children and adolescents transplantation is utilized as therapy after initial repairs or palliative procedures, especially in single ventricle patients undergoing Fontan palliations [16]. Single ventricle lesions, transposition of the great vessels and lesions requiring right outflow tract reconstruction are the most common lesions in patients who undergo cardiac transplantation for congenital heart disease (Fig. 30.7) [17]. Within the ISHLT database, congenital heart disease in the recent era (1996–2003; see Fig. 30.5) makes up a substantially smaller proportion of infant diagnoses when compared to the older era (1988–95). This phenomenon likely reflects a decreased utilization of transplantation as primary therapy for hypoplastic left heart syndrome with the improvement in outcomes with staged palliative surgery [18,19].

A trend to decreased utilization of transplantation for hypoplastic left heart syndrome has been noted within the PHTSG [20]. In the years 1993–95, hypoplastic left heart syndrome without previous surgery comprised approximately one-quarter of the patients listed for transplantation within the PHTSG database. This percentage dropped to 17% in the years 1996–98.

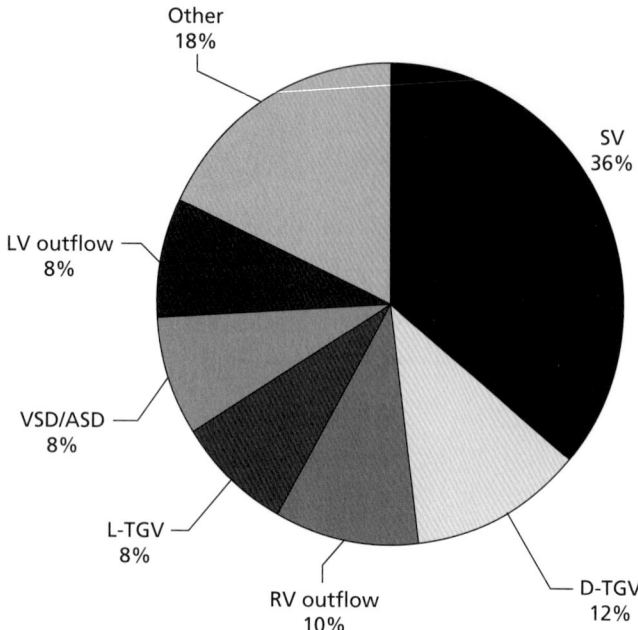

Fig. 30.7 Distribution of congenital heart lesions in patients greater than 6 months of age in the Pediatric Heart Transplant Study Group (PHTSG)/Cardiac Transplant Research Database (CTRD) database transplanted for congenital heart disease [17]. ASD, atrial septal defect; D-TGV, D-transposition of the great vessels; L-TGV, L-transposition of the great vessels; LV outflow, lesions with anomalies of left ventricular outflow; RV outflow, lesions with anomalies of right ventricular outflow; SV, single ventricle lesions; VSD, ventricular septal defect.

Cardiac transplantation is also utilized in patients with hypoplastic left heart syndrome who are failing after palliative surgery. Within the PHTSG, hypoplastic left heart syndrome with previous palliative surgery was the diagnosis in 5.3% of the patients listed for transplantation from 1993 to 1998 [20]. Patients with single ventricle lesions who have had previous Fontan or cavopulmonary anastomosis palliation have comprised approximately 5% of the transplanted patients within the PHTSG database [21,22]. When comparing an

earlier era (1993–97) [21] to a later era (1998–2001) [22] in the PHTSG, the number of patients listed for transplant with previous Fontan palliation and ultimately undergoing transplant has increased by 20–25%.

SEVERITY OF ILLNESS

Prior to 1999, pediatric heart transplant recipients in the USA were listed by the United Network for Organ Sharing (UNOS) as Status 1 (less than 6 months of age and/or in an intensive care unit on inotropic support) and Status 2 (everyone else). In 1999, Status 1 was subdivided into Status 1A and 1B [23] with Status 1A patients being the most severe, generally requiring mechanical support, artificial ventilation or high dose or multiple intravenous inotropic agents. Within the PHTSG database (Fig. 30.8), the average annual percentage of patients transplanted at UNOS Status 2 from 1993–98 was 27%. During the last 5 years (1999–2003) this has decreased to 16%. In 2002 and 2003, the percentage of PHTSG patients transplanted as Status 1A was 65% and 72%, respectively, compared to an average annual percentage of 57% from 1999 to 2001.

Figure 30.9 demonstrates the annual number of PHTSG patients who were transplanted while on extracorporeal membrane oxygenators (ECMO) or ventricular assist device (VAD) support prior to transplantation. Over the past 4 years (2000–03), the annual percentage of patients in the PHTSG transplanted from ECMO support has been 10% and from VAD support 6.5%. These figures represent a substantial increase compared to the 1993–99 figures, when the annual percentage of patients transplanted from ECMO support was 4.6% and from VAD support 3.6%.

SPECIAL POPULATIONS

The PHTSG database suggests that few pediatric patients are transplanted with a history of diabetes (5/1645); hepatitis (3/1645); or HIV infection (2/1645). Eighteen patients have

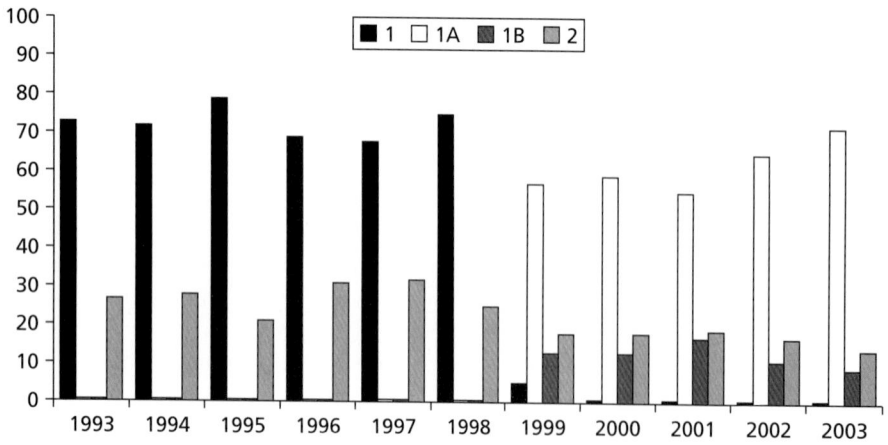

Fig. 30.8 Distribution of United Network for Organ Sharing (UNOS) listing status for pediatric heart transplant recipients within the Pediatric Heart Transplant Study Group (PHTSG).

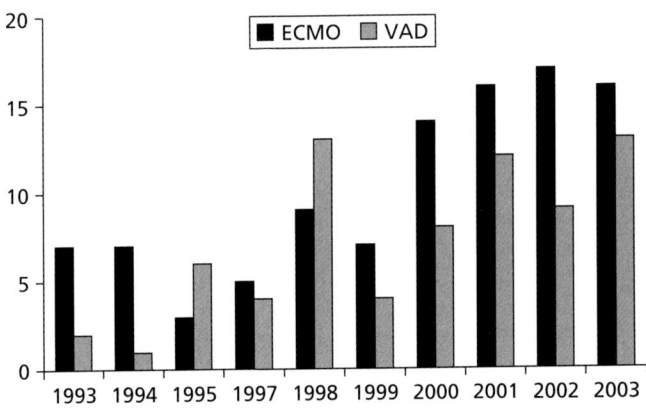

Fig. 30.9 Number of pediatric heart transplant recipients per year of transplantation undergoing transplantation while on extracorporeal membrane oxygenator (ECMO) or ventricular assist device (VAD) support in the Pediatric Heart Transplant Study Group (PHTSG) database.

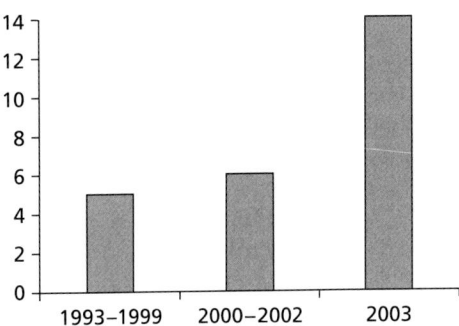

Fig. 30.10 Number of ABO-incompatible transplants performed within the Pediatric Heart Transplant Study Group (PHTSG) database.

been transplanted as a result of anthracycline toxicity from therapy for various neoplasms. Obesity at the time of listing or transplantation is a rare event among the pediatric patients in this database [24].

The presence of preformed antibodies to different HLA antigens in heart transplant recipients has traditionally been assessed by panel reactive antibody (PRA) screens. High PRA values (greater than 10%) have been associated with poor outcomes after transplantation [25,26]. Numerous strategies including prospective cross-matching, plasmapharesis and intravenous immunoglobulin have been utilized in this population, which is increasing in adult transplant recipients because of increasing utilization of VADs [27].

Aside from VADs, pediatric heart transplant candidates who have had previous congenital heart surgery using human homograft material will also develop high PRA values [28]. Within the PHTSG database, 8% of the patients with measured PRA values who were transplant recipients had PRA values of greater than 10% [29]. These high PRA values were significantly associated with patients with previous surgical palliation for hypoplastic left heart syndrome, with history of multiple sternotomies or with prior Fontan palliation.

Recent data [30,31] have suggested that cardiac transplantation with donor–recipient ABO incompatibility can be successfully performed in infants with the development of donor-specific B-cell tolerance. ABO-incompatible transplantation may offer an expansion of the donor pool for infant recipients. PHTSG data (Fig. 30.10) demonstrate a substantial increase in numbers of recipients transplanted with an ABO-incompatible donor. From 1993 to 1999 there were only five ABO-incompatible transplants performed. There were six performed between 2000 and 2002 and 14 performed in 2003.

CONCLUSIONS

Heart transplantation continues to be used for intractable cardiac failure from birth through adolescence. While the use of cardiac transplantation as primary therapy for hypoplastic left heart syndrome is decreasing, an increasing number of infants with cardiomyopathies are undergoing transplantation. Transplantation remains the final therapeutic option for pediatric patients deteriorating after congenital heart surgery, especially for patients born with a single ventricle. PHTSG data would suggest the severity of illness in pediatric heart transplant recipients is increasing at time of transplantation, and increasing numbers of pediatric patients are coming to transplant on ECMO or VAD mechanical circulatory support. Pediatric patients are being transplanted despite presensitization to multiple HLA antigens, and increasing experience is being obtained with ABO-incompatible heart transplantation in infants.

REFERENCES

1 Boucek MM, Edwards LB, Keck BM, et al. Registry for the International Society for Heart and Lung Transplantation: seventh official pediatric report, 2004. *J Heart Lung Transplant* 2004;**23**:933–47.
2 Trulock EP, Edwards LB, Taylor DO, et al. The Registry for the International Society for Heart and Lung Transplantation: twenty-first official adult heart transplant report. *J Heart Lung Transplant* 2004;**23**:804–15.
3 Mudge GH, Goldstein S, Addonizio LJ, et al. Task Force 3: recipient guidelines/prioritization. 24th Bethesda conference on cardiac transplantation. *J Am Coll Cardiol* 1993;**22**:21–31.
4 Costanzo MR, Augustine S, Bourge R, et al. Selection and treatment of candidates for heart transplantation. *Circulation* 1995;**92**:3593–612.
5 Fricker FJ, Addonizio L, Bernstein D, et al. Heart transplantation in children: indications. *Pediatr Transplant* 1999;**3**:333–42.

6 Shaddy RE, Tani LY, Gidding SS, et al. Beta-blocker treatment of dilated cardiomyopathy with congestive heart failure in children: a multi-institutional experience. *J Heart Lung Transplant* 1999;18:269–74.

7 Bruns LA, Kichuk Chrisant M, Lamour JM, et al. Carvedilol as therapy in pediatric heart failure: an initial multicenter experience. *J Pediatr* 2001;138:505–11.

8 Pohwani AL, Murali S, Mathier MM, et al. Impact of beta-blocker therapy on functional capacity criteria for heart transplant listing. *J Heart Lung Transplant* 2003;22:78–86.

9 Streiper M, Karpawich P, Frias P, et al. Initial experience with cardiac resynchronization therapy for ventricular dysfunction in young patients with surgically operated congenital heart disease. *Am J Cardiol* 2004;94:1352–4.

10 Rhee EK, Singh GK, Huddleston CB, Canter CE. Cardiac resynchronization therapy for moderate-to-severe pediatric heart failure: a pilot study (Abstract). *Circulation* 2004;110(Suppl 3):480.

11 Lipshultz SE, Sleeper LA, Towbin JA, et al. The incidence of pediatric cardiomyopathy in two regions of the United States. *N Engl J Med* 2003;348:1647–55.

12 Nugent AW, Daubeney PEF, Chondros P, et al. The epidemiology of childhood cardiomyopathy in Australia. *N Engl J Med* 2003;348:1639–46.

13 Cetta F, O'Leary P, Seward J, Driscoll D. Idiopathic restrictive cardiomyopathy in childhood: diagnostic features and clinical course. *Mayo Clin Proc* 1995;70:634–40.

14 Gewillig M, Mertens L, Moerman P, Dumoulin M. Idiopathic restrictive cardiomyopathy in childhood. *Eur Heart J* 1996;17:1413–20.

15 Rivenes SM, Kearney DL, Smith EO, Towbin JA, Denfield SW. Sudden death and cardiovascular collapse in children with restrictive cardiomyopathy. *Circulation* 2000;102:876–82.

16 Chen JM, Davies RR, Mital SR, et al. Trends and outcomes in transplantation for complex congenital heart disease: 1984–2004. *Ann Thorac Surg* 2004;78:1352–61.

17 Lamour JL, Kanter KR, Naftel DC, et al. The effect of age, diagnosis and previous surgery in 488 children and adults who undergo heart transplantation for congenital heart disease (Abstract). *J Am Coll Cardiol* 2005;45:322A.

18 Tweddell JS, Hoffman GM, Mussatto KA, et al. Improved survival of patients undergoing palliation of hypoplastic left heart syndrome: lessons learned from 115 consecutive patients. *Circulation* 2002;106(Suppl I):82–9.

19 Pizzaro C, Mroczek T, Malec E, Norwood WI. Right ventricle to pulmonary artery conduit reduces interim mortality after Stage 1

Norwood for hypoplastic left heart syndrome. *Ann Thorac Surg* 2004;78:1959–64.

20 Kichuk-Chrisant MR, Naftel D, Drummond-Webb J, et al. Fate of infants with hypoplastic left heart syndrome listed for cardiac transplant: a multi-center study (Abstract). *Circulation* 1999;100(Suppl I):99.

21 Bernstein D, Naftel DT, Hsu DT, et al. Outcome of listing for cardiac transplantation for failed Fontan: a multi-institutional study (Abstract). *J Heart Lung Transplant* 1999;18:69.

22 Bernstein D, Naftel D, Chin C, et al. Outcome of listing for cardiac transplantation (tx) for failed Fontan: a follow-up multi-institutional study (Abstract). *J Heart Lung Transplant* 2004;23:S162.

23 Van Meter CH, Heiney DA. Modifications to and implementation of UNOS policy 3.7 (Allocations of thoracic organs). UNOS policy communication. United Network for Organ Sharing, PO Box 13770, Richmond VA, December, 1998.

24 Ibrahim J, Canter CE, Chinnock RE, et al. Linear and somatic growth following pediatric heart transplantation (Abstract). *J Heart Lung Transplant* 2002;21:63.

25 Kobashigawa JA, Sabad A, Drinkwater D, et al. Pretransplant panel reactive-antibody screens: are they truly a marker for poor outcome after cardiac transplantation? *Circulation* 1996;94:II294–7.

26 Thompson JS, Thacker LR II, Takemoto S. The influence of conventional and cross-reactive group HLA matching on cardiac transplant outcome: an analysis from the United Network of Organ Sharing Scientific Registry. *Transplantation* 2000;69:2178–86.

27 Mehra M, Uber PA, Uber WE, Scott RL, Park MH. Allosensitization in heart transplantation: implications and management strategies. *Curr Opin Cardiol* 2003;18:153–8.

28 Hawkins JA, Hillman ND, Lambert LM, et al. Immunogenicity of decellularized cryopreserved allografts in pediatric cardiac surgery: comparison with standard cryopreserved allografts. *J Thorac Cardiovasc Surg* 2002;126:247–53.

29 Mahle WT, Naftel DC, Rusconi P, Edens RE, Shaddy RE. Panel-reactive antibody cross-reactivity and outcomes in the Pediatric Heart Transplant Study Group (Abstract). *J Heart Lung Transplant* 2004;23:S167.

30 West LJ, Pollock-BarZiv SM, Dipchand AI, et al. ABO-incompatible heart transplantation in infants. *N Engl J Med* 2001;344:793–800.

31 Fan X, Ang A, Pollock-BarZiv SM, et al. Donor-specific B-cell tolerance after ABO-incompatible infant heart transplantation. *Nat Med* 2004;10:1227–33.

31 Evaluation of the Candidate

Gerard J. Boyle

The success of heart transplantation surgery is dependent, perhaps above all else, upon a complete and thorough evaluation of the potential candidate [1]. The establishment of a center-specific "evaluation protocol" will identify some patients for whom alternative palliation may be more appropriate and others for whom transplantation is not a viable option. The evaluation of a candidate for heart transplantation must include assessment of long-term survival without transplantation, the patient's current quality of life, the possibility of further surgical or medical palliation and the inherent risks of the transplant surgery itself. A complete evaluation requires a multidisciplinary approach to assure the best outcome for the patient, as well as the most appropriate use of scarce donor organs (Table 31.1). In addition to the obvious need for evaluation by a pediatric cardiologist and cardiothoracic surgeon, evaluation of the candidate for heart transplantation must include a team approach including an infectious disease specialist, a psychiatrist/child psychologist, a transplant coordinator and a social worker. Complete evaluation is individualized according to the presentation and clinical status of each patient. For the newborn or young infant candidate, the involvement of a geneticist, neonatologist and metabolic disease specialist may be necessary. Individual candidates, usually outside the infant age group, may also benefit from a pretransplant evaluation by other services such as dentistry, nephrology, immunology, hematology-oncology and neurology. Increasingly, a genetic evaluation may contribute to the understanding of the candidate's suitability for transplantation and the possibility of their passing on an inheritable cardiac defect or myopathy. Patients who have experienced a prolonged period of debilitation prior to transplantation may derive benefit from the involvement of a nutritionist, physical and occupational therapist and child life specialist. Infants with congestive heart failure may require the services of a feeding specialist both before and after transplantation. It should also be noted that the transplant evaluation procedure is a "two-way process' " and that a key purpose of this process is for the family to evaluate the transplant center. Patient and family education forms a central part of the evaluation and is designed to allow the family to decide whether they wish to pursue transplantation as an option for their child.

ANATOMIC AND HEMODYNAMIC CONSIDERATIONS

The pretransplant evaluation by the pediatric cardiologist and surgeon must necessarily focus on elucidating the complete anatomy and physiology of the heart condition. Routine evaluation will include complete review of medical and surgical records along with basic cardiac studies such as a chest radiograph, echocardiogram, electrocardiogram and cardiac catheterization. Maximal exercise stress testing is helpful in many cases to obtain an objective measure of exercise performance [2]. This should be avoided, however, in patients with exercise-induced arrhythmias or syncope. In these cases, a 6-minute walk test can provide valuable and reproducible objective data [3,4]. Computed tomography of the chest, ventilation/perfusion scan, multiple gated acquisition (MUGA) scan, and magnetic resonance imaging are not routinely required but may be useful in certain cases where the complete anatomy and physiology cannot be determined by the routine studies outlined above.

Current surgical techniques have allowed patients with the most complex native and surgical cardiovascular anatomy to be transplanted [5–12]. Anatomic points of most interest to the surgeon include abnormalities of cardiac and visceral situs and associated anomalies of the systemic and pulmonary venous return [5,8,12]. Intracardiac anatomy is less important because the bulk of the cardiac mass will be explanted. Abnormalities in the relation of the great arteries usually pose few problems [5,6,9,10] but should be noted during the evaluation, as procurement of extended lengths of donor artery may facilitate reconstruction. The size and anatomy of the main and branch pulmonary arteries, including the presence of stenoses, distortions and nonconfluence, are of key importance to the success of heart transplantation [5–8,10,11]. Attention must also be given to the spatial relationship of vital cardiac structures to the sternum. After

Table 31.1 Evaluation of candidates for heart transplantation.

History and physical examination

Required consultations:
  Pediatric cardiologist
  Cardiovascular surgeon
  Cardiac anesthesiology
  Infectious disease specialist
  Psychiatrist or psychologist
  Transplant coordinator
  Transplant social worker

Additional consultations (as required), e.g. neonatology, genetics, neurology, dental, oncology, immunology, nephrology, nutritional services, physical/occupational therapy, developmental pediatrics, hospital financial consultant

Cardiac diagnostic studies:
  Chest radiograph
  Electrocardiogram
  Echocardiogram
  Cardiac catheterization
  Exercise test
  MUGA scan, ventilation/perfusion scan, chest CT or MRI (selected patients only)

Pulmonary function tests

Blood type (ABO), anti-HLA antibody screen, HLA typing,* complete blood count and white cell differential, platelet count, coagulation screen, blood urea nitrogen, serum creatinine, glucose, calcium, magnesium, liver function tests, lipid profile, brain natriuretic peptide

Serologic screening for antibodies to the following viruses: cytomegalovirus, Epstein–Barr, herpes simplex, human immunodeficiency, varicella, hepatitis A, B, C, D and measles; antibodies to *Toxoplasma gondii*

PPD/Mantoux placement

Update immunizations including hepatitis B, pneumoccocal and influenza (in season)

CT, computed tomography; HLA, human leukocyte antigen; MRI, magnetic resonance imaging; MUGA, multiple gated acquisition (scan); PPD, purified protein derivitive.
* HLA typing not routinely required prior to transplantation as donor–recipient HLA matching not routinely performed for thoracic transplantation.

multiple prior sternotomies for palliation of complex congenital heart disease, key structures such as right ventricular–pulmonary artery conduits or giant right atria (after Fontan procedure) may be adherent to the posterior aspect of the sternum. This can lead to inadvertent damage to a vital structure at the time of transplant. Computed tomography and magnetic resonance imaging are well suited to delineating these spatial arrangements.

Perhaps more important than anatomic considerations is the pretransplantation pulmonary vascular resistance [13–20]. Excessive fixed resistance will result in acute donor right ventricular failure and an inability to wean the patient from cardiopulmonary bypass. With this in mind, cardiac catheterization should be performed on all transplant candidates outside the neonatal period to determine the transpulmonary gradient, cardiac output and pulmonary vascular resistance.

The transpulmonary gradient (TPG) (in mmHg) is determined by subtracting the left atrial pressure (measured directly or inferred from the pulmonary capillary wedge pressure) from the pulmonary artery mean pressure. The pulmonary vascular resistance can then be calculated by dividing the TPG by the cardiac output. The resultant value is expressed in Wood units [13]. To make this value more relevant to the pediatric population, the TPG is divided by the cardiac output indexed to body surface area (BSA) and is expressed as the indexed pulmonary vascular resistance (PVRI) [13]. While elevated pulmonary vascular resistance is a recognized risk factor for increased early mortality after transplantation, children have survived heart transplantation at higher TPG and PVRI than their adult counterparts [17]. Adults with TPG $\geq$ 15 mmHg or PVR $\geq$ 5 Wood units are often considered unacceptable candidates for orthotopic heart transplantation [14]. When a child's baseline PVRI is elevated beyond these stated limits at the time of cardiac catheterization, they may still be considered for, and survive, transplant surgery if the pulmonary resistance exhibits reactivity to ventilatory and pharmacologic manipulation [13,16,17]. In cases where the PVRI exhibits reactivity, children have been considered acceptable candidates even with a TPG ≥ 15 mmHg when the PVRI is ≤ 10 indexed units [16–18]. Children with known or suspected elevation in PVRI should therefore have their airway secured via endotracheal intubation and be mechanically ventilated for the catheterization procedure. If high resistance is confirmed under baseline conditions, the patient should then be studied under conditions of hyperoxia ($FiO_2 = 1.00$) and hypocarbia ($PaCO_2 < 25–30$ mmHg). Either concurrently, or following these manipulations, the use of intravenous inotropes and vasodilators may help determine the reactivity of the pulmonary vascular bed [13,16,20]. Inhaled nitric oxide (up to 80 PPM) has also been used to help predict which patients may safely undergo heart transplantation [19]. Pediatric patients in whom the PVRI can be lowered to ≤ 10 indexed units, using the above approaches, are considered candidates for orthotopic heart transplantation at many experienced transplant centers [13,16,17,20].

LABORATORY INVESTIGATIONS

Careful pre-evaluation screening is important to ensure that all required pretransplant blood work is performed with one phlebotomy where practical. Blood typing is necessary to assure ABO compatibility with the transplanted organ. All patients, especially those with a history of previous blood transfusion or organ transplantation, should be tested for the presence of circulating preformed antibodies against human leukocyte antigens (HLA) [21,22]. The standard test for screening for pretransplantation humoral sensitization is a lymphocytotoxicity assay, the panel reactive antibody test (PRA). An elevated PRA (> 10%), after the addition of dithiothreitol to remove immunoglobulin M (IgM) antibodies, indicates recipient sensitization with IgG antibodies. Newer techniques for evaluation of anti-HLA antibodies appear more sensitive than PRA and include enzyme-linked immunosorbent assay (ELISA) and other HLA antigen-specific solid phase assays (see Chapter 4). In a sensitized patient, transplantation is most safely performed after a negative prospective cross-match between donor and recipient has been established. Routine HLA typing is not required at the time of evaluation in the non-sensitized patient because attempts to match donor and recipient for HLA class I or II antigens are impractical and are rarely performed in thoracic transplantation. Tissue typing is generally performed on the day of transplantation at the time of the retrospective donor-specific cross-match. For patients with an elevated PRA, full HLA typing should be performed at the time of evaluation. Knowledge of donor (when available) and recipient HLA typing, along with knowledge of unacceptable donor antigens, may allow for selection of suitable donor organs for the sensitized candidate when prospective cross-matching is not feasible. The involvement of a transplant immunologist or tissue typing specialist is strongly encouraged in the presence of preformed anti-HLA antibodies.

Other recommended laboratory studies are listed in Table 31.1. In addition to a complete blood count, electrolytes, liver and kidney function studies, a prothrombin time/partial thromboplastin time (PT/PTT) should be obtained. The determination of the brain natriuretic peptide (BNP) level has become a useful tool in stratifying the degree of congestive heart failure of the patient and thereby the urgency of a patient's candidacy [23]. The serologic studies to screen for prior infectious disease exposure and immunization efficacy should be performed at this time as well (see below).

INFECTIOUS DISEASE EVALUATION

Prior to transplantation, an infectious disease evaluation is important to identify infectious contraindications to transplantation, for reviewing immunization histories and in planning any special perioperative prophylaxis. In addition, it affords the family an opportunity to ask infectious disease related questions. Serologic testing for cytomegalovirus (CMV), Epstein–Barr virus (EBV) infection, varicella, herpes simplex virus, *Toxoplasma gondii*, human immunodeficiency virus (HIV), measles and hepatitis viruses A, B, C and D is recommended prior to transplantation. If the actual date of transplantation is more than 3 months after the initial evaluation, previously negative studies are repeated on the day of transplantation. Although CMV matching between donor and recipient is not routinely performed, knowledge of donor and recipient CMV serologic status allows the clinician to anticipate infection frequency and severity, and guides prophylaxis as well as the diagnostic evaluation of fever.

Prior infection with hepatitis C, while not an absolute contraindication to transplantation, presents an increased risk of reactivation of the hepatitis once immunosuppression has been instituted following transplantation [24–27]. Candidates with antibodies to hepatitis C should also have quantitative hepatitis C polymerase chain reaction performed and should be evaluated by a hepatologist. Frequently, severe heart failure results in modest elevations in bilirubin and liver enzymes. This may compound the problems of evaluating the extent of active hepatitis, and liver biopsy may be required in patients who are stable enough to tolerate this procedure.

The infectious disease evaluation should also include review of the immunization history. Those candidates in whom transplantation is not likely to be imminent should undergo an update of appropriate immunizations at the time of the pretransplant evaluation. Most vaccines are more efficacious when administered prior to immunosuppression. This is especially true for hepatitis B and pneumococcal vaccines. The availability of the conjugated pneumococcal vaccine has assisted in protecting children under 2 years of age. Measles–mumps–rubella (MMR) and varicella vaccines should also be administered prior to transplantation because the use of live viral vaccines after transplantation is currently discouraged. In the appropriate season, influenza vaccine should be given prior to transplantation. In addition, influenza vaccination is recommended for all household members to decrease potential exposure to the heart transplant candidate.

PSYCHIATRIC EVALUATION

A screening psychiatric and/or psychological examination of the patient and their family is beneficial to health care professionals and the patient [28]. A primary purpose of this evaluation is to identify patients and families at high risk for poor psychological outcome while waiting for transplantation and while adjusting to life after transplantation. This evaluation has not been shown to predict which patients or families will have difficulty complying with the rigorous post-transplant medication and follow-up regimens; however, issues that may interfere with compliance can be identified [29]. Intervention, where appropriate, can then be instituted prior to transplantation. It should be noted that the primary purpose of the psychiatric evaluation is not to seek to exclude individuals from transplantation, but to identify ways to help patients and families cope with the very stressful process of organ transplantation.

TRANSPLANT COORDINATOR AND SOCIAL SERVICES

The transplant coordinator will have contact with the referring center and family prior to the formal evaluation. This will help ensure that a complete evaluation is performed in an efficient and timely manner. This pre-evaluation planning helps to reduce the stress, physical and emotional, for both patient and family. The same coordinator will usually provide continuity of care during the waiting period prior to transplantation. The experienced coordinator contributes immeasurably to the success of transplantation in any given patient, as well as to the success of the transplant program itself.

Social service involvement is important for patients of any socioeconomic status. The maze of issues relating to insurance coverage, pre- and post-transplant financial commitments, transportation, and day-to-day living arrangements for patients and families, often in an unfamiliar setting, are best handled by the transplant social worker. These professionals also provide great insight into the psychosocial problems that are present, or may develop, in a given family.

EVALUATION OF THE INFANT CANDIDATE

In addition to hemodynamic and surgical considerations, infants present special circumstances and unique problems [30–32]. Lung maturity and pulmonary issues may warrant the early consultation of a pulmonologist. These patients often require the expertise of a neonatologist, working in conjunction with the cardiologist, for their daily management. The input of a geneticist and specialists in metabolic diseases and developmental medicine can often avoid transplantation of an infant with other severely disabling or lethal conditions, such as mitochondrial myopathy.

ONCOLOGIC EVALUATION

Patients who have survived a malignancy, but who present for transplantation after developing a cardiomyopathy, require the clearance of an oncologist. It has been stated that patients who are disease free 1 year after completing their chemotherapy regimen are acceptable transplant candidates [33]. However, this is very dependent on the type of tumor and the response to prior therapy. The input of an oncologist as part of the team evaluating the patient is crucial so that transplantation can be avoided or delayed in patients with high risk of disease recurrence.

SPECIAL CONSIDERATIONS

During the initial evaluation, questions and concerns may arise that call for the involvement of various subspecialists. The patient with end-stage heart failure and poor cardiac output may have borderline renal function on the basis of chronic renal hypoperfusion. Such chronic hypoperfusion can occasionally cause irreversible renal dysfunction and the early involvement of a pediatric nephrologist will be beneficial in these cases. More detailed pretransplant evaluation of renal status includes determination of creatinine clearance by 24-hour urine collection, estimation of glomerular filtration rate by radionuclide techniques and 24-hour urinary protein estimation in patients with proteinuria. Post-transplantation, improved cardiac output will improve renal blood flow, but recent cardiopulmonary bypass combined with introduction of nephrotoxic immunosuppressive drugs can result in deteriorating renal function and even acute renal failure [34,35].

A history of seizures or other concerns relating to the central or peripheral nervous system indicate the need for consultation with a neurologist to assist in the pre- and post-transplant evaluation and management [36,37]. Where there is a history of pretransplant central nervous system injury or seizure disorder, computed tomography or magnetic resonance imaging of the brain is indicated. This baseline imaging can prove very useful if repeat studies are indicated in the post-transplant period.

Liver dysfunction often accompanies severe congestive heart failure [38]. Routine determination of serum liver function studies and coagulation profiles can be used to judge the extent of dysfunction. Computed tomography may identify cirrhotic changes. Liver biopsy is rarely required, but may be warranted in long-term survivors of the Fontan procedure in whom there is concern about the development of cirrhosis. While most patients experience a complete reversal of liver dysfunction within days to weeks of their transplant, identification of liver dysfunction allows for modification in the dosage of post-transplant medications that are metabolized by the liver. It is also important to distinguish abnormal liver function tests resulting from severe heart failure from those brought about by hepatitis C or other viruses.

CONTRAINDICATIONS

While there are few true *absolute* contraindications to heart transplantation in the pediatric population, there are a few that must be adhered too. An acutely ill patient with an active severe infection is one. The presence of an uncontrolled infection, coupled with cardiopulmonary bypass surgery and the subsequent need for immunosuppression, combine to make for a patient with little or no chance of survival. Likewise, a patient with an active malignancy, or a patient recently treated for malignancy, is also more likely to be overcome by the malignancy when immunosuppressed. The presence of HIV infection, or a severe congenital or acquired immunodeficiency syndrome, is also considered an absolute contraindication to heart transplantation in children in most centers.

There are also several relative contraindications to transplantation that must be considered and objectively weighed at the time of transplant evaluation. Major systemic disorders and extracardiac abnormalities may impact quality of life and life expectancy after transplantation and must be considered objectively as part of the transplant evaluation. Finally, psychosocial factors that may impact on post-transplant survival, such as a history of non-adherence with medical therapy, psychological instability of the patient or the parent/primary caregiver or an inadequate social support system must all be considered as relative contraindications to transplant surgery in selected cases. Where these factors are remediable, all efforts should be made to do so and the patient reconsidered for transplantation once intervention has proven effective.

CONCLUSIONS

The complete evaluation of the pediatric heart transplant candidate involves a multidisciplinary approach. The best interest of the patient, and the best chance of a successful procedure with long-term survival, is served by an unbiased comprehensive evaluation. This requires that each patient undergo a standardized regimen of consultations and laboratory studies but which also has been thoughtfully individualized to the circumstances of each patient.

REFERENCES

1 Steinman T, Becker B, Frost A, *et al.* Guidelines for the referral and management of patients eligible for solid organ transplantation. *Transplantation* 2001;71:1189–204.

2 Ramos-Barbon D, Fitchett D, Gibbons W, *et al.* Maximal exercise testing for the selection of heart transplantation candidates: limitation of peak oxygen consumption. *Chest* 1999;115:410–7.

3 Opasich C, Pinna G, Mazza A, *et al.* Six-minute walk test performance in patients with moderate to severe heart failure. *Eur Heart J* 2001;22:488–96.

4 Kervio G, Ville N, Leclercq C, *et al.* Intensity and daily reliability of the six-minute walk test in moderate chronic heart failure patients. *Arch Phys Med Rehabil* 2004;85:1513–8.

5 Webber S, Fricker F, Michaels M, *et al.* Orthotopic heart transplantation in children with congenital heart disease. *Ann Thorac Surg* 1994;58:1664–9.

6 Chartrand C, Guerin R, Kangah M, Stanley P. Pediatric heart transplantation: surgical considerations for congenital heart diseases. *J Heart Lung Transplant* 1990;9:608–17.

7 Mayer J, Perry S, O'Brien P, *et al.* Orthotopic heart transplantation for complex congenital heart disease. *J Thorac Cardiovasc Surg* 1990;99:484–92.

8 Razzouk A, Gundry S, Chinnock R, *et al.* Orthotopic transplantation for total anomalous pulmonary venous connection associated with complex congenital heart disease. *J Heart Lung Transplant* 1995;14:713–7.

9 Reitz B, Jamieson S, Gaudiani V, Oyer P, Stinson E. Method for cardiac transplantation in corrected transposition of the great arteries. *Cardiovasc Surg* 1982;23:293–6.

10 Hsu D, Quaegebeur J, Michler R, *et al.* Heart transplantation in children with congenital heart disease. *J Am Coll Cardiol* 1995;26:743–9.

11 Cooper M, Fuzesi L, Addonizio L, *et al.* Pediatric heart transplantation after operations involving the pulmonary arteries. *J Thorac Cardiovasc Surg* 1991;102:386–95.

12 Doty D, Renlund D, Caputo G, Burton N, Jones K. Cardiac transplantation in situs inversus. *J Thorac Cardiovasc Surg* 1990;99:493–9.

13 Addonizio L, Gersony W, Robbins R, *et al.* Elevated pulmonary vascular resistance and cardiac transplantation. *Circulation* 1987;76(Suppl 5):52–5.

14 Murali S, Kormos R, Uretsky B, *et al.* Preoperative pulmonary hemodynamics and early mortality after orthotopic cardiac transplantation: the Pittsburgh experience. *Am Heart J* 1993;126:896–904.

15 Kawaguchi A, Gandjbakhch I, Pavie A, *et al.* Cardiac transplant recipients with preoperative pulmonary hypertension: evolution of pulmonary hemodynamics and surgical options. *Circulation* 1989;80(Suppl 3):90–6.

16 Gajarski R, Towbin J, Bricker J, *et al.* Intermediate follow-up of pediatric heart transplant recipients with elevated pulmonary vascular resistance index. *J Am Coll Cardiol* 1994;23:1682–7.

17 Addonizio L, Hsu D, Douglas J, *et al.* Cardiac transplantation in children with markedly elevated pulmonary vascular resistance. *J Heart Lung Transplant* 1995;12:S93.

18 Addonizio LJ, Gersony WM, Rose EA. Cardiac transplantation in children with high pulmonary vascular resistance. *Am Heart J* 1986;112:647.

19 Kieler-Jensen N, Ricksten S, Stenqvist O, *et al.* Inhaled nitric oxide in the evaluation of heart transplant candidates with elevated pulmonary vascular resistance. *J Heart Lung Transplant* 1994; 13:366–75.

20 Zales V, Pahl E, Backer C, *et al.* Pharmacologic reduction of pre-transplant pulmonary vascular resistance predicts outcome after pediatric heart transplantation. *J Heart Lung Transplant* 1993;12:965–73.

21 Weil R, Clarke D, Iwaki Y, *et al.* Hyperacute rejection of a transplanted human heart. *Transplantation* 1981;32:71–2.

22 Singh G, Thompson M, Griffith BP, *et al.* Histocompatibility in cardiac transplantation with particular reference to immunopathology of positive serologic cross-match. *Clin Immunol Immunopathol* 1983;28:56–66.

23 Mir T, Marohn S, Laer S, *et al.* Plasma concentrations of N-terminal pro-brain natriuretic peptide in control children from the neonatal to adolescent period and in children with congestive heart failure. *Pediatrics* 2002;110:e76.

24 Lake K, Smith C, Milford Laforest S, *et al.* Policies regarding the transplantation of hepatitis C-positive candidates and donor organs. *J Heart Lung Transplant* 1997;16:917–21.

25 Arbustini E, Dal-Bello B, Morbini P, *et al.* Factors increasing the risk of allograft vascular disease in heart transplant recipients. *G Ital Cardiol* 1997;27:985–99.

26 Bouthot B, Murthy B, Schmid C, Levey A, Pereira B. Longterm follow-up of hepatitis C virus infection among organ transplant recipients. *Transplantation* 1997;63:849–53.

27 Fishman J, Rubin R, Koziel M, Pereira B. Hepatitis C virus and organ transplantation. *Transplantation* 1996;62:147–54.

28 Uzark K, Sauer S, Lawrence K, *et al.* The psychosocial impact of pediatric heart transplantation. *J Heart Lung Transplant* 1992;11:1160–7.

29 Douglas J, Hsu D, Addonizio L. Noncompliance in pediatric heart transplant patients. *J Heart Lung Transplant* 1993;12:S92.

30 Webber S. Newborn and infant heart transplantation. *Curr Opin Cardiol* 1996;11:68–74.

31 Tweddell J, Canter C, Bridges N, *et al.* Predictors of operative mortality and morbidity after infant heart transplantation. *Ann Thorac Surg* 1994;58:972–7.

32 Bailey LL, Razzouk AJ, Wang N, Sciolaro CM, Chiavarelli M. Bless the babies: one hundred fifteen late survivors of heart transplantation during the first year of life. *J Thorac Cardiovasc Surg* 1993;105:805–15.

33 Armitage J, Kormos R, Griffith B, Fricker F, Hardesty R. Heart transplantation in children with malignant disease. *J Heart Lung Transplant* 1990;9:627–30.

34 Ruggenenti P, Perico N, Amuchastegui C, *et al.* Following initial decline, glomerular filtration rate stabilizes in heart transplant patients on chronic cyclosporine. *Am J Kidney Dis* 1994;24:549–53.

35 Greenberg A, Egel J, Thompson M, *et al.* Early and late forms of cyclosporine nephrotoxicity: studies in cardiac transplant recipients. *Am J Kidney Dis* 1987;9:12–22.

36 Martin A, Bricker J, Fishman M, *et al.* Neurologic complications of heart transplantation in children. *J Heart Lung Transplant* 1992;11:933–42.

37 Warnecke H, Scheuler S, Schliffka J, Hertza R. Neurologic complications after heart transplantation: the influence of immunosuppression. *Transplant Proc* 1987;19:2510–1.

38 Dunn G, Hayes P, Breen K, Scheneker S. The liver in congestive heart failure: a review. *Am J Med Sci* 1973;265:174–89.

32 Donor Evaluation, Surgical Technique and Perioperative Management

Frank A. Pigula and Steven A. Webber

DONOR EVALUATION

The success of the heart transplant operation is critically dependent on appropriate donor selection and optimal donor management. Evaluation of the donor heart begins with a careful review of the history. This includes donor age and sex, body size, cause of death, presence of any chest trauma, need for cardiopulmonary resuscitation, length of resuscitation and evaluation of the hemodynamic status of the donor (including blood pressure, heart rate and central venous pressure if available) (Table 32.1). The amount of inotropic support, and trends in usage over time, are also noted. A history of cardiopulmonary resuscitation is not, in itself, a contraindication to cardiac donation for pediatric recipients [1]. It must be recognized that brain death results in dramatic physiologic disturbances in the donor [2,3]. These include temperature instability with hypothermia, circulatory volume changes (most commonly depletion) and neuroendocrine dysfunction. There is depletion of circulating thyroxine, cortisol, insulin, glucagon and antidiuretic hormone (ADH).

To rule out structural abnormalities, a full M-mode, cross-sectional and Doppler echocardiographic study should be performed for all potential cardiac donors. Biventricular function, including ejection fraction, shortening fraction and valve function is assessed. Some degree of atrioventricular valvar regurgitation is common after brain death and mild degrees do not constitute a contraindication to organ donation. Pericardial effusion may be indicative of myocardial contusion, and should be excluded. A 12-lead electrocardiogram should be performed. Mild nonspecific ST and T wave changes are commonly present, and usually reflect central nervous system effects, electrolyte disturbances or hypothermia. These do not contraindicate organ donation. Interpretation of cardiac enzymes may be difficult in the setting of generalized trauma. However, the elevation in cardiac troponin I levels in donor serum appears to be a useful predictor for acute graft failure after infant heart transplantation [4], and these organs should be carefully scrutinized. Evaluation of adult donors for coronary artery disease by selective coronary arteriography is commonplace in adult transplantation. Use

of older donors (e.g. above 35 years of age) for pediatric recipients is associated with high risk of post-transplant coronary disease and poor long-term survival. Such donors are generally avoided.

Most centers avoid the use of donor hearts whose systolic function is more than mildly impaired with inotropic support (e.g. shortening fraction less than 26%, ejection fraction less than 50%). Although some groups have used donor hearts with greater degrees of systolic dysfunction, this strategy is

Table 32.1 Evaluation of the cardiac donor.

History
Donor age, height, weight and sex
Cause of brain death
History of cardiac arrest and length of resuscitation
Evidence of chest trauma
History of intravenous drug usage
Past history of cardiovascular disease
Distance from transplant center

Cardiovascular status
Heart rate, blood pressure, central venous pressure
Fluid balance
Blood gas
Types and doses of intravenous inotropes
Inotropic support increasing or decreasing

Cardiovascular testing
Electrocardiogram
Chest radiograph
Echocardiogram
Cardiac enzymes

Other testing
Infectious disease screen: CMV, EBV, *Toxoplasma gondii*, HIV-1, HIV-2, HTLV-1, HTLV-2, RPR, Hepatitis B and C
All culture results since admission to intensive care unit

CMV, cytomegalovirus; EBV, Epstein–Barr virus; HIV, human immunodeficiency virus; HTLV, human lymphotropic virus; RPR, rapid plasma reagin.

not without risk because primary graft failure is associated with high morbidity and mortality after pediatric orthotopic heart transplantation [5].

Size matching

Most centers avoid undersizing the donor below 75–80% of recipient weight. Below this, cardiac output of the donor may be insufficient to meet the needs of the recipient. Use of oversized donors is common. Most candidates will have marked cardiomegaly, leaving ample room within the chest for an oversized donor heart. Use of donor to recipient weight ratios of 2.5 : 1 is common in pediatric practice, and ratios of 3–4 : 1 have been successfully used, especially in newborn and infant candidates [6–8]. Marked oversizing is not without risk, as the incidence of delayed sternal closure increases. In infant recipients, donor to recipient weight ratios of greater than 2 have been associated with a more prolonged ventilatory course and increased risk of primary graft failure [9]. Oversized donor hearts may also give rise to a postoperative syndrome characterized by high output state associated with systemic hypertension, raised intracranial pressure and mental status changes [10].

It has been suggested that oversizing of donors may improve outcome when there is significant preoperative pulmonary hypertension in the recipient [11], although others have questioned the need for this [12,13]. Certainly, undersizing should be avoided in the presence of recipient pulmonary hypertension and in adults it has been shown that female donors are associated with higher perioperative mortality when recipient pulmonary vascular resistance is elevated [14].

Blood group and HLA typing

Heart transplantation is performed between donor and recipients with either identical or compatible blood groups. There appears to be no significant difference in outcomes between these two groups, so exact matching of blood groups is not necessary [15,16]. Recently, the Toronto group performed successful transplantation in young infants with "incompatible" blood groups [17]. This is feasible because naturally occurring anti-A and anti-B antibodies (isohemagglutinins) are not present in the newborn period and during early infancy and their development may be suppressed under immunosuppression or through the development of post-transplant B-cell tolerance [18]. The intermediate-term results of such a strategy appear promising [17], although long-term results in a large cohort of patients remains to be determined. This approach is not appropriate beyond infancy or once significant titers of candidate blood group isohemagglutinins have developed.

Donor human leukocyte antigen (HLA) typing is not routinely performed prior to heart transplantation and logistic issues prevent donor selection based on donor–recipient HLA matching. However, for candidates with preformed anti-HLA antibodies, knowledge of donor and recipient HLA type (along with knowledge of unacceptable donor HLA antigens) is often very useful. When it is not possible to perform a prospective donor-specific cross-match, this information may allow for the accurate prediction that a negative cross-match will occur. This may allow for successful transplantation of selected patients who are sensitized to HLA antigens.

Infectious disease issues in the donor

The evaluation of the donor for infections that may be transmitted with the heart is similar to that for other solid organ transplants (see Chapter 13). All donors should be screened for cytomegalovirus (CMV), Epstein–Barr virus (EBV) infection, human immunodeficiency viruses 1 and 2 (HIV-1, HIV-2), human lymphotropic viruses 1 and 2 (HTLV-1, HTLV-2) and hepatitis viruses A, B and C. Donors are also screened for syphilis and for antibodies to *Toxoplasma gondii*. Presence of antibodies to CMV, EBV or *T. gondii* do not constitute contraindication to transplantation but helps guide post-transplantation therapy and surveillance. Therefore, organs can be accepted even if the results of testing for these pathogens are not available pretransplantation. Evidence of donor retroviral infection (HIV or HTLV) is considered an absolute contraindication to heart transplantation. The presence of donor hepatitis B surface antigen is also usually considered an absolute contraindication to heart donation. The use of hepatitis C positive donors remains controversial [19–21]. Usually, only the antibody against hepatitis C is known at the time of donation. Although low recipient infection rates have been reported in some studies [19], it seems prudent to reserve transplantation of hepatitis C positive donors to critically sick cardiac candidates or to those who are themselves hepatitis C positive. Some regions are starting to screen donors for West Nile virus following reports of fatal donor-transmitted disease.

Donor management

A detailed discussion of management of the donor is outside the scope of this chapter. However, it is worth noting that careful donor management and good communication between the donor center and the recipient teams can often salvage organs that were originally deemed unusable. It is common to find that hypotensive pediatric donors are merely volume depleted and inotropic requirements often can be markedly reduced following correction of diabetes insipidus with use of vasopressin. Mildly depressed contractility may respond to use of triiodothyronine (T3). Following brief cardiopulmonary arrest, donor contractility will often recover quite quickly and, when feasible, serial echocardiograms should be performed to determine if donor cardiac function appears adequate for donation.

Cardiac preservation

For simplicity, it is convenient to divide cardiac preservation for transplantation into four separate phases: preharvest (donor management), cardioplegic arrest, storage and reperfusion. Important points of each phase must be adhered to optimize post-transplant organ function.

Cardioplegic arrest

Common to all solutions is the use of hypothermic cardioplegia. Because the fundamental effect of hypothermia on physiochemical solutions is to reduce molecular movement, the rate of enzymatic reactions leading to the degradation of intracellular energy is reduced.

Storage

Following cardioplegic arrest and surgical excision of the donor organ, the heart is placed in a container of cardioplegic solution, carefully secured, and placed on ice. This common technique is referred to as static storage. With an optimal temperature between 4° and 6°C, static storage provides reliable preservation for up to approximately 6 hours. However, there are reports of satisfactory results in hearts preserved up to 14 hours using this technique [22].

Reperfusion

Reperfusion is being recognized as an important, active stage of cardiac preservation. Multiple investigations have shown that after a period of ischemia, the myocardium is vulnerable to both myocardial and endothelial injury, manifest as functional impairment [23–27].

SURGICAL TECHNIQUES

Procurement of donor organ

A methodical and specific examination of the heart should be performed. Contractility can be assessed by gently elevating the apex of the heart. There should be uniform contractility, with a "corkscrew" or twisting displacement of the ventricular masses with each systole. Anatomic abnormalities should be looked for (e.g. persistent left superior vena cava).

Once all surgical teams are ready, the aorta is cross-clamped, the heart is vented by incising the inferior vena cava (IVC) and cold cardioplegia solution is infused. This, along with topical hypothermia, should result in prompt diastolic arrest of the heart. Once cardioplegia (15–20 mL/kg) is administered, excision of the heart proceeds from the IVC, superior vena cava (SVC), aorta, pulmonary artery and left atrial cuff. Once excised, the heart is placed in a container of cardioplegic solution, carefully secured and placed on ice as outlined above.

Graft implantation

While anatomic connections for heart transplantation in cardiomyopathies are routine, heart transplantation for congenital heart defects presents special surgical challenges. Over the last 10 years, however, experience with transplantation of congenital heart disease renders few anatomic combinations untransplantable. This section discusses the surgical approach to heart transplantation in the most common, and the most complex, anatomic arrangements found in congenital heart disease.

Biatrial technique

In 1960, Lower and Shumway [28] enumerated the basic surgical principles of orthotopic heart transplantation. The pioneering efforts led to the adoption of the biatrial anastomosis for cardiac transplantation. This technique has been applied to thousands of patients, of all ages, with excellent results.

Details of biatrial orthotopic heart transplantation have changed little since its introduction in 1960 (Fig. 32.1). The donor heart is inspected for valvular abnormalities, intracavitary thrombus and for the presence of a patent foramen ovale. After trimming the donor and recipient left atrial cuff, implantation begins with the left atrial anastomosis. Proper orientation of the donor heart in relation to pulmonary and systemic venous return is critical to avoid a torsion deformity of venous structures. Upon completion of the left atrial anastomosis, the right atrium is incised from the IVC towards the right atrial appendage, avoiding the sinoatrial (SA) node, and the donor right atrium is then anastomosed to the remnant of the recipient right atrium. At this juncture, we prefer to complete the aortic anastomosis. Methylprednisolone (15 mL/kg) is administered to the patient, the aortic cross-clamp removed and the patient rewarmed. The pulmonary artery anastomosis is then performed during cardiac reperfusion. With correction of calcium and electrolytes, cardiac function should be spontaneous and vigorous. Regardless, some form of inotropic support, usually in the form of dopamine or dobutamine, is preferable. If the patient is hypertensive on low-dose inotropic support, milrinone is preferred both for its inotropic as well as its vasodilatory effects.

Bicaval technique

Despite the great success of the biatrial technique, this is a non-anatomic technique that results in large atrial cavities. The resulting abnormal atrial geometry is thought to contribute to tricuspid valve dysfunction. Sinus node dysfunction, from surgical trauma or ischemia, has also been described. Beniaminovitz *et al.* [29] have shown improved echocardiographic indices

273

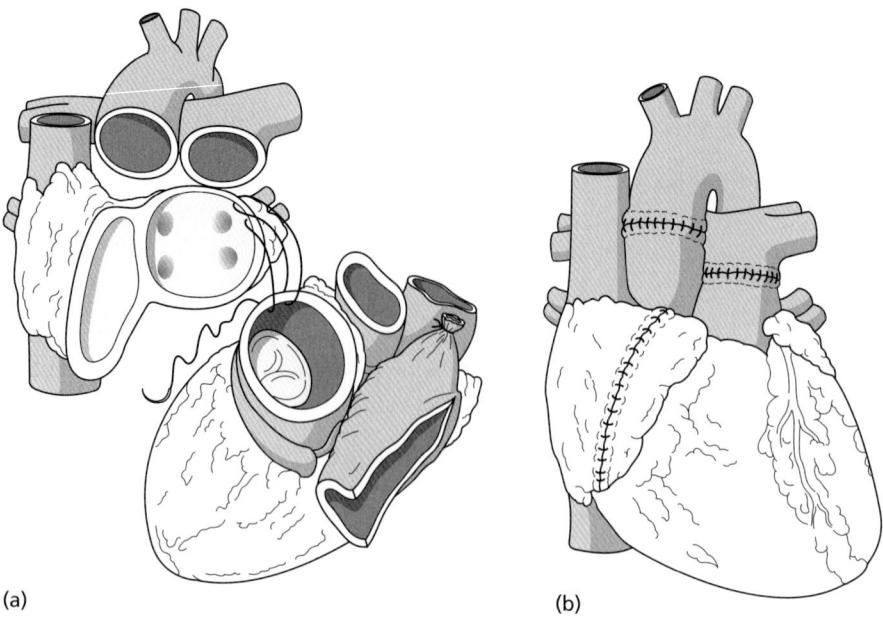

(a)   (b)

Fig. 32.1 Heart transplantation using biatrial anastomoses. (a) Recipient ventricular mass has been excised and left atrial anastomosis commences after proper graft alignment. (b) Completion.

of atrial function after bicaval anastomosis, with a trend toward less tricuspid regurgitation. In adults, Brandt *et al.* [30] concluded that preservation of the donor right atrial anatomy with the bicaval technique resulted in less atrial fibrillation and flutter than did the biatrial technique. Rothman *et al.* [31] undertook testing of the SA node after heart transplantation. They found evidence of SA node dysfunction in 14/32 (42%) patients undergoing biatrial anastomosis, while this was present in only 2/37 (5%) patients receiving bicaval anastomosis. They concluded that surgical trauma to the SA node, or its blood supply, was responsible. Finally, El Gamel *et al.* [32] have shown that the bicaval technique preserves the atrial contribution to cardiac output after transplantation.

For these reasons, we routinely perform bicaval anastomosis in children of all ages undergoing orthotopic heart transplantation (Fig. 32.2). Also, we have found that some specific forms of congenital heart disease lend themselves particularly well to the bicaval technique. For instance, patients who have previously undergone Mustard or Senning operations present with distorted atrial anatomy, with both cavae drawn to the midline. Excision of the intra-atrial baffle, leaving only the cavoatrial cuffs and pulmonary vein patch, simplify the operation conceptually as well as surgically.

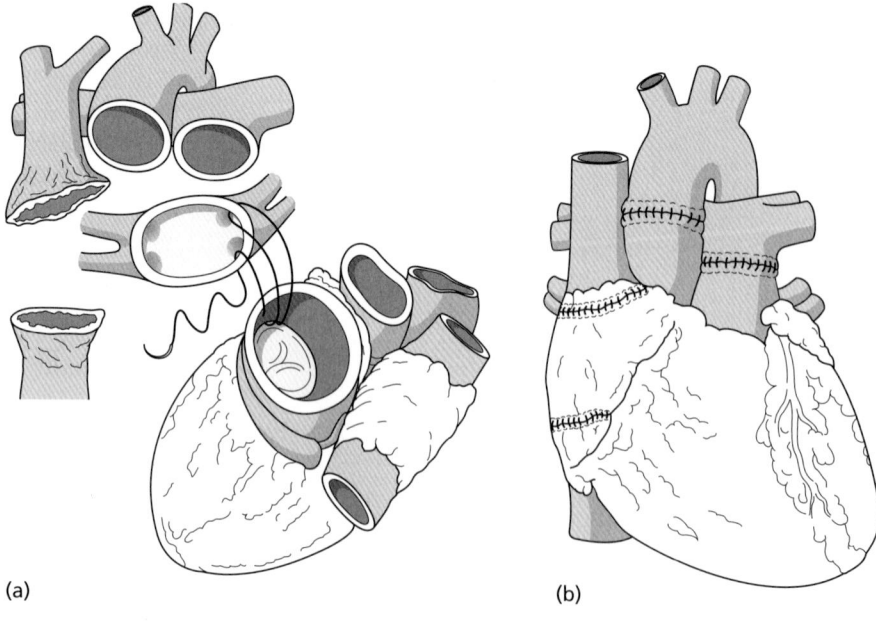

(a)   (b)

Fig. 32.2 Heart transplantation using the bicaval technique. (a) Generous cavoatrial cuffs remain. The left atrial cuff is trimmed and implantation proceeds from left atrium to inferior vena cava (IVC), superior vena cava (SVC), aorta and pulmonary artery. (b) Completion.

274

While the technique we use is similar to that described by Sarsam et al. [33] and El Gamel et al. [32], special attention to a number of details in the small patient must be observed. Orientation of the heart, relative to the pulmonary and systemic venous return, is critical. It is important to leave a generous cuff of right atrial tissue with both vena cavae. Great care is taken to orient the heart properly, using the orifice of the coronary sinus as a reference and placing it in the anatomic position. Because of the crenellated nature of the recipient cavoatrial cuff, it is important to splay out and display its edge to avoid suture line leaks.

The SVC anastomosis deserves special mention. Recipient cardiomegaly may displace the cavoatrial junction cephalad. In this case we have utilized a ring of donor aorta as an interposition graft to perform a tension-free anastomosis. Absorbable suture is also used for this anastomosis, leaving the front one-third incomplete. At this time, the aortic anastomosis is performed in a standard fashion. After steroids are administered, the heart and aorta are deaired, and the heart reperfused. By placing a small pump sucker into the right atrium via the incomplete SVC anastomosis, the pulmonary artery anastomosis can be completed while the heart is being perfused. The SVC anastomosis is then completed, and the patient weaned from cardiopulmonary bypass.

Cardiac transplantation for congenital heart disease

Transplantation for congenital heart disease is often performed after multiple palliative procedures, and can present formidable surgical challenges. The anatomic substrate can be broadly classified as abnormalities of the systemic venous return, of the pulmonary venous return and of the great vessels, including hypoplastic left heart syndrome. Surgical modifications of the two basic techniques, atrial and bicaval anastomosis, required for transplantation of these anatomic variants, are described.

Abnormalities of systemic venous return

Abnormalities of systemic venous return are among the most challenging anatomic variants to transplant. Fashioning unobstructed connections in a patient undergoing heart transplantation with dextrocardia with left-sided cavae requires special consideration and planning (Fig. 32.3). Unusual systemic venous anatomy often presents in the setting of visceral heterotaxy, and may include dextrocardia, single ventricle, bilateral or left SVC, and interrupted IVC with azygous continuation. Clearly, in these cases, surgical strategy must be altered to accommodate the anatomic substrate, and a variety of techniques have been devised.

In a recent report, Vricella et al. [34], from Loma Linda have published their experience with orthotopic heart transplantation in 15 infants and children with atrial situs inversus or heterotaxy syndrome. Technical points stressed were as follow:

1 oversewing left pulmonary vein orifices of the donor heart, with the opening of the left atrium more rightward than usual to accommodate the rotational malalignment;
2 leave abundant right atrial tissue with both cavae; and
3 incision of the left pericardium to allow rotation of the graft to approximate anatomic position.

The authors elected to perform these operations with single venous cannulation, under deep hypothermia using low flow or circulatory arrest as needed. While on low flow bypass, systemic venous return was handled with cardiotomy suction. After cardiectomy, the redundant cavoatrial cuff from the IVC was tubularized towards the right to allow connection with the donor right atrium. SVC return was accomplished by anastomosing the recipient innominate vein with the donor SVC, either in front of or behind the aorta. They reported one operative death from graft dysfunction, and three patients required some form of intervention for late SVC stenosis (2) or occlusion (1).

Thus, it is emphasized that recognition of the anatomic requirements in transplantation for complex congenital disease is essential. For these reasons, the donor heart should be procured with the complete SVC, innominate vein and aortic arch (including proximal descending aorta).

Abnormalities of the great arteries

In general, abnormalities of the great vessels are easily dealt with technically. As has been pointed out by Doty et al. [35], the relationship between the aorta and pulmonary artery, at the level of the pulmonary bifurcation, is quite constant. When both great vessels are present, the aorta is always anterior to the pulmonary artery. While technical modifications of the great artery anastomosis may be required, these are generally minor and easily accomplished. Thus, transplantation for transposition of the great arteries presents no special challenge with respect to great vessel anastomoses. The surgical challenge arises when previous palliative operations have resulted in discontinuous, shunted or banded pulmonary arteries, as discussed below.

Abnormalities of the pulmonary arteries

More and more children come to heart transplantation after multiple palliative operations have been performed. Often, these operations have involved the pulmonary arteries in the form of systemic-to-pulmonary shunts, cavopulmonary anastomosis or other procedures. In all cases, as much pulmonary artery as possible should be harvested, and the SVC should be included to the level of the innominate vein. When an extensive reconstruction is anticipated, the aortic arch and proximal descending aorta should be taken.

Most commonly, as is the case in bidirectional Glenn or Fontan operations, the cavopulmonary anastomosis is taken down, the pulmonary arteries are patched, and bicaval anastomoses are performed. Patch material may take the form of bovine pericardium, homograft, or donor or recipient

275

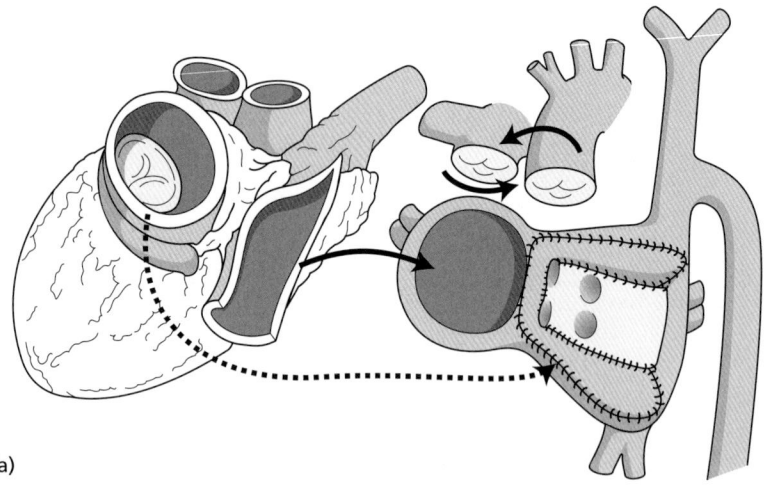

(a)

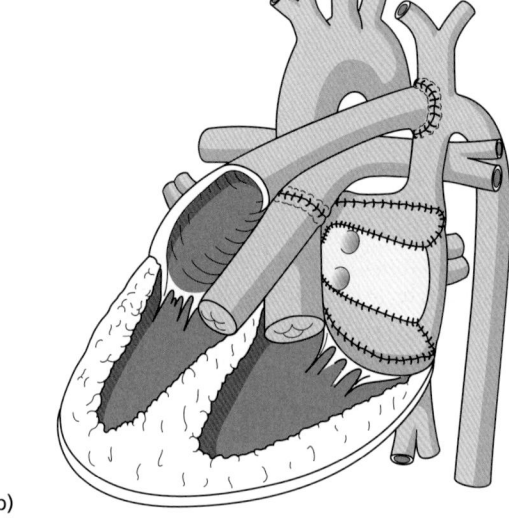

(b)

Fig. 32.3 Biatrial anastomoses in a patient transplanted for D-transposition of the great arteries and situs inversus following Mustard procedure. (a) Mustard baffle was preserved to direct systemic venous return to the donor right atrium. (b) Because of stenosis of the superior caval baffle, the donor superior vena cava (SVC) was anastomosed to the recipient SVC proximal to the baffle.

discard. Repair is best accomplished after recipient cardiectomy and before organ implantation.

In the case of discontinuous pulmonary arteries, the donor organ should be procured with the pulmonary bifurcation and pulmonary arteries intact (to the take off of the upper lobe branches) when possible (Fig. 32.4). Direct left and right pulmonary artery anastomoses are then performed. Alternatively, excess donor aorta can be used to connect the right and left pulmonary arteries prior to implantation.

Hypoplastic left heart syndrome
Techniques for transplantation of hypoplastic left heart deserve special mention. Because of the extensive arch hypoplasia, the donor surgeon must include the entire transverse and proximal descending aorta en bloc with the organ. While most centers perform transplantation of hypoplastic left heart syndrome (HLHS) under circulatory arrest, several techniques have been developed to minimize circulatory arrest time. The group from Loma Linda [36] has applied perfusion man-

agement techniques aimed at minimizing circulatory arrest times during transplantation of HLHS. Arterial cannulation is accomplished through the ductus arteriosus via the pulmonary artery. After ligation of the diminutive aorta, and clamping of the main pulmonary artery proximal to the arterial cannula, recipient cardiectomy is performed. Low flow cardiopulmonary bypass is maintained during the left and right atrial anastomoses. Systemic venous return is controlled using cardiotomy suction. However, circulatory arrest is still required for aortic arch reconstruction and the pulmonary artery anastomosis.

Newer techniques, such as regional low flow perfusion, can eliminate the need for circulatory arrest [37]. This technique employs a polytetrafluoroethylene tube graft (3.5 mm) anastomosed to the innominate artery, fashioned prior to bypass (Fig. 32.5), and has been well described. Vascular isolation of the brachiocephalic vessels and the descending aorta allows continued perfusion of the brain during cardiectomy as well as graft implantation. This technique provides physiologic

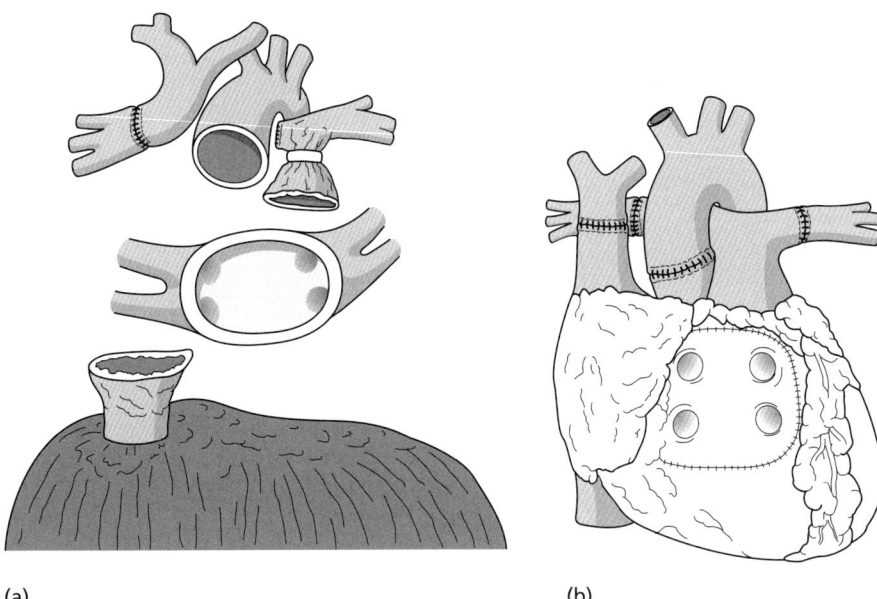

Fig. 32.4 Bicaval heart transplant in a child with discontinuous arteries, status post (s/p) right classic Glenn and pulmonary artery banding. (a) After recipient cardiectomy, inferior vena cava (IVC) cavoatrial cuff and left atrial button are prepared and the classic Glenn is taken down. (b) The donor organ is procured such that reconstruction of the pulmonary arteries is possible and a bicaval anastomosis is performed.

(a)

(b)

cerebral circulatory support, as well as significant somatic circulatory support, such that circulatory arrest can be avoided completely [38].

Heterotopic heart transplant

Heterotopic heart transplantation was introduced by Barnard in 1975 and has two primary indications [39]:

1 elevated and fixed pulmonary vascular resistance; and
2 undersized donor when immediate heart transplantation is required.

However, it must be emphasized that the point where pulmonary vascular resistance becomes an absolute contraindication to orthotopic heart transplantation remains ill-defined.

Technical details have been well described by Griffith *et al.* [40], and the largest pediatric experience, 12 patients, has been

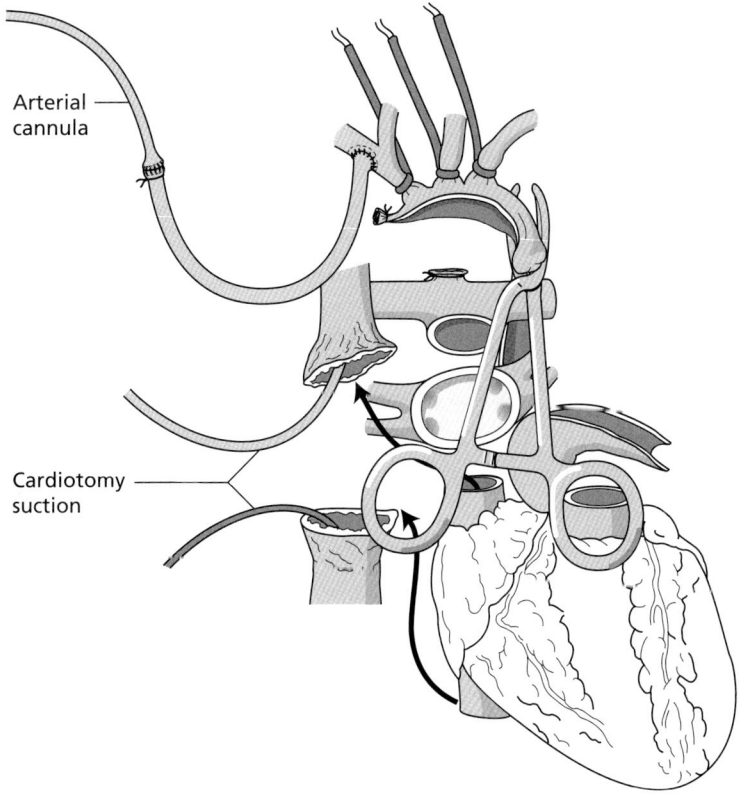

Arterial cannula

Cardiotomy suction

Fig. 32.5 Heart transplantation for hypoplastic left heart syndrome; technique for avoidance of circulatory arrest. The first step involves the anastomosis of a 3.5-mm polytetrafluoroethylene graft to the innominate artery. With control of the brachiocephalic vessels and the descending aorta, regional perfusion may be delivered via the graft and the innominate and right subclavian arteries. Thus, the entire transplant may be performed with circulatory support, avoiding the need for circulatory arrest completely. Upon decannulation the graft is oversewn.

reported by Khaghani *et al*. [41] from the Harefield Hospital program. At that institution, the indications for heterotopic transplant were undersized donor in four and elevated pulmonary vascular resistance in eight cases. All were operative survivors, with one early death from rejection. Despite these results, heterotopic heart transplantation has disadvantages: greater technical difficulty, potential pulmonary complications, thromboemboli emanating from the native heart, and difficulty obtaining endomyocardial biopsies for rejection surveillance. Because of these disadvantages, orthotopic heart transplantation remains the preferred technique.

POSTOPERATIVE MANAGEMENT

Many of the fundamental principles of early postoperative management after heart transplantation are similar to those for pediatric patients undergoing other procedures with cardiopulmonary bypass. This section focuses on aspects of care that are specific to the transplant recipient.

Cardiovascular considerations

Inotropic agents

Abnormalities in cardiac function are inevitable the result of the obligatory hypoxic or ischemic insult that the donor heart endures. Recovery of systolic function is usually rapid. Abnormalities in diastolic function, however, may persist for many weeks [42]. Most heart transplant recipients will benefit from low-dose inotropic support in the immediate postoperative period, although often this is only required for 2–3 days. The choice of inotrope will reflect both physician preference and hemodynamic factors such as heart rate, pulmonary vascular resistance and blood pressure. Low-dose dobutamine and isoproterenol are common choices. The latter is sometimes recommended because of its combined properties of chronotropy, inotropy and pulmonary vasodilatation. The addition of a combined vasodilator/inotropic agent such as milrinone is logical when there is low cardiac output and evidence of high systemic vascular resistance. Occasionally, particularly in infants with markedly oversized donors, the most dramatic way to improve cardiac function is to leave the chest open at the end of the transplant procedure.

Systemic hypertension

In contrast to the non-transplant cardiac surgical patient, systemic hypertension is common. Many factors contribute, including vigorous function of an oversized donor organ and use of high-dose corticosteroids. It is not unusual to observe quite severe systolic hypertension within 24 hours of a successful transplant procedure. If good ventricular function is confirmed by echocardiogram, rapid weaning of inotropic support is

performed. Where systemic resistance appears high, intravenous vasodilators are a logical choice. In the case of a vigorous oversized organ, some have advocated beta-blockade [43].

Pulmonary vascular resistance

The importance of pulmonary vascular resistance as a risk factor for acute donor right ventricular failure is discussed in detail elsewhere (see Chapter 31). If, on the basis of preoperative evaluation, there is a concern about elevated pulmonary vascular resistance, additional precautions should be taken. Nitric oxide is begun in the operating room with anesthetic induction, and is used to wean from cardiopulmonary bypass. Acidosis must be avoided and high levels of inspired oxygen are provided. Hyperventilation is performed and generous sedation is provided in the early postoperative period. If necessary, prostaglandin E_1 can also be used. The right heart may require significant inotropic support, and sometimes epinephrine may be required in addition to milrinone and dobutamine. If right ventricular dysfunction persists with poor cardiac output despite this level of support, then mechanical assistance should be provided (see below). If pulmonary vascular resistance is moderately elevated pretransplantation, (or if there is an acute elevation in resistance following bypass in a child with previously low resistance), then 24–48 hours of support will often enable the right ventricle to recover enough to support the circulation, despite elevated pulmonary pressures. If acute donor right heart failure reflects poor candidate selection (e.g. indexed pulmonary resistance greater than 10 units after vasodilator challenge), then recovery of right heart function is unlikely to occur.

Cardiac rate and rhythm

Postoperative tachyarrhythmias and bradyarrhythmias have been observed in children following heart transplantation [44]. Rhythm disturbances may be more common with high preoperative pulmonary vascular resistance [45]. The most common rhythm abnormality (other than sinus tachycardia) is sinus node dysfunction leading to sinus bradycardia, with or without an atrial or junctional escape rhythm. The denervated sinus node responds appropriately to exogenous chronotropic agents [46] and isoproterenol is useful in this respect. A simpler approach is atrial pacing, and all transplant recipients should have temporary pacing wires placed in the operating room. Sinus node dysfunction reflects ischemic and/or traumatic injury, but usually recovers in a few days [47]. Ventricular ectopy and non-sustained ventricular tachycardia are also quite common in the first week or two after transplantation. These presumably relate to the obligatory ischemia-reperfusion injury, and rarely require treatment.

The fresh cardiac allograft has limited ability to increase stroke volume, and therefore establishing an adequate heart rate is important for maintaining cardiac output. It is our practice to maintain a heart rate that reflects slight tachycardia for age. For instance, in an infant, a heart rate of 140–150 b/min would be maintained, and in a teenager a heart rate of at least at 100 b/min would be acceptable. We commonly employ atrial pacing to control the heart rate, though isoproterenol may also be used.

Primary graft failure

Failure to wean from cardiopulmonary bypass, or early postoperative graft failure, is a serious complication associated with high mortality. The term primary graft failure is often reserved for the finding of acute left ventricular or biventricular failure not caused by high pulmonary vascular resistance. Poor donor selection, very prolonged ischemic time, poor preservation technique and hyperacute rejection should all be considered. In our experience, the latter is extremely rare. When primary graft failure occurs (not resulting from hyperacute rejection), recovery is frequently possible if the circulation can be supported. This is usually achieved with extracorporeal membrane oxygenation (ECMO).

Respiratory support

The principles of respiratory support do not differ from those of other pediatric open heart procedures. Early extubation should be the goal. The patient who has required prolonged preoperative mechanical ventilation will usually need more prolonged ventilatory support postoperatively as retraining of respiratory muscles will be required. Infants with longstanding cardiomegaly will often have significant tracheobronchomalacia and persistent or recurrent pulmonary atelectasis is not unusual, especially of the left lower lobe.

Renal function

The combination of chronic heart failure, cardiopulmonary bypass and use of ciclosporin or tacrolimus all contribute to postoperative renal dysfunction. Oliguria is common. Fortunately, acute renal failure is rare in children and dialysis is seldom required. Persisting oliguria is managed with loop diuretics and low-dose dopamine (e.g. 3–5 µg/kg/min). We frequently administer a continuous furosemide infusion (up to 6 mg/kg/day), and augment this with infusion (continuous or bolus) of aminophylline, as a diuretic adjunct. These maneuvers are usually successful in stimulating an adequate urine output (> 1 mL/kg/hour). In some cases, particularly in neonates and infants, intravenous prostaglandin E_1 may also provide a diuretic effect.

Gastrointestinal considerations

Gastrointestinal complications are quite common early after pediatric heart transplantation [48]. All patients should receive intravenous and subsequently oral H_2 antagonists to decrease the risk of stress ulcers. These are usually continued until corticosteroids have been weaned to low doses or discontinued. The nasogastric tube is removed as soon as the patient is extubated and able to take oral feeds and medications. Attention is paid to providing optimal calories without use of excessive volumes because most patients will tend to retain fluid in the early postoperative period. Pancreatitis is not uncommon following transplantation and should be sought when there is abdominal pain or unexplained feeding intolerance. Immunosuppressive regimens that avoid the use of azathioprine and corticosteroids may reduce this complication.

Infection precautions

Infectious disease considerations are dealt with in detail elsewhere (see Chapter 12). During the first week after transplantation, invasive lines and drains are removed as soon as possible. A short course of antibiotics (e.g. 72 hours) is given as prophylaxis against mediastinal and wound infection. Usually a first generation cephalosporin will suffice. Broader staphylococcal coverage (e.g. vancomycin) is given if the patient has had a prolonged ICU stay and has multiple longstanding lines in place. Such lines are usually replaced in the operating room. Patients colonized with methicillin resistant *Staphylococcus aureus* (MRSA) are also covered with vancomycin. Oral nystatin is started in the ICU, along with ganciclovir, if indicated. Initiation of prophylaxis against *Pneumocystis carinii* can follow nearer to the time of hospital discharge.

Immunosuppression and early acute rejection

Immunosuppressive regimens are discussed elsewhere (see Chapter 34). In most centers, high-dose intravenous methylprednisolone (e.g. 15–20 mg/kg) is given in the operating room. A tapering course of corticosteroids is usually given over the next 1–2 weeks, with the majority of centers discharging patients on maintenance corticosteroid therapy [49]. However, there is increasing use of steroid-free immunosuppressive regimens in pediatric practice. Ciclosporin or tacrolimus is commenced generally within 24 hours of surgery. We usually wait 12–24 hours until good urine output has been established. If cytolytic induction therapy is used (most commonly polyclonal rabbit antithymocyte globulin), then there is less urgency to introduce a calcineurin inhibitor in the immediate post-transplant period. Ciclosporin or tacrolimus can then be commenced by the oral route rather than intravenously. Delay in commencement of these agents for 2–3 days (under coverage of induction therapy) may be particularly useful when urine output is low or renal function is deteriorating.

Careful daily assessment for signs of rejection are required, although severe rejection before 7–10 days is rare (except in the sensitized patient). Pallor, increasing tachycardia, abdominal pain, gallop rhythm and oliguria all are suggestive of severe rejection. Ideally, rejection is identified by echocardiography and/or surveillance biopsy before such signs develop. However, the tempo of rejection can be quite abrupt in the early post-transplant period and any deterioration in the patient's condition after initial recovery from surgery must be taken very seriously. If there is unequivocal evidence of new graft dysfuction, empiric treatment (usually consisting of bolus corticosteroids), or immediate endomyocardial biopsy, should be performed.

REFERENCES

1 de Begona JA, Gundry SR, Razzouk AJ, *et al.* Transplantation of hearts after arrest and resuscitation. Early and long-term results. *J Thorac Cardiovasc Surg* 1993;**106**:1196–201.

2 Novitzky D, Wicomb WN, Cooper DKC, *et al.* Electrocardiographic, haemodynamic and endocrine changes occurring during experimental brain death in the Chacma baboon. *Heart Transplant* 1984;**4**:63.

3 Darby JM, Stein K, Grenvik A, *et al.* Approach to management of the heart-beating 'brain dead' organ donor. *JAMA* 1989;**261**:2222–28.

4 Grant JW, Canter CE, Spray TL, *et al.* Elevated donor cardiac troponin I: A marker of acute graft failure in infant heart recipients. *Circulation* 1994;**90**:2618–21.

5 Boucek M, Novick R, Bennett L, *et al.* The Registry of the International Society of Heart and Lung Transplantation: Third official pediatric report, 1999. *J Heart Lung Transplant* 1999;**18**:1151–72.

6 Webber SA. Fifteen years of pediatric heart transplantation at the University of Pittsburgh: Lessons learned and future prospects. *Pediatr Transplant* 1997;**1**:8–21.

7 Razzouk AJ, Chinnock RE, Gundry SR, *et al.* Transplantation as a primary treatment for hypoplastic left heart syndrome: intermediate-term results. *Ann Thorac Surg* 1996;**62**:1–8.

8 Mitchell MB, Cambell DN, Clarke DR, *et al.* Infant heart transplantation: improved intermediate results. *J Thorac Cardiovasc Surg* 1998;**116**:242–52.

9 Tweddell JS, Canter CE, Bridges ND, *et al.* Predictors of operative mortality and morbidity after infant heart transplantation. *Ann Thorac Surg* 1994;**58**:972–7.

10 Fricker FJ, Armitage JM. Heart and heart-lung transplantation in children and adolescents. In: Emmanouilides GC, Riemenschneider TA, Allen HD, Gutgesell HP, eds. *Moss and Adams: Heart Disease in Infants, Children and Adolescents*, 5th edn. Williams and Wilkins, 1995:498.

11 Kawaguchi A, Gandjbakhch I, Pavie A, *et al.* Cardiac transplant recipients with preoperative pulmonary hypertension: evolution of pulmonary hemodynamics and surgical options. *Circulation* 1989;**80**(Suppl 3):90–6.

12 Costanzo-Nordin MR, Liao Y, Grusk BB, *et al.* Oversizing of donor hearts: beneficial or detremental? *J Heart Lung Transplant* 1991;**10**:717–30.

13 Gajarski R, Towbin J, Bricker JT, *et al.* Intermediate follow-up of pediatric heart transplant recipients with elevated pulmonary vascular resistance index. *J Am Coll Cardiol* 1994;**23**:1682–7.

14 Murali S, Kormos RL, Uretsky BF, *et al.* Preoperative pulmonary hemodynamics and early mortality after orthotopic cardiac transplantation: the Pittsburgh experience. *Am Heart J* 1993;**126**:896–904.

15 Shaddy RE, Naftel DC, Kirklin JK, *et al.* Outcome of cardiac transplantation in children: survival in a contemporary multi-institutional experience. *Circulation* 1996;**94**(Suppl 2):69–73.

16 Young JB, Naftel DC, Bourge RC, *et al.* Matching the donor and heart transplant recipient: clues for successful expansion of the donor pool. A multivariable, multi-institutional report. *J Heart Lung Transplant* 1994;**13**:353–65.

17 West LJ, Pollock-Barziv SM, Dipchand AI, *et al.* ABO-incompatible heart transplant in infants. *N Engl J Med* 2001;**344**:793–800.

18 Fan X, Ang A, Pollock-Barziv SM, *et al.* Donor-specific B-cell tolerance after ABO-incompatible infant heart transplantation. *Nat Med* 2004;**10**:1227–33.

19 Roth D, Fernandez JA, Babischkin S. Detection of hepatitis C virus infection among cadaveric organ donors: evidence of low transmission of disease. *Ann Intern Med* 1992;**117**:470–5.

20 Lake K, Smith C, Milford Laforest S, *et al.* Policies regarding the transplantation of hepatitis C-positive candidates and donor organs. *J Heart Lung Transplant* 1997;**16**:917–21.

21 Bouthot B, Murthy B, Schmid C, Levey A, Pereira B. Longterm follow-up of hepatitis C virus infection among organ transplant recipients. *Transplantation* 1997;**63**:849–53.

22 Obadia JF, Girard C, Ferrara R, *et al.* Long conservation organs in heart transplantation: postoperative results and long-term follow-up in fourteen patients. *J Heart Lung Transplant* 1997;**16**:256–9.

23 Murphy CO, Pan-Chih, Gott JP, Guyton RA. Coronary microvascular reactivity after ischemic cold storage and reperfusion. *Ann Thorac Surg* 1997;**63**:20–7.

24 Kevelaitis E, Nyborg NC, Menasché P. Coronary endothelial dysfunction of isolated hearts subjected to prolonged cold storage: patterns and contributing factors. *J Heart Lung Transplant* 1999;**18**:239–47.

25 Sawatari K, Kawata H, Assad RS, Mayer JE Jr. Effects of PO_2 level during initial reperfusion after hypothermic cardioplegia in neonatal lambs. *Circulation* 1990;**82**(Suppl 3):146A.

26 Fujiwara T, Kurtts T, Silvera M, Mayer JE. Physical and pharmacological manipulation of reperfusion conditions in neonatal myocardial preservation. *Circulation* 1988;**78**(Suppl 2):444A.

27 Sawatari K, Kadoba K, Bergner KA, Daitch JA, Mayer JE Jr. Influence of initial reperfusion pressure after hypothermic cardioplegic ischemia on endothelial modulation of coronary tone in neonatal lambs. Impaired coronary vasodilator response to acetylcholine. *J Thorac Cardiovasc Surg* 1991;**101**:777–82.

28 Lower RR, Shumway NE. Studies on orthotopic homotransplantation of the canine heart. *Surg Forum* 1960;**11**:18–25.

29 Beniaminovitz A, Savoia MT, Oz M, *et al.* Improved atrial function in bicaval versus standard orthotopic techniques in cardiac transplantation. *Am J Cardiol* 1997;**80**:1631–5.

30 Brandt M, Harringer W, Hirt SW, *et al.* Influence of bicaval anastomosis on late occurrence of atrial arrhythmia after heart transplantation. *Ann Thorac Surg* 1997;**64**:70–2.

31 Rothman SA, Jeevanandam V, Combs WG, *et al.* Eliminating bradyarrhythmias after orthotopic heart transplantation. *Circulation* 1996;**94**(Suppl 2):278–82.

32 El Gamel A, Yonan NA, Grant S, *et al*. Orthotopic cardiac transplantation: comparison of standard and bicaval Wythenshawe techniques. *J Thorac Cardiovasc Surg* 1995;**109**:721–30.

33 Sarsam MA, Campbell CS, Yonan NA, *et al*. An alternative surgical technique in orthotopic cardiac transplantation. *J Cardiac Surg* 1993;**8**:344–9.

34 Vricella LA, Razzouk AJ, Gundry SR, *et al*. Heart transplantation in infants and children with situs inversus. *J Thorac Cardiovasc Surg* 1998;**116**:82–9.

35 Doty DB, Renlund DG, Caputo GR, Burton NA, Jones KW. Cardiac transplantation in situs inversus. *J Thorac Cardiovasc Surg* 1990;**99**:493–9.

36 Vricella LA, Razzouk AJ, del Rio M, Gundry SR, Bailey LL. Heart transplant for hypoplastic left heart syndrome: modified technique for reducing circulatory arrest time. *J Heart Lung Transplant* 1998;**17**:1167–71.

37 Pigula FA, Siewers RD, Nemoto EM. Regional perfusion of the brain during neonatal aortic arch reconstruction. *J Thorac Cardiovasc Surg* 1999;**117**:1023–4.

38 Pigula FA, Gandhi SK, Siewers RD, *et al*. Regional low-flow perfusion provides somatic circulatory support during neonatal aortic arch surgery. *Ann Thorac Surg* 2001;**72**:401–6.

39 Barnard DN, Losman JG. Left ventricular bypass. *South Afr Med J* 1975;**49**:303–12.

40 Griffith BP, Kormos, RL, Hardesty RL. Heterotopic cardiac transplantation: current status. *J Cardiac Surg* 1981;**2**:283–9.

41 Khaghani A, Santini F, Dyke CM, *et al*. Heterotopic cardiac transplantation in infants and children. *J Thorac Cardiovasc Surg* 1997;**113**:1042–9.

42 Young JB, Leon CA, Short HD, *et al*. Evolution of hemodynamics after orthotopic heart and heart-lung transplantation: early restrictive patterns persisting in occult fashion. *J Heart Transplant* 1987;**6**:34–43.

43 Martin AB, Bricker T, Fishman M, *et al*. Neurologic complications of heart transplantation in children. *J Heart Lung Transplant* 1992;**11**:933–42.

44 Collins KK, Thiagarajan RR, Chin C, *et al*. Atrial tachyarrhythmias and permanent pacing after pediatric heart transplantation. *J Heart Lung Transplant* 2003;**22**:1126–33.

45 Gajarski R, Towbin J, Bricker J, *et al*. Intermediate follow-up of pediatric heart transplant recipients with elevated pulmonary vascular resistance index. *J Am Coll Cardiol* 1994;**23**:1682–7.

46 Quigg RJ, Rocco MB, Gauthier DF, *et al*. Mechanism of the attenuated peak heart rate response to exercise after orthotopic cardiac transplantation. *J Am Coll Cardiol* 1989;**14**:338–44.

47 Miyamoto Y, Curtiss EI, Kormos RL, *et al*. Bradyarrhythmia after heart transplantation: incidence, time course, and outcome. *Circulation* 1990;**82**(Suppl 4):313–7.

48 Rakhit A, Nurko S, Gauvreau K, Mayer JE, Blume ED. Gastrointestinal complications after pediatric cardiac transplantation. *J Heart Lung Transplant*. 2002;**21**:751–9.

49 Boucek MM, Edwards LB, Keck BM, *et al*. Registry of the International Society for Heart and Lung Transplantation: eighth official pediatric report, 2005. *J Heart Lung Transplant* 2005;**24**:968–82.

33 Pathology of the Cardiac Allograft

Maria Parizhskaya

The endomyocardial biopsy still remains the best method for detecting allograft rejection. An adequate sample should contain four to six pieces of endomycardium. The tissue should be fixed at the bedside in 10% buffered formalin. For histologic examination, biopsies are sectioned at a minimum of 10 levels with ribbons. Levels 3, 5, 7 and 9 are stained with hematoxylin and eosin (H&E). If necessary, one additional slide is stained with Masson trichrome or elastic trichrome.

Pathologic changes occurring within the first 10 days after heart transplantation include hyperacute cardiac rejection, reperfusion/ischemic injury and acute rejection [1]. Acute rejection may occur at any time after transplantation, although is most common within the first 6 months. The major limitation to long-term survival after heart transplantation is the development of chronic rejection (also known as graft vasculopathy or post-transplant coronary artery disease). This chapter deals with the pathology of acute and chronic rejection, as well as other pathologic conditions affecting the cardiac allograft.

HYPERACUTE REJECTION

Hyperacute rejection, mediated by preformed antibodies directed against major histocompatibility antigens on the vascular endothelium, is a rare event in cardiac transplant recipients [2]. We have not encountered cases of hyperacute rejection in our pediatric patient population. The histologic changes of hyperacute rejection consist of diffuse interstitial hemorrhage. Small vessels with fibrin thrombi and vessels with marginating neutrophils may be seen [1].

REPERFUSION/ISCHEMIC INJURY

Reperfusion/ischemic myocardial injury is commonly seen during the first 10 days after cardiac transplantation. It is more severe in patients whose donor hearts have had prolonged ischemic time. Histologically, it is characterized by interstitial edema and myocyte damage, usually without significant

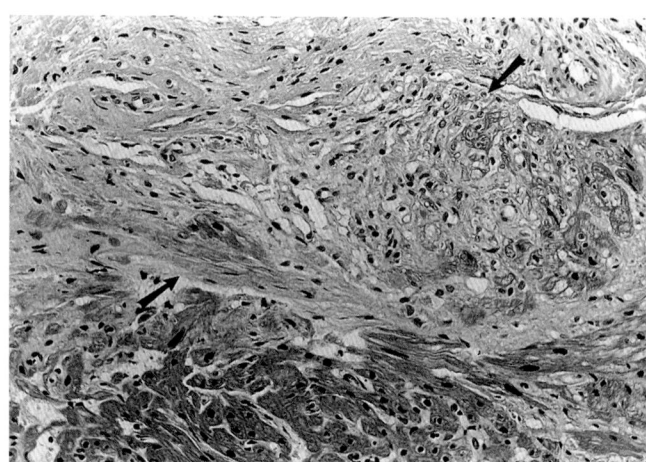

Fig. 33.1 Resolving ischemic injury. There has been myocyte dropout and replacement by loose connective tissue (arrows). Hemotoxylin and eosin (H&E), × 200.

inflammatory infiltrate. If inflammatory infiltrate is present it is neutrophilic rather than mononuclear. The resolving lesion demonstrates myocyte dropout and replacement by loose connective tissue containing rare mononuclear cells (Fig. 33.1).

ACUTE CELLULAR REJECTION

A standardized cardiac biopsy grading system for assessment of severity of acute cellular rejection is routinely employed [3]. This system was developed by the International Society for Heart and Lung Transplantation (ISHLT) and, while imperfect, is still used by most transplant centers for the grading of endomyocardial biopsy specimens (Table 33.1). A revision of the 1990 ISHLT classification system has recently been completed and simplifies the classification of low grade rejection [4]. This classification combines grades 1A, 1B and 2 under a single grade 1, mild acute cellular rejection. No distinction will be made between invasive and noninvasive

Table 33.1 Histological classification of acute cardiac allograft rejection. Criteria of the International Society for Heart and Lung Transplantation 1990 [3]; grades of the 2005 ISHLT revised classification are shown in parentheses [4].

Grade		(2005 revision [R])	Histologic findings
0	No rejection	(0 R)	No lymphocytic infiltrate
1A	Focal mild	(1 R)	Mild focal infiltrates without myocyte necrosis
1B	Diffuse mild	(1 R)	Diffuse mild infiltrate without myocyte necrosis
2	Focal moderate	(1 R)	Single large aggressive focus of inflammatory infiltrate
3A	Multifocal moderate	(2 R)	Multifocal aggressive infiltrates and/or myocyte necrosis
3B	Diffuse, borderline severe	(3 R)	Diffuse aggressive infiltrate with myocyte necrosis
4	Severe	(3 R)	Diffuse aggressive polymorphous infiltrate with myocyte necrosis and often with edema, hemorrhage and vasculitis

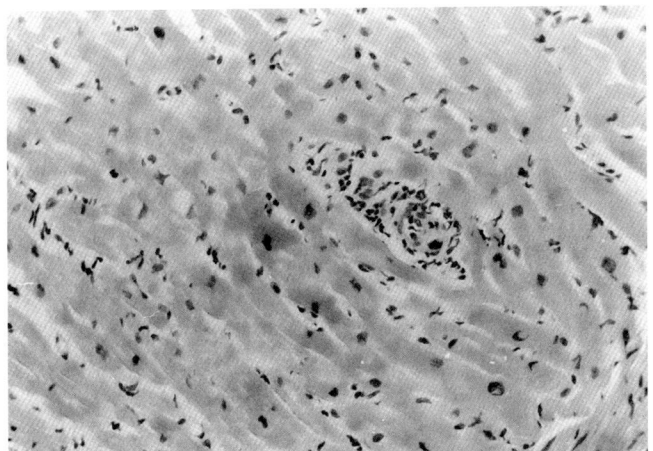

Fig. 33.2 Focal mild acute rejection, grade 1A. Lymphocytic infiltrate is limited to perivascular area. H&E, × 120.

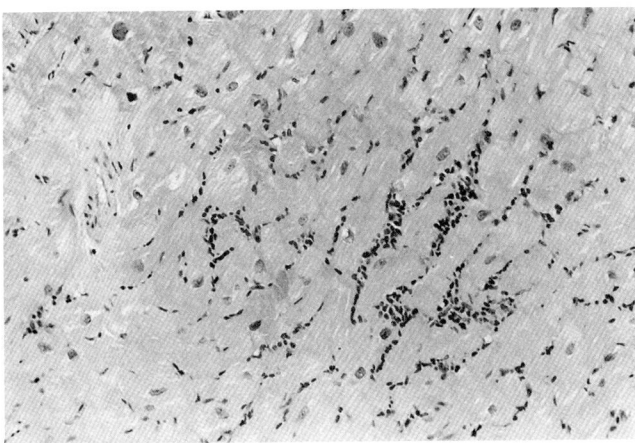

Fig. 33.3 Diffuse mild acute rejection, grade 1B. There are more diffuse perivascular and interstitial lymphocytic infiltrates without associated architectural changes. H&E, × 200.

Quilty lesions (see below), and greater emphasis is placed on the evaluation of antibody-mediated rejection [4]. The standard and revised grading system is described in more detail below.

Focal mild acute rejection, grade 1A (new grade 1R—revised)

Grade 1A is characterized by focal perivascular or interstitial lymphocytic infiltrates that cause no myocyte necrosis (Fig. 33.2).

Diffuse mild acute rejection, grade 1B (new grade 1R)

This grade represents more diffuse, perivascular and/or interstitial lymphocytic infiltrates with no myocyte necrosis (Fig. 33.3). In grades 1A and 1B one or more pieces of myocardium may be involved.

Focal moderate acute rejection, grade 2 (new grade 1R)

Grade 2 is used when there is a single, larger, sharply circumscribed focus of inflammatory infiltrate composed of small and activated lymphocytes with or without eosinophils (Fig. 33.4). In practice, many cases of so-called grade 2 rejection also have other occasional minor perivascular infiltrates. Some authors question the existence of grade 2 rejection [5]. Many of these cases may actually be deeply penetrating Quilty lesions (see below).

Multifocal moderate acute rejection, grade 3A (new grade 2R)

In grade 3A rejection, multifocal inflammatory infiltrates composed of small and activated lymphocytes with or without eosinophils are present (Fig. 33.5). The myofibers are often separated secondary to interstitial edema. Distortion

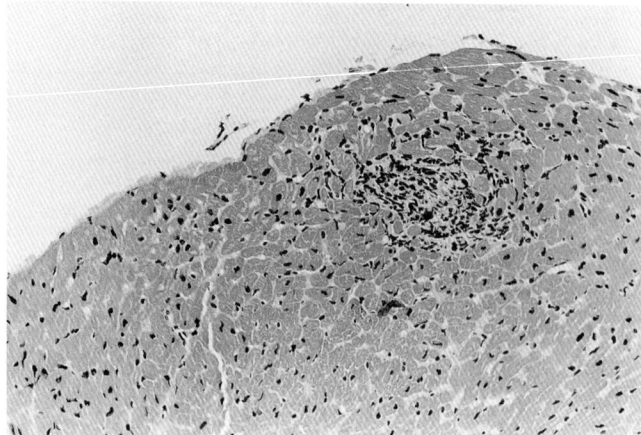

Fig. 33.4 Focal moderate acute rejection, grade 2. Lymphocytic infiltrate is limited to a single focus which is both perivascular and interstitial. H&E, × 200.

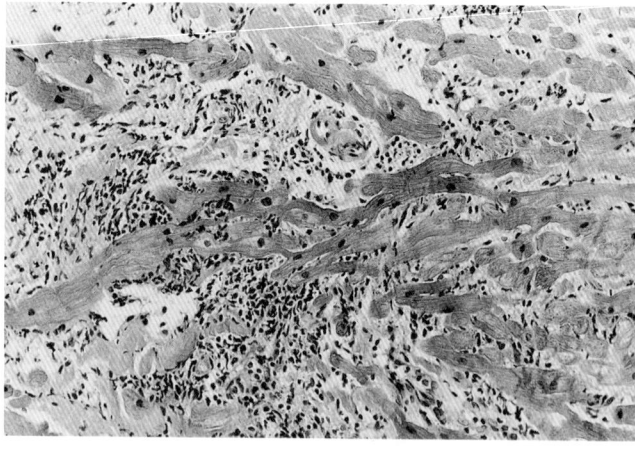

Fig. 33.6 Diffuse borderline severe acute rejection, grade 3B. There is diffuse inflammatory infiltrate accompanied by interstitial edema and distortion of individual myofibers. H&E, × 200.

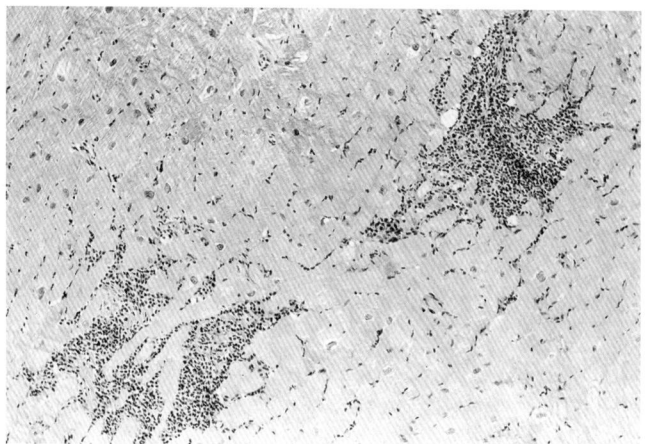

Fig. 33.5 Multifocal moderate acute rejection, grade 3A. There are multifocal lymphocytic infiltrates. H&E, × 60.

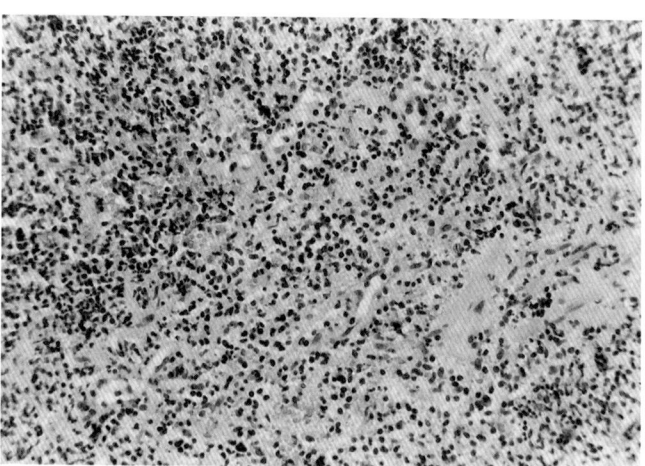

Fig. 33.7 Severe acute rejection, grade 4. There is dense polymorphous inflammatory infiltrate and patchy interstitial hemorrhage. H&E, × 120.

of individual myofibers, including myofiber branching and splitting, is frequently observed.

Diffuse borderline severe acute rejection, grade 3B (new grade 3R)

Grade 3B represents a diffuse inflammatory infiltrate, which involves several pieces of myocardium. The infiltrate is composed of activated and small lymphocytes admixed with eosinophils. A few neutrophils might be present. Hemorrhage is not usually seen, but interstitial edema and distortion of individual myofibers are prominent (Fig. 33.6). Like other authors [6,7], we have found myocyte necrosis difficult to identify in grades 3A and 3B. Therefore, our diagnosis is primarily based on the intensity of inflammation and associated architectural changes.

Severe acute rejection, grade 4 (new grade 3R)

In grade 4 rejection there is a diffuse polymorphous inflammatory infiltrate of activated lymphocytes, eosinophils and neutrophils. Myocyte necrosis, interstitial edema, hemorrhages and vasculitis are present (Fig. 33.7).

ACUTE HUMORAL REJECTION

Although T-cell-mediated rejection remains the most common form of acute rejection, humoral rejection is being increasingly recognized in patients with heart allografts. Detection of circulating antidonor antibodies (usually to donor HLA antigens) supports the diagnosis [8]. The morphology of humoral rejection is characterized by vascular dilatation with neutrophil accumulation and neutrophil adhesion to the activated vascular endothelium, as well as capillary deposition of complement fragment C4d [9]. The presence of capillary C4d is confirmed by either immunofluorescence on frozen sections or by immunoperoxidase staining of formalin-fixed paraffin-embedded endomyocardial tissue [8–11]. Capillary C4d deposits, however, have also been described in ischemic graft injury [12]. Therefore, positive C4d staining may not be unique for humoral rejection and further studies are necessary to clarify this issue.

CHRONIC REJECTION (GRAFT VASCULOPATHY, POST-TRANSPLANT CORONARY ARTERY DISEASE)

Concentric intimal proliferation leading to partial or total occlusion of the arterial lumen is a hallmark of chronic rejection (Fig. 33.8). In contrast to the eccentric, focal and often calcified lesions of naturally occurring atherosclerosis, the lesions in graft-induced coronary disease are concentric, rarely calcified and affect the entire length of the artery [1,13]. The intimal expansion is secondary to the proliferation of modified smooth muscle cells and accumulation of lipid-laden macrophages [1]. The internal elastic lamina shows mild damage and the media is usually not affected. Varying degrees of lymphocytic inflammation of the vessel wall may be present. Because chronic rejection primarily affects the larger coronary arteries, the diagnosis cannot reliably be made on endomyocardial biopsy. The presence of subendocardial infarcts and subendocardial fibrosis, however, may suggest an underlying coronary artery problem (Fig. 33.9).

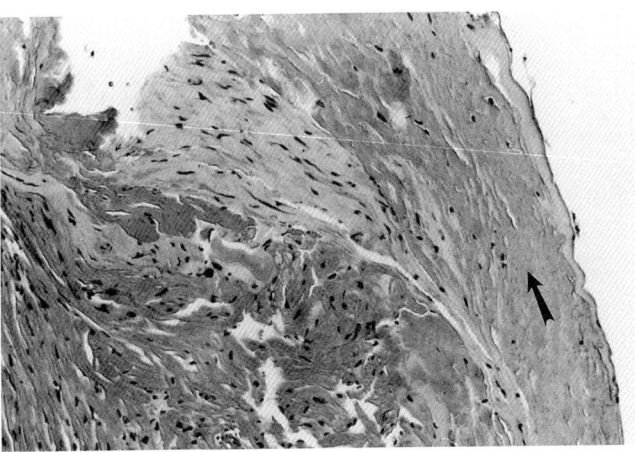

Fig. 33.9 The biopsy from a patient with known graft vasculopathy. Subendocardial necrotic myofibers (arrow) contrast with adjacent viable myocardial cells. H&E, × 100.

Other abnormalities in the cardiac allografts include Quilty lesions, previous biopsy sites and infections.

ENDOCARDIAL QUILTY LESION

The Quilty lesion is an endocardial or endomyocardial inflammatory infiltrate [1]. Both T and B lymphocytes are present and plasma cells and macrophages may also be observed, especially at the interface with the myocardium [14]. It is often well-vascularized with blood vessels lined by activated endothelium. In "noninvasive" Quilty lesions, the border between the endocardial infiltrate and the underlying myocardium is smooth (Fig. 33.10). In "invasive" Quilty lesions, the inflammatory infiltrate extends into the subadjacent myocardium, often causing distortion of individual myofibers

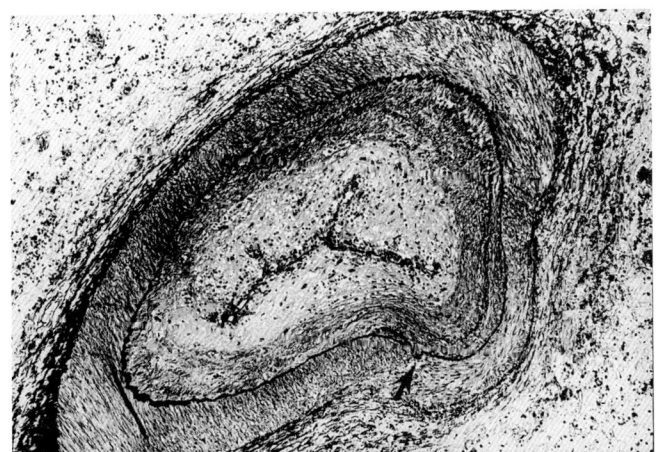

Fig. 33.8 Chronic rejection. The artery demonstrates near total luminal occlusion secondary to concentric intimal proliferation. The internal elastic lamina shows a small break (arrow). Mild perivascular and intimal lymphocytic infiltrate is present. Elastic trichrome, × 100.

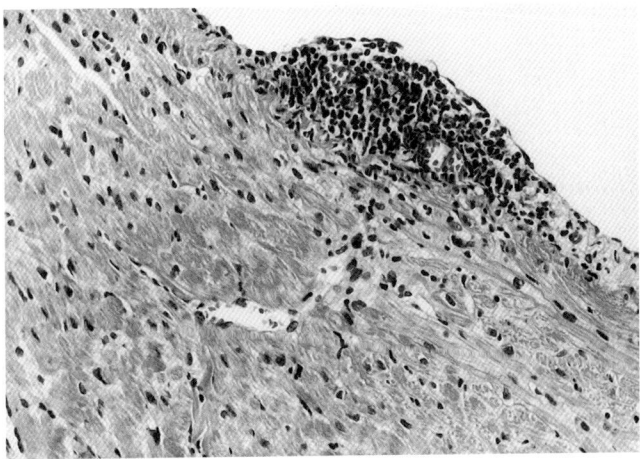

Fig. 33.10 "Noninvasive" Quilty lesion. The border between the endocardial infiltrate and the underlying myocardium is smooth. H&E, × 200.

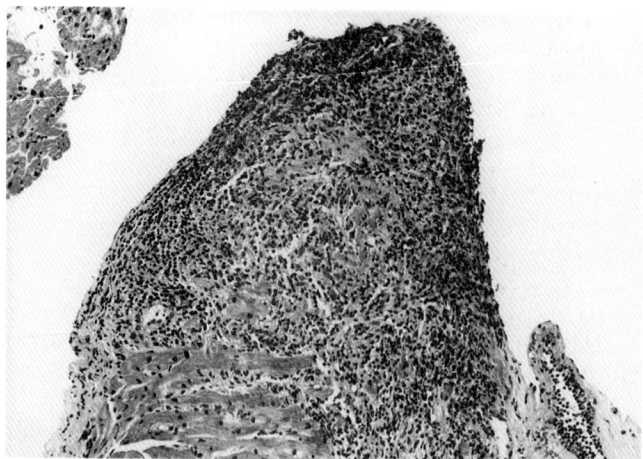

Fig. 33.11 "Invasive" Quilty lesion. The endocardial inflammatory infiltrate extends into the subadjacent myocardium. H&E, × 100.

and focal myocyte necrosis (Fig. 33.11). Quilty lesions that infiltrate the myocardium can be difficult to distinguish from acute rejection, especially if the endocardium is not visualized on the biopsy.

PREVIOUS BIOPSY SITES

Healing and healed biopsy sites are frequently encountered in biopsy specimens. They are typically seen in subendocardial locations. The histologic appearance depends on the age of the lesion. If a repeat biopsy is performed within a few days of the previous biopsy, necrotic myocytes with overlying thrombus are seen. A healing biopsy site is characterized by the presence of granulation tissue with scattered inflammatory cells and hemosiderin-laden macrophages (Fig. 33.12). Later on, the area of damage is replaced by a fibrotic scar.

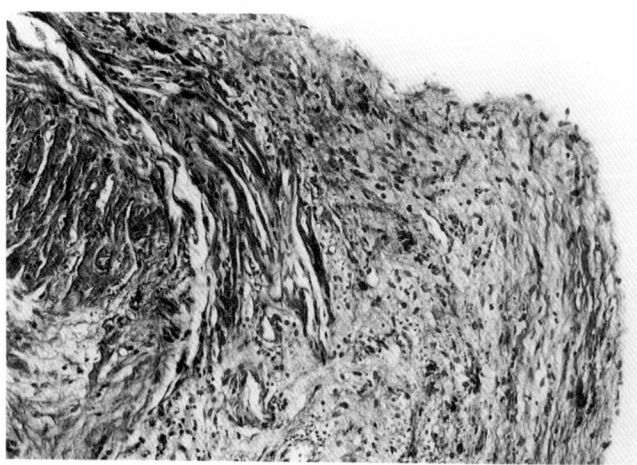

Fig. 33.12 Healing biopsy site. There is subendocardial granulation tissue with scattered inflammatory cells. Masson trichrome, × 100.

INFLAMMATION SECONDARY TO INFECTION

Infectious complications may occur at any time after cardiac transplantation. The most common infections that affect the heart during the early post-transplant period are cytomegalovirus (CMV) and infection by *Toxoplasma gondii* [1]. While bacterial and fungal infections are often associated with predominantly neutrophilic inflammation, the infiltrate seen in protozoal or viral infections may be reminiscent of acute rejection [15]. In CMV infection (Fig. 33.13) and toxoplasmosis (Fig. 33.14), the myocardium often contains a mixed inflammatory infiltrate with variable numbers of eosinophils. In an immunocompromised host, however, viral inclusions or *Toxoplasma* cysts may be seen in the absence of a significant inflammatory infiltrate. Epstein–Barr virus (EBV) myocarditis

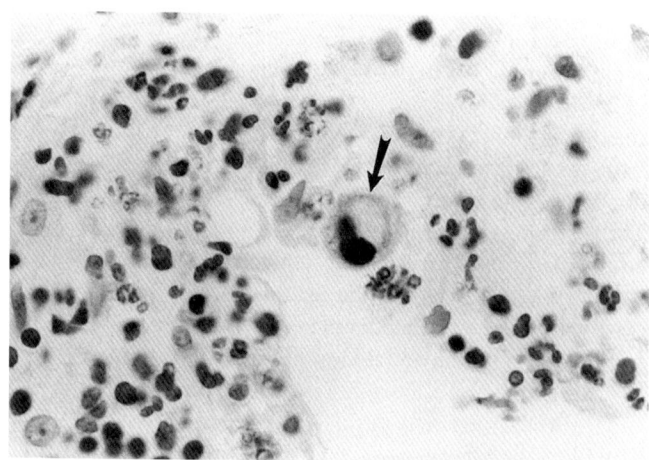

Fig. 33.13 Cytomegalovirus (CMV) endocarditis. The endocardium contains a mixed inflammatory infiltrate and a CMV inclusion (arrow). Anti-CMV, × 400.

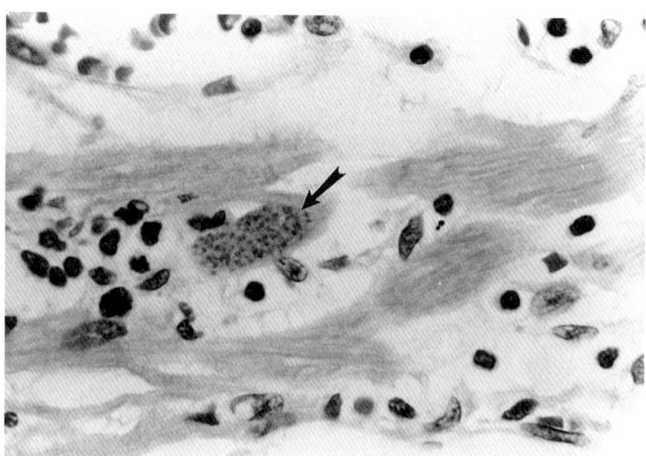

Fig. 33.14 *Toxoplasma gondii*. The myocardium contains *Toxoplasma* cyst (arrow) and mild inflammatory infiltrate. H&E, × 400.

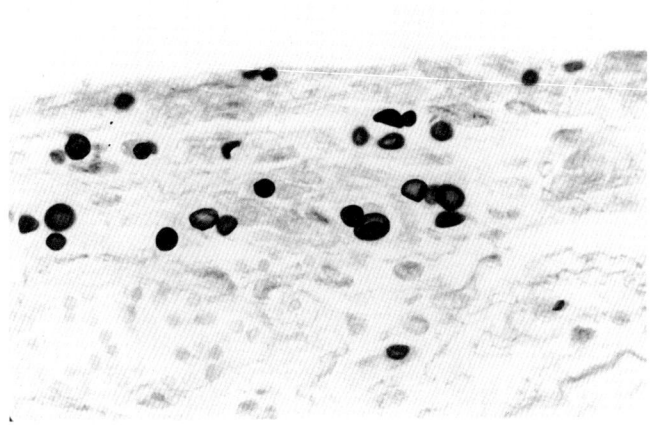

Fig. 33.15 Cryptococcal pericarditis. The epicardium contains yeast forms of *Cryptococcus neoformans*, which vary in size. Grocott, × 400.

may occur and is difficult to distinguish from acute rejection because both conditions present with lymphocytic infiltrate accompanied by interstitial edema. Immunostains for Epstein–Barr virus-related antigens (EBV LMP, EBV BZLF1) and *in situ* hybridization for EBV early RNA (EBER-1) may help to confirm viral myocarditis. Fungal infections may involve the transplanted heart. An example of cryptococcal endocarditis is illustrated in Figure 33.15.

REFERENCES

1 Billingham ME. The postsurgical heart: the pathology of cardiac transplantation. *Am J Cardiovasc Pathol* 1988;**1**:319–34.

2 Duquesnoy RJ, Cramer DV. Immunologic mechanisms of cardiac transplant rejection. *Cardiovasc Clin* 1990;**20**:87–103.

3 Billingham ME, Cary NR, Hammond ME, *et al.* A working formulation for the standardization of nomenclature in the diagnosis of heart and lung rejection: Heart Rejection Study Group. *J Heart Transplant* 1990;**9**:587–93.

4 Stewart S, Winters GL, Fishbein MC, *et al.* Revision of the 1990 working formulation for the standardization of nomenclature in the diagnosis of heart rejection. *J Heart Lung Transplant* 2005;**24**:1710–20.

5 Bell G, Lones M, Czer LSC, *et al.* Grade 2 cellular cardiac rejection: does it exist? *Lab Invest* 1994;**70**:26A.

6 Taylor SR, Yunis EJ, Fricker FJ. Cardiac transplantation in children. *Perspect Pediatr Pathol* 1991;**14**:60–93.

7 Sibley RK, Olivari MT, Ring WS, Bolman RM. Endomyocardial biopsy in the cardiac allograft recipient: a review of 570 biopsies. *Ann Surg* 1986;**203**:177–87.

8 Michaels PJ, Fishbein MC, Colvin RB. Humoral rejection of human organ transplants. *Springer Semin Immunopathol* 2003;**25**:119–40.

9 Duong Van Huyen JP, Fornes P, Guillemain R, *et al.* Acute vascular humoral rejection in a sensitized cardiac graft recipient: diagnostic value of C4d immunofluorescence. *Hum Pathol* 2004;**35**:385–8.

10 Behr TM, Feucht HE, Richter K, *et al.* Detection of humoral rejection in human cardiac allografts by assessing the capillary deposition of complement fragment C4d in endomyocardial biopsies. *J Heart Lung Transplant* 1999;**18**:904–12.

11 Chantranuwat C, Qiao JH, Kobashigawa J, *et al.* Immunoperoxidase staining for C4d on paraffin-embedded tissue in cardiac allograft endomyocardial biopsies: comparison to frozen tissue immunofluorescence. *Appl Immunohistochem Mol Morphol* 2004;**12**:166–71.

12 Baldwin WM III, Samaniego-Picota M, Kasper EK, *et al.* Complement deposition in early cardiac transplant biopsies is associated with ischemic injury and subsequent rejection episodes. *Transplantation* 1999;**68**:894–900.

13 Billingham ME. Pathology and etiology of chronic rejection of the heart. *Clin Transplant* 1994;**8**:289–92.

14 Kottke-Marchant K, Ratliff NB. Endomyocardial lymphocytic infiltrates in cardiac transplant recipients. *Arch Pathol Lab Med* 1989;**113**:690–8.

15 McManus BM, Winters GL. Pathology of heart allograft rejection. In: Kolbeck PC, Markin RS, McManus BM, eds. *Transplant Pathology*. Chicago: ASCP Press, 1994:197–217.

34 Post-Transplant Management

Shelley D. Miyamoto and Biagio A. Pietra

Heart transplantation is an effective therapy for children with end-stage heart disease. The overall survival of young heart recipients is now very good, with 1-year survival rates of approximately 90% and 5-year survival rates of 70–75% [1,2]. The standard for pediatric transplantation is higher than for adults, because 5, and even 10 year survival is not an acceptable goal in the scope of a child's life. In order to achieve not only short-term success, but decades long survival in children, optimal post-transplant management is critical. Animal studies suggest that graft-specific regulation is achievable and that if agents are used in the right sequence, dose and combination, operational tolerance and very long-term graft acceptance are possible. True transplantation tolerance is not yet possible in children, but is a feasible long-term goal especially for neonatal and young infant recipients. Postoperative management, immunosuppression, management of infectious issues and rejection surveillance and treatment are discussed.

POSTOPERATIVE INTENSIVE CARE UNIT MANAGEMENT

Although perioperative management of the heart transplant recipient is covered elsewhere in this book, the postoperative period is an extremely critical time and worth briefly mentioning here. The intensive care unit (ICU) is where the donor and recipient first encounter each other and the path of either destructive immunity (rejection) or nondestructive immunity (regulation) is begun. Although there are many factors we cannot control (donor and recipient genetics, immune memory, infectious history of either donor or recipient), there are many factors that we can control in the postoperative period that can impact late outcome. In addition, coordination and careful communication among the parents, primary care physicians, pediatric ICU and transplant teams will result in improved medical outcomes for this complex group of patients [3].

Foreign bodies (central venous lines, nasogastric and endotracheal tubes, and Foley catheters) are of particular import-

ance in this patient population, and should be minimized in an effort to lessen the risk of associated infections. Meticulous wound care and avoidance of postoperative wound infections are critical, as bacterial infection results in innate and antigen-specific immunity. This heightened state of the immune system lasts beyond the original infection. Donor antigen presented in temporal proximity to infection is more likely to result in destructive immunity. There is now direct evidence that heart transplant tolerance in animal models can be impaired by viral infection [4]. Bacteria can also directly activate the immune system in an antigen-independent fashion via Toll receptors which have been shown to influence allograft rejection [5]. The ultimate goal of postoperative management is to provide an environment that encourages nondestructive T-cell regulation while limiting antigen exposures that may predispose to destructive immunity.

POST-TRANSPLANT IMMUNOSUPPRESSION

The function of the immune system is to protect the host from foreign invaders (e.g. viruses, bacteria, fungi, parasites), or from transformed self (malignancy). The innate immune system is central in the repair of damaged tissue (healing). The immune system is constantly on the prowl looking for evidence of danger and is drawn to areas of injury and inflammation. Antigen is presented constantly, the result of which is either: (i) destructive immunity; or (ii) nondestructive immunity. The outcome, destructive versus nondestructive immunity, is largely dependent upon exceeding a threshold (quality and quantity of antigen plus costimulation) for a particular antigen. The threshold is variable and is influenced by many factors over which we have no control: the quality of antigen, the mismatch between donor and recipient, immunologic history of the recipient, etc. We cannot suppress the immune system of a patient to the point that no response is elicited by any antigen as this would result in the death of the recipient by infection or malignancy, and organ toxicities would also be unacceptable (e.g. renal failure). We must focus on the factors we can influence. Our goal should not be inhibition of all immune responses but rather to guide them to be nondestructive toward donor antigens, yet still respond to nonallogenic foreign antigens. Therefore, immunosuppression should be used judiciously and all stimuli to the immune system that may lead to destructive donor immunity minimized.

The goal of postoperative immunosuppressive regimens should be to influence the initial donor–recipient interaction down the path of nondestructive immunity and towards graft acceptance. Transition from postoperative immunosuppressive therapy to an outpatient regimen will be an easier and more successful endeavor if the early donor–recipient interaction is nondestructive.

Induction therapy

The choice to use induction therapy in the postoperative transplantation period is institution dependent and its utility debated within the transplant community. Antibody induction prevents T-cell activation, therefore allowing for modification of immunosuppressive protocols such that there is a decrease in the utilization of concomitant immunosuppressive medications (low or no calcineurin inhibition in the immediate post-transplantation period). If the intent of an induction protocol is active immune regulation to donor antigens, then high levels of calcineurin inhibitors can actually be immunologically counterproductive. Interestingly, in some animal models of cardiac allograft tolerance, the presence of cyclosporine during induction prevents long-standing tolerance [6]. In addition to the immune regulation advantages that antibody induction offers, it is also useful in patients with marginal hemodynamics and renal failure in whom the toxicity of calcineurin inhibitors can be avoided or decreased early after transplantation.

Although there are significant advantages to induction, the efficacy and safety of induction immunotherapy in pediatric heart transplantation remains controversial. Induction therapy may result in increased risk of severe infection and possibly increased risk of post-transplant lymphoproliferative disorders (PTLD). These risks will depend on the agents used and their dosage, the length of therapy and the amount of concomitant immunosuppression. Despite the paucity of efficacy data, the registry of the International Society for Heart and Lung Transplantation (ISHLT) shows that the use of all induction agents except OKT3 is rising [7]. Over 50% of pediatric heart transplant recipients now receive some form of induction therapy.

There are now several choices of induction agents (see Chapter 8). OKT3 is a monoclonal antibody against the lymphocyte–CD3 complex, which has been utilized for induction and treatment of severe acute rejection. It causes rapid peripheral T-cell depletion and cytokine release syndrome can be severe. Its use in adult and pediatric heart transplantation is declining. Daclizumab and basiliximab are also monoclonal antibodies but they target the α chain of the interleukin-2 (IL-2) receptor on activated T cells. Daclizumab has been shown to be an effective induction agent in cardiac transplantation [8–10]. Experience with basiliximab in heart transplantation is more limited. In a cohort of critically sick pediatric heart recipients, two doses of basiliximab were associated with low acute rejection rates despite intentional subtherapeutic dosing of calcineurin inhibitors in the immediate post-transplant period [11].

Polyclonal antibody preparations, such as equine or rabbit antithymocyte globulin (ATG), are an alternative to monoclonal preparations which have been used for many years. The most commonly used form of ATG is obtained from rabbits that have been immunized with human T cells. Polyclonal preparations have a theoretical advantage as they target multiple receptors on the T cell. These products are not as lytic as monoclonal antibodies such as OKT3, although peripheral T-cell counts do generally fall to very low levels. ATG in pediatric heart transplant patients appears to be safe [12–15]. Some groups advocate adjustment of the ATG dosage based on lymphocyte counts or on the basis of thrombocytopenia [13,14]. In a multicenter registry study, ATG induction in pediatric heart transplant recipients resulted in a lower rate of overall mortality and death resulting from rejection when compared with no induction or induction with OKT3 [15]. Most authorities conclude that polyclonal anti-T-cell antibody preparations appear superior to monoclonal depleting antibody preparations (OKT3) for induction in pediatric heart recipients, although no randomized trial has been performed to confirm this.

Intravenous immunoglobulin

In addition to antibody induction, some centers have used intravenous immunoglobulin (IVIG) preparations in the immediate post-transplantation period. IVIG is a good opsinogen, complementing the innate immune system's ability to destroy bacterial and viral infections. It can be helpful because of its anti-infectious properties but can also be immunoregulatory. IVIG can bind cytokines and other pro-inflammatory substances. It also contains anti-idiotypic antibodies that are potent inhibitors of human leukocyte antigen (HLA) specific alloantibodies *in vitro* and *in vivo*. This may be helpful in the patient who is sensitized pretransplantation against foreign HLA antigens. No randomized trials of perioperative use of IVIG have been performed following pediatric heart transplantation.

Maintenance immunosuppression

Following induction, patients must be transitioned to an immunosuppressive regimen that allows continuing immunosuppression/regulation with avoidance of graft rejection. The introduction of several new agents in the past decade has resulted in a number of potential immunosuppressive regimens,

Table 34.1 Maintenance immunosuppression regimens for pediatric heart transplant recipients.

Drug therapy regimens			
Drug class	Triple	Double	Single
Calcineurin inhibitor			
Cyclosporine	Yes	Yes	Yes
Tacrolimus			
Antimetabolite or antiproliferative			
Azathioprine	Yes	Yes	No
Mycophenolate mofetil			
Sirolimus/everolimus			
Corticosteroids			
Prednisone	Yes	No	No

none of which have been (or are likely to be) tested in randomized clinical trials in children.

The introduction of the calcineurin inhibitor (CNI), cyclosporine, in the early 1980s (the first oral agent to selectively target T-lymphocyte pathways) led to a dramatic reduction in acute rejection rates and improved graft and patient survival. A combination of cyclosporine, azathioprine and corticosteroids ("triple therapy") became the standard of care for pediatric and adult transplant recipients (Table 34.1). This regimen was used in 80–85% of patients in the 1980s to early 1990s [16].

CNIs remain the mainstay of maintenance immunosuppression. Most protocols begin CNIs in the early postoperative period, although some even start immediately pretransplantation. Intravenous preparations, delivered in a continuous infusion, are frequently used. Patients are typically converted to oral medication on postoperative day 3–5 when gastrointestinal function has returned. In addition to cyclosporine, tacrolimus (formerly knows as FK506) is gaining favor as an alternative CNI in many institutions [7]. In centers using induction therapy, it is common to delay introduction of CNIs for a few days. This may help optimize urine output and is a strategy frequently employed when pretransplant renal function is poor. Cyclosporine and tacrolimus have not been compared in large randomized trials in children after heart transplantation. One small (26 children) single-center randomized trial in pediatric heart transplantation has been performed, but was not powered to identify differences between immunosuppressive regimens [17]. A recent three-arm randomized trial of tacrolimus versus cyclosporine (along with corticosteroids and either sirolimus or mycophenolate mofetil [MMF] as adjunctive therapy) in adult heart transplantation showed lower acute rejection rates in tacrolimus treated patients [18]. There was also preliminary evidence of less early graft vasculopathy (post-transplant coronary artery disease or chronic rejection) in sirolimus treated patients.

Most centers use adjunctive therapy with an antimetabolite or antiproliferative agent in addition to a CNI (see Table 34.1). This allows for enhanced immunosuppressive efficacy, while reducing organ toxicities associated with single agents used in high dosages. Azathioprine is an antimetabolite that inhibits the growth and differentiation of immune cells – blocking the effect of cell-mediated immunity and decreasing antibody synthesis. Unfortunately, azathioprine affects all rapidly dividing cells and frequently leads to neutropenia. It also is less efficacious than other adjunctive agents that are now gaining favor. The mechanism of action of MMF is interruption of purine synthesis in lymphocytes, resulting in a diminished ability of recipient lymphocytes to respond to donor antigen. A phase III randomized trial in adults after cardiac transplantation showed a survival benefit for MMF over azathioprine [19].

The newest group of agents to be utilized as adjunctive therapies in heart transplantation is the proliferation signal or target of rapamycin (TOR) inhibitors. This group includes sirolimus and everolimus. There has been little experience with these agents in the pediatric population [20,21]. The main adverse effects have been hyperlipidemia, bone marrow suppression, mouth ulcers and poor wound healing. These agents do not demonstrate significant nephrotoxicity when used alone, but exacerbation of the nephrotoxicity caused by CNIs may occur if concomitant dose reduction of the primary immunosuppressant is not performed [22]. Life-threatening pulmonary toxicity, including pneumonitis, has also been reported with sirolimus after solid organ transplantation. The most interesting aspect of the use of TOR inhibitors is their possible role in the prevention of post-transplant coronary artery disease. Sirolimus and everolimus have antiproliferative effects on myointimal proliferation and theoretically could reduce, or prevent, graft vasculopathy in humans. Intravascular ultrasound (IVUS) studies in adults have demonstrated that coronary arterial intimal proliferation was less pronounced when MMF [19], everolimus [22] and sirolimus [23] were each compared with azathioprine in separate randomized clinical trials. MMF and sirolimus also promote donor-specific regulation in some animal models of tolerance induction whereas calcineurin inhibitors do not.

Steroids act in a nonspecific manner to affect the immune system in many different ways. Steroids prevent T-cell activation and prevent upregulation of several of the cytokine genes necessary to mount an alloimmune response [24]. Because of the significant adverse side-effects of corticosteroids in children, there has been a move to attempt to discontinue routine steroid use in maintenance immunosuppression [25,26]. Growth retardation, susceptibility to infection, impaired wound healing, hypertension and the development of a cushingoid appearance are some of the effects of long-term steroid use. In the current era, by eliminating chronic steroid use, a two-drug regimen usually includes a CNI in addition to the coadministration of either an antimetabolite or antiproliferative agent (e.g. MMF or sirolimus). It is likely that induction therapy is necessary if complete steroid avoidance is to be used post-transplantation. It is not known if a T-cell-depleting regimen is necessary or whether steroid avoidance can be routinely achieved with the use of an IL-2 receptor antagonist.

As the elucidation of immunosuppressive pathways continues to advance, many newer immunosuppressive agents will be developed that target specific critical pathways in the immune response to the allograft. These advances should lead to more focused immunosuppression, greater drug synergism, smaller doses of individual agents, steroid-sparing regimens and reduction in end-organ toxicities [27].

Infant recipients

Because of the immaturity and naivety of the neonatal immune system, young infant transplant recipients represent a unique population of patients and may be ideally suited for obtaining tolerance to their graft. For example, neonatal CD4+ T cells may be more easily influenced towards a phenotype that results in cytokine production that promotes antibody production and tolerance [28,29]. Single drug immunosuppression is possible in infant recipients with good results. Currently, approximately 70% of children transplanted at less than 2 years of age at Denver Children's Hospital are on single-drug immunotherapy.

ACUTE GRAFT REJECTION

The importance of acute rejection episodes becomes evident when causes of death after heart transplant are examined. Data from the ISHLT show that acute rejection is the most common cause of death between 30 days and 3 years after heart transplantation, accounting for almost 30% of all deaths [7]. The peak hazard, or instantaneous risk, for first rejection is 1–2 months after transplantation. By 1 year after transplantation, only 40% of pediatric heart recipients are free of acute rejection. Late acute rejection episodes (occurring beyond the first year after transplantation) appear to carry a particularly poor long-term prognosis. Understanding the risk factors for acute rejection is vital for designing effective strategies for surveillance and prevention. Older age at transplantation and recipient black race have been found to be consistent risk factors for acute rejection in children. The risk appears lowest in infant recipients.

Because moderate and severe graft rejection may occur in the absence of clinical symptoms, a highly effective monitoring system for rejection surveillance is critical. Unfortunately, no such system exists, and the optimal method of screening for rejection remains controversial. If graft dysfunction with hemodynamic compromise develops the outcome can be devastating, with up to 50% mortality reported in the year following the episode [30]. Interestingly, "rejection" with

hemodynamic compromise can often be associated with a low endomyocardial biopsy score [31]. This could be a result of sampling error of the biopsy, humoral (antibody-mediated) rejection or other poorly understood mechanisms of acute graft dysfunction. The challenge is to detect acute graft rejection at an early stage so that rejection therapy can be initiated in a timely fashion.

Detection of acute graft rejection

Some of the difficulty in accurately diagnosing and treating acute cellular rejection stems from the fact that the exact pathophysiologic mechanisms of rejection are not known. What is known is that T cells, and in particular CD4+ T cells, are required for rejection [32]. However, multiple cell lines and mechanisms are involved: the cytotoxic CD8 T-cell subpopulation and antibody producing B cells all contribute to the rejection process. Macrophages, natural killer cells and neutrophils are involved in the inflammatory response, while circulating cytokines also have a role. There is marked phenotypic variation in patient presentations of acute rejection. Not uncommonly, there is absence of a typical pathologic infiltrate on endomyocardial biopsy during episodes of rejection. Therefore, multiple different modalities of detecting graft rejection have been utilized in an attempt to offer comprehensive rejection surveillance.

Clinical assessment

Meticulous serial evaluation of the patient is of utmost importance for rejection surveillance. The onset of tachycardia or arrhythmias, rales, hepatosplenomegaly or a gallop rhythm should raise suspicion of graft rejection. Infants and young children may present with irritability, poor feeding, vomiting or lethargy [33]. Chest radiograph may demonstrate cardiomegaly, pulmonary edema and/or pleural effusions. The electrocardiogram may show reduced QRS voltages, change in QRS axis or arrhythmias. If there is high clinical index of suspicion, and suggestive echocardiographic changes of rejection (see below), rejection therapy is sometimes instituted without further (invasive) evaluation.

Role of cardiac catheterization

Cardiac catheterization for rejection surveillance remains an important tool because of the varied evaluations that can be performed with respect to graft function. Hemodynamic assessment including ventricular filling pressures, cardiac output and oxygen consumption can be helpful. Endomyocardial biopsies can be performed to provide tissue for histologic evaluation. Long after transplantation, acute graft dysfunction may be caused by post-transplant coronary artery disease (chronic rejection). Therefore, coronary artery assessment via angiography, coronary flow reserve and intravascular ultrasound can also be performed at the time of catheterization when indicated.

Historically, the endomyocardial biopsy has been considered the "gold standard" for diagnosing acute graft rejection. In the search for an objective measure of graft–host interactions, the endomyocardial biopsy was born [34]. However, because not all episodes of symptomatic rejection are associated with a positive biopsy, this tool is not universally reliable. So-called Quilty B lesions (endocardial infiltrates with myocardial extension) and residual inflammation from myocardium recovering from a previously treated rejection episode can result in diagnostic confusion [35]. False-negative biopsies can result from sampling error and from pathologist interpretation of the biopsy. In fact, a subset of patients with hemodynamic alterations consistent with rejection who subsequently respond to rejection therapy have minimal abnormalities on endomyocardial biopsy and lack a cellular infiltrate [31]. Additionally, as the time from transplantation increases, the incidence of classic acute biopsy-proven rejection decreases significantly [36]. Specifically, the utility of endomyocardial biopsy in diagnosing graft rejection in asymptomatic pediatric heart transplant patients beyond 1 year post-transplant is debatable [37]. In late follow-up, a selective approach to myocardial biopsies, on the basis of a change in clinical status or immunosuppressive medications, may be most appropriate [38].

Endomyocardial biopsy may be useful in the evaluation of humoral (antibody-mediated) rejection [39]. Immunoglobulin, complement and fibrin deposition can be confirmed with immunohistochemical staining of fresh biopsy specimens. In addition, immunoperoxidase staining for the complement product C4d can now be performed on paraffin sections, simplifying the diagnostic evaluation for humoral rejection on heart biopsies [40].

However, the costs and complications of cardiac catheterization cannot be underestimated. Limitations in peripheral venous access can make catheterization and biopsy challenging in children [35]. In particular, infant recipients present unique challenges with potential for higher risk of complications, especially when the biopsy procedure is performed from sites other than the internal jugular vein [41].

Role of echocardiography

The pediatric heart transplantation population has a great need for reliable noninvasive methods of rejection surveillance. The use of echocardiography in rejection surveillance has been validated in infant heart transplant recipients. Boucek *et al.* [42] prospectively evaluated infant heart transplant recipients and developed an echocardiographic scoring system for rejection which was correlated with endomyocardial biopsies. Multiple echocardiographic parameters need to be evaluated as there is not any single identifiable variable that can consistently predict graft rejection (our approach is outlined in Table 34.2). The utilization of this noninvasive surveillance tool, in addition to astute clinical assessments, can be effective in monitoring infant heart transplant recipients without the need for presumptive rejection therapy and frequent catheterization procedures.

Importantly, it should be noted that no prospective trials have compared outcomes among children who do, or do not, undergo invasive biopsy surveillance for acute rejection. However, excellent short- and medium-term outcomes have been reported from centers that do, and do not, rely on invasive

Table 34.2 Echocardiographic criteria for graft rejection. After Boucek *et al.* [42].

Echo parameter	Definition	Threshold	Weighted score
IVS thickening fraction	Percent change in IVS thickness from systole to diastole	< 25%	1
LVPW thickening fraction	Percent change in LVPW from systole to diastole	< 70%	2
LVEDV	Largest end-diastolic dimension	< 65%*	2
LVM	IVS and LVPW thickness measured by 2-D used for mass calculation	> 130%*	1
LVEDV/LVM		< 45%	1
Maximum velocity of LVPW thinning in diastole	Corrected for dimension	< 11 mm/s	1
Average velocity of LVPW thinning		< 25 mm/s	1
Average velocity of LV enlargement		< 60 mm/s	1
Mitral insufficiency		> 1+	1
		Total	11

IVS, interventricular septum; LVEDV, left ventricular end-diastolic volume; LVM, left ventricular mass; LVPW, left ventricular posterior wall.

* Percent of predicted normal based on body surface area.

Echocardiographic rejection grade (cumulative rejection score): Grade 1 (0), normal; Grade 2 (1–3), probably normal; Grade 3 (4–6), probable rejection; Grade 4 (7–11), rejection.

means of rejection surveillance. Multiple other noninvasive strategies for rejection surveillance are under investigation. Recent attempts to diagnose rejection based on gene expression profiling of peripheral blood leukocytes appear promising [43], with parallel studies underway in pediatric patients.

Treatment of acute graft rejection

In the presence of a high index of clinical suspicion, acute graft dysfunction (echocardiographic rejection score of ≥ 3) (see Table 34.2), or ISHLT endomyocardial biopsy grade ≥ 3A (or ≥ grade 2 in the new ISHLT classification), rejection therapy is indicated. Corticosteroids are first line therapy. High-dose intravenous methylprednisolone (10–20 mg/kg/day) for 3–4 days is administered. High-dose oral steroids are an alternative therapy, if the episode is felt to be mild.

If there is not a rapid improvement with intravenous steroids, if graft dysfunction progresses or if multiple recurrent episodes of acute rejection occur despite repeated bolus steroid therapy, cytolytic anti-T-cell antibody therapy is generally used. Rabbit ATG is the most commonly used agent, although some groups still use OKT3. If cytolytic therapy and increase in baseline maintenance immunosuppression fail to prevent recurrent rejection episodes, additional therapies may be required. Cyclosporine therapy may be discontinued and the patient transitioned to tacrolimus. Patients on azathioprine are often converted to MMF or sirolimus as adjunctive therapy. Oral corticosteroids are introduced or dosage increased. Methotrexate has also been utilized in patients with recurrent rejection episodes resistant to standard therapies. Careful monitoring for neutropenia and thrombocytopenia is performed.

Plasmapharesis has also been used successfully in patients who respond poorly to "standard" rejection therapy. In particular, these patients may have a humoral mechanism for their rejection with evidence of circulating donor-specific anti-HLA antibody and evidence for antibody deposition (IgG and/or complement) on endomyocardial biopsy. Plasmapharesis may also have a role in the elimination of proinflammatory cytokines and factors that promote either graft rejection or have direct myocardial depressive effects (e.g. TNF-α, IL-6). Typical plasmapharesis regimens involve a fivefold volume exchange and are often followed by adjunctive therapy with IVIG and/or cyclophosphamide or rituximab.

Two other therapeutic options for resistant or recurrent rejection are photopheresis and total lymphoid irradiation (TLI) [44,45]. Radiation affects all dividing cells and may be an effective immunomodulator during particularly severe episodes of rejection. Typical protocols utilize 80 cGy per treatment twice weekly for 10 treatments. In Denver, we have found TLI to be most efficacious if utilized in the first 6 months following transplantation in patients with multiple early and/or severe episodes of rejection [46]. Although these treatments are generally well tolerated, the long-term

consequences in children require further study. Long-term concerns about late lymphoma development have made this therapy a last resort in many centers.

CARDIAC ALLOGRAFT VASCULOPATHY

The terms chronic rejection and cardiac allograft vasculopathy (post-transplant coronary arterial disease) are often used synonymously. It should be noted, however, that chronic graft dysfunction is sometimes observed in the absence of evidence of coronary artery disease. This could be because of undiagnosed small vessel disease or mechanisms of graft dysfunction (e.g. progressive myocardial fibrosis) that might occur in the absence of coronary disease.

Cardiac allograft vasculopathy is the leading cause of death among late survivors of pediatric heart transplantation. It accounts for approximately 40% of deaths in the period 3–5 years after transplantation [7]. The pathology differs somewhat from that of ischemic heart disease in the normal adult population. Typical allograft coronary arterial disease consists of myointimal proliferation that is generally concentric and involves the entire length of the vessel, including intramyocardial branches. Eventually, luminal occlusion occurs. Both immune and nonimmune mechanisms likely contribute to the development of graft vasculopathy, although immune mechanisms are probably of central importance in young children.

The most detailed analysis of this problem in pediatric recipients comes from the Pediatric Heart Transplant Study (PHTS) [47]. The incidence of any angiographic evidence of coronary disease was 2%, 9% and 17% at 1, 3 and 5 years after transplantation, respectively, among 1222 children. Moderate to severe angiographic coronary disease was seen in 6% of children (compared with 15% in the comparable adult Cardiac Transplant Research Database) at 5 years after transplantation. In the PHTS analysis, older recipient age, older donor age (especially beyond 30 years) and greater number of episodes of rejection in the first year were the main risk factors for development of coronary arterial disease. These risk factors are similar to those reported in the ISHLT registry [7]. Late acute rejection episodes and noncompliance are also important risk factors [48,49].

Detection of cardiac allograft vasculopathy

Symptoms of ischemia are often absent, although some children will experience episodes of abdominal pain and/or chest pain, despite operative denervation of the heart [50]. Syncope and sudden death are also common presentations of graft coronary disease in children [49]. In the current era, the diagnosis is most often made during surveillance selective coronary angiography [47]. Dobutamine stress echocardiography has been explored as a screening method for cardiac allograft vasculopathy in children [51,52]. Mild degrees of coronary artery disease are unlikely to be detected, but dobutamine stress echocardiography may be a good tool for detecting disease sufficient to pose significant risk of graft failure, myocardial infarction or death. However, there are significant limitations of this technique that may limit its universal use; importantly, an experienced sonographer is needed to obtain accurate images and interpretation of the data must be performed by an experienced reviewer. Otherwise false-positive and false-negative results may be obtained.

Intravascular ultrasound has much greater sensitivity for this diagnosis, although experience in children is much more limited than in adults [53–55]. These studies have demonstrated that angiographically normal coronary arteries can have abnormal intimal thickening by IVUS evaluation. Coronary flow reserve (CFR) measurements may also aid in the detection of microvascular coronary disease. CFR is the ratio of hyperemic to baseline coronary flow before, and after, intracoronary infusion of a vasodilator (e.g. adenosine) and is an important indicator of small vessel disease. A low CFR (< 2.5) indicates the presence of distal microvascular endothelial dysfunction which would not be detectable by angiography. In adults, there is strong evidence that IVUS findings at 1 year are a powerful predictor of subsequent mortality, nonfatal cardiac events and the development of angiographic coronary disease [56]. Wider experience is required to fully establish the safety and clinical utility of IVUS studies in children.

Prevention and treatment of graft vasculopathy

Treating cardiovascular risk factors such as hyperlipidemia, hypertension and diabetes seems logical, although their importance in the development of graft vasculopathy in children is unclear. Many centers routinely use HMG-COA reductase inhibitors ("statins") post-transplantation. "Statins" have both lipid lowering, as well as anti-inflammatory, properties and there is increasing evidence that they may help prevent graft vasculopathy in heart transplant recipients [57,58]. Anecdotal reports, clinical trials in adults and experimental models in animals suggest that a large number of other nonimmunosuppressant therapies may also be potentially useful in preventing graft vasculopathy or its complications. These include angiotensin-converting enzyme inhibitors, antioxidants such as vitamin E, and aspirin. Diltiazem was once considered a promising therapy, but subsequent animal studies have demonstrated no effect of diltiazem on the suppression of intimal proliferation [59]. Because adherence to complex medical regimens is a significant challenge for many children and their families, it is hard to justify routine use of all these agents in the absence of proof of efficacy.

Evidence from animal work [60] and IVUS in adults suggest that coronary arterial intimal proliferation may be reduced when MMF [19], sirolimus [23] or everolimus [22] are used as part of the immunosuppressive regimen. IVUS is the best surrogate marker for the development of clinically important late graft vasculopathy and should be incorporated into all clinical trials of new immunosuppressive regimens [61]. The focus of assessment of new immunosuppressive regimens must shift from control of acute rejection to the prevention of late graft vasculopathy.

Unfortunately, no curative treatment exists for established coronary arterial disease. Coronary artery bypass grafting and coronary angioplasty and stenting have limited utility because of the diffuse and progressive nature of the disease [62]. In one randomized trial in adults, sirolimus slowed disease progression compared with continuation of standard immunosuppression [63]. Many programs are therefore adding sirolimus to the regimen of transplant recipients with newly diagnosed coronary artery disease [64,65].

The definitive treatment for progressive transplant coronary disease is retransplantation. The shortage of donors precludes this option for most recipients, especially for the older child who will be competing with adults for donor organs. Outcomes for late retransplantation (beyond 6 months) are similar to those for primary transplantation [66]. It should be noted, however, that transplant coronary artery disease can be stable over many years in pediatric patients treated aggressively [67]. It is therefore hard to know when children with coronary artery disease should be retransplanted. In general, the presence of severe angiographic disease and/or the development of systolic graft dysfunction are indications for evaluation for retransplantation.

INFECTIOUS ISSUES

The spectrum of infections after transplantation in children, and their prevention and treatment, is the focus of an earlier chapter. An increased prevalence of all forms of infection is seen compared with the general population of children. Most infections are caused by pathogens that also cause infection in the nonimmunocompromised host. Common examples include respiratory viruses, *Streptococcus pneumoniae*, and varicella virus. All infections that occur in nonimmunocompromised patients can cause greater disease severity in the recipient of a transplanted heart. Of particular note in this respect are cytomegalovirus (CMV) and Epstein–Barr virus (EBV) infection, which only rarely cause severe disease in the immunocompetent host. More rarely, opportunistic infections are seen such as that from *Pneumocystis jiroveci* (formerly *Pneumocystis carinii*). Although most infections are well tolerated, infection is second only to graft failure as the leading cause of death in the first 30 days after transplantation, and second only to rejection as the main cause of death during the remainder of the first post-transplant year [7].

The transplant physician must realize that infection of any etiology may have both short- and long-term effects in the transplant recipient. The short-term complications of serious

Table 34.3 Early postoperative cytomegalovirus (CMV) infection risk.

Donor	Recipient	Risk	Primary	Reinfection	Superinfection
–	–	Low	X		
–	+	Moderate		XX	XX
+	–	High	XXX		
+	+	Moderate		XX	XX

infections are generally self-evident. More subtle, but no less profound, is the long-term effect whereby donor graft antigens will be seen in the context of pathologic (infectious) antigens. This may lead to immunologic memory such that the threshold for destructive allograft immunity is lowered and the long-term prognosis affected. Intriguing data have recently been published showing that persistence of viral genome of various viruses (especially adenovirus) detected in the myocardium of heart biopsy samples by polymerase chain reaction (PCR) predicts the development of coronary disease and late graft loss in children [68].

Cytomegalovirus

Cytomegalovirus is a key pathogen responsible for infection-related morbidity and mortality in heart transplant recipients [69,70]. CMV testing in all donors and recipients is mandatory. Many infants less than 6 months of age will test positive for CMV but they have likely acquired the antibody passively from their mothers. Infection in adults is common (50–70% seropositive), and in normal hosts clinical disease is unusual. In the transplant recipient, infection can be primary, reactivation (secondary) or superinfection. A primary infection occurs in a patient who was previously seronegative. Reactivation, or secondary infection, occurs in a previously infected individual as a result of stress and/or immunosuppression. Reactivation of CMV is possible during the immediate postoperative period, especially during the induction phase of immunosuppression and during treatment for rejection when more aggressive immunosuppressive medications are utilized. A new strain of CMV can cause a superinfection in a previously infected individual (Table 34.3). The implications of infection are extensive as patients with CMV are predisposed to other opportunistic infections and are at increased risk for both acute graft rejection and late graft vasculopathy [71–73]. Therefore, preventing and controlling this infection are of paramount importance.

Patients in moderate and high-risk groups (see Table 34.3) should receive CMV prophylaxis in the post-transplant period. Intravenous gancyclovir should be used and some centers also use IVIG or CMV immunoglobulin. Intravenous acyclovir does not appear to have the same efficacy as intravenous gancyclovir [74,75]. Oral valgancyclovir is now being used in many centers for prevention of CMV infection after an initial period of treatment with intravenous gancyclovir. The optimal length of therapy remains to be determined and the pharmacokinetics of oral valgancyclovir in children are not well established. Another important advance in the prevention and management of CMV infection is the development of sensitive assays (most notably PCR) for the rapid diagnosis of active infection from peripheral blood samples.

Epstein–Barr virus

Epstein–Barr virus is another viral infection with significant implications in the pediatric heart transplant patient. In comparison to adult patients, a significant number of pediatric heart transplant recipients are seronegative for EBV at the time of transplantation and therefore are at risk for developing primary infection. Primary EBV infection is a key risk factor for the development of PTLD in the pediatric population. Detailed discussion regarding PTLD can be found in other areas of this text.

Other infections and antibiotic prophylaxis

A detailed review of all potential pathogens in post-transplant patients is beyond the scope of this chapter. Most protocols routinely include prophylaxis for *Pneumocystis jiroveci* (formerly *P. carinii*) with trimethoprim-sulfamethoxazole starting in the first 1–2 weeks after transplantation. Prophylaxis against *Candida* infection is also common in infants and young children. Oral nystatin is most commonly used but some centers will use an "azole" antifungal agent in high-risk patients such as those on post-transplant mechanical support or those requiring prolonged ventilation.

Some institutions utilize prophylaxis against *Toxoplasma gondii* infection in serologically negative recipients who are mismatched with a seropositive donor. This agent has tropism for cardiac muscle and is therefore of particular concern in the heart transplant recipient. Central nervous system infection has been fatal on occasion in pediatric heart transplant recipients. Prophylaxis with pyrimethamine is often used and ophthalmologic follow-up recommended in high-risk patients.

CONCLUSIONS

Pediatric heart transplantation remains a treatment option with good outcomes for infants and children with complex forms of congenital heart disease and in those with end-stage heart failure resulting from cardiomyopathy. Management of heart transplant recipients places a priority on realizing the impact of infections, invasive procedures and foreign body placement on immune stimulation and therefore ultimate transplantation outcome. Immunosuppression protocols are evolving with a general trend away from nonspecific immunosuppression. Agents that target specific aspects of the immune system may result in improved survival rates with less associated comorbidities. The optimal methods for rejection surveillance remain to be defined and acute rejection remains an important cause of death after transplantation. The prevention of chronic allograft vasculopathy will be key to the improvement of late outcomes. Pediatric heart transplantation has shown improving outcomes with each passing era and has an optimistic future given the continuing advancements in immunosuppressive therapy and the improved understanding of the mechanisms involved in graft rejection and acceptance.

ACKNOWLEDGMENT

Supported in part from NIH RO1 67977 01.

REFERENCES

1 Sweet SC, Wong HH, Webber SA, *et al*. Pediatric transplantation in the United States, 1995–2004. *Am J Transplant* 2006;**6**: 1132–52.

2 Blume ED. Current status of heart transplantation in children: update 2003. *Pediatr Clin North Am* 2003;**50**:1375–91.

3 Luikart H. Pediatric cardiac transplantation: management issues. *J Pediatr Nurs* 2001;**16**:320–31.

4 Williams MA, Onami TM, Adams AB, *et al*. Cutting edge: persistent viral infection prevents tolerance induction and escapes immune control following CD28/CD40 blockade-based regimen. *J Immunol* 2002;**169**:5387–91.

5 Goldstein DR, Tesar BM. Toll-like receptors and allograft rejection. *Am J Respir Crit Care Med* 2004;**169**:971; author reply 971–2.

6 Larsen CP, Elwood ET, Alexander DZ, *et al*. Long-term acceptance of skin and cardiac allografts after blocking CD40 and CD28 pathways. *Nature* 1996;**381**:434–8.

7 Boucek MM, Edwards LB, Keck BM, *et al*. Registry of the International Society for Heart and Lung Transplantation: eighth official pediatric report, 2005. *J Heart Lung Transplant* 2005; **24**:968–82.

8 Beniaminovitz A, Itescu S, Lietz K, *et al*. Prevention of rejection in cardiac transplantation by blockade of the interleukin-2 receptor with a monoclonal antibody. *N Engl J Med* 2000; **342**:613–9.

9 Kobashigawa J, David K, Morris J, *et al*. Daclizumab is associated with decreased rejection and no increased mortality in cardiac transplant patients receiving MMF, cyclosporine, and corticosteroids. *Transplant Proc* 2005;**37**:1333–9.

10 Chin C, Pittson S, Luikart H, *et al*. Induction therapy for pediatric and adult heart transplantation: comparison between OKT3 and daclizumab. *Transplantation* 2005;**80**:477–81.

11 Ford KA, Cale CM, Rees PG, Elliott MJ, Burch M. Initial data on basiliximab in critically ill children undergoing heart transplantation. *J Heart Lung Transplant* 2005;**24**:1284–8.

12 Lebeck LK, Chang L, Lopez-McCormack C, Chinnock R, Boucek M. Polyclonal antithymocyte serum: immune prophylaxis and rejection therapy in pediatric heart transplantation patients. *J Heart Lung Transplant* 1993;**12**:S286–92.

13 Parisi F, Danesi H, Squitieri C, *et al*. Thymoglobuline use in pediatric heart transplantation. *J Heart Lung Transplant* 2003; **22**:591–3.

14 Di Filippo S, Boissonnat P, Sassolas F, *et al*. Rabbit antithymocyte globulin as induction immunotherapy in pediatric heart transplantation. *Transplantation* 2003;**75**:354–8.

15 Boucek RJ Jr, Naftel D, Boucek MM, *et al*. Induction immunotherapy in pediatric heart transplant recipients: a multicenter study. *J Heart Lung Transplant* 1999;**18**:460–9.

16 Smith JM, Nemeth TL, McDonald RA. Current immunosuppressive agents: efficacy, side effects, and utilization. *Pediatr Clin North Am* 2003;**50**:1283–300.

17 Pollock-Barziv SM, Dipchand AI, McCrindle BW, Nalli N, West LJ. Randomized clinical trial of tacrolimus- vs cyclosporine-based immunosuppression in pediatric heart transplantation: preliminary results at 15-month follow-up. *J Heart Lung Transplant* 2005;**24**:190–4.

18 Kobashigawa JA, Miller LW, Russell SD, *et al*. Tacrolimus with mycophenolate mofetil (MMF) or sirolimus vs. cyclosporine with MMF in cardiac transplant patients: 1-year report. *Am J Transplant* 2006;**6**:1377–86.

19 Eisen HJ, Kobashigawa J, Keogh A, *et al*. Mycophenolate Mofetil Cardiac Study Investigators. Three-year results of a randomized, double-blind, controlled trial of mycophenolate mofetil versus azathioprine in cardiac transplant recipients. *J Heart Lung Transplant* 2005;**24**:517–25.

20 Lobach NE, Pollock-Barziv SM, West LJ, Dipchand AI. Sirolimus immunosuppression in pediatric heart transplant recipients: a single-center experience. *J Heart Lung Transplant* 2005;**24**: 184–9.

21 Sindhi R, Webber SA, Venkataramanan R, *et al*. Sirolimus for rescue and primary immunosuppression in transplanted children receiving tacrolimus. *Transplantation* 2001;**72**:851–5.

22 Eisen HJ, Tuzcu EM, Dorent R, *et al*. RAD B253 Study Group. Everolimus for the prevention of allograft rejection and vasculopathy in cardiac-transplant recipients. *N Engl J Med* 2003;**349**: 847–58.

23 Keogh A, Richardson M, Ruygrok P, *et al*. Sirolimus in *de novo* heart transplant recipients reduces acute rejection and prevents coronary artery disease at 2 years: a randomized clinical trial. *Circulation* 2004;**110**:2694–700.

24 Pietra BA. Transplantation immunology 2003: simplified approach. *Pediatr Clin North Am* 2003;**50**:1233–59.

25 Livi U, Caforio AL, Gambino A, *et al*. Cyclosporine-based steroid-free therapy in pediatric heart transplantation: long-term results. *Transplant Proc* 1998;**30**:1975–6.

26 Ferrazzi P, Fiocchi R, Gamba A, *et al*. Pediatric heart transplantation without chronic maintenance steroids. *J Heart Lung Transplant* 1993;**12**:S241–5.

27 Reddy SC, Laughlin K, Webber SA. Immunosuppression in pediatric heart transplantation: 2003 and beyond. *Curr Treat Options Cardiovasc Med* 2003;5:417–28.

28 Mosmann TR, Schumacher JH, Street NF, *et al.* Diversity of cytokine synthesis and function of mouse CD4⁺ T cells. *Immunol Rev* 1991;**123**:209–29.

29 Delespesse G, Yang LP, Ohshima Y, *et al.* Maturation of human neonatal CD4⁺ and CD8⁺ T lymphocytes into Th1/Th2 effectors. *Vaccine* 1998;**16**:1415–9.

30 Pahl E, Naftel DC, Canter CE, *et al.* Death after rejection with severe hemodynamic compromise in pediatric heart transplant recipients: a multi-institutional study. *J Heart Lung Transplant* 2001;**20**:279–87.

31 Mills RM, Naftel DC, Kirklin JK, *et al.* Heart transplant rejection with hemodynamic compromise: a multiinstitutional study of the role of endomyocardial cellular infiltrate. Cardiac Transplant Research Database. *J Heart Lung Transplant* 1997;**16**:813–21.

32 Pietra BA, Wiseman A, Bolwerk A, Rizeq M, Gill RG. CD4 T cell-mediated cardiac allograft rejection requires donor but not host MHC class II. *J Clin Invest* 2000;**106**:1003–10.

33 Chinnock RE, Baum MF, Larsen R, Bailey L. Rejection management and long-term surveillance of the pediatric heart transplant recipient: the Loma Linda experience. *J Heart Lung Transplant* 1993;**12**:S255–64.

34 Caves PK, Stinson EB, Graham AF, *et al.* Percutaneous transvenous endomyocardial biopsy. *JAMA* 1973;**225**:288–91.

35 Levi DS, DeConde AS, Fishbein MC, *et al.* The yield of surveillance endomyocardial biopsies as a screen for cellular rejection in pediatric heart transplant patients. *Pediatr Transplant* 2004;**8**:22–8.

36 Wagner K, Oliver MC, Boyle GJ, *et al.* Endomyocardial biopsy in pediatric heart transplant recipients: a useful exercise? (Analysis of 1169 biopsies). *Pediatr Transplant* 2000;**4**:186–92.

37 Boucek MM. Surveillance endomyocardial biopsy in pediatric heart transplantation: fashion or foible? *Pediatr Transplant* 2000;**4**:173–6.

38 White JA, Guiraudon C, Pflugfelder PW, Kostuk WJ. Routine surveillance myocardial biopsies are unnecessary beyond one year after heart transplantation. *J Heart Lung Transplant* 1995;**14**:1052–6.

39 Reed EF, Demetris AJ, Hammond E, *et al.* International Society for Heart and Lung Transplantation. Acute antibody-mediated rejection of cardiac transplants. *J Heart Lung Transplant* 2006;**25**:153–9.

40 Chantranuwat C, Qiao JH, Kobashigawa J, *et al.* Immunoperoxidase staining for C4d on paraffin-embedded tissue in cardiac allograft endomyocardial biopsies: comparison to frozen tissue immunofluorescence. *Appl Immunohistochem Mol Morphol* 2004;**12**:166–71.

41 Pophal SG, Sigfusson G, Booth KL, *et al.* Complications of endomyocardial biopsy in children. *J Am Coll Cardiol* 1999;**34**:2105–10.

42 Boucek MM, Mathis CM, Boucek RJ Jr, *et al.* Prospective evaluation of echocardiography for primary rejection surveillance after infant heart transplantation: comparison with endomyocardial biopsy. *J Heart Lung Transplant* 1994;**13**:66–73.

43 Deng MC, Eisen HJ, Mehra MR, *et al.*, CARGO Investigators. Noninvasive discrimination of rejection in cardiac allograft recipients using gene expression profiling. *Am J Transplant* 2006;**6**:150–60.

44 Kirklin JK, Brown RN, Huang ST, *et al.* Rejection with hemodynamic compromise: objective evidence for efficacy of photopheresis. *J Heart Lung Transplant* 2006;**25**:283–8. (Epub 2006, Jan 25.)

45 Kirklin JK, George JF, McGiffin DC, *et al.* Total lymphoid irradiation: is there a role in pediatric heart transplantation? *J Heart Lung Transplant* 1993;**12**:S293–300.

46 Pietra B, Mashburn WD, C *et al.* Total lymphoid irradiation (TLI) for treatment of resistant rejection in pediatric heart transplant patients. In: 15th Scientific Session of the International Society for Heart and Lung Transplantation. San Francisco, 1995.

47 Pahl E, Naftel DC, Kuhn MA, *et al.* Pediatric Heart Transplant Study. The impact and outcome of transplant coronary artery disease in a pediatric population: a 9-year multi-institutional study. *J Heart Lung Transplant* 2005;**24**:645–51.

48 Mulla NF, Johnston JK, Vander Dussen L, *et al.* Late rejection is a predictor of transplant coronary artery disease in children. *J Am Coll Cardiol* 2001;**37**:243–50.

49 Pahl E, Zales VR, Fricker FJ, Addonizio LJ. Posttransplant coronary artery disease in children: a multicenter national survey. *Circulation* 1994;**90**:II56–60.

50 Price JF, Towbin JA, Dreyer WJ, *et al.* Symptom complex is associated with transplant coronary artery disease and sudden death/resuscitated sudden death in pediatric heart transplant recipients. *J Heart Lung Transplant* 2005;**24**:1798–803.

51 Larsen RL, Applegate PM, Dyar DA, *et al.* Dobutamine stress echocardiography for assessing coronary artery disease after transplantation in children. *J Am Coll Cardiol* 1998;**32**:515–20.

52 Pahl E, Crawford SE, Swenson JM, *et al.* Dobutamine stress echocardiography: experience in pediatric heart transplant recipients. *J Heart Lung Transplant* 1999;**18**:725–32.

53 Ventura HO, Ramee SR, Jain A, *et al.* Coronary artery imaging with intravascular ultrasound in patients following cardiac transplantation. *Transplantation* 1992;**53**:216–9.

54 Costello JM, Wax DF, Binns HJ, *et al.* A comparison of intravascular ultrasound with coronary angiography for evaluation of transplant coronary artery disease in pediatric heart transplant recipients. *J Heart Lung Transplant* 2003;**22**:44–9.

55 Kuhn MA, Jutzy KR, Deming DD, *et al.* The medium-term findings in coronary arteries by intravascular ultrasound in infants and children after heart transplantation. *J Am Coll Cardiol* 2000;**36**:250–4.

56 Kobashigawa JA, Tobis JM, Starling RC, *et al.* Multicenter intravascular ultrasound validation study among heart transplant recipients: outcomes after five years. *J Am Coll Cardiol* 2005;**45**:1532–7.

57 Kobashigawa JA, Moriguchi JD, Laks H, *et al.* Ten-year follow-up of a randomized trial of pravastatin in heart transplant patients. *J Heart Lung Transplant* 2005;**24**:1736–40.

58 Mahle WT, Vincent RN, Berg AM, Kanter KR. Pravastatin therapy is associated with reduction in coronary allograft vasculopathy in pediatric heart transplantation. *J Heart Lung Transplant* 2005;**24**:63–6.

59 Takami H, Backer CL, Crawford SE, Pahl E, Mavroudis C. Diltiazem preserves direct vasodilator response but fails to suppress intimal proliferation in rat allograft coronary artery disease. *J Heart Lung Transplant* 1996;**15**:67–77.

60 Poston RS, Billingham M, Hoyt EG, *et al.* Rapamycin reverses chronic graft vascular disease in a novel cardiac allograft model. *Circulation* 1999;**100**:67–74.

61 Mehra MR, Benza R, Deng M, Russell S, Webber SA. Surrogate markers for late cardiac allograft survival. Proceedings of an AST/ASTS Sponsored NIH Consensus Conference, November 2001. *Am J Transplant* 2004;**4**:1184–91.

62 Tham EB, Yeung AC, Cheng CW, *et al.* Experience of percutaneous coronary intervention in the management of pediatric cardiac allograft vasculopathy. *J Heart Lung Transplant* 2005;**24**:769–73.

63 Mancini D, Pinney S, Burkhoff D, *et al.* Use of rapamycin slows progression of cardiac transplantation vasculopathy. *Circulation* 2003;**108**:48–53.

64 Eisen H, Kobashigawa J, Starling RC, Valantine H, Mancini D. Improving outcomes in heart transplantation: the potential of proliferation signal inhibitors. *Transplant Proc* 2005;**37**(Suppl):4–17.

65 Hummel M. Recommendations for use of Certican (everolimus) after heart transplantation: results from a German and Austrian Consensus Conference. *J Heart Lung Transplant* 2005;**24**(Suppl): S196–200; discussion S210–1.

66 Mahle WT, Vincent RN, Kanter KR. Cardiac retransplantation in childhood: analysis of data from the United Network for Organ Sharing. *J Thorac Cardiovasc Surg* 2005;**130**:542–6.

67 Pietra B, Boucek M. Coronary artery vasculopathy in pediatric cardiac transplant patients: the therapeutic potential of immunomodulators. *Paediatr Drugs* 2003;**5**:513–24.

68 Shirali GS, Ni J, Chinnock RE, *et al.* Association of viral genome with graft loss in children after cardiac transplantation. *N Engl J Med* 2001;**344**:1498–503.

69 Dummer JS, White LT, Ho M, *et al.* Morbidity of cytomegalovirus infection in recipients of heart or heart-lung transplants who received cyclosporine. *J Infect Dis* 1985;**152**:1182–91.

70 Patel R, Snydman DR, Rubin RH, *et al.* Cytomegalovirus prophylaxis in solid organ transplant recipients. *Transplantation* 1996;**61**:1279–89.

71 Grattan MT, Moreno-Cabral CE, Starnes VA, *et al.* Cytomegalovirus infection is associated with cardiac allograft rejection and atherosclerosis. *JAMA* 1989;**261**:3561–6.

72 Paya CV. Prevention of cytomegalovirus disease in recipients of solid-organ transplants. *Clin Infect Dis* 2001;**32**:596–603.

73 Valantine H. Cardiac allograft vasculopathy after heart transplantation: risk factors and management. *J Heart Lung Transplant* 2004;**23**(Suppl 1):S187–93.

74 Cole NL, Balfour HH Jr. *In vitro* susceptibility of cytomegalovirus isolates from immunocompromised patients to acyclovir and ganciclovir. *Diagn Microbiol Infect Dis* 1987;**6**:255–61.

75 Duncan SR, Grgurich WF, Iacono AT, *et al.* A comparison of ganciclovir and acyclovir to prevent cytomegalovirus after lung transplantation. *Am J Respir Crit Care Med* 1994;**150**:146–52.

35 Outcomes and Risk Factors

W. Robert Morrow and Richard E. Chinnock

Cardiac transplantation is a generally accepted approach to the treatment of end-stage heart disease in children with good early and intermediate survival reported from many institutions, multi-institutional studies and registries [1–16]. The number of centers in the USA and abroad that perform heart transplants in children is large but the total number of transplants performed each year is relatively small [12]. Consequently, the number of transplant procedures performed at any single institution averages five transplants per year, with very few centers performing more than 10 per year in pediatric recipients. The registry of the International Society for Heart and Lung Transplantation (ISHLT) records 5569 cardiac transplant procedures in children ranging from 11 in 1982 to 359 in 2002 [12], although the frequency of pediatric heart transplantation has declined slightly since a peak of 388 in 1993. Published experience demonstrates varying survival by center, patient age at transplant, diagnosis at listing and era of transplant in addition to a number of specific pretransplant risk factors. Important improvements in overall survival have been observed over time in both individual program experience and in registry and database reports (Annual Report of the Pediatric Heart Transplant Study Group, November 2004, unpublished data) [12]. In addition to mortality after transplantation, overall mortality for potential transplant recipients is significant prior to transplantation. Here we discuss survival of children who require primary heart transplantation inclusive of pretransplant mortality and risk factors for death before and after transplantation.

PRETRANSPLANT MORTALITY AND RISK FACTORS

Several studies have addressed pretransplant mortality in infants and children after listing for cardiac transplantation [16–24]. Mortality while waiting varies among institutions with reports ranging from 11% [8] to 30% [16,17]. McGiffin *et al.* [18], analyzing the Pediatric Heart Transplant Study (PHTS) experience (a prospective multi-institutional study of North American pediatric heart transplant centers initiated

in 1993), described for the first time the use of parametric competing outcomes analysis to study mortality while waiting in potential cardiac transplant recipients. In this study of 264 children listed for transplantation, ages ranged from 3 days to 17.9 years with a mean age of 4.7 years. Sixty percent of patients underwent transplantation by 6 months after listing, 23% died while waiting, 14% remained on the list awaiting transplantation and 4% improved and were removed from the list. In the Pittsburgh series [15], death while waiting was more likely to occur among blood type O recipients and those on ventilators, with the highest risk of death while waiting (33% of listed patients) occurring in candidates with both these risk factors. In the USA, the United Network for Organ Sharing (UNOS) policy now prioritizes allocation of blood type O donors to O recipients (discussed below) and this policy was designed to diminish the unfavorable allocation of O donors to recipients with other blood groups. At present, it is unclear whether this new allocation system addresses the concerns of distribution of O donors to non-O recipients, although preliminary evidence suggests no benefit in reduction of waiting time for type O recipients [24]. Death in children primarily occurs as a result of refractory heart failure, but sudden arrhythmic death is not uncommon.

The reports by Chiavarelli *et al.* [16] and Canter *et al.* [17] emphasized a higher pretransplant mortality of 25–30% among infants listed for transplantation. In a separate analysis of the PHTS database of infants (less than 6 months of age) who were listed for transplantation [19], nearly one-third died awaiting transplantation, although 60% did undergo transplantation by 6 months. Only 6% remained on the list awaiting transplantation at 1 year. Most infants listed for transplantation had hypoplastic left heart syndrome (HLHS) (70 of 118 patients, 59%) and were prostaglandin dependent, with the few surviving on the list having undergone interim Norwood palliation. The fate of infants listed for transplantation was largely determined by 3 months after listing. Risk factors for death while waiting among infants were the need for inotropic support at listing ($P = 0.02$), smaller size (weight) at listing ($P = 0.0007$) and recipient blood type O ($P = 0.003$). Similarly, risk factors for a longer time until transplantation were

299

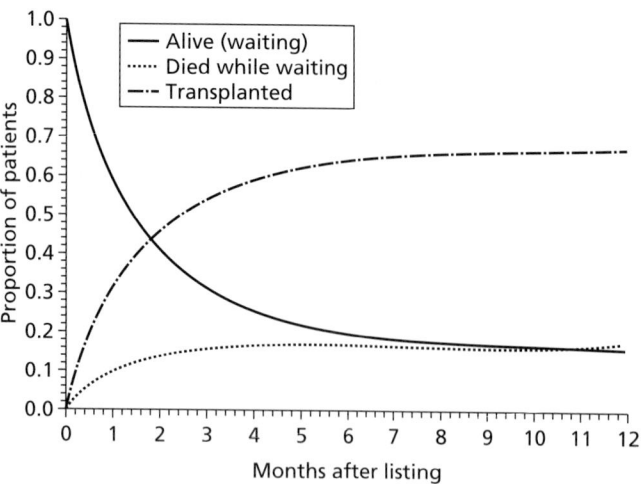

Fig. 35.1 Competing outcomes analysis of all 2375 patients listed for transplantation from January 1, 1993 through December 31, 2003 in the Pediatric Heart Transplant Study (PHTS) (*n* = 2375). The competing outcomes analysis provides a time-related parametric prediction of simultaneous mutually exclusive events. The sum of the proportions at any time after listing is equal to 1. The proportion of patients transplanted increases over time to 68% by 1 year after listing while the proportion who die increases to a maximum of 17% by 1 year.

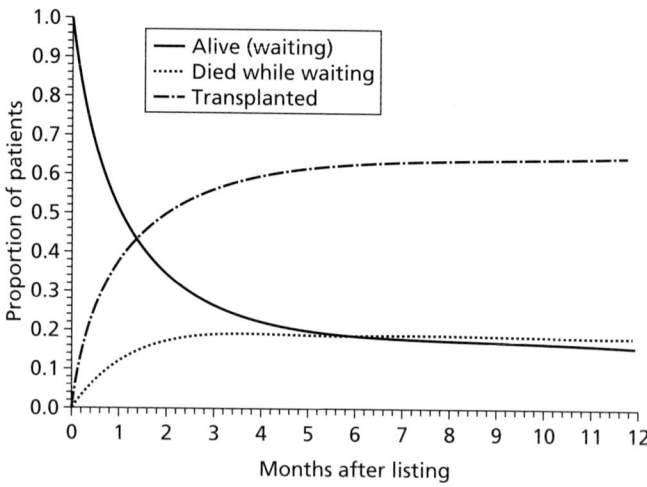

Fig. 35.2 A competing outcomes depiction for patients listed within the Pediatric Heart Transplant Study (PHTS) as United Network for Organ Sharing (UNOS) Status 1/1A (highest urgency status) from January 1, 1993 through December 31, 2003 (*n* = 643). Sixty-two percent survived to transplantation whereas 20% died waiting. Within 4–5 months after listing, all patients who were to receive a donor heart are predicted to have undergone transplantation and essentially all deaths while waiting are predicted to have occurred.

smaller size at listing (*P* = 0.001), blood type O (*P* = 0.0006) for patients with HLHS, and younger age at listing (*P* = 0.01) for patients without HLHS. Prostaglandin-dependent patients with HLHS were more likely to die waiting and less likely to undergo transplantation than infants without HLHS. Death in neonates, often patients with HLHS, may occur from heart failure, sepsis, necrotizing enterocolitis, restrictive atrial communication, as well as a variety of other causes.

The most recent analysis of the PHTS includes 2375 children listed from January 1993 through December 2003 for primary transplantation (Annual Report of the Pediatric Heart Transplant Study Group, November 2004, unpublished data). Of these, 38% were Status 1 (old allocation system), 27% were Status 1A and 6% were Status 1B. Twenty-six percent were Status 2 at listing. Overall, 22% had HLHS, 35% had other unoperated or operated congenital heart defects, and 43% had cardiomyopathy or myocarditis. In the competing outcome analysis of this entire PHTS experience (Fig. 35.1), mortality while waiting at 1 year was 17%, while 68% of patients survived to transplantation. This represents a small improvement in overall survival while waiting and survival to transplantation since the first analysis by McGiffin *et al.* [18]. For patients listed as Status 1 and 1A, 62% survived to transplantation and 20% died while waiting (Fig. 35.2). For children listed as Status 1B and 2, mortality while waiting by 1 year after listing was only 5–7%, leading some to question the appropriateness of listing patients as Status 2. However, many patients listed as Status 1B and 2 deteriorate while awaiting transplant and children listed as Status 1B

and 2 often have poor quality of life and failure to thrive. The UNOS urgency status system for heart transplantation is designed for organ allocation to those at greatest risk of dying. The favorable survival while waiting for Status 1B and 2 candidates implies that the urgency status system appears to be meeting its primary objective of prioritizing those patients most likely to die soon without transplantation. The PHTS data also demonstrate a notable improvement in survival prior to transplantation during the most recent era of analysis (1999–2003). Actuarial survival for those who remain on the list waiting for transplantation, excluding those who have undergone transplantation, was 64% at 1 year compared with approximately 38% in prior experience (Fig. 35.3). Chrisant *et al.* [22], also studying the PHTS dataset, has noted a recent improvement in survival following listing for transplant in infants with HLHS. This improvement in survival appears to be related to reduced competition for infant donor hearts as well as improved management of infants with HLHS awaiting transplantation [22,23]. There is no evidence of an increase in organ availability to account for this change.

SURVIVAL AND RISK FACTORS AFTER TRANSPLANTATION

A number of institutions have reported excellent early and intermediate survival in both infants and children following cardiac transplantation [1–11,13,15–17]. It is difficult to compare results between individual center and multicenter

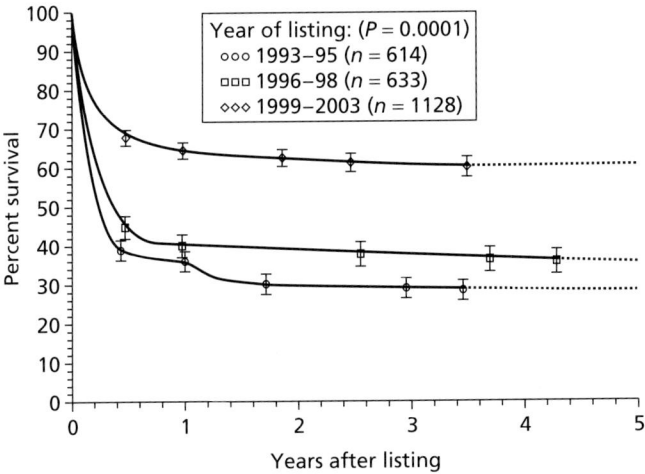

Fig. 35.3 Actuarial survival in pediatric patients 0–18 years of age in the Pediatric Heart Transplant Study (PHTS) who underwent listing for primary cardiac transplantation between January 1, 1993 to December 31, 2003 stratified by era of listing. There is a significant improvement in survival while waiting in the current era (1999–2003) compared with previous eras (1993–95, 1996–98). Patients were censored at time of transplant.

reports because of differences in recipient selection, era of transplant, evolving surgical experience, and differences in immunosuppressive and surveillance regimens. Moreover, survival data is often only reported stratified by era or by patient variables. Shaddy *et al.* [14] reported the initial PHTS survival experience and risk factor analysis among 191 children older than 1 year of age who underwent transplantation. Actuarial survival after transplant was 93% at 1 month and 82% at 1 year. By multivariable analysis, the major risk factor for death was the need for an assist device at the time of transplant (*P* = 0.02). Younger age was a significant risk factor for death in the multivariable analysis of this group of patients over 1 year of age at transplant. Patients in the 1–5 year age range had a 1-year actuarial survival of 74% compared with 86% for patients over 5 years of age at transplant. This observation of increased mortality in young children has been noted by others. Importantly, overall survival among Status 1 and 2 patients was not different.

In the Pittsburgh experience [15], an important risk factor for death in Status 1 patients was the requirement for a mechanical assist device prior to transplantation. In the pediatric age group, this usually means the use of extracorporeal membrane oxygenation (ECMO) although a variety of left ventricular assist devices are used including centrifugal pumps functioning as left ventricular assist devices as well as the Thoratec® and HeartMate® left ventricular assist devices in adolescents. Studies by a number of investigators have confirmed greater mortality in pediatric patients requiring mechanical assistance with ECMO [25–28], although an intermediate survival as great as 50% can be achieved. Stiller *et al.* [29] reported survival of 72% at 1 and 5 years following

bridge to transplant with the Berlin Heart pneumatic paracorporeal ventricular assist device. Survival in adolescents has also been reported using the DeBakey axial flow left ventricular assist device as a bridge to transplant [30].

Survival data reported by the ISHLT are in keeping with other multicenter studies and single institution experiences, with a 1-year survival of approximately 85% and a 4-year survival of 72% [12]. Fifteen-year actuarial survival for the earliest cohort of patients in the ISHLT registry (1982–88) is 40%. However, for this same cohort, actuarial survival at 4 years was 60%, whereas the actuarial survival at 4 years for the current era (1999–2002) is 72%. Most of this improved survival benefit is seen in the first year following transplant, with current 1-year survival of 90% compared with 75% in the era 1982–88. In fact, most of the benefit is seen within the first 6 months after transplantation. Risk factors for death at 1 year after transplantation were need for a ventilator prior to transplant and hospitalization prior to transplant, although the need for intravenous inotropic support and ECMO support were not risk factors for death. Interestingly, neither donor ischemic time nor transplant center volume were risk factors for death after transplantation, in contrast to previous analyses of the ISHLT registry data. The lack of a clear relation between center volume and survival was clarified in the study by Balfour *et al.* [31]. This report from the PHTS study group demonstrated that differences in survival at low volume centers did not persist with greater experience with transplantation, and hence experience, or the lack of it, and not annual volume, seems to be the key determinant of center specific mortality.

The most recent analysis of the PHTS data is in keeping with the ISHLT Registry report (Annual Report of the Pediatric Heart Transplant Study Group, November 2004, unpublished data). Of the 1644 transplanted patients, 39% were less than 1 year, 37% were between 1 and 12 years and 25% were greater than 12 years of age at transplant. Sixty-eight percent of patients were UNOS Status 1 or 1A. Overall, actuarial survival after transplantation for all age groups was 85% at 1 year and 75% at 5 years (Fig. 35.4a). One-year survival ranged from 82% in recipients less than 1 year of age at transplant to 88% in children more than 12 years of age. Neither urgency status at transplant nor ischemic time affected 5-year survival. However, survival in patients at PHTS centers was significantly better after 1996 compared with prior to that time (Fig. 35.4b). At this point, implementation of the new UNOS urgency status designation in January 2001 does not appear to have had any impact on post-transplant survival [24].

To summarize the two multi-institutional analyses above, improvements in survival after transplantation have occurred over recent years. A close examination of actuarial survival curves in the ISHLT and PHTS studies demonstrates that the greatest improvement in survival occurs within months following transplant while a constant hazard for death following transplant begins within 6 months of transplant.

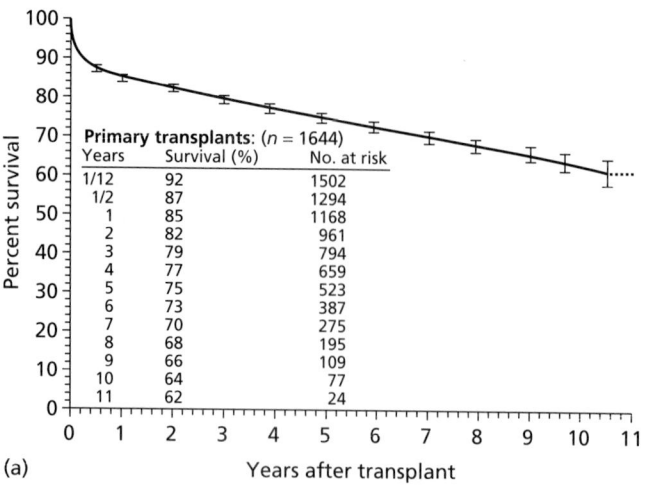

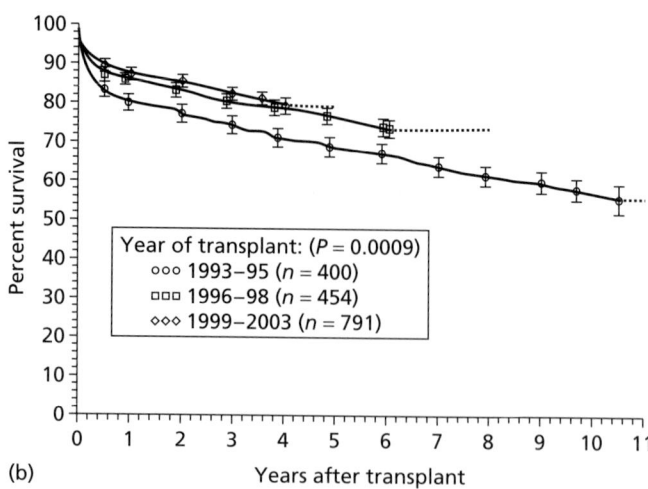

Primary transplants: (n = 1644)		
Years	Survival (%)	No. at risk
1/12	92	1502
1/2	87	1294
1	85	1168
2	82	961
3	79	794
4	77	659
5	75	523
6	73	387
7	70	275
8	68	195
9	66	109
10	64	77
11	62	24

(a) Years after transplant

(b) Years after transplant

Fig. 35.4 (a) Actuarial survival in the most current Pediatric Heart Transplant Study (PHTS) analysis (Annual Report of the Pediatric Heart Transplant Study Group, November 2004, unpublished data) among 1644 patients undergoing primary heart transplantation. A short early phase hazard for mortality is seen prior to 6 months post-transplant with an ongoing constant hazard for death thereafter. Survival is 85% at 1 year, 75% at 5 years and 64% at 10 years. (b) Survival after transplantation is significantly better after 1996 compared with before.

What is disturbing is the unchanged and continuing constant hazard for death after transplantation in both large multi-institutional experiences despite an era of transplantation and the associated improvements in management. In other words, recent advances in immunosuppression and medical management after transplant appear not to have affected intermediate and late mortality.

While it is important to know the risk of death before and after transplantation, patients and families are often most interested in knowing the chance of survival after listing, whether transplantation occurs or not. When one combines pre- and post-transplant mortality, that is death after listing regardless of transplantation, it is evident that the combined mortality before and after transplant is quite significant (Fig. 35.5a). In such an analysis, 1-year survival is 74%, 5-year survival is 66% and 10-year survival is 59%. More than half of the total mortality observed after listing occurs in the first year, irrespective of transplantation. However, improvement in 1-year survival after listing (irrespective of transplantation) improved over time, with 1-year survival after listing of 66% in the era 1993–95 to approximately 80% in the most recent era (1999–2003) (Fig. 35.5b).

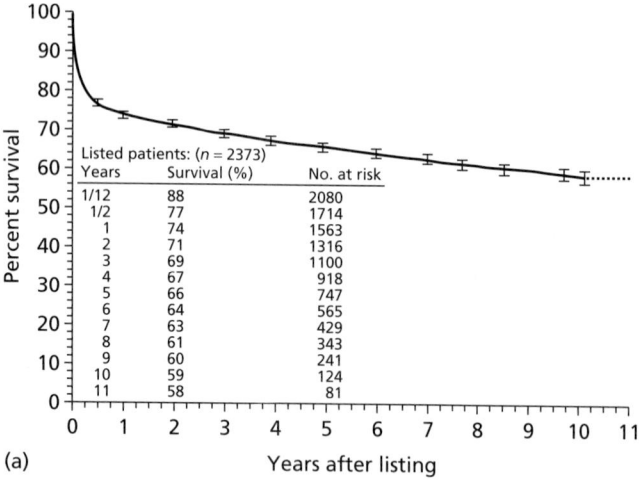

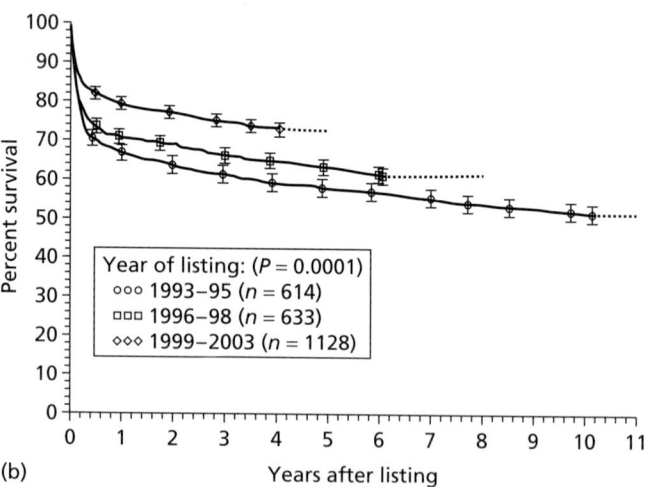

Listed patients: (n = 2373)		
Years	Survival (%)	No. at risk
1/12	88	2080
1/2	77	1714
1	74	1563
2	71	1316
3	69	1100
4	67	918
5	66	747
6	64	565
7	63	429
8	61	343
9	60	241
10	59	124
11	58	81

(a) Years after listing

(b) Years after listing

Fig. 35.5 (a) An actuarial depiction of survival irrespective of transplantation from the time of listing. Mortality in this analysis represents combined mortality while waiting and after transplantation. Survival after listing, whether transplanted or not, was 74% at 1 year, 66% at 5 years and 59% at 10 years. Most pretransplant mortality occurs in the first year after listing. Later mortality at 5 and 10 years reflects the cumulative effect of this early mortality, early post-transplant mortality, and the ongoing constant hazard for death after transplantation. (b) The effect of era on survival after listing irrespective of transplant. A significant improvement in survival after listing is demonstrated in the current era (1999–2003).

SURVIVAL IN INFANTS

Infant transplantation has always represented a special case of cardiac transplantation experience in children [1,5,13,16, 32–34]. A neonatal "window of opportunity" for organ transplantation has been proposed. The proposition is that there exists a decreased level of immunity during the newborn period, making engraftment and graft tolerance more likely the earlier a baby can receive his or her transplant [33]. Bailey et al. [1,5,13,16] reported the successful use of transplantation for infants with lethal heart disease and specifically for those with HLHS. Survival from the Loma Linda experience was 85% at 1 year and 80% at 5 years in 139 infants who underwent heart transplantation for a variety of diagnoses [1]. In a group with HLHS, survival was similar with a 5-year actuarial survival of 74% [16]. By far the most mortality was early, even perioperative, and was the result of early graft failure caused by primary graft dysfunction, pulmonary hypertension or technical factors. Others have reported excellent early survival in this age group [2]. Canter et al. [32] examined early survival after heart transplantation in the PHTS experience among infants less than 1 year at transplant. The majority of infants (66%) had HLHS. Survival was less than in older children, with 70% of infants surviving at 1 year compared with 82% in children older than 1 year. The peak hazard for death was within the first month post-transplant, with 16% of patients dying in this interval. Risk factors for death included a history of previous sternotomy (P = 0.0003) and a cause of donor death other than closed head trauma. Previous history of sternotomy in this age group implies a very recent attempt at repair and therefore represents a particularly high-risk group of patients for any intervention. Most deaths after transplantation occurred as a result of early graft failure or pulmonary hypertension. When combined, these two causes of death accounted for 75% of deaths in the infant age group. In the most recent PHTS analysis (Annual Report of the Pediatric Heart Transplant Study Group, November 2004, unpublished data), 1-year survival among infants less than 6 months of age at transplant was 80% at 1 year and 70% at 9 years post-transplant compared with older children where 1-year survival was 87% and 5-year survival was 66%. The 14 year Loma Linda University Medical Center infant heart transplantation experience offers the opportunity to study this important group of recipients in more detail [33].

Between November 1985 and December 2004, 412 infants and children underwent transplantation at Loma Linda University. Of these, 282 were transplanted during the first year of life. Within this experience, there have been 157 infants transplanted for HLHS, 76 in the first month of life and 81 from 1 month to 6 months of age. Patient and graft survival for newborn versus infant HLHS recipients is illustrated in Figure 35.6. Long-term patient survival for newborns was 77% at 10 years and 71% at 15 years and for infants was

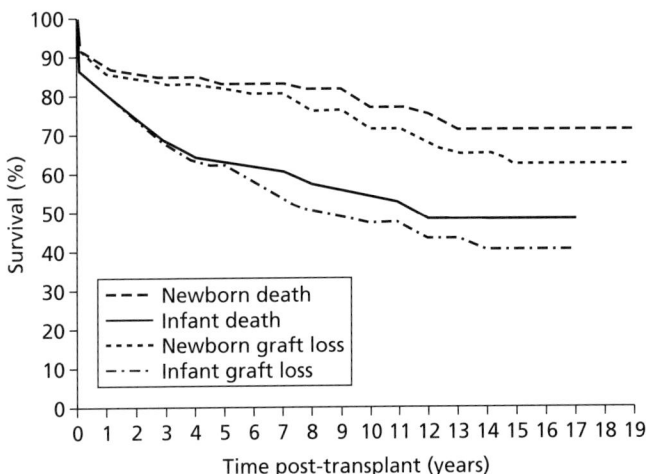

Fig. 35.6 Acutarial survival of infants following transplantation in the Loma Linda experience. Late survival is good and is better in those transplanted as neonates compared with older infants (see text for details).

54% and 48% at 10 and 15 years, respectively (P = 0.0029). Actuarial graft survival was 71% at 10 years and 62% at 15 years for newborns and 47% and 40% at 10 and 15 years, respectively, for infants (P = 0.0022). Graft loss, analyzed using age at transplant as a continuous variable, also shows that younger age at transplant was associated with a decreased risk of graft loss. Median age at transplantation for survivors was 24 days compared with 41.5 days for the non-survivors. Interestingly, graft loss during the first month (representing perioperative mortality) was similar.

To assess the contribution of immunologic factors, rejection history and graft loss resulting from rejection or post-transplant coronary artery disease were assessed. Interestingly, long-term actuarial freedom from rejection was 23% (10 years and above) for infants versus 8% (10 years and above) for newborns (P = 0.0038). However, actuarial freedom from graft loss resulting from rejection or post-transplant coronary artery disease was 67% at 10 years and 59% at 15 years for infants but 84% and 78% at 10 and 15 years, respectively, for newborns (P = 0.0094). Infection-related death was equivalent.

The reasons for differences in long-term survival are almost certainly multifactorial. However, earlier age at transplant is associated with improved patient and graft survival and is likely related to immunologic factors. This has implications for xenotransplantation and use of ABO-incompatible donors. A strategy that uses a prolonged waiting time before proceeding to xenotransplantation or accepting an ABO-incompatible donor could potentially disadvantage the neonatal recipient. West et al. [34] reported their experience with ABO-incompatible heart transplants in neonates and infants. Overall survival was 80%. Interestingly, these infants did not experience hyperacute rejection and the only deaths that occurred were not related to ABO incompatibility. Most patients did not develop antibody to donor blood group although two did without apparent graft damage.

TRANSPLANT FOR CONGENITAL HEART DISEASE

Patients with congenital heart disease account for more than half of all pediatric patients undergoing heart transplantation [12]. Survival in early experience with patients with congenital heart disease appeared to be lower than survival in patients with acquired heart disease [6,7]. However, more recent experience (Annual Report of the Pediatric Heart Transplant Study Group, November 2004, unpublished data) [35,36] suggests that there may be no significant difference in survival among children who undergo heart transplantation for a primary indication of congenital heart disease [12]. A pretransplant diagnosis of congenital heart disease was not an independent risk factor for death in the initial PHTS experience. It is important to distinguish between diagnoses and clinical status before or after surgical repair.

A special group of patients are those with a failed Fontan repair. These patients undergo transplantation for a variety of indications, the most common being protein losing enteropathy and right heart failure. Transplantation in this group can be performed with good survival (W.R. Morrow, D.C. Naftel, J. Kirklin, and the Pediatric Heart Transplant Study Group, unpublished data from PHTS Annual Report, November 1999) [37–39] and with anticipated improvement in protein losing enteropathy. However, in the series reported by Bernstein et al. [37] from the PHTS, 14% of patients died while waiting, with patients listed as Status 1 and those within 6 months of Fontan completion being at greater risk of death before transplant. Actuarial survival after transplant was 76% at 1 year and 63% at 5 years (Fig. 35.7). This survival was no different from patients with congenital heart disease older than 1 year at transplant and statistically poorer than survival in patients without congenital heart disease. Importantly, time since repair in this and other lesions seems to be important in predicting survival. Transplantation performed early after repair in an attempt to salvage patients is more likely to result in death compared with transplantation performed many years after repair. In contrast to all other diagnostic groups, the most common cause of death in patients transplanted for failed Fontan is infection. Clearly, appropriate patient selection is key to successful outcome and some patients with single ventricle physiology are better served by primary transplantation rather than attempts at surgical palliation with Fontan repair or revision of previous Fontan. Patients with protein losing enteropathy who have severe nutritional deficiency and wasting may be at greater risk of death from infection after transplantation because of immunodeficiency and poor healing associated with long-standing malnutrition. For survivors, resolution of protein losing enteropathy is the rule but

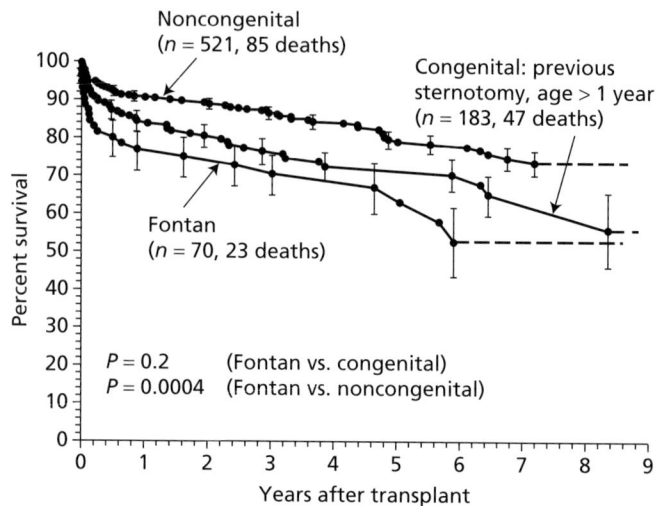

Fig. 35.7 Actuarial survival after transplantation in pediatric patients with and without congenital heart disease. Survival among 70 recipients with prior Fontan palliation was not statistically different from survival in other patients with congenital heart disease who were more than 1 year of age at transplant, but was significantly less than transplant recipients who did not have congenital heart disease. Data from the Pediatric Heart Transplant Study [PHTS], 1993–2001.

many have persistent hypoalbuminemia and protein loss for months following transplantation.

LATE SURVIVAL

Data is beginning to accumulate regarding long-term survival in pediatric heart transplant recipients. Late survival in the early Stanford experience was low, with a reported 10-year survival of 60% [8]. Importantly, the Stanford program pioneered heart transplantation in children and many patients in this series underwent transplantation prior to the cyclosporine era. The continuing occurrence of late rejection [41], rejection deaths (Table 35.1) [42,43], and the late appearance of coronary disease and coronary disease related deaths and retransplantation [12,44,45] raise concern about the ultimate fate of children who have undergone cardiac transplantation. Sigfusson et al. [45] analyzed survival from the experience of three institutions with long-term experience. In that analysis, actuarial survival of patients who had survived at least 5 years was 80% at 10 years post-transplant but 67% at 15 years, emphasizing ongoing mortality, primarily resulting from rejection and coronary disease. Only patients who had survived at least 5 years were included in the analysis and therefore these data do not reflect overall 10-year and 15-year survival. Webber [15] reported a 10-year survival of approximately 45% in a cohort of 37 patients transplanted between 1982 and 1989. This cohort represents one of the earliest reported

Table 35.1 Causes of death (*n* = 141) after transplantation among 683 recipients in the Pediatric Heart Transplant Study. From Frazier *et al.* [42] with permission.

Primary cause of death	*n*	%
Early graft failure	32	23
Rejection	26	18
Infection	29	21
Sudden	19	13
Non-specific graft failure	8	6
Malignancy	4	3
CAD/infarction	7	5
Other	16	11
Total	141	100

CAD, coronary artery disease.

experiences of pediatric heart transplantation. In the same report, Webber notes a much improved contemporary 4-year survival of more than 90%, implying the potential for much improved long-term survival in the current era. The ISHLT registry report gives a 15-year actuarial survival of approximately 45% for all ages [12]. The 10-year PHTS experience, cited above, confirms the presence of an ongoing constant phase of mortality (see Fig. 35.4a), which could result in a 15-year survival in the region of 45%. It is likely that improvement in early survival described above will translate to better long-term survival for patients transplanted in the current era, although strategies to prevent chronic rejection remain illusive. As noted above, the Loma Linda experience has demonstrated a better long-term survival in infants with HLHS transplanted as neonates [33]. More research is required to determine those immunologic factors that contribute to the apparent newborn advantage, in the hope that this state could be extended to other older recipients.

CONCLUSIONS

Lack of availability of donors continues to result in significant mortality while waiting among pediatric patients listed for heart transplantation, although most eventually undergo successful transplantation. In fact, this wait list mortality is virtually equal to the overall 5-year mortality after transplantation. Despite death while waiting in some patients, cardiac transplantation for infants and children with end-stage heart disease is effective and can provide good intermediate survival. Survival after transplantation in infants and children is equal to, if not better than, survival in adults. Long-term survival in children remains disappointing for those transplanted at least a decade ago. Young infant recipients appear to have a survival advantage, perhaps as a result of a relative degree of immune tolerance. Despite discouraging estimates of late

survival based on historical experience, early and intermediate survival is improving in recent studies at individual institutions and from the ISHLT registry and PHTS study group. This improving survival will probably result in improved long-term survival in future years. Development of new immunosuppressive agents and new strategies for immunosuppression may also significantly affect long-term survival by reducing the incidence and severity of acute and chronic rejection. In addition to improving surveillance and prevention of rejection, efforts to increase organ donation and strategies to increase the size of the organ donor pool, such as xenotransplantation and use of ABO-incompatible donors, are needed to reduce overall mortality significantly.

REFERENCES

1 Bailey LL, Razzouk AJ, Wang N, Sciolaro CM, Chiavarelli M. Bless the babies: one hundred and fifteen late survivors of heart transplantation during the first year of life. *J Thorac Cardiovasc Surg* 1993;**105**:805–15.

2 Canter CE, Moorhead S, Huddleston CB, Spray TL. Restrictive atrial communication as a determinant of outcome of cardiac transplantation for hypoplastic left heart syndrome. *Circulation* 1993;**88**(Suppl II):456–60.

3 Merrill WH, Frist WH, Stewart JR, *et al*. Heart transplantation in children. *Ann Surg* 1991;**213**:393–8.

4 Backer CL, Zales VR, Idriss FS, *et al*. Heart transplantation in neonates and in children. *J Heart Lung Transplant* 1992;**11**:311–9.

5 Bailey LL, Wood M, Razzouk A, Van Arsdel G, Gundry S. Heart Transplantation during the first 12 years of life. *Arch Surg* 1989;**124**:1221–6.

6 Armitage JM, Fricker FJ, del Nido P, *et al*. A decade (1982–1992) of pediatric cardiac transplantation and the impact of FK506 immunosuppression. *J Thorac Cardiovasc Surg* 1993;**105**:464–72.

7 Radley-Smith RC, Yacoub MH. Long-term results of pediatric heart transplantation. *J Heart Lung Transplant* 1992;**11**:S227–81.

8 Baum D, Bernstein D, Starnes VA, *et al*. Pediatric heart transplantation at Stanford: results of a 15-year experience. *Pediatrics* 1991;**88**:203–14.

9 Starnes VA, Bernstein D, Oyer PE, *et al*. Heart transplantation in children. *J Heart Lung Transplant* 1989;**8**:20–6.

10 Slaughter MS, Braunlin E, Bolman RM, Molina JF, Shumway SJ. Pediatric heart transplantation: results of 2- and 5-year follow-up. *J Heart Lung Transplant* 1992;**11**:311–9.

11 Turrentine MW, Kesler KA, Caldwell R, *et al*. Cardiac transplantation in infants and children. *Ann Thorac Surg* 1994;**57**:546–54.

12 Boucek MM, Edwards LB, Keck BM, *et al*. Registry for the International Society for Heart and Lung Transplantation: Seventh official pediatric report, 2004. *J Heart Lung Transplant* 2004;**23**:933–47.

13 Razzouk AJ, Chinnock RE, Gundry SR, *et al*. Transplantation as a primary treatment for hypoplastic left heart syndrome: intermediate-term results. *Ann Thorac Surg* 1996;**62**:1–8.

14 Shaddy RE, Naftel DC, Kirklin JK, *et al.* for the Pediatric Heart Transplant Study. Outcome of cardiac transplantation in children: survival in a contemporary multi-institutional experience. *Circulation* 1996;**94**(Suppl II):69–73.

15 Webber SA. 15 years of pediatric heart transplantation at the University of Pittsburgh: lessons learned and future prospects. *Pediatr Transplant* 1997;**1**:8–21.

16 Chiavarelli M, Gundry SR, Razzouk AJ, Bailey LL. Cardiac transplantation for infants with hypoplastic left heart syndrome. *JAMA* 1993;**270**:2944–7.

17 Canter CE, Moorhead S, Saffitz JE, *et al.* Steroid withdrawal in the pediatric heart transplant recipient initially treated with triple immunosuppression. *J Heart Lung Transplant* 1994;**13**: 74–80.

18 McGiffin DC, Naftel DC, Kirklin JK, *et al.* and the Pediatric Heart Transplant Study Group. Predicting outcome after listing for heart transplantation in children: comparison of Kaplan–Meier and parametric competing risk analysis. *J Heart Lung Transplant* 1997;**16**:713–22.

19 Morrow WR, Naftel DC, Chinnock R, *et al.* and the Pediatric Heart Transplant Study Group. Outcome of listing for heart transplantation in infants younger than six months: predictors of death and interval to transplantation. *J Heart Lung Transplant* 1997;**16**:1255–66.

20 Addonizio L, Naftel D, Fricker J, *et al.* and the Pediatric Heart Transplant Study Group. Risk factors for pretransplant outcome in children listed for cardiac transplantation: a multi-institutional study (abstract). *J Heart Lung Transplant* 1995;**14**:S48.

21 Morrow WR, Frazier EA, Naftel DC. Survival after listing for cardiac transplantation in children. *Prog Pediatr Cardiol* 2000;**11**:90–105.

22 Chrisant MR, Naftel DC, Drummond-Webb J, *et al.* and the Pediatric Heart Transplant Study Group. Fate of infants with hypoplastic left heart syndrome listed for cardiac transplantation: a multicenter study. *J Heart Lung Transplant* 2005;**24**:576–82.

23 Bourke KD, Sondheimer HM, Ivy DD, *et al.* Improved pretransplant management of infants with hypoplastic left heart syndrome enables discharge to home while waiting for transplantation. *Pediatr Cardiol* 2003;**24**:538–43.

24 Addonizio LJ, Zangwill SD, Rosenthal DN, *et al.* and the Pediatric Heart Transplant Study Group. Have changes in UNOS status system improved allocation in pediatric heart recipients? *J Heart Lung Transplant* 2005;**24**(Suppl 2):S64.

25 Del Nido P, Armitage JM, Fricker FJ, *et al.* Extracorporeal membrane oxygenation support as a bridge to pediatric heart transplantation. *Circulation* 1994;**90**:66–9.

26 Frazier EA, Faulkner SC, Seib PM, *et al.* Prolonged ECLS for bridging to transplant: technical and mechanical considerations. *Perfusion* 1997;**12**:93–8.

27 Fiser WP, Yetman AT, Gunselman RJ, *et al.* Pediatric arteriovenous extracorporeal membrane oxygenation (ECMO) as a bridge to cardiac transplantation. *J Heart Lung Transplant* 2003;**22**:770–7.

28 Gajarski RJ, Mosca RS, Ohye RG, *et al.* Use of extracorporeal life support as a bridge to pediatric cardiac transplantation. *J Heart Lung Transplant* 2003;**22**:28–34.

29 Stiller B, Hetzer R, Weng Y, *et al.* Heart transplantation in children after mechanical circulatory support with pulsatile pneumatic assest device. *J Heart Lung Transplant* 2003;**22**:1201–8.

30 Goldstein DJ. Worldwide experience with the MicroMed DeBakey Ventricular Assist Device as a bridge to transplantation. *Circulation* 2003;**108**(Suppl II):272–7.

31 Balfour I, Naftel D, Fricker J, *et al.* and the Pediatric Heart Transplant Study Group. Interaction of volume and era on survival of children listed for cardiac transplantation. *J Heart Lung Transplant* 2001;**20**:262.

32 Canter C, Naftel DC, Caldwell R, *et al.* and the Pediatric Heart Transplant Study Group. Survival and risk factors for death after cardiac transplantation in infants: a multi-institutional study. *Circulation* 1997;**96**:227–31.

33 Fortuna RS, Chinnock RE, Bailey LL. Heart transplantation among 233 infants during the first 6 months of life: the Loma Linda experience. Loma Linda Pediatric Heart Transplant Group. *Clin Transpl* 1999;263–72.

34 West LJ, Pollock-Barzu SM, Dipchand AI, *et al.* ABO-incompatible heart transplantation in infants. *N Engl J Med* 2001;**344**: 793–800.

35 Lamour JM, Kanter KR, Naftel DC, *et al.* The effect of age, diagnosis and previous surgery in 488 children and adults who undergo heart transplantation for congenital heart disease. *J Am Coll Cardiol* 2005;**45**:322A.

36 Hsu DT, Quaegebeur JM, Michler RE, *et al.* Heart transplantation in children with congenital heart disease. *J Am Coll Cardiol* 1995;**26**:743–9.

37 Bernstein D, Naftel DC, Hsu DT, *et al.* and the Pediatric Heart Transplant Study. Outcome of listing for cardiac transplantation for failed Fontan: a multi-institutional study (abstract). *J Heart Lung Transplant* 1999;**18**:69.

38 Carey JA, Hamilton JR, Hilton CJ, *et al.* Orthotopic cardiac transplantation for the failing Fontan circulation. *Eur J Cardiothorac Surg* 1999;**47**:47–56.

39 Michielon G, Parisi F, Di Carlo D, *et al.* Orthotopic heart transplantation for failing single ventricle physiology. *Eur J Cardiothorac Surg* 2003;**24**:502–10.

40 Gamba A, Merio M, Fiocchi R, *et al.* Heart transplantation in patients with previous Fontan operations. *J Thorac Cardiovasc Surg* 2004;**127**:555–62.

41 Webber SA, Naftel DC, Parker J, *et al.* and the Pediatric Heart Transplantation Study Group. Late rejection episodes more than 1 year after pediatric heart transplantation: risk factors and outcomes. *J Heart Lung Transplant* 2003;**22**:869–75.

42 Frazier EA, Naftel DC, Canter CE, *et al.* and the Pediatric Heart Transplant Study Group. Death after cardiac transplantation in children: who dies, when, and why? *J Heart Lung Transplant* 1999;**18**:69–70.

43 Pahl E, Naftel DC, Canter CE, *et al.* and the Pediatric Heart Transplant Study. Death after rejection with severe hemodynamic compromise in pediatric heart transplant recipients: a multi-institutional study. *J Heart Lung Transplant* 2001;**20**: 279–87.

44 Pahl E, Fricker FJ, Armitage J, *et al.* Coronary arteriosclerosis in pediatric heart transplant survivors: limitations of long-term survival. *J Pediatr* 1990;**116**:177–83.

45 Sigfusson G, Fricker FJ, Bernstein D, *et al.* Long-term survivors of pediatric heart transplantation: a multicenter report of sixty-eight children who have survived longer than five years. *J Pediatr* 1997;**130**:862–71.

Lung and Heart-Lung Transplantation

36 Historical Notes

Eric N. Mendeloff

As with other forms of solid organ transplantation, success with heart-lung and lung transplantation in the pediatric population was a natural extension of success with these procedures in adults. Therefore, to review the history of pediatric heart-lung and lung transplantation, one must review some of the landmarks in research and the events that led to successful transplantation of these organs in adults.

Notwithstanding the considerable interest in the area, progress with lung transplantation has lagged behind successes with other solid organ transplantation. Unlike other newly transplanted organs, the lung has an extensive surface area through which it interfaces and is directly exposed to viral and bacterial pathogens in the external environment. In addition to the vascular anastomoses that are inherent to other solid organ transplants, lung transplantation relies on successful creation and healing of bronchial anastomoses. The lung is unique among organ transplants in that its systemic arterial supply is not routinely attached at the time of implantation. This chapter aims to explain how factors such as these, which are peculiar to lung transplantation, provided unique challenges to pioneers in this field and how through careful experimentation a better understanding of these factors has been achieved. While our current level of expertise in the area of heart-lung and lung transplantation is substantial, vexing and substantial issues, particularly related to the occurrence of bronchiolitis obliterans, remain an important stumbling block in achieving long-term success.

The history of thoracic organ transplantation begins with the work of Alexis Carrel. Carrel was born and trained in Lyons, France and in 1901 worked with Jaboulay on sutureless vascular anastomoses and subsequently performed the first experimental renal transplant with Ullman in 1902. Carrel moved to the USA in 1904 to work in the Hull Physiological Laboratory at the University of Chicago in collaboration with Charles Claude Guthrie. Because of his pioneering work in the field of vascular anastomotic techniques, Carrel is known as the founding father of experimental organ transplantation and won the Nobel Prize in Physiology or Medicine in 1912. He then moved to the Rockefeller University in New York to become chief of the division of experimental surgery and in the 1930s collaborated with Charles Lindbergh on organ perfusion systems.

The importance and remarkable nature of the experimental work of Russian physiologist Vladimir Petrovich Demikhov is often overlooked. Born into a family of Russian peasants in 1916, Demikhov's father was killed a couple of years later in the Russian civil war [1]. Demikhov studied biology at Moscow University and was inspired by the philosophy and work of Pavlov, the famous Russian physiologist and Nobel Laureate. Despite circumstances of oppression and dogmatic control that existed in Russia at the time, Demikhov designed and implemented a series of operative achievements in canine models of cardiothoracic transplantation. Demikhov performed the first canine heart-lung transplant in 1946 and the first lung transplant in 1947. He performed both lobar and entire lung transplants and dealt with the bronchus either by performing direct anastomoses or by exteriorizing the bronchus to the chest wall. He demonstrated that viable lung function could be achieved without preservation of the bronchial arteries and nerves and was also the first to discover what would be a recurring theme that plagued early lung transplantation, complications of bronchial anastomoses. While these transplants were heterotopic, it is nonetheless remarkable that they were undertaken without the use of either hypothermia or cardiopulmonary bypass. He used more than 50 variations of transplantation in performing over 300 transplants. Given that Demikhov's work was performed without the assistance of cardiopulmonary bypass, it is all the more impressive both in its originality and breadth. Until his book *Experimental Transplantation of Vital Organs* was published in English in 1962, the contributions of Demikhov were not appreciated in the West [2].

Around the same time that Demikhov was performing his pioneering work, several other investigators achieved similar technologic milestones. Using a canine model, Metras in France reported successful whole left lung allotransplantation in which he not only preserved bronchial blood supply, but also performed the venous anastomosis using a cuff of left atrium [3]. In 1951, in an attempt to design an experiment to investigate the hypothesis that division of pulmonary autonomic nerves would interrupt reflex arcs that mediate asthmatic attacks, Juvenelle successfully performed canine right lung autotransplantation [4]. Over 10 years later (1964), with this same goal in mind, Meshalkin performed this same experimental procedure in humans; however, two of seven patients died of bronchial complications and the other five experienced rapid return of their asthma [5].

In 1953 at the Hahnemann Medical College in Pittsburgh, Wilford Neptune performed a series of heart-lung transplants in dogs in which he achieved survival of up to 6 hours. Up to that time, all cardiac transplants had been performed using individual pulmonary vein anastomoses and, in order to avoid this time-consuming process, Neptune decided to transplant the lungs too. As Demikhov had done, Neptune performed these transplants without cardiopulmonary bypass. He addressed the issues of graft preservation and recipient protection by placing both donor and recipient dogs in an ordinary beverage cooler [6]. The author states within the context of the article that with "the use of hypothermia we have been able to completely stop all circulation for periods of up to 30 minutes without subsequent morbidity or mortality." That same year Neptune performed 25 canine left lung allografts in which he demonstrated two important concepts. First, the use of steroids resulted in prolonged graft survival and, second, although bronchial anastomotic dehiscence was a frequent problem, it did not happen uniformly despite routinely sacrificing the bronchial arteries [7]. Over the next 5 years, Blumenstock and Hardy made important contributions by using different modes and combinations of immunosuppression to achieve improved graft survival [8,9].

In 1957, Webb and Howard [10] reported six successful canine orthotopic heart-lung transplants using cardiopulmonary bypass and achieving maximum survival of 22 hours, but without the dogs being able to resume spontaneous respiration. The authors concluded that "transplantation of the heart with both lungs will not be practical" and surmised that restoration of normal respiratory function could not be achieved in the presence of total denervation of the lungs. Four years later, their conclusion would be proved wrong as the Stanford group led by Shumway and Lower reported a series of six canine heart-lung transplants in which the recipients all resumed spontaneous respiration [11]. In the early 1960s, Lower and Shumway published several ground-breaking reports that took thoracic transplantation to the next level. Improvements in their technique included graft preservation by use of cardioplegia and immersion in 4°C iced saline, induction of moderate hypothermia in the recipient using both topical cooling as well as cardiopulmonary bypass, and implantation of the graft by a double atrial cuff technique. This latter modification was felt to reduce ischemic time [12]. Lower and Shumway studied the major obstacle imposed by graft rejection and recognized that immunologic barriers and not surgical technique were the greatest impediment to experimental and clinical thoracic transplantation.

Studies by Haglin et al. [13] on both dogs and primates helped clarify interspecies differences and some of the confounding results that had been achieved, and it no longer appeared that denervation of the lung would be a major obstacle to achieving successful lung transplantation. Almost 20 years later, Reitz et al. [14] published a landmark report on the surgical technique for heart-lung allotransplantation in monkeys using cyclosporine- and azathioprine-based immunosuppression. Both normal pulmonary function and long-term survival were achieved.

Thus, after years of intensive research in the laboratory by a multitude of investigators who had focused on organ preservation, technical aspects of transplantation, post-transplant respiratory physiology and methods of immunosuppression, the stage was set for clinical application. As difficult an issue as availability of donor organs is today, the situation was even worse in the early 1960s when thoracic transplantation was in its infancy and human transplatation was first being attempted. The definition of brain death had yet to be formalized so that in order to use a human donor, the accepted notion was that only cardiorespiratory arrest constituted death. Because transplantation of this nature was considered highly experimental, the recipient had to be a patient who was beyond salvage in almost every respect. Given this backdrop, the details surrounding the first human lung transplant performed by James Hardy and his team at the University of Mississippi in 1963 are truly startling. As documented in the article entitled "Lung Homotransplantation in Man," the first successful transplant recipient was a 58-year-old man with an obstructing left mainstem bronchial carcinoma [15]. In addition to the moral and ethical dilemma of the recipient being a convicted felon serving a life sentence, there are several interesting aspects of the clinical scenario that are worth mentioning. The donor presented to the emergency room with a massive myocardial infarction, cardiogenic shock and pulmonary edema. When the patient could not be resuscitated, consent for autopsy was obtained from the family and external cardiac massage and ventilation with endotracheal intubation were continued. A large dose of heparin was administered, the donor was transported to the operating suite and procurement was undertaken by halting the closed chest massage and performing a left thoracotomy. The pulmonary artery was perfused immediately with a considerable amount of cold heparinized glucose solution and the left mainstem bronchus was intubated and rhythmically inflated with 100% oxygen throughout the entire preservation interval. The authors noted that a considerable amount of frothy secretions were aspirated from the bronchus. Upon performing the thoracotomy for implantation, the recipient was found to have both metastatic carcinoma as well as an empyema. Nonetheless, the transplant proceeded, with a total ischemic time for the lung of 90 minutes. The patient survived the operation but eventually succumbed to renal failure 18 days following the transplant. While the recipient had the support of his native right lung following the transplant, it is nonetheless surprising that at the time of autopsy there was no gross or histologic evidence of allograft rejection. This is despite the fact that there was an ABO mismatch between the donor (type B) and the recipient (type A)! Considering our practices of lung procurement and transplantation today, it is enlightening, instructive and ironic to reflect back upon the details of this first transplant.

The world's first human lobar lung transplant was performed by Shinoi et al. [16] from Tokyo Medical College in 1966 and, while the patient eventually survived, the transplanted lobe was removed on postoperative day 18. The authors considered the transplant a success as it supplemented the patient's pulmonary function during a short period of time during which he was very sick and when his doctors felt that otherwise he would have succumbed to pulmonary insufficiency. This achievement by Shinoi et al. foreshadowed the eventual development of living donor lobar transplantation that would become an accepted modality some 25 years later. In 1968, Cooley performed the first clinical heart-lung transplant in a 2-month-old child. The patient survived only 14 hours and died from pulmonary insufficiency. Sporadic attempts at lung transplantation continued and in 1970 Wildevuur and Benfield [17] reviewed the accumulated world experience with 23 lung transplantations performed by 20 surgeons; only one patient had survived more than 30 days.

The Ad Hoc Committee of the Harvard Medical School to Examine the Definition of Brain Death was a landmark in transplantation in the late 1960s [18]. Not only did it expand the ability to harvest organs, but it also established ethical standards that would protect surgeons from accusations and litigation. With the perseverance of clinicians such as Norman Shumway and his team at Stanford, a modicum of success was achieved using steroids and azathioprine as the sole forms of immunosuppression. Four of seven adolescents transplanted by the Stanford group in the latter half of the 1970s survived for more than 10 years [19]. Other important advances in transplantation in the 1970s included improved selection of donors and recipients as well as improved methods of organ preservation allowing for distant procurement. Until 1977, potential donors were transferred, usually by aircraft, to major transplant centers such as Stanford so that brain death could be declared and procurement could be undertaken at the hospital in which the transplant was to take place. As this scheme was costly and very inconvenient for the donor families, the development of distant procurement in 1977 enabled a marked increase in the number of available donors. A landmark event in the 1970s was the isolation of a fungal extract with potent immunosuppressive properties that led to the discovery of the cyclic undecapeptide cyclosporine A. After being used in experimental heart transplantation as well as in clinical renal and hepatic transplantation, cyclosporine-based immunosuppression was used in the 1980s and resulted in a significant improvement in transplant survival.

By the late 1970s, another 13 unsuccessful human lung transplants had been reported, and while the future for achieving successful lung transplantation appeared bleak, several investigators continued to study the vexing issues that stood in the way of success. One of those issues was the major complications resulting from airway anastomotic healing, or lack thereof. Specifically, by the late 1970s, 16 of the 20 patients in the worldwide lung transplant experience who had survived more than 1 week had experienced major bronchial anastomotic complications that had caused or contributed to their eventual failure. While it was surmised that impaired bronchial healing was a multifactorial problem related to ischemia, rejection and the use of immunosuppressive medications, no structured encompassing approach to investigation of this issue in lung transplants had been undertaken. The group at the University of Toronto led by Pearson and Cooper methodically investigated this issue. Earlier work by Pearson in the 1960s had demonstrated that restoration of bronchial blood flow after division and reconnection of the bronchus required 2 weeks or more [20]. In 1981, using a canine model of left lung reimplantation and administering varying levels of immunosuppression, it became clear that steroids were the culprit responsible for reduced bronchial anastomotic breaking strength and increased incidence of disruption and necrosis of bronchial anastomoses [21]. As steroids had been employed universally in clinical lung transplants performed up to that time and were felt to be essential to achieving any type of meaningful long-term graft survival, these results caused significant consternation. These same type of experiments were then performed omitting steroids and using the newly available immunosuppressive agent cyclosporine. It was found that animals so treated had anastomotic tensile strength comparable to animals receiving no immunosuppression [22].

In an attempt to further address the role of ischemia in bronchial anastomotic breakdown, this same group performed several elegant experiments demonstrating that use of bronchial omentopexy resulted in the development of collaterals that achieved arterial circulation to the bronchus within 4 days [23]. Finally, these investigators performed lung allotransplants in dogs using bronchial omentopexy and immunosuppression with only cyclosporine and azathioprine. They achieved an 83% survival at 3 weeks, with no bronchial complications and with some animals surviving as long as 100 days [24]. With these encouraging experimental results, on November 7, 1983, the Toronto group performed the first long-term successful right lung transplant in a patient with end-stage pulmonary fibrosis. Initial immunosuppression consisted of cyclosporine and azathioprine with the addition of prednisone at 3 weeks, and this 58-year-old man was discharged from the hospital 6 weeks following the transplant. Success with single lung transplantation for pulmonary fibrosis stimulated interest in transplantation for other forms of lung pathology. Patients with end-stage septic pulmonary disease such as cystic fibrosis seemingly posed a contraindication to unilateral transplantation, and this led to bilateral lung transplantation. The first successful double lung transplant was performed in a 42-year-old woman with end-stage emphysema secondary to α_1-antitrypsin deficiency [25]. The first long-term successful heart-lung transplant had been performed by Reitz and Shumway 7 years earlier in March 1981 in a patient with primary pulmonary hypertension (PPH) [26]. Once success with double lung transplantation was established it became apparent that patients with PPH and interstitial lung disease had right heart failure that was reversible when exposed to a normal pulmonary vascular bed. These patients could have a single organ transplantation and thus avoid the acute and long-term problems associated with cardiac transplantation. This also allows the use of a donor heart for another recipient.

Lung transplantation was gradually applied in the pediatric population. The first reported pediatric lung transplant was performed at the University of Toronto in 1987 in a 16-year-old boy with familial pulmonary fibrosis (Joel D. Cooper, personal communication). According to the pediatric lung transplant registry of the International Society for Heart and Lung Transplantation (ISHLT) and United Network of Organ Sharing (UNOS) Scientific Registry data, by the end of 1991 only 41 pediatric lung transplants had been performed in the USA [27,28]. While cystic fibrosis and primary or secondary pulmonary hypertension remain the most common indications for transplantation in the pediatric population, over the years this modality has come to be employed for vastly different indications such as neonates dying from surfactant protein B deficiency. Further, following the report of the first living donor lobar lung transplant in 1990 [29], experience at the University of Southern California and at St. Louis Children's Hospital demonstrated that this is a viable option for children and small adults dying from intractable lung disease who would not survive the wait for cadaveric organs.

CONCLUSIONS

Achievement of successful human heart-lung and lung transplantation has been the result of a long and colorful progression of experimental and clinical advances. The first clinical heart-lung transplant and one of the first living donor lobar lung transplants were performed in pediatric patients. Thus, it gives us pause to reflect on the central role that pediatric transplantation has in the overall picture of thoracic organ transplantation. As transplantation can by no means be touted as a cure, many areas of investigation remain as a challenge and as a frontier for the physicians who care for these patients. While new immunosuppressive and immunomodulating agents have been introduced in the last decade such as tacrolimus, mycophenolate mofetil and daclizumab, how to induce actual graft tolerance remains at a relatively preliminary stage. As

the risks of awaiting thoracic organ transplantation exceed the risks of undergoing the procedure, the role of options such as a pediatric, totally implantable, artificial heart (currently unavailable), xenotransplantation, clinical application of stem cell biology and, most recently, exciting advances in transplantation across ABO barriers [30] remain frontiers in pediatric transplantation. The development of thoracic organ transplantation as a clinical tool for the treatment of heart and lung failure necessitated collective work of several generations of scientists and clinicians. Its current level of success represents a fusion of research from multiple disciplines including vascular and thoracic surgery, cardiology, immunology, pathology, medical ethics and engineering. From this review of some of the major scientific and clinical contributions that paved the way for the modern era, it can be seen that heart-lung and lung transplantation remain amongst the most visible success stories of 20th century medicine and it is likely that pediatric cardiopulmonary transplantation will remain in the forefront for years to come.

REFERENCES

1 Kostantinov IE. A mystery of Vladimir P. Demikhov: the 50th anniversary intrathoracic transplantation. *Ann Thorac Surg* 1998; **65**:1171–7.

2 Demikhov VP. *Experimental Transplantation of Vital Organs*. New York: Consultants Bureau Enterprises, 1962.

3 Metras H. Note preliminare sur la geffe totale du poumon chez le chien. *C R Acad Sci (Paris)* 1950;**231**:1176–8.

4 Juvenelle AA, Citret C, Wiles CE, Stewart JD. Pneumonectomy with reimplantation of the lung in the dog for physiologic study. *J Thorac Surg* 1951;**21**:111–5.

5 Meshalkin EN, Sergievskii VS, Feifilov GL, *et al*. First attempts at surgical treatment of bronchial asthma by the method of pulmonary autotransplantation. *Eksp Khir Anesteziol* 1964;**9**: 26–33.

6 Neptune WB, Cookson BA, Bailey CP, Appler R, Rajkowski F. Complete homologous heart transplantation. *Arch Surg* 1953; **66**:174–8.

7 Neptune WB, Weller R, Bailey CP. Experimental lung transplantation. *J Thorac Surg* 1953;**26**:275–89.

8 Blumenstock DA, Collins JA, Thomas ED, Ferrebee JW. Homotransplants of the lung in dogs. *Surgery* 1962;**51**:541–5.

9 Hardy JD, Eraslan S, Dalton ML Jr, Alican F, Turner MD. Reimplantation and homotransplantation of the lung: laboratory studies and clinical potential. *Ann Surg* 1963;**157**:707–18.

10 Webb WR, Howard HS. Cardio-pulmonary transplantation. *Surg Forum* 1957;**8**:313–7.

11 Lower RR, Stofer RC, Hurley EJ, Shumway NE. Complete homograft replacement of the heart an both lungs. *Surgery* 1961;**50**:842–5.

12 Lower RR, Shumway NE. Studies on orthotopic transplantation of the canine heart. *Surg Forum* 1960;**11**:18–25.

13 Haglin J, Telander RL, Muzzal RE, Kiser JC, Strobel CJ. Comparison of lung autotransplantation in the primate and dog. *Surg Forum* 1963;**14**:196–8.

14 Reitz BA, Burton NA, Jamieson SW, *et al.* Heart and lung transplantation: autotransplantation and allotransplantation in primates with extended survival. *J Thorac Cardiovasc Surg* 1980; 80:360–72.

15 Hardy JD, Webb WR, Dalton ML Jr, Walker GR Jr. Lung homotransplantation in man: report of the initial case. *JAMA* 1963;186:1065–74.

16 Shinoi K, Hayata Y, Aoki H, *et al.* Pulmonary lobe homotransplantation in human subjects. *Am J Surg* 1966;11:617–28.

17 Wildevuur RH, Benfield O. A review of 23 human lung transplantations by 20 surgeons. *Ann Thor Surg* 1970;9:489–515.

18 Ad Hoc Committee of the Harvard Medical School to Examine the Definition of Brain Death. A definition of irreversible coma. *JAMA* 1968;205:337–40.

19 Baum D, Kaye MP, Miller WW. Pediatric heart, heart-lung, and lung transplantation: historical perspective. *Prog Pediatr Cardiol* 1993;2:1–3.

20 Pearson FG, Goldberg M, Stone RM, *et al.* Bronchial arterial circulation restored after reimplantation of canine lung. *Can J Surg* 1970;13:243–50.

21 Lima O, Cooper JD, Peters WJ, *et al.* Effects of methylprednisilone and azathioprine on bronchial healing following lung transplantation. *J Thorac Cardiovasc Surg* 1981;82:211–5.

22 Goldberg M, Lima O, Morgan E, *et al.* A comparison between cyclosporine A and methylprednisilone plus azathioprine on bronchial healing following canine lung allotransplantation. *J Thorac Cardiovasc Surg* 1983;85:821–6.

23 Lima O, Goldberg M, Peters WJ, *et al.* Bronchial omentopexy in canine lung transplantation. *J Thorac Cardiovasc Surg* 1982; 83:418–21.

24 Dubois P, Choiniere L, Cooper JD. Bronchial omentopexy in canine lung allotransplantation. *Ann Thorac Surg* 1984;38:211–4.

25 Patterson GA, Cooper JD, Dark JH, *et al.* Experimental and clinical double lung transplantation. *J Thorac Cardiovasc Surg* 1988;95:70–4.

26 Reitz BA, Wallwork JL, Hunt SA, *et al.* Heart-lung transplantation: successful therapy for patients with pulmonary vascular disease. *N Engl J Med* 1982;306:557–64.

27 Boucek MM, Faro A, Novick RJ, *et al.* The registry of the international society for heart and lung transplantation: fourth official pediatric report – 2000. *J Heart Lung Transplant* 2001; 20:39–52.

28 1993 UNOS Annual Report of the US Scientific Registry of Transplant Recipients and the Organ Procurement and Transplantation Network. Transplant data: 1988–1991. Department of Health and Human Services, Health Resources and Services Administration, Office of Special Programs, Division of Transplantation, Rockville, MD; United Network for Organ Sharing, Richmond, VA; University Renal Research and Education Association, Ann Arbor, MI.

29 Goldsmith MF. Mother to child: first living donor lung transplant. *JAMA* 1990;49:55.

30 West LJ, Pollock-Barziv SM, Dipchand AI, *et al.* ABO-incompatible heart transplantation in infants. *N Engl J Med* 2001;344:793–800.

37 Recipient Characteristics

Eithne F. MacLaughlin

Lung and heart-lung transplantation is an option for some children with end-stage lung disease, idiopathic pulmonary arterial hypertension and other pulmonary vascular disorders that are often associated with congenital heart disease. Since the first pediatric lung transplants performed in the late 1980s, the number of procedures performed annually (as reported to the Registry of the International Society for Heart and Lung Transplantation) increased steadily to 84 recipients by the mid-1990s, but since 1999 has fallen to approximately 60–70 procedures per year (Fig. 37.1). The majority of these are performed in North America. Availability of donor organs remains a key issue in determining the number of procedures performed annually, and wait-list mortality remains high.

RECIPIENT CHARACTERISTICS

Age group

The indications for lung transplantation vary with the age group. In infants under 1 year of age, congenital heart disease and pulmonary vascular disease (including pulmonary vein

stenosis) account for the largest group, 60% of the recipients. Other diagnoses (e.g. surfactant protein B deficiency and interstitial lung disease) account for 20% of the recipients. Among recipients in the 1–10 year age group, cystic fibrosis is the most common diagnosis, accounting for 36% of cases, followed by idiopathic pulmonary arterial hypertension (IPAH) with 13%. Figure 37.2 shows the diagnoses of adolescent lung transplant recipients, who make up approximately three-quarters of pediatric lung transplant recipients; again cystic fibrosis is the most common underlying disorder [1].

The number of heart-lung transplants performed in children continues to decline from a peak volume in the late 1980s of over 40 per year to a low of nine in 2002 (Fig. 37.3) [2]. This is partly the result of a decline in availability of heart-lung blocks because of increased use of isolated heart transplants. Heart transplants are allocated in most regions preferentially over heart-lung transplants. Other factors include improved surgical technique for lung transplantation, alleviating some of the demand for heart-lung transplants [2]. In addition, it is now recognized that heart-lung transplantation is not generally required for the treatment of disorders such as cystic fibrosis and IPAH.

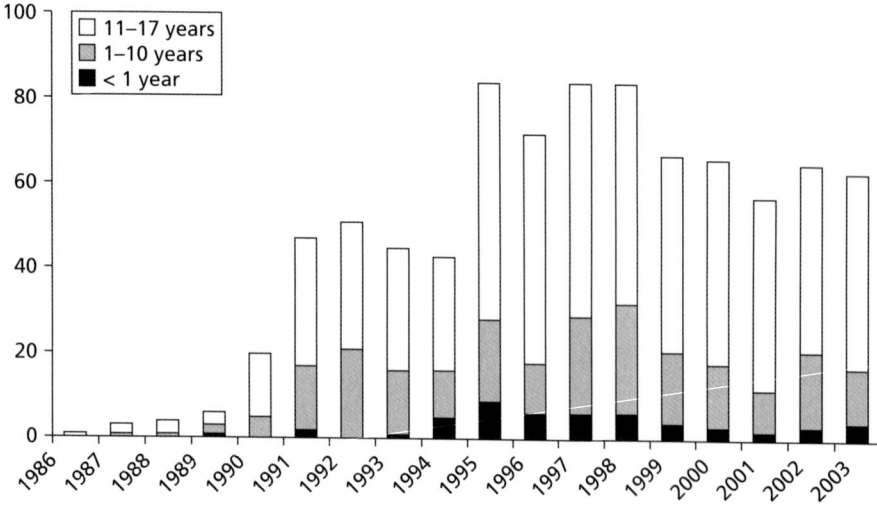

Fig. 37.1 Number of pediatric lung transplant procedures performed annually stratified by age. Data from the International Society for Heart and Lung Transplantation, 2005, with permission.

314

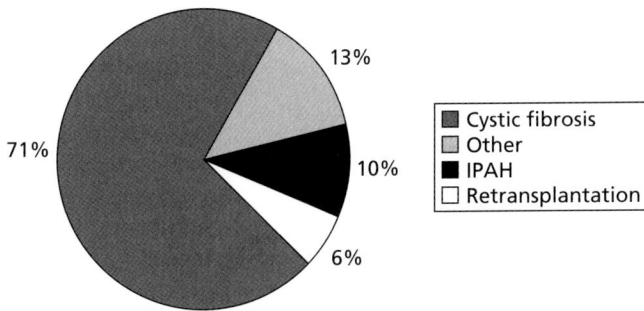

Fig. 37.2 Indications for lung transplantation in adolescents (aged 11–17 years). IPAH, idiopathic pulmonary arterial hypertension. Data adapted from the Registry of the International Society for Heart and Lung Transplantation, 2005.

Type of transplant

Heart-lung

Heart-lung transplantation is indicated for severe pulmonary vascular disease or pulmonary vascular anomalies with uncorrectable cardiac lesions. It is also indicated for end-stage lung disease associated with significant dysfunction of the left ventricle. In most cases of IPAH with right ventricular failure, isolated bilateral lung transplantation will lead to rapid resolution of right ventricular dysfunction. However, in selected cases of severe right ventricular failure and dysfunction, heart-lung transplantation may be the preferred procedure.

Double lung

Double or bilateral lung transplantation is the option of choice in children with end-stage lung disease and cardiopulmonary disorders when heart-lung transplant is not required. Double lung transplant gives the recipient a better pulmonary

reserve and larger pulmonary vascular bed than a single lung transplant. In patients with cystic fibrosis, double lung transplant is required because of bilateral lung infection in the native lungs. In children with IPAH, survival is better with double over single lung transplant and is the procedure of choice.

Single lung

Single lung transplant has been preformed in adolescents with pulmonary fibrosis but bilateral lung transplant is a better option when available.

Living donor lung

Living donor lobar lung transplantation is an option in a few transplant centers. The procedure was pioneered by Vaughn Starnes in the early 1990s [3]. This transplant procedure requires major resource mobilization which is presently only available in few centers worldwide. Living donor transplantation is a consideration for selected preteens and adolescents who meet standard criteria for lung transplantation and have suitable donors available [4]. Donor outcomes show low morbidity and no mortality [5]. Favorable outcomes have been reported in pediatric patients with cystic fibrosis and idiopathic pulmonary arterial hypertension [6–8].

Original disease

Cystic fibrosis

There are approximately 30 000 patients registered with the Cystic Fibrosis Foundation in the USA. The mean survival time is approximately 30 years. The majority of deaths are secondary to respiratory failure. Over 80% of cystic fibrosis patients receiving lung transplantation are over 18 years of age. Cystic fibrosis is the most common single etiology for lung transplant in the pediatric age group. In the 1980s

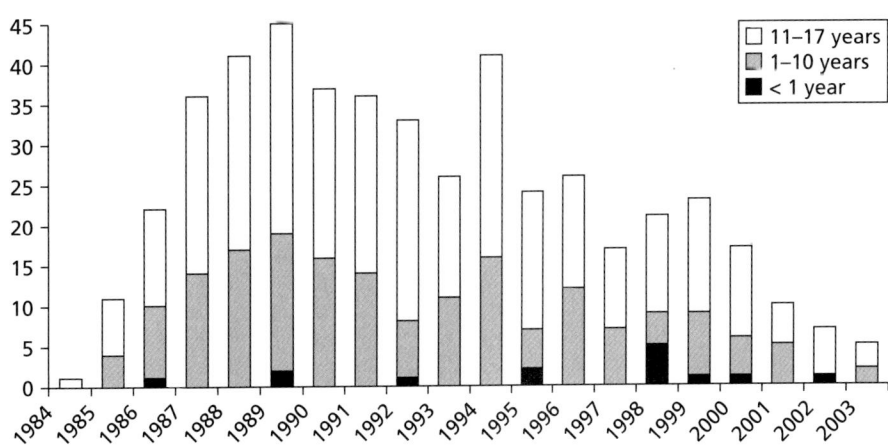

Fig. 37.3 Number of pediatric heart-lung transplants performed annually stratified by age. Data from the International Society for Heart and Lung Transplantation, 2005, with permission.

heart-lung transplant was first available, but since the late 1980s bilateral lung transplant is the usual procedure. Despite chronic bacterial colonization, cystic fibrosis lung transplant recipients have done as well, in terms of both short- and long-term survival, as other patients receiving lung transplantation [9]. The indications for referral and acceptance criteria are similar to other candidates, both adult and pediatric [10]. Timing of referral is based on several factors:

1 Waiting time anticipated for suitable donor. This may be 18 months to 2 years in many regions.

2 Expected survival time based on the individual patient's anticipated decline.

Several approaches have been suggested in the patient with cystic fibrosis, but progressive decline in pulmonary function to a forced expiratory volume in 1 second (FEV_1) of 30% and below remains a reasonable target for timing of evaluation and listing. Other factors that increase the risk for shortened survival are female sex, age less than 10 years, frequent hospitalization and inability to maintain weight. Special considerations need to be given to colonization or infection with pan-resistant organisms although this is not an absolute contraindication to lung transplantation. *Burkholderia cepacia* complex, in particular genomovar III, is associated with higher mortality [11–13]. *Aspergillus* colonization or infection is usually managed with appropriate antifungal therapy in the lung transplant candidate and recipient [14].

Idiopathic pulmonary arterial hypertension (primary pulmonary hypertension)

Early experience suggested a mean life expectancy of 2.8 years from the time of the initial diagnosis [15]. There has been a significant improvement in survival since the introduction of aggressive medical management including treatment with calcium channel blockade and/or epoprostenol. Patients who respond to these therapies have recently been shown to have a decrease in survival after 5 years of treatment. Lung transplantation remains an option for this group of patients [16]. New drugs are becoming available for the treatment of IPAH but their role for long-term treatment is unknown.

Pulmonary hypertension associated with congenital heart disease repaired or unrepaired

With the small number of heart-lung transplants available, lung transplant with repair of the cardiac lesion has been preformed in selected candidates, usually those with simple left-to-right shunts. Some patients with severe pulmonary arteriovenous malformations or inadequate vascular bed (usually with complex pulmonary atresia) may benefit from lung transplantation when they have severe functional limitation [17].

CONCLUSIONS

Lung and heart-lung transplantation is an option for children with end-stage lung disease and pulmonary vascular disease. Most pediatric transplants are performed in the adolescent age group, with cystic fibrosis being the most common indication. Among infants, congenital heart disease (including pulmonary vein stenosis) is the most common indication, but primary forms of lung disease such as surfactant protein B deficiency may also be treated with lung transplantation. Heart-lung transplantation has become a very rare procedure because of the poor availability of heart-lung blocks and the increasing use of lung transplantation for disorders previously treated with heart-lung transplantation.

REFERENCES

1 Boucek M, Edwards L, Keck B, *et al*. Registry for the International Society for Heart and Lung Transplantation: Seventh Official Pediatric Report, 2004. *J Heart Lung Transplant* 2004;**23**:933–47.

2 Boucek M, Edwards L, Keck B, *et al*. Registry for the International Society for Heart and Lung Transplantation: Sixth Official Pediatric Report, 2003. *J Heart Lung Transplant* 2003;**22**:636–52.

3 Starnes V, Barr M, Cohen R. Lobar transplantation: indications, technique and outcome. *J Thorac Cardiovasc Surg* 1994;**108**: 403–11.

4 Woo M. An overview of paediatric lung transplantation. *Paediatr Respir Rev* 2004;**5**:249–54.

5 Bowdish M, Barr M, Schenkel F, *et al*. A decade of living lobar lung transplantation: perioperative complications after 253 donor lobectomies. *Am J Transplant* 2004;**4**:1283–8.

6 Starnes V, Bowdish M, Woo M, *et al*. A decade of living lobar lung transplantation: recipient outcome. *J Thorac Cardiovasc Surg* 2004:**127**:114–22.

7 Starnes V, Woo M, MacLaughlin E, *et al*. Comparison of outcomes between living donor and cadaveric lung transplantation in children. *Ann Thorac Surg* 1999;**6**:2279–83.

8 Woo M, MacLaughlin E, Horn M, *et al*. Living donor lobar lung transplantation: the pediatric experience. *Pediatr Transplant* 1998;**2**:185–90.

9 Egan T, Detterbeck F, Mill M, *et al*. Improved results of lung transplantation for patients with cystic fibrosis. *J Thorac Cardiovasc Surg* 1995;**109**:24–35.

10 Steinman T, Becker B, Frost A, *et al*. Guidelines for the referral and management of patients for solid organ transplantation. *Transplantation* 2001;**71**:1189–204.

11 Aris R, Routh J, LiPuma J, Heath D, Gilligan P. Lung transplantation for cystic fibrosis patients with *Burkholderia cepacia* complex; survival linked to genomovar type. *Am J Respir Crit Care Med* 2001;**164**: 2102–6.

12 Chaparro C, Maurer J, Gutierrez C, *et al*. Infection with *Burkholderia cepacia* in cystic fibrosis: outcome following lung transplantation. *Am J Respir Crit Care Med* 2001;**163**:43–8.

13 Mahenthiralingam E, Baldwin A, Van Damme P. *Burkholderia cepacia* complex infection in patients with cystic fibrosis. *J Med Microbiol* 2002;**51**:533–8.

14 Dummer J, Lazarrashville N, Barnes J, Ninon M, Milstone A. A survey of anti-fungal management in lung transplantation. *J Heart Lung Transplant* 2004;**23**:1376–81.

15 D'Alonzo G, Barst R, Ayers S, *et al.* Survival in patients with primary pulmonary hypertension: results from a national prospective registry. *Ann Intern Med* 1991;**115**:343–9.

16 Yung D, Widlitz A, Rosenzweig E, *et al.* Outcomes in children with idiopathic pulmonary arterial hypertension. *Circulation* 2004;**110**:660–5.

17 Spray T. Lung transplantation in children with pulmonary hypertension and congenital heart disease. *Semin Thorac Cardiovasc Surg* 1996;**8**:286–95.

Lung transplantation should be considered in selected children with end-stage or progressive lung disease or pulmonary vascular disease for which there is no other therapy. The evaluation requires a multidisciplinary team approach that is tailored to each individual patient, family and underlying diagnosis.

The transplant evaluation provides an opportunity to determine the cause of respiratory insufficiency in those patients with end-stage lung disease of uncertain etiology. The evaluation process also identifies absolute contraindications that are not correctable or may be worsened by a lung transplant. If there are relative contraindications, appropriate strategies to address them and optimize the patient's outcome are developed. The evaluation also provides the surgical team with information that will help determine the ideal surgical approach.

Perhaps most importantly, the transplant evaluation provides the patient and family with an opportunity to learn about the procedure. Although a potentially life-saving procedure, lung transplantation remains fraught with possible complications and requires an unending commitment from patients and families. They must come away from the evaluation with a thorough understanding of the risks and benefits associated with a lung or heart-lung transplant.

Irrespective of underlying diagnosis, essential ingredients that all candidates should possess include:

1 A clear diagnosis or adequately delineated trajectory of illness despite optimal medical therapy that puts the individual child at risk of dying without a lung transplant.

2 An adequate array of family support personnel, almost always including at least one parent and an additional available person. If appropriate support is not available within the family, placement into medical foster care must be considered for lung transplantation to be an option. In some centers, placement into foster care is considered an absolute contraindication to transplantation.

3 Adequate access to transplant services and medications after transplantation including the ability to return regularly to the transplant center.

4 Adequate evidence of willingness and ability on the part of patient and parent to adhere to the rigorous therapy, daily monitoring and re-evaluation schedule after transplant.

GENERAL STUDIES

A number of studies and consultations are routinely performed during the transplant evaluation by most pediatric centers (Table 38.1).

Blood tests

Screening blood tests help rule out the presence of comorbidities that would impact a lung transplant recipient's outcome, such as renal or liver dysfunction. Blood typing is essential as lungs are transplanted based on ABO compatibility.

The presence of preformed, circulating anti-HLA antibodies increases the risk of hyperacute rejection, as well as recurrent acute rejection and chronic rejection. An elevated panel reactive antibody of more than 10% is a relative contraindication at most centers, but there are interventions, such as the pretransplant administration of high dose intravenous immunoglobulin and plasmapheresis, that may reduce pretransplant allosensitization. Additionally, rituximab (a chimeric human/mouse anti-CD20 monoclonal antibody) reduced anti-HLA antibodies in patients awaiting kidney transplantation [1] and is being tested in other organ candidates with preformed anti-HLA (human leukocyte antigen) antibodies. Post-transplantation, similar strategies, combined with perioperative antithymocyte globulin preparations and maintenance therapy with agents with anti-B-cell proliferative properties, may mitigate the development of antibody-mediated rejection [2,3].

Serologic studies screen for prior infectious exposures and immunization status. Management of patients post-transplant may vary substantially based on their serologic status. For instance, patients seronegative for cytomegalovirus (CMV) or Epstein–Barr virus (EBV) prior to transplant are at increased risk of developing specific complications post-transplantation, especially if the donor is seropositive.

Table 38.1 Recommended evaluation for pediatric lung and heart-lung transplant candidates.

Bloodwork
    Blood type (ABO)
    Complete blood count
    Coagulation studies (PT, INR and PTT)
    Complete biochemistries including electrolytes and liver and renal
        function tests
    Lipid profile
Serologies including CMV, EBV, HIV, hepatitis B and C, measles,
    varicella, herpes simplex, *Toxoplasma gondii*
    Anti-HLA antibody screen
    Arterial blood gas
Autoimmune screen (ANA, ANCA, rheumatoid factor, quantitative
    immunoglobulins for select patients)
Thyroid profile
Pulmonary function testing
Six minute walk test
Sputum culture and susceptibility testing
Tuberculin testing
Electrocardiogram
Cardiac catheterization (select candidates)
Imaging
    Chest radiograph
    Chest CT
    Sinus CT in patients with CF and immunodeficiency
    Ventilation/perfusion scan
    Echocardiogram
    Bone densitometry
Consultations with
    Cardiothoracic surgery
    Cardiology
    Infectious diseases
    Social services
    Psychology
    Nutrition
    Physical therapy
    Child life

ANA, antinuclear antibody; ANCA, antineutrophil cytoplasmic antibody; CF, cystic fibrosis; CMV, cytomegalovirus; CT, computed tomography; EBV, Epstein–Barr virus; HIV, human immunodeficiency virus; HLA, human leukocyte antigen; INR, international normalized ratio; PT, prothrombin time; PTT, partial thromboplastin time.

Microbiologic evaluation

Obtaining sputum or lower airway cultures in candidates with septic lung disease such as cystic fibrosis (CF) is essential. Chronic infection by *Burkholderia cepacia* or *Pseudomonas aeruginosa* in CF results in shorter survival [4,5]. Transplant centers may have different policies regarding transplantation based on the antibiotic susceptibility pattern of these organisms. It appears that patients transplanted with panresistant

P. aeruginosa have similar outcomes after transplantation to those patients who have sensitive organisms [6]. The key to treating these patients is being prepared with an appropriate antibiotic combination based on recent susceptibility and antibiotic synergy testing. However, the same is not true for infection with *B. cenocepacia* (previously genomovar III), in which 1-year survival following lung transplant is poor [7].

Tuberculin testing is mandatory as active infection with *Mycobacterium tuberculosis* is an absolute contraindication to transplantation. Patients with CF are at risk for airway colonization with nontuberculous mycobacteria (NTM), which is present in 7–24% of patients' sputum [8]. Although infection with NTM is not an absolute contraindication to transplantation, patients should be on appropriate antimycobacterial therapy prior to transplant [9,10].

Similar recommendations can be made for patients chronically colonized or infected with fungi. When treated appropriately, fungal infections, although common in lung transplant candidates, do not appear to increase post-transplant mortality [11].

Pulmonary function testing

Perhaps the most objective reliable measure of respiratory function, pulmonary function testing (PFT) can be performed in a child of any age. In specialized centers, smaller airway flows and lung volumes can be measured even in infants. However, because of the cost and inconvenience, the ability to perform infant PFT is not widespread. Thus, in some instances PFT may be as simple as obtaining an arterial blood gas to assess for hypercapnea and determine an alveolar–arterial oxygen gradient in an infant, to spirometric lung volume and diffusion capacity measurements in a patient capable of performing reproducible maneuvers. Persistent forced expiratory volumes in 1 second (FEV_1) of less than 30% predicted or rapid progressive deterioration in lung function warrants consideration for referral to a transplant center. Exercise testing such as the 6-minute walk test is also a reliable tool to assess the candidate's degree of respiratory dysfunction and need for a lung transplant evaluation [12].

For those candidates in respiratory failure, the need for mechanical ventilation prior to transplant portends lower survival rates post-transplant [13]. However, this may not be true in select populations such as those with CF [14]. The data from small recent studies do not seem to support the presumption that all mechanically ventilated patients pre-transplant have a lower incidence of survival compared with nonventilated patients, although they may potentially experience longer hospital stays post-transplant [15,16]. Outcomes may be acceptable in select groups of patients, such as infants who possess vast potential for rehabilitation, or those who are chronically ventilated but yet can successfully participate in pulmonary rehabilitation and physical therapy, or those who have been ventilated for only a short period of time.

Imaging

Radiographic examination is useful in assessing the degree of lung disease as well as possibly ascertaining an underlying etiology for the candidate's respiratory dysfunction, if unexplained. Most importantly, radiographic studies assist the surgeon in determining the best surgical technique and approach for the individual patient. Chest computed tomography (CT) provides information regarding the degree of pleural disease and adhesions [17]. Ventilation/perfusion scintillation scanning may predict a poorer outcome on the waiting list [18] and if the candidate undergoes a bilateral sequential lung transplant, it provides indispensable information as to which lung is to be replaced first. Aortography is helpful in assessing the extent of any collateral aortopulmonary circulation in cyanotic patients being considered for heart-lung transplantation.

Consultations

Specific consultations are required to complete a comprehensive transplant evaluation. This includes consultation with a psychologist and/or psychiatrist and a social worker familiar with the rigors of transplantation. It is vital to discover psychoaffective disorders that may impact outcomes. It is also important to identify patterns of nonadherence. In a study of pediatric heart and heart-lung transplant recipients, nearly one-third of the participants demonstrated unsatisfactory adherence to the treatment regimen [19]. Some pediatric transplant centers have instituted pretransplant contracts with patients with a history of nonadherence. If patients are able to meet the agreed goals, they are then conditionally listed for transplantation. An experienced social worker can assist with drawing up a pretransplant contract and following-up on adherence. A social worker familiar with the myriad of insurance, transportation and financial vagaries of transplantation is essential to patients and families.

Nutritional status impacts prognosis and a thorough nutritional evaluation is required to assess the risk or degree of nutritional failure. An abnormal body mass index (BMI) pretransplant in a group of adult and adolescent patients was associated with an increased risk of dying within 90 days of lung transplantation [20]. A nutritionist or dietitian should develop an intervention program to optimize a candidate's nutritional status.

A physical therapist can assess the candidate's potential for rehabilitation and devise a pretransplant plan to maximize conditioning. Other consultations will depend on the underlying disease state and/or the discovery of unexpected laboratory findings during the evaluation process. Patients being considered for heart-lung transplantation require consultation with a pediatric cardiologist experienced with pulmonary vascular disease. Patients with a history of malignancy should be evaluated by a pediatric oncologist for an assessment of risk of relapse.

DISEASE-SPECIFIC EVALUATION

Surfactant dysfunction syndromes

These include surfactant protein B (SPB) deficiency, associated with congenital alveolar proteinosis, which virtually always presents with severe acute respiratory failure in the first hours of life [21]. Other abnormalities of surfactant metabolism associated with progressive lung disease are surfactant protein C and ATP-binding cassette transporter A3 (ABCA3) mutations. Patients with these entities may present with congenital alveolar proteinosis (often less severe than SPB deficiency) or severe interstitial lung disease, usually with poor prognosis [22,23].

Specific indications

Confirmed surfactant dysfunction syndrome with unrelenting respiratory failure or progressive interstitial lung disease with respiratory insufficiency, unresponsive to medical interventions.

Specific contraindications

Extracorporeal membrane oxygenation (ECMO) dependence, cerebral hemorrhage and other organ insufficiency.

Timing of referral

Once a decision to pursue transplantation has been made, SPB deficient patients should be transferred to a transplant center as soon as possible. The prognosis for the other surfactant dysfunction syndromes is more variable and patients should be referred based on progressive unrelenting respiratory insufficiency.

Specific studies

Tracheal effluent or lung biopsy showing absence of SPB or abnormal surfactant protein C (SPC), genetic analysis confirming SPB mutation, or typical histopathology. In other disorders, genetic analysis of SPC and ABCA3 mutations by blood test, with or without open lung biopsy, should be performed.

Preoperative management

Ventilatory support in SPB deficiency, and optimize nutrition and growth. Rule out other complicating factors in older infants, including opportunistic infection and gastroesophageal reflux disease with aspiration. Many individuals with SPC mutations may benefit from anti-inflammatory therapy, which should be provided prior to referral for transplantation.

Idiopathic pulmonary hypertension

The specific entities leading to pulmonary vascular disease (PVD) and pulmonary hypertension in childhood include idiopathic (previously called "primary") pulmonary hypertension (IPH or PPH) [24], PVD associated with, or secondary to, congenital heart disease (CHD) and pulmonary vein abnormalities. These entities must be carefully distinguished. The presentation of infants with IPH is variable, but may consist of failure to thrive, diaphoresis, tachypnea and tachycardia [25]. After infancy, children may present with similar symptoms as adults including exercise intolerance, syncope and chest pain.

Specific indications

It is generally accepted that transplantation should be performed for patients who have failed or are failing medical management. Guidelines previously published for adults [26,27] include:
- New York Heart Association (NYHA) or World Health Organization (WHO) functional class III or IV despite pulmonary vasodilator therapy;
- low exercise tolerance with 6-minute walk test of less than approximately 350 m;
- uncontrolled syncope;
- hemoptysis; and
- right heart failure associated with the adverse hemodynamic markers of cardiac index of less than 2 L/min/m^2, right atrial mean pressure $\geq$ 12–15 mmHg, mixed venous oxygen saturation less than 60% and/or mean pulmonary artery pressure of more than 55 mmHg.

It is not clear if the same parameters are appropriate for pediatric patients. Studies in children suggested poorer survival with right atrial pressure of more than 7.4 mmHg, right ventricular end-diastolic pressure of more than 10.4 mmHg, decreasing cardiac index and with progressive elevation of pulmonary vascular resistance [28,29]. A model was generated to estimate the probability of death based on the product of mean right atrial pressure and pulmonary vascular resistance [29]. It should be noted, however, that both these studies consisted of heterogeneous patient populations. Others factors that may be taken into consideration include von Willebrand factor: antigen levels of more than 240% [30], elevated uric acid [31] and plasma brain natriuretic peptide (BNP) levels above 180 pg/mL, which correlated with poor survival [32].

Specific contraindications

Major comorbidities. Right ventricular dysfunction usually resolves rapidly following bilateral sequential lung trans-

plantation. For this reason, right ventricular dysfunction and failure is usually not a contraindication to lung transplantation.

Timing of referral

The natural history for IPH is generally progressive and fatal, although the outcome is highly variable, with some children having a very short life span while progression is considerably slower for others. Children with IPH often present late in the course of their disease with syncope and suprasystemic pulmonary arterial pressures. The National Institutes of Health PPH registry shows a median survival of 2.8 years for adults compared to 10 months for children [33], while another study suggests that there is no statistical difference in outcome between children and adults [28]. However, recent advances in therapy have dramatically changed the outcome of IPH in both adults and children [34,35]. Early referral should be considered for patients with NYHA class III or IV symptoms and for those with evidence of right heart failure without early response to vasodilator therapy. In infants or young children, it may be more difficult to classify their functional status and early referral seems appropriate when pulmonary pressures are at systemic level or above, despite aggressive medical therapy.

Specific studies

Identifiable etiologies such as collagen vascular disease, primary lung pathology, chronic thromboembolism and pulmonary vein obstruction must all be ruled out. Cardiac catheterization with assessment of pulmonary vasoreactivity is important in all patients, although it must be noted that failure to respond to acute vasodilator testing does not rule out potential response to chronic vasodilator therapy. A ventilation/perfusion scan is helpful to rule out thromboembolic disease. CT scan of the chest will rule out the presence of intrinsic lung disease or suspected pulmonary veno-occlusive disease. There should be a low threshold for polysomnography to assess for sleep disordered breathing with concomitant hypoxemia.

Preoperative management

Medical management of IPH may include vasodilators such as calcium-channel blockers, epoprostenol or its analogues, sildenafil and/or bosentan. Patients should also receive supplemental oxygen to prevent hypoxia, anticoagulation (warfarin or low molecular weight heparin), diuretic therapy as indicated, and nutritional support. Select patients may benefit from atrial septostomy, particularly when recurrent syncope has been documented.

Eisenmenger syndrome

Eisenmenger syndrome (ES) is a complex comprising CHD with a markedly elevated pulmonary vascular resistance and a right

321

to left shunt at the cardiac or great vessel level. Progressive cyanosis and hypoxia ensue. Poor prognosis correlates with worse NYHA classification, syncope, increased right atrial pressure, decreased cardiac index, increased pulmonary vascular resistance, falling Pao_2 and deteriorating renal function. Low cardiac output and high right atrial pressure were independent predictors of mortality in adults with ES [36]. Earlier age of onset is also associated with a poorer prognosis [37]. Similar to patients with IPH, serum uric acid is also a possible prognostic indicator in ES [38]. The survival advantage of transplantation remains the least clear for this group of patients, many of whom will live for years or even decades after diagnosis, despite severe cyanosis. Although pulmonary vasodilator therapy was first studied in patients with IPH, there are now trials commencing in patients with ES. Patients with progressive disease and severe symptoms will require consideration for heart-lung transplantation. Selected patients with simple cardiac lesions (e.g. atrial or ventricular septal defect, or patent arterial duct) can be considered as candidates for bilateral lung transplantation with cardiac repair. There is a final subgroup of patients with pulmonary atresia, ventricular septal defect and multiple aorto-pulmonary collaterals in whom there is an inadequate pulmonary vascular bed with or without segmental or global pulmonary hypertension [39]. Outcome for this group of patients is highly variable. In this population, transplantation is considered in selected patients with severe symptomatic cyanosis who are unsuitable for, or have failed, other palliative surgeries.

Specific indications

Progressive severe hypoxia, syncope or severely impaired quality of life.

Specific contraindications

Major comorbidities, multiple prior thoracotomies associated with extensive collateral circulation (high risk of uncontrolled perioperative bleeding).

Timing of referral

Trajectory of clinical illness progressing with unacceptable quality of life, recurrent life-threatening hemoptysis, cerebral vascular accident, deteriorating ventricular function and development of heart failure.

Specific studies

Full cardiovascular evaluation including complete anatomic evaluation, assessment of pulmonary vasoreactivity and assessment of aorto-pulmonary collateral circulation. Complete evaluation generally involves cardiac catheterization, echocardiography and radiographic imaging with CT or magnetic resonance imaging.

Preoperative management

Avoidance of dehydration, iron deficiency and extreme polycythemia. Trial of oxygen therapy and vasodilator therapy is considered in selected patients.

Pulmonary hypertension in repaired congenital heart disease

Pulmonary hypertension may also occur in patients with CHD that was previously corrected [39]. In the absence of right to left shunts, these patients will not be cyanosed and generally present with symptoms (and follow a clinical course) similar to those with IPH rather than ES. As for IPH, the development of right heart failure and syncope signal a poor prognosis. In the setting of a biventricular heart with adequate ventricular function, bilateral lung transplantation is the treatment of choice.

Other pulmonary vascular disorders

Some other pulmonary vascular disorders such as alveolar capillary dysplasia (ACD), pulmonary veno-occlusive disease (PVOD) and pulmonary vein stenosis are poorly responsive to medical or surgical management, with transplantation being the only option for long-term survival [40–44].

Timing of referral

Urgent, because these typically do not respond to medical management and have a very poor prognosis.

Specific studies

Cardiac catheterization for pulmonary vein stenosis, CT scan of chest for PVOD and open lung biopsy of ACD.

Preoperative management

Although there may be an occasional patient with PVOD who responds to pulmonary vasodilator therapy, the majority do not and vasodilator therapy may exacerbate the pulmonary edema because the obstruction is postcapillary. For patients with ACD, pulmonary vasodilator therapy (nitric oxide and prostacyclin) may prolong survival for a short time.

Cystic fibrosis

CF is a highly variable disease in which end-stage lung disease is the most common cause of death. Several models exist to help guide the clinician on when to consider referral of a patient with CF to a transplant center. Initial guidelines identified a greater risk for death in patients with FEV_1 of less than 30% predicted, with contributing factors including elevated $Paco_2$, decreased Pao_2, younger age, female gender and nutritional status [45]. More recently, Liou *et al.* [46] developed a predictive model using the CF Foundation registry for 5-year survival. This model was based on age, FEV_1, gender, weight-for-age z-score, pancreatic sufficiency, diabetes mellitus, *Staphylococcus aureus* infection, *Burkerholderia cepacia* complex infection and annual number of acute pulmonary exacerbations. A 2-year survival predictor model was also developed with univariate predictors including the number of hospitalizations or home intravenous antibiotics for exacerbations, *B. cepacia*, *P. aeruginosa*, weight percentile, FEV_1 percentage of predicted, height percentile and age [47].

Exercise parameters such as oxygen uptake at peak exercise are associated with overall mortality in patients with CF [48]. It was recently demonstrated that breathing reserve index at the lactate threshold correlated with poor survival [49]. Aurora *et al.* [50] developed a model for children which includes FEV_1, oxygen saturation during a 12-minute walk test, resting heart rate, age, gender, plasma albumin and hemoglobin as predictors of poor survival. Additional factors that may be taken into consideration include a decreased percentage ideal body weight, massive hemoptysis, presence of diabetes mellitus, pulmonary hypertension and more than 30% disparity in perfusion difference between lungs [18,51,52].

Specific indications

Progressive lung disease and disability despite optimal medical therapy, FEV_1 of less than 30% predicted.

Specific contraindications

Individual transplant centers have microbiologic contraindications, the most common of which is *B. cenocepacia*. Severe liver disease is a contraindication in some centers, while in others it may be an indication for combined lung-liver transplantation. Among surgical contraindications, pneumonectomy is often a contraindication, but pleurodesis is not an absolute contraindication in many centers.

Timing of referral

Other factors favoring early referral include increasingly frequent hospitalizations, often associated with inability to attend school, a decline or marked fluctuation in lung function including FEV_1 values less than 30% predicted, increasingly resistant microorganisms, hypoxemia and hypercapnia.

Specific studies

Chest radiographic studies, lung function studies, sputum microbiology, gastrointestinal and nutritional evaluation, evaluation of sinus disease, and consideration of bone densitometry to assess for osteoporosis.

Preoperative management

Continuation of an aggressive program of antimicrobial therapy together with nutritional supplementation and physical rehabilitation.

CONCLUSIONS

Long-term outcomes after lung or heart-lung transplantation are suboptimal, with 5-year survival rates of approximately 50%. A comprehensive multidisciplinary approach to the evaluation of the lung or heart-lung transplant candidate is crucial. The objective lung transplant evaluation determines if transplantation is the appropriate therapeutic option for each individual candidate and family, and provides the transplant team with the opportunity to prepare for potential complications prior to the procedure.

REFERENCES

1 Vierra CA, Agrawal A, Book BK, *et al.* Rituximab for reduction of anti-HLA antibodies in patients awaiting renal transplantation. I. Safety, pharmacodynamics, and pharmacokinetics. *Transplantation* 2004;**774**:542–8.

2 Bittner HB, Dunitz J, Hertz M, Bolman MR 3rd, Park SJ. Hyperacute rejection in single lung transplantation: case report of successful management by means of plasmapheresis and antithymocyte globulin treatment. *Transplantation* 2001;**71**: 649–51.

3 Leech SH, Rubin S, Eisen HJ, *et al.* Cardiac transplantation across a positive prospective lymphocyte cross-match in sensitized recipients. *Clin Transplant* 2003;**17**(Suppl 9):17–26.

4 Gibson RL, Burns JL, Ramsey BW. Pathophysiology and management of pulmonary infections in cystic fibrosis. *Am J Respir Crit Care Med* 2003;**168**:918–51.

5 Corey M, Farewell V. Determinants of mortality from cystic fibrosis in Canada, 1970–1989. *Am J Epidemiol* 1996;**143**: 1007 17.

6 Dobbin C, Maley M, Harkness J, *et al.* The impact of panresistant bacterial pathogens on survival after lung transplantation in cystic fibrosis: results from a single large referral centre. *J Hosp Infect* 2004;**56**:277–82.

7 Aris RM, Routh JC, LiPuma JJ, Heath DG, Gilligan PH. Lung transplantation for cystic fibrosis patients with *Burkholderia cepacia* complex: survival linked to genomovar type. *Am J Respir Crit Care Med* 2001;**164**:2102–6.

8 Olivier KN, Weber DJ, Wallace RJ Jr, *et al.* Nontuberculous mycobacteria. I. Multicenter prevalence study in cystic fibrosis. *Am J Respir Crit Care Med* 2003;**167**:828–34.

9 Fairhurst RM, Kubak BM, Shpiner RB, *et al.* Mycobacterium abscessus empyema in a lung transplant recipient. *J Heart Lung Transplant* 2002;**21**:391–4.

10 Baldi S, Rapellino M, Ruffini E, Cavallo A, Mancuso M. Atypical mycobacteriosis in a lung transplant recipient. *Eur Respir J* 1997;**10**:952–4.

11 Ruffini E, Baldi S, Rapellino M, *et al*. Fungal infections in lung transplantation: incidence, risk factors and prognostic significance. *Sarcoidosis Vasc Diffuse Lung Dis* 2001;**18**:181–90.

12 Kadikar A, Maurer J, Kesten S. The six-minute walk test: a guide to assessment for lung transplantation. *J Heart Lung Transplant* 1997;**16**:313–9.

13 Hertz MI, Taylor DO, Trulock EP, *et al*. The registry of the international society for heart and lung transplantation: nineteenth official report, 2002. *J Heart Lung Transplant* 2002;**21**:950–70.

14 Sood N, Paradowski LJ, Yankaskas JR. Outcomes of intensive care unit care in adults with cystic fibrosis. *Am J Respir Crit Care Med* 2001;**163**:335–8.

15 Baz MA, Palmer SM, Staples ED, *et al*. Lung transplantation after long-term mechanical ventilation: results and 1-year follow-up. *Chest* 2001;**119**:224–7.

16 Bartz RR, Love RB, Leverson GE, *et al*. Pre-transplant mechanical ventilation and outcome in patients with cystic fibrosis. *J Heart Lung Transplant* 2003;**22**:433–8.

17 Dosanjh A, Jones L, Yuh D, Robbins RC. Pleural disease in patients undergoing lung transplantation for cystic fibrosis. *Pediatr Transplant* 1998;**2**:283–7.

18 Stanchina ML, Tantisira KG, Aquino SL, Wain JC, Ginns LC. Association of lung perfusion disparity and mortality in patients with cystic fibrosis awaiting lung transplantation. *J Heart Lung Transplant* 2002;**21**:217–25.

19 Serrano-Ikkos E, Lask B, Whitehead B, Eisler I. Incomplete adherence after pediatric heart and heart-lung transplantation. *J Heart Lung Transplant* 1998;**17**:1177–83.

20 Madill J, Gutierrez C, Grossman J, *et al*. Nutritional assessment of the lung transplant patient: body mass index as a predictor of 90-day mortality following transplantation. *J Heart Lung Transplant* 2001;**20**:288–96.

21 Brasch F, Muller KM. Classification of pulmonary alveolar proteinosis in newborns, infants, and children. *Pathologe* 2004;**25**:299–309.

22 Shulenin S, Nogee LM, Annilo T, *et al*. ABCA3 gene mutations in newborns with fatal surfactant deficiency. *N Engl J Med* 2004;**350**:1296–303.

23 Tredano M, Griese M, Brasch F, *et al*. Mutation of SFTPC in infantile pulmonary alveolar proteinosis with or without fibrosing lung disease. *Am J Med Genet* 2004;**126A**:18–26.

24 Simmoneau G, Galie N, Rubin LJ, *et al*. Clinical classification of pulmonary hypertension. *J Am Coll Cardiol* 2004;**43**(12 Suppl S):5S–12S.

25 Rosenzweig EB, Widlitz AC, Barst RJ. Pulmonary arterial hypertension in children. *Pediatr Pulmonol* 2004;**38**:2–22.

26 Glanville AR, Estenne M. Indications, patient selection and timing of referral for lung transplantation. *Eur Respir J* 2003;**22**:845–52.

27 Pielsticker EJ, Martinez FJ, Rubenfire M. Lung and heart-lung transplant practice patterns in pulmonary hypertension centers. *J Heart Lung Transplant* 2001;**20**:1297–304.

28 Sandoval J, Bauerle O, Gomez A, *et al*. Primary pulmonary hypertension in children: clinical characterization and survival. *J Am Coll Cardiol* 1995;**25**:466–74.

29 Clabby ML, Canter CE, Moller JH, Bridges ND. Hemodynamic data and survival in children with pulmonary hypertension. *J Am Coll Cardiol* 1997;**30**:554–60.

30 Lopes AA, Maeda NY. Circulating von Willebrand factor antigen as a predictor of short-term prognosis in pulmonary hypertension. *Chest* 1998;**114**:1276–82.

31 Bendayan D, Shitrit D, Ygla M, *et al*. Hyperuricemia as a prognostic factor in pulmonary arterial hypertension. *Respir Med* 2003;**97**:130–3.

32 Leuchte HH, Holzapfel M, Baumgartner RA, *et al*. Clinical significance of brain natriuretic peptide in primary pulmonary hypertension. *J Am Coll Cardiol* 2004;**43**:764–70.

33 D'Alonzo GE, Barst RJ, Ayres SM, *et al*. Survival in patients with primary pulmonary hypertension: results from a national prospective registry. *Ann Intern Med* 1991;**115**:343–9.

34 Rich S, Kaufmann E, Levy PS. The effect of high doses of calcium-channel blockers on survival in primary pulmonary hypertension. *N Engl J Med* 1992;**327**:76–81.

35 Barst RJ, Rubin LJ, McGoon MD, *et al*. Survival in primary pulmonary hypertension with long-term continuous intravenous prostacyclin. *Ann Intern Med* 1994;**121**:409–15.

36 Oya H, Nagaya N, Uematsu M, *et al*. Poor prognosis and related factors in adults with Eisenmenger syndrome. *Am Heart J* 2002;**143**:739–44.

37 Daliento L, Somerville J, Presbitero P, *et al*. Eisenmenger syndrome: factors relating to deterioration and death. *Eur Heart J* 1998;**19**:1845–55.

38 Oya H, Nagaya N, Satoh T, *et al*. Haemodynamic correlates and prognostic significance of serum uric acid in adult patients with Eisenmenger syndrome. *Heart* 2000;**84**:53–8.

39 Mendeloff EN. Pediatric lung transplantation. *Chest Surg Clin N Am* 2003;**13**:485–504.

40 Tibballs J, Chow CW. Incidence of alveolar capillary dysplasia in severe idiopathic persistent pulmonary hypertension of the newborn. *J Paediatr Child Health* 2002;**38**:397–400.

41 Cassidy J, Smith J, Goldman A, *et al*. The incidence and characteristics of neonatal irreversible lung dysplasia. *J Pediatr* 2002;**141**:426–8.

42 Palmer SM, Robinson LJ, Wang A, *et al*. Massive pulmonary edema and death after prostacyclin infusion in a patient with pulmonary veno-occlusive disease. *Chest* 1998;**113**:237–40.

43 Palevsky HI, Pietra GG, Fishman AP. Pulmonary veno-occlusive disease and its response to vasodilator agents. *Am Rev Respir Dis* 1990;**142**:426–9.

44 Holcomb BW Jr, Loyd JE, Ely EW, Johnson J, Robbins IM. Pulmonary veno-occlusive disease: a case series and new observations. *Chest* 2000;**118**:1671–9.

45 Kerem E, Reisman J, Corey M, Canny GJ, Levison H. Prediction of mortality in patients with cystic fibrosis. *N Engl J Med* 1992;**326**:1187–91.

46 Liou TG, Adler FR, Fitzsimmons SC, *et al*. Predictive 5-year survivorship model of cystic fibrosis. *Am J Epidemiol* 2001;**153**:345–52.

47 Mayer-Hamblett N, Rosenfeld M, Emerson J, Goss CH, Aitken ML. Developing cystic fibrosis lung transplant referral criteria using predictors of 2-year mortality. *Am J Respir Crit Care Med* 2002;**166**(12 Pt 1):1550–5.

48 Moorcroft AJ, Dodd ME, Webb AK. Exercise testing and prognosis in adult cystic fibrosis. *Thorax* 1997;**52**:291–3.

49 Tantisira KG, Systrom DM, Ginns LC. An elevated breathing reserve index at the lactate threshold is a predictor of mortality in patients with cystic fibrosis awaiting lung transplantation. *Am J Respir Crit Care Med* 2002;**165**:1629–33.

50 Aurora P, Wade A, Whitmore P, Whitehead B. A model for predicting life expectancy of children with cystic fibrosis. *Eur Respir J* 2000;**16**:1056–60.

51 Vizza CD, Yusen RD, Lynch JP, *et al.* Outcome of patients with cystic fibrosis awaiting lung transplantation. *Am J Respir Crit Care Med* 2000;**162**(3 Pt 1):819–25.

52 Sharma R, Florea VG, Bolger AP, *et al.* Wasting as an independent predictor of mortality in patients with cystic fibrosis. *Thorax* 2001;**56**:746–50.

39 Donor Evaluation, Surgical Technique and Perioperative Management

Charles B. Huddleston

There are many components to the successful conduct of a transplant procedure. Likewise, failure to successfully accomplish any of these components will put the life of the patient in jeopardy. Given that the heart and lungs must function immediately to sustain the life of the patient, this is magnified in lung and heart-lung transplantation. This chapter discusses those critical elements of the relatively brief period of time in the life of a lung and heart-lung transplant patient, beginning with the few hours involved in donor evaluation and organ procurement, the transplant operation and immediate postoperative management. This will encompass approximately 4 days in total, a segment of time that can have a major impact on the days, months and years that follow.

DONOR EVALUATION

Inadequate numbers of donors continues to plague the entire transplant community in spite of quite extensive efforts put forth by a variety of local and national transplant organizations to boost public awareness of the problem and educate people on the benefits derived by recipients of this "gift of life." The waiting list for lung and heart-lung transplant recipients continues to grow while the number of donors remains stagnant. The situation for children (those under 18 years of age) is similar. The number of new pediatric lung candidates listed in the USA was 109 and 115 in 2000 and 2001; the number of transplants from cadaveric donors were 43 and 28 for the same 2 years, respectively. The heart-lung transplant statistics show the same trend, with nearly four times as many new patients listed as receiving transplants [1].

The donor shortage in organ transplantation in general is magnified in lung transplantation as only approximately 15–20% of organ donors have lungs that are suitable for procurement [1,2]. Lung injury may be related to the mechanism of brain death (e.g. trauma, drowning) or may be directly related to brain death itself (neurogenic pulmonary edema, consequences of mechanical ventilation and intensive care unit stay) [3]. There are certainly instances in which the management of the donor has led to apparent deterioration in lung function as management to optimize renal, hepatic or cardiac status may impact negatively on the pulmonary status [3]. As a corollary to that, there are clearly measures that can be taken to "resuscitate" the donor lungs so that they become suitable. These measures include aggressive pulmonary toilet including the use of bronchoscopy to clear secretions, judicious fluid management, aerosolized bronchodilators and optimal positive end-expiratory pressure [4]. High-dose steroid administration (15 mg/kg methylprednisolone) given relatively early in the donor management process may also be beneficial [5]. The "standard" criteria for acceptable lung donors are listed in Table 39.1. Those criteria for acceptable heart donors are presented elsewhere in this text and will not be presented here as they apply to heart-lung donors, except to say that the heart must have nearly normal function.

Matching size and blood type are the initial steps. Although ABO-incompatible transplants have been performed successfully for liver [6], kidney [7] and heart [8] transplants, this has occurred (and been reported) for lung transplantation only as an unintentional event [9]. It is conceivable that this could be applied for young infants in need of lung transplantation.

Table 39.1 Acceptable donor characteristics for cadaveric lung transplantation.

ABO compatible blood type
Height $\pm 25\%$ of recipient
Age < 55 years
Chest radiograph clear
$Pao_2 > 350$ mmHg with ventilator settings:
$\quad$ Fio$_2$ 1.0
$\quad$ Tidal volume 10 mL/kg
$\quad$ PEEP 5 cm H$_2$O
Smoking history < 20 pack-years
No history of chest trauma
No history of aspiration
No pre-existing history of lung disease
Sputum free of significant white cells and organisms on Gram stain

Fio$_2$, fraction of inspired oxygen; PEEP, positive end-expiratory pressure.

Donor size is obviously a major part of the donor evaluation for pediatric lung and heart-lung transplantation. In general, height is used as the preferred index for matching donors and recipients for lung transplantation and weight is used for heart transplantation. For heart-lung transplantation, height is probably a better indication of size match. Other indices of measurement, such as those taken from chest radiographs, are fraught with inaccuracies. Discrepancies in size are necessary to provide sufficient flexibility. Exactly how much flexibility is "allowable" remains unclear, but generally 25% above or below the recipient height should result in reasonable lung function when bilateral lung transplantation is the planned procedure. Single lung transplant generally should require a donor the same size or 25% taller. A slightly smaller donor for heart-lung transplantation may make the implant easier. These figures are somewhat arbitrary and reflect the experience of those involved in the field. Certainly, oversized lungs can be trimmed down, even to the extent of using only lobes on each side. How small the lungs from the donor can be is more difficult to judge. Transplanting very small lungs into a relatively large chest can result in lung dysfunction which resembles re-expansion pulmonary edema and the graft dysfunction may be severe.

Although the criteria for acceptable lung donors listed in Table 39.1 should provide a reasonable quality lung graft, many have challenged these and shown that so-called "marginal" donors result in equivalent short- and long-term results when compared with "ideal" donors. Marginal donors were those with age greater than 55 years, smoking history greater than 20 pack-years and abnormal chest radiograph (usually atelectasis) [4,10–13]. Although some of the donors in these series had an initial Pao$_2$ less than 300 on 100% oxygen, nearly all had achieved this level by the time of harvest. This value is probably still a significant goal to assure the appropriateness of the donor. In the face of these encouraging results with marginal donors, another series expressed a word of caution [14]. The important factor in the evaluation of a donor with marginal criteria is to individually assess the circumstances, the likelihood that there has been significant pulmonary injury, the anticipated ischemic time and the match with the recipient.

ORGAN HARVEST

Prior to arrival of the retrieval team, attention to pulmonary toilet and fluid management to keep the patient euvolemic are important. Flexible bronchoscopy and gross examination of the lungs and heart are performed by the retrieval team to confirm the suitability of the donor organs. Timing between the other harvest teams and the implanting team must be coordinated. When procuring lungs only, generally the harvest is performed separate from the heart, although some centers prefer to harvest the heart and lungs as a block and then separate on the back table. For heart-lung transplantation, the heart and lungs are removed *en bloc*.

A wide variety of solutions are utilized by various centers throughout the world for cardiac preservation. There are nearly as many different solutions utilized as there are transplant centers [15]. It is difficult to prove that significant differences exist with any of these solutions, although there is some suggestion that those with electrolyte composition described as "intracellular" – high potassium, low sodium concentration – have more favorable results. The pulmonary preservation solutions used most commonly are modified Euro-Collins solution, University of Wisconsin solution, low-potassium dextran and Celsior, the former two being intracellular and the latter two extracellular. Experimentally, it would appear that Celsior and low-potassium dextran solutions offer advantages over the others [16–18]. The volume of cardiac preservation given is approximately 30 mL/kg and that of the pulmonary preservation solution is 70 mL/kg. Following harvest of the lungs it is advisable to flush retrograde via the pulmonary veins by individually cannulating the veins [19]. At the very least, this will flush out a surprising amount of thrombus material that likely landed in the lungs as pulmonary emboli. This is not possible to accomplish with a heart-lung block.

Heart-lung procurement

The heart-lung block is taken all together for heart-lung transplantation [20]. The procedure is performed via a median sternotomy. The thymus is removed and the pleural and pericardial spaces are opened widely for visualization of the lungs and heart. The early dissection consists of mobilization of the venae cavae, aorta and main pulmonary artery. Next the trachea is exposed between the aorta and superior vena cava just cephalad to the right pulmonary artery. Ligation and division of the innominate vein may provide better exposure of this area. When the other organ procurement teams are ready, heparin is given in a dose of 3000 units/kg. Prostaglandin E$_1$ is injected into the main pulmonary artery in a dose of approximately 50–75 μg/kg. This provides vasodilatation of the pulmonary vasculature to more uniformly distribute the pulmonary preservative, but also causes hypotension. The superior vena cava is ligated, the inferior vena cava is divided just above the diaphragm, and the left atrial appendage is amputated. Within three or four heart beats the heart should be empty. The aorta is then cross-clamped and the preservation solutions are given. Topical cold saline and ice slush are placed on the heart and lungs. One must ascertain that the heart is decompressed and that the pulmonary preservation solution is flowing well through the left atrial appendage, eventually clearing of any blood. Ventilation should be maintained at a relatively slow rate with normal tidal volume during the infusion of the preservation solutions to encourage equal distribution throughout the lungs.

The ventilation is stopped with the beginning of the removal of the organs. The left lung is reflected to the donor's right and an incision in the posterior parietal pleura is made near the spine from the apex of the chest to a point just above the diaphragm. The inferior pulmonary ligament is divided so that all this tissue can be swept up into the mediastinum using both blunt and sharp dissection. The same is done for the right pleural space. The pericardium is taken down to the diaphragm. The esophagus is skeletonized and divided at the level of the diaphragm with a stapler. The aorta is divided proximally and distally. The proximal esophagus is divided again with the stapler. The ascending aorta is divided just below the clamp. The superior vena cava is divided. The inferior vena cava should have been divided already by this time. The trachea should be the only structure holding the heart-lung block in place. At this point the lungs are held in gentle inflation with a volume equal to approximately half the usual tidal volume with an inspired oxygen fraction (Fio_2) of approximately 0.4. The trachea is then occluded with a stapling device and divided proximal to that. The heart-lung block is placed in a container of the cold pulmonary preservation solution; this is placed in sequential bags with cold saline and slush and then all is placed in a cooler packed with ice for transport back to the recipient center.

Lung procurement

The procedure for retrieval of the lungs only requires co-operation between the heart and lung transplant teams to negotiate the division of the shared structures – the left atrium and the main pulmonary artery. Some centers remove the heart and lungs as a block and then separate the two organs on the back table. Most, however, remove the heart first and then proceed with removal of the lungs once the heart is out of the field [21]. The left atrial cuff necessary for the pulmonary venous anastomosis is 5 mm at most. Prostaglandin E_1 is administered, the superior vena cava is ligated, the inferior vena cava is divided and the left atrial appendage is amputated. The aorta is clamped and the pulmonary preservation solution is given via a large-bore cannula in the main pulmonary artery near the bifurcation. Ventilation is maintained with normal tidal volume. Care must be taken to assure that the cannula is not directed into one branch pulmonary artery preferentially. Once all the preservation solution has been administered as described above, the pulmonary artery is divided at the level of the bifurcation and the superior vena cava and aorta are divided. The heart is reflected superiorly and to the right to expose the entry of the left pulmonary veins. It is relatively straightforward to define the level of dividing the left atrium midway between the entry of the left pulmonary veins and the atrioventricular groove. The interatrial groove should be dissected to provide more length of left atrium anterior to the entry of the right-sided pulmonary veins to avoid cutting into these, particularly the right inferior

pulmonary vein. The division of the left atrium is then completed so that the heart can be removed from the field, leaving the lungs *in situ*. The lungs are then removed as described above, with the esophagus stapled and divided proximally and distally and the descending thoracic aorta divided proximally and distally. With the trachea dissected out circumferentially well above the carina, the lungs are gently inflated to approximately 15 cm H_2O pressure and an Fio_2 of 0.4 as the trachea is stapled. The trachea is divided proximal to the staple line. A clamp should be placed across the proximal trachea to avoid spilling tracheal secretions into the field as the abdominal organ procurement teams continue to work. The lungs are then placed in a bag containing some of the pulmonary preservation solution. This is then placed in two additional bags containing cold saline and sterile slush and all of this is placed in a cooler packed with ice.

TRANSPLANT OPERATION

Heart-lung procedure (Figs 39.1–39.3)

Heart-lung transplantation is generally performed via a median sternotomy. Dissection of the aorta, main pulmonary artery and venae cavae are carried out first. The pleural spaces are dissected free of any adhesions. In general, the transplant procedure is probably better carried out with caval anastomoses rather than right atrial anastomosis. However, the risk of stenosis in the superior vena cava for infants undergoing heart-lung transplantation mitigates for a right atrial anastomosis. There may also be special circumstances in which modifications of this procedure are necessary related to the presence of congenital anomalies. When the donor team is in the vicinity the patient is anticoagulated with heparin and cannulated for cardiopulmonary bypass. Generally speaking, the cannulation should be high in the aorta and superior vena cava and low in the inferior vena cava. The patient is cooled moderately and the aorta is clamped. The venae cavae are snared and the heart and then the lungs are removed. The aorta and pulmonary artery are divided and the anterior wall of the right atrium is opened. The atrial incision is carried down to the orifice of the coronary sinus inferiorly and around the right atrial appendage superiorly on to the roof of the right atrium. The left atrium is entered in the roof and that incision is carried around the left atrial appendage. The heart is then excised by dividing the remaining portion of the free wall of the left atrium and interatrial septum. If caval anastomoses are planned for the heart-lung implant, nearly all of the right atrium can be removed leaving sufficient cuff of tissue on the caval orifices for the anastomoses of the donor cavae. The back of the left atrium is removed and all of the mediastinal pulmonary arteries are removed except for a small button around the insertion of the ligamentum arteriosum. This is left to avoid injury to the recurrent laryngeal nerve. The pulmonary veins are dissected

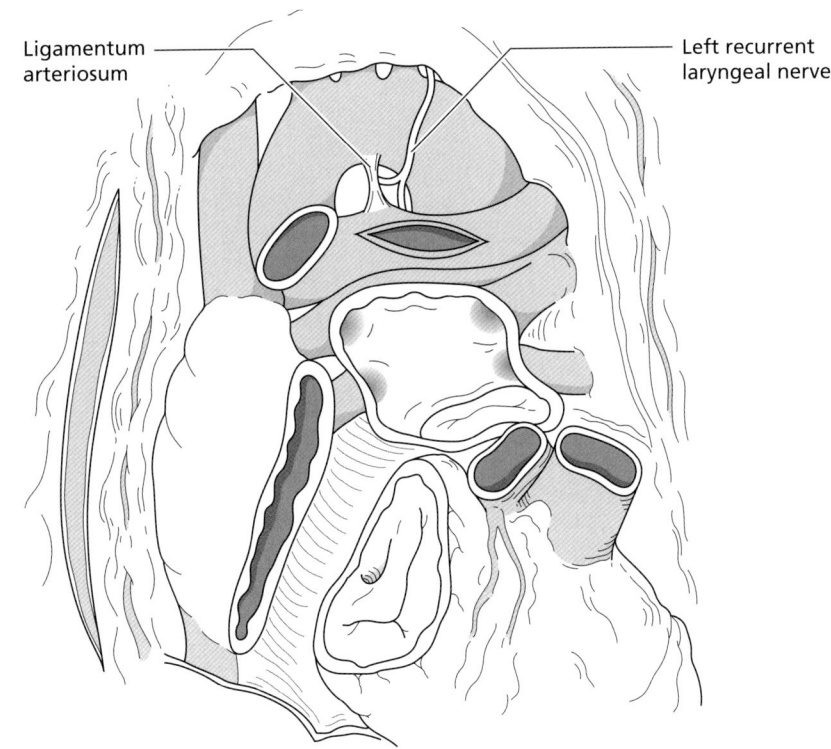

Fig. 39.1 Heart-lung transplantation is performed via a median sternotomy. The recipient heart is resected first followed by the resection of both lungs. To avoid injury to the recurrent laryngeal nerve, a portion of the back wall of the main pulmonary artery can be left behind as the recipient heart and lungs are excised. It is not necessary to ligate the pulmonary artery or vein branches during the recipient pneumonectomies. The mainstem bronchi are stapled on each side to avoid spillage of contaminated secretions into the chest.

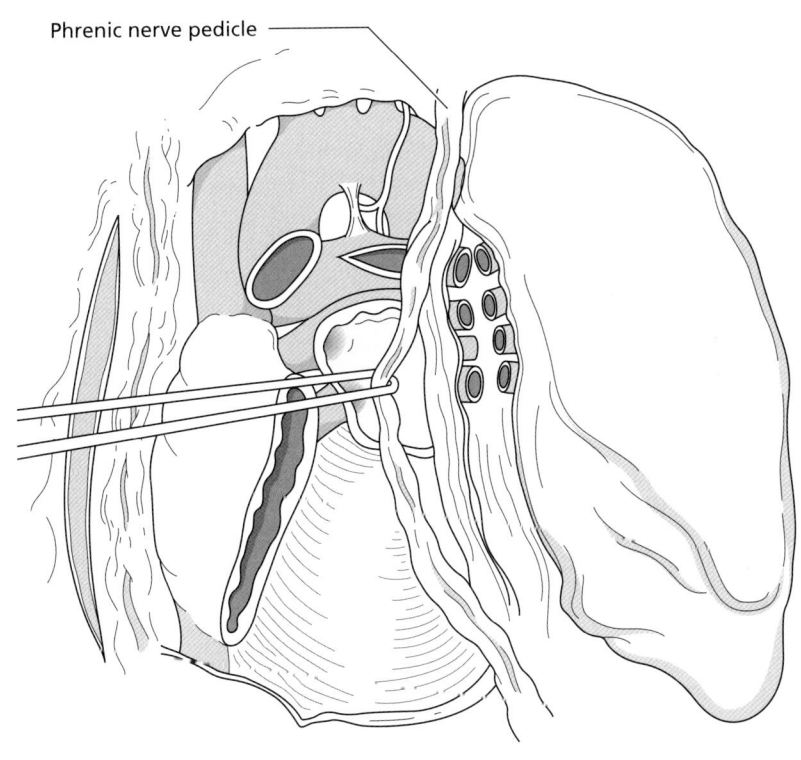

Fig. 39.2 Most of the pulmonary artery is removed, leaving a small island at the insertion of the ligamentum arteriosum so as to stay a safe distance from the recurrent laryngeal nerve. Nearly all the right and left atria are removed. The pulmonary artery and vein branches can be divided without ligating them; the bronchus is stapled and divided distal to that to remove the lung from the field. Phrenic nerve pedicles are created with a generous piece of pericardium on either side of each phrenic nerve to both preserve its blood supply and to guard against injury to the nerve itself. The remnants of the mainstem bronchi are dissected back to the trachea which is divided just above the carina.

back into the pleural spaces as are the pulmonary arteries, with care being taken to avoid injury to the phrenic nerves. The recipient bronchi are then dissected out. These are stapled and divided distally to remove each lung.

With both lungs and the heart removed from the chest, the next step is to dissect the bronchi back to the carina, avoiding the vagus nerve in the process. Phrenic nerve pedicles are created, staying well away from the nerve itself by leaving 1 cm

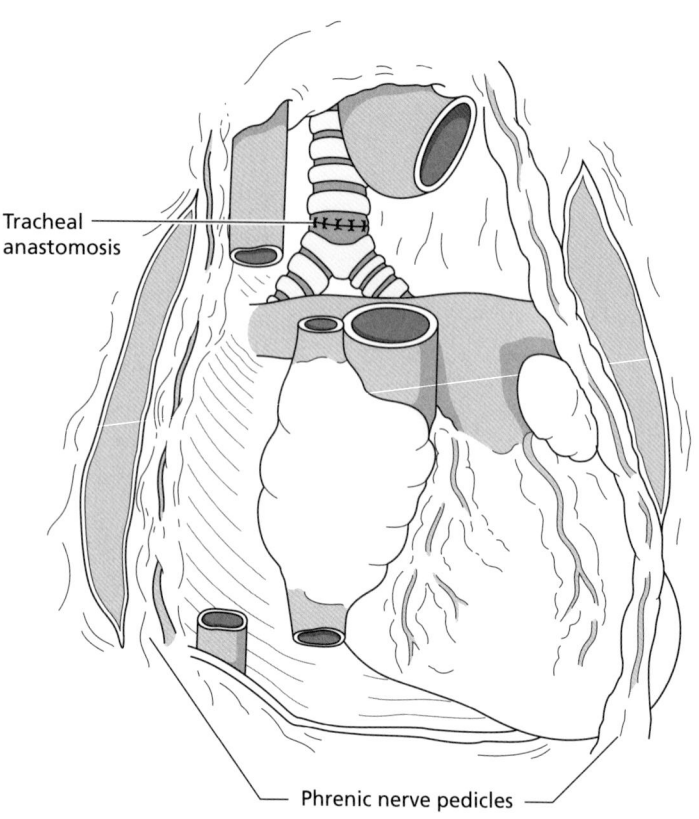

Tracheal anastomosis

Phrenic nerve pedicles

Fig. 39.3 The heart-lung block is positioned in the chest putting the right lung behind the right phrenic nerve pedicle and the left behind the other pedicle. Four anastomoses are required: trachea, aorta, superior vena cava (SVC) and inferior vena cava (IVC), in that order.

of pleura and pericardium on each side, from the level of the bronchus to the diaphragm. Meticulous hemostasis of the mediastinum and pleural spaces is carried out at this point as the exposure will never be better for this. Large collateral vessels are often present and will need to be accurately controlled.

The heart-lung block is brought up on to the table and the cuffs prepared appropriately. This consists of taking the staple line off the trachea leaving two or three cartilaginous rings of trachea above the donor carina, and trimming away excess pericardium. The venae cavae are trimmed to the appropriate lengths. The recipient trachea is divided just above the carina, removing the stapled mainstem bronchi. The lungs are then lowered into the pleural spaces behind the phrenic nerve pedicles, usually the right first and then the left. The tracheal anastomosis is performed in an end-to-end fashion with running monofilament suture. Although some surgeons prefer a combination of running and interrupted sutures for the tracheal anastomosis, the blood supply to the trachea is quite good on each side of the anastomosis and complications related to the running technique are extremely rare. The anterior portion of the tracheal anastomosis should be covered with some of the surrounding mediastinal tissue or pericardium so that this suture line will not be lying directly on the aortic suture line.

At this point a catheter is placed in the left atrial appendage (at the site previously amputated during the retrieval) using a pursestring stitch to secure it. Through this catheter cold saline is instilled to allow a means of de-airing the left-sided

cardiac structures as well as keeping the heart cool. Next, the aortic anastomosis is performed end-to-end with running monofilament suture. As this is being completed, the air in the left atrium and ventricle as well as that in the aortic root is evacuated through the open aortotomy. Just prior to completing this anastomosis the flow from the cardiopulmonary bypass circuit is reduced and the aortic cross-clamp removed to further de-air the aortic root. The anastomotic suture is then tightened and tied down. The catheter in the left atrial appendage is converted to a vent. The patient is rewarmed at this point and is kept in the Trendelenburg position until further de-airing is performed. The caval anastomoses are performed in an end-to-end fashion with monofilament fine suture, with care taken to avoid pursestringing the anastomoses (particularly the superior vena cava) usually by interrupting part of the suture line. Final de-airing is performed and the vent in the left atrium is removed. The lungs are gently inflated and held there at a relatively low inspiratory pressure to expand all atelectatic areas and then normal ventilation is resumed with a tidal volume of 10–15 mL/kg. The inspiratory pressure should remain less than 25 cm H_2O. Cardiopulmonary bypass is weaned and the cannulae removed. Temporary pacing wires are placed on the right atrium and ventricle. Chest tubes are placed in both pleural spaces; one is generally not placed in the mediastinum as the pleural spaces are widely opened with this procedure. The chest is then closed once hemostasis has been obtained.

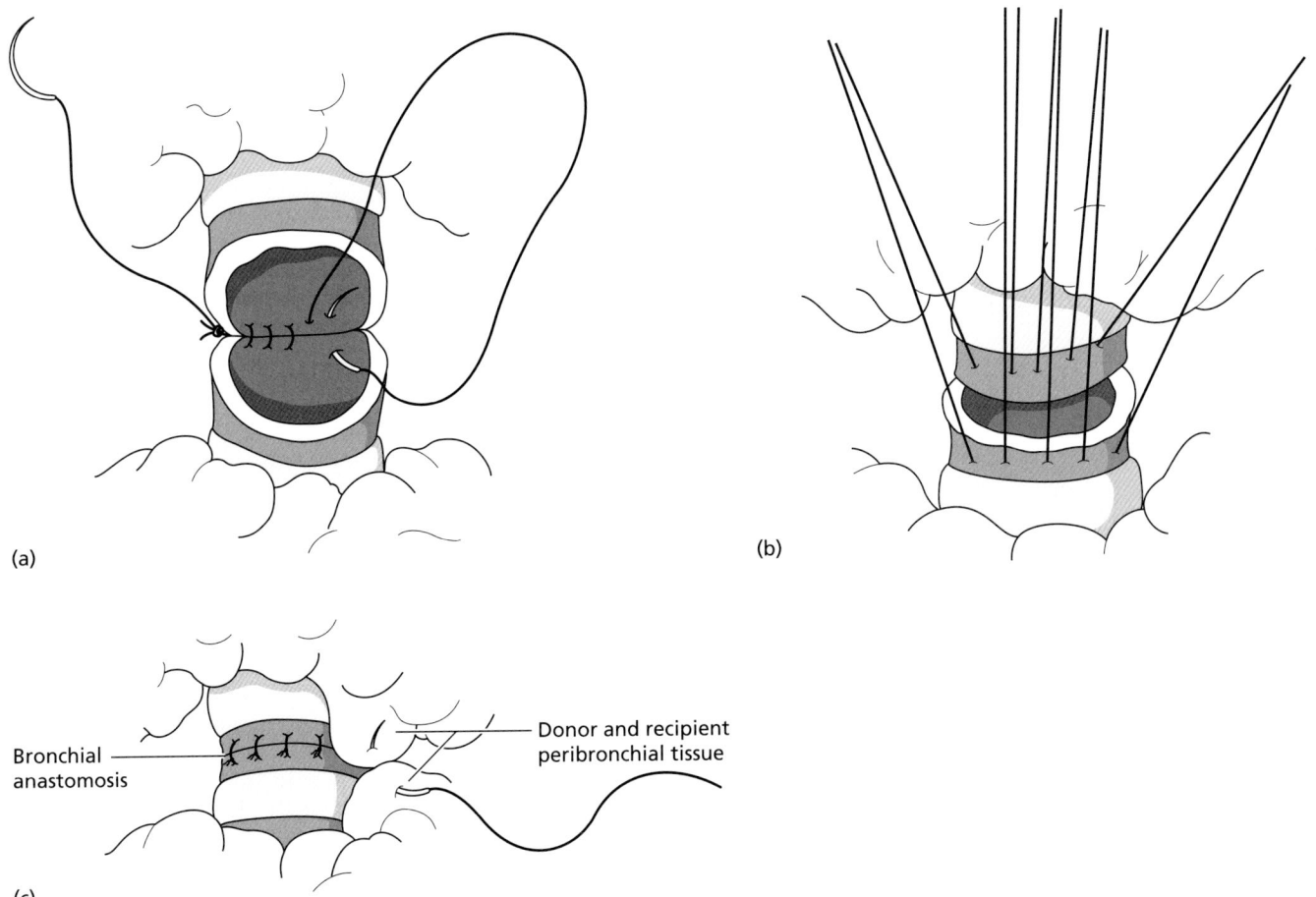

(a)

(b)

Bronchial anastomosis

Donor and recipient peribronchial tissue

(c)

Fig. 39.4 Lung transplantation is begun with the bronchial anastomosis, as illustrated in this series of figures. (a) The membranous portion of the bronchus is anastomosed with running suture and (b) the cartilaginous portion with interrupted simple sutures. (c) The bronchial anastomosis is covered with donor and recipient peribronchial tissue.

Lung transplant procedure (Figs 39.4–39.6)

Bilateral sequential lung transplant (rather than single lung transplant) is the procedure of choice in children, in large part because of concerns over the growth of the implanted lungs. This has supplanted the double lung transplant technique because of the ease of the procedure technically and fewer airway complications. The patient is positioned with the entire chest down to the mid-axillary line exposed and prepped. A bilateral trans-sternal anterior thoracotomy incision is made and the fourth intercostal space is entered. The internal mammary artery and vein on each side is ligated and divided. The sternum is transected at this level to create the so-called "clam shell" incision. The hilar regions are dissected out as much as possible; it is difficult to do much on the left side because of difficulty with exposure. Cardiopulmonary bypass is nearly always necessary for small children and teenagers because of the difficulty managing a single lumen endobronchial tube in relatively small airways. The pericardium is opened and the patient anticoagulated with heparin. The aorta and right atrium are cannulated for cardiopulmonary bypass.

As soon as the donor organs arrive, the patient is placed on cardiopulmonary bypass and the recipient pneumonectomies are performed. The pulmonary artery branches are ligated in relatively distal sites and divided. The pulmonary vein branches are handled in the same fashion. The inferior pulmonary ligament is divided and the remaining mediastinal tissue attached to the medial aspect of the lung is divided with the electrocautery. The bronchus is skeletonized to a limited extent and then occluded with a stapling device as far from the carina as possible. The bronchus is divided distal to this and the lung removed. This same procedure is carried out on the opposite side. The bronchial stump is mobilized back into the mediastinum for approximately 1 cm. The pulmonary artery on each side is also mobilized as much as possible. The pulmonary veins are mobilized within the pericardial sac. Dissection in the interatrial groove often provides additional left atrial tissue for ease of applying the vascular clamp to this area. If there is a need to repair a congenital cardiac lesion

331

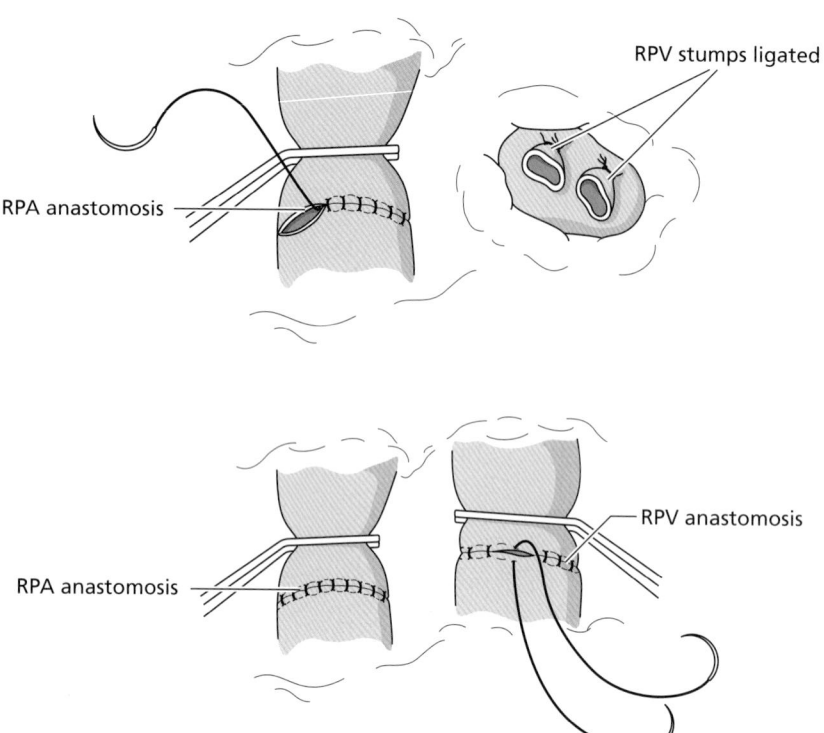

RPV stumps ligated

RPA anastomosis

Fig. 39.5 The ligated stumps of the recipient pulmonary arterial branches are removed at the level of the first upper lobe branch and the arterial anastomosis is performed in an end-to-end fashion with running monofilament suture. RPA, recipient pulmonary artery; RPV, recipient pulmonary vein.

RPV anastomosis

RPA anastomosis

Fig. 39.6 The interatrial groove on the right is dissected so that a vascular clamp can be easily applied to the left atrium to include the stumps of the divided recipient pulmonary veins. These are removed and the atrial tissue between the stumps is divided leaving a large opening for the pulmonary venous anastomosis. RPA, recipient pulmonary artery; RPV, recipient pulmonary vein.

such as a ventricular septal defect, that is performed at this time. Bicaval venous cannulation would have been necessary rather than a single venous cannula in the right atrium. With the recipient lungs out of the chest, there is no pulmonary venous return to the heart, providing a completely bloodless field to expeditiously repair the defect and then proceed with the lung transplant itself.

While the recipient pneumonectomies are being performed, the donor lungs are prepared on the back table by the harvesting team. The esophagus, aorta and excess pericardium are removed. The back wall of the left atrium is divided as is the mediastinal pulmonary artery at the bifurcation. The trachea is then removed by dividing the proximal bronchi. The proximal bronchi are cultured for bacteria, fungi and viruses. The bronchi are taken down to within two cartilaginous rings of the upper lobe orifice. This allows for enough room to place sutures for the anastomosis but makes the bronchus as short as possible for better collateral circulation to the anastomosis [22]. The blood supply to the bronchial anastomosis on the donor side is retrograde from the small collateral connections between the pulmonary and bronchial circulations at the level of the bronchioles. Care is taken to preserve the surrounding connective tissue near the divided end of the bronchus so that collateral circulation to this lymphatic tissue is maintained. The excess left atrial tissue is trimmed leaving 2–3 mm for the anastomosis. The pulmonary artery branches are trimmed well proximal to the first upper lobe branches.

The recipient bronchus is prepared by removing the staple line distally so that healthy bronchus is available for the anastomosis. The precise technique for the anastomosis has traditionally been a running absorbable suture for the membranous portion and interrupted sutures for the cartilaginous portion (Fig. 39.4a–c). Telescoping the donor into the recipient bronchus has been emphasized by some, but this is not universally accepted and may result in airway stenosis in small children. In fact, it appears that the precise method is not as critical as previously emphasized [23,24]. Covering the bronchial anastomosis has evolved from the use of omentum [25] to pericardial fat [26] to the peribronchial lymphatic tissue of the donor and recipient [27]. Some centers have employed direct bronchial revascularization as a means to avoid problems with airway healing [28]. However, this has not been widely accepted and there is some evidence to suggest that it is not at all advantageous [29]. Although success with bronchial healing has been achieved without wrapping at all, it seems logical to separate the bronchial and pulmonary artery anastomoses by something.

Following the bronchial anastomosis, the pulmonary artery connection is performed (Fig. 39.5). A vascular clamp is applied to the mediastinal portion of the recipient branch pulmonary artery and the ties applied previously are removed with the distal portion of the pulmonary artery. The anastomosis is performed in an end-to-end fashion with monofilament suture interrupted in two or three areas. Finally, another vascular clamp is applied to the margin of the left atrium to include the pulmonary vein stumps (Fig. 39.6). These stumps are removed and the orifices of the veins connected to produce a large opening. This anastomosis is also performed using monofilament suture material in an end-to-end fashion. Prior to completing the anastomosis, the clamp on the pulmonary artery is removed and the flow from the cardiopulmonary bypass circuit is turned down allowing blood to fill the right side of the heart and eject through the transplanted lung. This de-airs the venous side of the anastomosis. The lung is gently inflated to assist with evacuation of air through the open venous anastomosis. When this is completed, the vascular clamp is removed from the atrium and the venous suture line is tightened and tied down.

The second lung is implanted in the same fashion as the first. However, during the implant of the second lung the first is perfused in a controlled manner such that the pulmonary artery pressure remains around 20 mmHg systolic.

After the second lung has been implanted, the lungs are inflated to a pressure of approximately 20 cm H_2O and held there to expand all atelectatic areas. Ventilation is resumed with tidal volumes of approximately 10–15 mL/kg and the patient is weaned from cardiopulmonary bypass. Evaluation of the pulmonary venous anastomoses with transesophageal echocardiography is very useful at this point. Protamine is administered and the cannulae removed. Two chest tubes are placed in each pleural space: one anteriorly going to the apex and one posteriorly. Once hemostasis is assured, the chest is closed with wire for the sternum and heavy absorbable suture for the pericostal stitches.

POST-TRANSPLANT MANAGEMENT

The management of both the heart-lung transplant and the lung transplant patients is similar and aimed primarily at avoiding problems related to the lungs. Graft dysfunction of the lungs (referred to as reperfusion injury) is the most common postoperative complication of these transplant procedures. Although this may be an unavoidable consequence of events related to the donor selection, procurement process or recipient characteristics, careful management of issues as they arise may avoid major setbacks in the setting of minor problems. Overall, the management of these patients is similar to that for any patient undergoing a major cardiac procedure and involves:
1 pain control
2 fluid and hemodynamic monitoring
3 diuresis
4 wean mechanical ventilation
5 pulmonary toilet
6 nutrition
7 rehabilitation.
On top of all this, immunosuppression is initiated and surveillance for infection and rejection is ongoing.

All patients undergo flexible bronchoscopy and perfusion lung scans within 24 hours of the transplant procedure. These two tests will provide much information regarding the adequacy of all anastomotic connections. Flexible bronchoscopy

allows for not only an assessment of the patency of the bronchial anastomosis, but also the viability of the distal bronchial mucosa just beyond the suture line. Secretions are sampled at this time for microbiologic evaluation. A major imbalance in the percentage of flow to each lung on the perfusion scan should be investigated immediately with cardiac catheterization.

The hemodynamics must be carefully monitored and optimized. Low-dose inotropic support is often necessary. Filling pressures should be maintained at the lowest level possible to provide an adequate cardiac output. It is likely that the transplanted lungs will develop pulmonary edema at lower filling pressures than otherwise normal lungs because of the absence of functioning lymphatics as well as the temporary disruption of the usual membrane barriers to control intra-alveolar fluid. Diuretics are instituted early post-transplant as part of the overall theme of keeping the patients "dry."

Prostaglandin E_1 has been shown experimentally to provide some level of protection against reperfusion injury. It is given as a constant infusion at a rate of 0.025 µg/kg/minute [30]. Prostaglandin E_1 is also a pulmonary vasodilator. Nitric oxide is another agent that has demonstrated efficacy in prevention of graft dysfunction following lung transplantation [31]. Enhancing pulmonary blood flow will have a favorable impact upon blood flow to the bronchial anastomosis, promoting healing there. These drugs are given for 2 or 3 days post-transplant.

Bleeding is often a problem post-transplant because of the multiple suture lines involved as well as the dissection necessary. The use of aprotinin intraoperatively is now routine and has been shown to reduce bleeding [32]. Clotting studies are often abnormal in these patients post-transplant for a variety of reasons. Some come to the operating room on anticoagulants. Some have marginal hepatic function related to either heart failure or the underlying disease process (e.g. cystic fibrosis) resulting in reduced clotting factor production.

Infection, usually pneumonia, is a relatively common early complication of lung or heart-lung transplantation. The lung is the only solid organ exposed constantly to outside contamination. Many of these patients (especially those with cystic fibrosis) harbor resistant organisms in large quantities in the upper airways and sinuses. Immunosuppression is an important factor in the development of post-transplant infections. Secretions are poorly cleared because of impaired cilia function and loss of cough reflex. The selection of antibiotic prophylaxis post-transplant is based primarily on the organisms present on preoperative sputum cultures for those patients with cystic fibrosis, other septic lung disease or who are chronically ventilated. For all other patients, a first- or second generation cephalosporin is adequate. This is usually continued until all the chest drains have been removed.

Early extubation is always the goal post-transplant. This is primarily to avoid the consequences of microbiologic contamination, but also to allow for early ambulation and rehabilitation. Early extubation is complicated not only by the difficulty breathing and coughing related to postoperative pain, but also by the debilitated state most of these patients are in by the time they reach transplantation. Surfactant activity in the transplanted lungs is abnormal [33]. Division of the vagus nerve branches to the transplanted lung results in loss of the normal reflexes responsible for coughing and clearing secretions. Furthermore, there is a tendency for significant interstitial fluid in the lungs and pleural effusions related to loss of normal lymphatic drainage and whatever reperfusion injury occurs. The chest radiograph often shows evidence of pulmonary edema in the first week following transplantation [34]. Nonetheless, many patients will be able to be extubated within 48 hours of the transplant as long as the graft function itself is good. Measures to control pain, such as epidural catheters and low-dose narcotic agents are necessary to provide sufficient relief for the chest physiotherapy inevitably necessary for these patients.

Nutrition must be a priority as these patients are quite debilitated pretransplant. Many patients will need total parenteral nutrition because of the poor intestinal motility that frequently accompanies lung transplantation, probably related to injury to the vagus nerve. Enteral nutrition is initiated as soon as tolerated. Patients with cystic fibrosis have an added risk of developing distal intestinal obstruction syndrome related to impacted intestinal contents. This can be treated medically with intestinal lavage or hypaque enemas, although occasionally operative intervention is necessary [35]. Therefore, a regimen of cathartics begun soon after transplantation is recommended for these patients.

The number of problems and potential complications following lung or heart-lung transplantation in children are numerous. Any attempt at listing these would be incomplete. One must be extremely careful and diligent in the management of these patients. Early problems should be investigated thoroughly with a high index of suspicion. These children are very fragile and require treatment with drugs that have multiple side-effects. It is not at all uncommon for three or more subspecialists to be seeing these patients in consultation during their recovery. Thus, there is a major commitment required of the medical center to establish and maintain a successful lung and heart-lung transplant program.

LIVING DONOR LUNG TRANSPLANTATION

With the obvious disparity between available donors and recipients for lung transplantation, living donors have been utilized much as has occurred with kidney and liver transplantation. Living donor lung transplantation is generally considered when a potential recipient has declined to the point that he or she would not survive the anticipated waiting time for a cadaveric donor to become available. For living donor lung transplantation, two donors each supply a single lobe (the lower lobe) of either the right or left lung to serve as a whole lung for the recipient [36]. Nearly all these procedures are bilateral lung transplants. Most donors are blood relatives although they do not have to be. The donors are evaluated extensively for the presence of any underlying lung or other health problems. In addition, they are evaluated for psychologic issues that might come in to play after donation and transplantation. Matching donor and recipient size is difficult as there are generally few donors available for this procedure although the recipient should be significantly smaller than each donor. It is relatively easy to calculate the expected total lung capacity of the potential recipient and match it to the measured value for each donor, multiplied by 0.25, assuming that the lower lobe of each lung is approximately 25% of the total lung capacity. The harvest for these lobes is more complex because of the need to preserve the integrity of the bronchus, pulmonary artery and pulmonary vein for the remaining upper lobe [37]. Thus, the cuffs of the donor lobe are shorter, making the transplant procedure itself more difficult technically.

The results of living donor lung transplantation have been at least as good as lung transplantation using cadaveric donors. Although bronchiolitis obliterans appears less in the early years post-transplantation, it remains a significant late complication. The survival at 5 years post-transplantation is similar to that which has been accomplished with cadaveric lung transplantation, although the most common cause of death is infection rather than bronchiolitis obliterans [38]. Minor complications occur in approximately half of the donors and major complications in one-fourth. The major complications include atrial arrhythmias, pericardial effusions, persistent air leaks and pneumonia/atelectasis [39]. Although it may be appropriate to evaluate potential donors well in advance of the anticipated need for living donor lung transplantation, aggressive medical management of each potential recipient should be exhausted prior to embarking on this alternative form of transplant.

REFERENCES

1 2002 OPTN/SRTR Annual Report 1992–2001. HHS/HRSA/ OSP/DOT;UNOS;URREA.

2 Reilly PM, Grossman MD, Rosengard BR, *et al*. Lung procurement from solid organ donors: role of fluid resuscitation in procurement failures. *Chest* 1996;**110**:222S.

3 Novitzky D, Wicomb WN, Rose AG, *et al*. Pathophysiology of pulmonary edema following experimental brain death in the chacma baboon. *Ann Thorac Surg* 1987;**43**:288–94.

4 Gabbay E, Williams TJ, Griffiths AP, *et al*. Maximizing the utilization of donor organs offered for lung transplantation. *Am J Respir Crit Care Med* 1999;**160**:265–71.

5 Follette DM, Rudich SM, Babcock WD. Improved oxygenation and increased lung donor recovery with high-dose steroid administration after brain death. *J Heart Lung Transplant* 1998; **17**:423–9.

6 Mor E, Skerrett D, Manzarbeitia C, et al. Successful use of an enhanced immunosuppressive protocol with plasmapheresis for ABO-incompatible mismatched grafts in liver transplant recipients. Transplantation 1995;59:986–90.

7 Warren DS, Zachary AA, Sonnenday CJ, et al. Successful renal transplantation across simultaneous ABO incompatible and positive crossmatch barriers. Am J Transplant 2004;4:561–8.

8 West LJ, Pollock-Barziv SM, Dipchand AI, et al. ABO-incompatible heart transplantation in infants. N Engl J Med 2001;344:793–800.

9 Banner NR, Rose ML, Cummins D, et al. Management of an ABO-incompatible lung transplant. Am J Transplant 2004;4:1192–6.

10 Shumway SJ, Hertz MI, Petty MG, Bolman RM. Liberalization of donor criteria in lung and heart-lung transplantation. Ann Thorac Surg 1994;57:92–5.

11 Sundaresan S, Semenkovich J, Ochoa L, et al. Successful outcome of lung transplantation is not compromised by the use of marginal donor lungs. J Thorac Cardiovasc Surg 1995;109:1075–80.

12 Kron IL, Tribble CG, Kern JA, et al. Successful transplantation of marginally acceptable thoracic organs. Ann Surg 1993;217:518–24.

13 Follette D, Rudich S, Bonacci C, et al. Importance of an aggressive multidisciplinary management approach to optimize lung donor procurement. Transplant Proc 1999;31:169–70.

14 Pierre AF, Sekine Y, Hutcheon MA, et al. Marginal donor lungs: a reassessment. J Thorac Cardiovasc Surg 2002;123:421–8.

15 Demmy TL, Biddle JS, Bennett LE, et al. Organ preservation solutions in heart transplantation: patterns of usage and related survival. Transplantation 1997;63:262–9.

16 Rabanal JM, Ibanez AM, Mons R, et al. Influence of preservation solution on early lung function (Euro-Collins vs. Perfadex). Transplant Proc 2003;35:1938–9.

17 Muller C, Bittmann I, Hatz R, et al. Improvement of lung preservation: from experiment to clinical practice. Eur Surg Res 2002;34:77–82.

18 Thabut G, Vinatier I, Brugiere O, et al. Influence of preservation solution on early graft failure in clinical lung transplantation. Am J Respir Crit Care Med 2001;164:1204–8.

19 Wittwer T, Franke U, Fehrenbach A, et al. Impact of retrograde graft preservation in Perfadex-based experimental lung transplantation. J Surg Res 2004;117:239–48.

20 Baldwin JC. Heart-lung and lung graft preservation. In: Shumway SJ, Shumway NE, eds. Thoracic Transplantation. Cambridge: Blackwell Science, 1995: 71–6.

21 Sundaresan S, Trachiotis GD, Aoe M, Patterson GA, Cooper JD. Donor lung procurement: assessment and operative technique. Ann Thorac Surg 1993;56:1409–13.

22 Pinsker KL, Koerner SK, Kamholz SL, Hagstrom JW, Veith FJ. Effect of donor bronchial length on healing: a canine model to evaluate bronchial anastomotic problems in lung transplantation. J Thorac Cardiovasc Surg 1979;77:669–73.

23 Anderson MD, Kriett JM, Harrell J, et al. Techniques for bronchial anastomosis. J Heart Lung Transplant 1995;14:1090–4.

24 Aigner C, Jaksch P, Seebacher G, et al. Single running suture: the new standard technique for bronchial anastomoses in lung transplantation. Eur J Cardiothorac Surg 2003;23:488–93.

25 Cooper JD, Pearson FG, Patterson GA, et al. Technique of successful lung transplantation in humans. J Thorac Cardiovasc Surg 1987;93:173–81.

26 Emery RW, Arom KV, VonRueden T, Copeland JG. Use of the pericardial fat pad in pulmonary transplantation. J Card Surg 1990;5:145–8.

27 Meyers BF, Patterson GA. Technical aspects of adult lung transplantation. Semin Thorac Cardiovasc Surg 1998;10:213–20.

28 Norgaard MA, Olsen PS, Svendsen UG, Pettersson G. Revascularization of the bronchial arteries in lung transplantation: an overview. Ann Thorac Surg 1996;62:1215–21.

29 Khaghani A, Tadjkarimi S, al-Kattan K, et al. Wrapping the anastomosis with omentum or an internal mammary artery pedicle does not improve bronchial healing after single lung transplantation: results of a randomized clinical trial. J Heart Lung Transplant 1994;13:767–73.

30 Aoe M, Trachiotis GD, Okabayashi K, et al. Administration of prostaglandin E_1 after lung transplantation improves early graft function. Ann Thorac Surg 1994;58:655–61.

31 Struber M, Harringer W, Morschheuser T, et al. Inhaled nitric oxide as a prophylactic treatment against reperfusion injury of the lung. Thorac Cardiovasc Surg 1999;47:179–82.

32 Jaquiss RD, Huddleston CB, Spray TL. Use of aprotinin in pediatric lung transplantation. J Heart Lung Transplant 1995; 14:302–7.

33 Hohlfeld JM, Tiryaki E, Hamm H, et al. Pulmonary surfactant activity is impaired in lung transplant recipients. Am J Respir Crit Care Med 1998;158:706–12.

34 Anderson DC, Glazer HS, Semenkovich JW, et al. Lung transplant edema: chest radiography after lung transplantation: the first 10 days. Radiology 1995;195:275–81.

35 Minkes RK, Langer JC, Skinner MA, et al. Intestinal obstruction after lung transplantation in children with cystic fibrosis. J Pediatr Surg 1999;34:1489–93.

36 Starnes VA, Barr ML, Cohen RG, et al. Living-donor lung transplantation experience: intermediate results. J Thorac Cardiovasc Surg 1996;112:1284–91.

37 Cohen RG, Barr ML, Schenkel FA, et al. Living-related lobectomy for bilateral lobar transplantation in patients with cystic fibrosis. Ann Thorac Surg 1994;57:1423–8.

38 Starnes VA, Bowdish ME, Woo MS, et al. A decade of living lobar lung transplantation: recipient outcomes. J Thorac Cardiovasc Surg 2004;127:114–22.

39 Battafarano RJ, Anderson RC, Meyers BF, et al. Perioperative complications after living donor lobectomy. J Thorac Cardiovasc Surg 2000;120:909–15.

40 Pathology of the Lung Allograft

Paul S. Dickman

Lung allografts are routinely evaluated by transbronchial biopsy combined with bronchoalveolar lavage (BAL) [1–3]. Rarely, open lung biopsy is necessary for better delineation of pulmonary pathology in lung transplant patients. The disadvantage of the small size of transbronchial biopsy specimens is outweighed by the convenience and safety of the procedure. Valuable information is obtained from these specimens for monitoring rejection, infection and Epstein–Barr virus (EBV) associated complications, and to answer other clinical questions.

It is strongly recommended that at least five biopsy specimens be obtained for evaluation [3]. If biopsy material is required for evaluation of obliterative bronchiolitis (OB) or microbiologic studies, additional pieces of tissue may be necessary. Tissue for histopathologic study is fixed in neutral buffered formalin or other general purpose fixative. It may be helpful to shake the fixative container gently to facilitate penetration of fixative into air-filled spaces. Multiple levels of the biopsies are cut and at least three levels are stained with hematoxylin and eosin (H&E). Intervening levels should be stained with connective tissue stains (trichrome, periodic acid–Schiff [PAS], elastic). Grocott–Gomori methenamine-silver preparations for fungal and *Pneumocystis* organisms are used routinely, and stains for other microorganisms, such as Gram stain for bacteria and acid-fast stains for mycobacteria, should be used as required. Immunostains for suspected viruses, especially cytomegalovirus and adenovirus, may be critical.

PATHOLOGIC EVALUATION OF PULMONARY ALLOGRAFTS

Postoperative findings

Two types of immediate postoperative reactions are commonly seen. The *reimplantation response*, or "harvest effect," is characterized by interstitial and alveolar edema, sometimes accompanied by neutrophilic infiltrates. Cleared edematous areas surround septal bronchovascular and lymphatic structures. These findings most likely reflect ischemia (resulting from organ preservation or narrowed vascular anastomoses) or lack of lymphatic drainage, rather than rejection, and usually resolve spontaneously.

Diffuse alveolar damage (DAD) may occur, also related to graft ischemia. DAD corresponds to a clinical picture of acute respiratory distress syndrome. The findings of alveolar epithelial necrosis, capillary endothelial damage, protein exudation to form hyaline membranes, and interstitial inflammatory cell infiltrates are similar to the pattern seen in DAD in other clinical settings. Post-transplant DAD generally resolves but may progress to fibrosis.

Pathology of rejection

Effects of acute and/or chronic rejection are reflected in the biopsy specimens. As in other organs, both endothelial and epithelial cells are targets of mononuclear cell-mediated injury. Changes resulting from humoral rejection and reactions not involving lymphocytes are less well defined. The modified classification system for diagnosis of lung rejection provides standardized nomenclature [3].

A *Acute rejection.* Perivascular lymphocytic infiltrates involving arterioles and veins in alveolated lung parenchyma; capillaries and vessels in airway submucosa not included.

  0 No abnormality

  1 Minimal: infrequent infiltrates that are inapparent at low magnification

  2 Mild: infiltrates easily seen at low magnification, with subendothelial but not alveolar septal or airspace involvement; bronchioles may be involved

  3 Moderate: obvious dense infiltrates, with endotheliitis, interstitial infiltration and airspace involvement

  4 Severe: diffuse infiltrates accompanied by pneumocyte damage with hyaline membranes, hemorrhage and airspace neutrophils; necrosis, infarction or vasculitis may be present.

B *Airway inflammation.* Lymphocytic bronchitis/bronchiolitis. Grading (optional, at discretion of institution).

  0 No airway inflammation

  1 Minimal: rare mononuclear cells in airway submucosa

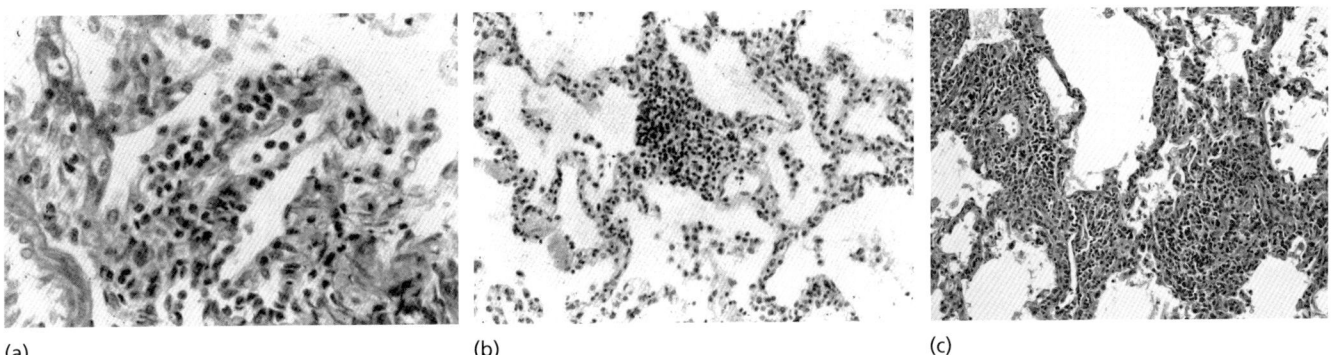

(a) (b) (c)

Fig. 40.1 Acute cellular rejection. (a) Grade A1 rejection. Sparse perivascular lymphocytic infiltrate does not extend into adjacent alveolar septa. (b) Grade A2 rejection. Perivascular lymphocytic infiltrates are visible at low power and involve multiple vessels. (c) Grade A3 rejection. Dense perivascular infiltrates may be confluent, with extensive alveolar septal involvement.

2 Mild: circumferential submucosal mononuclear cells and eosinophils; no epithelial lymphocytic inflammation or necrosis

3 Moderate: dense "band-like" submucosal mononuclear infiltrate with activated lymphocytes, eosinophils, epithelial necrosis, epithelial lymphocytic involvement

4 Severe: inflammation as in 3 with epithelial separation from basement membrane, ulceration, necrosis, fibrinopurulent exudates

X Ungradable: problems resulting from sampling, infection, orientation, etc.

C *Chronic airway rejection.*

1 Bronchiolitis obliterans: bronchioles are completely or partially occluded by dense fibrosis

(a) Active: fibrosis accompanied by inflammatory infiltrates

(b) Inactive: no inflammation present

D *Chronic vascular rejection.* Intimal fibrosis with luminal narrowing or occlusion.

Acute lung rejection manifests as perivascular lymphocytic infiltrates (Fig. 40.1a–c). Small and large activated lymphocytes surround and infiltrate parenchymal arterioles and veins and elevate endothelial cells. Peribronchiolar arteries are subsequently surrounded and infiltrated by lymphocytes. Later in the process there may be activation of bronchial-associated lymphoid tissue, bronchiolar and alveolar septal lymphocytic infiltration, and vascular fibrinoid necrosis. Alveolar lining cells may necrose, with serum leakage and hyaline membrane formation. In severe rejection, bronchiolar epithelium becomes necrotic and regenerative changes occur.

Airway inflammation occurs as lymphocytic bronchitis/bronchiolitis (LBB), without fibrous scarring (Fig. 40.2a,b). Lymphocytes involve the submucosa with or without mucosal infiltration, necrosis, ulceration or purulent exudates. Grading is left as an option at the discretion of individual institutions. Damage may also include glandular necrosis with squamous metaplasia. At times EBV infection may present as LBB; *in situ* hybridization for EBV EBER-1 RNA can distinguish between LBB resulting from rejection and EBV infection.

Chronic airway rejection is termed bronchiolitis obliterans (BO) or obliterative bronchiolitis (OB). It is defined as narrowing or occlusion of the bronchiolar lumen by fibrous scar tissue (Fig. 40.2c,d). This may be concentric or eccentric and extend into the alveolar interstitium. There is often destruction and loss of bronchiolar smooth muscle. OB may be accompanied by active lymphocytic inflammation with ongoing mucosal damage. The fibrous scarring seen in OB is most likely a reflection of multiple episodes of airway inflammation and is strongly associated with repeated bouts of acute rejection.

Chronic vascular rejection is manifested as fibrous thickening of the arterial and venous intima, similar to changes seen in arteries of heart and liver allografts (Fig. 40.2e). Mononuclear inflammation may accompany this fibrosis.

Biopsy specimens are graded using the letters and numbers in the above schema, accompanied by verbal summaries.

Biopsy findings of other post-transplant conditions

Infection causes major morbidity and mortality in transplant patients and may mimic rejection [4]. When grading rejection it may not be possible to exclude infection. Every effort should be made to identify possible infectious organisms by using special stains such as tissue Gram stain for bacteria, Grocott–Gomori methenamine-silver for fungi and *Pneumocystis*, and acid-fast stains for mycobacteria, as well as more specific immunostains when indicated. Viral infections are a frequent complication of pulmonary transplantation, and a search for viral inclusions is a routine part of the biopsy workup. In particular, cytomegalovirus and adenovirus are often found in these specimens (Fig. 40.3a,b). Immunostains for these and other organisms are extremely helpful. BAL fluid is used for cytologic study of cellularity and of pathogenic microorganisms, especially fungi and viruses. In BAL specimens one should expect to find pulmonary alveolar macrophages and variable numbers of lymphocytes, and bronchial or alveolar epithelial cells. When infection is present, neutrophils are

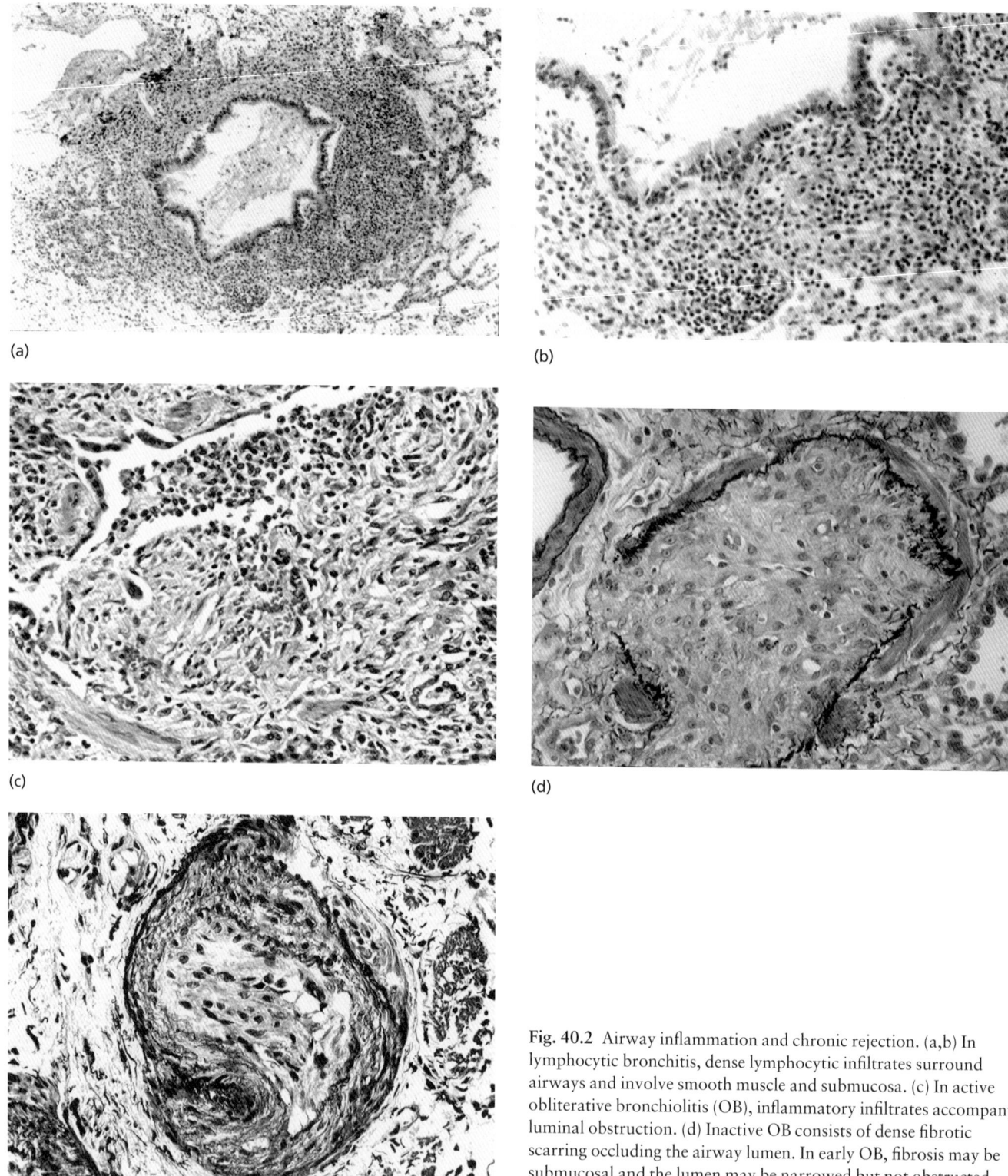

Fig. 40.2 Airway inflammation and chronic rejection. (a,b) In lymphocytic bronchitis, dense lymphocytic infiltrates surround airways and involve smooth muscle and submucosa. (c) In active obliterative bronchiolitis (OB), inflammatory infiltrates accompany luminal obstruction. (d) Inactive OB consists of dense fibrotic scarring occluding the airway lumen. In early OB, fibrosis may be submucosal and the lumen may be narrowed but not obstructed. (e) Vascular rejection consists of intimal fibrosis that partially or completely obstructs the lumen.

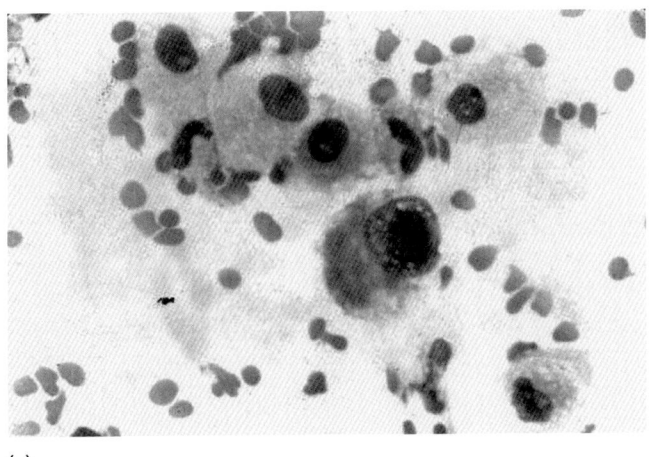

(a)

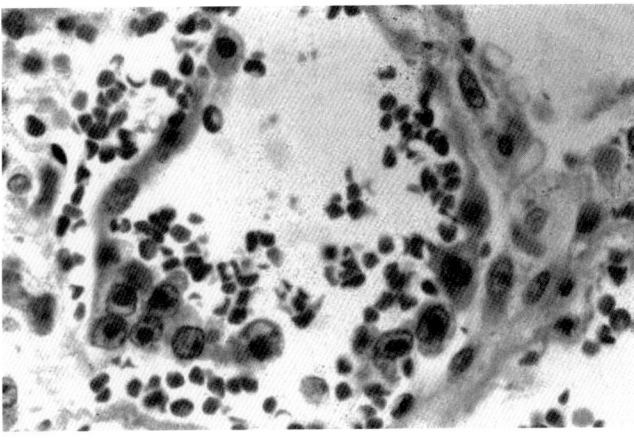

(b)

Fig. 40.3 Viral infection. (a) Cytomegalovirus infection in bronchoalveolar lavage (BAL) specimen is characterized by enlarged cells with intranuclear and cytoplasmic viral inclusions.

(b) Adenovirus-infected cells line an airway and have prominent intranuclear inclusions.

generally increased. Immunostains and microbiologic cultures of the BAL fluid permit characterization of bacteria, fungi and viruses that may not be observed in the small transbronchial biopsy specimen.

EBV-associated conditions are serious complications of transplantation (see Chapter 13) [5]. Manifestations in the lung biopsy specimen include benign lymphoid infiltrates that may be indistinguishable from LBB, and polymorphous or monomorphous post-transplant lymphoproliferative disease (PTLD). Classification of EBV-associated disorders is carried out according to criteria of the World Health Organization [6]. Evidence of EBV infection is most readily demonstrated using *in situ* hybridization for EBER-1 RNA.

PTLD is identified as interstitial, perivascular, and peribronchial or peribronchiolar infiltrates of mixtures of small lymphocytes, plasmacytoid lymphocytes and immunoblasts (see Chapter 13). Evaluation of the lesion is enhanced by molecular studies of immunoglobulin heavy-chain gene rearrangement and EBV clonality.

ACKNOWLEDGMENT

I am grateful to Dr. Ron Jaffe, Department of Pathology, Children's Hospital of Pittsburgh, for assistance with the illustrations.

REFERENCES

1 Yousem SA. Heart-lung transplantation. *Perspect Pediatr Pathol* 1989;**13**:82–104.
2 Yousem SA, Berry GJ, Brunt EM, *et al.* A working formulation for the standardization of nomenclature in the diagnosis of heart and lung rejection: lung rejection study group. *J Heart Transplant* 1990;**9**:593–601.
3 Yousem SA, Berry GJ, Cagle P, *et al.* Revision of the 1990 working formulation for the classification of pulmonary allograft rejection: Lung Rejection Study Group. *J Heart Lung Transplant* 1996;**15**: 1–15.
4 Kaditis AG, Phadke S, Dickman PS, *et al.* Mortality after pediatric lung transplantation: autopsies versus clinical impression. *Pediatr Pulmonol* 2004;**37**:413–8.
5 Randhawa PS, Jaffe R, Demetris AJ, *et al.* The systemic distribution of Epstein–Barr virus genomes in fatal post-transplantation lymphoproliferative disorders: an *in situ* hybridization study. *Am J Pathol* 1991;**138**:1027–33.
6 Harris NL, Swerdlow SH, Frizzera G, Knowles DM. Post-transplant lymphoproliferative disorders. In: Jaffe ES, Harris NL, Stein H, Vardiman JW, eds. *Pathology and Genetics of Tumours of Haematopoietic and Lymphoid Tissues, World Health Organization Classification of Tumours.* Lyon: IARC Press, 2001: 264–71.

41 Post-Transplant Management

Marlyn S. Woo

Since the earliest pediatric lung transplants, survival and graft function have steadily improved. However, the primary causes of allograft dysfunction in pediatric lung and heart-lung transplant patients have changed. During the early years of lung transplantation, hyperacute rejection, airway dehiscence, primary graft failure/dysfunction and infection were the chief causes of morbidity and mortality. While primary graft failure and infection continue to have a major impact on short- and long-term outcome, hyperacute rejection and airways dehiscence are no longer significant problems because of improved immunosuppression and surgical techniques. The pediatric recipient can expect to experience the same types of complications as his or her adult counterpart: the child who receives a lung or heart-lung transplant will be at risk for airway complications, infection, acute cellular rejection, bronchiolitis obliterans and malignancy (such as post-transplant lymphoproliferative disease). Recognition of these complications can be difficult. Pulmonary function tests (both standard and infant pulmonary mechanics; exercise stress testing), radiologic studies (e.g. chest radiograph, computerized axial tomography, magnetic resonance imaging, ventilation/perfusion studies) and oxygen saturation by pulse oximetry are noninvasive methods used to follow and to help determine the presence or absence of these pathologic processes. However, tissue biopsy (by transbronchial biopsy, percutaneous core needle biopsy or open lung procedure) remains the gold standard in diagnosing lung pathology in the pulmonary transplant patient.

The successful management of the pediatric lung and heart-lung transplant recipient involves not only early detection and recognition of potential complications, but close collaboration and prompt communication between members of the transplant team, the referring physician, the transplant patient and their family.

INTENSIVE CARE MANAGEMENT

Perioperative management is discussed in detail in Chapter 39. In brief, lung and heart-lung transplant patients after surgery are returned to the intensive care unit intubated and mechanic-ally ventilated. Depending on the type of transplant procedure (cadaveric versus living donor lobar), extubation can occur in 12–72 hours after uncomplicated surgery. Prolonged mechanical ventilatory support is associated with high central venous pressure (independent of poor myocardial function), poor right ventricular function, sepsis/infection, primary graft failure, neurologic complications (stroke, leukoencephalopathy secondary to hypomagnesemia or calcineurin inhibitor), phrenic nerve/diaphragm injury and hyperammonemia [1–3].

Chest tubes are placed at the end of cardiothoracic transplantation in order to remove air and pleural fluid. The number of chest tubes and the length of time they are kept in place depends on the patient's diagnosis (cystic fibrosis versus nonpurulent lung disease), type of transplant (cadaveric or living donor lobar) and size of the patient. In many centers, anterior and posterior tubes are placed on both sides of the chest of the bilateral lung transplant recipient. Some centers also place mediastinal tubes. The chest tubes are placed to suction and monitored for output as well as for the development of clots and blockage and amount of air leak. The amount of suction depends on the type of lung transplant; cadaveric recipients are often placed on conventional 20 cm H_2O. However, it has been reported that living donor lobar recipients may be difficult to ventilate if the suction is set at that level [4]. The size mismatch between the lobes and the thoracic cavity may contribute to this problem in living donor lobar patients [5]. Chest tubes are generally removed when there is no further air leak detected on water seal and there is minimal drainage. Centers vary on what they define as "minimal drainage" depending on the patient size and their experience: from < 200 to < 100 mL per 24 hours has been cited.

There are other differences in the postoperative management of cadaveric versus living donor lobar lung transplant patients. Living donor lobar patients typically require lower blood pressures, nitric oxide and milrinone infusion in the immediate postoperative period [6]. In addition, routine bronchoscopy with transbronchial biopsy should be avoided in living donor lobar lung transplant recipients, because of the increased risk of significant post-biopsy hemorrhage which can be life-threatening.

AIRWAY COMPLICATIONS

Bronchial dehiscence or air leak can occur soon after transplant surgery. Airway anastomotic dehiscence should be suspected when there are large air leaks from the chest tubes as well as by the presence of poor ventilation or blood gases in the lung transplant recipient. This complication is usually evident soon after admission to the intensive care unit and will only resolve with prompt surgical evaluation and repair. The most common cause of airway dehiscence is airway ischemia. Signs of airway ischemia include patchy areas of necrosis of the donor airway mucosa. There have been reports of airway dehiscence when sirolimus was used as one of the initial agents in lung transplant recipients [7,8]. Hence, routine use of sirolimus in the new lung transplant patient should be avoided when possible.

Flexible fiberoptic bronchoscopy is useful for monitoring the state of the airway anastomoses as well as for clearing airway secretions and obtaining cultures. While the airway is usually inspected at the end of the transplant surgery, timing of routine bronchoscopy varies from center to center. While several centers advocate routine bronchoscopy on the first postoperative day and then prior to extubation, others do not perform routine bronchoscopy in pediatric patients after lung transplant surgery.

Bronchial stenosis can occur as both an early and late post-lung transplant complication. Symptoms may be absent in mild cases but then wheezing and/or dyspnea may develop with progressive narrowing at the anastomotic site. On physical examination, there may be diminished breath sounds or air entry on the affected side or prolongation of the expiratory phase. Radiographically, atelectasis occurs distally to the stenosis and there may be an abrupt cut-off at the affected site. Although most stenoses are secondary to progressive fibrosis and narrowing at the region of the anastomosis, other etiologies include hematomas, "telescoping" of the bronchus during surgical implantation and infections (particularly *Aspergillus* sp.). Diagnosis is established by bronchoscopy with cultures. If infection is the cause of airway narrowing, aggressive antimicrobial therapy is essential. Extrusion of sutures at the anastomosis site may predispose to recurrent infections and airway narrowing. Reduction in immunosuppression may be necessary to eliminate the infectious agents. If stenosis is present, bronchial dilatation is recommended as initial treatment rather than stent placement. Incidence of significant airway complications ranges from 9% to 27% [9–11].

VASCULAR COMPLICATIONS

Vascular anastomotic complications can also occur in the recent lung transplant recipient. These complications are often associated with hypotension immediately after surgery. Arterial stenosis, venous thrombosis or stenosis, congestive heart failure and sepsis should be explored as possible causes of persistent or significant hypotension in the immediate postoperative period (Fig. 41.1). Thrombus formation at the left atrial anastomotic suture line or in the pulmonary veins is a devastating complication that can occur in the early

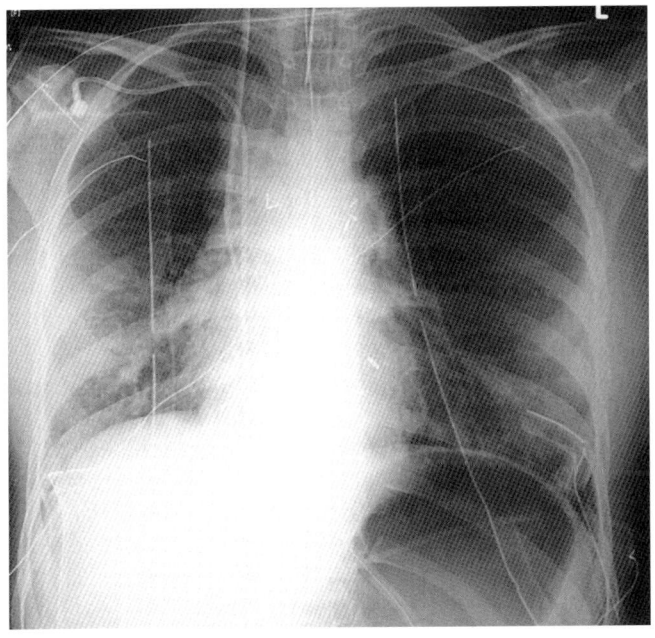

(a)

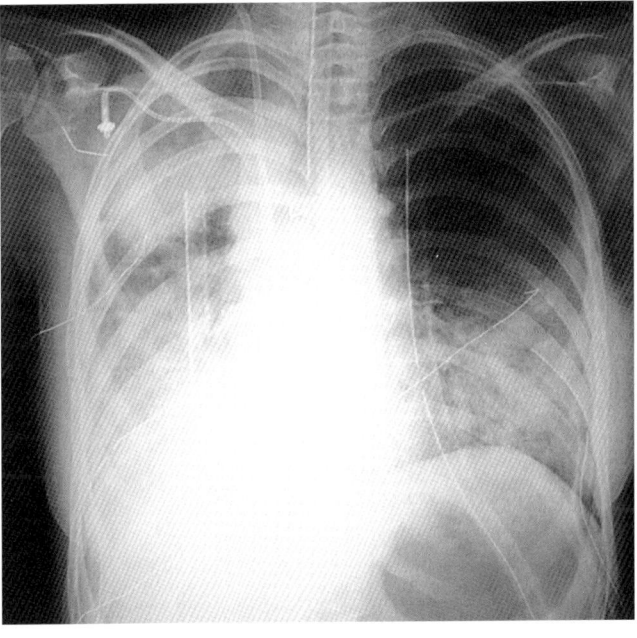

(b)

Fig. 41.1 Radiological progression of postoperative right pulmonary vein thrombosis: (a) admission; (b) six hours later.

postoperative period [12]. These pulmonary vein thromboses may also embolize to the systemic circulation and cause fatal cerebral emboli [13].

Transesophageal echocardiography should be used to evaluate the anastomosis and should be compared with the intraoperative studies. The microorganisms causing sepsis are most frequently from donor-derived bacteria. Hence, the transplant care team should pay close attention to the results of the Gram stains and cultures obtained from the donor bronchus.

NUTRITION

Most pediatric lung or heart-lung transplant recipients are malnourished at the time of transplant surgery. Total parenteral nutrition should be started within 24 hours of transplantation, even if it is anticipated that the patients will be successfully extubated within 24 hours. Even after successful extubation, most patients will be unable to take in sufficient calories by mouth. They will often have some pain as well as nausea and narcotic-induced intestinal dysmotility. Yet good nutrition is essential for wound healing, which is delayed as a result of immunosuppressive medications. If patients are stable after extubation, they can generally start on oral feeds within 12–24 hours. However, patients should be monitored for aspiration, postoperative ileus, gastroparesis (particularly in heart-lung transplant patients) and small bowel obstruction (cystic fibrosis patients) [14].

Monitoring nutritional status should not stop at hospital discharge; many pediatric lung and heart-lung transplant patients remain at risk for nutritional complications. Nutritional failure or malnutrition with weight loss, hypoalbuminemia and low serum protein levels are common in cystic fibrosis (CF) lung transplant patients. Obesity is a complication that can occur in previously sedentary, non-CF lung transplant children. The stigma of sudden weight gain, accompanied by stretch marks, can increase risk of depression and anxiety in the adolescent lung transplant patient. Hence, careful monitoring of weight and nutritional counseling should be provided to patients and their families at every transplant clinic visit.

INFECTION

The lifelong threat of infection begins in the perioperative period. For pediatric cadaveric lung and heart-lung recipients, infection is the major cause of morbidity and mortality during the first 6 months after surgery [15]. Denervation of the transplanted lung, immunosuppression, decreased mucociliary clearance, interruption of bronchial and lymphatic circulation, and impaired recruitment of antibody-forming cells in the transplanted lung combine to increase both the risk of

acquiring infection and the severity of infection once acquired [16,17]. Prevention rather than treatment of infections should be the primary aim of the medical care providers of the post-transplant patient. While it is common practice to place these patients in protective isolation, the use of gowns, gloves and visitor restrictions is center-dependent. The relative impact of these infection control practices as well as the benefit of particular dietary or beverage restrictions (e.g. bottled versus filtered water) has not been well studied. Other preventative measures, such as requiring sinus surgery in CF lung transplant candidates, have not been shown to affect short- or long-term outcome after lung transplantation.

The source of early infectious complications in the transplant recipient can often be traced back to organisms originating in the donor. It should be remembered that these donor organisms can include not only bacterial pathogens (*Pseudomonas, Staphylococcus, Burkholderia cepacia, Pneumocystis*), but serious viral (particularly cytomegalovirus and adenovirus) and fungal agents (*Aspergillus, Candida*) as well. However, if the lung transplant recipient's primary disease is CF, it is also likely that the infectious agents were pre-existing in the recipient's lower airways and/or sinuses. Treatment should be directed by infectious disease consultants and team members. If no organisms are identified, then intravenous vancomycin is usually given for the first 12–24 hours. For lung transplant recipients with CF, prior sputum and airway cultures and susceptibility testing should guide specific antibiotic regimens of at least two intravenous antibiotic agents. Prophylaxis against *Pneumocystic carinii* is usually started in the postoperative period. Co-trimoxazole (1 tablet on Monday-Wednesday-Friday) or aerosolized pentamidine (in patients with sulfa allergy) are the agents most commonly used to prevent *P. carinii* infection. Aerosolized antibiotics are usually not effective as treatment of pneumonia or infiltrates in these immunocompromised patients. However, it has been reported that aerosolized amphotericin (for treatment of *Aspergillus*) and aerosolized aztreonam (for treatment of *Burkholderia cepacia*) have been successful in treating affected lung transplant recipients.

In the perioperative period, mediastinitis and bloodstream infections are associated with increased mortality in the transplant patient. The best treatment for post-transplant mediastinitis must include not only appropriate antibiotic therapy, but also early aggressive débridement with substernal irrigation [18]. Bloodstream infections may occur as early or late complications after transplant surgery. These infections are most common within 30 days after lung transplant surgery [19]. The most commonly reported organisms isolated are *Staphylococcus, Pseudomonas aeruginosa* and *Candida*. Early bloodstream infections are associated with increased mortality risk in the first year after transplantation [19].

While the possibility for infectious complications is highest during the first months after transplantation, infection remains a significant risk for the rest of the patient's life. Several viral infections, particularly cytomegalovirus (CMV), Epstein–Barr virus (EBV) and human herpes virus type 6 (HHV6) infections are associated with increased risk for bronchiolitis obliterans syndrome, post-transplant lymphoproliferative disorders and dementia/encephalitis, respectively. Many transplant centers use quantitative polymerase chain reaction (PCR) to monitor viral loads of CMV and EBV post-transplantation.

At our center, outpatient lung transplant patients with fever and radiographic evidence of new pulmonary infiltrates are admitted and started on intravenous antibiotics based, whenever possible, on their previous culture and susceptibility results. If the patient is stable on intravenous antibacterial therapy, a bronchoscopy is performed within 24–48 hours for bronchoalveolar lavage and transbronchial biopsy. After definitive identification of infection, the antimicrobial agents are adjusted. Differential diagnosis of new infiltrates is dependent on the period of time after transplant surgery. In the perioperative period, reperfusion injury, vascular complications and pulmonary edema must be considered along with infection and acute cellular rejection. Patients with acute cellular rejection may also present with dyspnea, fever and radiographic infiltrates, including pleural effusions. Thus, it is not possible to definitively differentiate between infection and acute cellular rejection. In fact, both processes may be present simultaneously in the same patient. As therapy is different for these complications (antimicrobials versus bolus steroids), it is important to obtain tissue confirmation whenever feasible.

Transplant patients are at risk for acquiring opportunistic infections, not only *Pneumocystis carinii* and HHV6, but also atypical mycobacteria (*Mycobacteria avium*, *M. abscessus*) (Fig. 41.2) and *Bordetella bronchiseptica*. Depending on the geographic location, the atypical organisms will vary (e.g. coccidiomycosis, histoplasmosis, cryptococcus). Hence, the medical team needs to be aggressive in obtaining diagnostic cultures from bronchoalveolar lavage fluid and from affected tissue.

Prevention of infection should be the primary goal of the transplant team. Patients and their caregivers should be educated to avoid prolonged exposure to construction sites, contaminated water sources and obviously ill contacts. Timely immunization of pets (dogs, cats, birds) and patient routine immunizations (e.g. annual influenza A&B) are indicated. Use of appropriate filter masks in high-risk environments and cleansing of bathrooms and filters are the most common recommendations. Use of amphotericin aerosols or nasal spray may be used to prevent *Aspergillus* airway infections in the postoperative period.

PRIMARY GRAFT FAILURE/DYSFUNCTION

Primary graft failure/dysfunction is associated with high mortality risk. Also known as pulmonary reimplantation response and ischemia-reperfusion injury, primary graft failure

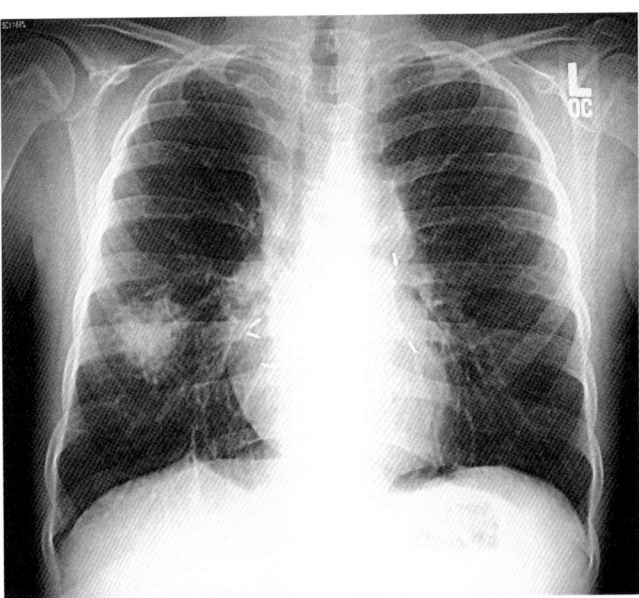

Fig. 41.2 *Mycobacterium avium* infection. Chest radiograph with right lung nodule found in an asymptomatic lung transplant recipient without prior history of mycobacterial infection. Computed tomography guided needle biopsy revealed *M. avium* and permitted successful treatment.

has been reported to occur in 13–35% of lung transplant recipients [20]. In some series, it is considered to rank above infection as the primary cause of morbidity and mortality [21]. Pathology is characterized by endothelial dysfunction, capillary leak and an intense neutrophilic inflammatory reaction. Clinical signs of ischemia-reperfusion injury occur within the first 24 hours after lung transplantation and include progressive deterioration in gas exchange, increased density on chest radiograph and increased pulmonary vascular resistance. Patients who develop reperfusion injury have higher morbidity (prolonged mechanical ventilation, hospital length of stay) and mortality [22]. There are also reports that lung transplant patients who survive ischemia-reperfusion injury have increased risk for developing subsequent obliterative bronchiolitis [23,24]. Factors such as cardiopulmonary bypass, prolonged graft ischemia time, high inflation during cold storage of the pulmonary graft, older donors, African American donors, donor female gender and recipient diagnosis of pulmonary hypertension have been reported to have variable impact on the development of primary graft failure in lung and heart lung patients [20,25–27]. Low-dose dopamine and dobutamine are often used for cardiovascular support as clinically indicated. Fluid restriction and diuretics, usually furosemide, are used to remove interstitial lung fluid from the newly transplanted lungs which are susceptible to pulmonary edema during reperfusion injury as well as from loss of lymphatic drainage. However, the medical team should carefully monitor strict intake and output to watch for signs of overly aggressive diuresis that may result in hypotension as well as prerenal azotemia. Extracorporeal membrane oxygenation has been shown to be an effective support for pediatric lung transplant patients with early severe graft dysfunction [28,29]. Other treatments, such as inhaled nitric oxide, have not been proven to prevent ischemia-reperfusion injury [30]. However, in one recent report, short-term use of a soluble complement receptor inhibitor may reduce the complications of reperfusion injury in lung transplant patients [31].

Hence, close monitoring and prevention are the keystones to management of primary graft failure. Treatment for primary graft failure often includes use of neuromuscular blockade and paralysis. However, use of muscle relaxants in combination with high doses of corticosteroids increases the risk of acute severe myopathy, which may persist for weeks and months after discontinuation of the agents [32,33].

ACUTE AND CHRONIC REJECTION

Risk of organ rejection begins at the time of transplant surgery. Lung transplant patients have a higher incidence of rejection than isolated heart, liver or kidney transplant recipients. In fact, early studies of heart-lung transplant patients noted a much higher incidence of rejection in the lungs than in the heart [34]. Rejection can be classified as hyperacute, acute or chronic. Histologic grading of pulmonary rejection is based upon the 1996 published guidelines produced by the Lung Rejection Study Group [35]. The histologic grades of acute rejection are based primarily on the intensity of the cellular infiltrate. The grading of pulmonary rejection is discussed in detail in the previous chapter. It is believed that T-cell lymphocytes are the primary effector cells of acute rejection. Acute rejection is diagnosed by both clinical and histopathologic criteria. However, after the early postoperative period, diagnosis of acute rejection should be based on evaluation of lung biopsy examination whenever possible.

Although hyperacute rejection is no longer common, lung transplant recipients are at high risk for acute cellular rejection within the first few months after transplant surgery. There are several hypotheses for this increased risk, including the extensive pulmonary vasculature with a large population of immunologically active cells (macrophages, lymphocytes, dendritic cells) as well as the fact that the lungs are exposed to antigens from the external environment. Signs of acute rejection can be similar to those of acute infection or reperfusion injury/pulmonary edema: drop in oxygenation, increased infiltrates (bilaterally in cadaveric recipients; unilateral in single lung recipients and often unilateral in living donor lobar patients), increase in pleural effusions, and even low-grade fever. In addition, inadvertent transplantation of blood-group incompatible organs should also be considered in cases of severe early rejection. Bronchoscopy with transbronchial biopsy should be performed for determination of infection versus rejection. If infection is eliminated as the primary cause of the clinical deterioration, then treatment should be initiated with pulsed steroids (methylprednisolone 10–15 mg/kg/day for 3 days). The majority of acute rejection episodes respond favorably to this conservative therapy (Fig. 41.3). If the rejection episode does not respond to steroids, options include use of the monoclonal antibody OKT3 or polyclonal antithymocyte globulin preparations.

Increased risk of acute cellular rejection and primary graft failure should be considered in those lung transplant recipients who received organs with long ischemic times or who have preformed donor-specific anti-HLA antibodies [36]. While pediatric cadaveric lung transplant patients are at higher risk for early acute rejection compared with children who receive living donor lobar procedures, there is no difference between the groups in overall incidence of acute rejection [37].

Bronchiolitis obliterans has been defined as the clinical syndrome of irreversible progressive airway obstruction in the pulmonary allograft caused by obliterative bronchiolitis (Fig. 41.4). While the terms "bronchiolitis obliterans" and "chronic rejection" are often used synonymously, it has been suggested that the term "chronic rejection" be applied only to those patients who have experienced frequent documented acute cellular rejection episodes [38]. Less confusion may occur if the term "recurrent acute rejection" is used to describe this latter phenomenon.

Bronchiolitis obliterans is rare within the first year after lung transplantation, but it can be identified in over half of cadaveric lung transplant recipients by 5 years after transplantation. Development of bronchiolitis obliterans is associated with increased frequency and severity of acute cellular rejection episodes and viral illnesses (such as CMV) [39]. It is the primary cause of morbidity and mortality in cadaveric recipients after the first year of transplant [40]. Clinically, the patient may complain of mild dyspnea and even wheezing. The wheezing may initially be reversible with aerosol bronchodilators, but later the airway obstruction is nonreversible. On physical examination, there is decreased air entry with "distant" breath sound, particularly at the bases. Radiographically, there is hyperinflation with loss of peripheral vascular markings (Fig. 41.5). Computerized tomography (CT) of the chest shows irregular distribution of hypolucency with air-trapping. Atelectasis and bronchiectasis are often present in advanced cases. While there are reports that use of tacrolimus, mycophenolate mofetil, sirolimus, methotrexate, total lymphoid irradiation, azithromycin and photophoresis have had some success at reducing the incidence or slowing bronchiolitis obliterans progression, there is currently no reliable therapy to treat this disease. Hence, the primary management is aimed at prevention of acute rejection and infection as well as treating conditions that increase the risk of bronchiolitis obliterans, such as gastroesophageal reflux. The ultimate long-term success of both adult and pediatric lung and heart-lung transplantation will depend on the identification of the mechanisms

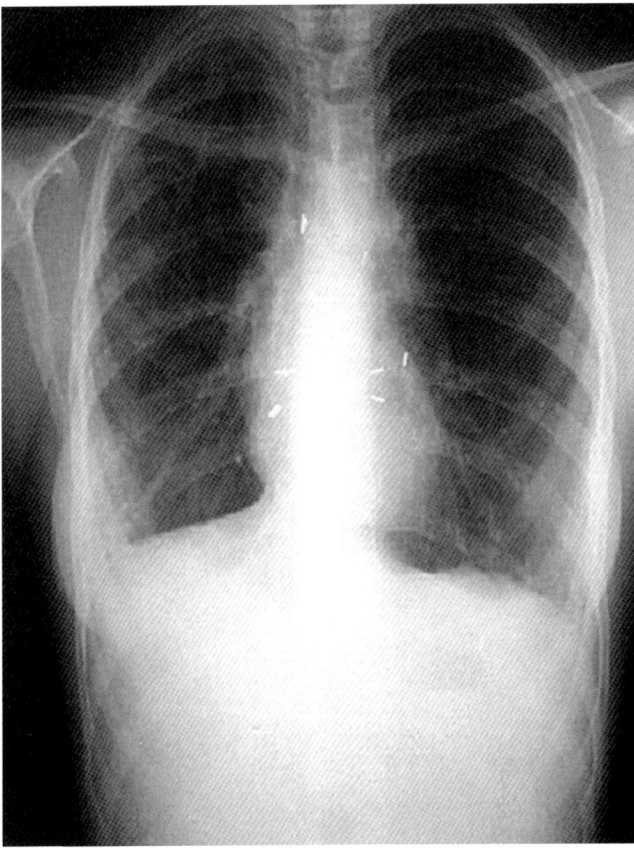

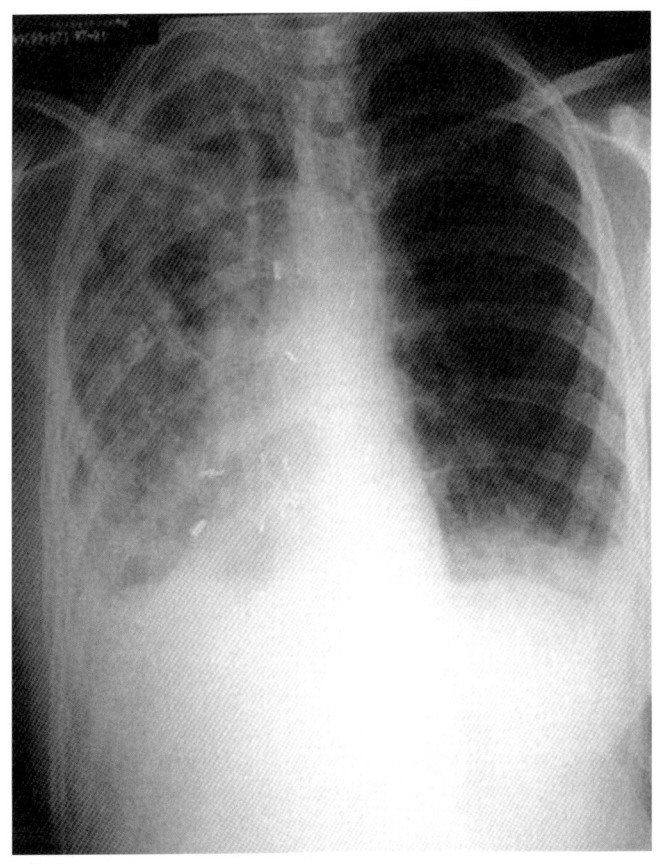

(a)

(b)

Fig. 41.3 Chest radiograph of acute cellular rejection before and after intravenous steroid bolus. (a) Acute cellular rejection with pleural effusion associated with low-grade fever. (b) Improvement in infiltrates and pleural effusion after 3 days of intravenous methylprednisolone 10 mg/kg/day.

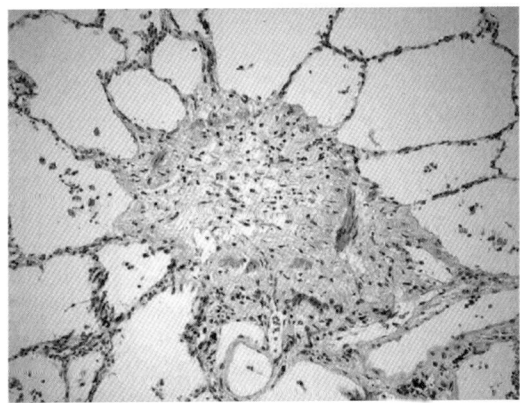

Fig. 41.4 Characteristic histologic findings of obliterative bronchiolitis. There is total fibrous obliteration of a small airway.

involved in the development and effective treatment of this process. At this time, retransplantation is the only known effective treatment option for severe bronchiolitis obliterans. However, survival is generally thought to be poor for lung transplant patients who require retransplantation because of bronchiolitis obliterans.

POST-TRANSPLANT LYMPHOPROLIFERATIVE DISEASE

Epstein–Barr virus mediated B-cell lymphocyte proliferation is thought to be the etiology of most post-transplant lymphoproliferative disorders (PTLD) in children. There is a wide range of disease manifestation: from mild (mononucleosis-type illness) to severe (poorly differentiated B-cell lymphoma). PTLD is discussed in detail in Chapter 13. Pediatric transplant patients have a higher incidence of PTLD because of their greater likelihood of being EBV-naïve at the time of transplant. It has been estimated that from 15% up to 19.5% of lung recipients will develop PTLD after 30 days post-transplant [9,41].

In the pediatric lung transplant recipient, the lung allograft is almost invariably involved and presentation is often with an asymptomatic mass identified on routine chest radiograph.

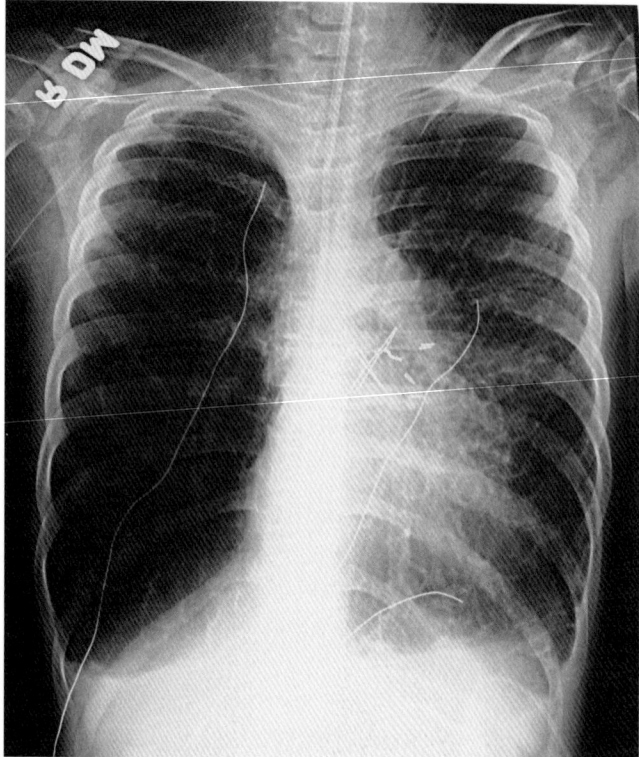

Fig. 41.5 Chest radiograph of a lung transplant patient with severe bronchiolitis obliterans and respiratory failure. There is marked hyperinflation with bilateral cystic lesions.

Other common sites of disease in the lung transplant recipient include peripheral lymph nodes and the gastrointestinal tract. The chest radiographic finding of a new mass in the lung should trigger an immediate investigation (Fig. 41.6). Symptoms of persistent sore throat, lymphadenopathy, chronic abdominal

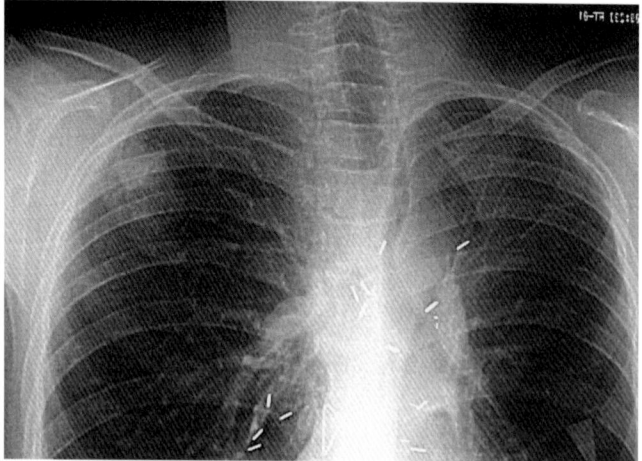

Fig. 41.6 Chest radiograph of post-transplant lymphoproliferative disease. A right upper lobe lesion was discovered on routine clinic chest radiograph in an asymptomatic patient.

pain, weight loss, vomiting, diarrhea, fever, anemia or gastrointestinal bleeding should also raise suspicion of the diagnosis of PTLD. Evaluation should include a CT scan with intravenous and oral contrast of the neck, chest and abdomen (including pelvis). EBV viral loads are usually very high at presentation. Diagnosis must be confirmed by tissue biopsy. Initial treatment is driven by clinical status and histology, but usually consists of reduction in immunosuppression. This has been less successful in the lung recipient than in pediatric kidney, liver and heart recipients, in part because of the high risk of rebound acute rejection and the development of chronic rejection. If there is no response to reduction in immunosuppression, then use of rituximab (anti-CD20 monoclonal antibody) or chemotherapy is indicated. Chemotherapy is used as first line treatment for aggressive histologies such as Burkitt lymphoma.

OTHER COMPLICATIONS

Colonic perforations have been reported in 3.3–8.6% of lung transplant patients. Although they may occur in the early to late post-transplant period, early perforations are thought to be secondary to perioperative hypoperfusion, increased intraluminal pressure from narcotics, use of bowel stimulants and high-dose immunosuppression [42,43].

Atrial fibrilllation or flutter are frequent complications that can prolong hospital stay and increase mortality risks in both pediatric and adult lung transplant populations. Incidence has been reported as high as 39% of adult lung transplant recipients [44]. It usually occurs 2–3 days after transplant surgery. Risk factors include advanced recipient age, pretransplant diagnosis of idiopathic pulmonary fibrosis, known coronary disease, enlarged left atrium and use of postoperative vasopressors. It may also be increased in patients who received bilateral lung transplantation.

Renal insufficiency is a common long-term complication which may have been present prior to transplant surgery or developed after transplant as a result of nephrotoxic calcineurin inhibitors and antibiotics. Risk of renal insufficiency and failure is increased in CF patients [45]. Reviewing patient medications and close monitoring of calcineurin inhibitor levels can help reduce risk for renal compromise. Poorly controlled hypertension increases the risk of renal complications. Hence, systemic hypertension should be treated aggressively.

Neurologic complications, such as tremor, headache and muscle weakness, are common in transplant patients mainly as side-effects of immunosuppressive medications [1]. CF patients are reported to be at increased risk for post-transplant seizures. A potentially devastating neurologic complication is drug-induced leukoencephalopathy. Early symptoms may include headache and photophobia but sudden onset of blindness, seizures and coma have also been cited as presenting signs. Diagnosis is confirmed by brain computerized axial tomography (non-enhancing areas of low attenuation in cerebral white matter) or magnetic resonance imaging (increased signal on T2-weighed images). Occipital lobes appear to be most commonly affected. Treatment is reduction in calcineurin inhibitor or changing immunosuppressive agents (e.g. changing cyclosporine to tacrolimus).

Other possible complications include systemic hypertension, post-transplant diabetes mellitus, hyperlipidemia, skin cancer, Kaposi sarcoma, osteoporosis and sensitivity to sun exposure or sunburn. Prevention and surveillance for these potential complications should be periodically reviewed with the transplant patient and family.

OUTPATIENT ROUTINE MANAGEMENT

Patient and family preparation for post-transplant outpatient care should begin as soon as the patient is stable after surgery and transferred to the hospital ward. Education concerning medications, complications and lifestyle changes should begin in the hospital and then be revisited at all routine post-transplant clinic visits. Patient and family should also receive instruction on how to contact the transplant team members and when it is appropriate to call the transplant group. At our institution, post-lung transplant patients are routinely evaluated by the transplant team (transplant physician, coordinator, social worker, psychologist) at least weekly for the first month after discharge from the hospital. If they are stable, then their routine transplant clinic visits are changed to every 2 weeks for the next month and then every 4–6 weeks until they are 1 year post-transplant surgery. Each routine clinic visit should include physical examination with vital signs, pulmonary function tests (at least spirometry) with a record of previous efforts, chest radiograph, and laboratory tests (including electrolytes, liver function tests, blood, urea and nitrogen, creatinine, glucose, magnesium).

In common with other solid organ transplant recipients, pediatric lung and heart-lung transplant patients are at risk for medical non-adherence. The highest risk group for medical non-adherence is the adolescent. Although this problem may develop very early in the post-transplant period, its risk increases with time after successful transplant surgery. Warning signs of increased patient risk for this problem include widely fluctuating immunosuppression medication blood levels, frequent appointment failures, poor communication and poor patient compliance with scheduled laboratory tests. Medical nonadherence, particularly nonadherence with medications, can lead to significant complications as well as death of the transplant recipient. Thus, it is important to address this potential problem frequently and monitor for possible signs of medical nonadherence. Close monitoring, patient and caregiver education and early referral to psychology or counseling services may help reduce the incidence of medical nonadherence.

The transplant clinic notes, in legible form, should be sent to the referring physician and/or the medical team who will be involved in the long-term care of the patient. As the patient approaches the 1-year anniversary of their transplant surgery, written guidelines for post-transplant follow-up and a clinical summary should be sent to the long-term care physician and clinic.

CONCLUSIONS

Successful management of the postoperative lung or heart-lung patient requires the coordinated efforts of the entire medical team. This team includes not only the transplant physicians and surgeons, but also the medical consultants, nurses, pharmacists and respiratory therapists. Open and frequent communication between all transplant team members as well as with the transplant patient themselves and their families provides the best chance of optimal outcomes for these high-risk and medically complex children.

REFERENCES

1 Kotloff RM, Ahya VN. Medical complications of lung transplantation. *Eur Respir J* 2004;23:334–42.
2 Pilcher DV, Scheinkestel CD, Snell GI, *et al.* High central venous pressure is associated with prolonged mechanical ventilation and increased mortality after lung transplantation. *J Thorac Cardiovasc Surg* 2005;129:912–8.
3 Ferdinande P, Bruyninckx F, Van Raemdonck D, Daenen W, Verleden G, Leuven Lung Transplant Group. Phrenic nerve dysfunction after heart-lung and lung transplantation. *J Heart Lung Transplant* 2004;12:105–9.
4 Haddy SM, Bremner RM, Moore-Jefferies EW, *et al.* Hyperinflation resulting in hemodynamic collapse following living donor lobar transplantation. *Anesthesiology* 2002;97:1315–7.
5 Starnes VA, Barr ML, Cohen RG, *et al.* Living-donor lobar lung transplantation experience: intermediate results. *J Thorac Cardiovasc Surg* 1996;112:1284–91.
6 Horn MV, Schenkel FA, Woo MS, Starnes VA. Pediatric recipients of living donor lobar lung transplants: post-operative care. *Prog Transplant* 2002;12:81–5.
7 King-Biggs MB, Dunitz JM, Park SJ, Savik SK, Hertz MI. Airway anastomotic dehiscence associated with use of sirolimus immediately after lung transplantation. *Transplantation* 2003;75:1437–43.
8 Groetzner J, Kur F, Spelsberg F, *et al.* Airway anastomosis complications in *de novo* lung transplantation with sirolimus-based immunosuppression. *J Heart Lung Transplant* 2004;23:632–8.
9 Armitage JM, Kurland G, Michaels M, *et al.* Critical issues in pediatric lung transplantation. *J Thorac Cardiovasc Surg* 1995;109:60–5.
10 Spray TL, Mallory GB, Canter CB, Huddleston CB. Pediatric lung transplantation: indications, techniques, and early results. *J Thorac Cardiovasc Surg* 1994;107:990–1000.

11 Sweet SC, Spray TL, Huddleston CB, *et al.* Pediatric lung transplantation at St. Louis Children's Hospital 1990–1995. *Am Rev Respir Crit Care Med* 1997;**155**:1027–35.

12 Schulman LL, Anandarangam T, Leibowitz DW, *et al.* Four-year prospective study of pulmonary venous thrombosis after lung transplantation. *J Am Soc Echocardiogr* 2001;**14**:806–12.

13 Watanabe MA, Homma S, Schulman LL. Fatal cerebral emboli in two recipients of lung transplants from one donor. *Transplantation* 2003;**75**:2157–8.

14 Sodhi SS, Guo JP, Maurer AH, *et al.* Gastroparesis after combined heart and lung transplantation. *J Clin Gastroenterol* 2002; **34**:34–9.

15 Green M, Avery RK, Preiksaitis J, eds. Guidelines for the prevention and management of infectious complications of solid organ transplantation. *Am J Transplant* 2004;**4**(Suppl 10):6–166.

16 Aeba R, Stout JE, Francalancia NA, *et al.* Aspects of lung transplantation that contribute to increased severity of pneumonia. *J Thorac Cardiovasc Surg* 1993;**106**:449–57.

17 Dowling RD, Zenati M, Yousem SA, *et al.* Donor transmitted pneumonia in experimental lung allografts: successful prevention with donor antibiotic therapy. *J Thorac Cardiovasc Surg* 1992;**103**:767–72.

18 Abid Q, Nkere UU, Hasan A, *et al.* Mediastinitis in heart and lung transplantation: 15 years experience. *Ann Thorac Surg* 2003;**75**:1565–71.

19 Danziger-Isakov LA, Sweet S, Delamorena M, *et al.* Epidemiology of bloodstream infections in the first year after pediatric lung transplantation. *Pediatr Infect Dis J* 2005;**24**:324–30.

20 Duarte AG, Lick S. Predicting outcome in primary graft failure. *Chest* 2002;**121**:1736–8.

21 Chatila WM, Furukawa S, Gaughan JP, Criner GJ. Respiratory failure after lung transplantation. *Chest* 2003;**123**:165–73.

22 King RC, Binns OA, Rodriguez F, *et al.* Reperfusion injury significantly impacts clinical outcome after pulmonary transplantation. *Ann Thorac Surg* 2000;**69**:1681–5.

23 Bando K, Paradis IL, Similo S, *et al.* Obliterative bronchiolitis after lung and heart-lung transplantation: an analysis of risk factors and management. *J Thorac Cardiovasc Surg* 1995;**110**:4–14.

24 Fiser SM, Tribble CG, Long SM, *et al.* Ischemia-reperfusion injury after lung transplantation increases risk of late bronchiolitis obliterans syndrome. *Ann Thorac Surg* 2002;**73**:1041–8.

25 Christie JD, Kotloff RM, Pochettino A, *et al.* Clinical risk factors for primary graft failure following lung transplantation. *Chest* 2003;**124**:1232–41.

26 Thabut G, Mal H, Cerrina J, *et al.* Graft ischemic time and outcome of lung transplantation: a multicenter analysis. *Am J Respir Crit Care Med* 2005;**171**:786–91.

27 Patel MR, Laubach VE, Tribble CG, Korn IL. Hyperinflation during lung preservation and increased reperfusion injury. *J Surg Res* 2005;**123**:134–8.

28 Kirshbom PM, Bridges ND, Myung RJ, *et al.* Use of extracorporeal membrane oxygenation in pediatric thoracic organ transplantation. *J Thorac Cardiovasc Surg* 2002;**123**:130–6.

29 Oto T, Rosenfeldt F, Rowland M, *et al.* Extracorporeal membrane oxygenation after lung transplantation: evolving technique improves outcomes. *Ann Thorac Surg* 2004;**78**:1230–5.

30 Meade MO, Granton JT, Matte-Martyn A, *et al.* A randomized trial of inhaled nitric oxide to prevent ischemia-reperfusion injury after lung transplantation. *Am J Respir Crit Care Med* 2003;**167**:1483–9.

31 Keshavjee S, Davis RD, Zamora MR, de Perrot M, Patterson GA. A randomized, placebo-controlled trial of complement inhibition in ischemia-reperfusion injury after lung transplantation in human beings. *J Thorac Cardiovasc Surg* 2005;**129**:423–8.

32 Hansen-Flaschen J, Cowen J, Raps EC. Neuromuscular blockade in the intensive care unit: more than we bargained for. *Am Rev Respir Dis* 1993;**147**:234–6.

33 Fisher JR, Baer RK. Acute myopathy associated with combined use of corticosteroids and neuromuscular blocking agents. *Ann Pharmacother* 1996;**30**:1437–45.

34 Conte JV Jr, Orens J. Lung transplantation. In: Kuo PC, Schroeder RA, Johnson LB, eds. *Clinical Management of the Transplant Patient*. London: Arnold, 2001: 169–200.

35 Yousem SA, Berry GJ, Cagle PT, *et al.* Revision of the 1990 working formulation for the classification of pulmonary allograft rejection: lung rejection study group. *J Heart Lung Transplant* 1996;**15**:1–15.

36 Reinsmoen NL, Nelson K, Zeevi A. Anti-HLA antibody analysis and crossmatching in heart and lung transplantation. *Transplant Immunol* 2004;**13**:63–71.

37 Woo MS, MacLaughlin EF, Horn MV, *et al.* Bronchiolitis obliterans is not the primary cause of death in pediatric living donor lobar lung transplant recipients. *J Heart Lung Transplant* 2001;**20**:491–6.

38 Heng D, Sharples LD, McNeil K, *et al.* Bronchiolitis obliterans syndrome: incidence, natural history, prognosis, and risk factors. *J Heart Lung Transplant* 1998;**17**:1255–63.

39 Sharples LD, Tamm M, McNeil K, *et al.* Development of bronchiolitis obliterans syndrome in recipients of heart-lung transplantation: early risk factors. *Transplantation* 1996;**61**:560–6.

40 Scott JP, Higgenbottam TW, Clelland C, *et al.* The natural history of obliterative bronchiolitis and occlusive vascular disease of patients following heart-lung transplantation. *Transplant Proc* 1989;**21**:2592–3.

41 Boyle GJ, Michaels MG, Webber SA, *et al.* Posttransplant lymphoproliferative disorders in pediatric thoracic organ recipients. *J Pediatr* 1997;**131**:309–13.

42 Maurer JR. The spectrum of colonic complications in a lung transplant population. *Ann Transplant* 2000;**5**:54–7.

43 Fenton JJ, Cicale MJ. Sigmoid diverticular perforation complicating lung transplantation. *J Heart Lung Transplant* 1997;**16**:681–5.

44 Nielsen TD, Bahnson T, Davis RD, Palmer SM. Atrial fibrillation after pulmonary transplant. *Chest* 2004;**126**:496–500.

45 Schindler R, Radke C, Paul K, Frei U. Renal problems after lung transplantation of cystic fibrosis patients. *Nephrol Dial Transplant* 2001;**16**:1324–8.

42 Outcomes and Risk Factors

Stuart C. Sweet

The first successful lung and heart-lung transplants were reported in the early 1980s [1,2]. Since that time, these procedures have become accepted therapies for end-stage pulmonary disease in adults. The most recent report of the registry of the International Society for Heart and Lung Transplantation (ISHLT) contains data on more than 20 000 lung and heart-lung transplants [3]. The success in adults led to the development of pediatric programs [4–6]. The most recent pediatric ISHLT report indicates that through 2002 there had been nearly 700 pediatric lung and heart-lung transplants [7]. Over the past several years, the number of pediatric lung transplants per year has decreased from more than 80 to 60. The St. Louis Children's Hospital/Washington University in St. Louis (SLCH) program has accounted for 20–30% of pediatric lung transplants each year during that period (Fig. 42.1).

This chapter reviews outcomes following lung transplant and, where possible, includes an analysis of risk factors. Because growth is an important component of pediatric medicine, a brief section on growth and development is also included. Some of the data included in the chapter are adapted from the most recent ISHLT registry reports [3,7]. Risk factor analysis is included where possible from data derived from the SLCH program.

SURVIVAL

Overall survival of pediatric lung transplant recipients is approximately 75% at 1 year, 55% at 3 years and 45% at 5 years [7]. These values are comparable to the adult experience [3] and to the SLCH center (Fig. 42.2). Compared with values reported in earlier registry reports, survival does not appear to have improved significantly over the past 5 years [8]. In a multivariate logistic regression analysis from the adult lung transplant experience, the most significant risk factors for 1 year mortality were repeat transplant, mechanical ventilation or intravenous inotropic support at transplant. Repeat transplant and mechanical ventilation were also risk factors for 5-year mortality [3]. Although an analysis of risk factors for survival is not included in the pediatric ISHLT registry reports [7], the SLCH experience suggests that pediatric patients have similar risk factors. Survival of patients undergoing retransplantation was significantly worse than patients undergoing primary transplant and multivariate analysis identified repeat transplant and mechanical ventilation as significant independent risk factors for death (Table 42.1). An additional risk factor unique to pediatrics, congenital heart disease with significant aortopulmonary collateral circulation, was also identified. Patients with parenchymal lung disease other than

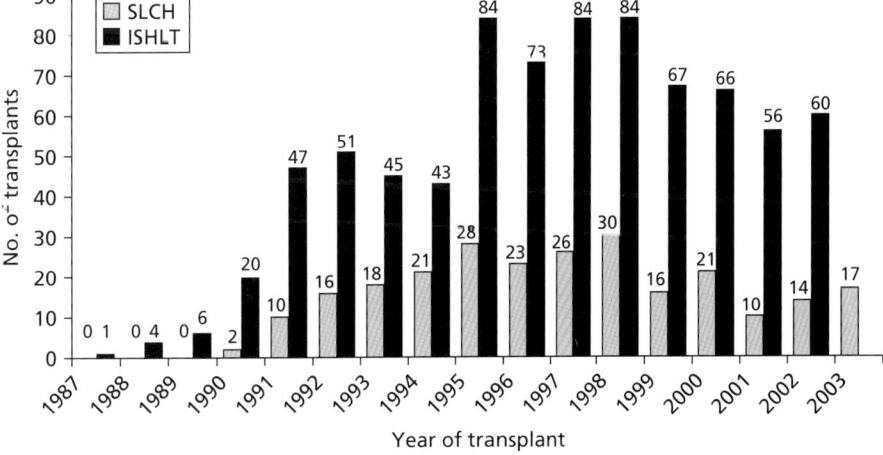

Fig. 42.1 Distribution of pediatric single and bilateral lung transplants by year of transplant. ISHLT, International Society for Heart and Lung Transplantation; SLCH, St. Louis Children's Hospital/Washington University in St. Louis. Modified from Boucek *et al.* [7] and from St. Louis Children's Hospital program.

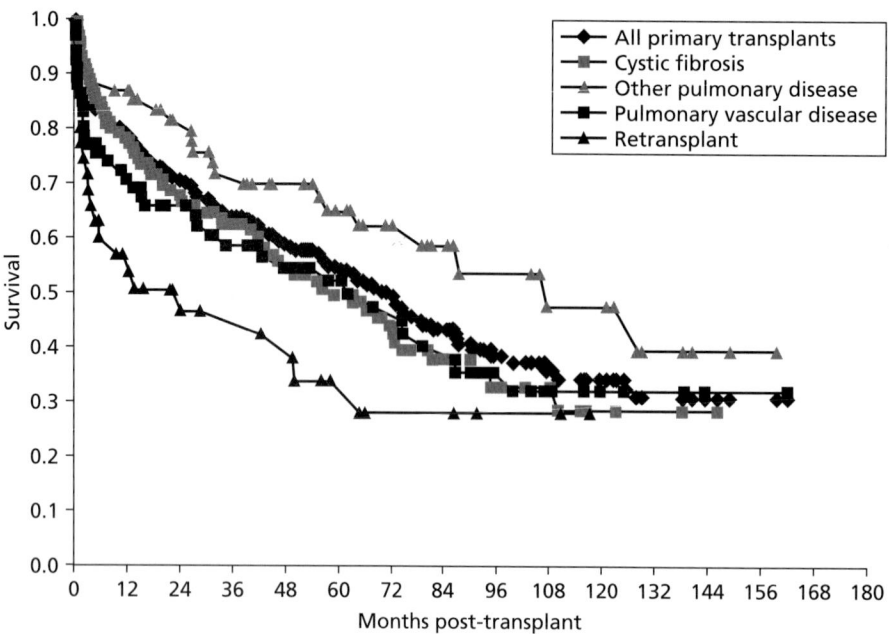

Fig. 42.2 Kaplan–Meier plot of survival post-transplantation stratified by diagnosis. Data from St. Louis Children's Hospital program through January 2004.

Table 42.1 Multivariate analysis of risk factors for survival after lung transplantation. Data from St. Louis Children's Hospital (SLCH) lung transplant program through January, 2000.

	Relative risk (95% CI)	P value
Significant variables		
Previous lung transplant	1.91 (1.04–3.51)	0.04
Significant AP collaterals	3.01 (1.34–6.74)	0.01
Ventilator at transplant	1.63 (1.01–2.62)	0.04
Insignificant variables		
Gender		0.61
Fungal colonization		0.36
Aspergillus colonization		0.06
Resistant *Pseudomonas*		0.39
Supplemental oxygen		0.18
$P_{CO_2} > 60$ mmHg		0.95
Ischemic time		0.15
Donor pulmonary infection		0.55
Prior thoracic surgery		0.77
CMV + donor or recipient		0.26

AP, aortopulmonary; CI, confidence interval; CMV, cytomegalovirus.

cystic fibrosis (CF) have typically had the best outcome at the SLCH center (Fig. 42.2). Although adult patients with CF have been reported to have a lower risk for 5-year mortality [9], this does not appear to be the case in pediatric recipients. This may be partly because CF patients comprise the majority of adolescent recipients (who have consistently poorer transplant outcomes compared with other age groups) [10]. Finally, mechanical ventilation does not appear to be a risk factor for infant recipients (unpublished observations), perhaps because the mechanism of respiratory failure in this population is less likely to be caused by progressive infection than in older children and adolescents.

Additional information regarding risk factors can be inferred by examining causes of death in the pediatric population (Fig. 42.3). Graft failure is the most common cause of death in the first 30 days after transplant. For the remainder of the first year, infection is the most common cause. Beyond 1 year post-transplant, obliterative bronchiolitis (OB), also known as bronchiolitis obliterans (BO), is responsible for the largest percentage of deaths [7]. Risk factors for these complications are discussed in detail below.

GRAFT FAILURE

The lungs are exquisitely sensitive to the ischemic injury that occurs as a result of the process of harvest and reimplantation. The response to injury following transplant is variable. It is typically manifested as noncardiogenic pulmonary edema with decreased lung compliance and poor oxygenation, requiring increased and prolonged ventilator support. Estimates of the incidence of significant pulmonary dysfunction related to this ischemic injury range from 13% to 35% [11,12]. The reasons for this wide range of incidence are not entirely clear. The most likely explanation is lack of uniformly accepted criteria. However, the role of donor factors (cause of death, presence of subclinical pulmonary injury, time from brain death to organ harvest), as well as recipient factors (use of cardiopulmonary bypass, presence of chronic infection/inflammation) remains to be elucidated. An extensive literature exists investigating

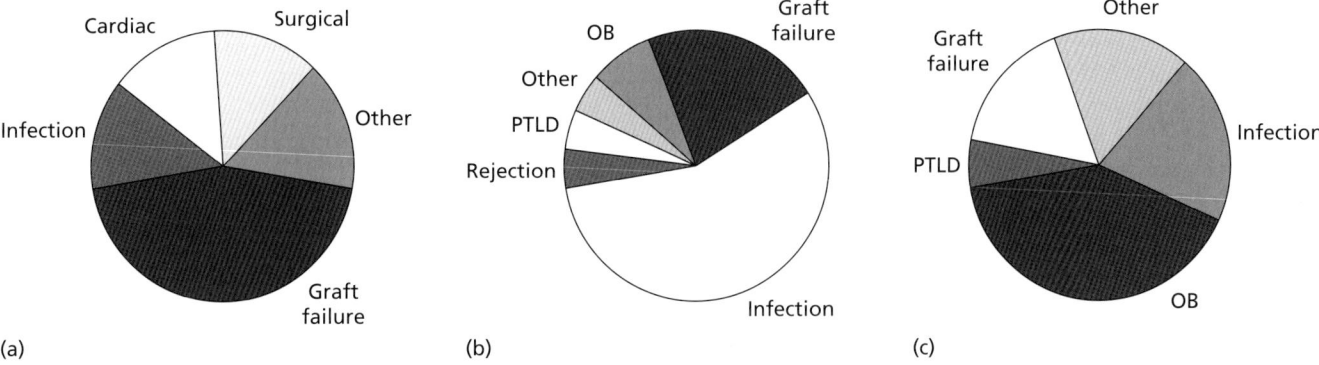

Fig. 42.3 Causes of death after pediatric lung transplantation by time after transplant: (a) 0–30 days; (b) 30 days to 1 year;

(c) > 1 year. OB, bronchiolitis obliterans; PTLD, post-transplant lymphoproliferative disorder. Modified from Boucek *et al.* [7].

Table 42.2 Multivariate analysis of risk factors for early graft dysfunction. Adapted from Sweet *et al.* [79].

	Relative risk (95% CI)	*P* value
Significant variables		
On ventilator at transplant	5.29 (2.06–13.60)	0.0005
Average ischemic time (hours)	1.40 (1.14–1.72)	0.001
Insignificant variables		
Pretransplant WBC	1.05 (0.99–1.12)	0.09
Pretransplant P_{CO_2}	2.13 (0.87–5.20)	0.10
Pretransplant creatinine	0.55 (0.21–1.45)	0.23
Explant shows abscess	1.01 (0.99–1.03)	0.62
On ECMO at transplant	1.20 (0.19–7.62)	0.84

CI, confidence interval; ECMO, extracorporeal membrane oxygenation; WBC, white blood count.

the factors responsible for early graft dysfunction (EGD) and are well summarized in a recent review [13]. For pediatric recipients, multivariate analysis of risk factors for EGD at the SLCH center identified (not unexpectedly) that ischemic time was a significant risk factor. In addition, patients receiving mechanical ventilation at the time of transplant were also at increased risk (Table 42.2). The reason for increased risk in the latter category remains to be elucidated. In addition to the risk of early mortality, a retrospective analysis from a single center suggests that EGD may be an independent risk factor for the development and progression of OB [14].

INFECTION

Lung transplant recipients remain at risk for infectious complications throughout the entire post-transplant course. Infectious complications are described in detail in elsewhere in this volume; here we focus on infections that have a clear impact on survival.

In the immediate post-transplant period, two categories of infection can impact survival. First, patients with significant pulmonary infection, most commonly those with CF, likely have seeding of their bloodstream with bacterial organisms and toxins during lung explantation. In these patients, bacteremia and, rarely, frank sepsis may occur in spite of the routine use of empiric antibiotics to cover organisms colonizing the recipient airway. Because of the poor outcomes in these instances, some centers include evidence of sepsis or systemic inflammatory response syndrome in the list of contraindications to lung transplant.

The second category of early infection that can lead to catastrophic consequences is an acute viral infection present in the donor or recipient at the time of transplant, particularly in infants and small children who may have a limited repertoire of antiviral immune responses. Bridges *et al.* [15,16] have reported that viral infections, particularly adenovirus, were a major cause of morbidity in the series of infants transplanted at SLCH and the Children's Hospital of Philadelphia.

Infections continue to contribute to mortality beyond the immediate post-transplant period. The availability of ganciclovir and valganciclovir has significantly decreased the incidence of cytomegalovirus (CMV) disease, but CMV infection remains a potential source of significant morbidity and rarely mortality. CMV viremia was identified as a risk factor for death or retransplant in a single-center pediatric experience [17]. CMV has also been implicated as a risk factor for OB (see below). Primary infection with Epstein–Barr virus (EBV) is associated with the development of post-transplant lymphoproliferative disorders (PTLD). In pediatric lung and heart-lung recipients, PTLD remains a challenging clinical problem and accounts for nearly 20% of deaths beyond 5 years [7,18,19]. PTLD is discussed in detail elsewhere in this volume.

Although patients may develop bacterial lower respiratory tract infection at any point following transplant, multiple factors place patients at increased risk in the early post-transplant period. This is likely because of a combination of poor mucus clearance and impaired immune function. Ciliary function may be impaired as a result of early graft dysfunction. Mucosal integrity can be interrupted as a result of mucosal sloughing just distal to the mainstem bronchial anastomoses. Cough may be impaired because of postoperative pain, and diaphragm function may be impaired as a result of phrenic nerve injury. In addition, in patients whose nutritional status is poor at the time of transplantation, immune function may be at a nadir in this window of time. Finally, especially when an antibody induction regimen is used, immunosuppression will likely be at a maximum during this time. Colonization with difficult-to-treat organisms, primarily *Burkholderia cenocepacia* (formerly known as *Burkholderia cepacia*, genomovar III) has been identified a risk factor for mortality in adult populations [20–22]. Anecdotal experience of the author suggests that infection with pan-resistant *Pseudomonas aeruginosa* and other Gram-negative rods also poses significant risk.

Fungal infections, particularly with *Aspergillus*, can lead to catastrophic outcomes. Infection at the site of the bronchial anastomosis can cause dehiscence. Because of the proximity of the pulmonary arteries to this region, extension of the infection has the potential to lead to exsanguination. For these reasons, isolation of *Aspergillus* prior to transplant has been considered a contraindication to lung transplant at some centers. More recently, centers have adopted prophylactic regimens in the peritransplant period [23,24]. The availability of newer agents effective against *Aspergillus* but less nephrotoxic than amphotericin B, such as voriconazole and caspofungin, has made this approach more appealing.

BRONCHIOLITIS OBLITERANS

The primary reason lung transplantation has not achieved long-term survival rates comparable to other solid organ transplants is OB. Approximately half of lung transplant recipients are diagnosed with OB by 5 years after transplant. More than 40% of deaths occurring beyond 1 year post-transplant are a direct or indirect result of OB [7]. Actuarial freedom from OB for pediatric recipients is 83% at 1 year and 61% at 3 years [7]. These values are not significantly different than those reported for the SLCH program in 1998 [25]. The etiology of OB remains elusive in spite of a growing body of basic science and clinical research.

Bronchiolitis obliterans is diagnosed on the basis of the presence in lung biopsy of lymphocytic infiltration, fibromyxoid airway deposits, subepithelial fibrosis and total fibrous obliteration of the bronchioles [26–28]. OB is a focal process. Therefore, transbronchial biopsy may not be sufficient to establish a diagnosis [29]; even open lung biopsy is not 100% sensitive [30]. Therefore a corresponding clinical syndrome, "bronchiolitis obliterans syndrome (BOS)", was established to describe the otherwise unexplained development of an obstructive decrease in pulmonary function [31]. OB should be suspected with BOS grade 1 or greater (reflecting a decline in forced expiratory volume in 1 second [FEV_1] greater than 20% from the post-transplant best). Because of growth issues for pediatric recipients, the percent predicted rather than absolute values for FEV_1 and forced vital capacity (FVC) values may be used in calculating the BOS grade [32].

Additional details of diagnosis and therapy are provided elsewhere in this volume; here, we focus on population analyses leading to identification of risk factors. Although there are many theories regarding the etiology of OB, the most comprehensive hypothesis suggests that OB is caused by a combination of airway epithelial injury (potential sources include ischemia, infection, immunologic injury and perhaps mechanical stress) coupled with aberrant repair, perhaps related to increases in profibrotic cytokines such as transforming growth factor β [33] or platelet-derived growth factor [34].

Acute rejection is the most consistently identified risk factor for OB, supporting a role for immune-mediated injury [35]. At highest risk were patients experiencing more frequent [36] or more severe [26] acute rejection episodes. Smaller studies suggest that lymphocytic bronchitis and bronchiolitis [37] are also risk factors. Other data supporting immune-mediated injury include the observation that OB was less likely in patients with decreased donor alloreactivity (on the basis of peripheral microchimerism and absence of donor antigen reactivity in bronchoalveolar lavage (BAL) lymphocytes [38,39]) or HLA mismatches [40]. There is a growing body of literature implicating anti-HLA antibodies in the etiology of OB [41–47]. A systematic review of the risk factors for OB was recently published by Sharples *et al.* [48].

A univariate analysis of the risk factors for OB in the SLCH population [25] identified acute rejection (two episodes of grade A2 or greater), prolonged ischemic time (more than 3 hours), low cyclosporine levels (less than 200 ng/mL twice, at least 14 days apart) and age over 3 years at the time of transplant. Multivariate analysis identified acute rejection and ischemic time as independently significant (Table 42.3). In addition, Ibrahim *et al.* [49] reported decreased incidence of chronic graft dysfunction in young children receiving thoracic organ transplants at the SLCH programs. For infant lung transplant recipients, this may be a result of a lower incidence of acute rejection [50]. Living donor lobar transplant recipients also have a lower incidence of OB, (perhaps related to shorter ischemic times) [51].

Infection may have a role in the development of OB, either directly, through injury to the airway epithelium, or indirectly, through effects on the immune response. The most often studied infection is CMV [41,52–55]. A single-center study concluded that CMV prophylaxis with ganciclovir reduced the incidence of OB in the first year post-transplant [56]. Indirect evidence suggests a role for community-acquired viral infections in the development of OB [57,58]. Evidence for bacterial infections as a risk factor OB is less convincing [48,52,57,59]. Nonetheless, chronic lower respiratory tract

Table 42.3 Multivariate analysis of risk factors for bronchiolitis obliterans. Adapted from Sharples *et al.* [36].

	Relative risk (95% CI)	*P* value
Significant variables		
Acute rejection grade ≥ A2	1.25 (1.11–1.40)	0.0001
Average ischemic time (hours)	1.51 (1.08–2.12)	0.017
Insignificant variables		
Age at transplant		0.40
Low cyclosporine levels		0.735
PTLD		0.65
CMV disease		0.84

CI, confidence interval; CMV, cytomegalovirus; PTLD, post-transplant lymphoproliferative disorder.

infection is a common complication of OB [60]. Infection may be exacerbated by the augmented immunosuppression used to treat OB and is a common cause of morbidity and mortality [61]. Finally, a single retrospective report found that airway injury as a result of chronic aspiration was a risk factor for OB [62]. This finding was supported by finding that patients with reflux had improved lung function after fundoplication [63].

Animal models for OB remain suboptimal. An exhaustive review of this literature is beyond the scope of this discussion. However, one can find studies that support roles for both immune-mediated injury and profibrotic growth factors [64–66]. Two studies concluded that an intact airway epithelium was necessary to prevent OB [67.68]. Finally, animal models using immunosuppressive regimens that include anti-proliferative agents have prompted the use of rapamycin and its analogs as OB therapy [69,70]. Efficacy has not yet been demonstrated for these agents for prevention or treatment of OB in humans.

In summary, OB remains the major barrier to long-term success of lung transplantation. It is worth emphasizing that the future of lung transplantation hinges on improved understanding, prevention and therapy for OB.

GROWTH

Whether transplantation will facilitate growth is an ongoing concern in pediatric solid organ recipients [71]. This is one reason for reduction in immunosuppression dosages, particularly corticosteroids, in the first year after transplant. Pediatric lung transplant recipients can achieve effective somatic growth; in one longitudinal study the overall rate of somatic growth was approximately 64% of the predicted values [50]. Several infants transplanted at SLCH who are doing well more than 4 years post-transplant have achieved growth parameters in the normal range.

Whether the transplanted lungs will grow commensurate with the patient is a unique concern of pediatric lung transplantation, but is difficult to assess. Pulmonary function measurements following lung transplant can return to the normal range in infants [72] and older children [50]. Lungs transplanted into immature animals can grow [73,74], and using serial imaging studies in a small retrospective study it was noted that airway growth did occur [75]. In humans, however, assessment for alveolar growth is difficult. Routine pulmonary function measurements primarily assess volumes. Therefore, increases in FEV_1 and FVC may indicate increased volume of each alveolar unit rather than alveolar growth or increased surface area for gas exchange. Measurement of the diffusing capacity of carbon monoxide (DLCO) provides a better estimate of gas exchange surface area, but is not readily measurable in infants. However, a single-center study in pediatric recipients of cadaveric and living donor transplants did not show an appreciable increase in DLCO [76]. Further study is needed to clarify these findings.

FUTURE CONSIDERATIONS

In summary, lung transplant is a viable alternative for pediatric patients with end-stage pulmonary parenchymal and vascular disease. Long-term survival rates are, however, well below those for heart and other solid organ transplants and have not improved appreciably over the past 5 years. The key risk factors identified include ventilation at transplant (a risk factor for early graft dysfunction and overall mortality), infection and OB. Retransplantation becomes an issue because of the poor overall survival, and unfortunately is an independent risk factor for poor outcome. Reducing transplants of patients on ventilators will require earlier referral for transplant and continued judicious use of living donor transplant. It is to be hoped that recent refinements to allocation policy in the USA, designed to provide organs to patients based in part on need, will also reduce the number of patients transplanted while on a ventilator. Addressing morbidity and mortality related to infection will require careful patient selection and continued adjustment of prophylactic and therapeutic strategies. For example, the availability of synergy testing of antibiotic combinations against multiresistant Gram-negative organisms has improved our ability to control these infections [77,78]. Improved outcomes following retransplantation await prospective identification of the most suitable candidates. OB remains the key factor limiting long-term survival; unfortunately, the incidence of OB in pediatrics has also has remained constant over the past 5 years. A better understanding of the etiology of OB, coupled with earlier diagnosis and more effective therapy, is needed. Hopefully, ongoing research efforts will address these issues and allow lung transplantation as a therapeutic option for children with fatal lung disease to move beyond palliation and closer to cure.

REFERENCES

1 Reitz BA, Wallwork JL, Hunt SA, *et al*. Heart-lung transplantation: successful therapy for patients with pulmonary vascular disease. *N Engl J Med* 1982;**306**:557–64.

2 Toronto Lung Transplant Group. Unilateral lung transplantation for pulmonary fibrosis. *N Engl J Med* 1986;**314**:1140–5.

3 Trulock EP, Edwards LB, Taylor DO, *et al*. The Registry of the International Society for Heart and Lung Transplantation: twenty-first official adult lung and heart-lung transplant report, 2004. *J Heart Lung Transplant* 2004;**23**:804–15.

4 Smyth RL, Higenbottam TW, Scott JP, *et al*. Early experience of heart-lung transplantation. *Arch Dis Child* 1989;**64**:1225–9.

5 Starnes VA, Marshall SE, Lewiston NJ, *et al*. Heart-lung transplantation in infants, children, and adolescents. *J Pediatr Surg* 1991;**26**:434–8.

6 Spray TL, Mallory GB, Canter CB, Huddleston CB. Pediatric lung transplantation: indications, techniques, and early results. *J Thorac Cardiovasc Surg* 1994;**107**:990–9.

7 Boucek MM, Edwards LB, Keck BM, *et al*. Registry for the International Society for Heart and Lung Transplantation: seventh official pediatric report, 2004. *J Heart Lung Transplant* 2004;**23**:933–47.

8 Boucek MM, Faro A, Novick RJ, *et al*. The Registry of the International Society of Heart and Lung Transplantation: third official pediatric report, 1999. *J Heart Lung Transplant* 1999;**18**:1151–72.

9 Trulock EP, Edwards LB, Taylor DO, *et al*. The Registry of the International Society for Heart and Lung Transplantation: twentieth official adult lung and heart-lung transplant report, 2003. *J Heart Lung Transplant* 2003;**22**:625–35.

10 Magee JC, Bucuvalas JC, Farmer DG, *et al*. Pediatric transplantation. *Am J Transplant* 2004;**4**(Suppl 9):54–71.

11 Christie JD, Bavaria JE, Palevsky HI, *et al*. Primary graft failure following lung transplantation. *Chest* 1998;**114**:51–60.

12 Christie JD, Kotloff RM, Pochettino A, *et al*. Clinical risk factors for primary graft failure following lung transplantation. *Chest* 2003;**124**:1232–41. [See comment]

13 de Perrot M, Liu M, Waddell TK, Keshavjee S. Ischemia-reperfusion-induced lung injury. *Am J Respir Crit Care Med* 2003;**167**:490–511.

14 Fiser SM, Tribble CG, Long SM, *et al*. Ischemia-reperfusion injury after lung transplantation increases risk of late bronchiolitis obliterans syndrome. *Ann Thorac Surg* 2002;**73**:1041–7.

15 Bridges ND, Mallory GB, Huddleston CB, Canter CE, Spray TL. Lung transplantation in infancy and early childhood. *J Heart Lung Transplant* 1996;**15**:895–902.

16 Bridges ND, Spray TL, Collins MH, Bowles NE, Towbin JA. Adenovirus infection in the lung results in graft failure after lung transplantation. *J Thorac Cardiovasc Surg* 1998;**116**:617–23.

17 Danziger-Isakov LA, DelaMorena M, Hayashi RJ, *et al*. Cytomegalovirus viremia associated with death or retransplantation in pediatric lung-transplant recipients. *Transplantation* 2003;**75**:1538–43.

18 Boyle GJ, Michaels MG, Webber SA, *et al*. Post-transplantation lymphoproliferative disorders in pediatric thoracic organ recipients. *J Pediatr* 1997;**131**:309–13.

19 Cohen AH, Sweet SC, Mendeloff E, *et al*. High incidence of post-transplant lymphoproliferative disease in pediatric patients with cystic fibrosis. *Am J Respir Crit Care Med* 2000;**161**:1252–5.

20 Chaparro C, Maurer J, Gutierrez C, *et al*. Infection with *Burkholderia cepacia* in cystic fibrosis: outcome following lung transplantation. *Am J Respir Crit Care Med* 2001;**163**:43–8.

21 De SA, McDowell A, Archer L, *et al*. *Burkholderia cepacia* complex genomovars and pulmonary transplantation outcomes in patients with cystic fibrosis. *Lancet* 2001;**358**:1780–1.

22 Aris RM, Routh JC, LiPuma JJ, Heath DG, Gilligan PH. Lung transplantation for cystic fibrosis patients with *Burkholderia cepacia* complex: survival linked to genomovar type. *Am J Respir Crit Care Med* 2001;**164**:2102–6.

23 Calvo V, Borro JM, Morales P, *et al*. Antifungal prophylaxis during the early postoperative period of lung transplantation. Valencia Lung Transplant Group. *Chest* 1999;**115**:1301–4.

24 Drew RH, Dodds AE, Benjamin DK Jr, *et al*. Comparative safety of amphotericin B lipid complex and amphotericin B deoxycholate as aerosolized antifungal prophylaxis in lung-transplant recipients. *Transplantation* 2004;**77**:232–7.

25 Huddleston CB, Sweet SC, Cohen AH, Mallory GB. Bronchiolitis obliterans after pediatric lung transplantation. *J Heart Lung Transplant* 1998;**17**(supplement).

26 Berry GJ, Brunt EM, Chamberlain D, *et al*. A working formulation for the standardization of nomenclature in the diagnosis of heart and lung rejection: Lung Rejection Study Group. The International Society for Heart Transplantation. *J Heart Transplant* 1990;**9**:593–601.

27 Yousem SA, Suncan SR, Ohori NP, Sonmez-Alpan E. Architectural remodeling of lung allografts in acute and chronic rejection. *Arch Pathol Lab Med* 1992;**116**:1175–80.

28 Yousem SA, Berry GJ, Cagle PT, *et al*. Revision of the 1990 working formulation for the classification of pulmonary allograft rejection: Lung Rejection Study Group. *J Heart Lung Transplant* 1996;**15**:1–15.

29 Cagle PT, Brown RW, Frost A, Kellar C, Yousem SA. Diagnosis of chronic lung transplant rejection by transbronchial biopsy. *Mod Pathol* 1995;**8**:137–42.

30 Weill D, McGiffin DC, Zorn GL Jr, *et al*. The utility of open lung biopsy following lung transplantation. *J Heart Lung Transplant* 2000;**19**:852–7.

31 Cooper JD, Billingham M, Egan T, *et al*. A working formulation for the standardization of nomenclature and for clinical staging of chronic dysfunction in lung allografts. International Society for Heart and Lung Transplantation. *J Heart Lung Transplant* 1993;**12**:713–6.

32 Estenne M, Maurer JR, Boehler A, *et al*. Bronchiolitis obliterans syndrome 2001: an update of the diagnostic criteria. *J Heart Lung Transplant* 2002;**21**:297–310.

33 El Gamel A, Sim E, Hasleton P, *et al*. Transforming growth factor β (TGF-β) and obliterative bronchiolitis following pulmonary transplantation. *J Heart Lung Transplant* 1999;**18**:828–37.

34 Hertz MI, Henke CA, Nakhleh RE, *et al*. Obliterative bronchiolitis after lung transplantation: a fibroproliferative disorder associated with platelet-derived growth factor. *Proc Natl Acad Sci USA* 1992;**89**:10 385–9.

35 Boehler A, Kesten S, Weder W, Speich R. Bronchiolitis obliterans after lung transplantation: a review. *Chest* 1998;**114**:1411–26.

36 Sharples LD, Tamm M, McNeil K, *et al*. Development of bronchiolitis obliterans syndrome in recipients of heart-lung transplantation: early risk factors. *Transplantation* 1996;**61**:560–6.

37 Reichenspurner H, Girgis RE, Robbins RC, *et al.* Stanford experience with obliterative bronchiolitis after lung and heart-lung transplantation. *Ann Thorac Surg* 1996;**62**:1467–72.

38 Zeevi A, Rabinowich H, Yousem SA, *et al.* Presence of donor-specific alloreactivity in histologically normal lung allografts is predictive of subsequent bronchiolitis obliterans. *Transplant Proc* 1991;**23**:1128–9.

39 McSherry C, Jackson A, Hertz MI, *et al.* Sequential measurement of peripheral blood allogeneic microchimerism levels and association with pulmonary function. *Transplantation* 1996;**62**: 1811–8.

40 Chalermskulrat W, Neuringer IP, Schmitz JL, *et al.* Human leukocyte antigen mismatches predispose to the severity of bronchiolitis obliterans syndrome after lung transplantation. *Chest* 2003;**123**:1825–31.

41 Smith MA, Sundaresan S, Mohanakumar T, *et al.* Effect of development of antibodies to HLA and cytomegalovirus mismatch on lung transplantation survival and development of bronchiolitis obliterans syndrome. *J Thorac Cardiovasc Surg* 1998;**116**:812–20.

42 Sundaresan S, Mohanakumar T, Smith MA, *et al.* HLA-A locus mismatches and development of antibodies to HLA after lung transplantation correlate with the development of bronchiolitis obliterans syndrome. *Transplantation* 1998;**65**:648–53.

43 SivaSai KS, Smith MA, Poindexter NJ, *et al.* Indirect recognition of donor HLA class I peptides in lung transplant recipients with bronchiolitis obliterans syndrome. *Transplantation* 1999; **67**:1094–8.

44 Reznik SI, Jaramillo A, SivaSai KS, *et al.* Indirect allorecognition of mismatched donor HLA class II peptides in lung transplant recipients with bronchiolitis obliterans syndrome. *Am J Transplant* 2001;**1**:228–35.

45 Lu KC, Jaramillo A, Mendeloff EN, *et al.* Concomitant allorecognition of mismatched donor HLA class I- and class II-derived peptides in pediatric lung transplant recipients with bronchiolitis obliterans syndrome. *J Heart Lung Transplant* 2003;**22**:35–43.

46 Jaramillo A, Smith MA, Phelan D, *et al.* Temporal relationship between the development of anti-HLA antibodies and the development of bronchiolitis obliterans syndrome after lung transplantation. *Transplant Proc* 1999;**31**:185–6.

47 Jaramillo A, Smith MA, Phelan D, *et al.* Development of ELISA-detected anti-HLA antibodies precedes the development of bronchiolitis obliterans syndrome and correlates with progressive decline in pulmonary function after lung transplantation. *Transplantation* 1999;**67**:1155–61.

48 Sharples LD, McNeil K, Stewart S, Wallwork J. Risk factors for bronchiolitis obliterans: a systematic review of recent publications. *J Heart Lung Transplant* 2002;**21**:271–81.

49 Ibrahim JE, Sweet SC, Flippin M, *et al.* Rejection is reduced in thoracic organ recipients when transplanted in the first year of life. *J Heart Lung Transplant* 2002;**21**:311–8.

50 Sweet SC, Spray TL, Huddleston CB, *et al.* Pediatric lung transplantation at St. Louis Children's Hospital, 1990–1995. *Am J Respir Crit Care Med* 1997;**155**:1027–35.

51 Woo MS, MacLaughlin EF, Horn MV, *et al.* Bronchiolitis obliterans is not the primary cause of death in pediatric living donor lobar lung transplant recipients. *J Heart Lung Transplant* 2001;**20**:491–6.

52 Bando K, Paradis IL, Similo S, *et al.* Obliterative bronchiolitis after lung and heart-lung transplantation: an analysis of risk factors and management. *J Thorac Cardiovasc Surg* 1995;**110**:4–13.

53 Keenan RJ, Lega ME, Dummer JS, *et al.* Cytomegalovirus serologic status and postoperative infection correlated with risk of developing chronic rejection after pulmonary transplantation. *Transplantation* 1991;**51**:433–8.

54 Keller CA, Cagle PT, Brown RW, Noon G, Frost AE. Bronchiolitis obliterans in recipients of single, double, and heart-lung transplantation. *Chest* 1995;**107**:973–80.

55 Kroshus TJ, Kshettry VR, Savik K, *et al.* Risk factors for the development of bronchiolitis obliterans syndrome after lung transplantation. *J Thorac Cardiovasc Surg* 1997;**114**:195–202.

56 Duncan SR, Grgurich WF, Iacono AT, *et al.* A comparison of ganciclovir and acyclovir to prevent cytomegalovirus after lung transplantation. *Am J Respir Crit Care Med* 1994;**150**:146–52.

57 Billings JL, Hertz MI, Savik K, Wendt CH. Respiratory viruses and chronic rejection in lung transplant recipients. *J Heart Lung Transplant* 2002;**21**:559–66.

58 Hohlfeld J, Niedermeyer J, Hamm H, *et al.* Seasonal onset of bronchiolitis obliterans syndrome in lung transplant recipients. *J Heart Lung Transplant* 1996;**15**:888–94.

59 Husain S, Singh N. Bronchiolitis obliterans and lung transplantation: evidence for an infectious etiology. *Semin Respir Infect* 2002;**17**:310–4.

60 Metras D, Viard L, Kreitmann B, *et al.* Lung infections in pediatric lung transplantation: experience in 49 cases. *Eur J Cardiothorac Surg* 1999;**15**:490–4.

61 Estenne M, Hertz MI. Bronchiolitis obliterans after human lung transplantation. *Am J Respir Crit Care Med* 2002;**166**:440–4.

62 Berkowitz N, Schulman LL, McGregor C, Markowitz D. Gastroparesis after lung transplantation: potential role in postoperative respiratory complications. *Chest* 1995;**108**:1602–7.

63 Davis RD Jr, Lau CL, Eubanks S, *et al.* Improved lung allograft function after fundoplication in patients with gastroesophageal reflux disease undergoing lung transplantation. *J Thorac Cardiovasc Surg* 2003;**125**:533–42.

64 Boehler A, Chamberlain D, Kesten S, *et al.* Lymphocytic airway infiltration as a precursor to fibrous obliteration in a rat model of bronchiolitis obliterans. *Transplantation* 1997;**64**:311–7.

65 Kallio E, Koskinen P, Buchdunger E, Lemstrom K. Inhibition of obliterative bronchiolitis by platelet-derived growth factor receptor protein-tyrosine kinase inhibitor. *Transplant Proc* 1999; **31**:187.

66 Kelly KE, Hertz MI, Mueller DL. T-cell and major histocompatibility complex requirements for obliterative airway disease in heterotopically transplanted murine tracheas. *Transplantation* 1998;**66**:764–71.

67 Ikonen TS, Brazelton TR, Berry GJ, Shorthouse RS, Morris RE. Epithelial re-growth is associated with inhibition of obliterative airway disease in orthotopic tracheal allografts in non-immunosuppressed rats. *Transplantation* 2000;**70**:857–63.

68 King MB, Pedtke AC, Levrey-Hadden HL, Hertz MI. Obliterative airway disease progresses in heterotopic airway allografts without persistent alloimmune stimulus. *Transplantation* 2002; **74**:557–62.

69 Salminen US, Alho H, Taskinen E, *et al.* Effects of rapamycin analogue SDZ RAD on obliterative lesions in a porcine heterotopic bronchial allograft model. *Transplant Proc* 1998;**30**:2204–5.

70 Fahrni JA, Berry GJ, Morris RE, Rosen GD. Rapamycin inhibits development of obliterative airway disease in a murine heterotopic airway transplant model. *Transplantation* 1997;**63**:533–7.

71 Fine RN. Growth following solid-organ transplantation. *Pediatr Transplant* 2002;**6**:47–52.

72 Cohen AH, Mallory GB Jr, Ross K, *et al.* Growth of lungs after transplantation in infants and in children younger than 3 years of age. *Am J Respir Crit Care Med* 1999;**159**:1747–51.

73 Binns OA, DeLima NF, Buchanan SA, *et al.* Mature pulmonary lobar transplants grow in an immature environment. *J Thorac Cardiovasc Surg* 1997;**114**:186–94.

74 Ibla JC, Shamberger RC, DiCanzio J, *et al.* Lung growth after reduced size transplantation in a sheep model. *Transplantation* 1999;**67**:233–40.

75 Ro PS, Bush DM, Kramer SS, *et al.* Airway growth after pediatric lung transplantation. *J Heart Lung Transplant* 2001;**20**:619–24.

76 Sritippayawan S, Keens TG, Horn MV, *et al.* Does lung growth occur when mature lobes are transplanted into children? *Pediatr Transplant* 2002;**6**:500–4.

77 Saiman L, Mehar F, Niu WW, *et al.* Antibiotic susceptibility of multiply resistant *Pseudomonas aeruginosa* isolated from patients with cystic fibrosis, including candidates for transplantation. *Clin Infect Dis* 1996;**23**:532–7.

78 Lang BJ, Aaron SD, Ferris W, Hebert PC, MacDonald NE. Multiple combination bactericidal antibiotic testing for patients with cystic fibrosis infected with multiresistant strains of *Pseudomonas aeruginosa. Am J Respir Crit Care Med* 2000;**162**: 2241–5.

79 Sweet SC, Berlinski A, Mendeloff EN, Mallory GB Jr, Huddleston CB. Early graft dysfunction in pediatric lung transplant recipients. *J Heart Lung Transplant* 1999(supplement).

Intestinal Transplantation

43 Historical Notes

Jorge Reyes

The beginning of the 21st century has ushered in almost 15 years of success with clinical transplantation of the intestine; however, this has come after 40 years of elusive success and frequent setbacks. The history of intestinal transplantation in many ways mimics that of other organs. The paradigm established by Medawar [1] that disruption of the alloactivated T-cell response could result in prolongation of allograft survival allowed for the thoughtful development of surgical technique, preservation technology and immunosuppressive protocols which led to successful clinical trials of kidney, liver, heart, lung and pancreas transplantation. However, this technology was not readily applicable to the intestine.

Ironically, the proposed barriers to success are factors that make the intestine a uniquely successful organ. Essentially, the intestine is perpetually exposed to the external environment and, as such, possesses various lymphoid aggregates (in the lamina propria, Peyer patches and mesenteric lymph nodes) throughout its entire length; this is known as the gut-associated lymphoid tissue (GALT). Experimental studies in the 1950s noted such a lymphoid capacity as distinctly "immunogenic," and responsible for the uncontrollable nature of intestinal allograft rejection; it was thought the same response would also facilitate graft-versus-host disease (GVHD). Such an event in the context of an "external environment" containing bacteria, fungi, viruses, toxins and allergens could easily translocate through the disrupted mucosa causing significant surgical and clinical complications with infection, graft loss and death.

Consequently, intestinal transplantation had to wait, not only for the development of solid clinical platforms for multi-organ transplantation, but also, most importantly, for a better understanding of immunosuppression and the immunologic events that have led to success with other organs. These historic strides have followed three intimately related paths: surgical technique and the development of intestinal grafts in their various forms; the evolution of immunosuppressive management; and the development of the concept of intestinal failure (IF).

The development of intestinal grafts in their various forms began with the experimental canine models of Lillehei *et al.* [2] in 1959 (studying autografts and allografts), and Starzl and Kaupp [3] in 1960 (studying the transplantation of the intestine as part of a multivisceral graft), providing technical and immunologic observations that prompted the largely unsuccessful clinical trials after 1964 [4]. Despite experimental insights into the significance of the gut-associated lymphoid population, immunosuppression was dogmatic and followed the available drug therapies of the day, which in the 1960s were performed under azathiaprine and/or steroid immunosuppression, and then subsequently in the 1980s using cyclosporine and/or steroid regimens; these trials were largely unsuccessful [5,6]. However, the cyclosporine-based regimens of the 1980s reported limited success (survival measured in months) utilizing multivisceral, combined liver and intestine, and isolated intestine allografts. Many of these cases utilized the routine depletion of intestinal graft lymphocytes by infusing the donor with an antithymocyte globulin prior to procurement and also *ex vivo* radiation of the intestinal allografts. This strategy was utilized in 1987 with the recipient of a multivisceral graft, which provided limited nutrition supporting survival for 6 months [7]. In 1988, Deltz *et al.* [8] transplanted an isolated intestinal allograft from a living donor, achieving nutritional autonomy for 56 months. A significant variation of the multivisceral graft was established with the "composite liver and intestine graft," which provided even further extension of the survival of these patients, as demonstrated by Grant *et al.* [9] and later Margreiter *et al.* [10]. The only survivor from the cyclosporine era at the present time is a cadaveric isolated intestinal recipient performed by Goulet *et al.* in 1989 [11].

The emergence in 1987 of tacrolimus allowed for better control of rejection of all organs, and changed the course of clinical intestinal transplantation. This was achieved thanks to better control of rejection, and consequent fewer overall drug toxicities and infections. The introduction of this drug for intestinal transplantation occurred after 1990, and rapidly led to a rise in the number of successful intestinal transplants performed [12]. This first series of successful cases performed under tacrolimus helped to enhance our knowledge of the gut-associated lymphocytes in the intestine and demonstrated the interaction between the immune system of the recipient and the donor immunocytes contained in the transplanted allograft; this has been postulated as a two-way paradigm of transplantation immunology [13]. These lymphocyte populations are highly mobile and can be found in the recipient peripheral blood soon after intestinal transplantation. Consequently, this interaction between donor and recipient lymphocytes (host-versus-graft and graft-versus-host) is exemplified with intestinal transplantation to a greater extent than with any other solid organ transplant. Host-versus-graft has been the predominant reaction, which has precipitated a higher level of immunoreactivity and rejection with graft loss after intestinal transplantation. The reverse reaction, graft-versus-host disease, although described both in animal models and clinical small bowel transplantation, has not been of clinical significance when compared with other transplant-related events after intestinal transplantation.

The gains accrued during the subsequent decade have been slow and incremental. The initial enthusiasm of the early 1990s was blunted as a result of gradual patient losses from recurrent rejection, and also the toxicity of high levels of immunosuppressive therapy that these patients required. Further increments in survival would only come with improvements in drug therapy, which have included interleukin-2 receptor antagonist, sirolimus and, most recently, the thymoglobulin protocols.

Our understanding of the patient population for which intestinal transplantation is most indicated has also evolved since the early clinical trials of intestinal transplantation in the 1960s. Most patients considered for such a procedure were suffering from short gut after losing significant lengths of their native intestinal tract; short gut syndrome remained the appropriate terminology. The clinical failures of intestinal transplantation in the 1960s were serendipitously accompanied by the introduction of total parenteral nutrition (TPN), which remained the standard of care for short gut syndrome for over three decades. However, it effectively paralleled the temporizing benefits that hemodialysis demonstrated in patients with renal failure, whereby established survival introduced a new set of morbidities which were predominantly a consequence of TPN (liver disease), catheter sepsis and loss of venous access. TPN was used for a host of disease entities, which included short gut syndrome, motility disorders and absorptive disorders of the intestine, many of which went on to develop these complications. Such patients are presently referred to as having IF. This concept introduced new approaches to the management of patients with IF, by applying multidisciplinary integrated care to this host of diseases, and also defining the criteria for intestinal transplantation, which was the basis for its present applications.

The subsequent chapters incorporate and expand on this course of history. Improving survival has now enabled workers in this field to pursue pressing questions of native gut immunology, function and quality of life.

REFERENCES

1 Medawar PB. The behavior and fate of skin allografts and skin homografts in rabbits. *J Anat* 1944;**78**:176–99.
2 Lillehei RC, Goott B, Miller FA. The physiologic response of the small bowel of the dog to ischemia including prolonged *in vitro* preservation of the bowel with successful replacement and survival. *Ann Surg* 1959;**150**:543–60.
3 Starzl TE, Kaupp HA Jr. Mass homo-transplantation of abdominal organs in dogs. *Surg Forum* 1960;**11**:28–30.
4 Grant D. Intestinal transplantation: current status. *Transplant Proc* 1989;**21**:2869–71.
5 Watson AJ, Lear PA. Current status of intestinal transplantation. *Gut* 1989;**30**:1771–82.
6 McAlister VC, Grant DR. Clinical small bowel transplantation. In: Grant DR, Wood RF, eds. *Small Bowel Transplantation*. London: Edward Arnold, 1994: 122.
7 Starzl TE, Rowe MI, Todo S, *et al.* Transplantation of multiple abdominal viscera. *JAMA* 1989;**261**:1449–57.
8 Deltz E, Schroeder P, Gebhardt H, *et al.* Successful clinical small bowel transplantation: report of a case. *Clin Transplant* 1989;**21**:89–91.
9 Grant D, Wall W, Mimeault R, *et al.* Successful small bowel/liver transplantation. *Lancet* 1990;**335**:181–4.
10 Margreiter R, Konigsrainer A, Schmid T, *et al.* Successful multivisceral transplantation. *Transplant Proc* 1992;**24**:1226–7.
11 Goulet O, Revillon Y, Brousse N, *et al.* Successful small bowel transplantation in an infant. *Transplantation* 1992;**53**:940–3.
12 Todo S, Tzakis AG, Abu-Elmagd K, *et al.* Cadaveric small bowel and small bowel-liver transplantation in humans. *Transplantation* 1992;**53**:369–76.
13 Starzl TE, Demetris AJ, Trucco M, *et al.* Cell migration and chimerism after whole-organ transplantation: the basis of graft acceptance. *Hepatology* 1993;**17**:1127–52.

44 Recipient Characteristics

Jean F. Botha and Debra L. Sudan

Intestinal transplantation has become the therapy of choice for children experiencing life-threatening complications of intestinal failure. The success of intestinal transplantation has lagged behind that of other solid organ transplants as a consequence of technical and immunologic failures. Recent advances in surgical technique, the introduction of tacrolimus, and refinements in patient and donor selection have allowed for improved patient and graft survival. Recent approval of payment for intestinal transplantation by the Health Care Funding Agency for Medicare patients is testimony of the evolution of intestinal transplantation from an experimental procedure to an accepted form of therapy for intestinal failure (Medicare Coverage Policy Decisions, Intestinal and Multivisceral Transplantation, CAG-00036, October 4, 2004).

Total parenteral nutrition (TPN) has revolutionized the treatment of children with intestinal failure. TPN allows normal growth and development in most children while intestinal adaptation takes place. Current survival rates for children and young adults on home TPN are 90% and 75% at 1-year and 5-years, respectively [1]. While TPN currently remains the mainstay of therapy for children with intestinal failure, some patients still succumb to complications of the therapy including liver disease, loss of central venous access and sepsis. It is for these patients that intestinal transplantation can be a life-saving treatment.

CAUSES OF INTESTINAL FAILURE

Intestinal failure (IF) is defined as the reduction of gut mass below the minimum necessary for digestion and absorption of nutrients and fluids required for maintenance in adults and growth in children [2]. The causes of intestinal failure can be broadly classified into three categories:
1 Anatomic loss of intestine (i.e. short bowel syndrome), which accounts for the majority of cases of IF.
2 Motility disorders, either neuropathic diseases such as Hirschsprung disease or myopathic diseases such as chronic intestinal pseudo-obstruction syndrome (CIPOS).
3 Congenital disease of the intestinal epithelium such as micro-

Table 44.1 Common causes of short bowel syndrome in infants.

Prenatal	Postnatal
Jejuno-ileal atresia	Necrotizing enterocolitis
Gastroschisis and omphalocele	Midgut volvulus
Midgut volvulus	Vascular thrombosis

villous inclusion disease and epithelial dysplasia or tufting enteropathy.

Short bowel syndrome

Short bowel syndrome occurs in the prenatal period as a result of jejuno-ileal atresia, midgut volvulus and abdominal wall defects such as gastroschisis and omphalocele. In neonates, necrotizing enterocolitis, midgut volvulus and vascular thrombosis are the most frequent causes (Table 44.1). Most infants survive extensive small bowel resection and the prognosis for these patients depends on the length and function of the remnant bowel. Infants with less than 35 cm of small bowel and an absent ileocecal valve are likely to remain TPN dependent. In addition, infants who tolerate less than 50% of their caloric requirement enterally are also less likely to achieve enteral autonomy [3]. These infants have a high risk of developing TPN-related complications and early referral to a specialist center is desirable as liver disease progresses rapidly in such patients [4].

Motility disorders

Intestinal aganglionosis

For children suffering from near total intestinal aganglionosis (long-segment Hirschsprung disease) there is no medical or surgical therapy to improve intestinal function and TPN dependency is inevitable. Intestinal transplantation therefore offers the only realistic chance of long-term survival and enteral autonomy [5,6]. Isolated intestinal transplantation should be considered before the onset of liver disease. Inclusion of the colon with the graft has previously been reported to be associated with a higher mortality and therefore has not been standard of care. A recent report from the Paris group suggests that inclusion of the right colon with the allograft followed by an abdominal pull-through procedure 6 months to 1 year after the transplant resulted in a satisfactory functional outcome and perhaps this issue should be re-examined [7].

Chronic intestinal pseudo-obstruction syndrome

CIPOS represents a heterogeneous array of conditions that manifest as severe impairment of intestinal motility in the absence of mechanical obstruction. Broadly speaking, CIPOS can be characterized as neuropathic, myopathic or a combination of the two. The clinical presentation is also highly variable and there may be involvement of extra intestinal organs such as the bladder and the central nervous system [8–10]. Abdominal pain from intestinal distention and fluid losses from chronic vomiting resulting from intestinal dysmotility are common features of CIPOS. The disease can afflict different portions of the gastrointestinal tract and patients may benefit from a variety of decompressive procedures such as ileostomy or even ileorectal anastomosis in patients with predominantly colonic disease [4]. Reports suggest that 20–25% of these children will become TPN dependent and intestinal transplantation now represents a viable alternative for these patients, many of whom have a poor quality of life [8]. Our own experience with transplantation for children with CIPOS demonstrates that successful intestinal transplantation provides these children with good quality of life [11]. An ongoing debate for this group of children is whether or not to resect or leave intact the native stomach. Our program has never used the donor stomach as part of the graft with good functional outcome, but others advocate this despite the risks of severe gastroparesis.

Congenital enterocyte disorders

Children with secretory diarrhea as a result of congenital disorders of enterocyte development are generally recommended to undergo intestinal transplantation before the onset of liver disease or loss of intravenous access. Excessive fluid and electrolyte losses occur as a result of intractable diarrhea for which there is no medical treatment. Life-long TPN is expected, but is often associated with severe metabolic disturbances. Early referral and pre-emptive transplantation currently offers the best chance of survival [12].

Microvillous inclusion disease

Microvillous inclusion disease (MID) appears to be inherited as an autosomal recessive trait, with a poor expectation for long-term survival [13]. The pathogenesis is thought to be brought about by a defect in membrane trafficking leading to failure of development of the enterocyte brush border and plasma membrane. Electron microscopy reveals sparse or absent microvilli on the apical membrane and microvillous inclusions in the cytoplasm of the enterocyte [14]. Intestinal transplantation for MID has been reported by Ruemmele et al. [15], alone or in combination with the liver, with patient and graft survival over 80% at 3 years, which was in stark contrast to the survival rate of a subgroup of MID patients not transplanted. Our own experience is similar and we therefore offer MID patients pre-emptive transplantation with a combined liver/intestinal allograft. In our early experience we offered isolated intestinal transplantation, but currently believe that the liver is involved with the disease after one MID patient continued to experience cholestasis after weaning from TPN. We subsequently performed an isolated liver transplant 4 years after successful isolated small bowel transplant in this young boy with MID, because of cirrhosis, progressive jaundice and intractable pruritus. When MID is suspected in a child, early referral to a transplant center is recommended, as transplantation for these patients is highly successful.

Intestinal epithelial dysplasia

Also known as "tufting enteropathy," intestinal epithelial dysplasia (IED) is associated with a defect in the basement membrane. The condition is characterized histologically by the presence of epithelial "tufts," varying degrees of villous atrophy and crypt hyperplasia. Clinical presentation with excessive watery diarrhea is similar to that of MID and is also thought to be inherited in an autosomal recessive pattern [16,17]. As with MID, there is no medical treatment for IED and children with this condition should also be considered for intestinal transplantation before the onset of complications of TPN.

INDICATIONS FOR TRANSPLANTATION

While survival rates for small bowel transplantation are steadily improving, the level of success has not yet reached that of kidney transplantation, where quality of life is a major indication for transplantation [18]. While it is often reported that the results of intestinal transplantation are not as good as those seen with home TPN, it is difficult to make this comparison as the patient population undergoing intestinal transplantation is generally in considerably poorer medical condition than those remaining on home TPN [19]. Despite increasing survival rates after transplantation, timing of transplantation remains a matter of debate and currently is limited to patients who are experiencing one or more of the following life-threatening complications of IF.

Liver disease

Patients with IF can have a broad spectrum of liver disease, ranging from mild cholestasis to cirrhosis [20]. The mechanism of IF-associated liver disease remains poorly understood but appears to be a result of gut dysfunction rather than a toxic effect of TPN. The presence of hyperbilirubinemia, splenomegaly, thrombocytopenia and gastrointestinal bleeding suggests that the liver disease in not reversible and combined liver/small bowel transplantation is necessary [21]. In other patients, however, it is often difficult to predict whether or not liver disease is reversible. Fishbein *et al.* [22] recently reported the resolution of bridging fibrosis after isolated intestinal transplantation, similar to that reported by Iyer *et al.* [23] after salvage of native gut.

Vascular thrombosis

Impending loss of intravenous access is a major indication for intestinal transplantation. Loss of venous access has been defined as thrombosis of two or more of the major venous access sites (subclavian and internal jugular). We avoid use of the femoral veins in infants until absolutely necessary, because of the high risk of septic complications. This definition may seem somewhat conservative but late referral when all intravenous access has been exhausted is a contraindication for transplantation. Consideration of long-term anticoagulation should be given in any patient with permanent intestinal failure and any major vascular thrombosis.

Sepsis

Sepsis can be related to the central line itself or to bacterial overgrowth leading to bacterial translocation, and accounts for substantial morbidity and mortality [24]. Infections with low morbidity that are easily treated do not represent failure of TPN and an attempt should be made to treat the infection without removal of the central venous catheter. Children with life-threatening infections and infections with multidrug-resistant organisms should be evaluated for transplantation [25].

Other indications

Although infrequently reported, intestinal transplantation has been performed for locally invasive abdominal tumors such as desmoid tumors and neuroendocrine tumors that encase the root of the mesentery necessitating extensive small bowel resections to achieve tumor clearance [26,27]. Patients with a nonreconstructible gastrointestinal tract with or without biliopancreatic fistulae have also been shown to benefit from early intestinal transplantation before signs of failure of TPN [28].

WAITING LIST AND ORGAN ALLOCATION

Patients listed for combined liver and small intestine allografts have a waiting list mortality between 30% and 50%, with infants being at greatest risk. The mortality rate for intestinal transplant recipients exceeds the waiting list mortality for all other organ types [29]. When reviewing the United Network for Organ Sharing (UNOS) database for the period 1997–2001, Fryer *et al.* [30] confirmed that 36% of patients listed for combined liver and small intestine transplantation died on the waiting list during this period. This is in contrast to the wait list mortality for liver-only recipients of 14%. The major cause of death in intestinal transplant candidates is systemic sepsis. These patients are at particular risk of developing infectious complications because of the presence of central venous catheters, bacterial overgrowth and translocation, stomas, enteral tubes and diarrhea. These unique risk factors for mortality are not incorporated into the organ allocation scheme [12,30].

The UNOS Liver/Intestine committee recognizes that liver and small intestine transplant candidates are not well served by the current organ allocation scheme. Recent adjustments to the Model for End-Stage Liver Disease and Pediatric End-Stage Liver Disease (MELD/PELD) policy have been made to address this issue; currently combined liver/small bowel candidates receive an automatic MELD/PELD upgrade corresponding to a 10% increase in mortality (Fig. 44.1).

These changes to MELD/PELD policy alone are unlikely to resolve the inequalities in organ distribution for patients requiring intestinal transplantation and it remains a challenge to obtain suitable organs for these unique patients.

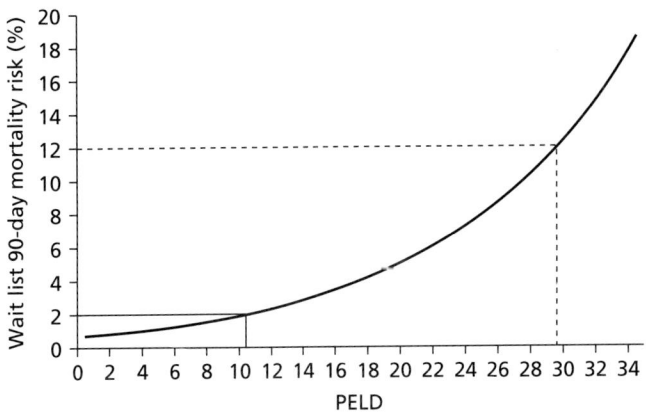

Fig. 44.1 Example of the model for end-stage liver disease (MELD) and pediatric end-stage liver disease (PELD) 10% 3-month mortality risk adjustment for intestinal transplant candidates. A biological PELD score of 10 equates to a 3-month mortality risk of 2%, an additional 10% will adjust the PELD score to 29.

REFERENCES

1 Howard L, Malone M. Current status of home parenteral nutrition in the United Sates. *Transplant Proc* 1996;**28**:2691.

2 Fleming CR, Remington M. Intestinal failure. In: Hill GL, ed. *Nutrition and Surgical Patient*. New York: Churchill Livingstone, 1981: 219–35.

3 Kaufman SS, Loseke CA, Lupo JV, *et al.* Influence of bacterial overgrowth and intestinal inflammation on duration of parenteral nutrition in children with short bowel syndrome. *J Pediatr* 1997; **131**:356–61.

4 Goulet O, Allegri A, Colomb V, *et al.* Growth and nutritional status after intestinal transplantation in children. *J Pediatr Gastroenterol Nutr* 2000;**31**(Suppl 2):S165.

5 Saxton ML, Ein SH, Hophner J, *et al.* Near total intestinal aganglionosis: long term follow-up of a morbid condition. *J Pediatr Surg* 2000;**35**:669–72.

6 Sharif K, Beath SV, Kelly DA, *et al.* New perspective for the management of near-total or total intestinal aganglionosis in infants. *J Pediatr Surg* 2003;**38**:25–8.

7 Yann R, Yves A, Dominique J, *et al.* Improved quality of life by combined transplantation in Hirschsprung's disease with a very long aganglionic segment. *J Pediatr Surg* 2003;**38**:422–4.

8 Goulet O, Jobert-Giraud A, Michel JL, *et al.* Chronic intestinal pseudoobstruction syndrome in pediatric patients. *Eur J Pediatr Surg* 1999;**9**:83–9.

9 Masetti M, Rodriguez MM, Thompson JF, *et al.* Multivisceral transplantation for megacystis microcolon intestinal hypoperistalsis syndrome. *Transplantation* 1999;**68**:228–32.

10 Masetti M, Di Benedetto F, Cautero N, *et al.* Intestinal transplantation for chronic intestinal pseudo-obstruction in adult patients. *Am J Transplant* 2004;**4**:826–9.

11 Iyer K, Kaufman S, Sudan D, *et al.* Long-term results of intestinal transplantation for pseudo-obstruction in children. *J Pediatr Surg* 2001;**36**:174–7.

12 Kaufman SS. Small bowel transplantation: selection criteria, operative techniques, advances in specific immunosuppression, prognosis. *Curr Opin Pediatr* 2001;**13**:425–8.

13 Phillips AD, Jenkins P, Raafat F, *et al.* Congenital microvillous atrophy: specific diagnostic features. *Arch Dis Child* 1985;**60**:136–40.

14 Bell SW, Kerner JA Jr, Sibley RK. Microvillous inclusion disease: the importance of electron microscopy for diagnosis. *Am J Surg Pathol* 1991;**15**:1157–64.

15 Ruemmele FM, BindlL, Woelfle J, *et al.* Recurrent episodes of necrotizing enterocolitis complicating congenital microvillous atrophy. *Dig Dis Sci* 2001;**46**:1264–9.

16 Reifen RM, Cutz E, Griffiths AM, *et al.* Tufting enteropathy: a newly recognized clinicopathological entity associated with refractory diarrhea in infants. *J Pediatr Gastroenterol Nutr* 1994;**18**:379–85.

17 Kaufman SS, Atkinson JB, Bianchi A, *et al.* Indications for pediatric intestinal transplantation: a position paper of the American Society of Transplantation. *Pediatr Transpl* 2001;**5**:80.

18 Langnas AN. Advances in small-intestine transplantation. *Transplantation* 2004;**77**(9 Suppl):S75–8.

19 Quigley EM. Small intestinal transplantation: reflections on an evolving approach to intestinal failure. *Gastroenterology* 1996; **110**:2009–12.

20 Braxton C, Lowry SF. Parenteral nutrition and liver dysfunction: new insight? [Editorial]. *J Parenter Enteral Nutr* 1995;**19**:3–4.

21 Sudan DL, Kaufman SS, Shaw BW Jr, *et al.* Isolated intestinal transplantation for intestinal failure. *Am J Gastroenterol* 2000; **95**:1506–15.

22 Fishbein TM, Kaufman SS, Florman SS, *et al.* Isolated intestinal transplantation: proof of clinical efficacy. *Transplantation* 2003; **76**:636–40.

23 Iyer K, Horslen S, Torres C, *et al.* Histology is not predictive of functional liver recovery in parenteral-nutrition associated liver dysfunction (Abstract). *Pediatr Transpl* 2003;**7**:69.

24 Messing B, Crenn P, Beau P, *et al.* Long-term survival and parenteral nutrition dependence in adult patients with short bowel syndrome. *Gastroenterology* 1999;**117**:1043.

25 Kaufman S, Atkinson JB, Bianchi A, *et al.* Indications for pediatric intestinal transplantation: a position paper of the American Society of Transplantation. *Pediatr Transpl* 2001;**5**:80–7.

26 Misiakos EP, Pinna A, Kato T, *et al.* Recurrence of desmoid tumor in a multivisceral transplant patient with Gardner's syndrome. *Transplantation* 1999;**67**:1197–9.

27 Calne RY, Pollard SG, Jamieson NV, *et al.* Intestinal transplant for recurring mesenteric desmoid tumour. *Lancet* 1993;**342**: 58–9.

28 Shuster B, Bond G, Martin L, *et al.* Acute irreversible intestinal failure and early intestinal transplantation: indications and survival outcomes (Abstract). *Transplantation* 2004;**78**:23.

29 Gilroy R, Sudan D. Liver and small bowel transplantation: therapeutic alternatives for the treatment of liver disease and intestinal failure. *Semin Liver Dis* 2000;**20**:437.

30 Fryer J, Pellar S, Ormond D, *et al.* Mortality in candidates waiting for combined liver-intestine transplants exceeds that for other candidates waiting for liver transplants. *Liver Transpl* 2003;**9**:748–53.

45 Evaluation of the Candidate

Stuart S. Kaufman

By present standards, life-threatening intolerance of parenteral nutrition (PN) with permanent intestinal failure is the indication for considering intestinal transplantation. The first objective in the evaluation of a patient for an intestinal transplant is to determine if transplantation is the most appropriate means of ending PN. The next objectives are to determine if transplantation can be performed with a reasonable probability of success based on evaluation of other vital organ systems and whether additional organs should be included in the allograft. Further evaluation includes a consideration of the ability of the family to care for an intestinal transplant recipient and what additional resources they may require.

DETERMINING ORGANS TO BE TRANSPLANTED

Assessment of the gastrointestinal tract
(Table 45.1)

Patients with short bowel syndrome

The immediate goal of evaluation is verification that the patient with short bowel syndrome is experiencing life-threatening complications from PN, usually progressive liver disease or

Table 45.1 Questions to be asked in assessment of the gastrointestinal tract for intestinal transplant.

---

1 Can the patient be expected to require PN indefinitely? Based on:
  Available anatomic information (operative reports, X rays)
  Actual enteral nutrient absorption
2 Are there any medical or surgical measures that may improve tolerance of enteral nutrition short of transplantation?
3 Will the native stomach and duodenum function adequately with an intestinal transplant?
4 Will the native colon function adequately in continuity with an intestinal transplant?

PN, parenteral nutrition.

progressive loss of venous access, and has no meaningful chance to end therapy [1]. Evaluation begins with an estimation of the length of remnant small bowel and colon, usually by review of operative reports, supplemented with contemporaneous contrast imaging studies. Next, anatomic information is compared with historical feeding tolerance. Permanence of PN is frequently obvious, as the typical patient often has an estimated jejunum length of no more than 40 cm, no ileum or ileocecal valve, and partial colon; by referral, PN supplies most if not all calories, as previous attempts to end therapy has been unsuccessful [2].

Some patients retain more bowel than is customarily associated with permanent PN but do not tolerate enteral feeds as expected. Contrast radiography may identify marked intestinal dilatation that warrants considering remedial surgical procedures such as tapering enteroplasty or intestinal lengthening before proceeding with transplant [3]. If endoscopic small bowel biopsy reveals an essentially normal mucosa in a nondilated bowel, the implication is that the shortened gut is already functioning at maximum efficiency; low D-xylose absorption supports this conclusion. Conversely, chronic enteritis implies that a trial of anti-inflammatory or antibiotic therapy is appropriate, possibly in conjunction with enteroplasty when associated with gut dilatation and stasis, before concluding that transplantation performed as soon as practicable is the only realistic therapeutic option. When intractable vomiting resulting from gastroparesis and/or duodenal stasis without demonstrable mechanical bowel obstruction is present, a multivisceral allograft that includes the stomach as well as intestine must be considered. Confirmatory nuclear imaging may be useful.

Less commonly, patients referred for intestinal transplant have obvious end-stage liver disease associated with PN (see below) but seem to "tolerate" substantial enteral calories, raising the possibility of an isolated liver transplant in anticipation of completing intestinal adaptation in the future [4]. This situation most likely applies to patients who will end PN based on customary anatomic criteria and a current PN requirement not exceeding one-third of estimated total energy expenditures. In our experience, expressing PN requirements in this fashion is more realistic than as a fraction of total caloric intake (enteral and parenteral), because the latter does not consider that a substantial fraction of enteral feeding may not be absorbed [5]. When PN delivers more than 50% of estimated energy needs, then further attempts at intestinal rehabilitation are likely to be fruitless, irrespective of the absolute quantity of enteral feeding.

Other important points to consider include the following. Chronic or recurrent PN-associated pancreatitis may be present and undermine attempts to end PN despite seemingly adequate intestinal anatomy [6]. Determination of fecal excretion of pancreatic enzymes such as chymotrypsin or elastase may guide a trial of replacement therapy before discounting ability of the gastrointestinal tract to complete adaptation. A history of overt or occult gastrointestinal bleeding is germane to identification of portal hypertension and is also a clue to persistent bowel disease (e.g. occult perforation) which, if unrecognized, may complicate the intestinal transplant. Severe intractable abdominal pain is not ordinarily a feature of pediatric short bowel syndrome, and narcotic dependence may exaggerate intrinsic intestinal dysfunction. Although some patients with chronic pancreatitis or gallbladder disease experience chronic recurring pain, considerable caution should be exercised when this symptom is the ostensible reason for referral. Münchausen syndrome by proxy and other major psychologic disturbances in a transplant candidate, a parent, or both, may be present that makes transplantation either inappropriate or relatively contraindicated until coassociated psychologic problems are identified and treated [7,8].

Patients with functional intestinal failure

Considerations in evaluation of patients with an established diagnosis of functional intestinal failure (i.e. pseudo-obstruction or congenital secretory diarrhea) differ somewhat from those of patients referred for intestinal transplantation because of complicated anatomic short bowel syndrome. In the former group, the underlying diagnosis is likely to have been established before referral by definitive investigations, and the decision to proceed with transplant is based on assessment of the threat to the life of the patient. In those patients with evolving liver disease and progressive reduction in central venous access, both the permanent character of PN and the impending nature of PN failure may be readily apparent, in which case a recommendation for transplant is straightforward [7,9]. Review of feeding history, upper gastrointestinal imaging and previous antro-duodenal manometry may clarify whether all or most of the native stomach should be retained or whether donor stomach should be included in the composite allograft. Recommending transplantation becomes less clear when a history consistent with deteriorating life quality is the reason for referral, particularly in patients with pseudo-obstruction. In this setting, evaluation focuses on objectively delineating time away from school, hospitalizations due to

Table 45.2 Questions to be asked for determination of whether simultaneous liver transplant is indicated.

1 Has the infant remained icteric (bilirubin > 3–6 mg/dL and climbing) despite enteral feeding? Has the child become icteric suddenly after a prolonged period of PN?
2 Does the icteric patient have a remnant small bowel so short as to predict permanent PN?
3 Has the patient begun to experience stoma bleeding after a prolonged period without this symptom?
4 Does the patient have marked liver *and* spleen enlargement?
5 Is the platelet count falling (< 100 000–150 000/μL) in the absence of recent sepsis?

catheter-associated bloodstream infection and fluid–electrolyte disturbances, need for gastrointestinal decompression, and abdominal pain that has a pathophysiologic etiology.

Assessment of the liver (Table 45.2)

History

Importance of assessing PN-associated liver disease and liver failure is emphasized by the fact that approximately half of all pediatric intestinal transplants include liver in the composite allograft [10]. The key objective is determination of whether liver disease that may have been the primary rationale for referral is likely to be reversed by initiating (or resuming) total enteral nutrition with an isolated intestinal transplant. If evaluation suggests that liver disease has already progressed to end stage, which remains a common occurrence, combined liver and intestinal transplant is mandated. In practice, distinguishing reversible from irreversible liver disease can be difficult [11]. A combination of historical features, physical examination, common laboratory tests, imaging studies and, possibly, histology, are needed to determine the severity of hepatocellular synthetic dysfunction and portal hypertension. From a historical perspective, duration and severity of hyperbilirubinemia are a primary consideration; hyperbilirubinemia since birth and recent appearance following prolonged PN are particularly worrisome in infants and older children, respectively [12]. Status of the intestinal tract is also of primary relevance, because a very short remnant small bowel and minimal tolerance of enteral nutrition predict progressive and irreversible disease [2]. A history of severe abdominal sepsis at the time of initial bowel resection is generally important, serving as an independent predictor of liver failure, as may recurrent catheter-associated sepsis. Transfusion-grade gastrointestinal bleeding, particularly that emanating from gastrostomies, enterostomies and colostomies, implies that portal hypertension is severe and liver disease advanced regardless of all other historical and physical findings.

Physical examination

Features of physical examination that distinguish reversible from end-stage liver disease are less apparent when liver disease coexists with intestinal failure as compared with when it does not. Clinically important ascites and esophagogastric varices are unusual, presumably because these cardinal features of end-stage liver disease require both high portal vein resistance owing to liver disease *per se* and increased portal vein blood flow, the majority of which comes from the superior mesenteric vein [13,14]. Following massive midgut resection and commensurate reduction in superior mesenteric vein flow, splenic vein circulation alone appears insufficient to produce significant portosystemic shunting. However, increased intrahepatic resistance readily produces congestive splenomegaly and gastroenteropathy which, together with hyperbilirubinemia and severe hepatosplenomegaly, become the clinical hallmarks of the condition. Superficial abdominal wall veins may be prominent because of the additive effect of shunting produced by compression of the inferior vena cava by an enlarged liver. Subtle clinical features suggestive of hepatic encephalopathy, particularly disordered sleeping habits and idiopathic irritability, are very late findings as is fetor hepaticus. These findings sharply contrast with those in patients with intestinal failure but no advanced liver disease, in whom icterus is mild or absent, and the spleen, if enlarged at all, rarely projects below the umbilicus.

Laboratory tests

Certain blood tests are useful when assessing the need for liver transplant concurrent with intestinal transplant. Limited prospective data imply that stable or worsening hyperbilirubinemia, as mild as 3–6 mg/dL, that persists for 6 months after neonatal bowel resection and is unimproved by some enteral nutrition warrants inclusion of liver in the composite allograft, particularly when associated with worsening splenomegaly and functional hypersplenism [15]. A platelet count below 100 000/μL is particularly indicative of end-stage disease in the absence of recent sepsis or other cause of bone marrow suppression [16]. Fasting hypoglycemia, abnormal coagulation tests, elevated plasma ammonia concentration and neutropenia resulting from hypersplenism are indicative of late referral. Climbing serum aminotransferase levels may be of prognostic significance in adults [12] but their significance is less clear in children and, similarly, gamma glutamyl transferase (GGT) is often low in relation to aminotransferase levels in the setting of total ileal resection and little or no enterohepatic recirculation of bile salts.

Relative few prospective data are available concerning the role of liver biopsy in evaluation. In general, presence of up to grade 2 fibrosis (portal expansion with early bridging) suggests reversible disease and the feasibility of isolated intestinal transplant, while grade 3 fibrosis (advanced bridging) or grade 4 fibrosis (fully established cirrhosis) support an impression of irreversible disease [15]. In practice, grade 2 changes on needle biopsy are often demonstrated when all other clinical and laboratory findings suggest irreversible disease, implying that structural deterioration of the liver can be delayed in comparison with deteriorating liver function. Conversely, relatively advanced fibrosis does not absolutely prove the need for a liver allograft, particularly if features of portal hypertension are not prominent [3]. Radiologic evaluation of the abdomen has a limited role in assessment of the liver. Ultrasound is most useful to quantify splenomegaly in ambiguous cases. Portal vein flow usually remains antegrade even with severe portal hypertension, although a peaked hepatic arterial waveform is often seen. Magnetic resonance (MR) or computed tomographic (CT) angiography are relevant to technical planning for combined liver and intestinal transplantation for the purposes of quantifying liver volume and verifying patency of key vessels including the inferior vena cava.

Assessment of other organs (Table 45.3)

Vascular anatomy

Progressive central vein occlusion resulting from repeated catheterization occurs commonly in patients committed to prolonged PN therapy, usually within the setting of recurrent catheter-related bloodstream infection. Declining vascular access that threatens continuation of PN in a patient likely to require it indefinitely is a common indication for intestinal transplantation in patients beyond infancy. Maintenance of central venous access is mandatory during transplant surgery and up to several months thereafter, even with a successful operation [1]. Consequently, at evaluation for transplant, existing central vein patency must be determined in order to verify that the transplant is technically feasible and that post-transplant catheter replacement necessitated by catheter malfunction or sepsis will be possible. MR venography (MRV) with coronal three-dimensional reconstruction has largely supplanted conventional contrast venography for this purpose (Fig. 45.1). MRV overcomes the limitations of Doppler ultrasonography in patients likely to have had catheterizations repeatedly in the past in two ways. First, unlike ultrasound, MRV images very proximal vessels within the thorax including brachiocephalic veins that may be occluded despite patency

Table 45.3 Radiologic imaging in intestinal transplant evaluation.

Upper gastrointestinal series with small bowel follow-through
Contrast enema
Abdominal ultrasonography
Magnetic resonance venography and abdominal imaging
X-ray and/or computed tomography of the chest
Echocardiography

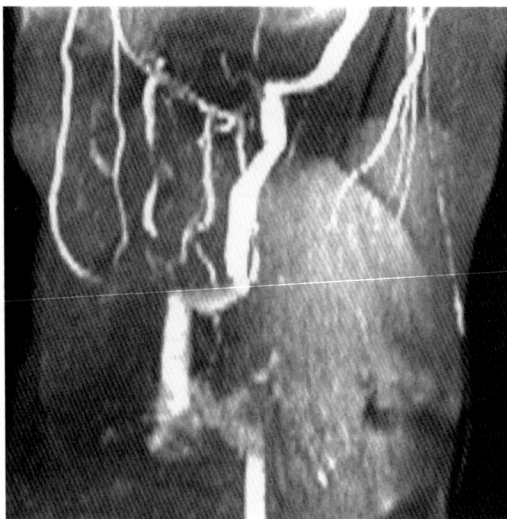

Fig. 45.1 Magnetic resonance venogram demonstrating occluded right internal jugular vein with collateral circulation and patent left internal jugular vein.

of more distal vessels. Second, ultrasound may fail to distinguish multiple unusable collateral vessels that form around a thrombosed original central vein, leading to a mistakenly optimistic view of available venous access.

Demonstration of numerous occluded vessels in a pediatric transplant candidate, particularly if subjectively increased compared with the number of previous catheter replacements or catheter-related septic episodes, should prompt a search for primary thrombophilia [17]. Because most congenital thrombophilic disorders are based in the liver, evaluation is particularly important in candidates for an isolated intestinal transplant, as the defect will persist after transplant. However, clinically suspicious findings in candidates for a combined liver and intestinal transplant also require evaluation because of the genetic implications of a positive diagnosis.

The customary criterion for performing an intestinal transplant based on declining central vein access is 50% loss of usual sites, jugular and subclavian in infants, and jugular, subclavian and femoral in older children [18]. Individual transplant centers have their own requirements concerning the minimum number of remaining access sites necessary to perform the operation. Regrettably, some patients have lost all standard venous access at referral, receiving PN via such tenuous routes as translumbar or transhepatic vein placed by interventional radiologic services [19]; in this situation, many established centers will undertake an isolated intestinal transplant, albeit reluctantly, because transplantation will not disturb the catheter. In contrast, transplant centers often reject patients needing a liver and intestine or multivisceral transplant because of the relatively prolonged recovery following a more complex operation and the unavailability of the transhepatic approach during the transplant.

Pulmonary function

A history of respiratory tract disease mandates assessment of pulmonary reserve in candidates for intestinal transplantation, because significant respiratory pathology may increase the risk of intraoperative complications and intractable postoperative mechanical ventilation. The most common cause of respiratory insufficiency in pediatric patients with intestinal failure is bronchopulmonary dysplasia associated with prematurity. Much less frequently, congenital malformations (e.g. pulmonary hypoplasia associated diaphragmatic hernia and midgut malrotation) are responsible [20]. Factors that increase the risk of, or contraindicate, transplantation include oxygen dependence, reactive airway disease and radiologic findings that suggest fibrosis and chronic atelectasis. Chest X-ray, chest CT and echocardiography are generally indicated, and pulmonary function tests may be useful if available. Chronic oxygen dependence (room air saturation less than 92–93%) resulting from chronic lung disease is probably the most common reason to decline transplant, particularly if sufficient to cause pulmonary hypertension and right ventricular hypertrophy [14]. Portopulmonary hypertension severe enough to contraindicate transplant is a rare occurrence in patients with liver disease associated with intestinal failure [21].

Cardiac function

Formal cardiac evaluation is appropriate when evaluating pediatric candidates for intestinal transplantation because of long-standing central venous catheterization and frequent catheter-associated bloodstream infections that increase the risk of occult or overt valvular disease. Premature infants may present with a persistently patent ductus arteriosus, severity of which may not be appreciated in the absence of formal testing; repair before the transplant may be desirable. Identification of hyperdynamic circulation and ventricular hypertrophy, which are common when liver disease is advanced, is important, although their relation to development of posttransplant hypertrophic cardiomyopathy under corticosteroid and tacrolimus therapy remains unclear [22,23].

Renal function

Intestinal failure places affected patients, including children, at risk of acquired renal insufficiency. Contributory factors include repeated exposure to nephrotoxic drugs, especially aminoglycoside antibiotics, and chronic underhydration inherent to the condition [24]. Patients with PN-associated cholestasis may be at particular risk as liver disease worsens. Recognizing renal insufficiency in infants may be challenging, because plasma urea nitrogen and creatinine concentrations are relatively insensitive measures. Severe sepsis may expose underlying renal insufficiency. Ultrasound or CT of the kidneys is an essential part of evaluation to detect renal atrophy, nephrocalcinosis, hydronephrosis or more subtle indications of renal disease. In the presence of ambiguous findings, nuclear renal imaging may be useful. Abnormal renal function detected during evaluation may indicate kidney transplantation, which is most often the case when intestinal failure results from pseudo-obstruction [25]. Significant but less extreme renal dysfunction may prompt consideration of less nephrotoxic immunosuppressive regimens.

Neurodevelopmental assessment

Developmental delays are commonly observed in children referred for intestinal transplantation and are usually the consequence of extreme prematurity and chronic postnatal illness. Less frequently, congenital disorders such as syndromic Hirschsprung disease and metabolic diseases produce both neurologic and gastrointestinal dysfunction of variable severity; intractable diarrhea or pseudo-obstruction may lead to consideration of a transplant [26,27]. Regardless of etiology, developmental delays and related neurologic disorders may be severe enough to contraindicate transplant. CT or MR brain imaging is most useful to detect structural abnormalities when there is a possibility of a genetic or metabolic disorder. Cerebral atrophy is commonly seen irrespective of etiology of intestinal failure and often does not correlate with intellectual development postoperatively. Testing of visual acuity and hearing are helpful to document existing deficits resulting from prematurity and drug toxicity so that they will not be wrongfully attributed to the transplant itself and to guide rehabilitation therapy. No precise guidelines exist as to the degree of disability that contraindicates an intestinal transplant. In general, the usual tenet that the patient should be sufficiently functional as to benefit from a difficult but life-saving intervention prevails.

Psychosocial status

Poor social functioning is often apparent in families of infants with intestinal failure, because prematurity, young parent age and a disadvantaged background are commonly present. Inclusion of a social worker in the transplant team is essential to evaluate the ability of families to care for an intestinal transplant recipient [28]. The key predictor of success after transplant is successful family care before referral. Worrisome events before transplant include a delay in initial hospital discharge because of an inadequate home environment, lack of consistent back-up care providers, a consistent need for health care personnel in the home to perform relatively mundane tasks such as connecting and disconnecting PN infusions, and previous involvement of child protective agencies. Frequent hospitalizations for catheter-related bloodstream infection and other problems with the central venous catheter are also of concern as is a history of prolonged confinement to a subacute or chronic care facility when there is no specific medical reason to justify it. If there are indications that a parent or family is not able to provide the complex, demanding and prolonged care needed following an intestinal transplant, the transplant team is obliged to ascertain whether sufficient social, medical and legal resources can be mobilized to achieve success at home or in an alternate venue. In the event that an adequate framework for post-transplant home care cannot be constructed, then transplantation may be inappropriate.

MISCELLANEOUS FACTORS TO BE CONSIDERED IN EVALUATION

Transfusion and infection history

A history of repeated transfusions of red cells and platelets is typical among patients undergoing evaluation for intestinal transplant in light of the common history of numerous previous operations and gastrointestinal bleeding. Multiple transfusions promote production of anti-HLA antibodies, a high titer of which is associated with a positive lymphocytotoxic cross-match and an adverse outcome in intestinal transplantation [29]. Some centers routinely screen for pre-formed anti-HLA antibodies using the panel reactive antibody (PRA) test during evaluation, because detection of a high level of antibody may indicate therapy to inactivate or remove these antibodies before and after the transplant [30,31]. Recurring catheter-related bloodstream infections in patients with intestinal failure also promote colonization with organisms that are relatively resistant to antimicrobial therapy, including methicillin-resistant staphylococci, vancomycin-resistant enterococci, extended spectrum beta-lactamase-producing coliforms and unusual fungi. Screening for these organisms during evaluation by sampling of the nasal cavity, rectum or stool facilitates modification of perioperative prophylactic antibiotic regimens and patient isolation practices.

Immune status

It is important to determine susceptibility of an intestinal transplant candidate to certain primary infections and reactivation of latent infections that can run an unusually severe course in the setting of intense immunosuppressive therapy. Worthy of assessment are herpes simplex (encephalitis), cytomegalovirus (CMV, massive intestinal bleeding and perforation), Epstein–Barr virus (EBV, post-transplant lymphoproliferative disease) and *Toxoplasma gondii* (sepsis/encephalitis) [32,33]. Demonstrating susceptibility to some infections emphasizes the importance of vaccination (or revaccination) before transplant (e.g. to varicella, measles, mumps, rubella, hepatitis A and B viruses). Inoculation against pneumococcal species is particularly important if a multivisceral transplant, which requires splenectomy, is anticipated.

Table 45.4 Suggested immunologic testing in intestinal transplant evaluation.

For patients less than 1 year of age
Maternal CMV total or IgG antibody
Maternal EBV VCA and EBNA IgG antibody
Maternal HCV antibody
Maternal HSV IgG antibody
Maternal RPR
Maternal *Toxoplasma* IgG antibody
HAV IgM antibody
HBs Ag, HBs Ab, and HBc IgM antibody
HIV 1 and 2 antibody
CMV urine shell viral culture

For all patients older than 1 year of age
CMV total antibody
EBV VCA and EBNA IgG antibody
HIV 1 and 2 antibody
HAV total antibody
HBsAg, HBs Ab and HBc total antibody
HCV antibody
HSV IgG antibody
Measles IgG antibody
Mumps IgG antibody
Rubella IgG antibody
RPR
Toxoplasma IgG antibody
VZV IgG antibody
Plant TST and control

CMV, cytomegalovirus; EBNA, Epstein–Barr virus nuclear antigen; EBV, Epstein–Barr virus; HAV, hepatitis A virus; HBc, hepatitis B core; HBs Ab, hepatitis B surface antibody; HBs Ag, hepatitis B surface antigen; HCV, hepatitis C virus; IgG, immunoglobulin G; IgM, immunoglobulin M; RPR, rapid plasma regain; TST, tuberculin skin test; VCA, viral capsid antigen; VZV, varicella zoster virus.

Age of the patient interferes with identification of previous infection and/or immunity. Particularly in patients under the age of 1 year, which comprises a substantial number of pediatric intestinal transplant candidates, immunoglobulin G (IgG) against various pathogens may be of transplacental origin and therefore only suggests rather than confirms previous infection. Viruria confirms CMV infection in infants with detectable CMV IgG. Similarly, detection of DNA sequences of CMV or EBV using polymerase chain reaction technology confirms infection when serologic findings are ambiguous or indeterminate. A schema for immunologic testing before intestinal transplant is depicted in Table 45.4.

CONCLUSIONS

Evaluation of a patient potentially needing an intestinal transplant consists of verifying that the patient does, in fact,

have intestinal failure (i.e. a permanent requirement for PN due to gastrointestinal dysfunction), and that intractable complications of PN threaten survival on this therapy. Once the medical need for intestinal transplantation is established, the next step is to identify other organs that that should be included in a composite allograft, usually the liver. Finally, the evaluation must determine whether the patient is sufficiently stable medically to survive the operation and has a reasonable chance of receiving appropriate care by an active and willing family.

REFERENCES

1 Iyer KR. Organ transplantation for intestinal failure. *J Parenter Enteral Nutr* 2002;**26**(5 Suppl):S49–54.

2 Kaufman SS, Fishbein TM. Intestinal failure: outcomes. In: Walker WA, Goulet O, Kleinman RE, *et al.*, eds. *Pediatric Gastrointestinal Disease.* Hamilton, ON: BC Decker; 2004;782–8.

3 Iyer KR, Horslen S, Torres C, Vanderhoof JA, Langnas AN. Functional liver recovery parallels autologous gut salvage in short bowel syndrome. *J Pediatr Surg* 2004;**39**:340–4.

4 Horslen SP, Sudan DL, Iyer KR, *et al.* Isolated liver transplantation in infants with end-stage liver disease associated with short bowel syndrome. *Ann Surg* 2002;**235**:435–9.

5 Jeppesen PB, Mortensen PB. Intestinal failure defined by measurements of intestinal energy and wet weight absorption. *Gut* 2000;**46**:701–6.

6 Rovera GM, Sigurdsson L, Reyes J, *et al.* Immunoreactive trypsinogen levels in pediatric patients with intestinal failure awaiting intestinal transplantation. *Clin Transplant* 1999;**13**: 395–9.

7 Sigurdsson L, Reyes J, Kocoshis SA, *et al.* Intestinal transplantation in children with chronic intestinal pseudo-obstruction. *Gut* 1999;**45**:570–4.

8 Hyman PE, Bursch B, Beck D, DiLorenzo C, Zeltzer LK. Discriminating pediatric condition falsification from chronic intestinal pseudo-obstruction in toddlers. *Child Maltreat* 2002; **7**:132–7.

9 Iyer K, Kaufman S, Sudan D, *et al.* Long-term results of intestinal transplantation for pseudo-obstruction in children. *J Pediatr Surg* 2001;**36**:174–7.

10 Intestinaltransplant.org [homepage on the Internet]. Toronto: The Intestinal Transplant Registry [updated 2004 Oct 28]. Available from: http://www.intestinaltransplant.org

11 Kaufman SS, Gondolesi GE, Fishbein TM. Parenteral nutrition associated liver disease. *Semin Neonatol* 2003;**8**:375–81.

12 Chan S, McCowen KC, Bistrian BR, *et al.* Incidence, prognosis, and etiology of end-stage liver disease in patients receiving home total parenteral nutrition. *Surgery* 1999;**126**:28–34.

13 Ohnishi K, Sato S, Pugliese D, *et al.* Changes of splanchnic circulation with progression of chronic liver disease studied by echo-Doppler flowmetry. *Am J Gastroenterol* 1987;**82**:507–11.

14 Silver MM, Bohn D, Shawn DH, *et al.* Association of pulmonary hypertension with congenital portal hypertension in a child. *J Pediatr* 1992;**120**(2 Pt 1):321–9.

15 Beath SV, Needham SJ, Kelly DA, *et al.* Clinical features and prognosis of children assessed for isolated small bowel or

combined small bowel and liver transplantation. *J Pediatr Surg* 1997;**32**:459–61.

16 Bueno J, Ohwada S, Kocoshis S, *et al.* Factors impacting the survival of children with intestinal failure referred for intestinal transplantation. *J Pediatr Surg* 1999;**34**:27–32.

17 van Ommen CH, Heijboer H, Buller HR, *et al.* Venous thromboembolism in childhood: a prospective two-year registry in the Netherlands. *J Pediatr* 2001;**139**:676–81.

18 Kaufman SS, Atkinson JB, Bianchi A, *et al.* American Society of Transplantation. Indications for pediatric intestinal transplantation: a position paper of the American Society of Transplantation. *Pediatr Transplant* 2001;**5**:80–7.

19 Sharif K, de Ville de Goyet J, Beath SV, Protheroe S, John P. Transhepatic Hickman line placement: improving line stability by surgically assisted radiologic placement. *J Pediatr Gastroenterol Nutr* 2002;**34**:561–3.

20 Rescorla FJ, Shedd FJ, Grosfeld JL, Vane DW, West KW. Anomalies of intestinal rotation in childhood: analysis of 447 cases. *Surgery* 1990;**108**:710–5.

21 Buhler L, Charbonnet P, Majno P, *et al.* Small intestine graft in Switzerland: indications and potential recipients. *Schweiz Med Wochenschr Suppl* 1997;**89**:46S–50S. [In French.]

22 Chang RK, McDiarmid SV, Alejos JC, Drant SE, Klitzner TS. Echocardiographic findings of hypertrophic cardiomyopathy in children after orthotopic liver transplantation. *Pediatr Transplant* 2001;**5**:187–91.

23 Jarzembowski TM, John E, Panaro F, *et al.* Reversal of tacrolimus-related hypertrophic obstructive cardiomyopathy 5 years after kidney transplant in a 6-year-old recipient. *Pediatr Transplant* 2005;**9**:117–21.

24 Buyukgebiz B, Arslan N, Ozturk Y, Soylu A, Kavukcu S. Complication of short bowel syndrome: an infant with short bowel syndrome developing ammonium acid urate urolithiasis. *Pediatr Int* 2003;**45**:208–9.

25 Loinaz C, Mittal N, Kato T, *et al.* Multivisceral transplantation for pediatric intestinal pseudo-obstruction: single center's experience of 16 cases. *Transplant Proc* 2004;**36**:312–3.

26 Masumoto K, Arima T, Izaki T, *et al.* Ondine's curse associated with Hirschsprung disease and ganglioneuroblastoma. *J Pediatr Gastroenterol Nutr* 2002;**34**:83–6.

27 Nishino I, Spinazzola A, Papadimitriou A, *et al.* Mitochondrial neurogastrointestinal encephalomyopathy: an autosomal recessive disorder due to thymidine phosphorylase mutations. *Ann Neurol* 2000;**47**:792–800.

28 Brook G. Quality of life issues: parenteral nutrition to small bowel transplantation – a review. *Nutrition* 1998;**14**:813–6.

29 Wu T, Abu-Elmagd K, Bond G, Demetris AJ. A clinicopathologic study of isolated intestinal allografts with preformed IgG lymphocytotoxic antibodies. *Hum Pathol* 2004;**35**:1332–9.

30 Tschernia A, LeLeiko NS, Grima K, *et al.* Anti-HLA antibody removal by extracorporeal immunoadsorption in two hyperimmunized pediatric patients awaiting hepatointestinal transplantation. *Transplant Proc* 2002;**34**:900–1.

31 Glotz D, Antoine C, Julia P, *et al.* Desensitization and subsequent kidney transplantation of patients using intravenous immunoglobulins (IVIg). *Am J Transplant* 2002;**2**:758–60.

32 Reyes J, Mazariegos GV, Bond GM, *et al.* Pediatric intestinal transplantation: historical notes, principles and controversies. *Pediatr Transplant* 2002;**6**:193–207.

33 Elliot DL, Tolle SW, Goldberg L, Miller JB. Pet-associated illness. *N Engl J Med* 1985;**313**:985–95.

46 Donor Evaluation, Surgical Technique and Perioperative Management

Thomas M. Fishbein and Cal S. Matsumoto

Intestinal transplantation has evolved from an experimental procedure with limited success to standard of care for patient with intestinal and parenteral nutrition failure, achieving outcomes commensurate with other solid organ transplants [1,2]. Paramount to achieving the success of intestinal and multivisceral organ transplant procedures has been the refinement of donor organ selection criteria, graft procurement and transplantation techniques [3]. Early graft failures and deaths resulting from technical and donor-related complications have been minimized using the techniques described here, leaving the current challenge largely of optimizing immunologic and infection management strategies [4,5].

INITIAL DONOR EVALUATION

The evaluation of deceased donor organs for intestinal and multivisceral transplantation is similar to that used with other solid organs. Assessment of appropriate serologic typing, hemodynamic stability, adequate tissue oxygenation, maintenance of electrolyte balance and an optimal physiologic environment are all tenets of donor management common to the intestinal or multivisceral donor. Specific donor information of special significance to intestinal or multivisceral donor evaluation which must be sought include the following criteria.

ABO compatibility

In general, identical blood group matching is preferred for intestinal transplantation, although the clinical situation of the recipient will dictate the possible use of (nonidentical) ABO-compatible blood types. Critically ill liver-intestine or multivisceral recipients may receive ABO-compatible blood types, but this practice is generally discouraged in isolated intestine recipients. This is because of the large passenger lymphoid load included in the allograft, which may cause hemolytic reactions after transplantation [6,7].

Size

Size matching is of critical importance for successful intestinal

and multivisceral donor evaluation. Short-bowel recipients frequently suffer loss-of-domain of the abdominal cavity. This leads to the need for appropriately size-matched donor organs to allow abdominal closure after transplantation. Careful physical examination and evaluation of remaining small bowel and colon either radiographically or by other means will help determine optimal donor size. Preoperative radiographic liver volume determination may be helpful for liver-intestine and multivisceral recipients. Parenteral nutrition associated liver disease (PNALD) generally leads to significant hepatomegaly and splenomegaly. Explantation of the diseased liver results in acquired abdominal domain. In multivisceral transplant recipients with large cholestatic livers and splenomegaly from chronic portal hypertension, consideration should be given to the increased abdominal space gained during the recipient total abdominal exenteration. Some literature suggests that the ideal donor to recipient weight ratio should be between 50% and 67% to allow adequate abdominal wall closure after transplantation [8]. Poor size matching will result in a large proportion of recipients left with an open abdomen requiring prosthetic mesh or other techniques for closure, and limiting success rates.

Donor age

There are no specific restrictions to donor age. However, one study suggested that adult intestinal allografts from donors less than 50 years of age demonstrated improved survival [9,10]. Additionally, reports of necrotizing enterocolitis occurring in the allograft after transplantation suggest that neonatal donors may be of higher risk for small pediatric recipients [11]. We generally do not accept donors of less than 2 weeks of age, and do not employ donor organs recovered from premature infants.

Cardiac arrest

In general, donors who have suffered cardiac arrest with the institution of cardiopulmonary resuscitation yield poor intestinal allografts. Intestinal blood flow is physiologically shunted to other essential organs during the resuscitation period, rendering the intestine ischemic. With the reinstitution of cardiac activity, vasoactive hemodynamic support is usually required, further contributing to a prolonged ischemic state. Biopsy of the terminal ileum may reveal ischemic mucosal injury at the time of organ procurement. Pediatric donors who have had arrest may either demonstrate ileus or pass bloody bowel movements, suggesting ischemic enteropathy with sloughing of intestinal mucosa. These signs should be assessed before considering any donor with cardiac arrest and would mitigate against use of the bowel.

Circulatory collapse

Management of donor circulatory collapse, whether from a hypovolemic state resulting from diabetes insipidus or neurogenic shock, requires active participation of the intestinal donor surgeon well prior to the procurement operation. The intestine is very sensitive to ischemia and care must be taken to avoid underperfusion. Massive resuscitation with crystalloid fluids commonly results in intestinal tissue edema, which can impair peristalsis, make the intestinal graft unnecessarily engorged and potentially cause microcirculatory injury. Red blood cell transfusion is used for volume replacement, and colloids are preferable to decrease tissue edema. Alpha adrenergic agonists such as norepinephrine are potent vasoconstrictors and, if persistent, will lead to ischemic intestinal injury. Dopamine is preferred for hemodynamic support if feasible. Ideally, donors are volume resuscitated and alpha range adrenergic pressors discontinued prior to organ recovery. It is important to obtain information regarding dose and duration of each vasopressor to assess the degree of intestinal ischemia. Prolonged alpha range pressor support continuing to the time of allocation should discourage intestinal recovery.

Evaluation of the donor intestinal tract

A thorough history of the donor's gastrointestinal tract can yield important information regarding the quality of the graft. Specifically, a history of inflammatory bowel disease or irritable bowel syndrome, previous gastrointestinal operations, recent viral gastroenteritis, chronic diarrhea, pediatric feeding intolerance, chronic malabsorption or hematochezia are all indicators of poor intestinal graft quality. Pediatric donors should be evaluated for exposure to viral pathogens prior to death. Enteral feeding during donor hospitalization is an important factor that must be addressed upon notification of donor availability. Gastric tube feeding is desired to promote gut mucosal stimulation prior to graft recovery. Affirmation of bowel sounds is a good clinical indicator of gut integrity and overall motility.

Pediatric donors with clinical presentations consistent with central nervous system decompensation and death of unknown etiology should be considered carefully; undiagnosed metabolic disorders or viral syndromes should be carefully excluded as far as possible by consideration of brain imaging (demyelination) or spinal fluid results.

Abdominal trauma

Donors who have suffered abdominal trauma require additional scrutiny. Computed tomography (CT), if already performed, should be evaluated for any possibility of abdominal visceral injury. Deceleration injury may cause unrecognized or subclinical injuries to the mesenteric root, duodenal hematoma, tears of the liver at the falciform, or injury to the jejunum at the ligament of Treitz. Pancreatic and duodenal injuries make a donor poorly suited for intestinal donation. If a CT scan has not been previously obtained and if there is any doubt of abdominal visceral injury such as unexplained anemia, flank hematoma or free air, a CT scan should be obtained at the donor hospital.

Infection

Careful inquiry should be made as to recent viral or bacterial exposure of the donor or donor family members within the past 30 days. Particular attention is given to screening the donor for any recent gastrointestinal or respiratory viral symptoms that may be transmitted to the recipient.

Selective digestive decontamination

Some centers, ours included, prefer to decontaminate the intestinal allograft at the time of procurement. This can be performed with an antibacterial solution placed through the nasogastric tube at the time of acceptance of the donor, redosing intermittently until procurement.

Lymphocytotoxic cross-matching

Positive lymphocytotoxic cross-match has been associated with a higher rate and increased severity of intestinal allograft rejection. Some centers choose not to perform intestinal transplantation in this setting. Our preference is for a negative T-lymphocyte cross-match to be confirmed prior to implantation for isolated intestinal transplantation. This may require institution of a protocol for treatment of sensitization prior to transplantation for some patients. Because of the protective effect of the liver over other organs from injury related to preformed antibody, we do not employ negative T-lymphocyte cross-match prior to implantation of liver-containing allografts.

Intestinal procurement

Intestinal procurement is generally performed in the setting of multiple organ retrieval by several procurement teams.

Careful coordination between teams is critical for success. Items specific to intestinal donor procurement that should be discussed and agreed upon prior to the donor operation are as follow:

1 Type of flush solution.

2 Pretreatment of intestinal graft with lymphocyte depleting antibody.

3 Technique of extraction (en bloc vs. individual).

4 Sharing of arterial and venous conduits. If pancreas, intestine and liver grafts are being procured by separate hospital teams, a plan to share quality iliac and femoral vessels grafts must be in place. For pediatric donors, we utilize the descending thoracic aorta, transposed to the infrarenal position. This is easily accomplished in the setting of heart procurement. For isolated intestinal transplantation with systemic drainage, a segment of external iliac artery and vein will suffice for extension grafts, even if the pancreas is also being procured. The iliac bifurcation graft will retain sufficient length as only a short segment is required for the bowel graft.

DONOR SURGICAL TECHNIQUE

Isolated intestine donor technique

The standard sternum to pubis incision is made with care not to injure the bowel upon entering the abdomen. On many occasions, either because of the nature of injury or the preoperative state of the donor, the intestine may be dilated or edematous and may closely abut the abdominal wall. A nasogastric tube should be placed to decompress the stomach and upper gastrointestinal tract. Immediately upon entering the abdomen, another dose of selective gut decontaminant may be administered.

The liver is mobilized in the usual fashion. The isolated intestine donor operation historically precluded the use of the pancreas from the same donor; however, with close coordination between liver, pancreas and intestinal procurement teams, successful procurement of individual organs can be safely achieved [12].

A broad Cattell maneuver and Kocher maneuver are performed and the aorta and inferior vena cava are exposed behind the intestinal mesentery up to the superior mesenteric artery. The abdominal aorta is encircled distally for eventual aortic cannulation and flush. The gastrocolic omentum is divided, and the left colon is mobilized such that the base of the mesentery is also mobilized with division of the ligament of Treitz. The mesentery of the colon is then dissected, exposing right, middle and left colic vessels. The tail of the pancreas is mobilized with the spleen, exposing the left side of the aorta and the origin of the mesenteric vessels. The proximal jejunum is then divided with a stapling device. The small intestinal luminal contents should then be advanced down

into the colon. Care must be taken while manually advancing luminal contents to prevent serosal injury of the sometimes fragile graft. A quick total abdominal colectomy is then performed, ligating the previously exposed vessels, and the colon is stapled at the pelvic brim and removed to eliminate portal venous drainage of the colon, which will become ischemic. The donor is then systemically heparinized and prepared for the flush through the distal aorta. No portal flush is used, to avoid obstruction of intestinal venous outflow and edema. After the flush, performed with suprahepatic caval venting, the pancreas may be split along the axis of the mesenteric vessels. A Carrel patch is taken with the entire intestine and root of the mesentery. The origin of the portal vein is divided at the confluence, leaving the orifice of the splenic vein with the intestinal side to be used as a patch if required. The liver is then excised in the standard fashion and flushed on the back table through the portal vein. The pancreas and bowel are retrieved en bloc to remove the pancreas on the back table, and the pancreas may be used for islets.

If the pancreas is also to be transplanted from the donor, we dissect the base of the small bowel mesentery *in situ* prior to the flush. The mesentery is isolated upon a moist lap pad, and the mesenteric vessels are isolated below the inferior pancreaticoduodenal artery and vein, which provide necessary flow to the pancreas allograft. The middle colic vessels and first jejunal arcade usually require ligation. Care should be taken not to injure the major jejunal vein, which usually courses behind the superior mesenteric artery to join the ileocolic vein high in the base of the small bowel mesentery. Small vascular clamps are placed on the superior mesenteric artery and vein after the flush, and these vessels are transected. The pancreatic sides are oversewn with small nonabsorbable sutures individually and the bowel graft is again flushed on the back table. The pancreas and liver are then removed in the usual fashion. In the event that an aberrant right hepatic artery or aberrant common hepatic artery is encountered from the superior mesenteric artery (SMA), care must be taken to avoid injury to these vessels and the SMA must be divided distally to the origin of the aberrant vessel. When this is encountered, good quality iliac or common femoral artery and vein extension grafts are required for implantation of the small bowel graft.

The back table procedure entails cleaning and ligation of ganglion tissue that will bleed above the Carrel patch. In some cases, placement of iliac or femoral arterial and venous conduits onto the graft vessels will be required. We have found this to facilitate transplantation when the pancreas has been procured for transplantation. Finally, the base of the mesentery is examined for leaks by flushing with University of Wisconsin (UW) solution. An alternative technique of removing the entire liver, pancreas, small bowel and spleen en bloc for separation on the back table (as for combined organ procedures) may also be used [13].

Liver-intestine donor technique

Donor management and operation begin as for isolated intestinal transplantation [14]. The gallbladder is incised and the biliary tract is flushed with saline. After broad Cattell and Kocher maneuvers, the tail of the pancreas and spleen are mobilized from the retroperitoneum, with care taken to avoid injury of the superior mesenteric vessels or the inferior pancreaticoduodenal arcade. The proximal duodenum is then dissected at the level of the pylorus and divided with a stapling device. Care must be taken during this process to inspect the gastrohepatic liagament to avoid injury to an aberrant left hepatic artery if present. After advancement of intraluminal contents distally, removal of the colon and systemic heparinization, the flush is performed with only aortic cannulation. Suprahepatic caval venting is performed. By retracting the spleen medially, pancreas and the small bowel in a cold lap pad, a Carrel patch or circumferential segment of aorta can then easily be taken, containing the origins of the celiac and superior mesenteric arteries. Care must be taken not to injure the takeoff of renal arteries. If the kidneys are not being used (often the case with small pediatric donors), the entire aorta may be removed with the graft. We remove the entire aorta from iliac bifurcation to proximal descending aorta in the small pediatric donor; this requires the diaphragm to be split at the time of extraction. Then, the entire pancreas, spleen, small intestine and liver are removed en bloc with intact inferior vena cava and duodenum. The back table procedure requires resection of the distal pancreas to the left of the mesenteric vessels, oversewing or stapling the pancreatic remnant. The splenic artery must be ligated, but the gastroduodenal and inferior pancreaticoduodenal arteries are preserved, feeding the head of pancreas and duodenum to be transplanted with the allograft. If the pancreas is diminutive, no reduction is necessary. In infant donors, the small caliber of the aorta at the level of the SMA and celiac artery makes aortic inflow to the graft suitable. This can be performed using the supraceliac, infrarenal or a transposed thoracic aortic segment used as a conduit to the distal donor aorta (Figs 46.1–46.3). The vena cava of the graft is then prepared as for isolated liver transplantation.

Multivisceral donor technique

Donor procurement is fundamentally the same as in the liver-intestine procurement except that variable amounts of the stomach and colon will be preserved with the graft. Recipients with disorders of motility and gastric dysfunction may benefit from inclusion of the stomach in the allograft. Recipients with severe chronic pancreatitis may benefit from inclusion of the entire pancreas. Some children may rarely require concomitant renal transplantation. In this case, one or both pediatric kidneys can be kept in continuity with the allograft, with either the distal or the thoracic allograft aorta used for inflow. The fundamental technical alterations are preservation of the left gastric artery, careful preservation of the gastroepiploic arcade when removing the colon, and enteric division of the proximal stomach, rather than the pylorus or jejunum. The abdominal viscera are then removed en bloc with the vena cava and the same Carrel patch, or intact aorta, as for liver-intestine procurement.

RECIPIENT PREOPERATIVE MANAGEMENT

Preoperatively, adequate vascular access must be established. This is often challenging for intestinal transplantation when the indication is vanishing vascular access for parenteral nutrition. It is common to encounter patients with thrombosis of both the inferior and superior vena cava [15]. Placement of translumbar, azygous or transhepatic access, intraoperative placement of retrohepatic vena caval access and other techniques may be required. Parenteral nutrition lines that have sustained prior infections may be used intraoperatively and removed at the conclusion. Antibiotic coverage should be guided by documented recent infections. Management by an anesthesia team familiar with complex liver transplantation is a minimal critical requirement for success, as blood loss and reperfusion stressors may be substantial with intestinal, and particularly multiorgan transplantation.

RECIPIENT SURGICAL TECHNIQUE

Isolated intestine

Isolated intestinal transplantation is described by the technique of vascular reconstruction used, the two general techniques being either "mesenteric/portal" or "systemic." The surgical approach is determined by the underlying recipient intestinal disease, the health of the recipient's liver and anatomic considerations that may influence the surgeon [16]. This is usually accomplished through a generous midline incision (see Fig. 46.1).

Mesenteric vascular reconstruction

For candidates receiving an isolated intestinal allograft for functional disorders (infantile diarrhea or motility disorder), the native small bowel is usually in place. In this instance, blood flow through the mesenteric vessels is preserved, and they are of adequate caliber and quality for supply to the graft. Implantation can therefore be performed using these vessels prepared in the same manner as for isolated intestinal donor procurement. The jejunum is divided 10–20 cm distal to the ligament of Treitz, which is broadly mobilized. The

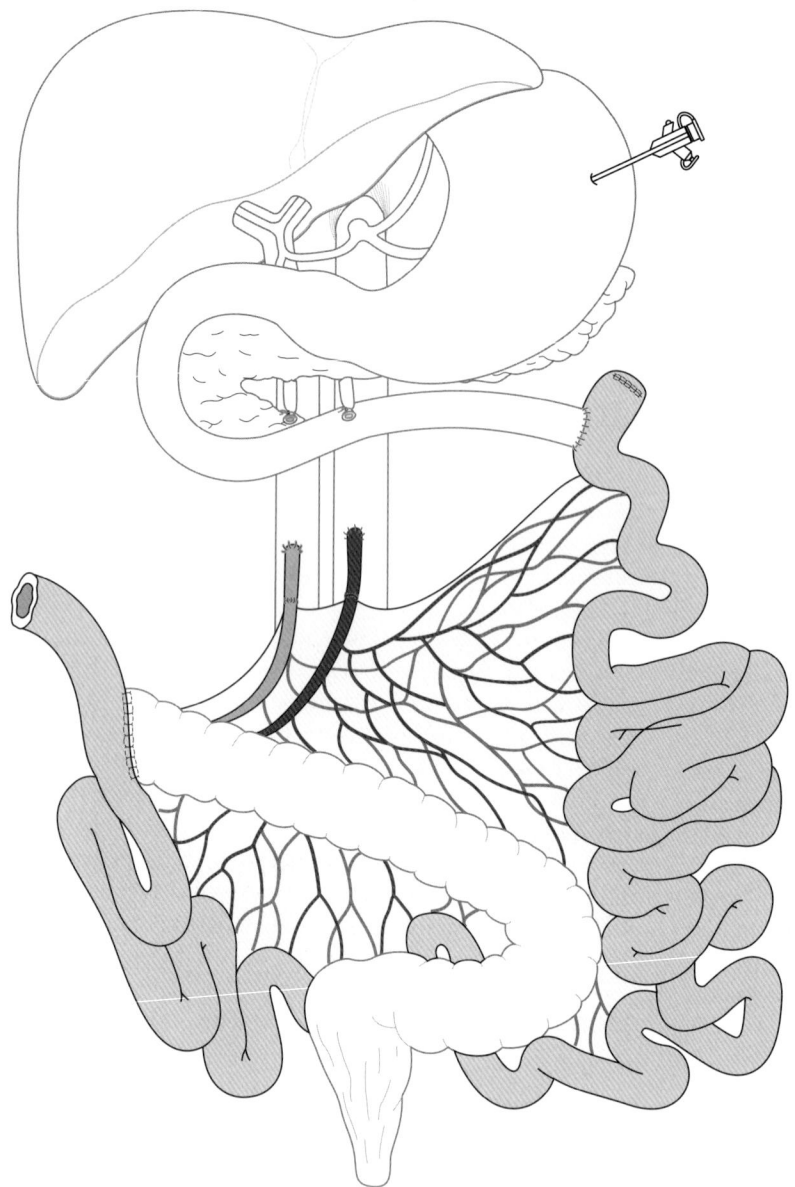

(a)

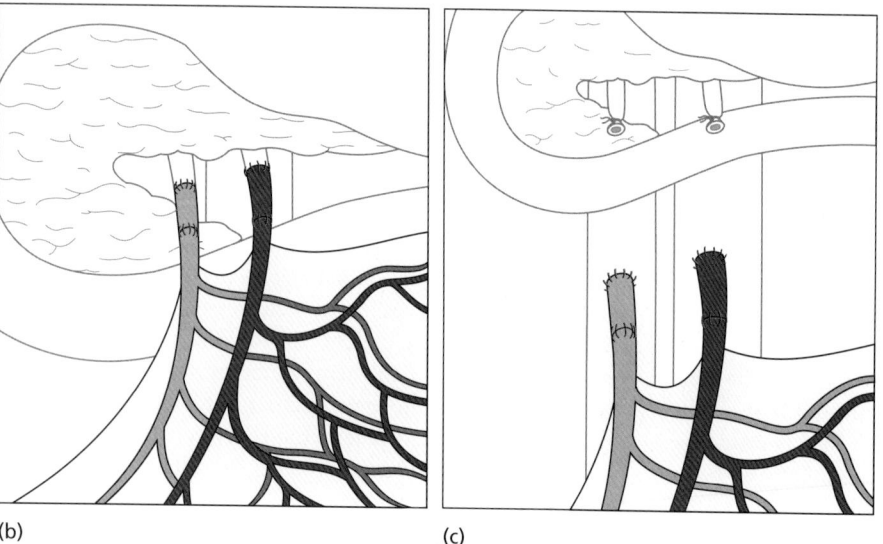

(b)

(c)

Fig. 46.1 (a) Isolated intestinal transplantation using systemic drainage employing short extension vascular grafts. Graft shown in tint, with native viscera not tinted. Proximal enteric continuity is jejunojejunostomy, and distal chimney ileocolostomy. Panels (b) and (c) demonstrate mesenteric (portal) and systemic vascular reconstructions.

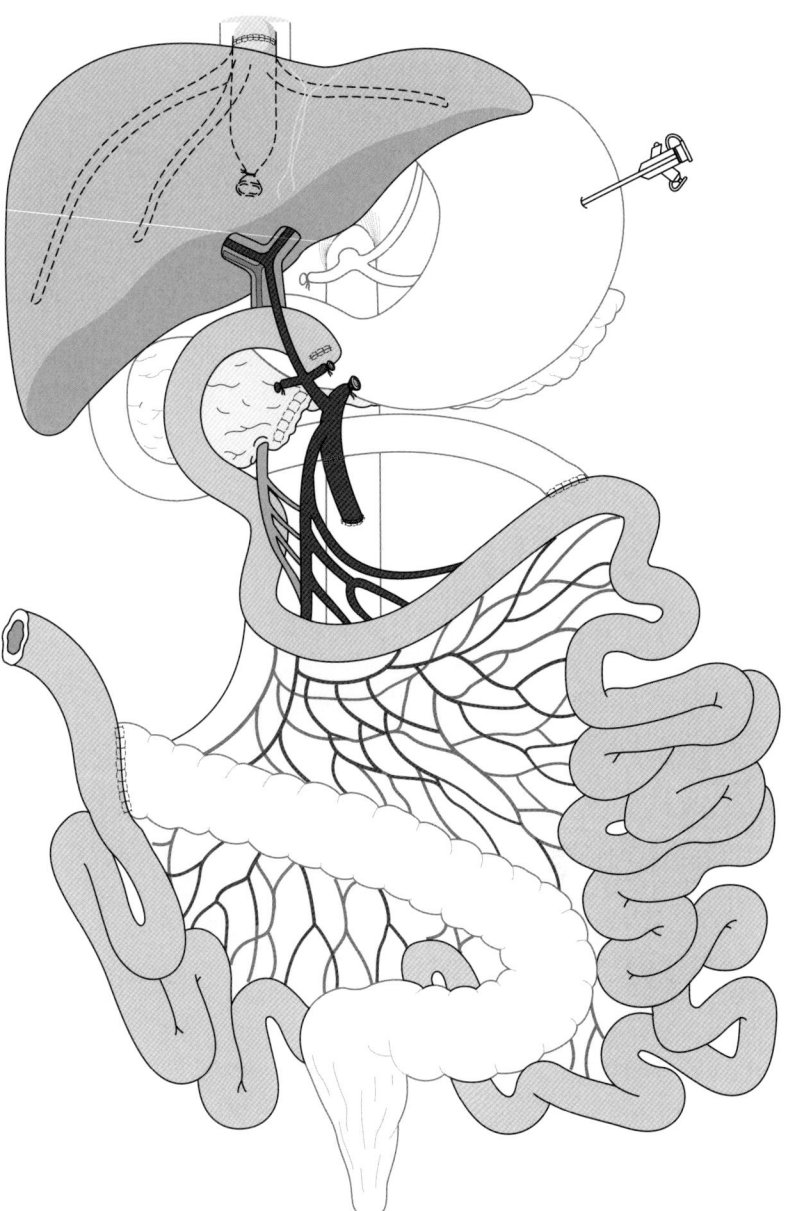

(a)

Fig. 46.2 (a) Schematic of composite liver-intestinal transplantation using the duodenal preservation technique. Panel (b) highlights the use of thoracic aorta transposed to the infrarenal aorta of the recipient as an interposition conduit to infrarenal aorta of the donor allograft. Allograft is tinted, with native viscera not tinted. Gastrointestinal reconstruction similar to as in Fig. 46.1, and portocaval shunt not shown, deep to porta hepatis of the donor organs.

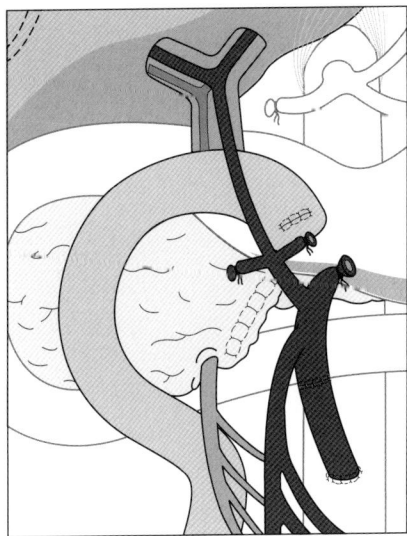

(b)

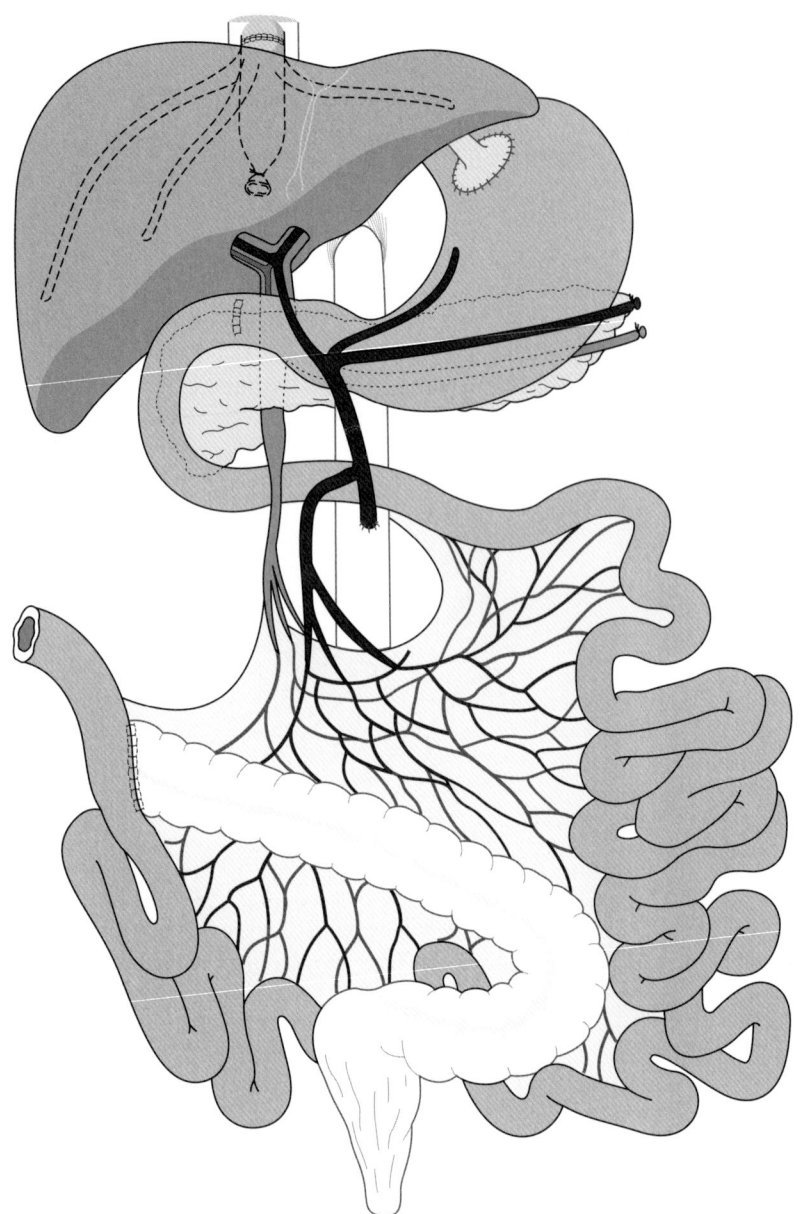

(a)

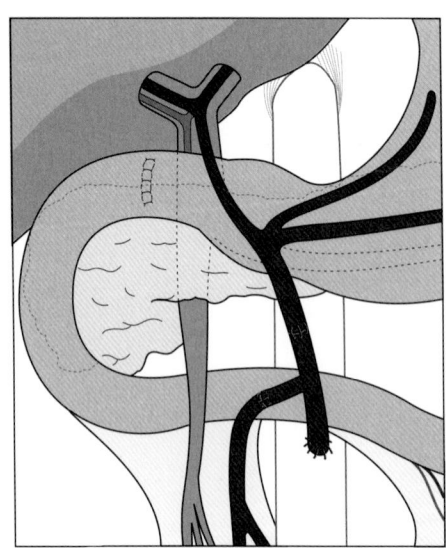

(b)

Fig. 46.3 (a) Multivisceral transplantation performed with piggyback venous drainage, and the use of a bifurcating iliac artery inflow conduit from the recipient infrarenal aorta. Gastrogastric anastomosis and standard distal reconstruction are employed, in addition to a plyoroplasty, as a result of denervation of the stomach. Panel (b) highlights vascular reconstruction.

arcade to the proximal jejunum is preserved, and the distal bowel is suspended atop a moist lap. If the colon is intact, the middle colic vessels are ligated, the right and transverse colon mobilized and the left transverse or descending colon divided. We always mobilize or remove the splenic flexure of the colon to assure endoscopic access to the ileum from below after closure of the stoma. The superior mesenteric vein is located laterally and dissection of the base of the mesentery is undertaken to skeletonize the vessels. These tissues should all be ligated to avoid lymphatic or chylous ascites after transplantation [17]. Small vascular clamps may be used to control the superior mesenteric artery and vein, dividing them distally and preserving long cuffs for anastomosis. In the case where the donor pancreas was also procured from the bowel donor, the SMA is short and extension vessels are helpful to avoid tension on the base of the small bowel mesentery. Again, the main superior mesenteric vein (SMV) should be used above the confluence of jejunal and ileal branches, which may be quite close to the duodenal sweep.

In short-bowel patients, the superior mesenteric vein sometimes cannot be exposed, as the base of the mesentery may be contracted after multiple prior resections. The venous anastomosis is rarely to the lateral wall of the portal vein in piggyback fashion, dissecting this vein free from the posterior porta hepatis, and placing an extension graft of iliac vein onto this in end-to-side fashion [18]. We have only rarely employed this technique and discourage routine use, as outcomes with systemic drainage are equivalent and are accomplished with greater ease. However, the technique can be useful in cases of inferior vena cava thrombosis.

The bowel can be brought to the field after extension grafts are placed on the recipient vessels, and the base of the mesentery placed in a transverse plane aligning the donor and recipient vessels. The assistant may use a cold moist lap pad to both flatten the base of the mesentery as well as prevent bowel loops from entering the field. The vessels are anastomosed end-to-end, and reperfusion accomplished without heparinization. Fixation of the base of the mesentery transversely and without kinking of the vessels is critical to avoid volvulus or traction on the mesenteric vessels.

Systemic vascular reconstruction

This technique is more commonly employed for patients with short-bowel syndrome, particularly those with total or near total loss of jejunum and ileum. In this disease state, the mesenteric vessels are often small in caliber, lacking good inflow. However, this is not always the case, and when a smaller donor with commensurately small vessels is being used, mesenteric drainage may be easily accomplished.

The recipient operation requires exposure of the infrarenal aorta for anastomosis of the arterial graft. This must be performed in a tension-free manner, as the weight of the bowel

filled with secretions can lead to traction from the aorta to the pelvis or lead to decreased flow and thrombosis. The venous anastomosis is end-to-side to the anterior wall of the vena cava, as with a portocaval shunt. This is best accomplished after removal of an ellipse of vena cava to avoid narrowing. We prefer aortic inflow and caval drainage for patients who have demonstrated significant liver cholestasis, fibrosis or ultra-short bowel syndrome [19]. It is easy to accomplish, and in cases where intestinal transplantation is indicated because of progressive liver disease, avoids drainage of the bowel graft into the possibly high pressure portal circulation. The bowel graft is again oriented with the mesentery flat to the retroperitoneum and sewn either directly to the aorta and vena cava or, as is our preference, to short extension grafts already placed to these vessels. The mesentery is then fixed to the retroperitoneum to avoid internal hernia, volvulus or traction on the vessels, care being taken to avoid the ureters. Systemic drainage has not been shown to yield inferior nutritional results, as some had initially predicted [20–22].

Another technique is required when systemic drainage is being used in a patient with thrombosis of the inferior vena cava. This is not infrequently encountered, as a result of multiple femoral accesses for parenteral nutrition. In this case, ligation and division of a few low caudate veins allows placement of an extension graft of iliac or femoral vein on the suprarenal vena cava. This is accomplished with placement of a partially occluding clamp, then the extension graft is tunneled behind the mobilized duodenum and head of pancreas, to lie next to the infrarenal aortic anastomosis. We have found this easier to accomplish than piggyback drainage to the portal vein.

Enteral continuity is established proximally and distally in conjunction with an ileostomy, using either a loop diverting ileostomy or a proximal ileocolostomy in a "chimney" fashion, to provide access for surveillance allograft biopsy. These stomas also allow future ileostomy closure to be performed as a relatively minor operation. Placement of tubes for intestinal access can be accomplished with gastric, jejunal or combined tubes. These are placed to avoid prolonged need for nasogastric suction and facilitate early feeding.

Liver-intestine transplantation (see Fig. 46.2)

This is most commonly accomplished using an en bloc allograft with duodenal preservation. This technique allows for transplantation of the biliary system and hepatic arterial branches without disruption and may be advantageous in small pediatric patients with tiny vascular and biliary structures which are otherwise easily injured [23–25]. The recipient is explored through a midline incision with bilateral subcostal extension, usually placed lower on the abdominal wall than for liver transplantation to provide improved lower abdominal exposure. Initial dissection of the liver hilum allows ligation of the hepatic artery and common bile duct. The portal vein is then skeletonized and the infrahepatic vena cava is isolated for construction of a portacaval shunt. Thereafter, the liver is dissected from the cava as for piggyback liver transplantation. The infrarenal or supraceliac aorta is then exposed for anastomosis. Particularly among patients whose disease was inflammatory (i.e. necrotizing enterocolitis), adhesions may be great, and care must be taken to avoid significant bleeding during this phase of the operation. Mobilization of the recipient duodenum is important to exposure of the infrarenal aorta. An aortic extension graft (either donor thoracic aorta or a bifurcation iliac artery graft) can then be placed on the infrarenal aorta to facilitate inflow to the graft. Alternatively, some prefer to use supraceliac aorta, with direct anastomosis of the donor supraceliac aorta. This is easiest to expose during the anhepatic phase. The hepatic veins can then be clamped and the liver removed. Because the native foregut is preserved, a portacaval shunt must be performed to provide venous outflow for these organs when the composite liver-bowel graft is transplanted [26,27]. An end-to-side portacaval shunt is most easily constructed during the anhepatic phase. With relief of the portal hypertension, the adhesions from multiple prior operations can be lysed with care to avoid enterotomy, which can be disastrous. The graft is brought to the table and the suprahepatic caval anastomosis is performed as in piggyback liver transplantation. The Carrel patch can then be anastomosed either directly to the aorta or, preferably, to the interposition conduit of donor thoracic aorta or bifurcating iliac artery. The stump of the splenic vein may be used for venting preservation solution, and if this is planned, the surgeon should isolate and prepare the splenic vein orifice during the back table procedure [28]. Cholecystectomy is performed in the usual fashion. Enteral continuity is re-established with either jejunojejunostomy after removal of most proximal recipient small bowel, anastomosis being performed distal to the ligament of Treitz of the allograft. Distal anastomosis is accomplished as with isolated intestinal allografting. This is the most difficult of the intestinal transplant procedures.

In some cases it may be preferable to place separate liver and intestinal allografts rather than employing the en bloc allograft technique [29]. Severe portal hypertension and dense adhesions may make the aortic exposure required for combined transplantation difficult. Placement of the liver prior to aortic exposure can facilitate transplantation when faced with this difficulty. The piggyback liver transplant is performed, and the isolated intestinal transplant procedure with systemic drainage is then performed.

Multivisceral transplantation (see Fig. 46.3)

This transplant procedure is different in that the entire splanchnic circulation is removed; no portacaval shunt or bypass can be employed. The pancreas and spleen, the root of the intestinal mesentery, the stomach and the liver are removed together, preserving vena cava continuity. Thus, the recipient operation is similar to the multivisceral donor operation itself. The steps include mobilization of the liver from the retrohepatic vena cava to allow piggyback placement of the allograft. No portal dissection is required. Next, the gastroesophageal junction is identified and the proximal stomach divided with a stapling device. This exposes the supraceliac aorta, sometimes allowing the celiac to be identified. However, this is most easily found proceeding from the left with a medial visceral rotation, allowing isolation of the base of the celiac and superior mesenteric arteries. Cattell and Kocher maneuvers (if the colon is intact) allow exposure of the right side of the SMA, and mobilization of the entire base of the intestinal mesentery. The left colon is divided, taking care to preserve the left colic artery and inferior mesenteric arteries, as no collateral flow from the SMA will exist after exenteration. Vascular clamps can then be placed on the base of the two arteries, and they may be transected. The hepatic veins are clamped and divided. The patient is then functionally anhepatic, and the stomach, pancreas, spleen, small bowel and right colon and liver are removed together, preserving the inferior vena cava for piggyback allograft implantation. This venous piggyback anastomosis is performed first, aligning the graft. Inflow must be brought to both the celiac and superior mesenteric arteries. Two inflow vascular anastomoses may be used, either using the native celiac artery and SMA end-to-end with the same donor structures (our preferred method), using an iliac bifurcating graft to these vessels from either the supraceliac or infrarenal aorta after ligation of the native vessels, or through a single anastomosis of infrarenal aorta of the donor allogaft end-to-side to the infrarenal aorta of the recipient. Preservation of the cuff of native stomach allows for a gastrogastric two-layer anastomosis, rather than an esophagogastric anastomosis. We have encountered no anastomotic leakage with this technique [30]. Pyloroplasty is required to provide gastric emptying of the denervated stomach. Distal enteral continuity is re-established with ileostomy construction and colon anastomosis as described above. Transplantation of the stomach may result in either gastric stasis or mild dumping, and some form of gastric decompression tube is mandatory, usually with a combined gastrostomy-jejunostomy tube to allow early feeding into the graft jejunum.

PERIOPERATIVE MANAGEMENT

Patients will require intensive care unit (ICU) care immediately after transplant. They will generally remain intubated in the early postoperative period, although isolated intestinal transplant patients may be extubated early. In the first 24 hours, the transplanted intestine will usually produce minimal stool, but third space losses can be significant, requiring aggressive hydration. If kidneys are transplanted with the graft, the urine output should be replaced on an hourly basis accordingly. If the urine output exceeds 500 mL/h, then the replacement volume should be commensurately decreased. Finally, pulmonary artery catheter pressures or transthoracic echocardiography may be employed to help guide fluid management at the discretion of the critical care team. The intestinal vasculature is sensitive to vasoconstrictive agents, particularly alpha adrenergic agents, and these should be avoided. Sepsis syndrome that requires such intervention usually indicates the need for reoperation because of vascular compromise or perforation. Because the graft is exteriorized with an ileostomy, blood flow to the graft may be assessed with Doppler flow at the bedside, rather than ultrasound duplex, which is made difficult by overlying bowel gas. A bedside nurse may employ a fetal Doppler hourly to assure good waveform, as would be performed for a vascularized free flap.

Electrolyte imbalances must be corrected aggressively with intravenous delivery. The transplanted bowel often exhibits calcium and magnesium malabsorption with high ileostomy outputs, although this usually does not develop until after the institution of enteral nutrition. Water, sodium and bicarbonate may be lost in large quantities with high ileostomy outputs. This may lead to a characteristic metabolic acidosis requiring sodium bicarbonate added to the intravenous or enteral formula for correction. Hypomagnesemia will potentiate tacrolimus-related neurotoxicity and should be avoided.

Intravenous broad-spectrum antibiotics should be continued early after transplantation or until the first biopsy confirms mucosal integrity of the transplanted bowel. Antibiotic use after this time should be guided by culture and sensitivities, or by the results of such studies in the late pretransplant period in the case of patients with recurrent bouts of line-related sepsis. Selective digestive decontamination may also be continued during this time and discontinued when enteral feedings are begun via the jejunal access tube. Mechanical ventilation is discontinued according to standard measures used by the critical care team, in conjunction with the transplant surgeon and a view of the future course of the particular patient. Some patients will have lost the right of domain of the abdominal cavity and will return to the ICU closed with a prosthetic mesh, with the plan of sequential abdominal lavage and staged closure. A dedicated line for parenteral nutrition should be maintained during the ICU stay, as the average time to the achievement of complete enteral nutrition after intestinal transplantation is approximately 1 month [1,16]. We generally institute feeding 5 days after transplantation if no reoperation is planned, and early graft function is adequate, judged by initiation of stomal output.

CONCLUSIONS

Intestinal transplantation is a very technically demanding field, requiring intimate knowledge of advanced techniques in both liver transplantation and gastrointestinal surgery. Some degree of individualization of procedures is required, based on each recipient's gastrointestinal anatomy, function and vascular complications of parenteral nutrition. Appropriate technical and logistic planning will minimize unnecessary complications and avert technical failures.

REFERENCES

1 Grant D, Abu-Elmagd K, Reyes J, et al. 2003 report of the intestine transplant registry: a new era has dawned. Ann Surg 2005;241:607–13.

2 Intestinal Transplant Registry (ITR); www.intestinaltransplant.org/ accessed Feb 1, 2005.

3 Fishbein TM, Gondolesi GE, Kaufman SS. Intestinal transplantation for gut failure. Gastroenterology 2003;124:1615–28.

4 Fishbein TM. The current state of intestinal transplantation. Transplantation 2004;78:175–8.

5 Fishbein TM, Matsumoto CS. Regimens for intestinal transplant immunosuppression. Curr Opin Organ Transpl 2005;10:120–3.

6 Panaro F, DeChristopher PJ, Rondelli D, et al. Severe hemolytic anemia due to passenger lymphocytes after living-related bowel transplant. Clin Transplant 2004;18:332–5.

7 Sindhi R, Landmark J, Shaw B, et al. Combined liver/small bowel transplantation using a blood group compatible but non-identical donor. Transplantation 1996;61:1782–3.

8 Kato T, Ruiz P, Thompson J, et al. Intestinal and multivisceral transplantation. World J Surg 2002;26:226–37.

9 Abu-Elmagd K, Bond G, Reyes J, et al. Intestinal transplantation: a coming of age. Adv Surg 2002;36:65–101.

10 Hanto D, Fishbein TM, Pinson CW, et al. Liver and intestine transplantation: summary analysis, 1994–2003. Am J Transplant 2005;5(4 Pt 2):916–33.

11 Khan FA, Kato T, Berho M, et al. Graft failure secondary to necrotizing enterocolitis in multi-visceral transplantation recipients: two case reports. Pediatr Transplant 2000;4:215–20.

12 Abu-Elmagd K, Fung JJ, Bueno J, et al. Logistics and techniques for procurement of intestinal, pancreatic, and hepatic grafts from the same donor. Ann Surg 2000;232:680–7.

13 Boggi U, Vistoli F, DelChiaro M, et al. A simplified technique for the en bloc procurement of abdominal organs that is suitable for pancreas and small bowel transplantation. Surgery 2004;135: 629–41.

14 Sindhi R, Fox IJ, Heffron T, et al. Procurment and preparation of human isolated small intestinal grafts for transplantation. Transplantation 1995;60:771–3.

15 Mims TT, Fishbein TM, Feierman DE. Management of a small bowel transplant with complicated central venous access in a patient with asymptomatic superior and inferior vena cava obstruction. Transplant Proc 2004;36:388–91.

16 Fishbein TM, Kaufman SS, Florman SS, et al. Isolated intestinal transplantation: proof of clinical efficacy. Transplantation 2003; 76:636–40.

17 Reyes J, Bueno J, Kocoshis S, et al. Current status of intestinal transplantation in children. J Pediatr Surg 1998;33:243–54.

18 Tzakis A, Todo S, Reyes J, et al. Piggyback orthotopic intestinal transplantation. Surg Gynecol Obstet 1993;176:297–8.

19 Fishbein T, Schiano T, Jaffe D, *et al.* Isolated intestinal transplantation in adults with nonreconstructible GI tracts. *Transplant Proc* 2000;**32**:1231–2.

20 Shaffer D, Diflo T, Love W, *et al.* Immunological and metabolic effects of caval versus portal drainage in small bowel transplantation. *Surgery* 1988;**104**:518–24.

21 Berney T, Kato T, Nishida S, *et al.* Portal versus systemic venous drainage of small bowel allografts: comparative assessment of survival, function, rejection and bacterial translocation. *J Am Coll Surg* 2002;**195**:804–13.

22 Reyes J, Mazariegos GV, Bond G, *et al.* Pediatric intestinal transplantation: historical notes, principles and controversies. *Pediatr Transplant* 2002;**6**:193–207.

23 Sudan D, Iyer K, Deroover A, *et al.* A new technique for combined liver/small intestinal transplantation. *Transplantation* 2001;**72**:1846–8.

24 Bueno J, Abu-Elmagd K, Mazariegos G, *et al.* Composite liver–small bowel allografts with preservation of donor duodenum and hepatic biliary system in children. *J Pediatr Surg* 2000;**35**:291–5; discussion 295–6.

25 Kato T, Romero R, Verzaro R, *et al.* Inclusion of entire pancreas in the composite liver and intestinal graft in pediatric intestinal transplantation. *Pediatr Transplant* 1999;**3**:210–4.

26 Grant D, Wall W, Mimeault R, *et al.* Successful small bowel/liver transplantation. *Lancet* 1990;**335**:181–4.

27 Starzl T, Rowe M, Todo S, *et al.* Transplantation of multiple abdominal viscera. *JAMA* 1989;**261**:1449–57.

28 Fishbein T, Facciuto M, Harpaz N, *et al.* A simple blood flush technique and mannitol promote hemodynamic stability and avoid reperfusion injury in isolated intestinal transplantation. *Transplant Proc* 2000;**32**:1313–4.

29 Fishbein TM, Florman SS, Gondolesi GE, Decker R. Noncomposite simultaneous liver and intestinal transplantation. *Transplantation* 2003;**75**:564–5.

30 Kato T, Tzakis A, Selvaggi G, *et al.* Surgical techniques used in intestinal transplantation. *Curr Opin Organ Transpl* 2004;**9**:207–13.

47 Pathology of the Intestinal Allograft

Maria Parizhskaya and Ronald Jaffe

Small bowel allograft mucosal biopsy remains the only method to confirm clinically suspected acute rejection. An adequate sample should contain at least two mucosal fragments from unremarkable appearing bowel and up to four from abnormal mucosa. The tissue should be fixed in 10% buffered formalin, embedded in paraffin, cut at 4 μm, with levels 2, 4 and 6 stained with hematoxylin and eosin. Immunohistochemical stains can be obtained when there is a clinical suspicion of viral infection or when the histology is suggestive. Comparison with previous biopsies and correlation with endoscopic and laboratory findings, and immunosuppression levels, is essential because there is a significant morphologic overlap between different conditions involving the intestinal allograft.

Pathologic changes typically occurring within the first couple of weeks after small bowel transplantation include preservation/ischemic injury and acute rejection. Acute rejection and infectious complications, however, may emerge at any time during the post-transplant course. The major limitation to long-term survival after small bowel transplantation is the development of chronic rejection (graft vasculopathy). This chapter discusses the pathology of acute and chronic rejection, as well as infections and other conditions not uncommonly affecting the intestinal allograft.

PRESERVATION/ISCHEMIC INJURY

Preservation/ischemic injury is most common in the first 7–10 days after intestinal transplantation. It is characterized by surface epithelial denudation, loss or flattening of villi, regenerative epithelial changes, mild neutrophilic and macrophage infiltration of the superficial lamina propria and surface epithelium, and usually only mild crypt cell apoptosis [1,2]. It should be kept in mind, however, that none of these features are pathognomonic of preservation/ischemic injury and they may be encountered in other conditions, including acute cellular rejection and infections. A clinical history (i.e. cold ischemia time, surgical complications, stool cultures) and comparison with morphologic findings in the properly fixed reperfused donor small bowel help make the correct diagnosis in early post-transplant biopsies.

ACUTE HUMORAL REJECTION

Acute humoral rejection resulting from the presence of high levels of preformed immunoglobulin G (IgG) lymphocytotoxic antibodies can cause damage in the first few weeks after transplantation. Congestion with neutrophil margination and fibrin-platelet thrombi are seen [3]. The documented examples of humoral rejection, accompanied by serological evidence of circulating anti-HLA antibodies have been infrequent in our pediatric population, seen more commonly after retransplantation. The vessels have activated endothelium, marginated neutrophils and there are commonly small platelet or platelet-fibrin thrombi in the vessels. The C4d is widely represented in almost all capillaries, not just in the larger vessels which may have some staining even in the unaffected allograft (see Plate 47.1, facing page 384).

ACUTE CELLULAR REJECTION

In acute cellular rejection, the ileum is most commonly affected and morphologic changes tend to be distributed unevenly along the intestinal allograft. Acute cellular rejection is characterized by a varying combination of deep crypt cell apoptosis, mixed cell infiltrate and crypt epithelial injury. Although crypt cell apoptosis is considered a cardinal feature of acute rejection, it is not unique and may be seen in conditions such as preservation/ischemic injury, infections and even delayed fixation [1]. According to Wu *et al.* [4], six or more apoptotic bodies per 10 crypts are required for the diagnosis of mild acute rejection. Several apoptotic bodies can be present in a single crypt and predominantly deep portions of the crypts are affected [1,2]. Apoptotic activity in rejection involves the epithelial cells; apoptotic debris from infiltrating leukocytes should not be considered. Dropout of adjacent epithelial cells is a powerful indicator of mild or early rejection (see Plate 47.2a, facing page 384). The inflammatory infiltrate usually comprises a heterogeneous population of blastic and small lymphocytes and plasma cells admixed with lesser numbers of eosinophils and neutrophils. The intensity of inflammation varies from case to case, and in some patients crypt cell apoptosis predominates over the inflammatory component. As was noticed by Lee *et al.* [2], later rejection episodes (more than 100 days post-transplant) tend to show lesser cellular infiltration and greater apoptosis than earlier episodes. Crypt injury varies with the severity of acute rejection and manifests as necrosis of epithelial cells, crypt destruction and eventual loss of crypts. Cryptitis may occur but crypt abscesses are rarely observed [2]. In moderate acute rejection, mucosal damage is more extensive, confluent areas of crypt cell apoptosis are present [4] and focal ulceration is sometimes seen. Crypts with intraluminal sloughed necrotic cells and destroyed crypts are commonly encountered (see Plate 47.2b, facing page 384). In the appropriate clinical and endoscopic setting, severe acute rejection is characterized by extensive mucosal ulceration with loss of normal epithelial structures (see Plate 47.2c, facing page 384) [1,2]. Other changes seen in acute cellular rejection may include endothelial cell prominence, stromal edema, vascular congestion and varying degrees of villous blunting. A lack of regenerative changes is more characteristic of acute rejection but regenerative changes may appear as rejection is treated (see Plate 47.2d, facing page 384) [5].

CHRONIC REJECTION (CHRONIC GRAFT VASCULOPATHY)

The mucosal biopsy diagnosis of chronic vascular rejection can be difficult because the affected vessels, the distal branches of the mesenteric arteries, and the larger arteries of the subserosa and submucosa are not routinely sampled (see Plate 47.3a–c, facing page 384). The possibility of underlying arteriopathy, however, can sometimes be inferred from the presence of secondary "early" and "late" mucosal changes in the small bowel biopsies (Table 47.1).

The specificity of the individual morphologic changes of early and late chronic rejection is low, and must be augmented by finding repeated and progressive changes. As with other grafts, it can be difficult to distinguish between residual damage/repair from acute rejection and "early" chronic rejection. When persistent ischemic changes develop, chronic rejection should be considered as well as other causes of intestinal ischemia (e.g. vascular anastomotic problems, recurring volvulus or intussusception, adhesions).

The mucosal histopathology should be correlated with endoscopic and radiographic features of chronic rejection, which include loss of mucosal folds, focal ulcers and mural thickening, and pruning of the mesenteric arterial tree [7]. Clinical features that suggest the diagnosis of chronic rejec-

Table 47.1 Criteria for possible chronic rejection in mucosal biopsies [6].

"Early" changes (nonspecific, "inflammatory")
Patchy mild fibrosis of lamina propria
Focal loss of the crypts of Lieberkühn
Deep portions of the crypts of Lieberkühn do not reach muscularis mucosae

"Late" changes (vascular/ischemic)
Loss of villous architecture
Chronic ulcers with exudate and granulation tissue
Widespread loss of the crypts of Lieberkühn
Crypts of Lieberkühn with pyloric gland metaplasia
Mucosal fibrosis

tion include persistent diarrhea with nonhealing ulcers and repeated bouts of suboptimally controlled acute rejection. Thus, endoscopic, radiographic and clinical findings, and sometimes full-thickness intestinal biopsies should be used to establish the diagnosis. The biopsies should be taken at the mesenteric attachment where the vascular arcade is located (see Plate 47.3a,c, facing page 384).

Examination of full-thickness biopsies and resected intestinal allografts reveals the previously described "late" mucosal alterations, neural hyperplasia, as well as irregularly distributed arterial changes in the submucosa, subserosa and in the mesentery immediately adjacent to the bowel wall (see Plate 47.3d, facing page 384) [6,8]. Large and medium-sized arteries are preferentially involved. The arterial changes consist of graft atherosclerotic-type lesions with eccentric intimal hyperplasia, sometimes accompanied by intimal and medial foam cell deposition. Concentric fibrous intimal thickening and medial hypertrophy characteristic of hypertensive-type arterial lesions are also observed [6].

INFECTIONS

A variety of infections may affect the intestinal allograft, including adenovirus, cytomegalovirus (CMV), rotavirus, Epstein–Barr virus (EBV), Norwalk virus, *Clostridium difficile*, *Giardia* and cryptosporidium. Rotavirus, adenovirus and *Clostridium difficile* may emerge at any time after transplantation. Adenovirus and rotavirus enteritis, however, appear to be seasonal rather than immunosuppression dependent. CMV and EBV infections are related to immunosuppression and both are unusual in the first post-transplant month.

Adenovirus enteritis is characterized by proliferative changes of the surface epithelium with nuclear inclusions (see Plate 47.4a, facing page 384). Three types of nuclear changes can be seen in adenovirus infection [5,9]. Eosinophilic inclusion bodies may fill the entire nucleus and displace the chromatin to the periphery. There may be slightly enlarged,

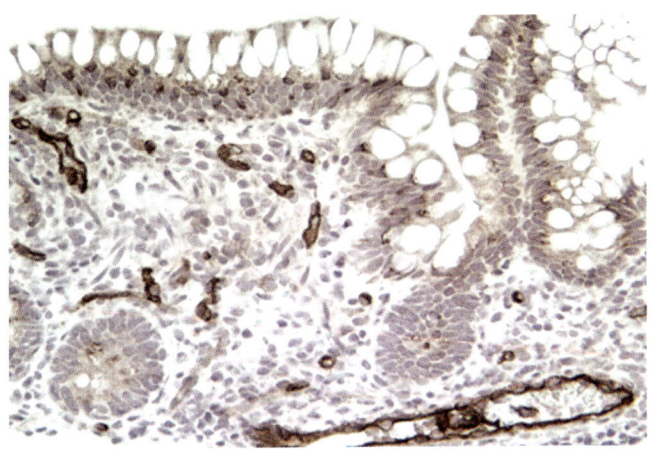

Plate 47.1 Humoral rejection. A diffuse deposition of C4d in all capillaries in the patient who is 11 days after retransplantation with high panel reactive antibodies (C4d immunostain).

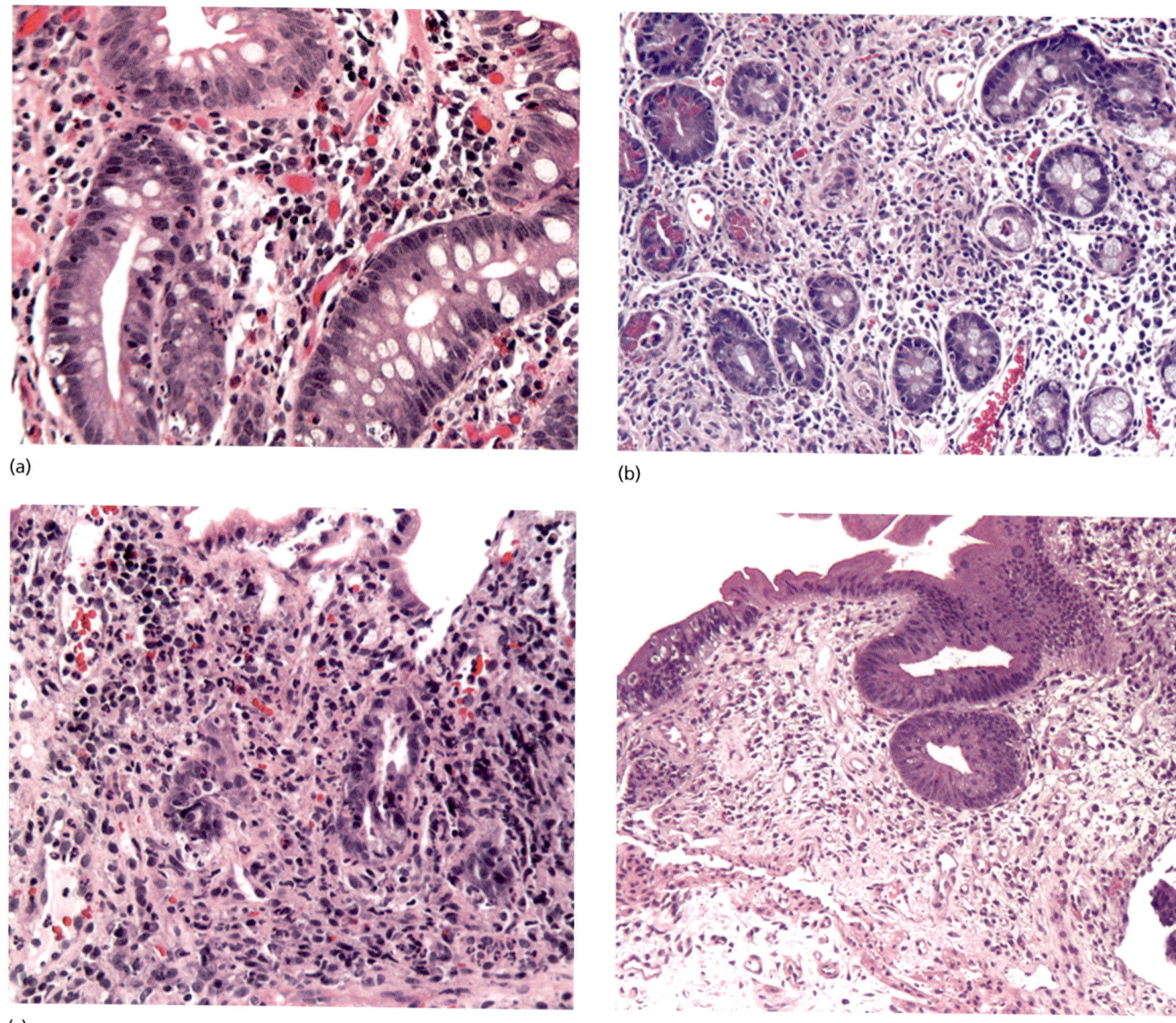

(a)

(b)

(c)

(d)

Plate 47.2 (a) Mild cellular rejection. The intestinal crypts are preserved but apoptotic epithelial activity is most marked in the deep portions of the crypts with loss of adjacent cells. (b) Moderate cellular rejection. Crypt loss is documented with cellular debris and crypts with apoptotic activity elsewhere. (c) Severe cellular rejection. Extensive crypt loss is accompanied by sloughing of surface epithelium and a neutrophilic presence. Apoptotic activity is still visible in the epithelial remnants. (d) Regeneration following severe rejection. The surface has largely re-epithelialized and there is rudimentary crypt regeneration. The lamina propria has a granulation-type quality.

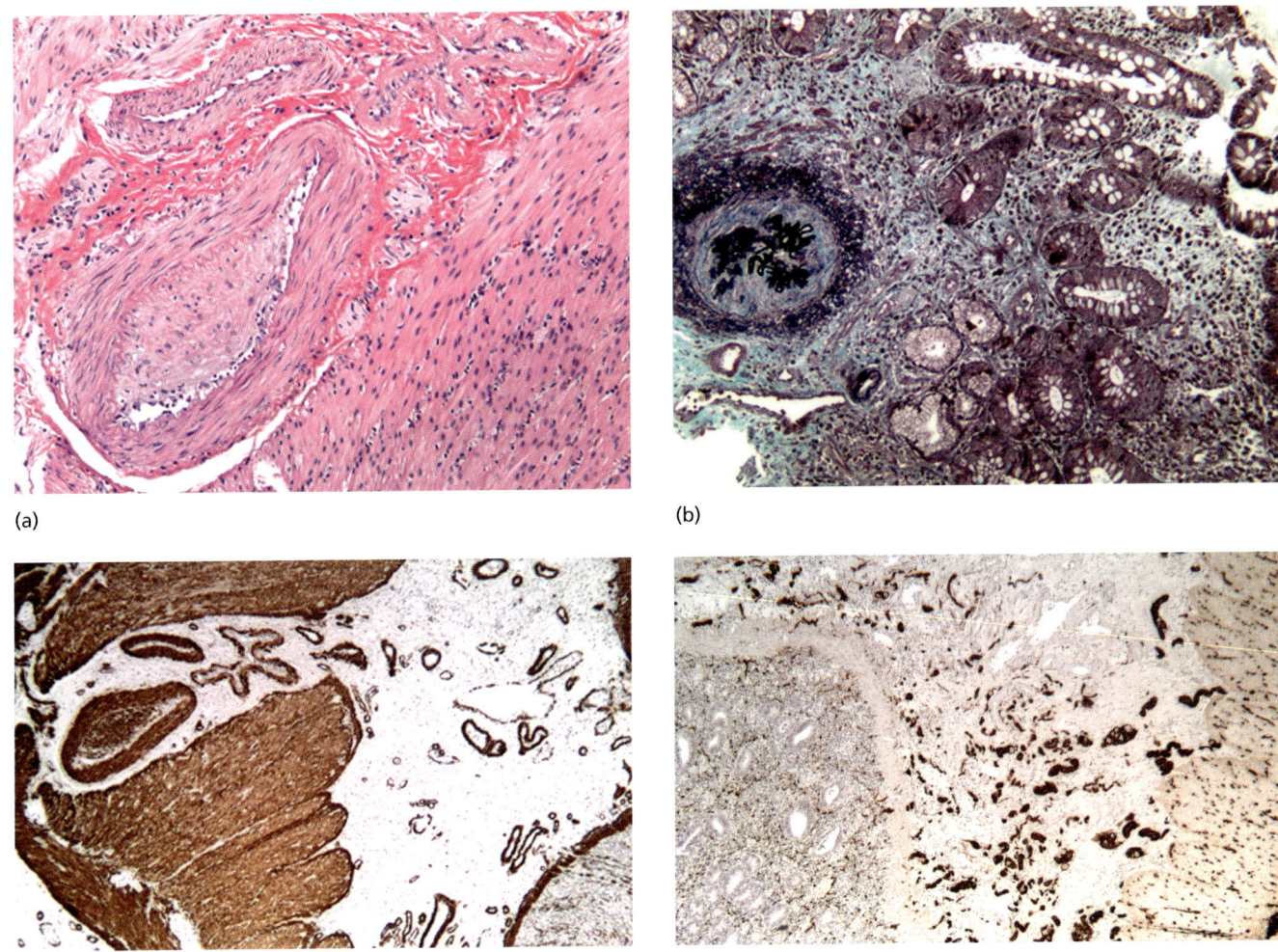

(a)

(b)

(c)

(d)

Plate 47.3 (a) Chronic vascular rejection. A deep penetrating branch of the arterial arcade has a large subintimal plaque. (b) Chronic vascular rejection. Arterial changes, such as this badly damaged artery in a distorted submucosa, are unusual in mucosal biopsies. (Elastic-Trichrome). (c) Chronic vascular rejection.

An actin immunostain shows the subintimal occlusion of the deep penetrating vessels, but the submucosal vessels are unaffected. (d) Chronic rejection. Neural hyperplasia can be extreme, but is not restricted to chronic rejection in the allograft. (S100).

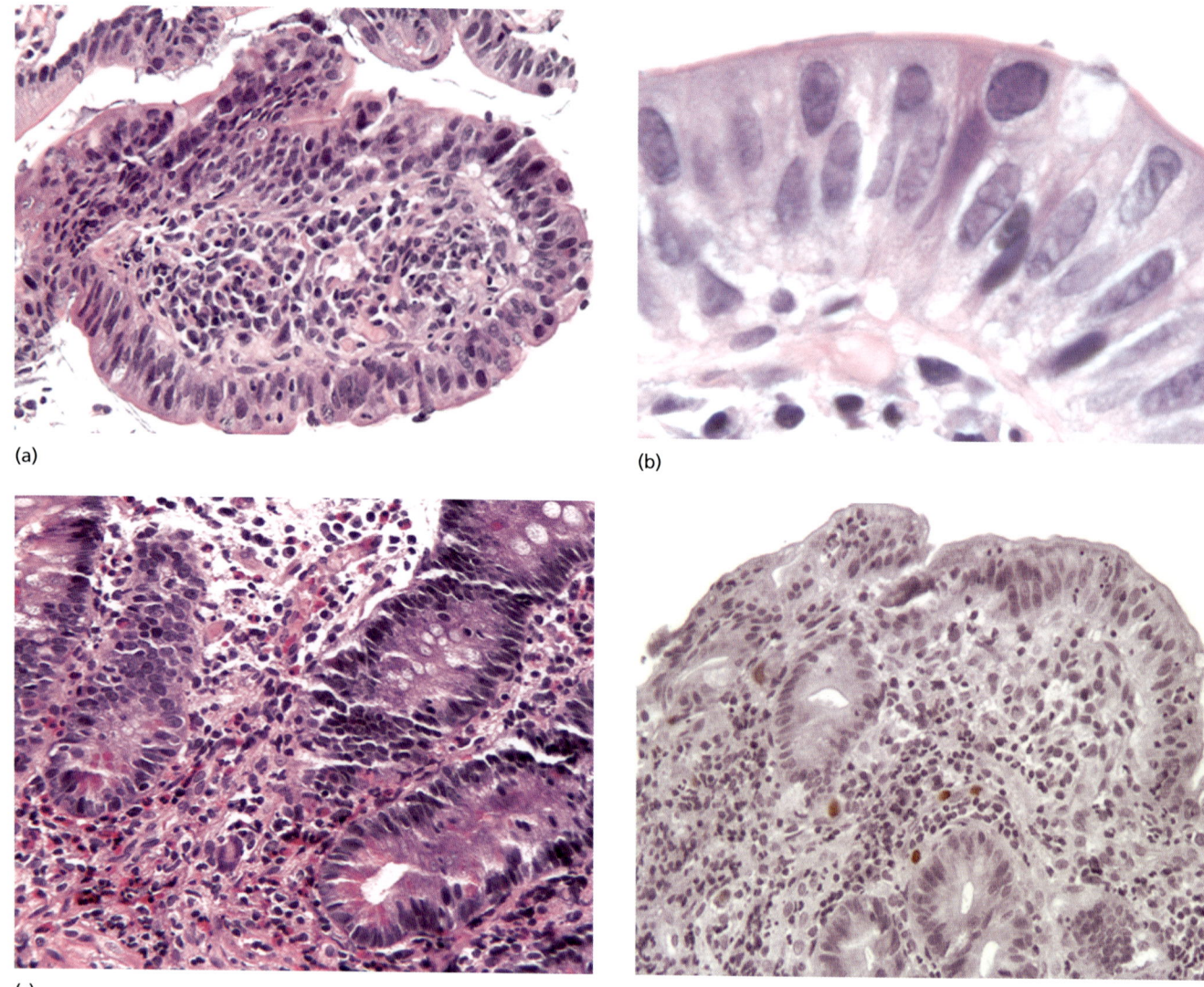

(a)

(b)

(c)

(d)

Plate 47.4 (a) Adenovirus. The loss of the monotonous nuclear arrangement in this unusually heavily infected case is a low-power clue to adenovirus. Enlarged nuclei contain adenovirus inclusions. (b) Adenovirus. The most distinctive of the various inclusions is a waxy eosinophilic or light purple with accentuation of the nuclear membrane. Unfortunately there are many artifacts with a similar appearance, including drying artifact. (c) Cytomegalovirus. The finding is often subtle and the inflammatory response local when the infection is not overwhelming. (d) Cytomegalovirus. Immunostain for early antigen (nuclear) can reveal more virus in smaller, nontransformed cells and gives an indication of viral production.

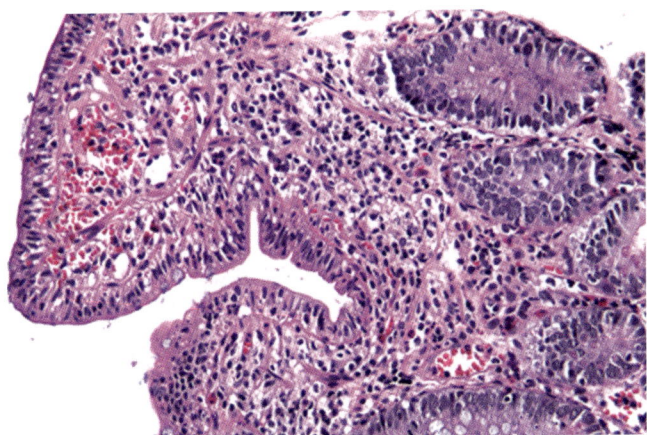

Plate 47.5 Rotavirus. There is an "enteritis" with an increase in the number of intraepithelial inflammatory cells, regenerative changes and an increase in lamina propria cells. Rotavirus enzyme linked immunosorbent assay (ELISA) was positive and the subsequent biopsies were normal with no change in therapy.

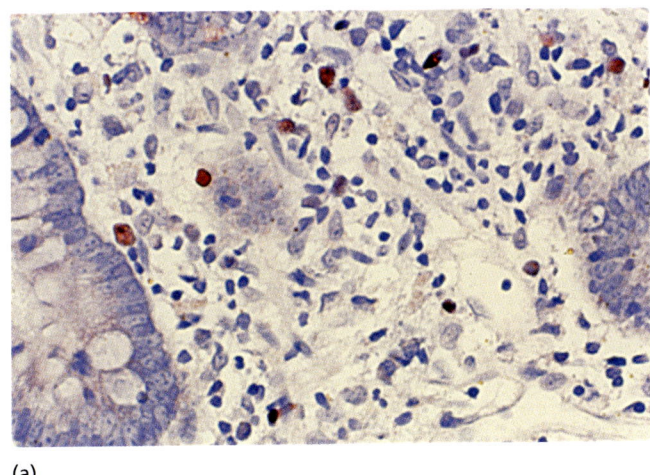

(a)

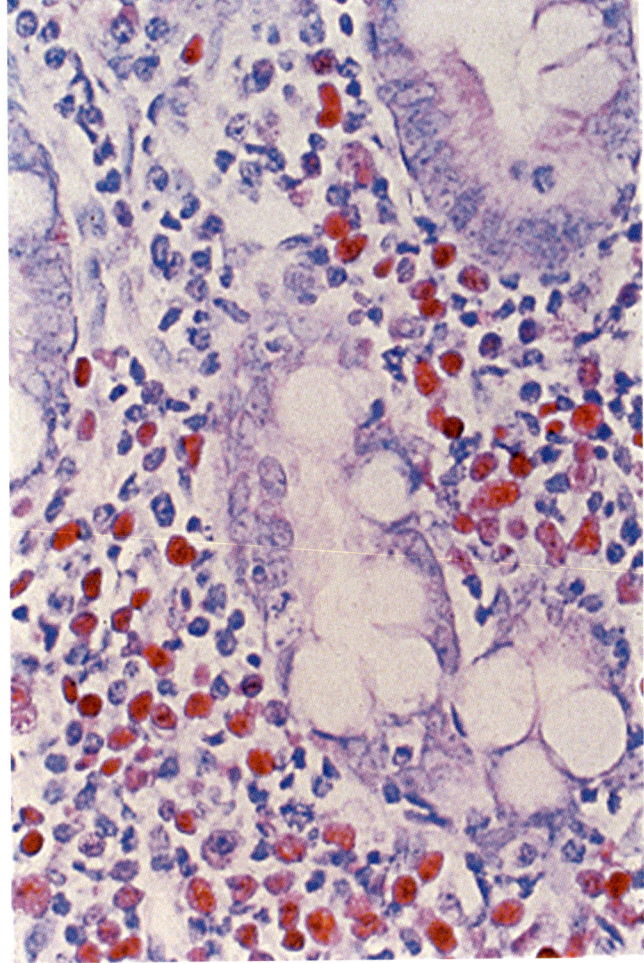

(b)

Plate 47.6 (a) Epstein–Barr virus (EBV) infection. EBER-1 probe in an otherwise normal allograft biopsy, without infiltrate, but with high blood EBV-polymerase chain reaction (PCR), shows scattered staining nuclei consistent with a low-grade EBV infection. (b) EBV infection. EBER-1 probe in an allograft biopsy with stromal lymphocytosis but no mass, shows many EBER-1 staining nuclei, consistent with a high-grade EBV infection.

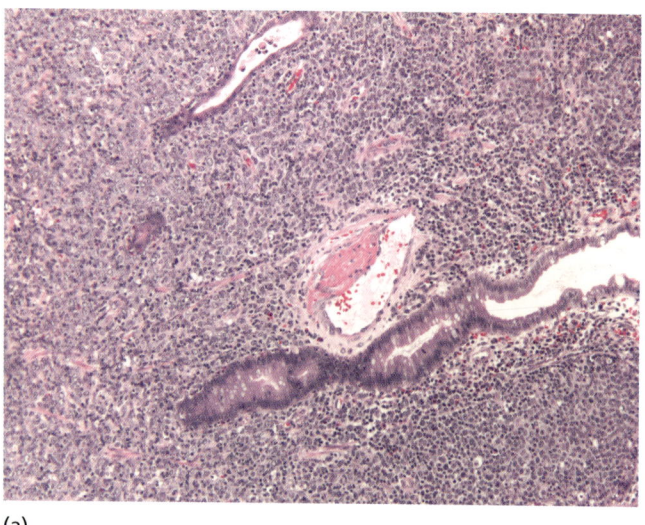

(a)

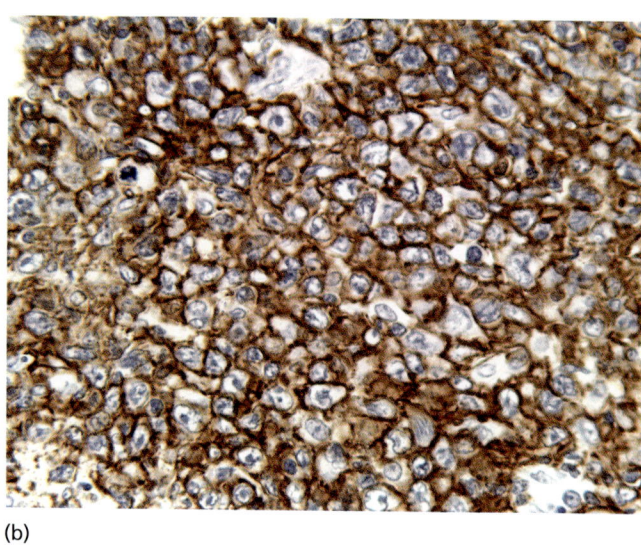

(b)

Plate 47.7 (a) Posttransplant lymphoproliferative disease (PTLD). A mass lesion has a monomorphous character (left) while the lamina propria has a more mixed population. (b) PTLD. CD20 immunostain reveals the monotonous high-level expression on the lesional cells.

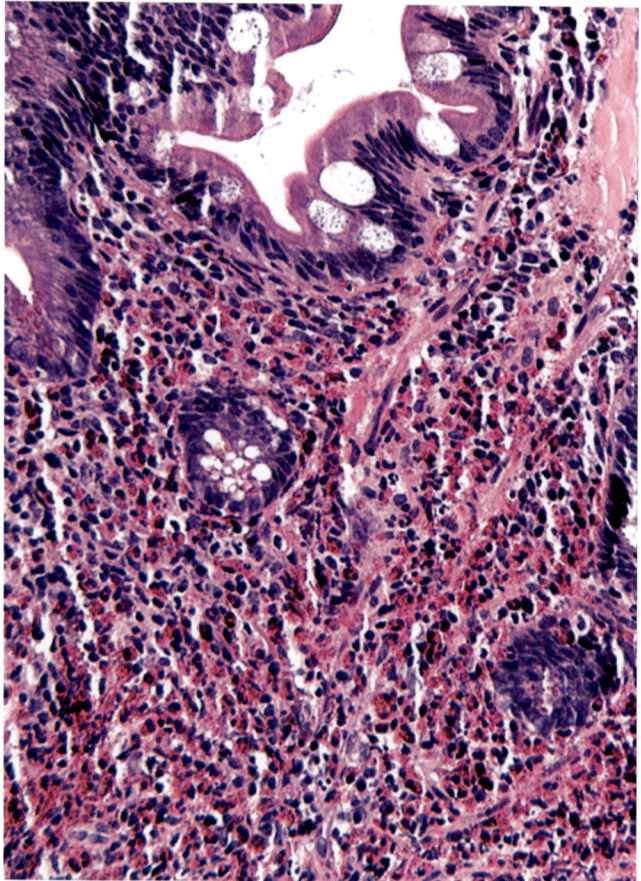

Plate 47.8 Eosinophilia. Eosinophilia is a common finding in the allograft. The implication is not always clear. In this instance, there were 30% circulating eosinophils and clinical manifestations of allergy.

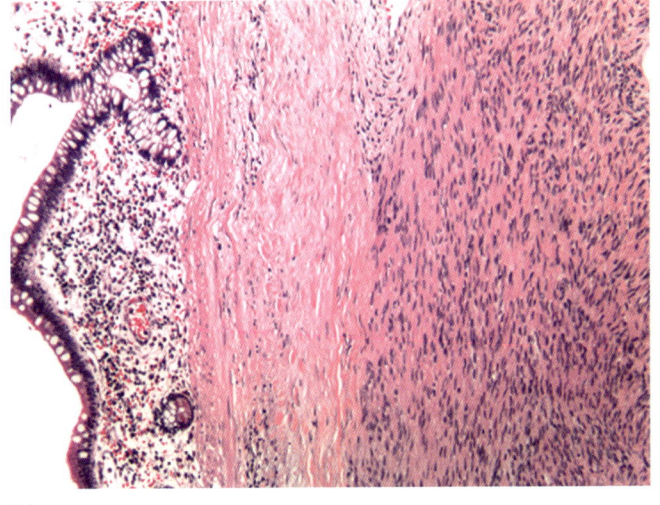

(a)

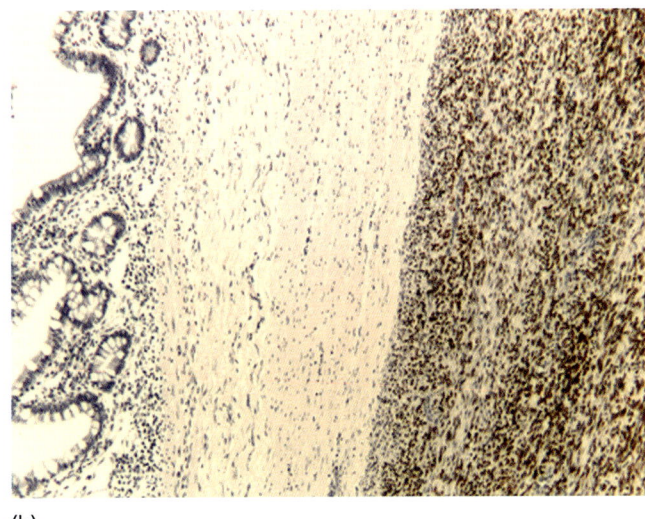

(b)

Plate 47.9 (a) Spindle cell lesion. A nodular lesion has a spindle cell, smooth-muscle appearance and the overlying mucosa is attenuated.

(b) Spindle cell lesion. An EBER-1 probe shows the nuclear staining, confined to the smooth muscle cells.

homogeneous, basophilic nuclei without a well-defined nuclear membrane (smudge cells) (see Plate 47.4b, facing page 384). Eosinophilic inclusions may be surrounded by a halo and a distinct nuclear membrane. Other features of adenovirus enteritis include regenerative epithelial changes (i.e. mucin depletion, nuclear hyperchromatism, increased mitoses), a predominantly plasmacytic infiltrate and usually mild apoptosis preferentially involving the superficial portions of the crypts [5].

In CMV enteritis, a mild to moderate neutrophilic infiltrate in the lamina propria is usually associated with mild neutrophilic cryptitis (see Plate 47.4c,d, facing page 384). As in adenovirus infection, crypt cell apoptosis may be seen in the immediate proximity of virus and in severe untreated CMV infection ulceration may develop. CMV nuclear and cytoplasmic inclusions may involve endothelial, stromal and, less often, epithelial cells.

In our experience, rotavirus enteritis is sometimes characterized by surface epithelial changes, predominantly neutrophilic inflammation, and paucity of crypt cell apoptosis (see Plate 47.5, facing page 384). The surface epithelium is altered in places by vacuolar changes and loss of goblet cells, particularly at the tips of the villi, which are often flattened or even effaced. Mild lymphocytic and neutrophilic infiltration of the surface epithelium may be present. The lamina propria shows predominantly neutrophilic infiltrate, but lymphocytes and plasma cells may be increased in numbers. Regenerative epithelial changes may be observed, but crypt cell apoptosis is sparse.

The incidence of EBV infection in pediatric small intestinal transplant recipients is higher than reported for any other solid organ group [10]. Low-grade EBV infections may precede the development of post-transplant lymphoproliferative disease (PTLD). On light microscopy, EBV infection should be suspected when the lamina propria is more cellular than usual because of increased numbers of small lymphocytes associated with varying numbers of plasma cells and occasional large transformed lymphoid cells. However, the crypts remain intact and epithelial cell apoptosis is rare. Nuclear staining with *in situ* hybridization for EBV early RNA transcript (EBER-1) confirms the presence of EBV. In EBV infection, the number of EBER-positive lymphoid cells is usually less than 15 per field (see Plate 47.6a,b, facing page 384) [10].

A prolonged diarrhea and enteritis secondary to Norwalk virus have been recently described in pediatric small bowel transplant recipients [11]. The interval between transplantation and the clinical presentation varied from 17 to 326 days. The pathologic changes in the allograft and native small bowel included villous blunting, crypt hyperplasia, predominantly lymphoplasmacytic infiltrate with small numbers of admixed neutrophils, disarray and apoptosis of the surface epithelium and a significant amount of apoptotic debris in the superficial lamina propria. Crypt cell apoptosis was increased

in some patients, raising the question of superimposed acute rejection.

The differential diagnosis between acute rejection and infection can be difficult. In general, a "mixed" cell infiltrate is more characteristic of acute rejection and a "predominant" (i.e. plasmacytic, lymphocytic, neutrophilic) infiltrate is more suggestive of an infectious process. In an immunocompromised host, however, the "expected" inflammatory response may be either minimal or absent. The presence of regenerative changes in the face of active epithelial damage should alert the pathologist to the possibility of infection because lack of regeneration is more characteristic of the acute rejection process. Although some crypt cell apoptosis is seen in infectious enteritis, the presence of significant apoptosis involving predominantly deep portions of the crypts should raise the question of a concomitant acute rejection.

POST-TRANSPLANT LYMPHOPROLIFERATIVE DISEASE

PTLD is closely associated with EBV infection [12,13]. In "polymorphous PTLD" the intestinal lamina propria shows a mass that contains a diffuse heterogeneous proliferation of lymphoid cells, including small and large cleaved and noncleaved lymphocytes, immunoblasts, as well as plasmacytoid and plasma cells. In contrast to conventional EBV infection, the PTLD infiltrate distorts the normal crypt architecture and is usually associated with a nodule, a mass or an ulceration that is visible on endoscopy. The lesions of "monomorphous PTLD" are composed of sheets of large transformed immunoblasts (see Plate 47.7a,b, facing page 384). They are often malignant appearing with areas of necrosis and essentially indistinguishable from large cell lymphoma. These ulcerated lesion(s) are also recognizable on endoscopy. In both "polymorphous" and "monomorphous" PTLDs the number of EBER-positive lymphoid cells is more than 15 per field [10].

OTHER PROBLEMS AND PITFALLS

Although isolated cases of acute cellular rejection show predominantly eosinophilic infiltrate, the presence of significant numbers of eosinophils in the intestinal allograft should raise the question of allergic enteritis. The biopsies from the native gastrointestinal tract may be helpful, as well as laboratory tests (e.g. peripheral blood eosinophil count, serum IgE) (see Plate 47.8, facing page 384).

The intestinal biopsy, taken close to the anastomosis shortly after transplantation, may reveal fibrinoid vascular necrosis and bring up acute humoral rejection in the differential diagnosis. A lack of histologic features that are traditionally associated with humoral rejection (i.e. vascular thrombosis, endothelial cell activation, erythrocyte extravasation and neutrophil margination), as well as negative immunofluorescence, negative pretransplant panel reactive antibodies and the knowledge of the biopsy site may make the distinction easier.

Intestinal ulcers are common in small bowel transplant recipients. Examples include blind loop ulcers and anastomotic ulcers. The ulcers may also accompany acute and chronic rejection, viral infections and ischemia. Crypt cell apoptosis is always increased in the vicinity of the ulceration and hence it is important to assess the degree of apoptosis in nonulcerated areas to avoid a false diagnosis of acute rejection. For the same reason, biopsies of the stoma are discouraged because stoma may undergo a variety of secondary changes, including apoptosis and ulceration.

Smooth muscle tumors containing EBV may arise in the allograft and native gastrointestinal tract (see Plate 47.9a,b, facing page 384) [10,14]. These tumors typically occur in a setting of prior or ensuing diagnosis of PTLD. The smooth muscle tumors are composed of fascicles of spindled cells, which show cytoplasmic staining with muscle-specific and smooth muscle actins and nuclear staining with EBER-1 probe.

A primary intestinal allograft carcinoma with both neuroendocrine and undifferentiated components has been reported [8]. This carcinoma was of donor origin by *in situ* hybridization for X and Y chromosomes and demonstrated a variable expression of cytokeratins (AE1/AE3), PGP 9.5 and synaptophysin, but EBV presence was not detected by EBER-1 probe.

REFERENCES

1 White FV, Reyes J, Jaffe R, Yunis EJ. Pathology of intestinal transplantation in children. *Am J Surg Pathol* 1995;**19**:687–98.

2 Lee RG, Nakamura K, Tsamandas AC, *et al.* Pathology of human intestinal transplantation. *Gastroenterology* 1996;**110**: 1820–34.

3 Wu T, Abu-Elmagd K, Bond G, Demetris AJ. A clinicopathologic study of isolated intestinal allografts with preformed IgG lymphocytotoxic antibodies. *Hum Pathol* 2004;**35**:1332–9.

4 Wu T, Abu-Elmagd K, Bond G, *et al.* A schema for histologic grading of small intestine allograft acute rejection. *Transplantation* 2003;**75**:1241–8.

5 Parizhskaya M, Walpusk J, Mazariegos G, Jaffe R. Enteric adenovirus infection in pediatric small bowel transplant recipients. *Pediatr Dev Pathol* 2001;**4**:122–8.

6 Parizhskaya M, Redondo C, Demetris A, *et al.* Chronic rejection of small bowel grafts: pediatric and adult study of risk factors and morphologic progression. *Pediatr Dev Pathol* 2003; **6**:240–50.

7 Demetris AJ, Murase N, Lee RG, *et al.* Chronic rejection: a general overview of histopathology and pathophysiology with emphasis on liver, heart, and intestinal allografts. *Ann Transplant* 1997;**2**:27–44.

8 Noguchi S, Reyes J, Mazariegos G, *et al.* Pediatric intestinal transplantation: the resected allograft. *Pediatr Dev Pathol* 2002; **5**:3–21.

9 Yunis EJ, Atchison RW, Michaels RH, DeCicco FA. Adenovirus and ileocecal intussusception. *Lab Invest* 1975;**33**:347–51.

10 Finn L, Reyes J, Bueno J, Yunis E. Epstein–Barr virus infections in children after transplantation of the small intestine. *Am J Surg Pathol* 1998;**22**:299–309.

11 Morotti RA, Kaufman SS, Fishbein TM, *et al.* Calicivirus infection in pediatric small intestine transplant recipients: pathological considerations. *Hum Pathol* 2004;**35**:1236–40.

12 Ho M, Miller G, Atchison RW, *et al.* Epstein–Barr virus infections and DNA hybridization studies in posttransplant lymphoma and lymphoproliferative lesions: the role of primary infection. *J Infect Dis* 1985;**152**:876–86.

13 Ho M, Jaffe R, Miller G, *et al.* The frequency of Epstein–Barr virus infection and associated lymphoproliferative syndrome after transplantation and its manifestations in children. *Transplantation* 1988;**45**:719–27.

14 Lee ES, Locker J, Nalesnik M, *et al.* The association of Epstein–Barr virus with smooth-muscle tumors occurring after organ transplantation. *N Engl J Med* 1995;**332**:19–25.

48 Post-Transplant Management

Erick Hernandez, Tomoaki Kato, Andreas G. Tzakis and John F. Thompson

The outcome after intestinal transplantation has improved markedly over the past decade. Initially considered as an experimental procedure, it is now accepted as a life-saving method in the treatment of patients with intestinal failure. However, the postoperative management after intestinal transplantation remains one of the most challenging and demanding tasks in transplantology. Acute rejection remains a serious complication for these patients [1]. The difficulties in maintaining an appropriate balance between the control of acute rejection and infections requires careful attention to detail and prompt evaluation and treatment for optimal outcomes. Improved outcomes after transplantation depends on several factors, including early identification and referral of patients with intestinal failure in need of intestinal transplantation, the emergence of better surgical techniques, the use of new immunosuppression regimens and the management of its associated complications. A multidisciplinary approached is required in the follow-up of these patients. Here we describe the most important aspects to consider in their care.

IMMUNOSUPPRESSION

The most critical aspect of successful outcome in intestinal transplantation is adequate immunosuppression. Many approaches have been investigated over the past 15 years but some of these approaches have not been productive. Recent advances have resulted in markedly improved outcomes. There is still no consensus among the large centers in post-intestinal transplant immunosuppression protocols but each of the large centers has experienced continued improvement in their clinical outcomes after intestinal transplantation. A significant landmark was the introduction of tacrolimus (Prograf®, Fujisawa Healthcare) in 1989 by the University of Pittsburgh group [2,3]. It was believed that the use of this strong calcineurin inhibitor made intestinal transplantation a reality for human patients. However, tacrolimus and steroids alone were still not satisfactorily controlling rejection during the early postoperative period; therefore, several induction agents, including cyclophosphamide and OKT3, were utilized

in the early 1990s [4,5]. When mycophenolate mofetil (MMF, CellCept®, Roche) became available, it was added to the immunosuppression regimen for patients undergoing intestinal transplantation, but without significant clinical benefits.

The introduction of interleukin-2 (IL-2) receptor antibodies in the late 1990s further improved patient and graft survival [6,7]. The use of these antibodies (daclizumab, Zenapax®, Roche; basiliximab, Simulect®, Novartis) in combination with tacrolimus and steroids did confer adequate protection against rejection. However, the improvement in outcome could not be attributed solely to the use of these antibodies because postoperative monitoring, patient selection and surgical techniques were also improving at the same time.

New immunosuppression strategies were introduced in 1999 by several large transplant centers in North America. The first noteworthy trial was started by the University of Pittsburgh. The intestinal graft was irradiated *ex vivo* so as to eliminate passenger graft mature lymphocytes in the intestinal graft in an attempt to modulate post-transplantation immune reactions [8,9]. This group also adopted a novel approach using antithymocyte globulin as an induction agent with satisfactory results. The University of Miami group, at about the same time, started utilizing as induction agent alemtuzumab (Campath-1H), a monoclonal antibody directed against the CD52 surface marker on the surface of mature lymphocytes and monocytes, while at the same time eliminating the need for steroid maintenance therapy [10,11]. The experience in the use of Campath-1H, however, was mostly limited to the adult population. In children, our results have been mixed, with significant morbidity related to non-rejection complications in children less than 4 years of age [7,11–13]. We have therefore currently restricted the use of Campath-1H to patients 4 years and older.

Currently, the approach in our center consists of a triple therapy approach: tacrolimus, corticosteroids and daclizumab (Table 48.1). Tacrolimus administration is initially intravenous, then enterally or orally when the intestinal graft returns to function. The tacrolimus intravenous dose is 0.02–0.05 mg/kg/day; the oral dose is 0.05–0.3 mg/kg/day. The goal is to achieve a target through level of 15–20 ng/mL in the first month

Table 48.1 Routine immunosuppression protocols for pediatric intestinal transplant recipients.

	Induction	Maintenance
Steroids (methylprednisolone)	20 mg/kg/dose i.v. in OR, then: 25 mg i.v. q 6 hr times 4 doses 20 mg i.v. q 6 hr times 4 doses 15 mg i.v. q 6 hr times 4 doses 10 mg i.v. q 6 hr times 4 doses 10 mg i.v. q 12 hr times 2 doses 10 mg i.v./p.o. q 24 hr	Wean as clinically indicated to stop steroids 6–12 months post-transplant
Daclizumab	2 mg/kg i.v. in OR, then: 2 mg/kg i.v. on arrival to ICU 2 mg/kg i.v. day 7, 14 POD 2 mg/kg i.v. q 2 weeks for 3 months 1 mg/kg i.v. q 2 weeks for 3 months	
Tacrolimus	0.02–0.05 mg/kg/dose i.v. over 24 hr when GI tract functional, 0.05 mg/kg/dose divided b.i.d. (trough levels 8–12 ng/mL)	0.05 mg/kg/dose divided b.i.d. (trough levels 15–20 ng/mL)

GI, gastrointestinal; ICU, intensive care unit.

of treatment and 8–12 ng/mL in the subsequent 2 months. Corticosteroids are given in a standard manner, as a bolus of methylprednisolone i.v., followed by weaning cycle and maintenance dose, with tentative weaning starting 6 months after transplant. Daclizumab is given as induction agent perioperatively at a dose of 2 mg/kg before and after reperfusion, followed by a protocol-based infusion schedule, is given every 2 weeks for 3 months, then the dose is decreased to 1 mg/kg biweekly for another 3 months.

Tacrolimus has been recognized to cause renal insufficiency as well as hypertrophic cardiomyopathy. In addition, the risk of renal insufficiency is increased because of fluid and electrolyte losses from the ostomy as well as additional nephrotoxic drugs both pre- and post-transplantation. Therefore, attention must be given to ongoing monitoring of these potential complications of the present immunosuppression protocols.

Acute cellular rejection is treated with steroid cycle, optimizing tacrolimus blood levels and OKT3 when indicated. Sirolimus (rapamycin) has been used for persistent rejection or when tacrolimus has to be reduced or withdrawn because of related nephrotoxicity or neurotoxicity [7,14].

NUTRITIONAL THERAPY IN THE POSTOPERATIVE PERIOD

Total parenteral nutrition (TPN) is required in the first 3–6 weeks after transplantation [15,16]. The total caloric and fluid requirements are calculated according to the patient's preoperative weight and metabolic demands. However, studies determining the caloric requirements of these patients in the immediate postoperative period are needed. The macronutrient requirements are based on the patient's metabolic rate. Ideally, this should be measured at the patient's bedside. However, in clinical practice, data are usually extrapolated from studies in critically ill children with other clinical conditions. Therefore, calories are usually provided at approximately the patient's recommended daily allowance (RDA) for age and preoperative weight. Additional fluid requirements, plasma and blood products are supplemented as indicated by the patient's clinical condition. A close observation of the patient's glucose levels is important, because corticosteroids predispose the patient to hyperglycemia. In case of hyperglycemia, the glucose concentration of the TPN infusion is adjusted or insulin is added to the infusate. The protein requirement is 1.5 times the RDA for age (2.0–3.0 g/kg/day). Ammonia level and renal function should be closely monitored to adjust the patient's protein infusion. Intravenous fat emulsions are used for calories and to prevent fatty acid deficiency; no more than 40% of the total caloric intake should be administered by intravenous fat [17,18]. The patient must be reassessed on a daily basis, taking into consideration their clinical status and need for mechanical ventilation, as well as serum ammonia, blood, urea, nitrogen (BUN), glucose and lipid profile.

Enteral feeding is usually initiated on the tenth day post-transplantation if the clinical condition is stable [19]. Once the enteral route becomes an adequate nutritional source for the patient, we start cycling and weaning of TPN. The TPN infusion is discontinued when the patient is receiving 100% of his or her caloric requirement through the enteral route. A gastric or gastrojejunal tube is placed at the time of transplantation and the enteral infusion is delivered continuously through the jejunal port while the gastric port is left to drainage, if necessary. An age-appropriate free amino acid, moderate fat content formula (e.g. Neocate®/SHS North America, Gaithersburg, MD or Pediatric Vivonex®/Sandoz, Minneapolis, MN) should be used for initial enteral feeding. Enteral feeding is initially advanced slowly, usually not more than 5 mL/hour each day, according to the volume of the patient's ostomy output and presence of reducing substances in the output. Fat soluble vitamins (ADEK) supplementation is required because of the relative fat malabsorption in the immediate post-transplant period [17,18]. Consideration should also be given to supplementation with zinc.

When the child is stable and tolerating enteral feeds, solid food is introduced according to the child's age and preference. The transition to full oral intake may take months to years because many of these patients have a feeding aversion [20]. Therefore it is important to utilize an experienced pediatric speech and swallow therapist. On the other hand, some children quickly start eating a normal diet of their newly discovered favorite foods. There are few studies examining the absorptive capacity of the transplanted gastrointestinal tract, including pancreatic and gastric function. Studies suggest that these children do not exhibit catch-up linear growth but do progress in both height and weight [16,21]. Longitudinal follow-up of growth and micro- and macronutrient status is important to optimize long-term outcomes.

COMPLICATIONS

Rejection

Acute cellular rejection of the intestinal allograft is a common problem. Between 70 and 90% of patients will experience at least one episode of rejection in the immediate postoperative period [1]. Acute cellular rejection is more common in the first year post-transplantation, but it might appear thereafter at any time, requiring close surveillance of the graft. Rejection can progress rapidly from mild to severe [22]. Severe rejection carries a poor prognosis, with only 20% long-term survival in our experience. There are no reliable serum markers or physical signs or symptoms that can aid in the diagnosis of rejection accurately. However, recent evidence suggests that serum citrulline levels might help identify patients with mild rejection [23]. Serial endoscopy remain the most effective way of checking for rejection. An enterostomy (ileostomy) is of vital importance to achieve this task. Ileoscopies with biopsies are performed in our patients 2–3 times a week during the first month after transplant, subsequently once a week in the following 1–2 months, and when clinically indicated (Table 48.2). Several biopsies during each endoscopic session are preferable, because mucosal changes of rejection can appear in a patchy distribution and are frequently not appreciated grossly during the ileoscopy. Because the length of the

Table 48.2 Frequency of endoscopic surveillance after intestinal transplantation.

Postoperative period	Frequency
Weeks 0–4	Every 2–4 days
Weeks 5–12	Weekly
Month 4–6 or until stoma closure	Monthly
During rejection episodes	Every 2–4 days

ileum usually visualized is less than 10 cm, we do not routinely use sedation during this procedure. Sampling of the tissue close to the anastomotic suture line or the ostomy should be avoided because postoperative change in these areas may be confusing in the diagnosis of rejection.

Zoom videoendoscopy magnifies the view of the intestinal mucosa more than 100 times. This new technique facilitates analysis of the intestinal villus anatomy and can facilitate early and accurate recognition of the mucosal changes seen during rejection [24]. We have developed a scoring system of mucosal abnormalities of rejection visualized by zoom endoscopy, including assessment of villous blunting, villous length, villous erythema, background mucosal erythema and mucosal friability (Table 48.3). The larger size of the zoom endoscope precludes its use in patients less than 2 years of age.

The early pathologic signs of rejection are increased cellularity (mixed lymphocyte infiltrate) of the lamina propria and crypt apoptosis [22]. Moderate signs of rejection occur with the appearance of villous blunting in addition to cryptitis, increased lymphocytic infiltration of the lamina propria and confluent crypt apoptosis [22]. Worsening rejection leads to the loss of the mucosal architecture with total villous disappearance and sloughing of the intestinal epithelium (severe rejection) [25]. Because the endoscopic changes from viral enteritis might resemble those from rejection, it is always imperative to review the histologic specimens to confirm the clinical impression [19]. Clinical signs of rejection appear later than endoscopic or pathologic changes of the intestinal epithelium. The earliest manifestation is an increase in ostomy output; as rejection progresses, other signs such as fever, bloody diarrhea, sepsis, abdominal pain and distention might become more apparent.

Early treatment is indicated for rejection prior to the development of severe rejection (Table 48.4). However, it is our experience that subtle changes of early rejection should be followed closely by daily endoscopies with biopsies to determine if these changes will resolve with minor adjustments in immunosuppression rather than immediately pursuing a treatment protocol with OKT3. Rejection may be treated by increasing the dose of tacrolimus to achieve a 12-hour trough level close to 20 ng/mL, plus the use of corticosteroid boluses. OKT3 is indicated if there is no histologic or clinical improvement after the increase in baseline treatment. Subacute or chronic rejection is a transmural inflammation of the allograft

Table 48.3 Scoring system for analysis of transplant intestinal mucosa using zoom endoscopy.

Villus height

Normal	0
Mildly shortened	1
Moderately shortened	2
Flat	3

Villus blunting

Normal	0
Mildly blunted	1
Moderately blunted	2
Flat	3

Villus congestion

Normal vascular pattern	0
Mildly congested	1
Moderately congested	2
Severely congested	3

Background mucosal erythema

No erythema	0
Mild erythema	1
Moderate erythema	2
Severe erythema	3

Mucosal friability

Normal	0
Easily bleeds with biopsy	1
Easily bleeds with scope	2
Continuous oozing	3

Score range: 0–15

0	No rejection
1–5	Indeterminate (grade 1)
6–10	Mild (grade 2)
>10	Moderate–severe (grade 3–4)

intestine, characterized by villous atrophy and fibrosis of the mucosa, submucosa and muscle layers. These patients may present with signs of malabsorption or obstruction.

GRAFT-VERSUS-HOST DISEASE

Graft-versus-host disease (GVHD) is an unusual but potentially serious complication of intestinal transplantation [26,27]. As a result of the high load of hematopoietic cells present in the allograft intestine, this complication is more com-monly present in intestinal transplant recipients than in any other type of solid organ transplantation. The organs affected are usually the skin and lungs and the native gastrointestinal tract. Clinical manifestations of GVHD in intestinal transplant recipients include low-grade fever, skin rash and pulmonary insufficiency [28,29]. We routinely perform skin biopsy in any patient with an unexplained skin rash to make an early diagnosis of GVHD. GVHD may progress to severe desquamating skin rash, colitis in native colon and/or pulmonary disease. The treatment of severe GVHD remains problematic.

INFECTIONS

In an immunosuppressed patient with an inadequate intestinal barrier, the incidence of infection is quite problematic [1]. Infections are the most common cause of morbidity and mortality in these patients. Indwelling central catheters or postoperative complications such as bowel strictures, perforations or anastomotic leaks are also predisposing factors for infection. Bacterial infection, most commonly *Escherichia coli*, *Staphylococcus* sp., *Enterococcus faecium*, *Enterobacter cloacae*, *Klebsiella*, *Proteus* and *Pseudomonas aeruginosa* are

Table 48.4 Treatment according to severity of rejection episode.

	Mild	Moderate	Severe
Steroids (methylprednisolone)	20 mg/kg/dose i.v., then: 25 mg i.v. q 6 hr times 4 doses 20 mg i.v. q 6 hr times 4 doses 15 mg i.v. q 6 hr times 4 doses 10 mg i.v. q 6 hr times 4 doses 10 mg i.v. q 12 hr times 2 doses 10 mg i.v./p.o. q 24 hr	20 mg/kg/dose i.v., then 10 mg i.v./p.o. q 24 hr	20 mg/kg/dose i.v., then 10 mg i.v./p.o. q 24 hr
Tacrolimus	Increase dosage to reach trough levels of 15–20 ng/mL	Increase dosage to reach trough levels of 15–20 ng/mL	Increase dosage to reach trough levels of 15–20 ng/mL
OKT3		2.5–5 mg i.v. q 24 hr for 7–14 days	2.5–5 mg i.v. q 24 hr for 14 days (consider explant if refractory)

the most frequent organisms isolated in patients with sepsis [29–31]. Once sepsis is suspected, it is important to obtain peripheral as well as central line cultures. The initiation of broad-spectrum antibiotics is warranted if the index of suspicion for sepsis is high. The appropriate antibiotic is selected based on the result of the culture's antibiograms. Fungal line sepsis with yeast, especially *Candida* species, is also common. *Aspergillus* infections have not been a major problem in our experience.

Viral infections are often serious and life-threatening. Cytomegalovirus (CMV), Epstein–Barr virus (EBV), adenovirus, respiratory syncytial virus (RSV), herpes simplex virus and rotavirus infections have contributed to significant morbidity and mortality in these patients [32]. We have also observed atypical mycobacterial and cryptosporidial infections in our patients [33]. A polymerase chain reaction (PCR) from the allograft intestinal biopsies and from a serum sample of the patient is useful in the diagnosis of viral infections. The clinical manifestations of these viral infections depend on the organ involved. Complications such as pneumonitis, gastroenteritis, encephalitis, hepatitis, bone marrow suppression and viremia are some of the manifestations associated with viral infections. Synagis® (MedImmune, Gaithersburg, MD) is used as prophylaxis against RSV in children under 2 years of age. This approach has reduced the morbidity and mortality of RSV significantly in our experience. Adenovirus is a serious problem which manifests primarily as enteritis or pneumonitis and should be aggressively treated by a decrease in immunosuppresion [34]. Adenovirus can also be isolated from the patient's stools. The symptoms, endoscopic appearance and pathology of these viral infections, particularly adenovirus, must be distinguished from rejection.

CMV infection is a common problem among intestinal transplanted patients [1,25,29]. The incidence of primary CMV infection or reactivation in these patients is close to 30%. Prophylaxis or early detection appears to be quite effective against severe CMV infection. In our center the prophylaxis protocol consists in the use of ganciclovir therapy for 6 months and anti-CMV immunoglobulin (CytoGam®, Genesis Bio-Pharmaeuticals, Hackensack, NJ) infusions, given every other day for 1 month and then every 2 weeks for 3 more months (Table 48.5).

Post-transplant lymphoproliferative disorders (PTLD) related to EBV-mediated B-cell proliferation is another common and serious complication [35–37]. This condition is more frequently seen in patients with recently acquired EBV infection and in younger patients. Compared with other solid organ transplantations, the incidence of PTLD is highest among intestinal transplanted patients, mostly because of the high level of immunosuppression in this group. The symptoms are sometime subtle and very nonspecific. PTLD may involve the lymphoid tissue such as tonsils and lymph nodes, including thoracic and abdominal, or the intestinal allograft. A high index of suspicion is warranted. Hypoalbuminemia is a useful laboratory parameter suggestive of intestinal PTLD. An early diagnosis by either endoscopy or computerized tomography is imperative. We perform upper and lower endoscopy with any clinical change in the patient or if the child has converted to a positive blood EBV PCR or rising EBV PCR quantitation. Endoscopic appearance of PTLD includes nodularity or focal ulceration with raised margins. However, a grossly normal endoscopic appearance does not rule out early PTLD and therefore biopsy specimens should be carefully reviewed for signs of EBV infection. Intestinal biopsies can show characteristic atypical lymphocytes associated with lymphoid nodules. EBER stain is positive for EBV-containing lymphocytes. The serum PCR as well as PCR from the patient's allograft is also helpful in the diagnosis of PTLD. The treatment involves the use of ganciclovir and CytoGam, plus a reduction of the immunosuppression. Rituximab (Rituxan® Genentech, South San Francisco, CA) has also been very useful in the treatment of PTLD [38,39].

CONCLUSIONS AND FUTURE DIRECTIONS

The post-transplant management of children who have undergone intestinal transplantation remains a great challenge. Furthermore, advances in the management of these children proceeds forward at a rapid pace. Attention to detail is absolutely critical both in the immediate postoperative period as well as in their long-term management. Changes in clinical condition of the child (e.g. fever, rash, cough, increase in ostomy or stool output, blood in stool or lymphadenopathy)

Table 48.5 Cytomegalovirus (CMV) prophylaxis in intestinal transplant recipients.		First 4 weeks	4 weeks–6 months
	Ganciclovir	5 mg/kg/dose i.v. q 12 hr when p.o. tolerated Valcyte 10–15 mg/kg/dose q 24 hr	Valcyte 10–15 mg/kg/dose q 24 hr
	CytoGam®	100 mg/kg/dose i.v. q 48 hr	150 mg/kg/dose i.v. q 2 weeks for 2 months, then 100 mg/kg/dose i.v. q 4 weeks for 2 months

must be addressed immediately. Early detection and treatment of rejection and opportunistic infection has dramatically improved the outcome of these children. Concerns about long-term renal and cardiac toxicity of tacrolimus, as well as PTLD, highlight the need for newer and safer immunosuppression regimens. Newer treatment protocols for the prevention, treatment and detection of intestinal rejection will undoubtedly continue to improve the outcome and quality of life of these children.

REFERENCES

1 Fishbein TM, Gondolesi GE, Kaufman SS. Intestinal transplantation for gut failure. *Gastroenterology* 2003;**124**:1615–28.

2 Lee KK, Stangl MJ, Todo S, *et al.* Comparison of short-term immunosuppressive therapy with cyclosporine and FK 506 in small-bowel transplantation. *Transplant Proc* 1990;**22**:2485–6.

3 Hoffman AL, Makowka L, Banner B, *et al.* The use of FK-506 for small intestine allotransplantation: inhibition of acute rejection and prevention of fatal graft-versus-host disease. *Transplantation* 1990;**49**:483–90.

4 Kocoshis SA. Small bowel transplantation in infants and children. *Gastroenterol Clin North Am* 1994;**23**:727–42.

5 Tzakis AG, Nery JR, Thompson J, *et al.* New immunosuppressive regimens in clinical intestinal transplantation. *Transplant Proc* 1997;**29**:683–5.

6 Carreno MR, Kato T, Weppler D, *et al.* Induction therapy with daclizumab as part of the immunosuppressive regimen in human small bowel and multiorgan transplants. *Transplant Proc* 2001;**33**:1015–7.

7 Nishida S, Levi D, Kato T, *et al.* Ninety-five cases of intestinal transplantation at the University of Miami. *J Gastrointest Surg* 2002;**6**:233–9.

8 Murase N, Ye Q, Lee RG, *et al.* Immunomodulation of intestinal transplant with allograft irradiation and simultaneous donor bone marrow infusion. *Transplant Proc* 1999;**31**: 565–6.

9 Murase N, Ye Q, Nalesnik MA, *et al.* Immunomodulation for intestinal transplantation by allograft irradiation, adjunct donor bone marrow infusion, or both. *Transplantation* 2000;**70**: 1632–41.

10 Selvaggi G, Weppler D, Tzakis A. Liver and gastrointestinal transplantation at the University of Miami. *Clin Transpl* 2003;255–66.

11 Tzakis AG, Kato T, Nishida S, *et al.* Alemtuzumab (Campath 1H) combined with tacrolimus in intestinal and multivisceral transplantation. *Transplantation* 2003;**75**:1512.

12 Garcia M, Weppler D, Mittal N, *et al.* Campath-1H immunosuppressive therapy reduces incidence and intensity of acute rejection in intestinal and multivisceral transplantation. *Transplant Proc* 2004;**36**:323–4.

13 Kato T, Gaynor JJ, Selvaggi G, *et al.* Intestinal transplantation in children: a summary of clinical outcomes and prognostic factors in 108 patients from a single center. *J Gastrointest Surg* 2005;**9**: 75–89.

14 Fishbein TM, Florman S, Gondolesi G, *et al.* Intestinal transplantation before and after the introduction of sirolimus. *Transplantation* 2002;**73**:1538–42.

15 Dionigi P, Alessiani M, Ferrazi A. Irreversible intestinal failure, nutrition support, and small bowel transplantation. *Nutrition* 2001;**17**:747–50.

16 Nucci AM, Barksdale EM Jr, Beserock N, *et al.* Long-term nutritional outcome after pediatric intestinal transplantation. *J Pediatr Surg* 2002;**37**:460–3.

17 Schulz RJ, Dignass A, Pascher A, *et al.* New dietary concepts in small bowel transplantation. *Transplant Proc* 2002;**34**:893–5.

18 Kaufmann SS, Lyden ER, Brown CR, *et al.* Disaccharidase activities and fat assimilation in pediatric patients after intestinal transplantation. *Transplantation* 2000;**69**:362.

19 Sudan DL, Kaufman SS, Byers W, *et al.* Isolated intestinal transplantation for intestinal failure. *Am J Gastroenterol* 2000;**95**: 1506.

20 Silver HJ, Castellanos VH. Nutritional complications and management of intestinal transplant. *J Am Diet Assoc* 2000;**100**: 680–9.

21 Iyer K, Horslen S, Iverson A, Sudan D, *et al.* Nutritional outcome and growth of children after intestinal transplantation. *J Pediatr Surg* 2002;**37**:464–6.

22 Ruiz P, Bagni A, Brown R, *et al.* Histological criteria for the identification of acute cellular rejection in human small bowel allografts: results of the pathology workshop at the VIII International Small Bowel Transplant Symposium. *Transplant Proc* 2004;**36**:335–7.

23 Pappas PA, Tzakis AG, Saudubray JM, *et al.* Trends in serum citrulline and acute rejection among recipients of small bowel transplants. *Transplant Proc* 2004;**36**:345–7.

24 Kato T, O'Brien CB, Berho M, *et al.* Improved rejection surveillance in intestinal transplant recipients with frequent use of zoom-video endoscopy. *Transplant Proc* 2000;**32**:1200.

25 Ishii T, Mazariegos GV, Bueno J, *et al.* Exfoliative rejection after intestinal transplantation in children. *Pediatr Transplant* 2003;**7**:185–91.

26 Todo S, Tzakis AG, Abu-Elmagd K, *et al.* Intestinal transplantation in composite visceral grafts or alone. *Ann Surg* 1992;**216**: 223–33.

27 Goulet O, Jan D, Brousse N, *et al.* Intestinal transplantation. *J Pediatr Gastroenterol Nutr* 1997;**25**:1–11.

28 Grant D, Wall W, Mimerault R. Successful small bowel-liver transplantation. *Lancet* 1990;**335**:181–4.

29 Misiakos EP, Kato T, Levi D, *et al.* Pediatric small bowel transplantation. In: Tejani A, Harmon WE, Fine R, eds. *Pediatric Solid Organ Transplantation*. Munksgaard, 2000:447–60.

30 Grant D. Current results of intestinal transplantation: International Intestinal Transplant Registry. *Lancet* 1996;**347**:1801–3.

31 Guaraldi G, Cocchi S, De Ruvo N, *et al.* Outcome, incidence, and timing of infections in small bowel/multivisceral transplantation. *Transplant Proc* 2004;**36**:383–5.

32 Delis S, Kato T, Ruiz P, *et al.* Herpes simplex colitis in a child with combined liver and small bowel transplant. *Pediatr Transplant* 2001;**5**:374–7.

33 Delis S, Tector J, Kato T, *et al.* Diagnosis and treatment of *Cryptosporidium* infection in intestinal transplant recipients. *Transplant Proc* 2002;**34**:951–2.

34 McLaughlin GE, Delis S, Kashimawo L, *et al.* Adenovirus infection in pediatric liver and intestinal transplant recipients: utility of DNA detection by PCR. *Am J Transplant* 2003;**3**:224–8.

35 Niv Y, Mor E, Tzakis AG. Small bowel transplantation: a clinical review. *Am J Gastroenterol* 1999;**94**:3126–30.

36 Goulet O, Jan D, Lacaille F, *et al*. Intestinal transplantation in children: preliminary experience in Paris. *JPEN J Parenter Enteral Nutr* 1999;23(5 Suppl):S121–5.

37 Grant D. Intestinal transplantation: 1997 report of the international registry. Intestinal Transplant Registry. *Transplantation* 1999;**67**:1061–4.

38 LeVasseur R, Ganjoo J, Green M. Lymphocyte subsets may discern treatment effects in children and young adults with post-transplant lymphoproliferative disorder. *Pediatr Transplant* 2003; 7:370–5.

39 Berney T, Delis S, Kato T, *et al*. Successful treatment of post-transplant lymphoproliferative disease with prolonged rituximab treatment in intestinal transplant recipients. *Transplantation* 2002; **74**:1000–6.

49 Outcomes and Risk Factors
Douglas G. Farmer

Intestinal transplantation (ITx) has become a clinical reality over the past decade. Experience has been gained in a few centers worldwide leading to nearly 1000 such transplants being performed to date. The indications for this procedure have become more established as have the surgical techniques and postoperative management. In this chapter, the current outcomes are examined with a focus on large center experience and pooled data sets such as those from the Intestinal Transplant Registry (ITR) and the United Network for Organ Sharing/Organ Procurement and Transplant Network (UNOS/OPTN). Attention is focused on standard outcome measurements as well as others less often considered. Risk factors contributing significantly to these outcomes are also discussed.

DATA SETS

The following data sets were analyzed for this chapter:
1 ITR [1–3] represents the largest single source of data regarding ITx recipients. Nearly all patients worldwide who have undergone an intestinal transplant procedure since 1985 have been voluntarily submitted to this registry. As of the last update in May 2003, 61 worldwide centers have submitted 923 patients who have undergone 989 intestinal transplants including 606 children. This data set indicates that the peak number of intestinal transplants per year occurred in 2001 and 2002 when approximately 140 transplants per year were performed.
2 UNOS/OPTN [4] represents a second pooled registry source of data that is formulated through the mandated submission of all ITx candidate and recipient data in the USA. Data collected from the website includes data as of January 14, 2005. The data set includes 1317 total candidates (176 in 2004) and 936 total recipients (126 in 2004) transplanted since 1990. This data set includes 586 children who have been transplanted since 1990.
3 Individual single center reports were also used as data sources. Only publications from centers reporting large cohorts of patients undergoing ITx were used. The center reports used are from the University of Pittsburgh [5–7],

the University of Miami [8,9], the University of Nebraska [10], the Mount Sinai Medical Center in New York [11,12], Hopital Necker-Enfants Malades, Paris, France [13,14] and the University of California, Los Angeles (UCLA) [15,16].

PRETRANSPLANT MORTALITY

The most common parameter used to judge outcome is typically post-transplant survival. However, when examining overall outcomes after any transplant, it is important to examine wait-list mortality: the percentage of patients deemed appropriate candidates for ITx who die without receiving a transplant. The first data to address this issue were published by Fryer *et al.* [17]. In this study, data from UNOS/OPTN were gathered regarding patients listed for intestinal transplants and compared with those listed for liver transplants during the interval 1993–2001. The annual mortality rate of candidates listed for liver-intestinal transplants exceeded that for candidates of liver transplants in every year examined. The death rate was particularly high in candidates aged less than 17 years. In examining the most recent data from UNOS [2], the risk of death without a transplant remains significant. As of UNOS/OPTN data from January 14, 2005, there were 176 candidates removed from the intestinal transplant list in 2004. Forty-three (24%) were removed for reasons of "death" or "too sick to transplant," whereas 120 (68%) were removed because of transplantation. The pediatric population remains most at risk as 58.5% of those removed for reasons of "death" were less than 17 years of age. Clearly, this represents a significant problem that is not accounted for in the interpretation of post-transplant outcome data.

POST-TRANSPLANT PATIENT SURVIVAL

Without a doubt, the survival of patients after ITx has improved over the past decade. Table 49.1 outlines the patient survival statistics from the data sources analyzed. The overall 1- and 5-year survival rates range between 40–88% and

Table 49.1 Patient survival. The patient survival reported in the data sources analyzed are shown.

Ref.	Center	Year	n	1-year (%)	3-year (%)	5-year (%)	Comment
3	ITR	1996	69	83	40	–	SBT
3	ITR	1996	83	66	40	–	LSBT
3	ITR	1996	28	59	43	–	MVT
2	ITR	1999	113	68	48	43	SBT
2	ITR	1999	130	61	40	40	LSBT
2	ITR	1999	30	43	40	38	MVT
2	ITR	1999	–	64	–	–	SBT 1995–97
2	ITR	1999	–	64	–	–	LSBT 1995–97
2	ITR	1999	–	64	–	–	MVT 1995–97
4	USA	2004	77	62–83	33–80	51–60	Pediatric
13	Paris	2002	39 GFT/36 PT	77	77	–	Pediatric
11	Mt Sinai	2002	37 GFT/34 PT	74	–	–	Total
11	Mt Sinai	2002	14	87	–	–	SBT
11	Mt Sinai	2002	20	63	–	–	MVT
12	Mt Sinai	2003	28 GFT/26 PT	88	88	–	SBT
16	UCLA	2001	21 GFT/17 PT	63	55	–	Total
15	UCLA	2004	37 GFT/33 PT	77	–	52	Total
8	Miami	2002	16	84	–	–	SBT 1997–2002
8	Miami	2002	28	40	–	–	LSBT all
8	Miami	2002	40	48	–	–	MVT all
8	Miami	2005	124 GFT/108 PT	59	–	41	Pediatric
6	Pittsburgh	1998	104 GFT/98 PT	72	–	48	Total
5	Pittsburgh	2001	165 GFT/155 PT	75	–	54	Total
5	Pittsburgh	2001	93	78	–	63	> 1994
7	Pittsburgh	2002	89 GFT/84 PT	74	59	56	Pediatric
7	Pittsburgh	2002	50	77	68	64	Pediatric > 1994

GFT, intestinal transplant graft; ITR, Intestinal Transplant Registry; LSBT, combined liver-small bowel transplants; MVT, multivisceral transplants; n, patient number; PT, patient; SBT, isolated small bowel transplants; UCLA, University of California Los Angeles.

28–60%, respectively. Centers with multiple reports demonstrate that the most recent experience is associated with improved survival rates. Furthermore, the highest early survival rates are seen in recipients of isolated intestinal grafts. The most common cause of patient loss is sepsis or multisystem organ failure.

There are many factors that have contributed to these improvements. Several of the most obvious include early referral for transplantation, which generally translates into candidates who are in a better medical condition at the time of transplantation. No single statistic reflects this trend better than pretransplant location of the recipients. In the ITR data set, 73% of all recipients were at home at the time of transplant in the group transplanted since 2001. A decade ago, performing an intestinal transplant on a patient from home was unusual. Other factors contributing to improved outcome include a reduction in rejection rates and infection rates as discussed below, standardization of surgical techniques and less toxic immunotherapeutic regimens. Experience also has been shown to have a role. In the most recent ITR data, transplant centers with experience in more than 10 intestinal

transplants had significantly better outcomes than those with experience in less than 10 intestinal transplants.

POST-TRANSPLANT GRAFT SURVIVAL

A summary of the graft survival from the data sources is shown in Table 49.2. The overall 1- and 5-year survival rates range between 37–78% and 34–54%, respectively. Again, several trends are noted including a tendency toward higher reported survival rates in the more recent experiences as well as with isolated intestinal grafts. The most common cause of graft loss is rejection.

RISK FACTORS

Rejection

Rejection of the transplanted intestine has perhaps been the major obstacle to successful application of this procedure in

Table 49.2 Graft survival. The patient survival reported in the data sources analyzed are shown.

Ref.	Center	Year	n	1-year (%)	3-year (%)	5-year (%)	Comment
3	ITR	1996	69	60	30	–	SBT
3	ITR	1996	83	60	40	–	LSBT
3	ITR	1996	28	52	40	–	MVT
2	ITR	1999	–	50	–	–	SBT 1995–97
2	ITR	1999	–	62	–	–	LSBT 1995–97
2	ITR	1999	–	62	–	–	MVT 1995–97
4	USA	2004	77	56.5–77	31–73	41–54	Pediatric
13	Paris	2002	39 GFT/36 PT	46	31	–	Pediatric
11	Mt Sinai	2002	37 GFT/34 PT	64	–	–	Total
11	Mt Sinai	2002	16	73	–	–	SBT
11	Mt Sinai	2002	21	58	–	–	MVT
12	Mt Sinai	2003	28 GFT/26 PT	78	71	–	SBT
16	UCLA	2001	21 GFT/17 PT	73	55	–	Total
15	UCLA	2004	37 GFT/33 PT	64	–	34	Total
8	Miami	2002	16	72	–	–	SBT 1997–2002
8	Miami	2002	28	37	–	–	LSBT
8	Miami	2002	40	40	–	–	MVT
6	Pittsburgh	1998	104 GFT/98 PT	64	–	40	Total
5	Pittsburgh	2001	165 GFT/155 PT	65	–	45	Total
7	Pittsburgh	2002	89 GFT/84 PT	67	53	47	Pediatric

GFT, intestinal transplant graft; ITR, Intestinal Transplant Registry; LSBT, combined liver-small bowel transplants; MVT, multivisceral transplants; n, patient number; PT, patient; SBT, isolated small bowel transplants; UCLA, University of California Los Angeles.

humans and success of the procedure was rarely seen until the clinical introduction of tacrolimus in the late 1980s [18]. This agent, which was both potent and readily absorbed in the gastrointestinal tract, facilitated successful ITx. Still, rejection rates remained high and graft loss secondary to rejection was common. As evidence, the results from the 1997 ITR, which included 260 recipients, indicated that rejection occurred in 73% [2]. A review of the data sources reveals that the rates of acute rejection are as high as 93%. The 2003 ITR data reported that rejection is responsible for 62% of all grafts removed and 11% of all patient deaths. Using more recent immunotherapeutic regimens such as induction interleukin 2 receptor antagonist [19], antithymocyte globulins [20] and alemtuzumab [21], rejection rates have been reduced to 43%, 44% and 19%, respectively. Chronic rejection has been a very much underdiagnosed and underappreciated entity. It has been conservatively diagnosed in approximately 9% of intestinal transplant recipients [22].

Infectious complications

Infection still remains a formidable problem after ITx. Not surprisingly, this group of patients is at high risk for infections. Most have had significant infectious complications in the past and many have antimicrobial resistant organisms colonizing the skin, respiratory and gastrointestinal tracts.

Furthermore, the relatively heavy degree of immunosuppression needed to prevent rejection renders these patients susceptible to infectious complications. Compounding this issue is the fact that the transplant procedure itself is high risk for infectious complications – a lengthy abdominal operation that involves both vascular and gastrointestinal procedures. Rejection of the intestine can also be associated with bacterial translocation – a fact that further exacerbates the problem. The most recent ITR data emphasizes these points with the diagnoses of "sepsis" and "multisystem organ failure" as the cause of death in 48.3% of cases. An increasingly recognized cause of graft loss and morbidity has been infectious enteritis including cytomegalovirus (CMV), adenovirus, *Clostridium difficile* and *Cryptosporidium* [23].

Cytomegalovirus

Not surprisingly, infection with CMV is a common cause of morbidity and mortality after ITx as this virus is a common pathogen for both the liver and the intestine and is also a common pathogen in immunosuppressed patient populations. The data sources used for this study report tissue-invasive infection rates as high as 36%. One of the early reports regarding CMV infection in pediatric ITx reflects these findings [24,25]. Additionally, CMV infections have been a significant cause of graft loss in most series.

One of the major advances in this field has been the control of CMV infections using prophylaxis and pre-emptive therapies. While protocols have varied, prophylaxis is generally accomplished through the administration of either ganciclovir or CMV immunoglobulin. At UCLA, we give intravenous ganciclovir for a total of 100 days after transplantation followed by conversion to oral acyclovir [26]. Using this protocol, there has been no tissue-invasive CMV seen during the first 100 days after ITx. Pre-emptive therapy against CMV infection has also gained widespread acceptance. Again, while protocols vary, most centers regularly test the blood of recipients for viral DNA or early antigens, thereby diagnosing the early onset of CMV viremia [26]. When early viremia is detected, treatment with ganciclovir or CMV immunoglobulin is then initiated to prevent tissue-invasive disease. Using this protocol at UCLA, there has only been a 6% incidence of tissue-invasive CMV infection and there has been no associated graft or patient loss.

Epstein–Barr virus and post-transplant lymphoproliferative disorders

Like CMV, Epstein–Barr virus (EBV) and post-transplant lymphoproliferative disorders (PTLD) have also been a major problem after ITx. Examining the data sources reveals that the incidence after pediatric ITx ranges from 10% to 44%. The ITR data indicate that lymphoma is the cause of graft loss in 2.2% of pediatric intestinal transplants and the cause of death in 6% of all patients after the procedure.

A real improvement in outcome has been seen with the initiation of similar protocols of prophylaxis and pre-emptive therapy against EBV infection (see section on Cytomegalovirus above) [26]. Using these protocols, the negative predictive value associated with the absence of EBV viremia has been shown [27]. Furthermore, at UCLA, the incidence of frank PTLD after intestinal transplantation is 2%.

NUTRITIONAL AUTONOMY

Nutritional autonomy is an important benchmark by which the success of ITx should be judged. Because of the many technical, immunologic and infectious obstacles historically encountered after ITx, this benchmark has been frequently relegated to a single line at the end of a publication regarding independence from parenteral nutrition (PN). Further complicating data interpretation is the fact that centers report nutritional autonomy rates variably as surviving patients off PN, discharged patients off PN, and most recent experiences with PN autonomy. As shown in Table 49.3, the reported rates of nutritional autonomy from the data sources range between 77% and 95%.

There are few reports detailing nutritional autonomy, growth and nutritional parameters after ITx. The University

Table 49.3 Nutritional autonomy. The rates of parenteral nutrition independence after intestinal transplantation as defined by cessation of parenteral nutrition in the data sources analyzed are shown.

Ref.	Center	Year	n	Total (%)
3	ITR	1996	180 GFT/170 PT	78
2	ITR	1999	273 GFT/260 PT	77
1	ITR	2003	989 GFT/923 PT	80
13	Paris	2002	39 GFT/36 PT	95
16	UCLA	2001	16	81
12	Mt Sinai	2003	28 GFT/26 PT	81
6	Pittsburgh	1998	104 GFT/98 PT	91
5	Pittsburgh	2001	76 PT	93
7	Pittsburgh	2002	89 GFT/84 PT	87

GFT, intestinal transplant graft; ITR, Intestinal Transplant Registry; n, patient number; PT, patient; UCLA, University of California Los Angeles.

of Pittsburgh has several relevant brief reports regarding post-transplant nutrition. Rovera et al. [28] reported the nutritional status of 23 children post-transplant, demonstrating improved serum and anthropometric indices. In a later study of 24 children after ITx [29], Nucci et al. [29] showed a positive trend in z-scores for weight and height only in 39% and 22% of patients, respectively. Serum growth factors were then examined by Nucci et al. [30] in five children post-transplant, showing a normalization of serum insulin-like growth factor 1 in all patients and insulin-like growth factor binding protein 3 in three of five patients. Linear growth failure was common in this small group. Lastly, Rovera et al. [31] studied the nutritional outcome of 22 adult intestinal transplant recipients. At 12 months, 77% remained free of PN with nutritional indices that did not differ significantly from pre-transplant measurements.

There are several reports from the University of Nebraska detailing nutritional outcomes after ITx. Kaufman et al. [32] examined 22 children post-transplant and found no disaccharidase deficiencies on biopsy, normal dietary lipid absorption but impaired vitamin E absorption. Sudan et al. [33] administered a questionnaire and examined nutritional outcome in 31 patients more than 1 year after ITx. Thirty-five percent required a period of supplemental PN after achieving nutritional autonomy. Half of the children demonstrated normal growth while 11% maintained pretransplant growth failure and 15% demonstrated catch-up growth. Iyer et al. [34] examined 21 children more than 1 year after ITx with functioning allografts and showed that the median time to nutritional autonomy was 29 days (range, 18–54 days) and all were off PN. Examination of z-scores for both linear growth and weight revealed persistant linear growth retardation up to 2 years after ITx and persistant weight gain without evidence of catch-up. Therefore, the detailed studies from both of these centers reveal a mixed picture regarding nutritional outcomes after ITx, although the small numbers of patients limit conclusions. Disappointingly, catch-up growth is not common and could be related to the severe pre-existing growth failure or the immunosuppressive medication and complications seen after ITx.

QUALITY OF LIFE

Similar to the status of nutritional outcomes, there are sparse data available on quality of life (QOL) after ITx. One indirect indicator of QOL is length of hospitalization and rehospitalizations. While there are no available data on the latter, results from the data sources indicate that while length of hospital stay of ITx has decreased, lengthy hospitalizations are still the rule. The average length of stay ranges between 39.9 ± 32.9 and 84.4 ± 60.9 days [5]. The ITR data indicate the length of stays vary based on type of graft, with recipients of isolated intestinal transplants having the shortest duration (55.1 ± 65 days) while recipients of multivisceral grafts have the longest (72.6 ± 79 days). The ITR also attempts to capture a QOL index by using a modified Karnofsky performance score. The results as submitted by the health care providers reveals that approximately 85% of 383 intestinal transplant survivors function in the 90–100% category: overall well, with only minor symptoms and resuming normal activities. Other variables impacting QOL such as the number of medications needed on a daily basis, laboratory draws, clinic visits and the need for special care of central venous catheters, ostomies and feeding tubes have not been studied in detail [7].

There are several small publications dedicated to QOL after ITx. Sudan *et al.* [33] reported on 31 patients and, in addition to the nutritional findings discussed above, found that 63% of children required special services such as speech or physical therapy and 84% have returned to level-appropriate school or work. The mean number of hospital readmissions was 2.3 ± 1.1. Sudan *et al.* [35] also reported that pediatric ITx recipients perceive physical and psychologic functioning at a level similar to normal school-aged children. Rovera *et al.* [36] administered a QOL Inventory to three living donor intestinal recipients and found significant improvement in measured indices. A similar although not as uniform result was reported by Cameron *et al.* [37].

COSTS

There are very few data published on costs after ITx. The University of Nebraska reported in 2002 that the median cost is $275 000, with a range of $77 000–1 800 000 [10]. It is unclear if this represents only the initial hospitalization cost or charges. As more insurance providers are now involved in this procedure, further data should be forthcoming.

CONCLUSIONS

Without a doubt, the outcomes after ITx have improved substantially over the past decade. Classic outcome parameters such as survival must be interpreted in light of data indicating a high pretransplant mortality in candidates listed for the procedure. Nevertheless, post-transplant standard outcome measures such as patient and graft survival show a marked improvement. Risk factors for poor outcome include post-transplant major infectious episodes and rejection episodes, both of which are the leading causes of patient and graft loss, respectively. Reduction in rejection rates through the use of induction immunotherapies and in the incidences of CMV and EBV infection through the use of prophylactic and pre-emptive therapy protocols have contributed to improved outcomes. Now that simply achieving survival is no longer the only acceptable outcome measure, efforts must be targeted toward assessing quality of nutritional outcomes, QOL measurements and transplant-associated costs.

REFERENCES

1 www.intestinaltransplant.org
2 Grant D. Intestinal transplantation: 1997 report of the international registry. Intestinal Transplant Registry. *Transplantation* 1999;**67**:1061–4.
3 Grant D. Current results of intestinal transplantation. The International Intestinal Transplant Registry. *Lancet* 1996;**347**: 1801–3.
4 www.OPTN.org
5 Abu-Elmagd K, Reyes J, Bond G, *et al*. Clinical intestinal transplantation: a decade of experience at a single center. *Ann Surg* 2001;**234**:404–16.
6 Abu-Elmagd K, Reyes J, Todo S, *et al*. Clinical intestinal transplantation: new perspectives and immunologic considerations. *J Am Coll Surg* 1998;**186**:512–25.
7 Reyes J, Mazariegos GV, Bond GM, *et al*. Pediatric intestinal transplantation: historical notes, principles and controversies. *Pediatr Transplant* 2002;**6**:193–207.
8 Kato T, Gaynor JJ, Selvaggi G, *et al*. Intestinal transplantation in children: a summary of clinical outcomes and prognostic factors in 108 patients from a single center. *J Gastrointest Surg* 2005;**9**:75–89.
9 Nishida S, Levi D, Kato T, *et al*. Ninety-five cases of intestinal transplantation at the University of Miami. *J Gastrointest Surg* 2002;**6**:233–9.
10 Langnas A, Chinnakotla S, Sudan D, *et al*. Intestinal transplantation at the University of Nebraska Medical Center: 1990 to 2001. *Transplant Proc* 2002;**34**:958–60.
11 Fishbein T, Kaufman S, Schiano T, *et al*. Intestinal and multi-organ transplantation: the Mount Sinai experience. *Transplant Proc* 2002;**34**:891–2.
12 Fishbein TM, Kaufman SS, Florman SS, *et al*. Isolated intestinal transplantation: proof of clinical efficacy. *Transplantation* 2003; **76**:636–40.

13 Goulet O, Lacaille F, Colomb V, et al. Intestinal transplantation in children: Paris experience. *Transplant Proc* 2002;**34**:1887–8.

14 Jan D, Michel JL, Goulet O, et al. Up-to-date evolution of small bowel transplantation in children with intestinal failure. *J Pediatr Surg* 1999;**34**:841–3.

15 Farmer DG, McDiarmid SV, Edelstein S, et al. Improved outcome after intestinal transplantation at a single institution over 12 years. *Transplant Proc* 2004;**36**:303–4.

16 Farmer DG, McDiarmid SV, Yersiz H, et al. Outcome after intestinal transplantation: results from one center's 9-year experience. *Arch Surg* 2001;**136**:1027–31.

17 Fryer J, Pellar S, Ormond D, Koffron A, Abecassis M. Mortality in candidates waiting for combined liver-intestine transplants exceeds that for other candidates waiting for liver transplants. *Liver Transplant* 2003;**9**:748–53.

18 Todo S, Tzakis A, Reyes J, et al. Clinical small bowel or small bowel plus liver transplantation under FK 506. *Transplant Proc* 1991;**23**:3093–5.

19 Farmer DG, McDiarmid SV, Edelstein S, et al. Induction therapy with interleukin-2 receptor antagonist after intestinal transplantation is associated with reduced acute cellular rejection and improved renal function. *Transplant Proc* 2004;**36**:331–2.

20 Farmer DG. Clinical immunosuppression for intestinal transplantation. *Curr Opin Organ Transplant* 2004;**9**:214–9.

21 Garcia M, Weppler D, Mittal N, et al. Campath-1H immunosuppressive therapy reduces incidence and intensity of acute rejection in intestinal and multivisceral transplantation. *Transplant Proc* 2004;**36**:323–4.

22 Parizhskaya M, Redondo C, Demetris A, et al. Chronic rejection of small bowel grafts: pediatric and adult study of risk factors and morphologic progression. *Pediatr Dev Pathol* 2003;**6**: 240–50.

23 Ziring D, Tran R, Edelstein S, et al. Infectious enteritis after intestinal transplantation: incidence, timing, and outcome. *Transplantation* 2005;**79**:702–9.

24 Bueno J, Green M, Kocoshis S, et al. Cytomegalovirus infection after intestinal transplantation in children. *Clin Infect Dis* 1997;**25**:1078–83.

25 Manez R, Kusne S, Green M, et al. Incidence and risk factors associated with the development of cytomegalovirus disease after intestinal transplantation. *Transplantation* 1995;**9**: 1010–4.

26 Farmer DG, McDiarmid SV, Winston D, et al. Effectiveness of aggressive prophylatic and preemptive therapies targeted against cytomegaloviral and Epstein–Barr viral disease after human intestinal transplantation. *Transplant Proc* 2002;**34**:948–9.

27 Green M, Bueno J, Rowe D, et al. Predictive negative value of persistent low Epstein–Barr virus viral load after intestinal transplantation in children. *Transplantation* 2000;**70**:593–6.

28 Rovera GM, Strohm S, Bueno J, et al. Nutritional monitoring of pediatric intestinal transplant recipients. *Transplant Proc* 1998;**30**:2519–20.

29 Nucci AM, Barksdale EM Jr, Beserock N, et al. Long-term nutritional outcome after pediatric intestinal transplantation. *J Pediatr Surg* 2002;**37**:460–3.

30 Nucci AM, Reyes J, Yaworski JA, et al. Serum growth factors and growth indices pre- and post-pediatric intestinal transplantation. *J Pediatr Surg* 2003;**38**:1043–7.

31 Rovera GM, Schoen RE, Goldbach B, et al. Intestinal and multivisceral transplantation: dynamics of nutritional management and functional autonomy. *JPEN J Parenter Enteral Nutr* 2003;**27**:252–9.

32 Kaufman SS, Lyden ER, Brown CR, et al. Disaccharidase activities and fat assimilation in pediatric patients after intestinal transplantation. *Transplantation* 2000;**69**:362–5.

33 Sudan DL, Iverson A, Weseman RA, et al. Assessment of function, growth and development, and long-term quality of life after small bowel transplantation. *Transplant Proc* 2000;**32**: 1211–2.

34 Iyer K, Horslen S, Iverson A, et al. Nutritional outcome and growth of children after intestinal transplantation. *J Pediatr Surg* 2002;**37**:464–6.

35 Sudan D, Horslen S, Botha J, et al. Quality of life after pediatric intestinal transplantation: the perception of pediatric recipients and their parents. *Am J Transplant* 2004;**4**:407–13.

36 Rovera GM, Sileri P, Rastellini C, et al. Quality of life after living related small bowel transplantation. *Transplant Proc* 2002;**34**: 967–8.

37 Cameron EA, Binnie JA, Jamieson NV, Pollard S, Middleton SJ. Quality of life in adults following small bowel transplantation. *Transplant Proc* 2002;**34**:965–6.

Special Issues after Pediatric Transplantation

50 Growth and Puberty

Franz Schaefer

The realization of a patient's genetic growth potential is one of the key objectives of organ transplantation in pediatric patients with solid organ failure. In theory, the restoration of full organ function should permit catch-up growth and a normal onset and progress of puberty. However, the recovery of growth and development following organ transplantation is commonly incomplete, and to date final adult height is below target in a major proportion of patients who received an allograft in their childhood years. This review details the factors affecting post-transplant growth and the current strategies to improve growth and development following solid organ transplantation.

GROWTH RETARDATION AND DELAYED PUBERTAL DEVELOPMENT IN CHRONIC ORGAN FAILURE

Chronic organ failure in children leads to alterations of growth and development. Consequently, retarded growth and delayed puberty are common in pediatric solid organ recipients at the time of grafting. Skeletal maturation and the onset of puberty is commonly delayed commensurate with growth retardation.

Registry and large single center surveys have provided information about the average growth deficit at time of transplantation in solid organ recipients. The natural history of growth in children end-stage renal disease (ESRD) is characterized by a gradual deviation from the normal growth channel by 0.2–0.5 standard deviation (SD) per year in infancy and mid-childhood, a marked deceleration of growth in the late prepubertal period and a pubertal growth spurt that is delayed by 1.5–2 years and is of subnormal size and duration, resulting in a 50% reduction of cumulative pubertal height gain compared with healthy children (see Schaefer and Mehls [1] for review). Fortunately, growth failure in chronic renal insufficiency and ESRD can be prevented and treated by aggressive nutritional management and recombinant human growth hormone (rhGH) therapy. The intense therapeutical attention to growth failure has resulted in improved growth

patterns in the pretransplant phase. In the annual reports of the North American Pediatric Renal Transplant Cooperative Study Registry (NAPRTCS), mean standardized height at the time of first kidney transplantation has increased from –2.2 SD in 1987 to –1.5 SD in 1999 [2].

As pediatric liver diseases most commonly occur in infancy, severe malnutrition and rapid growth failure are common sequelae of liver failure. Indeed, failure to thrive is considered one of the indications for elective liver transplantation in patients with disorders such as biliary atresia or Alagille syndrome. The mean pretransplant height of 569 patients enrolled into the Studies of Pediatric Liver Transplantation (SPLIT) registry was –1.3 SD [3]. Single center studies from UCLA [4], the University of Chicago [5] and the UK [6] comprising 236, 294 and 107 pediatric recipients, respectively, reported a mean baseline height of –1.7, –1.6 and –1.2 SD.

In children with end-stage liver disease, growth retardation is usually inversely correlated with age, supporting the notion that liver failure is more critical to the nutrition-dependent growth phase of infancy. The crucial role of nutrition is also underlined by the severe growth retardation observed in the majority of infants with short bowel syndrome requiring isolated small bowel or combined liver-small bowel transplantation [7]. In contrast, patients acquiring end-stage liver disease in post-infantile life more commonly undergo rescue liver transplantation because of acute conditions such as fulminant hepatitis or intoxications, without preceding growth failure. A third group of patients with liver failure is comprised of syndromal disorders with hepatic involvement. In these children, chronic liver failure may be one of several factors contributing to severe growth retardation. A genetic disposition for small stature has been suggested in Alagille or Byler syndrome; intrauterine growth retardation occurs in 50% of patients affected with these disorders and normalization of liver function by transplantation does not appear to induce catch-up growth [8–10].

Growth is also suboptimal in patients with severe cardiac disease awaiting transplantation. Impaired tissue oxygenation can cause impaired intestinal motility and nutrient malabsorption, acidosis, increased energy expenditure and even ischemic injury to the hypothalamo-pituitary axis with resultant insufficiencies of one or more of the hormones promoting growth and development [11].

FACTORS AFFECTING POST-TRANSPLANT GROWTH AND DEVELOPMENT

Kidney transplantation

Post-transplant growth and development has been studied most systematically in renal allograft recipients. While a wide variety of growth patterns after kidney transplantation has been reported by individual centers, ranging from progressive growth failure to almost complete catch-up growth [12–26], most reports are in agreement about the main determinants of post-transplant growth. These are the age and the degree of stunting at time of transplantation [15,16,26–29], the level of allograft function and the modalities of glucocorticoid treatment.

The potential for post-transplant catch-up growth appears to be inversely related to the *age at transplantation*. Excellent catch-up growth is unanimously observed in infants [15,27–30]. The critical age beyond which a significant improvements in height SD were no longer observed was 2 [28], 6 [27,29], 7 [15], 10 [31] and 12 years [25] in different studies. Pubertal growth seems to benefit least from renal transplantation. As in dialyzed patients, the onset of puberty and the pubertal growth spurt are delayed in renal allograft recipients by approximately 2 years. Although a distinct acceleration of height velocity occurs, total pubertal height gain is subnormal because of a shortened duration of the pubertal growth spurt [32]. An inverse relationship between pubertal peak height velocity and cumulative glucocorticoid intake has been observed [32,33].

In addition to the impact of age, the change in standardized height following renal transplantation is closely correlated to the *height at time of grafting* [30,34]. Hence, the general principle of catch-up growth "by demand" (i.e. the tendency of an organism to return to a predetermined growth channel after removal of growth-inhibitory conditions) holds also true for renal allograft recipients.

Post-transplant growth appears to be very sensitive to the *function of the allograft*. Whereas native kidney function only affects linear growth when glomerular filtration rate (GFR) is consistently reduced to less than 30 mL/min/1.73 m^2, post-transplant growth velocity is significantly reduced at any GFR below 60 mL/min/1.73 m^2 [14,27]. Multivariate analyses have confirmed that the growth-suppressive effects of poor graft function is independent of glucocorticoid dosage [22,25].

In view of the profound growth-suppressive endocrine and metabolic effects of *glucocorticoids* (see below), there is little doubt that this component of immunosuppressive medica-

tion has a major role in post-transplant growth. Results from clinical trials using modified steroid administration, complete steroid withdrawal or even primary steroid avoidance protocols have provided compelling evidence that glucocorticoids affect catch-up growth in renal transplant recipients (see below). On the other hand, surprisingly few studies found a consistent correlation between steroid dosage and the post-transplant change in standardized height [12,33]. The lack of a consistent correlation between glucocorticoid dose and post-transplant growth may be explained by a nonlinear "threshold" relationship, and by the large interindividual variability of glucocorticoid resorption and pharmacokinetics. Indeed, the area under the serum methylprednisolone concentration curve was superior to the administered glucocorticoid dose in predicting post-transplant growth rates [35].

After more than three decades of pediatric renal transplantation, several thousand patients worldwide have achieved *final adult height*. This provides the opportunity to assess the ultimate completeness of post-transplant catch-up growth, and to analyze the eventual impact of the modulatory factors mentioned above on the ultimate endpoint of longitudinal growth. In the past 5 years, final height has been assessed in three single center studies and one registry report [32,34, 36,37]. Adult height was found to be below the normal range in 25–41% of all patients who developed ESRD and underwent kidney transplantation during childhood. Significant but incomplete post-transplant catch-up growth was noted in the single center studies. In 237 children reported to the NAPRTCS registry who had received a graft at age ≤ 12 years, mean final height SD was exactly identical to standardized height at the time of transplantation, indicating no overall catch-up growth in the pediatric renal transplant population as a whole [37]. As found for early post-transplant growth in the studies cited above, final height was inversely related to the age at transplantation; significant catch-up growth was limited to prepubertal patients. The most severely stunted patients exhibited the most marked post-transplant growth improvement, and renal graft function was an additional independent predictor of final height. The height attained at time of transplantation remained the most significant predictor of final height, illustrating the limited overall potential for post-transplant catch-up growth in the ESRD population. In addition, an average prednisone dosage in excess of 0.15 mg/kg/day was independently associated with a retarded final height in the NAPRTCS analysis [37].

Liver transplantation

Post-transplant catch-up growth is observed in 40–50% of liver allograft recipients [5,8,38]. In the 560 pediatric liver allograft recipients followed in the SPLIT registry, a slight increase in mean standardized height from −1.3 to −1.1 was noted [3]. As in kidney transplantation, age and the degree of stunting at time of transplantation are the most important predictors of post-transplant catch-up growth [5,38]. Young infants usually exhibit substantial catch-up growth [4,5,38,39], whereas older children perform less well. The best growth recovery was seen in infants aged less than 1 year. In 204 recipients aged 0–1 year reported to the SPLIT registry, the mean standardized height improved from −1.8 at transplant to −1.3 at 18 months post-transplant.

The primary hepatic diagnosis appears to impact on post-transplant growth potential. McDiarmid et al. [4] noted an increase in height z-score of +0.7 at 5 years post-transplant for recipients with biliary atresia compared with a decrease by −1.0 for those with fulminant hepatic failure and −0.9 in those whose primary disease was a tumor [39]. Lacking catch-up growth was also noted in recipients with Alagille syndrome and familial cirrhosis [6,39]. The differences in post-transplant growth performance could either be because of persistent differences in post-transplant growth conditions, or simply reflect the different preferential age at which end-stage liver disease typically occurs.

Long-term growth outcome appears to be favorable in liver allograft recipients. McDiarmid et al. [4] noted an improvement in standardized height from −1.7 SD at baseline to −1.4 SD at 5 years post-transplant in 236 children, Viner et al. [6] an increase from −1.2 to −0.84 SD at 7 years in 107 recipients, and Fouquet et al. [39] an increase from −1.4 to −0.47 SD 10 years post-transplant in 80 children with biliary atresia. Hence, the majority of pediatric liver allograft recipients reach a height in the normal range.

The long-term growth preformance of liver allograft recipients appears to be crucially determined by maintenance steroid administration (see below) and graft function [4,5,40,41]. In immunologically nonproblematic patients with good liver function who can be weaned off steroids entirely, nearly complete catch-up growth is common [4,42,43].

Heart transplantation

Varying growth patterns have been observed in cardiac allograft recipients, ranging from progressive growth retardation to impressive catch-up growth. The early propagation of steroid-free immunosuppressive protocols in this area of organ transplantation has provided evidence that maintenance glucocorticoid therapy is the most important determinant of the long-term growth performance in pediatric cardiac allograft recipients.

In an analysis of 78 pediatric heart allograft recipients receiving low-dose maintenance glucocorticoids (2.4 mg/m^2 at 12 months) subnormal height velocity was observed in 48, 26 and 22% of patients in the first, second and third post-transplant year, respectively, resulting in a progressive deterioration of standardized height [44]. This was accompanied by a significant bone age delay in 65–74% of the population. The retardation of growth and skeletal maturation was most marked in those children transplanted before 7 years and in

those with cardiomyopathy. While progressive bone age delay has also been noted in previous studies [45,46], a rather stable degree of growth retardation was observed in most assessments of populations receiving maintenance glucocorticcoid immunosuppression [45–47].

These results contrast with an impressive catch-up growth seen with steroid-free immunosuppressive regimens. A small group of heart transplant recipients in Newcastle, UK, followed for more than 1 year without maintenance corticosteroid therapy exhibited an increase in standardized height from a mean of −2.15 at baseline to −1.15 [48]. Similarly, in 77 infants transplanted at less than 6 months of age who received no maintenance corticosteroid therapy, catch-up growth was almost universally observed during the first post-transplant year [49]. Interestingly, factors predicting subnormal height at 5 years post-transplant in a population free of maintenance steroid immunosuppression included prolonged hospitalization during the first post-transplant year, frequent late rejection and below-average parental stature.

Lung transplantation

Few data are available on growth following lung transplantation in children. A single paper, from St. Louis Children's Hospital, reports on 88 recipients of a lung transplant [50]. At transplantation the mean height of the recipients was 72% of normal and at the time of the report it was 64%.

Intestinal transplantation

A single report describes the post-transplant growth performance in children undergoing intestinal with or without liver transplantation [7]. In a cohort of 46 children, 35 retained a functioning small-bowel graft for an average of 3 years without any need for additional parenteral nutrition. Immunosuppression was maintained with tacrolimus and prednisone. Despite usually young age at transplantation (median 3.7 years), no catch-up growth was noted. Median height SD was stable around −1.8 throughout the first 2 years post-transplant.

ENDOCRINE MECHANISMS OF GLUCOCORTICOID-INDUCED GROWTH FAILURE

In the post-infantile period, longitudinal growth is mainly driven by the hormones of the somatotropic and, during puberty, of the gonadotropic hormone axis. These endocrine systems appear to be affected to a major degree by glucocorticoid immunosuppression in pediatric allograft recipients.

In children after renal transplantation, growth plates appear responsive to stimulation via the somatotropic axis as suggested by a positive correlation between growth hormone (GH) pulse amplitudes and height velocity [51]. However, pituitary GH secretion is variably reduced, most likely because of a stimulatory effect of chronic glucocorticoid therapy on hypothalamic somatostatin synthesis and release [52]. Hence, some children receiving post-transplant glucocorticoid medication appear to be partially GH deficient. During normal puberty, augmented pulsatile gonadotropin secretion stimulates sex hormone secretion. The increase of circulating sex steroid concentrations elicits the pubertal growth spurt, both by direct action on the growth plate and by stimulating pulsatile GH secretion. In kidney transplant recipients, the pubertal surge of gonadotropin secretion appears intact but, at least in boys, sex steroid levels rise insufficiently [51]. This is associated with a blunted augmentation of GH pulses and a subnormal pubertal height gain [18,51].

In addition to suppressing GH secretion, experimental and clinical evidence suggest that glucocorticoid exposure may suppress GH action on the target organ level. Hepatic GH receptor expression is dose dependently reduced by growth suppressive doses of methylprednisolone treatment in rats [53,54] and circulating GH binding protein, reflecting hepatic GH receptor content, is low in pediatric kidney allograft recipients [18,55,56]. The steroid-induced alterations of GH secretion and action would imply reduced availability of insulin-like growth factor 1 (IGF-1), the principal downstream mediator of GH. Indeed, reduced IGF-1 gene transcription has been demonstrated in glucocorticoid treated animals [54,57]. Surprisingly, plasma IGF-1 levels in glucocorticoid-treated renal allograft recipients are in the normal range [18,55,56]. This discrepancy may be explained by additional steroid-induced alterations of IGF-1 mRNA stability, post-trancriptional processing and secretion of IGF-1 peptide or increased plasma half-life by altered IGF-1 binding protein composition [55]. In contrast to the normal immunoreactive plasma IGF-1 concentrations, IGF *bioactivity* was found significantly suppressed in patients on glucocorticoid treatment [55,58]. It has been suggested that glucocorticoids may induce the production of IGF inhibitors [58]. These putative IGF inhibitors appear to have a molecular weight of 12–20 kD, but have not been characterized any further to date.

In addition to these endocrine effects, glucocorticoids interfere with growth and endochondrial ossification by multiple mechanisms on the level of the growth plate chondrocyte. They inhibit proliferation, suppress autocrine/paracrine IGF-1 synthesis, downregulate chondrocyte GH and IGF-1 receptor expression and interfere with the sulfation and mineralization of epiphyseal cartilage matrix [59,60].

STRATEGIES TO OPTIMIZE POST-TRANSPLANT GROWTH

Glucocorticoid treatment has profound effects on endocrine functions and growth performance in pediatric allograft reci-

pients, but also on multiple other systems including body composition, lipid metabolism, bone mineralization and blood pressure regulation. The severe consequences of steroid-related side-effects for long-term health and quality of life have stimulated the search for alternatives to daily methylprednisolone therapy in pediatric organ transplant recipients [61].

Modification of steroid therapy

Registry results and evidence from clinical trials suggest that improved longitudinal growth can be achieved without any risk for long-term graft function when the same total dose of corticosteroids is applied in an alternate-day rather than a daily fashion [20,25]. In the NAPRTCS registry, alternate-day steroid regimens (performed in 17% of all transplant recipients) predicted a positive change in height SD during the first 2 years post-transplant independently of the absolute corticosteroid dosage. In both studies, a gain in standardized height by 0.5 SD was observed with alternate-day steroid regimens, in contrast with an unchanged height SD observed on daily steroids. A recent analysis of long-term (5–7 years) growth performance in 30 infantile renal allograft recipients receiving alternate-day steroids demonstrated nearly complete catch-up growth, from −1.9 to −0.4 SD, in children aged 2–5 years at time of transplantation, and stable growth at a mean height of −1.1 SD in children who received a graft at age less than 2 years [30]. Eighty-one percent of all patients exhibited some degree of catch-up growth. Because of its well-established safety, alternate-day administration is the preferred mode of steroid therapy in many experienced centers beyond the first post-transplant year in immunologically unproblematic allograft recipients. In the NAPRTCS registry, 26% of all children beyond the fourth year post-transplant are on alternate-day steroid treatment [62].

Deflazacort, a prednisolone derivative, has been proposed as an alternative steroid agent with a potentially more favorable side-effect profile at equivalent anti-inflammatory dosage [63]. Two pilot studies switching pediatric kidney allograft recipients from daily methylprednisolone to deflazacort suggested a distinct improvement of obesity, bone mineralization and dyslipidemia, but observed only marginal effects on longitudinal growth [64,65]. The lack of availability of deflazacort in large parts of the world impedes further assessment of this compound.

Steroid withdrawal

In the first two decades of pediatric *kidney* transplantation, complete steroid withdrawal has been problematic because steroid-free immunosuppressive protocols based on cyclosporine A (CsA) and azathioprine alone resulted in deterioration of renal function in at least 50% of children [19,66]. Nonetheless, several uncontrolled small-scale studies suggested that if successful, steroid withdrawal may result in significant catch-up growth [17,23,67]. More recently, the advent of more potent immunosuppressive agents has increased the therapeutic window for steroid withdrawal in kidney transplantation. Tacrolimus-based immunosuppressive protocols provide an option to reduce the need for glucocorticoids in pediatric renal transplantation. Long-term steroid withdrawal is possible in 70% of pediatric allograft recipients receiving tacrolimus [68]. In 52 children weaned off steroids 6 months post-transplant, mean height had increased from −2.41 to −1.31 SD after 3 years [69]. Furthermore, mycophenolate-mofetil (MMF) has largely replaced azathioprine in the past decade, particularly in CsA-based protocols. Using CsA microemulsion in combination with MMF, Höcker et al. [70] successfully discontinued glucocorticoids in the second post-transplant year in 20 selected patients with major side-effects of steroid therapy, stable graft function and not more than one preceding rejection episode. After 4 years of follow-up, height had increased from −1.60 to −1.0 SD, compared with an unchanged standardized height in a matched control group on continued daily methylprednisolone (4.3 mg/m^2). Catch-up growth was limited to six prepubertal children who improved from −2.24 to −0.77 SD, whereas pubertal patients had no significant benefit from steroid withdrawal with respect to growth. Other sequelae of steroid therapy such as obesity and hypertension were considerably improved.

Steroids are still a cornerstone of immunosuppression in the vast majority of pediatric *liver* transplantation programs. Several uncontrolled [71] and one controlled study [72] evaluated the concept of steroid withdrawal in pediatric liver allograft recipients. In five uncontrolled studies attempting steroid withdrawal at 3–58 months post-transplant with concomitant CsA therapy, acute rejection episodes occurred in 7–27%, chronic rejection in 4–13% and graft loss or patient death in 3–13% of the recipients. In contrast, McDiarmid et al. [72], weaning steroids with very rigid inclusion criteria in 23 patients at a mean interval of 3.5 years post-transplant, a 6% acute rejection rate and no resultant chronic rejection, graft loss or patient death were noted. Unfortunately, no significant benefit of steroid withdrawal on linear growth compared with a control group on continued steroid therapy was observed. In three studies attempting steroid withdrawal within the first post-transplant year using concomitant tacrolimus immunosuppression, the incidence of acute rejection varied from 14% to 29% [71]. Reding [71] compared the impact of steroid withdrawal on linear growth in recipients receiving either CsA or tacrolimus. Within 12 months of steroid discontinuation, standardized height slightly worsened with CsA (−0.2 to −0.4 SD) compared with a modest improvement in the tacrolimus group (−0.2 to +0.3 SD). The observed difference could be a result of the much shorter steroid exposure in the patients receiving tacrolimus (weaned on average 1.2 years post-transplant) compared with those treated with CsA (weaned 5–6 years post-transplant).

In pediatric *heart* transplantation, steroids are commonly discontinued early in the post-transplant period; more than 50% of heart allograft recipients are on steroid-free maintenance immunosuppression 12 months post-transplant [73]. In an analysis of 25 infants who underwent heart transplantation at less than 3 months of age [74], growth performance was compared in 18 patients weaned off steroids 7 months post-transplant with eight patients continued on steroid therapy. There was no difference in standardized height at follow-up between the eight patients maintained on low-dose steroids and the 18 who underwent steroid withdrawal. However, the overall post-transplant growth performance in this group of cardiac allograft recipients was rather poor. The mean standardized height worsened from −1.08 at transplant to −1.8 at 4 years post-transplant.

Steroid avoidance

With the increasing number of new potent and selective immunosuppresive agents, complete steroid avoidance has become a realistic option in pediatric organ transplantation. In addition to the advantage of eliminating all side-effects of glucocorticoid treatment from the beginning, data from animal models suggest that the steroid avoidance strategy may even facilitate the induction of tolerance against allogenic tissue.

Steroid avoidance protocols have been pioneered in *cardiac* transplantation. Almost universal catch-up growth has been observed in pediatric heart transplant recipients. In one large series, only 12% of recipients were below the 5th height percentile 5 years after transplantation [49].

The Stanford group recently reported their very favorable experience of steroid-free *kidney* transplantation in 50 children who received a combination of tacrolimus and MMF or sirolimus, complemented by interleukin 2 (IL-2) receptor blockade during the first 6 post-transplant months [75]. After a mean of 22 months follow-up, acute rejection had occurred in only 8% of the children, compared with 32% in historic matched control patients on a steroid-based regimen. Growth was superior in the steroid-free group. This was most marked in infants younger than 5 years, who gained 1.72 ± 0.83 SD within the first 12 post-transplant months compared with an unchanged mean standardized height in the steroid-treated controls.

A similar immunosuppressive protocol has recently been applied by the pediatric *liver* transplant program in Brussels, Belgium. Twenty children receiving combined tacrolimus and basiliximab were compared with 20 matched historic controls treated with tacrolimus and steroids. The tacrolimus-basiliximab group exhibited higher rejection-free survival rates and significantly better growth rates in the first year after transplantation. The slight growth retardation (−0.57 SD) at time of transplantation was completely caught up within 6 months post-transplant in the steroid-free patients, whereas growth recovered at a slower pace in the steroid-treated children [75].

Growth hormone treatment

Chronic administration of rhGH has proven remarkably successful in the treatment of growth failure in children with chronic renal insufficiency, and resulted in a steady increase of height SD at the time of transplantation in pediatric allograft recipients over the past 15 years. Hence, rhGH treatment has been considered as an alternative to modification or withdrawal of steroid treatment in growth-retarded renal allograft recipients who do not exhibit post-transplant catch-up growth.

Experimental support for this concept has been provided by animal studies showing that the growth-depressing effects of glucocorticoid treatment are compensated by rhGH administration [76,77], mediated in part by stimulation of circulating or local IGF-1 synthesis [78–80].

Numerous uncontrolled trials have suggested a growth-promoting effect of rhGH in children with renal allografts over up to 3 years of therapy [55,56,81–87], with a median annual standardized height increment of 0.5 SD during the first 2 years' treatment. Four randomized controlled trials have provided confirmatory evidence of the short-term (6–12 months) efficacy of rhGH in renal allograft recipients [88–91], and a recent long-term growth assessment in 513 pediatric post-transplant patients and 2263 untreated controls followed in the NAPRTCS registry suggested an increased cumulative height gain and a superior final height (-1.83 ± 0.14 vs. -2.63 ± 0.05 SD) associated with rhGH treatment [31].

Successful growth stimulation was also achieved by rhGH treatment in seven *liver* allograft recipients on prednisolone. In the first treatment year, annual growth velocity increased from 3.9 to 8.2 cm, and median height from –2.7 to –2.1 SD [92].

It has been argued that rhGH may not only antagonize the growth inhibitory, but also the immunosuppressive effects of glucocorticoids. Two large controlled trials and the registry analysis of pediatric renal allograft recipients were powered to evaluate any changes in the risk of rejection and graft failure during rhGH treatment. While none of the studies found an increase in the overall incidence of rejection episodes or the rate of renal function decline, the prospective trials noted an increased risk of subsequent rejection episodes in those patients who had more than one rejection prior to treatment.

CONCLUSIONS

In conclusion, while large individual variation of growth and pubertal development exists in solid organ allograft recipients, as of today many allograft recipients grow up to become undersized adults. Major determinants of post-transplant growth and development are the age at transplantation, long-term graft function, the nature of the underlying disorder and steroid-based immunosuppression. With the currently available immunosuppressive armament, complete withdrawal or even primary avoidance of steroids appears to be possible in the majority of children undergoing solid organ transplantation, at least in recipients without a history of severe or recurrent rejection episodes. However, the growth-promoting efficacy and immunologic safety of minimized steroid exposure remain to be demonstrated in carefully designed comparative trials including age-matched control groups receiving alternateday steroid therapy. Also, the optimal timing of steroid withdrawal still needs to be established. GH treatment may be an alternative to steroid withdrawal in patients with a history of allograft rejection. The transduction of these approaches into routine clinical practice should allow improved catch-up growth and a normal final adult height in many allograft recipients.

REFERENCES

1 Schaefer F, Mehls O. Endocrine and growth disorders in chronic renal failure. In: Avner ED, Niaudet P, Harmon WE, eds. *Pediatric Nephrology*, 5th edn. Baltimore, MD: Lippincott Williams & Wilkins, 2004: 1313–45.

2 North American Pediatric Renal Transplant Cooperative Study (NAPRTCS). *2001 Annual Report*. Rockville, MD: Emmes Corporation, 2001.

3 Studies of Pediatric Liver Transplantation (SPLIT). *Annual Report, 2000*. Rockville, MD: EMMES Corporation, 2000.

4 McDiarmid S, Gornbein J, DeSilva P, *et al.* Factors affecting growth after pediatric liver transplantation. *Transplantation* 1999;67:404–11.

5 Bartosh SM, Thomas SE, Sutton MM, Brady LM, Whitington PF. Linear growth after pediatric liver transplantation. *J Pediatr* 1999;135:624–31.

6 Viner RM, Forton JTM, Cole TJ, *et al.* Growth of long-term suvivors of liver transplantation. *Arch Dis Child* 1999;80:235–40.

7 Iyer K, Horslen S, Iverson A, *et al.* Nutritional outcome and growth of children after intestinal transplantation. *J Pediatr Surg* 2002;37:464–6.

8 Burdelski M, Nolkemper D, Ganschow R, *et al.* Liver transplantation in children: long-term outcome and quality of life. *Eur J Pediatr* 1999;158:S34–42.

9 Quiros-Tejeira RE, Ament ME, Heyman MB, *et al.* Does liver transplantation affect growth pattern in Alagille syndrome? *Liver Transpl* 2000;6:582–7.

10 Arvay JL, Zemel BS, Gallagher PR, *et al.* Body composition of children aged 1 to 12 years with biliary atresia or Alagille syndrome. *J Pediatr Gastroenterol Nutr* 2005;40:146–50.

11 Hathout EH, Chinnock RE. Growth after heart transplantation. *Pediatr Transplant* 2004;8:97–100.

12 DeShazo CV, Simmons RL, Berstein SM, *et al.* Results of renal transplantation in 100 children. *Surgery* 1974;76:461–3.

13 Potter DE, Holliday MA, Wilson SJ, Salvatierra JO. Alternate day steroids in children after renal transplantation. *Transplant Proc* 1975;7:79.

14 Pennisi AJ, Costin G, Phillips LS, *et al*. Linear growth in long-term renal allograft recipients. *Clin Nephrol* 1977;8:415–21.

15 Ingelfinger JR, Grupe WE, Harmon WE, Fernbach SK, Levey RH. Growth acceleration following renal transplantation in children less than 7 years of age. *Pediatrics* 1981;68:255–9.

16 Bosque M, Munian A, Bewick M, Haycock G, Chantler C. Growth after renal transplants. *Arch Dis Child* 1983;58:110–4.

17 Offner G, Hoyer PF, Jüppner H, Krohn HP, Brodehl J. Somatic growth after kidney transplantation. *Am J Dis Child* 1987;141:541–6.

18 Rees L, Greene SA, Adlard P, *et al*. Growth and endocrine function after renal transplantation. *Arch Dis Child* 1988;63:1326–32.

19 Reisman L, Lieberman KV, Burrows L, Schanzer H. Follow-up of cyclosporine-treated pediatric renal allograft recipients after cessation of prednisone. *Transplantation* 1990;49:76–80.

20 Broyer M, Guest G, Gagnadoux M-F. Growth rate in children receiving alternate-day corticosteroid treatment after kidney transplantation. *J Pediatr* 1992;120:721–5.

21 Kaiser BA, Polinsky MS, Palmer JA, *et al*. Growth after conversion to alternate-day corticosteroids in children with renal transplants: a single-center study. *Pediatr Nephrol* 1994;8:320–5.

22 Hokken-Koelega AC, Van Zaal MA, de Ridder MA, *et al*. Growth after renal transplantation in prepubertal children: impact of various treatment modalities. *Pediatr Res* 1994;35:367–71.

23 Chao SM, Jones CL, Powell HR, *et al*. Triple immunosuppression with subsequent prednisolone withdrawal: 6 years' experience in paediatric renal allograft recipients. *Pediatr Nephrol* 1994;8:62–9.

24 Ellis D. Clinical use of tacrolimus (FK-506) in infants and children with renal transplants. *Pediatr Nephrol* 1995;9:487–94.

25 Jabs K, Sullivan EK, Avner ED, Harmon WE. Alternate-day steroid dosing improves growth without affecting graft survival or long-term graft function. A report of the North American Pediatric Renal Transplant Cooperative Study. *Transplantation* 1996;61:31–6.

26 Tejani A, Cortes L, Sullivan EK. A longitudinal study of the natural history of growth post-transplantation. *Kidney Int* 1996;53:103–8.

27 Tejani A, Fine R, Alexander S, Harmon W, Stablein D. Factors predictive of sustained growth in children after renal transplantation. The North American Pediatric Renal Transplant Cooperative Study. *J Pediatr* 1993;122:397–402.

28 Helling TS, Nelson PW, Reed L, *et al*. A seven year experience with kidney transplantation for pediatric end stage renal disease. *Mol Med* 1994;91:33–7.

29 Kohaut EC, Tejani A. The 1994 annual report of the North American Pediatric Renal Transplant Cooperative Study. *Pediatr Nephrol* 1996;10:422–34.

30 Qvist E, Marttinen E, Rönnhom K, *et al*. Growth after renal transplantation in infancy or early childhood. *Pediatr Nephrol* 2002;17:438–43.

31 Fine RN, Stablein D. Long-term use of recombinant human growth hormone in pediatric allograft recipients: a report of the NAPRTCS Transplant Registry. *Pediatr Nephrol* 2005;20:404–8.

32 Nissel R, Brazda I, Feneberg R, *et al*. Effect of renal transplantation in childhood on longitudinal growth and adult height. *Kidney Int* 2004;66:792–800.

33 Schaefer F, Seidel C, Binding A, *et al*. Pubertal growth in chronic renal failure. *Pediatr Res* 1990;28:5–10.

34 Englund MS, Tyden G, Wikstad I, Berg UB. Growth impairment at renal transplantation: a determinant of growth and final height. *Pediatr Transplant* 2003;7:192–9.

35 Sarna S, Hoppu K, Neuvonen PJ, Laine J, Holmberg C. Methylprednisolone exposure, rather than dose, predicts adrenal suppression and growth inhibition in children with liver and renal transplantation. *J Clin Endocrinol Metab* 1997;82:75–7.

36 Rodriguez-Soriano J, Vallo A, Quintela MJ, Malaga S, Loris C. Predictors of final adult height after renal transplantation during childhood: a single-center study. *Nephron* 2000;86:266–73.

37 Fine RN, Ho M, Tejani A. The contribution of renal transplantation to final adult height: a report of the North American Pediatric Renal Transplant Cooperative Study (NAPRTCS). *Pediatr Nephrol* 2001;16:951–6.

38 Renz JF, de Roos M, Rosenthal P, *et al*. Post-transplantation growth in pediatric liver recipients. *Liver Transpl* 2001;7:1040–55.

39 Fouquet V, Alves A, Branchereau S, *et al*. Long-term outcome of pediatric liver transplantation for biliary atresia: a 10-year follow-up in a single center. *Liver Transpl* 2005;11:152–60.

40 Lopez-Espinosa J, Yeste D, Iglesias J, *et al*. Analysis of growth during prepubertal years in long-term survivors after pediatric orthotopic liver transplantation. *J Pediatr Endocrinol Metab* 2004;17:1221–9.

41 Superina R, Zangari A, Acal L. Growth in children following liver transplantation. *Pediatr Transplant* 1998;2:70–5.

42 Kelly D. Nutritional factors affecting growth before and after liver transplantation. *Pediatr Transplant* 1997;1:80–4.

43 Orii T, Ohkohchi N, Koyamada N, *et al*. Growth of pediatric patients with biliary atresia after liver transplantation: influence of age at transplantation and steroid administration. *Transplant Proc* 2000;32:2210–2.

44 Cohen A, Addonizio LJ, Softness B, Lamour JM, McMahon DJ. Growth and skeletal maturation after pediatric cardiac transplantation. *Pediatr Transplant* 2004;8:126–35.

45 De Broux E, Huot CH, Chartrand S, Vobecky S, Chartrand C. Growth and pubertal development following pediatric heart transplantation: a 15-year experience at Ste-Justine Hospital. *J Heart Lung Transplant* 2000;19:825–33.

46 Baum MF, Cutler DC, Fricker FJ, Trimm RF, Mace J. Session VII: physiologic and psychological growth and development in pediatric heart transplant recipients. *J Heart Lung Transplant* 1991;10:848–55.

47 Lebidois J, Kachaner J, Vouhe P, Sidi D, Tamisier D. Heart transplantation in children: mid-term results and quality of life. *Eur J Pediatr* 1992;151:S59–64.

48 Au J, Gregory JW, Colquhoun IW, *et al*. Paediatric cardiac transplantation with steroid-sparing maintenance imunosuppression. *Arch Dis Child* 1992;67:1262–6.

49 Chinnock R, Baum M. Somatic growth in infant heart transplant recipients. *Pediatr Transplant* 1998;2:30.

50 Sweet SC, Spray T, Huddleston CB. Pediatric lung transplantation at St. Louis Children's Hospital, 1990–95. *Am J Respir Crit Care Med* 1997;155:1027–35.

51 Schaefer F, Hamill G, Stanhope R, Preece MA, Schärer K. Cooperative study on pubertal development in chronic renal failure: pulsatile growth hormone secretion in peripubertal patients with chronic renal failure. *J Pediatr* 1991;119:568–77.

52 Wehrenberg WB, Janowski BA, Piering AW. Glucocorticoids: potent inhibitors and stimulators of growth hormone secretion. *Endocrinology* 1990;**126**:3200–3.

53 Tönshoff B, Eden S, Weiser E, *et al.* Reduced hepatic growth hormone (GH) receptor gene expression and increase in plasma GH binding protein in experimental uremia. *Kidney Int* 1994; **45**:1085–92.

54 Gabrielsson BG, Carmignac DF, Flavell DM, Robinson ICAF. Steroid regulation of growth hormone (GH) receptor and GH binding protein messenger ribonucleic acids in the rat. *Endocrinology* 1995;**133**:2445–52.

55 Tönshoff B, Haffner D, Mehls O, *et al.* German Study Group for Growth Hormone Treatment in Chronic Renal Failure. Efficacy and safety of growth hormone treatment in short children with renal allografts: three year experience. *Kidney Int* 1993;**44**: 199–207.

56 van Dop C, Jabs KL, Donohue PA, *et al.* Accelerated growth rates in children treated with growth hormone after renal transplantation. *J Pediatr* 1992;**120**:244–50.

57 Luo J, Murphy LJ. Dexamethasone inhibits growth hormone induction of insulin-like growth factor-I (IGF-I) messenger ribonucleic acid (mRNA) in hypophysectomized rats and reduces IGF-I mRNA abundance in the intact rat. *Endocrinology* 1989; **125**:165–71.

58 Unterman TG, Phillips LS. Glucocorticoid effects on somatomedins and somatomedin inhibitors. *J Clin Endocrinol Metab* 1985;**61**:618–26.

59 Silbermann M, Maor G. Mechanisms of glucocorticoid-induced growth retardation: impairment of cartilage mineralization. *Acta Anatomica* 1978;**101**:140–9.

60 Jux C, Leiber K, Hügel U, *et al.* Dexamethasone inhibits growth hormone (GH)-stimulated growth by suppression of local insulin-like growth factor (IGF)-I production and expression of GH- and IGF-I receptor in cultured rat chondrocytes. *Endocrinology* 1998;**139**:3296–305.

61 Reding R, Webber SA, Fine R. Getting rid of steroids in pediatric solid-organ transplantation? *Pediatr Transplant* 2004;**8**:526–30.

62 Benfield MR, Sullivan EK, Stablein DM, Tejani A. The 1997 Annual Renal Transplantation in Children Report of the North American Pediatric Renal Transplant Cooperative Study (NAPRTCS). *Pediatr Transplant* 1999;**3**:152–67.

63 Ferraris J, Fainstein Day P, Balzaretti M, *et al.* Effect of therapy with a new glucocorticoid, deflazacort, on growth velocity and thyroid function in renal transplantation. *Pediatr Nephrol* 1992; **6**:C140.

64 Ferraris JR, Pasqalini T, Legal S, *et al.* The Deflazacort Study Group. Effect of deflazacort versus methylprednisone on growth, body composition, lipid profile, and bone mass after renal transplantation. *Pediatr Nephrol* 2000;**14**:682–8.

65 Schärer K, Feneberg R, Klaus G, *et al.* Experience with deflazacort in children and adolescents after renal transplantation. *Pediatr Nephrol* 2000;**14**:457–63.

66 Ingulli E, Sharma V, Singh A, Suthanthiran M, Tejani A. Steroid withdrawal, rejection and the mixed lymphocyte reaction in children after renal transplantation. *Kidney Int Suppl* 1993;**43**: S36–9.

67 Klare B, Strom TM, Hahn H, *et al.* Remarkable long-term prognosis and excellent growth in kidney-transplant children under cyclosporine monotherapy. *Transplant Proc* 1991;**23**:1013–7.

68 Chakrabarti P, Wong HY, Scantlebury VP, *et al.* Outcome after steroid withdrawal in pediatric renal transplant patients receiving tacrolimus-based immunosuppression. *Transplantation* 2000; **70**:760–4.

69 Ellis D. Growth and renal function after steroid-free tacrolimus-based immunosuppression in children with renal transplants. *Pediatr Nephrol* 2000;**14**:689–94.

70 Höcker B, John U, Plank C, *et al.* Successful withdrawal of steroids in pediatric renal transplant recipients receiving cyclosporine A and mycophenolate mofetil treatment: results after four years. *Transplantation* 2004;**78**:228–34.

71 Reding S. Steroid withdrawal in liver transplantation. *Transplantation* 2000;**70**:405–10.

72 McDiarmid S, Farmer DA, Goldstein LI, *et al.* A randomized prospective trial of steroid withdrawal after liver transplantation. *Transplantation* 1995;**60**:1443.

73 Boucek MM, Edwards LB, Keck BM, *et al.* The registry of the International Society of Heart and Lung Transplantation: Fifth official pediatric report, 2001 to 2002. *J Heat Lung Transplant* 2002;**21**:827–40.

74 Hirsch R, Huddleston CB, Mendeloff EN, Sekarski TJ, Canter TE. Infant and donor organ growth after heart transplantation in neonates with hypoplastic left heart syndrome. *J Heart Lung Transplant* 1996;**15**:1093–100.

75 Reding R, Gras J, Sokal E, Otte JB, Davies HF. Steroid-free liver transplantation in children. *Lancet* 2003;**362**:2068–70.

76 Selye H. Prevention of cortisone overdosage effects with the somatotropic hormone (STH). *Am J Physiol* 1952;**171**:381–4.

77 Kovàcs G, Fine RN, Worgall S, *et al.* Recombinant human growth hormone prevents catabolic effects of methylprednisolone in the healthy and uremic organism. *Kidney Int* 1991;**40**: 1032–40.

78 Tomas FM, Knowles SE, Owens PC. Insulin-like growth factor I (IGF-I) variants are anabolic in dexamethasone treated rats. *Biochem J* 1992;**282**:91–7.

79 Mehls O, Tönshoff B, Kovacs G, *et al.* Interaction between glucocorticoids and growth hormone. *Acta Paediatr Suppl* 1993; **388**:77–82.

80 Kovacs GT, Oh J, Kovacs J, *et al.* Growth promoting effects of growth hormone and IGF-I are additive in experimental uremia. *Kidney Int* 1996;**49**:1413–21.

81 Johannson G, Janssens F, Proesmans W. Treatment with genotropin in short children with chronic renal failure, either before active replacement therapy or with functioning renal transplants: an interim report on five European studies. *Acta Paediatr Scand* 1990;**370**:36–42.

82 Fine RN, Yadin O, Nelson PA, *et al.* Recombinant human growth hormone treatment of children following renal transplantation. *Pediatr Nephrol* 1991;**5**:147–51.

83 van Es A. Growth hormone treatment in short children with chronic renal failure and after renal transplantation: combined data from European clinical trials. *Acta Paediatr Scand* 1991;**379**:42–8.

84 Hokken-Koelega AC, Stijnen T, de Jong RC, *et al.* A placebo-controlled, double-blind trial of growth hormone treatment in prepubertal children after renal transplant. *Kidney Int Suppl* 1996;**53**:S128–34.

85 Rees L, Rigden SPA, Ward G, Preece MA. Treatment of short stature in renal disease with recombinant human growth hormone. *Arch Dis Child* 1990;**65**:856–60.

86 Hokken-Koelega AC, de Jong RC, Donckerwolcke RA, Groothoff JW, Wolff ED. Use of recombinant human growth hormone (rhGH) in pubertal patients with CRI/dialysis/post-transplant: Dutch data. Dutch Study Group on Growth in Children with Chronic Renal Disease. *Br J Clin Pract Symp Suppl* 1996;**85**:5–6.

87 Hokken-Koelega AC, Stijnen T, de Ridder MA, *et al.* Growth hormone treatment in growth-retarded adolescents after renal transplant. *Lancet* 1994;**343**:1313–7.

88 Hokken-Koelega ACS, Stijnen T, de Jong RC, *et al.* A placebo-controlled double-blind trial of growth hormone treatment in prepubertal children with renal allografts. *Kidney Int* 1996; **49**(Suppl):S128–34.

89 Maxwell H, Rees L, for the British Association for Paediatric Nephrology. Randomised controlled trial of recombinant human growth hormone in prepubertal and pubertal renal transplant recipients. *Arch Dis Child* 1998;**79**:481–7.

90 Guest G, Berard E, Crosnier H, *et al.* Effects of growth hormone in short children after renal transplantation. *Pediatr Nephrol* 1998;**12**:437–46.

91 Fine RN, Stablein D, Cohen AH, Tejani A, Kohaut E. Recombinant human growth hormone post-renal transplantation in children: a randomized controlled study of the NAPRTCS. *Kidney Int* 2002;**62**:688–96.

92 Rodeck B, Kardoff R, Melter M, Ehrich JH. Improvement of growth after growth hormone treatment in children who undergo liver transplantation. *J Pediatr Gastroenterol Nutr* 2000;**31**: 286–90.

51 Cognitive Development

Erik Qvist, Hannu Jalanko and Christer Holmberg

Most children who undergo solid organ transplantation (TX) have suffered from a chronic illness, which may affect their cognitive development [1]. Failure of a major organ, such as the liver, kidney or heart, often leads to neuropsychologic sequelae with cognitive deficits [2]. Many children suffer from additional disabilities that will increase the risk, particularly if the underlying disease or treatment affects the developing brain. Growth retardation, often connected with malnutrition, is common in organ failure and may affect neurodevelopment and cognitive function [3]. Thus, in very young children, a less favorable developmental outcome may be expected with early onset of the disease and longer duration of end-stage organ failure [4]. With improved survival after organ transplantation, the number of children surviving into adulthood increases, and the issue of their cognitive development is of paramount importance.

Numerous standardized tests assess cognitive development and many are useful in comparing development within a population (e.g. pre- and post-transplantation). However, the value of this information is limited when comparing different populations, age groups and treatment regimens, with a vast number of confounding factors. The heterogeneity of patients and small sample sizes in the studies make it difficult to draw definitive conclusions on the impact of interventions such as transplantation on cognitive development [4]. Coping skills and psychosocial adjustment of the children and their parents affect cognitive performance, a circumstance that is usually difficult to assess [5,6]. One of the easiest measures of cognitive performance is school performance (i.e. the number of transplanted children who are attending age-appropriate regular classes), which gives information comparable to employment figures in adults. Many studies compare their results with historical data and most children perform better than historical controls.

However, for a comprehensive analysis of cognitive performance, standardized tests for global intelligence, achievement (for detecting specific impairment, e.g. mathematical and language deficits) and neuropsychologic evaluation, including adequate control groups, should be administered [4]. Understandably, such reports are scarce in the literature. Most of the experience has been gathered from patients with chronic renal failure (CRF), dialysis treatment and after kidney TX.

KIDNEY TRANSPLANTATION

Cognitive performance

Children with a severe renal disease from birth are vulnerable to neurologic complications, and the first reports were extremely disappointing. Progressive encephalopathy, characterized by developmental delay, microcephaly, hypotonia, seizures, dyskinesia and electroencephalogram (EEG) abnormalities, was described in children with untreated CRF as well as in patients on dialysis. This unfavorable outcome presumably had a multifactorial etiology resulting from toxic effects of uremia, malnutrition, aluminum toxicity and from the psychosocial complications associated with a severe chronic illness [7–10].

TX has subsequently been shown to improve neurodevelopmental outcome in both adults and children and to ameliorate many of the adverse effects of CRF [11–14]. In the report by Davis *et al.* [11], 12 of 18 children under 3 years of age improved from mild delay to normal mental development when tested before and after TX. Cognitive performance may still be inferior compared with healthy children, as was shown in a multicenter study by Brouhard *et al.* [15]. Sixty-one percent of the transplant patients attended regular full-time school classes compared with 83% of their healthy siblings. The average intelligence quotient (IQ) and the scoring on achievement tests were significantly lower for the patients than for their siblings [15]. In the European Dialysis and Transplant Association (EDTA) registry report, 16% of children who had renal replacement therapy had entered special schools for the handicapped [16]. Davis [17] reported the long-term educational status of children with CRF since infancy. In that report, 76% attended full-time regular classes and 14% attended full-time special classes. In children with CRF since infancy and TX under 5 years of age, attendance at a special school (21%) after TX was mainly dependent on additional comorbidity (such as brain ischemia) [18]. Englund *et al.* [19] reported a normal school attendance of 94% in children who had survived more than 10 years after TX.

Although kidney function is restored after TX, some of the perturbations in the developing brain caused by CRF and its complications may not be reversible. Neurodevelopmental outcome after TX must therefore be viewed also incorporating the pre-TX history. Much of the progress in the neurodevelopmental outcome of small children with CRF is not solely attributable to TX. Vigorous nutritional support, treatment of uremic complications and elimination of aluminum have contributed to more favorable outcomes [20–24]. Also, the improved management of patients on dialysis has been important [21,24,25] and the survivors show a superior neurodevelopmental outcome compared with historical controls. In a report by Ledermann *et al.* [25], 14 of 16 infants achieved normal developmental milestones or attended mainstream school. In another report by Warady *et al.* [24], 94% of children, who had been on peritoneal dialysis in infancy, attended school full time in age-appropriate classes.

There are conflicting data on whether cognitive performance differs in dialysis and transplant patients [15,26,27]. Lawry *et al.* [26] found no significant differences in intelligence scores between patients undergoing dialysis and after TX (although lower in the dialysis patients), but performance in achievement tests for mathematics and language were significantly better in the TX patients compared with dialysis patients. In the multicenter study by Brouhard *et al.* [15], there were no significant differences between dialysis and transplant patients in achievement tests on spelling, arithmetic or reading or in intelligence tests. However, 75% of the transplant patients were under 10 years of age when CRF was diagnosed, compared with only 27% in the dialysis group. Both groups had lower intelligence scores and lower achievement scores compared with age-matched siblings [15]. Mendley and Zelko [14] studied children using refined computer-based neuropsychologic assessments during dialysis and after TX and found improvement in several measurements, such as in mental processing speed and working memory. This was consistent with the finding of Kramer *et al.* [13], who investigated adults, analyzing specific electroencephalogram potentials as a marker of mental processing speed. The results improved after TX.

Risk factors

There are several possible risk factors affecting outcome and cognitive performance of children with CRF (Table 51.1). The improved management of these patients has improved their neurodevelopmental outcome compared with historical controls. Adequate nutrition and dialysis treatment are of supreme importance, particularly in infants and small children. Early onset and longer duration of CRF affecting the developing brain are major risk factors for an inferior cognitive outcome [4,12,15]. Aluminum intoxication is an

Table 51.1 Risk factors for an impaired cognitive development in chronic renal failure.

Disease-specific
    Other organ (e.g. brain) manifestations
Age
Nutrition
Uremia
    Multifactorial etiology
Aluminum toxicity
Hypertension/hemodynamic crises
Seizures
Severe infections
Disability that affects learning
    e.g. hearing handicap
Chronic severe illness/hospitalization
Drugs

iatrogenic problem caused mainly by the use of aluminum compounds for phosphate binding. Severe neurologic complications were reported in the 1980s in relation to the oral intake of aluminum in patients with CRF [10,28]. Aluminum toxicity has been shown to cause encephalopathy, metabolic bone disease and microcytic anemia [29]. Subsequently, many reports have attributed an improved neurodevelopmental outcome in CRF, at least in part, to avoiding aluminum, although this aspect has not been specifically studied [20,24]. It is still unclear which uremic factors are deleterious for cognitive performance [30]. It is also unclear if the uremia causes global or more specific impairment of some parts of cognitive functioning [12,14,18].

The most common neurologic complications seen in adult renal transplant recipients are cerebrovascular events [31]. Their risk increases with age and is not a major complication in children after TX [32], with the exception of children with coagulation problems [18,33]. There are few studies in which neuroradiologic investigations have been performed routinely after renal TX. Ischemic lesions in the border-zone or watershed regions of the brain were reported in up to 54% of small children after renal TX (usually visible only with magnetic resonance imaging [MRI]) [33]. However, the findings did not affect neurodevelopmental outcome in most of the children [18]. The timing of their appearance could not be assessed in the study because pre-TX radiology included only computed tomography (CT) scans that do not detect these changes easily [18,33].

Brain atrophy was originally reported in up to 60% of children with CRF, including patients undergoing dialysis and after TX [34–36]. However, Elzouki *et al.* [20] observed a prevalence of 23%, and the authors attributed the improved neurologic outcome to the policy of avoiding aluminum therapy and giving vigorous nutritional support. Severe dilatation of the brain ventricles was also found to be reversible after TX in a report by Valanne *et al.* [33]. Thus, the ventricle dilatation did not represent true atrophy but a reversible contraction of brain tissue caused for example by disturbances of electrolyte and fluid balance, hypoproteinemia or medication [33]. The high prevalence of atrophy reported in earlier studies may, at least partially, be explained by these factors.

In epidemiologic studies, hypertension has been the most important risk factor for stroke [37]. Hypertensive crises prior to TX were also a risk factor for later inferior neurodevelopmental outcome in the study by Qvist et al. [18]. Elevated blood pressure was found in up to 59% of children with stable renal function at a mean of 34 months after TX, measured by 24-hour ambulatory blood pressure monitoring [38]. Accordingly in the report by the North American Pediatric Renal Transplant Cooperative Study Registry (NAPRTCS), 58% were using antihypertensive medication 5 years after TX [39]. Thus, it is important to treat hypertension adequately both pre- and post-TX.

Severe arterial hypertension is often associated with seizures [36,40,41]. In a report by McEnery et al. [41], seizures occurred in 31% of children, either before or after TX. Eighteen percent of the patients had documented seizures after TX and 5% required anticonvulsive treatment in a report by Awan et al. [40]. In the NAPRTCS report of 1997, 6% of living donor recipients and 10% of cadaver donor recipients had anticonvulsant therapy after TX [32]. Children with seizures after renal TX usually have a good prognosis and a good long-term neurologic outcome [41], unless the seizures are secondary to intracerebral pathology [18].

Hearing loss is frequent in renal diseases and after renal TX [42]. Mancini et al. [43] documented sensorineural hearing loss (SNHL) in 47% after TX and Qvist et al. [18] observed an incidence of 20%. Congenital nephropathies and the use of ototoxic drugs were shown to carry an increased risk of SNHL [43]. Hearing loss has also been reported after administration of various immunosuppressive drugs, including cyclosporine A (CsA) [44]. Hearing disability or handicap was reported in 8% of patients in the EDTA registry including both dialysis and TX patients [45]. This was consistent with the two single-center reports above where a hearing aid was required in 7% and 9% of the patients [18,43].

CsA is potentially neurotoxic and a decline in cognitive performance in adult heart transplant patients was related to the cumulative dose of CsA [46]. Schwartz et al. [47] performed CT and MRI on patients who had neurologic findings attributed to CsA therapy, and found that the radiologic appearance was identical to that seen in hypertensive encephalopathy. The neurotoxicity may equally be a problem with tacrolimus [48].

LIVER TRANSPLANTATION

Patient survival after pediatric liver TX has improved, with survival rates over 80% [49,50]. Liver transplant recipients may have a different neurodevelopmental and cognitive outcome according to their liver disease. A previously healthy child transplanted because of acute liver failure is different from an infant suffering from a congenital disease such as biliary atresia which constitutes over 40% of patients in registry reports [49]. The increased risk for an inferior outcome in small children has been shown in several studies [51,52]. Thus, there is a major concern that small children will have an inferior neurodevelopmental outcome, regardless of a successful TX. Chronic liver disease may lead to neurologic complications [53]. Although the accumulation of cerebrotoxic substances (e.g. bilirubin and ammonia) is harmful [54], correlation of their levels with cognitive development after TX has not yielded consistent results [51]. Correlation of post-TX development with low albumin (which also reflects poor nutritional status) and poor growth before TX has been more convincing [51,55]. Correction of malnutrition seems to have had a major impact on improved neurodevelopmental outcome after liver TX in infants and small children [51,55].

A substantial number of liver transplanted children are considered to have inferior cognitive performance. In the study by Wayman et al. [51], 35% (TX at less than 2 years of age) were considered developmentally delayed 1 year after TX. The degree of disability had been even higher 3 months after TX, which underlines the importance of long-term follow-up [51,55]. Eighteen percent were found to be mentally deficient (IQ scores below 70) and the mean scores for the whole group were in the low average range in the long-term report by Kennard et al. [56]. The outcome is usually better if older children are included in the studies [57,58]. Schulz et al. [58] reported that the majority of their liver transplant children scored within the normal range on cognitive tests (half of the children were living related recipients). However, performances were lower compared with healthy controls, which has been confirmed in other studies [59]. Some specific cognitive problems have been more frequent than others, particularly visuospatial impairment and language problems [51,60]. Krull et al. [61] compared liver transplanted children with matched children with cystic fibrosis. Transplant patients had lower IQ and performance scores on language measures.

In a report of 56 pediatric living related liver recipients who had survived more than 3 years after TX, 82% led normal daily lives with daily school attendance [62]. Millar et al. [63] have reported that all their school-age survivors attended school normally. In another report, more than 1 year after TX, all except one of 26 children were attending a normal school [64]. Stone et al. [65] also reported a 100% school attendance in 20 children with a follow-up up to 10 years after TX. Two-thirds of them did not have any special education needs [65]. Törnqvist et al. [66] studied long-term adjustment after liver TX in 146 children. School attendance after TX was not substantially affected. However, most of the transplanted children had higher problem scores compared with healthy children, although most were within the normal range. Thus, it seems that rehabilitation, in terms of education and school attendance, is good in survivors after pediatric liver TX. Awareness of the children's need for special attention may, however, be underestimated. Kennard *et al.* [56] recognized learning problems in 26% of long-term survivors of pediatric liver TX, but only 38% of them had received special education services.

HEART AND/OR LUNG TRANSPLANTATION

In many studies, children have shown cognitive performance within normal limits after heart TX, albeit inferior to controls [67,68]. The two major patient groups requiring heart TX are children with cardiomyopathy and those with complex congenital heart defects. Neurodevelopmental outcome and cognitive performance may be very different in an infant with a congenital heart defect compared with a previously healthy adolescent with an acquired cardiomyopathy.

Cognitive development has been shown to be inferior for infants after heart TX. In the study by Baum *et al.* [69], 67% scored within normal limits and 13–23% were significantly delayed as assessed by the Bayley mental and psychomotor developmental indexes. The underlying disease seems to affect outcome and children with cyanotic congenital heart defects may not improve their cognitive performance even after a successful TX [70,71]. Chronic hypoxia, as in cyanotic congenital heart diseases, is expected to have some impact on cognitive brain function [70]. Surgery of congenital heart defects using circulatory arrest may also increase the risk of brain damage [72] and congenital heart disease may involve congenital defects of the brain [73]. Thus, the impact of age is difficult to assess. As stated above, the age at TX is confounded by the severity of the disease and the underlying diagnosis.

Neurologic complications have occurred in 10–50% of children [74–76]; however, most of them are mild. Persistent neurologic sequelae were reported in only 4% by Bauer *et al.* [74]. The incidence of neurologic complications was higher during the early years of heart TX and lower in a later cohort, as reported by Martin *et al.* [76]. Survival also improved and it may be assumed that both results reflect the improved results experienced in heart TX and patient management with time [76]. Forty-five percent of 135 children had neurologic complications after lung TX in a report by Wong *et al.* [77]. Seizures occurred in 27% but encephalopathy, headache, depression and focal neurologic deficits were also documented [77]. Many of the seizures were caused by CsA toxicity and the long-term prognosis accordingly not necessary inferior [77].

School performance and cognitive development have been shown to be within normal limits in many studies, but inferior compared with normal children [68]. In a follow-up study of 47 heart TX and 34 heart-lung TX recipients, including children with congenital heart defects, cardiomyopathy and cystic fibrosis, the results were compared with matched healthy children. As a group, the transplant children performed within normal limits but significantly lower than the control group. Children with congenital heart defects consistently performed at a lower level than the other children with cardiomyopathy and cystic fibrosis, although the differences did not reach statistical significance [68].

CONCLUSIONS

It is to be expected that cognitive performance after solid organ TX in children will improve in the future. Management, both before and after TX, becomes better all the time. However, it is possible that more patients with severe diseases affecting cognitive development are incorporated in transplant programs in the future. It is of paramount importance to assess continuously the neurodevelopmental outcome and cognitive performance in transplanted children in order to identify avoidable or treatable risk factors.

REFERENCES

1 Cadman D, Boyle M, Szatmari P, Offord DR. Chronic illness, disability, and mental and social well-being: findings of the Ontario Child Health Study. *Pediatrics* 1987;**79**:805–13.

2 Farmer ME. Cognitive deficits related to major organ failure: the potential role of neuropsychological testing. *Neuropsychol Rev* 1994;**4**:117–60.

3 Fine RN. Growth following solid-organ transplantation. *Pediatr Transplant* 2002;**6**:47–52.

4 Fine RN, Alonso EM, Fischel JE, *et al.* Pediatric transplantation of the kidney, liver and heart: summary report. *Pediatr Transplant* 2004;**8**:75–86.

5 Wallander JL, Varni JW. Effects of pediatric chronic physical disorders on child and family adjustment. *J Child Psychol Psychiatry* 1998;**39**:29–46.

6 Lavigne JV, Faier-Routman J. Correlates of psychological adjustment to pediatric physical disorders: a meta-analytic review and comparison with existing models. *J Dev Behav Pediatr* 1993;**14**:117–23.

7 Geary DF, Fennell RS, Andriola M, *et al.* Encephalopathy in children with chronic renal failure. *J Pediatr* 1980;**97**:41–4.

8 McGraw ME, Haka-Ikse K. Neurologic-developmental sequelae of chronic renal failure in infancy. *J Pediatr* 1985;**106**:579–83.

9 Rotundo A, Nevins TE, Lipton M, *et al.* Progressive encephalopathy in children with chronic renal insufficiency in infancy. *Kidney Int* 1982;**21**:486–91.

10 Sedman AB, Wilkening GN, Warady BA, Lum GM, Alfrey AC. Encephalopathy in childhood secondary to aluminum toxicity. *J Pediatr* 1984;**105**:836–8.

11 Davis ID, Chang PN, Nevins TE. Successful renal transplantation accelerates development in young uremic children. *Pediatrics* 1990;**86**:594–600.

12 Fennell RS 3rd, Rasbury WC, Fennell EB, Morris MK. Effects of kidney transplantation on cognitive performance in a pediatric population. *Pediatrics* 1984;**74**:273–8.

13 Kramer L, Madl C, Stockenhuber F, et al. Beneficial effect of renal transplantation on cognitive brain function. Kidney Int 1996;49:833–8.

14 Mendley SR, Zelko FA. Improvement in specific aspects of neurocognitive performance in children after renal transplantation. Kidney Int 1999;56:318–23.

15 Brouhard BH, Donaldson LA, Lawry KW, et al. Cognitive functioning in children on dialysis and post-transplantation. Pediatr Transplant 2000;4:261–7.

16 Ehrich JH, Rizzoni G, Broyer M, et al. Rehabilitation of young adults during renal replacement therapy in Europe. 2. Schooling, employment, and social situation. Nephrol Dial Transplant 1992;7:579–86.

17 Davis ID. Pediatric renal transplantation: back to school issues. Transplant Proc 1999;31:61S–2S.

18 Qvist E, Pihko H, Fagerudd P, et al. Neurodevelopmental outcome in high-risk patients after renal transplantation in early childhood. Pediatr Transplant 2002;6:53–62.

19 Englund M, Berg U, Tyden G. A longitudinal study of children who received renal transplants 10–20 years ago. Transplantation 2003;76:311–8.

20 Elzouki A, Carroll J, Butinar D, Moosa A. Improved neurological outcome in children with chronic renal disease from infancy. Pediatr Nephrol 1994;8:205–10.

21 Holtta T, Ronnholm K, Jalanko H, Holmberg C. Clinical outcome of pediatric patients on peritoneal dialysis under adequacy control. Pediatr Nephrol 2000;14:889–97.

22 Kari JA, Gonzalez C, Ledermann SE, Shaw V, Rees L. Outcome and growth of infants with severe chronic renal failure. Kidney Int 2000;57:1681–7.

23 Ledermann SE, Shaw V, Trompeter RS. Long-term enteral nutrition in infants and young children with chronic renal failure. Pediatr Nephrol 1999;13:870–5.

24 Warady BA, Belden B, Kohaut E. Neurodevelopmental outcome of children initiating peritoneal dialysis in early infancy. Pediatr Nephrol 1999;13:759–65.

25 Ledermann SE, Scanes ME, Fernando ON, et al. Long-term outcome of peritoneal dialysis in infants. J Pediatr 2000;136: 24–9.

26 Lawry KW, Brouhard BH, Cunningham RJ. Cognitive functioning and school performance in children with renal failure. Pediatr Nephrol 1994;8:326–9.

27 Fukunishi I, Honda M. School adjustment of children with end-stage renal disease. Pediatr Nephrol 1995;9:553–7.

28 Andreoli SP, Bergstein JM, Sherrard DJ. Aluminum intoxication from aluminum-containing phosphate binders in children with azotemia not undergoing dialysis. N Engl J Med 1984;310: 1079–84.

29 Sedman A. Aluminum toxicity in childhood. Pediatr Nephrol 1992;6:383–93.

30 Moe SM, Sprague SM. Uremic encephalopathy. Clin Nephrol 1994;42:251–6.

31 Adams HP Jr, Dawson G, Coffman TJ, Corry RJ. Stroke in renal transplant recipients. Arch Neurol 1986;43:113–5.

32 Benfield MR, McDonald R, Sullivan EK, Stablein DM, Tejani A. The 1997 Annual Renal Transplantation in Children Report of the North American Pediatric Renal Transplant Cooperative Study (NAPRTCS). Pediatr Transplant 1999;3:152–67.

33 Valanne L, Qvist E, Jalanko H, Holmberg C, Pihko H. Neuroradiologic findings in children with renal transplantation under 5 years of age. Pediatr Transplant 2004;8:44–51.

34 Schnaper HW, Cole BR, Hodges FJ, Robson AM. Cerebral cortical atrophy in pediatric patients with end-stage renal disease. Am J Kidney Dis 1983;2:645–50.

35 Steinberg A, Efrat R, Pomeranz A, Drukker A. Computerized tomography of the brain in children with chronic renal failure. Int J Pediatr Nephrol 1985;6:121–6.

36 Trompeter RS, Smith RL, Hoare RD, Neville BG, Chantler C. Neurological complications of arterial hypertension. Arch Dis Child 1982;57:913–7.

37 MacMahon S, Peto R, Cutler J, et al. Blood pressure, stroke, and coronary heart disease. Part 1. Prolonged differences in blood pressure: prospective observational studies corrected for the regression dilution bias. Lancet 1990;335:765–74.

38 Sorof JM, Poffenbarger T, Portman R. Abnormal 24-hour blood pressure patterns in children after renal transplantation. Am J Kidney Dis 2000;35:681–6.

39 Sorof JM, Sullivan EK, Tejani A, Portman RJ. Antihypertensive medication and renal allograft failure: a North American Pediatric Renal Transplant Cooperative Study report. J Am Soc Nephrol 1999;10:1324–30.

40 Awan AQ, Lewis MA, Postlethwaite RJ, Webb NJ. Seizures following renal transplantation in childhood. Pediatr Nephrol 1999;13:275–7.

41 McEnery PT, Nathan J, Bates SR, Daniels SR. Convulsions in children undergoing renal transplantation. J Pediatr 1989;115: 532–6.

42 Bergstrom L, Thompson P. Hearing loss in pediatric renal patients. Int J Pediatr Otorhinolaryngol 1983;5:227–34.

43 Mancini ML, Dello Strologo L, Bianchi PM, Tieri L, Rizzoni G. Sensorineural hearing loss in patients reaching chronic renal failure in childhood. Pediatr Nephrol 1996;10:38–40.

44 Arinsoy T, Akpolat T, Ataman M, et al. Sudden hearing loss in a cyclosporin-treated renal transplantation patient. Nephron 1993;63:116–7.

45 Rizzoni G, Ehrich JH, Broyer M, et al. Rehabilitation of young adults during renal replacement therapy in Europe. 1. The presence of disabilities. Nephrol Dial Transplant 1992;7:573–8.

46 Grimm M, Yeganehfar W, Laufer G, et al. Cyclosporine may affect improvement of cognitive brain function after successful cardiac transplantation. Circulation 1996;94:1339–45.

47 Schwartz RB, Bravo SM, Klufas RA, et al. Cyclosporine neurotoxicity and its relationship to hypertensive encephalopathy: CT and MR findings in 16 cases. AJR Am J Roentgenol 1995;165: 627–31.

48 Scott LJ, McKeage K, Keam SJ, Plosker GL. Tacrolimus: a further update of its use in the management of organ transplantation. Drugs 2003;63:1247–97.

49 Studies of Pediatric Liver Transplantation (SPLIT). Year 2000 outcomes. Transplantation 2001;72:463–76.

50 Burdelski M, Nolkemper D, Ganschow R, et al. Liver transplantation in children: long-term outcome and quality of life. Eur J Pediatr 1999;158(Suppl 2):S34–42.

51 Wayman KI, Cox KL, Esquivel CO. Neurodevelopmental outcome of young children with extrahepatic biliary atresia 1 year after liver transplantation. J Pediatr 1997;131:894–8.

52 Stewart SM, Uauy R, Waller DA, *et al*. Mental and motor development, social competence, and growth one year after successful pediatric liver transplantation. *J Pediatr* 1989;**114**:574–81.

53 Hall WA, Martinez AJ. Neuropathology of pediatric liver transplantation. *Pediatr Neurosci* 1989;**15**:269–75.

54 Butterworth RF. Effects of hyperammonaemia on brain function. *J Inherit Metab Dis* 1998;**21**(Suppl 1):6–20.

55 van Mourik ID, Beath SV, Brook GA, *et al*. Long-term nutritional and neurodevelopmental outcome of liver transplantation in infants aged less than 12 months. *J Pediatr Gastroenterol Nutr* 2000;**30**:269–75.

56 Kennard BD, Stewart SM, Phelan-McAuliffe D, *et al*. Academic outcome in long-term survivors of pediatric liver transplantation. *J Dev Behav Pediatr* 1999;**20**:17–23.

57 Atkison PR, Ross BC, Williams S, *et al*. Long-term results of pediatric liver transplantation in a combined pediatric and adult transplant program. *CMAJ* 2002;**166**:1663–71.

58 Schulz KH, Wein C, Boeck A, Rogiers X, Burdelski M. Cognitive performance of children who have undergone liver transplantation. *Transplantation* 2003;**75**:1236–40.

59 Adeback P, Nemeth A, Fischler B. Cognitive and emotional outcome after pediatric liver transplantation. *Pediatr Transplant* 2003;**7**:385–9.

60 Stewart SM, Hiltebeitel C, Nici J, *et al*. Neuropsychological outcome of pediatric liver transplantation. *Pediatrics* 1991;**87**:367–76.

61 Krull K, Fuchs C, Yurk H, Boone P, Alonso E. Neurocognitive outcome in pediatric liver transplant recipients. *Pediatr Transplant* 2003;**7**:111–8.

62 Asonuma K, Inomata Y, Uemoto S, *et al*. Growth and quality of life after living-related liver transplantation in children. *Pediatr Transplant* 1998;**2**:64–9.

63 Millar AJ, Spearman W, McCulloch M, *et al*. Liver transplantation for children: the Red Cross Children's Hospital experience. *Pediatr Transplant* 2004;**8**:136–44.

64 Chin SE, Shepherd RW, Cleghorn GJ, *et al*. Survival, growth and quality of life in children after orthotopic liver transplantation: a 5 year experience. *J Paediatr Child Health* 1991;**27**:380–5.

65 Stone RD, Beasley PJ, Treacy SJ, Twente AW, Vacanti JP. Children and families can achieve normal psychological adjustment and a good quality of life following pediatric liver transplantation: a long-term study. *Transplant Proc* 1997;**29**:1571–2.

66 Törnqvist J, Van Broeck N, Finkenauer C, *et al*. Long-term psychosocial adjustment following pediatric liver transplantation. *Pediatr Transplant* 1999;**3**:115–25.

67 Stewart SM, Kennard BD, Waller DA, Fixler D. Cognitive function in children who receive organ transplantation. *Health Psychol* 1994;**13**:3–13.

68 Wray J, Long T, Radley-Smith R, Yacoub M. Returning to school after heart or heart-lung transplantation: how well do children adjust? *Transplantation* 2001;**72**:100–6.

69 Baum M, Chinnock R, Ashwal S, *et al*. Growth and neurodevelopmental outcome of infants undergoing heart transplantation. *J Heart Lung Transplant* 1993;**12**:S211–7.

70 Wray J, Sensky T. Congenital heart disease and cardiac surgery in childhood: effects on cognitive function and academic ability. *Heart* 2001;**85**:687–91.

71 Wray J, Radley-Smith R. Developmental and behavioral status of infants and young children awaiting heart or heart-lung transplantation. *Pediatrics* 2004;**113**:488–95.

72 Wypij D, Newburger JW, Rappaport LA, *et al*. The effect of duration of deep hypothermic circulatory arrest in infant heart surgery on late neurodevelopment: the Boston Circulatory Arrest Trial. *J Thorac Cardiovasc Surg* 2003;**126**:1397–403.

73 Glauser TA, Rorke LB, Weinberg PM, Clancy RR. Congenital brain anomalies associated with the hypoplastic left heart syndrome. *Pediatrics* 1990;**85**:984–90.

74 Bauer J, Thul J, Kramer U, *et al*. Heart transplantation in children and infants: short-term outcome and long-term follow-up. *Pediatr Transplant* 2001;**5**:457–62.

75 Lynch BJ, Glauser TA, Canter C, Spray T. Neurologic complications of pediatric heart transplantation. *Arch Pediatr Adolesc Med* 1994;**148**:973–9.

76 Martin AB, Bricker JT, Fishman M, *et al*. Neurologic complications of heart transplantation in children. *J Heart Lung Transplant* 1992;**11**:933–42.

77 Wong M, Mallory GB Jr, Goldstein J, Goyal M, Yamada KA. Neurologic complications of pediatric lung transplantation. *Neurology* 1999;**53**:1542–9.

52 Psychosocial Adaptation and Adherence

Eyal Shemesh

Recipients of solid organ transplantation can expect dramatically improved survival [1–6]. The transplant operation offers improved quality of life (QOL) in recipients [7] compared with the pretransplant status. Cognitive abilities, psychosocial indices and QOL are generally acceptable post-transplant and are comparable to or better than these indices in children who suffer from chronic medical illnesses [8–17]. While the psychosocial and emotional (as well as medical) benefits of organ transplantation are substantial, organ transplantation is best viewed as a "trade off" of a life-threatening serious medical illness with a less severe, but still serious and chronic medical condition [18]. The transplant recipient still faces life-threatening situations as a routine part of the post-transplant course (i.e. infections). The recipient needs to adjust to the limitations and consequences of living with a chronic medical condition, which include the need to take immunosuppressant medications, and routine or emergent medical visits or hospitalizations. Positive psychosocial adjustment to this "post-transplant condition" is extremely important on the way to ensure adherence to medical recommendations and improved QOL as well as graft survival [19].

Solid organ transplant operations (including liver, lung, heart, kidney, small intestine) differ in their procedures, length, the degree of relief they offer and the intensity of follow-up that they require. Yet there is some evidence that pediatric transplant recipients react emotionally in a similar manner to different kinds of transplantation [20,21]. For the sake of brevity as well as coherence, this chapter does not make a distinction between adjustment to different kinds of transplants and discusses them as one entity. This is undoubtedly an oversimplified approach. Also for the sake of brevity, I discuss emotional reactions in children as one group, although developmental differences between children of different ages can be enormous. Finally, I will not specifically discuss children who are a priori disabled or suffer a serious developmental or mental disorder pretransplant (i.e. mentally retarded individuals or individuals with documented psychiatric disease).

One of the main mechanisms by which poor adjustment affects post-transplant outcome is through nonadherence to treatment recommendations [19]. Because nonadherence to medications is of particular interest in pediatric transplant recipients (who need to take immunosuppressants for the rest of their lives in most cases), this chapter is divided into two main components: psychosocial (and psychiatric) considerations in adjustment to the post-transplant phase, and adherence to medical recommendations.

PSYCHOSOCIAL ADJUSTMENT

Any solid organ transplant operation involves the experience of pain, and the risks of the operation and anesthesia. The pretransplant diagnosis as well as the operation itself and its immediate aftermath can be emotionally traumatic [21–24]. In addition, the long-term adjustment following a transplant operation includes the need to cope with an altered body and body image because of a disfiguring scar (although there is also potential improvement in body figure and image because of reduced ascites or edema after some types of transplantation). Recipients also need to take medications and follow an appointment and evaluation schedule, and they live under the constant threat of rehospitalization, rejection and even potential death. This chapter is divide into reactions that are noted in the immediate aftermath of transplantation (first 2 months) in children who had a transplant and their parents, and those that are encountered after that.

Stress reactions immediately after transplantation

Following the transplant operation, the immediate recovery phase includes the experience of pain, discomfort and, at times, delirium or even brief psychotic episodes that may be caused by the effects of anesthetics, pain medications and other medications (such as high doses of corticosteroids). These reactions are not the subject of this chapter, because they are caused by the immediate effects of the biologic interventions rather than by a psychologic adjustment. Other reactions, encountered shortly after transplantation, can be

Table 52.1 Potential immediate post-transplant stress-related reactions in the child (recipient).

Type of stress reaction	Specific symptoms
Acute stress disorder	Extreme anxiety/nervousness, a "state of shock", dissociative phenomena (i.e. excessive "daydreaming" or confusion at certain situations)
Post-traumatic stress symptoms	Anxiety, hypervigilance, hostility (associated feature), avoidance of reminders of the stressor (i.e. does not want to come to clinic), intrusive thoughts about the event (i.e. "can't shake" the memory of what happened)
Depressive symptoms	Does not enjoy things as much as before, sleeping problems, eating problems, sadness, crying, suicidal ideation (in severe cases), irritability (especially in younger children), lack of concentration
Separation–anxiety disorder	Child is not willing to leave the parent, gets extremely angry, anxious or agitated when the parent leaves or even is talking about leaving the child. Note – some of these symptoms almost invariably happen and may be normal and self-contained post-transplant
Increased conflict levels (family/caretakers)	Irritability in communicating with family, "inability to accept" explanations, tension between family members, divorce (in extreme cases), lack of sleep
Adjustment disorder	Depressed mood, irritability, anxiety, behavioral problems, etc. that appear after the stressor (the transplant) and do not meet full criteria for another psychiatric disorder

related to the emotional state that follows transplantation, and include symptoms of acute stress disorder, post-traumatic stress disorder, adjustment disorder, depressive disorders and anxiety disorders [18,21–26]. In families, immediate post-transplant reactions could range from happiness and increased energy through fatigue and exhaustion, and may include communication problems and conflict. It is important to note that none of these need to be present – most transplant recipients recover well and do not develop any psychiatric disorder. Furthermore, although there are no longitudinal data about the progression of psychiatric symptoms in pediatric transplant recipients, data from other medical illnesses [27] and other kind of traumas [28] strongly suggest that nonspecific stress reactions are mostly self-contained. Nevertheless, the practitioner should note these symptoms and follow them; a significant proportion of patients who display severe stress symptoms will eventually develop a fully fledged psychiatric disorder [29]. Potential stress-related symptoms are summarized in Table 52.1. In extreme cases of anxiety, fear or depressed mood, it is important to assess the patient for the existence of suicidal thoughts and ensure a safe environment, and also assess for pre-existing mental health conditions including past reactions to traumatic events. A consultation with a specialist (i.e. a psychiatrist) is probably warranted at this stage. Treatment may include supportive psychotherapy; however, it is not clear what the term "supportive psychotherapy" includes, and there are no controlled studies that assess its efficacy in this, or even similar, settings. Cognitive–behavioral therapy (CBT) has been shown to be effective for the treatment of depressive and anxiety disorders in children [30], including post-transplant (anecdotally [24]). CBT has not been rigorously studied in medically ill children

and is hard to administer in an inpatient setting. If needed, it may be useful to prescribe short-term anxiolytic medications in consultation with the medical team. In cases with active psychotic symptoms or behavioral disruption, short-acting antipsychotics can also be prescribed on a limited basis. With regards to antidepressant medications – selective serotonin reuptake inhibitors (SSRIs) or tricyclic antidepressants (TCAs), our group rarely if ever uses these classes of medications in the immediate post-transplant phase, because of the limited efficacy of antidepressants in children [31]. Finally, as in any traumatic event, it is important not to neglect physical support to the patient and family, including referrals for financial aid if possible, age-appropriate education about the transplant, and pain management.

The family

A child's medical illness may be associated with more traumatic stress symptoms in a parent than even the stress associated with a parent's own life-threatening acute medical illness [32,33]. Symptoms of emotional trauma have been well-documented in parents of children who had a transplant [20,21]. Table 52.2 summarizes potential emotional reactions of parents and families in the immediate post-transplant period. The parent's physical needs (sleep, food) should be met in order to allow the parent to provide ongoing support for the child. Immediately post-transplant, the transplant team may wish to congratulate the parent for having gotten the transplant, but it is also a time to emphasize that it is a long-term challenge. As in any situation where increased distress is experienced, family relations may be strained as well as relationships with the medical team. Within the family as

419

Table 52.2 Potential immediate post-transplant stress-related reactions in the parent of a child recipient.

Type of reaction	Specific symptoms
Acute stress disorder	Same as in the child (see Table 52.1)
Post-traumatic stress symptoms	Anxiety, inability to deal with the child's needs because of "paralysis" when approaching elements of his or her care, sleep problems, inability to concentrate, intrusive thoughts about the event or about "losing" the child
Depressive symptoms	Sleeping problems, eating problems, sadness, inability to concentrate, inability to enjoy things or activities
Increased conflict levels (family/caretakers)	Irritability in communicating with family, "inability to accept" explanations, tension between family members, divorce (in extreme cases), hostility towards caretakers/staff
Adjustment disorder	Depressed mood, irritability, anxiety, that appear after the stressor (the transplant) and do not meet full criteria for another psychiatric disorder in the parent

well as the medical teams, open and consistent communication is important so as to minimize friction [34]. Specific emphasis should also be given to assess and address sibling reactions (even if parents do not bring the issue up). There are studies that document increased conflict levels in families of children who are treated in intensive care settings [34], but interventions to reduce conflict have not been rigorously studied post-transplant. The lack of concrete evidence should not, however, be a reason to fail to address specific aspects that may exacerbate conflict. These may include pre-existing family pathology, psychopathology, medical illness in another family member, the degree of acuity of the child's condition, and lack of resources and social supports. In the author's experience, the role of the psychiatrist in facilitating the family's adjustment in the immediate post-transplant phase is very limited. Emphasis should be given to social work and nursing interventions.

Long-term adjustment

Long-term adjustment in solid organ transplant recipients includes the adjustment to a life-long physical threat, the need to take medications, sometimes inability to bear children, adjustment to altered body appearance (the transplant scar, change in weight) and sometimes physical disability. Adjustment to the post-transplant "state" is ongoing, children never "grow out" of the adjustment phase, and each developmental stage brings new challenges. For example, a previously "well-adjusted" child may become nonadherent, depressed or anxious as adolescence approaches with its specific developmental challenges [19]. Most children manage to adjust well to the transplant and its aftermath; only a minority have clinically significant psychiatric disorders [17,24]. The medical team should be aware of the need to reassess the degree of coping at each developmental stage, and of the particular challenges that may arise. Financial hardship may become more apparent or significant as the

child becomes an older adult. Children may develop new psychopathology (depression, post-traumatic stress), or present with an exacerbation of pre-existing psychopathology. Children who had a transplant, especially adolescents, may engage in risk-taking beha-viors [19] that may have devastating consequences in these patients (i.e. binge-drinking, smoking).

"Good post-transplant adjustment" cannot be defined precisely and is individual to each patient. Coping styles vary, and as long as they are not dysfunctional, different styles can lead to good adjustment. The role of the clinician in long-term management of post-transplant adjustment in recipients is related to several key issues:

1 *Continuous assessment*: of psychopathology, increased distress, increase in psychosocial stressors.

2 *Ongoing education*: different levels of cognitive abilities require different levels of education. Therefore, it should never be assumed that a given child "knows enough" about the illness. Each medical encounter is an opportunity to assess and reassess the child's knowledge of his or her illness and its treatment and provide age-appropriate education.

3 *Intervene early*: if psychopathology, increased level of distress, or increased level of stressors are identified.

4 *Use a multidisciplinary approach*: involve physicians (including psychiatrists if appropriate), social workers, psychologists, educators, community resources, etc. as needed.

Specific treatment modalities (other than education) include social work interventions within the community and family, individual psychotherapy, psychotropic medications and group treatment including post-transplant support groups. The clinician should tailor the interventions to the patient's needs rather than offer it to all or most patients. Thus, it is not necessarily good practice to advocate supportive group treatments for all children, as some children may not benefit from this modality. Similarly, it is not advisable to prescribe anxiolytics to all transplant survivors. An individualized eclectic approach is recommended.

Long-term adjustment in families

As is the case with the child, the patient's family goes through different developmental stages, and faces different challenges at different times. Attention to the family's developmental stage is important. Newly divorced parents, parents who have lost their jobs, or parents who relocate to a different neighborhood, face different challenges after the index event. These events should therefore be looked for and initiate a discussion or even in-depth assessment – if needed – by the medical team. New and distressing events may put an extra burden on already stressed families and be the reason for a drastic change in their level of supervision or support of the child. This may lead to medical as well as emotional consequences in the transplant recipient. Families also need to adjust to the child's different developmental needs and emerging emotional symptoms when applicable. The family should therefore be assessed and treated in tandem with the child, using the same general principles presented above.

Summary

A transplant operation is the first step in a long journey of ongoing adjustment to a life with increased possibilities but also increased distress and ongoing challenges. It is useful to identify key tasks in short- as well as long-term adjustment and address them. Short-term problems may involve more dramatic presentations; long-term adjustment is ongoing and is the key to successful survival. The clinician caring for the pediatric transplant survivor has many options in facilitating this adjustment. Interventions should be used in tandem with an ongoing assessment. Psychosocial adjustment is an ongoing task. Most patients and families are able to overcome the enormous challenges associated with a transplant operation and are able to enjoy healthy and productive lives. Clinicians should strive to identify those patients and families who face temporary or permanent difficulties and offer appropriate treatment at the right time.

ADHERENCE TO MEDICAL RECOMMENDATIONS

While a transplant operation typically offers far better prognosis and quality of life, it is not an absolute "cure" in the sense that it implies a life-long need to adhere to medical recommendations, including taking medications with significant potential side-effects (e.g. immunosuppressants). The transplant recipient faces the challenge of recognizing the need for long-term medical care and adherence to medications post-transplant. Adherence to medical recommendations is frequently not ideal in the pediatric age group [19,24,35–37] and nonadherence is one of the leading causes of organ rejection, hospital admissions and death post-transplant [19,37,38]. Yet the assessment and treatment of nonadherence is rarely approached in a systematic way in clinical practice [39].

This section briefly discusses elements related to the assessment and improvement of adherence in pediatric transplant recipients. Although adherence is needed to a variety of recommendations (including clinic visits, nutrition, life-style recommendations), I will concentrate on adherence to prescribed medications in this chapter, because this form of adherence is the best-studied to date in pediatric transplant recipients. I emphasized the section on assessment, because the detection of nonadherence is the most crucial step in its eventual treatment – once it is known that a patient is not taking the medications, there are many interventions that can be proposed or tried. The limited scope of this chapter allows only a brief discussion of the potential treatment options.

Assessment of adherence to medications

It is difficult to know whether a patient takes his or her medications or not. There is no gold standard for the measurement of adherence [39–41], and each proposed method has its shortcomings. Nonadherence is dynamic in nature [42]. A patient may present as nonadherent at one point in time and adherent at another. Therefore, any method used to measure adherence must be applied over time rather than at only one time point. Specific comments about methods that could be used are given below.

Self-report
When compared with objective measures of adherence, data suggest that self-reports are not a sensitive or reliable way to assess adherence [39,40].

Pill counts
A patient may engage in a variety of behaviors that would invalidate this method as a measure of adherence. For example, a patient may remove pills but not take them, or take the correct number of pills at an incorrect time [42]. Routine use of this method is time-consuming.

Electronic event monitoring devices
Electronic event monitoring devices (e.g. MEMS Caps, a product of AARDEX/APREX©) are pill boxes with electronic caps that register each opening of the device (for dispensation of a pill). Dedicated software translates the pill box readings into an output chart that gives information about the number and timing of openings. Although this method has been described as the state-of-the-art adherence monitoring method post-transplant [43], it is not free of bias. Patients may open the pill box but not remove a pill, or they may discard the pill after removing it. Electronic monitoring provides a way to ascertain precisely when a bottle was opened. However, data are lacking about the importance of this precise information. It is possible that taking an immunosuppressant 10 hours

as opposed to 12 hours apart does not really constitute a significant adherence problem. The precise threshold at which timing becomes important is not well defined. Finally, the use of electronic monitoring was not validated in predicting clinical outcomes in children who had a transplant.

Prescription refill rates

In order to use this method, the clinician needs to be able to communicate with the pharmacy, or pharmacies, that the patient is using [44]. Patients are likely to request a refill a few days before they run out of their medications, and refilling a prescription is not synonymous with having taken the previously prescribed dose. Hence, prescription refill rates are an objective but crude method of detection.

Medication blood levels

The use a blood level drawn only once may be misleading. This is because some fluctuation is permissible and expected. Therefore, an evaluation of the *fluctuation of medication blood levels over time* is a better predictor of nonadherence [24], except in the very rare case of a patient who never takes the medication (this patient will have a consistent level of zero without any fluctuation). A higher standard deviation of medication blood levels (SD), and therefore more fluctuation between individual measures, was shown to be consistent with a panel assessment of adherence in pediatric liver transplant recipients [24] and with adherence-specific medical outcome [39]. It is important to note that this method assumes that medication blood levels are closely related to intake. This was shown to be the case for tacrolimus, but is not true for cyclosporine [39]. Hence, fluctuations in cyclosporine blood levels cannot be used as a reliable adherence detection method.

Metabolites

These are levels of a medication's degradation or metabolic products. Metabolite levels of azathioprine have been used to assess the degree of adherence to this medication [45]. The benefit of using this method is that metabolites accumulate over time, and hence their level reflects the level of medication intake over a period of time, not just recent intake. This method may be less sensitive than others in that only a significant deviation from the prescribed regimen will be detected. It is also usually quite expensive. Further, drug metabolism may be affected by factors other than intake (e.g. level of activity of an enzyme that is responsible for the metabolite that is being measured), and may therefore differ between patients.

Clinician's assessment of adherence

Although used in a few adherence studies, this was not shown to be a particularly reliable method for the detection of nonadherence [39]. It may be more reliable in the most severe cases [24].

Treatment of nonadherence to medications

Who is nonadherent?

In pediatric transplant recipients, the first major question in treating nonadherence is who the treatment should focus on. It is obvious that a 16-month-old "nonadherent" child would benefit from intervention targeted almost exclusively at the parents, whereas a 19-year-old college student who is living alone should probably be the focus of intervention (not the parents). In practice, various degrees of assessment and treatment of parent and child are usually warranted; neither should be completely "forgotten."

What should be done in identified cases?

Treatment of nonadherence is best conceptualized as a stratified effort. It should begin with preventative efforts that are aimed at every patient and are expected to improve adherence in the clinic or practice as a whole. The preventative effort should also create a mechanism for early identification of nonadherence that needs to be further addressed. Specialized treatment strategies for identified or suspected cases that have not improved by using the general preventative model should then be offered.

Preventative measures

The hallmarks of this part of an effort to improve adherence are:

1 Creation of a systematic method to assess patient's adherence as a part of the general clinical care (e.g. routinely asking about it, routine medication blood level determinations)
2 Provision of general and specific education about medication-taking
3 Prospective assessment of risk factors that are known or suspected to be related to nonadherence, and addressing these risk factors as they become known and before nonadherence develops.

Patient and/or parent education

Education about the illness should be provided to all patients during the routine medical management of their illness. This section addresses a more intensive educational approach intended for confirmed or suspected nonadherent patients. The components of this approach are the *assessment* of the patient's (and parent's) actual understanding of the prescribed regimen, its administration and the reasons for it, the *correction* of any misinformed notions that are discovered, and an *open discussion* about the ways the medication is being taken, how can it be better integrated into a patient's lifestyle, and what concessions or resources are needed in order to make medication-taking possible. Thus, education is an interactive process in which the clinician tries to identify the cognitive and procedural needs of the patient and address them. Educational approaches have been shown to have limited but significant effects on adherence [46,47]. Because they are relatively straightforward and not labor-intensive, they should be attempted in most cases as a first line of treatment. However, education alone is not sufficient in many instances [48].

Specialized treatments

Nonadherence can be managed in several ways once diagnosed, or even when suspected but not confirmed. Available treatment strategies can be grouped into those that focus on patient education and awareness, on the adherence behavior itself and those that seek to improve risk factors (such as psychopathology, poor social supports) that are considered to be the main reason for nonadherence in a particular patient. These specialized treatment strategies can be time-consuming and sometimes require a highly skilled individual to deliver them. However, the provision of such care may have a profound impact on adherence and outcome in selected patients. A comprehensive review of risk factors for nonadherence and specialized treatment strategies is beyond the scope of this chapter and the reader is encouraged to refer to other texts for this purpose [19,39–41].

SUMMARY AND CONCLUSIONS

A transplant operation, while life-saving, is similar to a long-term medical illness in that it involves the need for ongoing medical care. The most important message of this chapter is that psychosocial adjustment following transplantation is a long-term process that needs to be monitored and addressed as a regular part of post-transplant care to improve graft survival. Problems in adjustment may become apparent at any time post-transplant – even years after an uneventful recovery – and the practitioner should recognize and address them as soon as possible. With proper care, positive psychosocial adjustment, as well as good adherence to medical recommendations, can usually be accomplished.

REFERENCES

1 Tagge EP, Campbell DA Jr, Dafoe DC, et al. Pediatric renal transplantation with an emphasis on the prognosis of patients with chronic renal insufficiency since infancy. *Surgery* 1987;**102**:692–8.

2 Roberts MS, Angus DC, Bryce CL, Valenta Z, Weissfeld L. Survival after liver transplantation in the United States: a disease-specific analysis of the UNOS database. *Liver Transpl* 2004;**10**:886–97.

3 Kaufman SS. Small bowel transplantation: selection criteria, operative techniques, advances in specific immunosuppression, prognosis. *Curr Opin Pediatr* 2001;**13**:425–8.

4 Beath SV, Needham SJ, Kelly DA, et al. Clinical features and prognosis of children assessed for isolated small bowel or combined small bowel and liver transplantation. *J Pediatr Surg* 1997;**32**:459–61.

5 Nagral S, Muiesan P, Vilca-Melendez H, et al. Liver transplantation for extra hepatic biliary atresia. *Tohoku J Exp Med* 1997;**181**:117–27.

6 Klare B, Strom TM, Hahn H, et al. Remarkable long-term prognosis and excellent growth in kidney-transplant children under cyclosporine monotherapy. *Transplant Proc* 1991;**23**:1013–7.

7 Taylor R, Franck LS, Gibson F, Dhawan A. A critical review of the health-related quality of life of children and adolescents after liver transplantation. *Liver Transpl* 2004;**11**:51–60.

8 Schulz KH, Wein C, Boeck A, Rogiers X, Burdelski M. Cognitive performance of children who have undergone liver transplantation. *Transplantation* 2003;**75**:1236–40.

9 Avitzur Y, De Luca E, Cantos M, et al. Health status ten years after pediatric liver transplantation: looking beyond the graft. *Transplantation* 2004;**78**:566–73.

10 Freier MC, Babikian T, Pivonka J, et al. A longitudinal perspective on neurodevelopmental outcome after infant cardiac transplantation. *J Heart Lung Transplant* 2004;**23**:857–64.

11 Cole CR, Bucuvalas JC, Hornung RW, et al. Impact of liver transplantation on HRQOL in children less than 5 years old. *Pediatr Transplant* 2004;**8**:222–7.

12 Sudan D, Horslen S, Botha J, et al. Quality of life after pediatric intestinal transplantation: the perception of pediatric recipients and their parents. *Am J Transplant* 2004;**4**:407–13.

13 Pollock-BarZiv SM, Anthony SJ, Niedra R, Dipchand AI, West LJ. Quality of life and function following cardiac transplantation in adolescents. *Transplant Proc* 2003;**35**:2468–70.

14 Manificat S, Dazord A, Cochat P, et al. Quality of life of children and adolescents after kidney or liver transplantation: child, parents and caregiver's point of view. *Pediatr Transplant* 2003;**7**:228–35.

15 Bucuvalas JC, Britto M, Krug S, et al. Health-related quality of life in pediatric liver transplant recipients: a single-center study. *Liver Transpl* 2003;**9**:62–71.

16 Midgley DE, Bradlee TA, Donohoe C, Kent KP, Alonso EM. Health-related quality of life in long-term survivors of pediatric liver transplantation. *Liver Transpl* 2000;**6**:333–9.

17 Wray J, Radley-Smith R. Depression in pediatric patients before and 1 year after heart or heart-lung transplantation. *J Heart Lung Transplant* 2004;**23**:1103–10.

18 Stuber ML. Psychiatric aspects of organ transplantation in children and adolescents. *Psychosomatics* 1993;**34**:379–87.

19 Rianthavorn P, Ettenger RB, Malekzadeh M, Marik JL, Struber M. Noncompliance with immunosuppressive medications in pediatric and adolescent patients receiving solid-organ transplants. *Transplantation* 2004;**77**:778–82.

20 Young GS, Mintzer LL, Seacord D, et al. Symptoms of posttraumatic stress disorder in parents of transplant recipients: incidence, severity, and related factors. *Pediatrics* 2003;**111**:e725–31.

21 Stuber ML, Shemesh E, Saxe GN. Posttraumatic stress responses in children with life-threatening illnesses. *Child Adolesc Psychiatr Clin N Am* 2003;**12**:195–209.

22 Walker AM, Harris G, Baker A, Kelly D, Houghton J. Post-traumatic stress responses following liver transplantation in older children. *J Child Psychol Psychiatry* 1999;**40**:363–74.

23 Stukas AA Jr, Dew MA, Switzer GE, et al. PTSD in heart transplant recipients and their primary family caregivers. *Psychosomatics* 1999;**40**:212–21.

24 Shemesh E, Lurie S, Stuber ML, *et al.* A pilot study of posttraumatic stress and nonadherence in pediatric liver transplant recipients. *Pediatrics* 2000;**105**:E29.

25 Rothenhausler HB, Ehrentraut S, Kapfhammer HP, *et al.* Psychiatric and psychosocial outcome of orthotopic liver transplantation. *Psychother Psychosom* 2002;**71**:285–97.

26 Dew MA, Kormos RL, DiMartini AF, *et al.* Prevalence and risk of depression and anxiety-related disorders during the first three years after heart transplantation. *Psychosomatics* 2001;**42**:300–13.

27 Bennett P, Conway M, Clatworthy J, Brooke S, Owen R. Predicting post-traumatic symptoms in cardiac patients. *Heart Lung* 2001;**30**:458–65.

28 Yehuda R, ed. *Treating Trauma Survivors with PTSD.* American Psychiatric Press, 2002.

29 Harvey AG, Bryant RA. The relationship between acute stress disorder and posttraumatic stress disorder: a 2-year prospective evaluation. *J Consult Clin Psychol* 1999;**67**:985–8.

30 Compton SN, March JS, Brent D, *et al.* Cognitive–behavioral psychotherapy for anxiety and depressive disorders in children and adolescents: an evidence-based medicine review. *J Am Acad Child Adolesc Psychiatry* 2004;**43**:930–59.

31 Jureidini JN, Doecke CJ, Mansfield PR, *et al.* Efficacy and safety of antidepressants for children and adolescents. *BMJ* 2004;**328**:879–83.

32 Shemesh E, Newcorn JH, Rockmore L, *et al.* Comparison of parent and child reports of emotional trauma symptoms in pediatric outpatient settings. *Pediatrics* 2005;**115**:E582–9.

33 Shemesh E, Keshavarz R, Leichtling NK, *et al.* Pediatric emergency department assessment of psychological trauma and posttraumatic stress. *Psychiatr Serv* 2003;**54**:1277–81.

34 Studdert DM, Burns JP, Mello MM, *et al.* Nature of conflict in the care of pediatric intensive care patients with prolonged stay. *Pediatrics* 2003;**112**:553–8.

35 Lurie S, Shemesh E, Sheiner PA, *et al.* Non-adherence in pediatric liver transplant recipients: an assessment of risk factors and natural history. *Pediatr Transplant* 2000;**4**:200–6.

36 Ringewald JM, Gidding SS, Crawford SE, *et al.* Nonadherence is associated with late rejection in pediatric heart transplant recipients. *J Pediatr* 2001;**139**:75–8.

37 Molmenti E, Mazariegos G, Bueno J, *et al.* Noncompliance after pediatric liver transplantation. *Transplant Proc* 1999;**31**:408.

38 Butler JA, Roderick P, Mullee M, Mason JC, Peveler RC. Frequency and impact of nonadherence to immunosuppressants after renal transplantation: a systematic review. *Transplantation* 2004;**77**:769–76.

39 Shemesh E, Shneider BL, Savitzky JK, *et al.* Medication adherence in pediatric and adolescent liver transplant recipients. *Pediatrics* 2004;**113**:825–32.

40 Shemesh E. Adherence to medical regimens. In: Walker WA, *et al.* eds. *Walker's Pediatric Gastrointestinal Disease*, 4th edn. Ontario, Canada: BC Decker, 2004.

41 Shemesh E. Non-adherence to medications following pediatric liver transplantation. *Pediatr Transplant* 2004;**8**:600–5.

42 Johnson SB. Measuring adherence. *Diabetes Care* 1992;**15**:1658–67.

43 De Geest S, Abraham I, Dunbar-Jacob J. Measuring transplant patients' compliance with immunosupressive therapy. *West J Nurs Res* 1996;**18**:595–605.

44 Galt KA, Backes J, Sondag LD. Identifying noncompliance by combining refill audits with telephone follow-up. *Am J Health Syst Pharm* 2000;**57**:219–20.

45 Rumbo C, Emerick KM, Emre S, Shneider BL. Azathioprine metabolite measurements in the treatment of autoimmune hepatitis in pediatric patients: a preliminary report. *J Pediatr Gastroenterol Nutr* 2002;**35**:391–8.

46 Bender BG. Overcoming barriers to nonadherence in asthma treatment. *J Allergy Clin Immunol* 2002;**109**(Suppl):S554–9.

47 Becker DM, Allen JK. Improving compliance in your dyslipidemic patient: an evidence-based approach. *J Am Acad Nurse Pract* 2001;**13**:200–7.

48 Katz RC, Ashmore J, Barboa E, *et al.* Knowledge of disease and dietary compliance in patients with end-stage renal disease. *Psychol Rep* 1998;**82**:331–6.

53 Pregnancy

Vincent T. Armenti, Michael J. Moritz and John M. Davison

The first successful post-transplant pregnancy occurred in a kidney recipient in 1958 (reported in 1963), who had received a kidney from her identical twin and delivered a healthy baby boy by cesarean section without apparent adverse effects on her transplant [1]. Since then, thousands of successful pregnancy outcomes in all types of recipients have been reported. Concerns of recipients and their caregivers are centered on the effects of immunosuppressive medications on fetal development as well as the effects of pregnancy on transplant function. From the experience gained over the years, it has become the consensus that in the presence of stable graft function and with stable maintenance immunosuppressive regimens, pregnancy is reasonably well tolerated, with most pregnancies resulting in successful outcomes for mother and newborn. No specific pattern of malformations has been noted in the newborns of solid organ recipients.

In general, reports have not distinguished between recipients who were transplanted as adults and those transplanted during childhood or adolescence.

The National Transplantation Pregnancy Registry (NTPR), established in 1991, studies the outcomes of female recipients who have had pregnancies and male recipients who have fathered pregnancies. Data are collected via questionnaires, telephone interviews and hospital records. Data include follow-up on the recipient, graft and offspring. The NTPR is an ongoing voluntary retrospective database-centered study. The UK Transplant Register, also a national database pregnancy registry, was initiated in 1997 but is currently not actively enrolling recipients [2].

This report from the NTPR describes the pregnancy outcomes of female transplant recipients who received a solid organ transplant when less than 21 years old. The analysis includes kidney, liver, liver-kidney, heart and lung recipients. No recipients in the registry received a pancreas-kidney or heart-lung transplant prior to age 21. To date, the NTPR has not received reports of pregnancy in a small bowel recipient. Included in Table 53.1 is the total number of female recipients reported to the registry and Table 53.2 lists recipients transplanted under age 21 who later had pregnancies.

Immunosuppressive regimens in the 1960s and into the

Table 53.1 The National Transplantation Pregnancy Registry (NTPR): pregnancies in all female transplant recipients (January 2005).

Organ	Recipients	Pregnancies	Outcomes*
Kidney	716	1097	1125
Liver	111	187	189
Liver-kidney	4	6	7
Pancreas-kidney	38	56	58
Heart	33	54	54
Heart-lung	3	3	3
Lung	14	15	15
Total	919	1418	1451

* Includes twins and triplets.

Table 53.2 The National Transplantation Pregnancy Registry (NTPR): pregnancies in female transplant recipients transplanted under age 21 (May 2005).

Organ	Recipients	Pregnancies	Outcomes*
Kidney	294	391	396
Liver	43	73	73
Liver-kidney	2	4	5
Heart	13	21	21
Lung	1	1	1
Total	353	490	496

* Includes twins and triplets.

early 1980s were azathioprine- and prednisone-based until cyclosporine became the mainstay of immunosuppressive therapy. Subsequently, newer agents and newer combinations of immunosuppressive medications have been introduced. As a background to the outcomes of pregnancies in each of the recipient groups, it is worthwhile to first review the immunosuppressive medications with regard to their potential reproductive toxicity.

COMMONLY USED IMMUNOSUPPRESSIVE AGENTS AND PREGNANCY EXPOSURE

Prior to the early 1980s, experience in pregnancy was based on exposure to azathioprine-based regimens. With the introduction of calcineurin inhibitors and newer immunosuppressives, clinicians are now faced with drugs for which there are limited pregnancy outcome data. The Food and Drug Administration (FDA) classification of safety during pregnancy provides information on prior experience with pregnancy in humans. Most drugs used during pregnancy, however, do not have clear pregnancy safety guidelines, even given the FDA categories. The FDA categories are as follows:

A There are controlled studies and no risk identified
B There is no evidence of risk in humans
C Human risks cannot be ruled out, either because of limited clinical controlled studies or potential adverse events in animal studies
D Positive evidence of human risk
X Contraindicated

Approximately 3–5% of children manifest birth defects and when major and minor birth defects are considered together, they approach approximately 10% of the general population. Immunosuppressive agents used during pregnancy with available pregnancy information are listed in Table 53.3 [3]. With respect to corticosteroids, a survey of the literature of over 400 nontransplant mothers exposed to cortisone had pregnancy outcomes analyzed with an overall malformation rate of 3.5% [4]. When used at high doses in animal studies, corticosteroids have been identified as agents that can cause cleft palate and have been implicated in increasing the risk of premature rupture of membranes as well as adrenal insufficiency in newborns [5–6]. They are classified as Category B agents: low teratogenic risk.

In comparison, thousands of pregnancy outcomes have been reported and analyzed with azathioprine as the primary immunosuppressant at doses 2–3 times higher than its subsequent use as an adjunctive, rather than as a primary drug. At the higher doses, problems identified in newborns included thymic atrophy, leukopenia, anemia, thrombocytopenia, transient chromosomal aberrations and reduced immunoglobulin levels, as well as infections and sepsis [7–10]. No predominant structural malformations have been identified. While animal studies suggested a teratogenic risk, this has not been supported by clinical outcome data [11]. Despite its clinical record, azathioprine is classified category D.

The calcineurin inhibitors cyclosporine and tacrolimus are listed as Category C agents and for each of the agents, toxicities noted in animal studies were at higher doses than those in the therapeutic range. Early reports of pregnancy outcomes with cyclosporine exposure raised concerns about its safety but there have been no patterns or increased incidence of malformations in subsequent studies to indicate any increased teratogenic risk [12]. With regard to tacrolimus, a higher transient perinatal hyperkalemia has been noted but, like cyclosporine, no specific teratogenicity was seen [13].

In contrast to the calcineurin inhibitors, there is concern with the use of mycophenolate mofetil (MMF, CellCept®) during pregnancy, based on reproductive toxicity studies in animals. Developmental toxicities, malformations, intrauterine death or intrauterine growth retardation were noted in rats and rabbits at doses of MMF that, based on body surface area, appear to be within clinical doses [14]. On the basis of these studies therefore, there is a possibility of increased teratogenic risks in humans, although it too is listed as a Category C drug. Limited clinical data are available as yet and in a recent NTPR review of 21 pregnancies (11 spontaneous abortions, 10 livebirths) in kidney recipients with MMF exposure, two of 10 liveborns had birth defects reported. Of these recipients with exposure to MMF, five were transplanted less than 21 years (one liveborn with malformations) [3,15]. Although not a pediatric recipient, a case report from

Drug	Animal reproductive data	Pregnancy category*
Corticosteroids (prednisone, methylprednisolone, others)	Y	B
Azathioprine (Imuran®)	Y	D
Cyclosporine (Sandimmune®, Neoral®, others)	Y	C
Tacrolimus, FK506 (Prograf®)	Y	C
Antithymocyte globulin (ATG, Atgam®, Thymoglobulin®)	N	C
Orthoclone (OKT3)	N	C
Mycophenolate mofetil (CellCept®)	Y	C
Mycophenolic acid (MPA, Myfortic®)	Y	C
Basiliximab (Simulect®)	Y	B
Daclizumab (Zenapax®)	N	C
Sirolimus (Rapamune®)	Y	C

Table 53.3 The Food and Drug Administration (FDA) pregnancy categories for commonly used immunosuppressive drugs in transplantation.

* FDA categories briefly defined: B, no fetal risk, no controlled studies; C, fetal risk cannot be ruled out; D, evidence of fetal risk.

France (not included in NTPR data) reported a conception occurring while on MMF, tacrolimus and prednisone resulting in elective termination of a fetus with multiple anomalies. At 18 weeks, the pregnancy was discovered and MMF was discontinued and azathioprine started. On ultrasound at 22 weeks, multiple malformations were noted and the pregnancy was electively terminated. At autopsy, malformations included: cleft lip and palate, micrognathia, ocular hypertelorism, microtia, external auditory duct atresia and complete agenesis of the corpus callosum [16]. Comorbid factors, other medications and genetic background must also be considered in assessing the teratogenic risk of MMF in transplant recipients.

Sirolimus (Rapamune®) is also listed as Category C. In animal reproductive studies, decreased fetal rates and delayed ossification of skeletal structures were reported but no teratogenicity noted. When administered in animal reproductive studies in combination with cyclosporine, increased fetal mortality was noted as evidenced by increased numbers of resorptions and decreased numbers of liveborns [17]. Clinical data are limited [3]. No female pediatric recipient reported a conception while on sirolimus.

No animal reproductive studies have been conducted for OKT3, Thymoglobulin or daclizumab. Basiliximab is listed as Category B as there was no maternal toxicity, embryo toxicity or teratogenicity noted in animal studies during organogenesis [18]. Because these agents are used for induction and/or rejection treatment, their role with regard to pregnancy is far more limited; however, longer term use (e.g. for 1 year) of daclizumab and basiliximab has begun.

KIDNEY TRANSPLANT RECIPIENTS

Surveys of the literature from the 1970s and 1980s summarized thousands of successful post-transplant pregnancies in women on azathioprine-based immunosuppression. Overall, there was a spontaneous abortion rate of approximately 14%, with therapeutic terminations in approximately 20% of conceptions. It was estimated that for conceptions that continued beyond the first trimester, more than 90% were successful. There was some impairment of renal function in approximately 15% of pregnancies, while in others there was evidence of transient deterioration, with or without proteinuria. Hypertension was evident in approximately 30% of these pregnancies and preterm delivery was noted in 45–60%, with fetal growth restriction in approximately 20%. No predominant or frequent anomalies were noted in the newborns [19].

Registry data from the NTPR since 1991 as well as additional case and center reports, have catalogued pregnancies in the cyclosporine era. The incidence of preterm deliveries is similar, with a higher incidence of hypertension, but with no frequent or predominant malformations in the newborn. Regarding the question of whether pregnancy itself adversely affects graft function, two well-designed case–control studies

suggested that in the presence of stable graft function, pregnancy is well tolerated with perhaps a minor deleterious effect of pregnancy [20,21]. NTPR data have shown slightly increased postpartum serum creatinine when compared with baseline prepartum serum creatinine. Another group noted that deterioration occurred when there was evidence of prepregnancy chronic rejection [22]. Two extensive analyses of the primary immunosuppressives cyclosporine and tacrolimus were recently published [23,24]. From the Mother Risk Program in Toronto, the overall prevalence of malformations in the study population of cyclosporine-exposed offspring was 4.1% [23]. Similar outcomes have been noted in NTPR data [25]. In 100 pregnancies analyzed from tacrolimus-treated recipients, there were no specific patterns of malformations noted in the newborns. Four of the 71 liveborns (5.6%) had evidence of structural malformation [24]. Thus, the consensus with respect to pregnancy post-kidney transplantation is that while there are a significant number of premature deliveries, there are no specific structural problems in the newborn and the majority of recipients tolerate pregnancy with respect to graft function.

Outcomes of kidney recipients in the NTPR who were transplanted before age 21 years are shown in Tables 53.4–53.10, categorized by immunosuppressive regimen and by age at transplant. The majority of pregnancies reported to the registry in the pediatric transplanted age group resulted in liveborns, from 74% to 87% of outcomes. Mean gestational age ranged from 36 to 37 weeks and mean birthweight ranged from 2493 to 2575 g. Of note, there were no acute rejections during pregnancy in the Neoral®-treated group, and a lower incidence of pre-eclampsia in the tacrolimus-treated group.

Graft loss within 2 years of delivery occurred in 12 cyclosporine-treated recipients (13%), none in the Neoral treated group and four recipients (25%) in the tacrolimus-treated group. In those with graft loss, the mean transplant-to-conception interval was 4.0 years in the cyclosporine-treated recipients and 4.2 years in the tacrolimus-treated recipients. Prepregnancy mean serum creatinine levels were 1.8 ± 0.5 mg/dL in the cyclosporine treated versus 1.6 ± 0.8 mg/dL in the tacrolimus treated with a range of 1.0–2.8 mg/dL. Transplant-to-conception interval ranged from 1.1 to 10.2 years. One recipient in the tacrolimus-treated group suffered graft loss during pregnancy with a serum creatinine level of 11 mL/dL just prior to dialysis, which accounts in part for the higher mean serum creatinine level during pregnancy in the tacrolimus-treated group.

Listed in Table 53.11 are structural malformations in the newborns of calcineurin inhibitor treated recipients. Shown in Tables 53.12–53.14 are the outcomes of 159 recipients and 190 pregnancy outcomes in recipients on azathioprine/prednisone regimens. Mean gestational age and birth weights are greater when compared with the calcineurin inhibitor regimens, and of note is a lower incidence of maternal hypertension. There were two rejections and 7% of recipients reported graft loss within 2 years of delivery. Eighty-eight

	CsA*	Neoral†	Tacrolimus‡
Maternal factors			
Transplant to conception interval	4.2 years	7.1 years	4.3 years
Hypertension during pregnancy	57%	65%	53%
Diabetes during pregnancy	2%	3%	5%
Infection during pregnancy	27%	27%	41%
Rejection episode during pregnancy§	2%	0%	11%
Pre-eclampsia	27%	52%	21%
Mean serum creatinine (mg/dL)			
Before pregnancy	1.4	1.3	1.2
During pregnancy	1.4	1.3	2.0
After pregnancy	1.7	1.4	1.7
Graft loss within 2 years of delivery	13%	0%	25%
Outcomes (n)§	(150)	(37)	(19)
Therapeutic abortions	9%	0%	0%
Spontaneous abortions	10%	11%	16%
Ectopic	1%	0%	0%
Stillborn	5%	3%	11%
Livebirths	77%	87%	74%
Livebirths (n)	(114)	(32)	(14)
Mean gestational age	36 weeks	37 weeks	36 weeks
Premature (< 37 weeks)	49%	50%	36%
Mean birthweight	2493 g	2531 g	2575 g
Low birthweight (< 2500 g)	46%	47%	43%
Cesarean section	54%	48%	50%
Newborn complications	39%	28%	50%
Neonatal deaths *n* (%) (within 30 days of birth)	1 (1)	0	0

Table 53.4 The National Transplantation Pregnancy Registry (NTPR): outcomes in female kidney pediatric recipients (age less than 21 years at time of transplant).

* CsA: Sandimmune® brand cyclosporine (90 recipients, 147 pregnancies).
† Neoral® brand cyclosporine (29 recipients, 35 pregnancies).
‡ Tacrolimus Prograf® (16 recipients, 19 pregnancies).
§ Includes twins, triplets.

Recipient age (years)	No. liveborn	Conception age (years)	Mean		
			TI* (years)	Gestational age (weeks)	Birth weight (g)
5–10	3	24.8	8.1	38.0	2504
10–15	21	23.2	4.3	36.5	2464
15–20	92	24.5	4.1	36.0	2486

Table 53.5 The National Transplantation Pregnancy Registry (NTPR): female kidney recipients – cyclosporine treated, outcomes in relation to age (age less than 21 years at time of transplant).

* TI, transplant to conception interval (calculated from most recent transplant prior to the estimated date of conception).

percent of the regimens included azathioprine/prednisone, with 3% azathioprine alone and 9% prednisone alone (one recipient on no immunosuppression).

There are three offspring of kidney recipients who themselves had kidney transplants and whose mothers were maintained on azathioprine and prednisone during their pregnancies. The first mother required a transplant as a result of glomerulonephritis (GN) at age 12 years and became pregnant 6 years after transplant. Her child was born with hypoplastic kidneys and required a transplant at age 9 years. The second mother was transplanted at age 17 years and became pregnant 12 years after transplant. Her child required a transplant at age 15 years due to Alport's syndrome. The third mother was transplanted at age 15 years because of GN and became pregnant 15 years post-transplant. Her child required a transplant at age 9 years as a result of GN.

Table 53.6 The National Transplantation Pregnancy Registry (NTPR): female kidney recipients – cyclosporine treated, outcomes in relation to age (age less than 21 years at time of transplant).

Recipient age (years)	No. liveborn	Percent premature	Mean premature gestational age (weeks)	Percent with low birth weight	Mean low birth weight (g)	Percent newborn complications
5–10	3	33	35.0	33	2353	33
10–15	21	43	33.8	62	2136	33
15–20	92	52	33.6	45	1808	41

Table 53.7 The National Transplantation Pregnancy Registry (NTPR): female kidney recipients – Neoral treated, outcomes in relation to age (age less than 21 years at time of transplant).

Recipient age (years)	No. liveborn	Conception age (years)	Mean TI* (years)	Mean Gestational age (weeks)	Mean Birth weight (g)
5–10	2	26.61	18.7	36.0	1814
10–15	7	24.10	6.0	36.3	2438
15–20	22	27.00	7.4	36.8	2613

* TI, transplant to conception interval (calculated from most recent transplant prior to the estimated date of conception).

Table 53.8 The National Transplantation Pregnancy Registry (NTPR): female kidney Recipients – Neoral treated, outcomes in relation to age (age less than 21 years at time of transplant).

Recipient age (years)	No. liveborn	Percent premature	Mean premature gestational age (weeks)	Percent with low birth weight	Mean low birth weight (g)	Percent newborn complications
5–10	2	0	–	100	1844	50
10–15	7	57	34	57	1921	29
15–20	22	48	35	41	2036	23

Table 53.9 The National Transplantation Pregnancy Registry (NTPR): female kidney recipients – tacrolimus treated, outcomes in relation to age (age less than 21 years at time of transplant).

Recipient age (years)	No. liveborn	Conception age (years)	Mean TI* (years)	Mean Gestational age (weeks)	Mean Birth weight (g)
5–10	0	–	–	–	–
10–15	5	25.8	4.5	37.1	2822
15–20	9	26.8	4.1	35.2	2438

* TI, transplant to conception interval (calculated from most recent transplant prior to the estimated date of conception).

Table 53.10 The National Transplantation Pregnancy Registry (NTPR): female kidney recipients – tacrolimus treated, outcomes in relation to age (age less than 21 years at time of transplant).

Recipient age (years)	No. liveborn	Percent premature	Mean premature gestational age (weeks)	Percent with low birth weight	Mean low birth weight (g)	Percent newborn complications
5–10	0	–	–	–	–	–
10–15	5	50	33.7	40	2098	60
15–20	9	44	32.1	44	1367	56

Table 53.11 The National Transplantation Pregnancy Registry (NTPR): reported birth defects in offspring of calcineurin inhibitor treated pediatric female kidney recipients (n = 160).

Defect	Regimen
Kidney recipient offspring	
Atrial septal defect	Sandimmune, azathioprine
Kidney hypoplasia	Sandimmune, prednisone
Metatarsus adductus	Sandimmune, azathioprine and prednisone
Cleft lip and palate, microtia	Tacrolimus, MMF and prednisone

MMF, mycophenolate mofetil.

Included in the cyclosporine (Sandimmune®) group are two recipients who reported biopsy-proven acute rejection during pregnancy. No recipients maintained on Neoral reported acute rejection during pregnancy. Two recipients maintained on tacrolimus reported acute rejection during pregnancy, including one case with an exposure to MMF. Additionally, in a small percentage of cases, recipients reported rejection (not biopsy proven), chronic rejection or recurrent disease. The cases of biopsy proven rejection during pregnancy are discussed below.

The *first recipient* received a kidney transplant at age 19 years for GN and had a third pregnancy 4.5 years post-transplant. Her first two post-transplant pregnancies resulted in a livebirth and a miscarriage. Her prepregnancy serum

Table 53.12 The National Transplantation Pregnancy Registry (NTPR): female pediatric recipients treated with azathioprine/prednisone (159 recipients, 190 pregnancy outcomes).

Maternal factors	
Transplant to conception interval	7.9 years
Hypertension during pregnancy	28%
Diabetes during pregnancy	3%
Infection during pregnancy	11%
Rejection episode during pregnancy	4%
Pre-eclampsia	26%
Graft loss within 2 years of delivery	7%
Outcomes (n)	(190)
Therapeutic abortions	3%
Spontaneous abortions	11%
Ectopic	2%
Stillbirth	2%
Livebirths	83%
Livebirths (n)	(158)
Mean gestational age	37 weeks
Premature (< 37 weeks)	39%
Mean birthweight	2809 g
Low birthweight (< 2500 g)	31%
Cesarean section	57%
Newborn complications	30%
Neonatal deaths (within 30 days of birth)	0

Recipient age (years)	No. liveborn	Conception age (years)	Mean TI* (years)	Mean Gestational age (weeks)	Mean Birth weight (g)
5–10	6	20.6	11.9	35.5	2648.5
10–15	44	24.0	9.4	37.1	2679.0
15–20	107	25.6	7.0	37.3	2878.0

Table 53.13 The National Transplantation Pregnancy Registry (NTPR): female kidney recipients – noncyclosporine-treated, outcomes in relation to age (age less than 21 years at time of transplant).

* TI, transplant to conception interval (calculated from most recent transplant prior to the estimated date of conception).

Table 53.14 The National Transplantation Pregnancy Registry (NTPR): female kidney recipients – noncyclosporine-treated, outcomes in relation to age (age less than 21 years at time of transplant).

Recipient age (years)	No. liveborn	Percent premature	Mean premature gestational age (weeks)	Percent with low birth weight	Mean low birth weight (g)	Percent newborn complications
5–10	6	66.7	34.4	16.7*	1600	33
10–15	44	44.0	34.6	41.0	2092	30
15–20	107	36.0	34.4	27.0	2113	31

* One child.

creatinine was 2.0 mg/dL. The recipient was maintained on cyclosporine, azathioprine and prednisone. She had no hypertension, diabetes or infections during pregnancy. She had a graft biopsy at 14 weeks gestation for a serum creatinine of 4.0 mg/dL, which demonstrated acute and chronic rejection, treated with methylprednisolone and plasmapheresis. A therapeutic termination was performed at 20 weeks. The recipient lost her graft 8 weeks post-pregnancy.

The *second recipient* with a rejection was transplanted at age 17 years because of lupus nephritis. She had two post-transplant pregnancies, the second occurred 1.7 years post-transplant. She was maintained on cyclosporine, azathioprine and prednisone. She had no hypertension, diabetes or infections during pregnancy. At 8 weeks gestation a graft biopsy was performed for an increase in serum creatinine which revealed acute cellular rejection, treated with methylprednisolone. There was a question of noncompliance. A therapeutic termination was performed at 22 weeks. Graft loss occurred at 10 weeks post-pregnancy.

A *third recipient* was transplanted at age 13 years for reflux nephropathy. She had two post-transplant pregnancies; one livebirth and one therapeutic termination. Her third post-transplant pregnancy occurred at 10 years post-transplant while maintained on Neoral, azathioprine and prednisone. It was reported that she stopped her medications. At 4 weeks gestation she had a biopsy for an increase in serum creatinine showing acute rejection, treated with OKT3 and radiation therapy. Her maintenance immunosuppresion was changed to tacrolimus. She had a miscarriage at 6 weeks. Graft loss occurred at 3 months post-pregnancy.

The last case of rejection during pregnancy includes the case with exposure to MMF. The recipient was transplanted at age 17 for hemolytic uremic syndrome and had graft loss secondary to chronic rejection. She was retransplanted at age 29 years and 4.2 years later conceived while taking tacrolimus, MMF and prednisone. At 24 weeks, a biopsy-proven acute rejection was documented and she required dialysis. The rejection was treated with steroids, antithymocyte globulin (Thymoglobulin®) and a change from MMF to sirolimus. During the rejection she received prophylactic ganciclovir. At 31 weeks, a 1531-g infant was delivered with a cleft lip and palate and microtia, defined as a smallness of the auricle of the ear with a blind or absent external auditory meatus.

Two kidney recipients reported complications of cytomegalovirus (CMV) in their offspring. One recipient had a liveborn with hearing loss ascribed to CMV; she did not have documented CMV viremia during pregnancy. The other recipient had a stillbirth at 29 weeks and in the autopsy report CMV was noted; again, active CMV viremia was not documented during pregnancy.

There were five recipients with pregnancies while on Sandimmune who died after pregnancy. Two recipients died with kidney function, one each of myocardial infarction and cardiac arrhythmia. Three recipients died without kidney function, one of respiratory arrest after return to dialysis, another of complications after a kidney retransplant and the third recipient died of complications from pancreatitis.

LIVER TRANSPLANT RECIPIENTS

The first series of 17 female liver recipients' pregnancies from the group in Pittsburgh [26] has been followed by a number of case and center reports [13,27–30]. No specific malformation patterns have been noted among the newborns. Issues of concern in the mothers have related to worsening graft function in the presence of chronic rejection and/or hepatitis. Shown in Tables 53.15–53.17 are the outcomes of those liver recipients entered into the NTPR who had been transplanted under age 21 years, categorized by age at transplant and by immunosuppression. Structural malformations are listed in Table 53.18.

Mean gestational ages ranged from 36 to 37 weeks and mean birthweights from 2629 to 2813 g. Hypertension during pregnancy ranged from 18% in the tacrolimus group to 40% in the cyclosporine group. Recipients with graft loss are shown in Table 53.19.

There are also four recipients who reported four pregnancies with four livebirths while maintained on Gengraf®. The mean gestational age of the infants was 37 weeks and the mean birthweight was 2885 g. One infant was born at 31 weeks with a birthweight of 1786 g; at last follow-up the infant was healthy and developing well. There were no rejections reported during pregnancy and at last follow-up all four mothers reported adequate graft function.

No recipients maintained on Neoral and tacrolimus reported biopsy-proven acute rejection during pregnancy. One recipient with three pregnancies reported rejection during two of her three post-transplant pregnancies while taking Sandimmune and prednisone. She was transplanted at age 19 years for hepatitis C. During all three pregnancies she reported hepatitis flares. Her first pregnancy occurred 1.2 years post-transplant. She had biopsy-proven acute rejection treated with methylprednisolone at 16 weeks. She delivered a 39-week, 2920-g infant. She also reported rejection after this pregnancy. Her second pregnancy occurred 2 years post-transplant and ended in a spontaneous abortion. During the third pregnancy 3.7 years post-transplant, she reported rejection, again treated with methylprednisolone at 7–8 weeks. The pregnancy was terminated at 8 weeks. The recipient had another rejection post-termination with worsening graft function and 4 months later she was retransplanted. She died 7 months later.

There were five maternal deaths among the liver recipients. Three occurred in the Sandimmune group, including the recipient detailed above. The other deaths occurred in one Neoral and one tacrolimus-treated recipients. Another cyclosporine recipient had three post-transplant pregnancies and died 0.8 years after her third pregnancy of worsening

Table 53.15 The National Transplantation Pregnancy Registry (NTPR): female liver pediatric recipients (age less than 21 years at time of transplant).*

	CsA[†]	Neoral[‡]	Tacrolimus[§]	No immunosuppression[¶]
Maternal factors				
Transplant to conception interval	4.1 years	9.4 years	3.9 years	9.4 years
Hypertension during pregnancy	40%	23%	18%	0%
Diabetes during pregnancy	3%	0%	6%	0%
Infection during pregnancy	45%	23%	33%	0%
Rejection episode during pregnancy	6%	0%	0%	0%
Pre-eclampsia	22%	20%	20%	0%
Graft loss	20%	13%	0%	0%
Outcomes (n)	(35)	(13)	(17)	(5)
Therapeutic abortions	23%	0%	6%	0%
Spontaneous abortions	11%	15%	6%	20%
Ectopic	0%	0%	0%	0%
Stillborn	3%	0%	6%	0%
Livebirths	63%	85%	82%	80%
Livebirths (n)	(22)	(11)	(14)	(4)
Mean gestational age	36 weeks	37 weeks	37 weeks	39 weeks
Premature (< 37 weeks)	46%	40%	41%	50%
Mean birthweight	2629 g	2686 g	2813 g	2892 g
Low birthweight (< 2500 g)	41%	36%	29%	25%
Cesarean section	30%	27%	36%	50%
Newborn complications	32%	27%	36%	25%
Neonatal deaths *n* (%) (within 30 days of birth)	0	0	0	0

* Recipients may have had pregnancies on more than one regimen.

[†] CsA: Sandimmune® brand cyclosporine (20 recipients, 35 pregnancies).

[‡] Neoral: Neoral® brand cyclosporine (8 recipients, 13 pregnancies).

[§] Tacrolimus: (13 recipients, 17 pregnancies).

[¶] No immunosuppression: (2 recipients, 5 pregnancies).

Table 53.16 The National Transplantation Pregnancy Registry (NTPR): female liver recipients (age less than 21 years at time of transplant).

			Mean		
Recipient age (years)	No. liveborn	Conception age (years)	TI* (years)	Gestational age (weeks)	Birth weight (g)
< 5	1	23.0	3.3	35.0	2495
5–10	1	22.0	14.5	38.0	3289
10–15	3	20.3	8.9	37.5	2259
15–20	49	24.0	5.7	36.9	2768

* TI, transplant to conception interval (calculated from most recent transplant prior to the estimated date of conception).

Table 53.17 The National Transplantation Pregnancy Registry (NTPR): female liver recipients (age less than 21 years at time of transplant).

Recipient age (years)	No. liveborn	Percent premature	Mean premature gestational age (weeks)	Percent with low birth weight	Mean low birth weight (g)	Percent newborn complications
< 5	1	100	35.0	100.0	2495	100.0
5–10	1	0	0.0	0.0	–	–
10–15	3	67	35.0	66.7	1942	66.7
15–20	49	41	33.4	31.0	1803	29.0

Table 53.18 The National Transplantation Pregnancy Registry (NTPR): reported birth defects in offspring of pediatric female liver recipients (n = 55).

Defect	Regimen
Liver recipient offspring	
Pyloric stenosis	Sandimmune and prednisone
Hypospadias	Sandimmune and prednisone

Table 53.19 The National Transplantation Pregnancy Registry (NTPR): seven female liver recipients with graft loss (age less than 21 years at time of transplant).

	Original liver disease	Pregnancy no.	Transplant to conception interval (years)
1	Fulminant hepatitis B	3	2.90
2	Hepatitis C	3	3.70
3	Trauma	3	9.00
4	Unknown	1	0.42
5	Unknown (later thought to be autoimmune)	2	10.00
6	Drug abuse	1	3.20
7	Hepatitis C	3	10.7
Mean			5.7 ± 4.1 years

hepatitis. One recipient after three pregnancies (two spontaneous abortions and one livebirth) died of sepsis 3.7 years postpartum. She required dialysis beginning 2 years postpartum. The Neoral-treated recipient had two post-transplant pregnancies and died 9 months postpartum of vanishing bile duct syndrome while awaiting retransplant. The tacrolimus-treated recipient died 2.1 years postpartum of recurrent hepatitis B.

LIVER-KIDNEY TRANSPLANT RECIPIENTS

Two recipients were transplanted as children and reported pregnancies. The first recipient transplanted for oxalosis became pregnant 1.3 years after transplant while on Sandimmune, prednisone and azathioprine. She had no complications during pregnancy and at 38 weeks had a cesarean section for a breech presentation and a 2665-g infant was delivered with no neonatal complications. The recipient died 4.5 years postpartum of a probable accidental drug overdose with satisfactory liver and kidney function at that time.

The second recipient had three pregnancies with one set of twins. She was transplanted with a kidney only for autoimmune disease but 4 years later received a liver-kidney because of autoimmune hepatitis. Her first pregnancy occurred 3.9 years post second transplant while maintained on Sandimmune and

azathioprine. She reported no complications and at 37 weeks a 3402-g infant was delivered. The second pregnancy was on Neoral and azathioprine, occurred 7.9 years post-transplant, and was a twin pregnancy. She reported pre-eclampsia, was induced and delivered 3033- and 2665-g infants at 37 weeks. The third pregnancy occurred 10.4 years after transplant while on Neoral, azathioprine and prednisone. She was induced at 35 weeks, delivering a 2551-g infant with mild respiratory distress and an increased bilirubin treated with phototherapy. All the children are reported healthy and developing well. Approximately 2 months postpartum the recipient had a liver biopsy demonstrating chronic rejection and her immunosuppression was changed to tacrolimus and MMF.

HEART TRANSPLANT RECIPIENTS

Outcomes in heart recipients under age 21 years are summarized in Table 53.20 [31]. There were 13 recipients with 21 pregnancies. Reasons for transplantation included cardiomyopathy (two), transposition of the great vessels (one), viral myocarditis (three), idiopathic dilated cardiomyopathy (three) and postpartum cardiomyopathy (four). Included in Table 53.21 are the rejections reported during female heart recipient pregnancies. Many were below the threshold for treatment and pregnancy

Table 53.20 The National Transplantation Pregnancy Registry (NTPR): pediatric female heart transplant recipients (13 recipients, 21 pregnancies).

Maternal factors	
Transplant to conception interval	4.5 years
Hypertension during pregnancy	42%
Diabetes during pregnancy	5%
Infection during pregnancy	10%
Rejection episode during pregnancy	42%
Pre-eclampsia	5%
Graft loss within 2 years of delivery	0%
Outcomes (n)	(21)
Therapeutic abortions	14%
Spontaneous abortions	14%
Ectopic	5%
Stillbirth	5%
Livebirths	62%
Livebirths (n)	(13)
Mean gestational age	37 weeks
Premature (< 37 weeks)	46%
Mean birthweight	2860 g
Low birthweight (< 2500 g)	39%
Cesarean section	36%
Newborn complications*	38%
Neonatal deaths (within 30 days of birth)	0%

* No structural malformations reported.

Table 53.21 The National Transplantation Pregnancy Registry (NTPR): pediatric female heart recipients – rejection during pregnancy.

Recipient	Rejection grade	Treatment	Current graft status	Outcome
1 (pregnancy no. 1)	2	Prednisone		TA
1 (pregnancy no. 2, two biopsies)	2; 2	None; none	Death due to cardiogenic shock 5.5 years after pregnancy no. 2	40 week, 3813 g
2	Moderate	Methylprednisolone	Adequate	33 week, 2240 g
3 (pregnancy no. 2)	1A	None		M
3 (pregnancy no. 3)	2	None	Reduced function	30 week, 1673 g
4	2	Methylprednisolone	Adequate	34 week, 2381 g
5	Mild	Increase in oral prednisone	Adequate	32 week, 2523 g
6	3A	Oral steroid pulse	Adequate	40 week, 2495 g
7 (two biopsies)	1B; 1A	Increase Neoral; none	Adequate	S

M, miscarriage; S, stillbirth; TA, therapeutic abortion.

and maternal graft outcome was adequate in most cases. There were three deaths among the heart recipients including recipient number 1 in Table 53.21. Two of the other recipients died 3 years postpartum, one with congestive heart failure, acute rejection and a question of noncompliance, the other of sepsis after a heart retransplant and kidney transplant.

LUNG TRANSPLANT RECIPIENTS

There is only one female lung recipient who reported a pregnancy after being transplanted at the age of 20.7 years for cystic fibrosis [32]. She became pregnant 1.2 years post-transplant maintained on Neoral, prednisone and azathioprine. She had no rejection prepregnancy. There was no hypertension, diabetes or infection reported during pregnancy. At 24 weeks she developed shortness of breath and a biopsy revealed a grade II rejection treated with methylprednisolone for 3 days. At 30 weeks, labor followed induction because of worsening lung function. A 1077-g infant was delivered and was treated for necrotizing enterocolitis and adrenal suppression. At last follow-up, the child was healthy and developing well. The recipient's lung function decreased because of chronic rejection and she died 1.6 years postpartum.

OTHER SOLID ORGAN RECIPIENTS (PANCREAS/KIDNEY, HEART/LUNG)

No pregnancies have been reported to the registry in recipients transplanted under age 21 years for pancreas-kidney or for heart-lung. Of note, in the adult pancreas transplant recipients reported to the registry, there has been good glycemic control during pregnancy, although there does appear to be a slightly higher percentage of graft loss and/or rejection when compared to kidney-only recipients.

MANAGEMENT AND SUMMARY

Within each organ recipient group, there are a small percentage of cases where problems arise, whether rejection, graft dysfunction or graft loss within 2 years of pregnancy. In some cases there is peripartum graft dysfunction that would appear to be related to pregnancy events. Malformation risk in the newborn does not appear to be significantly different from the background malformation rate in the general population. Continuing efforts to identify pregnancy risks are in progress, especially in light of newer immunosuppressive regimens.

Management of the transplant recipient during pregnancy should be interdisciplinary and involve close collaboration between the high-risk obstetrician and transplant personnel. Issues that must be considered include: allograft function, immunosuppressive medications, regimens, management of hypertension, allograft rejection, maternal infection, pre-eclampsia and other obstetric issues, including decision on timing and mode of delivery. It is the general recommendation that antenatal visits be every 2 weeks up to 32 weeks and weekly thereafter. From a counseling standpoint, general guidelines have advised recipients to wait a period of at least 1 year post-transplant to allow for establishment of good, stable graft function (e.g. serum creatinine level less than 2 mg/dL for renal recipients), lowering immunosuppressive medications to maintenance levels, and re-establishment of good general health (including control of blood pressure, lipids and bone metabolism). Stable graft function means absence of chronic rejection and recurrent disease (e.g. for renal recipients no proteinuria, for liver recipients control of viral hepatitis). During pregnancy in renal recipients, in addition to routine laboratory studies, it is recommended that a 24-hour creatinine clearance and protein excretion be checked monthly, in addition to liver function tests, calcium and phosphate levels at 6-week intervals, herpes simplex virus titers checked in each trimester if the initial titer is negative, and calcineurin inhibitor levels as well as other drug levels as appropriate. Recipients should be monitored for maternal CMV infection by detection of CMV antigenemia or viremia in the mother. Amniotic fluid analysis can be used if suspicion warrants [33].

Surveillance of graft function must be an issue during pregnancy as rejections have occurred in a small number of cases reported to the registry. In the majority of cases, calcineurin inhibitor doses have either been increased or kept the same, with regular checking of levels during pregnancy. It is common for drug levels to drop during pregnancy given the gestational increase in plasma volume and changes in drug metabolism. Graft function, however, should not be expected to deteriorate during pregnancy and elevation of creatinine and/or abnormalities in liver function or other evidence of graft dysfunction should be investigated. Patients should be managed with the high incidence of pre-eclampsia in mind. Prophylactic antibiotics are recommended to cover delivery with cesarean section undertaken for obstetric indication only. In the presence of adequate stable graft function, a favorable outcome can generally be anticipated for mother and newborn.

With regard to breastfeeding, there is much controversy in the literature because of newborn exposure to immunosuppressives transferred via breast milk. Some recipients have chosen to breastfeed. Issues regarding its appropriateness remain under investigation [34,35].

Continued study through entries to the NTPR as well as case reports and center reports will help the practitioner in the care of these recipients, especially with the introduction of newer immunosuppressive regimens.

ACKNOWLEDGMENTS

The National Transplantation Pregnancy Registry acknowledges the cooperation of all transplant recipients and over 200 centers in North America who have contributed their time and information to the registry. The authors would like to thank Lisa Coscia, RN, BSN, CCTC for her assistance in the preparation of this manuscript.

The National Transplantation Pregnancy Registry is supported by grants from Novartis Pharmaceuticals Corp., Astellas Pharma US, Inc., Roche Laboratories, Inc., and Wyeth Pharmaceuticals, Inc.

REFERENCES

1 Murray JE, Reid DE, Harrison JH, et al. Successful pregnancies after human renal transplantation. N Engl J Med 1963;269: 341–3.

2 Davison JM, Redman CWG. Pregnancy post-transplant: the establishment of a UK registry. Br J Obstet Gynaecol 1997;104: 1106–7.

3 Armenti VT, Radomski JS, Moritz MJ, et al. Report from the National Transplantation Pregnancy Registry (NTPR). In: Cecka JM, Terasaki PI, eds. Outcomes of Pregnancy after Transplantation. Clinical Transplants 2004. Los Angeles, CA: UCLA Immunogenetics Center, 2005: 103–19.

4 Fraser FC, Sajoo A. Teratogenic potential of corticosteroids in humans. Teratology 1995;51:45–6.

5 Fraser FC, Fainstat TD. The production of congenital defects in the offspring of pregnant mice treated with cortisone: a progress report. Pediatrics 1951;8:527–33.

6 Hou S. Pregnancy in transplant recipients. Med Clin North Am 1989;73:667–83.

7 Registration Committee of the European Dialysis and Transplant Association. Successful pregnancies in women treated by dialysis and kidney transplantation. Br J Obstet Gynaecol 1980;87:839–45.

8 Penn I, Makowski EL, Harris P. Parenthood following renal and hepatic transplantation. Transplantation 1980;30:397–400.

9 Rudolph J, Schweizer RT, Bartus SA. Pregnancy in renal transplant patients. Transplantation 1979;27:26–9.

10 Davison JM. Dialysis, transplantation, and pregnancy. Am J Kidney Dis 1991;17:127–32.

11 Friedman JM, Polifka JE. The Effects of Drugs on the Fetus and Nursing Infant: a handbook for health care professionals. Baltimore, MD: John Hopkins University Press, 1996.

12 Pickrell MD, Sawers R, Michael J. Pregnancy after renal transplantation: severe intra-uterine growth retardation during treatment with cyclosporin A. BMJ 1988;296:825.

13 Jain A, Venkataramanan R, Fung JJ, et al. Pregnancy after liver transplantation under tacrolimus. Transplantation 1997;64: 559–65.

14 Roche Laboratories. Mycophenolate mofetil package insert. Nutley, NJ: Roche Laboratories.

15 Pérgola PE, Kancharla A, Riley DJ. Kidney transplantation during the first trimester of pregnancy: immunosuppression with mycophenolate mofetil, tacrolimus and prednisone. Transplantation 2000;71:94–7.

16 Le Ray C, Coulomb A, Elefant E, et al. Mycophenolate mofetil in pregnancy after renal transplantation: a case of major fetal malformations. Obstet Gynecol 2004;103:1091.

17 Wyeth-Ayerst Pharmaceuticals. Sirolimus package insert. Philadelphia, PA: Wyeth Laboratories.

18 Novartis Pharmaceuticals. Basiliximab package insert. East Hanover, NJ: Novartis Pharmaceuticals Corporation.

19 Davison JM. Pregnancy in renal allograft recipients: problems, prognosis and practicalities. In: Lindheimer MD, Davison JM, eds. Balliere's Clin Obstet Gynaecol. 8. London, UK: Bailliere Tindall, 1994: 501–27.

20 First MR, Combs CA, Weiskittel P, Miodovnik M. Lack of effect of pregnancy on renal allograft survival or function. Transplantation 1995;59:472–6.

21 Sturgiss SN, Davison JM. Effect of pregnancy on the long-term function of renal allografts: an update. Am J Kidney Dis 1995; 26:54–6.

22 Kozlowska-Boszko B, Lao M, Gaciong Z, et al. Chronic rejection as a risk factor for deterioration of renal allograft function following pregnancy. Transplant Proc 1997;29:1522–3.

23 Oz BB, Hackman R, Einarson T, Koren G. Pregnancy outcome after cyclosporine therapy during pregnancy: a meta-analysis. Transplantation 2001;71:1051–55.

24 Kainz A, Harabacz I, Cowlrick IS, Gadgil SD, Hagiwara D. Review of the course and outcome of 100 pregnancies in 84 women treated with tacrolimus. *Transplant* 2000;**70**:1718–21.

25 Armenti VT, Radomski JS, Moritz MJ, *et al.* Report from the National Transplantation Pregnancy Registry (NTPR): outcomes of pregnancy after transplantation. In: Cecka JM, Terasaki PI, eds. *Clinical Transplants 2001*. Los Angeles, CA: UCLA Immunogenetics Center, 2002;97–105.

26 Scantlebury V, Gordon R, Tzakis A, *et al.* Childbearing after liver transplantation. *Transplantation* 1990;**49**:317–21.

27 Laifer SA, Darby MJ, Scantlebury VP, Harger JH, Caritis SN. Pregnancy and liver transplantation. *Obstet Gynecol* 1990;**76**: 1083–8.

28 Ville Y, Fernandez H, Samuel D, Bismuth H, Frydman R. Pregnancy in liver transplant recipients: course and outcome in 19 cases. *Am J Obstet Gynecol* 1993;**168**:896–902.

29 Molmenti EP, Jain AB, Marino N, *et al.* Liver transplantation and pregnancy. *Clin Liver Dis* 1999;**3**:163–74.

30 Armenti VT, Herrine SK, Radomski JS, Moritz MJ. Pregnancy after liver transplantation. *Liver Transplant* 2000;**6**:671–85.

31 Branch KR, Wagoner LE, McGrory CH, *et al.* Risks of subsequent pregnancies on mother and newborn in female heart transplant recipients. *J Heart Lung Transplant* 1998;**17**:698–702.

32 Gertner G, Coscia L, McGrory C, Moritz M, Armenti V. Pregnancy in lung transplant recipients. *Prog Transplant* 2000; **10**:109–12.

33 Armenti VT, Moritz MJ, Davison JM. Medical management of the pregnant transplant recipient. *Adv Ren Replace Ther* 1998; **5**:14–23.

34 Nyberg G, Haljamäe U, Frisenette-Fich C, Wennergren M, Kjellmer I. Breast-feeding during treatment with cyclosporine. *Transplantation* 1998;**65**:253–5.

35 Thiagarajan KD, Easterling T, Davis C, *et al.* Breast-feeding by a cyclosporine treated mother. *Obstet Gynecol* 2001;**97**:816–7.

54 Gynecologic Issues

Gina S. Sucato and Pamela J. Murray

The improved survival of pediatric recipients of solid organ transplants has prompted increased attention to quality of life issues. These include attainment of normal growth, involvement in romantic relationships and the desire to control fertility. In adolescent females, issues such as pubertal development and menstruation, contraception and routine gynecologic health care are typically addressed by the patient's primary care provider or gynecologist. However, the complexity of the adolescent transplant recipient's medical care necessitates close collaboration between all health care providers caring for the patient. This chapter focuses on the gynecologic health care and contraceptive needs of female adolescent solid organ transplant recipients.

MENSTRUATION

Among pediatric transplant recipients, pubertal delay is common and girls experience menarche 2–3 years later than average. Van Diemen-Steenvoorde *et al.* [1] studied children who received a renal transplant prior to puberty and found the average chronologic age of menarche was 15.3 years (range 13.4–17.7 years; *n* = 13). At menarche, the mean bone age was 12.9 years, comparable to the average chronologic age at which menarche typically occurs in healthy girls [1]. Similarly, Viner *et al.* [2] found that girls who were prepubertal when they received their liver transplant reached menarche at a mean age of 14.4 years (range 12.1–17.5; *n* = 18) [2]. Few data exist about the timing of menarche in heart or other solid organ transplant patients [3], but it is likely to be similarly delayed.

Among women who develop organ failure after puberty, menstrual dysfunction is common prior to transplantation, ranging from amenorrhea (absent menses) to menometrorrhagia (heavy and irregular bleeding) [4–6]. For example, among 13 postmenarchal adolescents with chronic renal failure, all had oligomenorrhea (few menses) or secondary amenorrhea [7]. However, studies indicate that pretransplant menstrual cycle dysfunction frequently resolves subsequent to transplantation. In a study of 72 South Korean women, the

proportion who reported regular menses dropped from 75% to 24% after they developed renal failure. After renal transplantation, 47% reported regular menses, taking an average of 7 months to recover "regular menstruation" [5]. Similar findings have been reported among adolescents. Among seven patients who underwent renal transplantation in pubertal stage IV or V, six reinitiated their menses within 8 months after transplant [7].

As with renal transplantation, regular cycles frequently resume after liver transplantation. Mass *et al.* [8] surveyed 82 adult female recipients of liver transplantation. Among the women younger than 45 years, 95% resumed menstrual bleeding within 1 year after transplant. These findings are congruent with smaller studies that have also found prompt resumption of menses after liver transplantation [9–11]. Acute vaginal bleeding requiring gynecologic consultation may be more common in the first 15 postoperative days, or during periods of acute rejection [12]. Otherwise, menstrual regularity does not correlate with organ function of a transplanted kidney [13] or liver [8].

Menstrual disorders in adolescent transplant recipients

No studies have specifically addressed the occurrence of dysmenorrhea, premenstrual syndrome or dysfunctional uterine bleeding in adolescent transplant recipients. However, there is no reason to believe that transplant recipients would be spared from these common menstrual disorders. Evaluation by the patient's primary care provider or gynecologist can proceed in the same manner as for healthy adolescents, with additional consideration of any ongoing or residual effects of the underlying diagnosis and ongoing medication use.

The mainstay of treatment for dysmenorrhea is periodic administration of nonsteroidal anti-inflammatory agents, and premenstrual syndrome responds best to treatment with selective serotonin reuptake inhibitors. However, it is common practice for the treatment of both these conditions to be augmented with combined oral contraceptive pills (COCs), which are also frequently used to treat dysfunctional uterine bleeding. Combination hormonal therapy will be discussed in detail below, in the framework of providing birth control.

ROMANTIC AND SEXUAL RELATIONSHIPS

Normal adolescent development includes an evolving sense of self that incorporates sexual identity and romantic relationships. However, adolescents with chronic disease may have fewer opportunities for social interaction and sexual experimentation, and they may be perceived as having fewer romantic and sexual desires than healthy adolescents [14]. Melzer et al. [15] found that 38% of adolescents with renal transplants had ever had a boyfriend or girlfriend compared with 75% of their healthy peers, and only 13% had experienced intercourse compared with 65% of the healthy matched control group. In another study, Henning et al. [16] compared young adults (14–29 years) with juvenile onset diabetes to those with end-stage renal disease, most with stable functioning kidney grafts. Those with renal disease reported fewer significant romantic relationships and more sexual problems, and were more likely to believe their disease had adversely affected their social life, specifically because of short stature, obesity and other side-effects of medication.

Nonetheless, it should be assumed that young transplant recipients, like other chronically ill adolescents, are often sexually active. In adults, the sexual dysfunction and loss of libido associated with end-stage kidney or heart disease often resolves after transplantation [17,18]. Some adolescent recipients may become sexually active for the first time with the improvement in health status that occurs post-transplant, and may, given their medical condition, underestimate their own fertility [5,19]. However, neither transplantation nor immunosuppressant medications decreases fertility [18] and conception has been seen as early as 3 weeks after a liver transplant [20]. However, it is generally recommended that pregnancy in transplant recipients should be avoided for at least the first 6–12 months after transplantation [4,20,21].

Adolescent transplant recipients may find it difficult to discuss contraceptive needs with health care providers. This can be especially challenging because parents may remain present during all medical encounters. Furthermore, subspecialty physicians have been found to underestimate the proportion of their female adolescent patients with chronic disease who are sexually active [22] and in need of contraception. It is critical that transplant team providers make it routine to talk privately and confidentially with all of their adolescent transplant recipients. Early identification of adolescents who are considering or who are already sexually active may prevent an unplanned pregnancy. Patients desiring pregnancy should obtain preconceptual care from an obstetrician with expertise in this area. Patients wishing to avoid pregnancy should use a highly effective method of birth control [23]. Because many clinics that usually provide confidential care,

such as federally funded family planning clinics, may not be comfortable providing contraception to medically complicated patients, it may be useful for the transplant team to maintain a list of reproductive health care providers to whom they refer young patients for contraceptive care, or to develop their own expertise in this area.

CONTRACEPTIVE METHOD CHOICE

For each individual patient, the risks of any given contraceptive method must be weighed against the significant adverse psychosocial and health risks of a mistimed pregnancy. Sexually active women may choose from hormonal methods that contain both estrogen and a progestin or only a progestin, and barrier/mechanical methods such as intrauterine devices (IUDs), condoms, diaphragms or cervical caps. In the event of an episode of unprotected sex, emergency contraception provides an opportunity to prevent pregnancy.

There are limited data to guide the provision of contraception to adolescent transplant recipients, and one cannot generalize from studies that have included many adult women, in whom sterilization is a popular option. In studies of adult renal [19] and liver [8] transplant recipients, 60% and 24%, respectively, opted for personal or partner sterilization. Sterilization is typically not recommended for minors; in many states minors who are competent to make their own medical decisions are prohibited from consenting for sterilization [24]. Therefore, for adolescents who are not abstinent, the most effective contraceptive method is likely to be a hormonal method. Important considerations when prescribing a contraceptive method include the risk of adverse events and the side-effect profile associated with the method, and how these relate to the specific vulnerabilities of the transplanted organ and the patient's underlying condition. Potential drug interactions must also be carefully assessed and avoided.

Extremely reliable contraception can be provided using a combination of estrogen and progestin, the prototype of which is the oral birth control pill. Combined hormonal contraception is also currently available in the form of weekly patches, and a vaginal ring worn for 3 weeks at a time. Hormonal contraception containing only progestin can be delivered as progestin-only pills, or as injectable depo medroxyprogesterone acetate.

Combined hormonal contraception

The combined oral contraceptive pill (COC) contains a combination of a synthetic progestin and "low dose" (20–35 µg) estrogen (ethinyl estradiol). The most serious complications attributable to COCs are thromboembolic and cardiovascular conditions. Therefore, COCs should not be used in patients with hypercoagulability risk factors, a personal or strong family history of thromboembolic disease [25], a history of migraine with focal neurologic signs, or risk factors for cardiovascular disease such as hypertension, or a history of stroke or coronary artery disease. Among heart transplant recipients, coronary artery disease is a known complication of the transplant procedure. It is found in 40% of transplant recipients by 2–5 years after transplantation, and its presence is a contraindication to oral contraceptive pills [26]. In addition, transplant recipients are at risk of developing hypertension as a side-effect of immunosuppressant use. The World Health Organization considers hypertension (greater than 160 mmHg systolic or 100 mmHg diastolic) a contraindication to the use of COCs [27]. However, the benefits of COC use may outweigh the risks for some women whose hypertension is medically controlled. Other contraindications to COCs include estrogen-sensitive cancers [27] and active liver disease (see below).

There have been many investigations of the effects of COC use on the liver. Patients with ongoing liver dysfunction may not adequately metabolize estrogen because sex steroids are made water-soluble in the liver before they can be excreted by the kidneys [28]. In addition, estrogen has a well-documented cholestatic action, and is not recommended for patients with jaundice or biliary tree problems [29]. Hepatocellular adenoma has been associated with COC use (3.4 cases per 100 000 users). Although these uncommon tumors have been reported to rupture and bleed, they are otherwise benign, and regress when COC use is discontinued [30]. The use of COCs does not cause liver cancer [31]. Another concern is the rare occurrence of thrombosis in the hepatic circulation [30], presumably related to the thrombogenic effects of estrogen in patients with underlying risks for hypercoagulability.

Because of the concerns listed above, and the importance of the liver for sex hormone metabolism, some authors consider COCs relatively contraindicated for liver transplant recipients [20,32]. However, with the exceptions of the uncommon complications noted above, in the absence of ongoing liver disease, COCs have minimal impact on liver function [30]. With careful attention to comorbid conditions and drug interactions, COCs can be safely prescribed after transplantation of the liver [31] or kidney. Excretion of steroid metabolites is primarily renal with minimal fecal excretion [33]. As a result, patients with renal dysfunction will have increased levels of circulating steroid metabolites. However, this has little impact on the levels of active sex steroids [28]. In summary, for those transplant recipients who have established normal organ function and are stable at least 6–8 months post-transplant, combined hormonal contraceptives can be considered for patients who do not have other contraindications to the use of low-dose estrogen [19,21,26]. There are no additional contraindications to the progestin component.

There are two relatively new contraceptive methods that also contain a combination of estrogen and a progestin: Evra®, a skin patch that contains ethinyl estradiol 0.75 mg

and norelgestromin 6.00 mg; and NuvaRing, a vaginal ring that delivers ethinyl estradiol 15 μg and etonogestrel 120 μg/day. These methods differ from COCs in that neither is orally administered and thus they bypass first pass metabolism in the intestinal wall and liver. However, their content and mechanism of action are sufficiently similar to COCs that, until further data are available, they should be used with the same precautions that apply to COCs.

Drug interactions with COCs

COCs can interact with many medications used by transplant recipients, and their use mandates careful surveillance, both to avoid drug toxicities [34] and to maintain the effectiveness of all prescribed medications (Table 54.1) [35]. This chapter is intended to provide general guidance regarding contraceptive prescribing. It is not exhaustive; individual patient care decisions may require consultation with a clinical pharmacologist.

COCs and immunosuppressants

It is important to carefully monitor immunosuppressant concentrations in the blood for all patients also using COCs [4]. COCs inhibit the P450 3A4 pathway [36], and their use may increase the bioavailability of other medications that are metabolized through this pathway, such as cyclosporine [34], tacrolimus and sirolimus [37]. COCs also decrease the clearance of some steroids, causing up to a 30% increase in the plasma concentration of prednisolone [38], and requiring close monitoring for corticosteroid side-effects [39]. To date, there are limited data on COC interactions with newer immunosuppressant agents. The standard regimen for COCs is 21 days of hormonal pills followed by a 7-day hormone-free interval. Because COCs change immunosuppressant levels, patients on COCs can use them continuously, without a hormone-free interval, to avoid monthly fluctuations in drug levels. Issues related to continuous pill use in adolescents have been reviewed elsewhere [40], and patient handouts related to continuous pill use can be found on the Internet (e.g. http://www.youngwomenshealth.org/conthormpills.html).

COCs and other medications

The use of COCs has little impact on most of the other medications commonly used by transplant recipients. However, for patients using diuretics it should be noted that the new progestin drospirenone has a weak spironolactone-like effect that may increase potassium levels. Antihypertensives and antacids are unlikely to have significant impact on contraceptive choice, with the exception that hypertension is a contraindication to COC use. Among the cholesterol lowering medications, lipophilic statins may increase blood levels of steroid hormones so side-effects should be monitored closely.

Table 54.1 Immunosuppressant side-effects and interactions with hormonal contraception. From Sucato and Murray [35] with permission.

Type of medication	Drug interactions	Side-effects influencing contraception	Contraceptive considerations
Corticosteroids (Prednisone)	COCs may increase plasma levels: monitor for increased corticosteroid side-effects	Hypertension	Hypertension is a contraindication to COC use
		Diabetes	Low dose pills have minimal impact on glucose metabolism
		Weight gain Osteoporosis	Monitor weight and bone density carefully if DMPA is used
Azathioprine (Imuran)		Liver toxicity	Liver dysfunction interferes with estrogen metabolism
Mycophenolate mofetil (CellCept)		Diarrhea Vomiting	Severe gastrointestinal disturbance could decrease COC absorption
Cyclosporine Tacrolimus (Prograf, FK506)	Hormonal contraceptives may increase levels: monitor blood levels closely	Hypertension Hyperlipidemia Hyperkalemia	Severe hypertension is a contraindication to COC use COCs have minimal effect on lipids Drospirenone (a progestin with weak spironlactone-like activity) is contraindicated with hyperkalemia
		Diabetes	Low dose pills have minimal impact on glucose metabolism
		Headache	Headache can be a side-effect of steroid hormones, monitor headache frequency*
Sirolimus (Rapamune)	Hormonal contraceptives may increase levels: monitor blood levels closely	Hyperlipidemia	COCs have minimal effect on lipids

* If headaches increase after initiation of contraceptive method, or neurologic symptoms accompany migraine headache, consider changing method.
COC, combined oral contraceptive pill; DMPA, depo medroxyprogesterone acetate.

There has been long-standing concern that antibiotic use decreases COC effectiveness. However, there is no strong evidence linking decreased COC effectiveness with the use of any antibiotic except rifampin [41]. Nonetheless, COC metabolism varies among individuals, and American Medical Association policy advises counseling women about the small risk of interactions with antibiotics that could cause COC failure. A back-up method should be provided to women who are uncomfortable with this risk or who have breakthrough bleeding while also using antibiotics [41]. The back-up method most commonly chosen is a male condom, providing an opportunity to remind adolescents that the combination of hormonal and barrier methods provides the most effective prevention of both pregnancy and infection. In addition to rifampin, concurrent use of any medications that induce hepatic metabolism through cytochrome P450 3A4 (e.g. anticonvulsants and griseofulvin) may accelerate the elimination of ethinyl estradiol and many of the progestins [41] and thereby decrease the effectiveness of hormonal contraception. In order to maintain contraceptive effectiveness in these patients, it may be necessary to change to a pill regimen containing higher doses of both the estrogen and the progestin components.

Progestin-only contraception

For patients who have contraindications to estrogen, consider using a progestin-only method. Progestins have minimal if any effect on the liver [42]. Although drug interactions with progestin-only methods are uncommon, monitoring cyclosporine levels is advisable [43]. Progestin-only contraception is currently available orally, as an intramuscular injection or as part of an intrauterine system.

Progestin-only pills (POPs, also known as "mini-pills") work primarily by thickening cervical mucus, not by inhibiting ovulation. Because of the timing of this effect, it is generally recommended that pills be taken between 4 and 22 hours before coitus usually takes place. Because of the importance of even small variations in the timing of pill administration and the continued potential for ovulation, POPs are much less effective than combined COCs. Therefore, POPs are not typically recommended as a first choice contraceptive in healthy adolescents. Nonetheless, they can be considered for the selected adolescent transplant recipient who has already demonstrated excellent medication adherence.

Depo medroxyprogesterone acetate

Depo medroxyprogesterone acetate 150 mg (DMPA) provides exceptionally effective pregnancy protection, in part because it is less user-dependent; it is delivered as an intramuscular injection every 11–13 weeks. DMPA use in adolescents can be limited by its associated side-effects. It frequently causes irregular bleeding, especially early in use, and can result in weight gain of 5 pounds or more per year.

DMPA has also been associated with decreased bone density [44], an important concern for transplant patients, many of whom may already be osteoporotic [45–48]. This does not rule out DMPA as a possible contraceptive method for transplant recipients. However, patients who choose DMPA should be encouraged to exercise and to maintain adequate intake of calcium and vitamin D. Physicians should consider increased monitoring of bone density and periodic monitoring of estradiol levels. In some centers, healthy women are encouraged to take physiologic estrogen replacement if their estradiol level drops below 30 pg/mL [49].

Intrauterine devices

Intrauterine devices (IUDs) are rarely used in healthy adolescents because of the increased risk of IUD expulsion in nulliparous women [50], and concerns that IUDs would increase the risk of pelvic infection and infertility in a population whose sexual behaviors already put them at high risk for pelvic inflammatory disease (PID). However, current data link pelvic infection to risk factors for sexually transmitted infections rather than the presence of an IUD [51,52], and dispel the concern that IUDs cause infertility [51–54]. In addition, the World Health Organization does not consider nulliparity a contraindication to IUD placement [50,55]. However, IUDs are considered relatively contraindicated for use by transplant recipients because of immunocompromise and the concern for infection [4,19,20,26,32,56]. Recent work evaluating the use of copper IUDs in human immunodeficiency virus-infected women in Nairobi [57,58] appears promising. However, these results are insufficient to use as a basis to recommend IUD use in transplant recipients.

Barriers

Many experts consider barrier contraception to be the safest option for transplant patients [4,20,21,26]. Condoms decrease the risk of sexually transmitted disease, and should be recommended for use by all adolescents. However, for healthy adolescent patients who are sexually active, condoms are rarely recommended as the sole method of pregnancy prevention, even when used in conjunction with spermicide, because of the high failure rate. For women younger than 20 years old, contraceptive failure of condoms during the first year of typical use ranges from 10% to 53% [59]. Diaphragms and cervical caps are rarely used by adolescents, have unacceptably high failure rates and require intravaginal insertion that may be unacceptable or difficult for many adolescents. For an older adolescent, condoms and spermicide, especially in conjunction with a diaphragm or cervical cap, can provide adequate pregnancy prevention. However, this will rarely be the contraceptive method preferred by the adolescent or her parent.

Emergency contraception

Pregnancy can be prevented as late as 5 days after an episode of unprotected sexual intercourse by using emergency contraception [60]. In adolescents, emergency contraception is provided with high-dose progestin (Plan B®). Alternatively, higher doses of common oral contraceptive pills containing estrogen and progestin can also be used. (Dosing and other information about emergency contraception can be found on the Internet, e.g. http://www.plannedparenthood.org/EC/index.html.) There are no known contraindications to the use of emergency contraception, which can prevent up to 85% of pregnancies that would have otherwise occurred [61].

The progestin-only regimen is preferred because of its improved effectiveness and lower incidence of side-effects. It consists of two doses of levonorgestrel (0.75 mg each), 12 hours apart, or as a single large dose (levonorgestrel 1.5 mg) [62]. The safety and effectiveness of progestin-only emergency contraception is outstanding, and many experts advocate for its over-the-counter availability. Until this occurs, all potentially sexually active adolescents, including those not yet sexually active and those already using a reliable method of birth control, should be educated about emergency contraceptive pills, and provided with an advance prescription for emergency contraception to have immediately available should the need arise. Preparation is important because the sooner emergency contraception is used, the more effective it is in preventing pregnancy [63]. This is especially important for transplant recipients given the excess risks associated with unplanned pregnancies in this population. After a patient uses emergency contraception, a reproductive health care visit should be scheduled 2 weeks later to test for pregnancy and sexually transmitted infection and to discuss ongoing contraceptive method choice.

Other than the barrier methods, no contraceptive method is without some risk. Therefore the patient's transplant team and her reproductive health provider must work in collaboration to help the patient choose an acceptable, safe and effective contraceptive method (Table 54.2). In many cases, the risks of unintended pregnancy, with the associated psychosocial, hormonal and physiologic effects, outweigh the risks of

Table 54.2 Contraceptive method advantages and disadvantages. From Sucato and Murray [35] with permission.

Contraceptive method	Advantages	Disadvantages
Combined hormonal methods	Patch and ring do not require daily administration Good menstrual cycle control	Pills require daily administration Contraindicated with active liver dysfunction, coronary artery disease, hypertension Possible drug interactions
Emergency contraception	Effective after sexual intercourse No contraindications	Not effective as an ongoing contraceptive method
Progestin-only pills	Few drug interactions	Less effective than COCs Require carefully timed daily administration
DMPA	Very effective Administered every 11–13 weeks	Side-effects include weight gain, osteoporosis and irregular bleeding
Intrauterine system or IUD	Very effective	Little experience in transplant recipients Theoretic increased risk of infection with immunosuppression
Surgical sterilization	Permanent and very effective	Often not available to minors Difficult to reverse

COC, combined oral contraceptive pill; DMPA, depo medroxyprogesterone acetate; IUD, intrauterine device.

hormonal contraception. As long as the transplanted organ is functioning normally, all hormonal methods can be considered. However, deterioration of organ function or episodes of rejection would require re-evaluation and consideration of substituting a barrier method, at least temporarily.

SEXUALLY TRANSMITTED INFECTION

Infectious complications are a significant cause of morbidity and mortality in solid organ transplant recipients [64,65]. Sexually active adolescents are at high risk for sexually transmitted infections (STIs), which can be difficult to eradicate in immunosuppressed patients. Therefore it is imperative to always obtain a confidential history and patients who are found to be sexually active should be given specific referrals to clinicians who provide comprehensive reproductive health care, confidentially if necessary.

Routine reproductive health care for the sexually active adolescent should include screening for STIs, including specific laboratory testing for gonorrhea and *Chlamydia*, the two most common bacterial STIs. Screening should occur every 6 months or whenever there are complaints of vaginal discharge, dysuria or other genitourinary symptoms. Although recurrent urinary tract infection is common among pediatric renal transplant recipients [65], dysuria can also be the only presenting symptom of *Chlamydia* infection and the other STIs that may occur simultaneously.

Reproductive health care providers, while awaiting laboratory results, should have a low threshold for empiric treatment of STIs in immunosuppressed adolescents with genitourinary symptoms, especially if the patient has a new partner, or other epidemiologic, clinical or microscopic findings suggestive of an STI. Early treatment of cervicitis may decrease the risk of developing pelvic inflammatory disease, a polymicrobial infection of the upper genital tract that can be complicated by the formation of a tubo-ovarian abscess. Tubo-ovarian abscess can present with relatively mild symptoms in immunosuppressed women, and there are reports of tubo-ovarian abscesses resulting from uncommon organisms (*Pseudomonas aeruginosa* and *Aspergillus*) [66,67].

In addition to bacterial STIs, adolescents also commonly acquire viral sexually transmitted diseases. With current immunization guidelines, prior to transplant most adolescents will have been immunized against hepatitis B and possibly hepatitis A. In the future, a vaccine for herpes simplex virus may also be available [68].

There are encouraging new data about a vaccine that reduces the incidence of HPV-16, and HPV-16-related cervical intraepithelial neoplasia in women [69]. Transplant recipients are more likely than immunocompetent patients to have high-risk oncogenic HPV subtypes 16 and 18 [70] and have substantially increased risk of anogenital neoplasia [71]. To improve early detection and prevent invasive anogenital cancer, some authors advocate cervical Papanicolaou (Pap) smears every 6 months and yearly colposcopy [72]. Unfortunately, many transplant recipients do not obtain even routine Pap smears [8,73]. Careful attention to the presence of sexual activity in adolescents and provision of the necessary gynecologic health care can be life-saving in young female transplant recipients.

Table 54.3 Gynecologic issues of the adolescent recipient of a solid organ transplant. Adapted from Sucato and Murray [35] with permission.

Key concepts for gynecologic care
Menarche is often delayed
Menstrual irregularity is common prior to transplant, but often normalizes afterward
Menstrual disorders should be evaluated as they would in a healthy patient, with special attention to the transplanted organ and current medications
Hormonal contraceptive methods can be used to treat menstrual disorders and to provide contraception
Sexual activity and fertility are likely in adolescent transplant recipients
A confidential history is the key to identifying reproductive health care needs
Encourage condoms
Screen for sexually transmitted infections every 6 months, and in the presence of genitourinary symptoms
Treat empirically if index of suspicion for infection is high
Perform Papanicolaou smears at least yearly
Maintain a low threshold for colposcopy
Vaccinate against sexually transmitted infections before transplant whenever possible

CONCLUSIONS

Advances in the field of transplant medicine are providing adolescent recipients with improved quality of life and increased opportunities for normal social and sexual relationships. As a result, adolescent females require careful attention to their gynecologic and reproductive health (Table 54.3). Anticipating the onset of sexual activity before it occurs may help prevent a mistimed pregnancy by providing or prescribing condoms and emergency contraception in advance. In addition, a transplanted solid organ, provided it has normal function, is not a contraindication to progestin-only or combined hormonal contraception. With careful monitoring of immunosuppressant levels and close clinical follow-up, any of the new delivery systems of combined estrogen and progestin could be used by solid organ transplant recipients. Use of extended cycles of combined hormonal contraception may minimize the impact of drug interactions with immunosuppressants.

REFERENCES

1 van Diemen-Steenvoorde R, Donckerwolcke RA, Brackel H, Wolff ED, de Jong MC. Growth and sexual maturation in children after kidney transplantation. *J Pediatr* 1987;**110**:351–6.

2 Viner RM, Forton JT, Cole TJ, *et al.* Growth of long-term survivors of liver transplantation. *Arch Dis Child* 1999;**80**:235–40.

3 de Broux E, Huot CH, Chartrand S, Vobecky S, Chartrand C. Growth and pubertal development following pediatric heart transplantation: a 15-year experience at Ste-Justine Hospital. *J Heart Lung Transplant* 2000;**19**:825–33.

4 Laifer SA, Guido RS. Reproductive function and outcome of pregnancy after liver transplantation in women. *Mayo Clin Proc* 1995;**70**:388–94.

5 Kim LH, Chun CJ, Kang DM, Kwak J. Kidney transplantation and menstrual changes. *Transplant Proc* 1998;**30**:3057–9.

6 Phocas I, Sarandakou A, Kassanos D, *et al.* Hormonal and ultrasound characteristics of menstrual function during chronic hemodialysis and after successful renal transplantation. *Int J Gynaecol Obstet* 1992;**37**:19–28.

7 Ferraris JR, Domene HM, Escobar ME, *et al.* Hormonal profile in pubertal females with chronic renal failure: before and under haemodialysis and after renal transplantation. *Acta Endocrinol (Copenh)* 1987;**115**:289–96.

8 Mass K, Quint EH, Punch MR, Merion RM. Gynecological and reproductive function after liver transplantation. *Transplantation* 1996;**62**:476–9.

9 Cundy TF, O'Grady JG, Williams R. Recovery of menstruation and pregnancy after liver transplantation. *Gut* 1990;**31**:337–8.

10 Parolin MB, Rabinovitch I, Urbanetz AA, *et al.* Impact of successful liver transplantation on reproductive function and sexuality in women with advanced liver disease. *Transplant Proc* 2004;**36**:943–4.

11 de Koning ND, Haagsma EB. Normalization of menstrual pattern after liver transplantation: consequences for contraception. *Digestion* 1990;**46**:239–41.

12 Nicholas SL, Rulin MC. Acute vaginal bleeding in women undergoing liver transplantation. *Am J Obstet Gynecol* 1994;**170**:733–6.

13 Ghazizadeh S, Lessan-Pezeshki M, Mahdavi M, Razeghi E, Seifi S. Menstrual problems among kidney transplant recipients. *Transplant Proc* 2003;**35**:2720–1.

14 Valencia LS, Cromer BA. Sexual activity and other high-risk behaviors in adolescents with chronic illness: a review. *J Pediatr Adolesc Gynecol* 2000;**13**:53–64.

15 Melzer SM, Leadbeater B, Reisman L, Jaffe LR, Lieberman KV. Characteristics of social networks in adolescents with end-stage renal disease treated with renal transplantation. *J Adolesc Health Care* 1989;**10**:308–12.

16 Henning P, Tomlinson L, Rigden SP, Haycock GB, Chantler C. Long term outcome of treatment of end stage renal failure. *Arch Dis Child* 1988;**63**:35–40.

17 Ghahramani N, Behzadi A, Gholami S, *et al.* Postrenal transplant improvement of sexual function. *Transplant Proc* 1999;**31**:3144.

18 Cupples SA. Cardiac transplantation in women. *Crit Care Nurs Clin North Am* 1997;**9**:521–33.

19 O'Donnell D. Contraception in the female transplant recipient. *Dial Transplant* 1986;**15**:610–2.

20 Laifer SA, Darby MJ, Scantlebury VP, Harger JH, Caritis SN. Pregnancy and liver transplantation. *Obstet Gynecol* 1990;**76**: 1083–8.

21 Riely CA. Contraception and pregnancy after liver transplantation. *Liver Transpl* 2001;**7**(Suppl 1):S74–6.

22 Britto MT, Rosenthal SL, Taylor J, Passo MH. Improving rheumatologists' screening for alcohol use and sexual activity. *Arch Pediatr Adolesc Med* 2000;**154**:478–83.

23 Lessan-Pezeshki M, Ghazizadeh S, Khatami MR, *et al.* Fertility and contraceptive issues after kidney transplantation in women. *Transplant Proc* 2004;**36**:1405–6.

24 Smith S. Legal issues in treating minors. In: Sanfilippo J, Muram D, Dewhurst J, Lee P, eds. *Pediatric and Adolescent Gynecology.* Philadelphia: WB Saunders, 2001: 513–26.

25 Creinin MD, Lisman R, Strickler RC. Screening for factor V Leiden mutation before prescribing combination oral contraceptives. *Fertil Steril* 1999;**72**:646–51.

26 Kossoy LR, Herbert CM III, Wentz AC. Management of heart transplant recipients: guidelines for the obstetrician-gynecologist. *Am J Obstet Gynecol* 1988;**159**:490–9.

27 Hatcher R, Guillebaud J. The pill: combined oral contraceptives. In: Hatcher R, Trussell J, Stewart F, *et al.*, eds. *Contraceptive Technology.* New York: Ardent Media, 1998: 405–66.

28 Faigle J, Schenkel L. Pharmacokinetics of estrogens and progestogens. In: Fraser I, Jansen R, Lobo R, Whitehead M, eds. *Estrogens and Progestogens in Clinical Practice.* London: Churchill Livingstone, 1998: 273–94.

29 Goldzieher J. Effects on other tissues. In: Fraser I, Jansen R, Lobo R, Whitehead M, eds. *Estrogens and Progestogens in Clinical Practice.* London: Churchill Livingstone, 1998: 825–9.

30 Connell E. Clinical aspects of oral contraception. In: Fraser I, Jansen R, Lobo R, Whitehead M, eds. *Estrogens and Progestogens in Clinical Practice.* London: Churchill Livingstone, 1998: 555–77.

31 Dourakis SP, Tolis G. Sex hormonal preparations and the liver. *Eur J Contracept Reprod Health Care* 1998;**3**:7–16.

32 Blumenfeld Z, Enat R, Brandes JM, Baruch Y. Gonadotropin-releasing hormone analogues for dysfunctional bleeding in women after liver transplantation: a new application. *Fertil Steril* 1992;**57**:1121–3.

33 Longcope C. Metabolism of estrogens and progestogens. In: Fraser I, Jansen R, Lobo R, Whitehead M, eds. *Estrogens and Progestogens in Clinical Practice.* London: Churchill Livingstone, 1998: 89–94.

34 Deray G, Le Hoang P, Cacoub P, *et al.* Oral contraceptive interaction with cyclosporin. *Lancet* 1987;**1**:158–9.

35 Sucato G, Murray P. Gynecologic issues of the adolescent female solid organ transplant recipient. *Pediatr Clin North Am* 2003;**50**: 1521–42.

36 Bush WW. Overview of transplantation immunology and the pharmacotherapy of adult solid organ transplant recipients: focus on immunosuppression. *AACN Clin Issues* 1999;**10**:253–69.

37 Gaston RS. Maintenance immunosuppression in the renal transplant recipient: an overview. *Am J Kidney Dis* 2001;**38**(Suppl 6):S25–35.

38 Gustavson LE, Legler UF, Benet LZ. Impairment of prednisolone disposition in women taking oral contraceptives or conjugated estrogens. *J Clin Endocrinol Metab* 1986;**62**:234–7.

39 Seidegard J, Simonsson M, Edsbacker S. Effect of an oral contraceptive on the plasma levels of budesonide and prednisolone and the influence on plasma cortisol. *Clin Pharmacol Ther* 2000;**67**:373–81.

40 Sucato G, Gold M. Extended cycling of oral contraceptive pills for adolescents. *J Pediatr Adolesc Gynecol* 2002;**15**:325–7.

41 Dickinson BD, Altman RD, Nielsen NH, Sterling ML. Drug interactions between oral contraceptives and antibiotics. *Obstet Gynecol* 2001;**98**:853–60.

42 McCann MF, Potter LS. Progestin-only oral contraception: a comprehensive review. *Contraception* 1994;**50**(Suppl 1)):S1–195.

43 Mastrobattista JM, Katz AR. Pregnancy after organ transplant. *Obstet Gynecol Clin North Am* 2004;**31**:415–28, vii.

44 Scholes D, LaCroix AZ, Ichikawa LE, Barlow WE, Ott SM. Injectable hormone contraception and bone density: results from a prospective study. *Epidemiology* 2002;**13**:581–7.

45 Braith RW, Howard C, Fricker FJ, Mitchell M, Edwards DG. Glucocorticoid-induced osteopenia in adolescent heart transplant recipients. *J Heart Lung Transplant* 2000;**19**:840–5.

46 Chesney RW, Rose PG, Mazess RB. Persistence of diminished bone mineral content following renal transplantation in childhood. *Pediatrics* 1984;**73**:459–66.

47 Boot AM, Nauta J, Hokken-Koelega AC, *et al.* Renal transplantation and osteoporosis. *Arch Dis Child* 1995;**72**:502–6.

48 el Husseini AA, el Agroudy AE, Wafa EW, *et al.* Bone mineral density in live related kidney transplant children and adolescents. *Int Urol Nephrol* 2004;**36**:95–100.

49 Hatcher R. Depo-provera, norplant, and progestin-only pills (minipills). In: Hatcher R, Trussell J, Stewart F, *et al.*, eds. *Contraceptive Technology.* New York: Ardent Media, 1998:467–510.

50 Nelson AL. The intrauterine contraceptive device. *Obstet Gynecol Clin North Am* 2000;**27**:723–40.

51 Darney PD. Time to pardon the IUD? *N Engl J Med* 2001;**345**: 608–10.

52 Lee NC, Rubin GL, Borucki R. The intrauterine device and pelvic inflammatory disease revisited: new results from the Women's Health Study. *Obstet Gynecol* 1988;**72**:1–6.

53 Hubacher D, Lara-Ricalde R, Taylor DJ, Guerra-Infante F, Guzman-Rodriguez R. Use of copper intrauterine devices and the risk of tubal infertility among nulligravid women. *N Engl J Med* 2001;**345**:561–7.

54 Kronmal RA, Whitney CW, Mumford SD. The intrauterine device and pelvic inflammatory disease: the Women's Health Study reanalyzed. *J Clin Epidemiol* 1991;**44**:109–22.

55 Stewart G. Intrauterine devices. In: Hatcher R, Trussell J, Stewart F, *et al.*, eds. *Contraceptive Technology.* New York: Ardent Media, 1998: 545–88.

56 Zerner J, Doil KL, Drewry J, Leeber DA. Intrauterine contraceptive device failures in renal transplant patients. *J Reprod Med* 1981;**26**:99–102.

57 Morrison CS, Sekadde-Kigondu C, Sinei SK, *et al.* Is the intrauterine device appropriate contraception for HIV-1-infected women? *BJOG* 2001;**108**:784–90.

58 Sinei SK, Morrison CS, Sekadde-Kigondu C, Allen M, Kokonya D. Complications of use of intrauterine devices among HIV-1-infected women. *Lancet* 1998;**351**:1238–41.

59 Fu H, Darroch JE, Haas T, Ranjit N. Contraceptive failure rates: new estimates from the 1995 National Survey of Family Growth. *Fam Plann Perspect* 1999;**31**:56–63.

60 Rodrigues I, Grou F, Joly J. Effectiveness of emergency contraceptive pills between 72 and 120 hours after unprotected sexual intercourse. *Am J Obstet Gynecol* 2001;**184**:531–7.

61 Grimes DA, Raymond EG. Emergency contraception. *Ann Intern Med* 2002;**137**:180–9.

62 von Hertzen H, Piaggio G, Ding J, *et al*. Low dose mifepristone and two regimens of levonorgestrel for emergency contraception: a WHO multicentre randomised trial. *Lancet* 2002;**360**: 1803–10.

63 Task Force on Postovulatory Methods of Fertility Regulation. Randomised controlled trial of levonorgestrel versus the Yuzpe regimen of combined oral contraceptives for emergency contraception. *Lancet* 1998;**352**:428–33.

64 Munoz SJ. Long-term management of the liver transplant recipient. *Med Clin North Am* 1996;**80**:1103–20.

65 Green M, Michaels MG. Infectious complications of solid-organ transplantation in children. *Adv Pediatr Infect Dis* 1992;**7**:181–204.

66 El Khoury J, Stikkelbroeck MM, Goodman A, *et al*. Post-menopausal tubo-ovarian abscess due to *Pseudomonas aeruginosa* in a renal transplant patient: a case report and review of the literature. *Transplantation* 2001;**72**:1241–4.

67 Kim SW, Nah MY, Yeum CH, *et al*. Pelvic aspergillosis with tubo-ovarian abscess in a renal transplant recipient. *J Infect* 2001;**42**:215–7.

68 Stanberry LR, Spruance SL, Cunningham AL, *et al*. Glycoprotein-D-adjuvant vaccine to prevent genital herpes. *N Engl J Med* 2002;**347**:1652–61.

69 Koutsky LA, Ault KA, Wheeler CM, *et al*. A controlled trial of a human papillomavirus type 16 vaccine. *N Engl J Med* 2002; **347**:1645–51.

70 Brown MR, Noffsinger A, First MR, Penn I, Husseinzadeh N. HPV subtype analysis in lower genital tract neoplasms of female renal transplant recipients. *Gynecol Oncol* 2000;**79**:220–4.

71 Sillman FH, Sentovich S, Shaffer D. Ano-genital neoplasia in renal transplant patients. *Ann Transplant* 1997;**2**:59–66.

72 Ozsaran AA, Ates T, Dikmen Y, *et al*. Evaluation of the risk of cervical intraepithelial neoplasia and human papilloma virus infection in renal transplant patients receiving immunosuppressive therapy. *Eur J Gynaecol Oncol* 1999;**20**:127–30.

73 Zeldin GA, Maygers J, Klein A, Thuluvath PJ. Vaccination, screening for malignancy, and health maintenance of the liver transplant recipient. *J Clin Gastroenterol* 2001;**32**:148–50.

55 Transition to Adult Care

Janet McDonagh and Deirdre Kelly

The survival rate for child and adolescent recipients of solid organ transplantation is 80% over 15 years. The challenge of developing of transitional care for these young people is based on effective collaboration at the pediatric–adult interface and is a major challenge for pediatric and adult providers alike in the 21st century.

During adolescence and early adulthood, a young person requiring solid organ transplantation during childhood potentially negotiates several transitions – from adolescence to adulthood, education to employment, family life to independent living, as well as from pediatric to adult health care. Although such transitions are interdependent, this chapter concentrates primarily on the transition in health care, with acknowledgment of the interweaving of the other transitions. This reflects the holistic concept of health care transition, which has been defined as "a multi-faceted, active process that attends to the medical, psychosocial and educational/vocational needs of adolescents as they move from child to adult centered care" [1]. The aims of transition are detailed in Table 55.1.

Transitional care for young people with special health care needs (SHCN) has gained increasing recognition on the international adolescent health agenda [2–6]. The majority of policy statements, guidelines and reviews acknowledge the noncategorical generic nature of many transitional care issues facing such young people [1–9]. Many authors report unmet transitional care needs of such young people [10–27],

although perspectives vary as to the relevance, importance and concern of such needs [18,19, 22]. With the increasing numbers of young people with solid organ transplants now surviving into adulthood, transitional care is an important quality issue for pediatric and adult care providers.

THE KEY PLAYERS IN TRANSITION

Transition is, by definition, a team effort, potentially involving a significant number of people (Table 55.2) between whom effective communication is vital to ensure coordination. The perspectives of the young person, their caregivers and the health care providers are considered below.

The young person's perspective

Central to transition are the young people themselves. Young people with cystic fibrosis and a lung transplant reported wanting to set and attain meaningful long-term goals and expressed a need to control as many aspects of their lives as possible – important concepts within transitional care [18] and in keeping with the definition of transitional care [1].

Models of care
In terms of actual service provision, young people have also expressed definite opinions. In models of care where young

Table 55.1 Aims of transition.

1 To provide high-quality coordinated uninterrupted health care that is patient-centered, age and developmentally appropriate, future-focused, culturally competent, flexible, responsive and comprehensive
2 To promote skills in communication, decision making, assertiveness, self-care, self-determination and self-advocacy
3 To enhance sense of control and interdependence in health care
4 To maximize lifelong functioning and potential
5 To support the parent(s)/guardian of the young person during transition and in particular to enhance their advocacy skills

Table 55.2 The key players in transition.

Young person and their family
Peers
Professionals
   Primary health care
   Secondary/tertiary health care
Education services
Vocational services
Social services
Voluntary agencies

people continue as adults to see the same doctors, they want their care to become more "adult-like" [18,25]. Although there is currently no evidence that particular models of transitional care are more effective than others [10,28], young people with a range of chronic illnesses have reported preference for at least meeting the adult team prior to transfer [14–17,20,25]. Such practices have been associated with improved adherence to appointments in young adulthood [20,21]. This practice also serves to communicate the reassuring message to the young person and their family that the pediatric and adult teams are working together and facilitates a conducive environment for experiential training in transitional care for professionals from both teams.

Information

Young people requiring solid organ transplantation during childhood have had a different childhood and adolescence compared with their "healthy peers" by virtue of their transplant. The impact of the pretransplant condition on their adolescent development (physical, psychosocial and cognitive) needs to be considered [9]. One such area is the relationship of information provision and cognitive development. Salient, age and developmentally appropriate information is an integral part of self-management and informed consent. The range of information requested by young people is potentially wide and often extends beyond the medical aspects of the condition, in keeping with their desire for health professionals to acknowledge their lives beyond the health care setting [29,30]. Provision and delivery of such information requires an understanding of adolescent cognitive development, characterized by the evolution of adult-like abstract thinking and a more complete personal identity. The pretransplant condition and transplant experience may affect cognitive development because of the impact of drug side-effects, pain, fatigue, school absence, etc. Assessment of the stage of cognitive development and the relative impact of the chronic illness is important in planning health and disease education, decision-making and self-care for such young people. If the young person has had their primary disease since early childhood, much of the initial "onset" disease education may have been primarily directed to the parents. Disease education must be taught, assessed, retaught and reassessed, acknowledging the changing cognitive development of growing children (e.g. for young adolescents, "here-and-now" concrete examples are more developmentally appropriate than abstract "if, then" discussions). Immediate rather than future motivators should be used in adherence and self-management skills training. Having a full understanding of their illness and being involved in medical decisions was rated as important by over two-thirds (69%) of young adult survivors of a pediatric dialysis and transplantation program, and as the most helpful coping strategy overall by 36% [31]. Disclosure issues (e.g. to potential partners, teachers, employers) have also been highlighted as an important component of transitional

care by young people [22,25] and implicit to disclosure is knowledge of the condition.

Disease education

If the young person has had their primary disease since early childhood, much of the initial disease education may have been primarily directed to the parents. Disease education must be retaught, acknowledging the changing cognitive development of the growing child. The use of age-appropriate literature and a skilled play worker or teacher are invaluable to help the young person to understand and accept difficult issues such as having a dead person's organ, or facing a lifetime of medical monitoring and medication [32].

A requirement for successful transition is an understanding of and an ability of the young person to describe the signs and symptoms requiring urgent medical attention. Appropriate literature is vital, as well as easy access to medical care, which may be more daunting in an adult unit [13,14]. Information regarding drugs should extend beyond the importance of adherence and side-effect profile and monitoring, and include rationale, benefits as well as risks, etc.

Self-advocacy skills

One of the stated aims of transition is to promote skills in self-advocacy (see Table 55.1). Aspects of self-advocacy in health care include being confident in seeing professionals independently from their parents when they choose to do so, a full understanding of the condition and its management, involvement in decision making, self-medication, adherence, independent living skills and knowledge of accessing the health service. Acknowledging that adolescents are essentially "new users" of health services [4] is a useful concept to support the need for skills training in this area, their parents having previously accessed health care on their behalf. Communicating with health professionals is a key skill in developing self-advocacy and should be nurtured by the health care team where possible. Evidence suggests, however, that young people may have little opportunity to practice with health professionals who either fail to listen to their cues or favor unidirectional strategies which tend to silence the young person who may not feel able to interrupt (see below) [33].

Confidentiality is the main attribute of an adolescent-friendly practice according to young people [34], and if it is not assured may influence how young people access health care [35]. Young people with chronic illnesses have reported that the presence of parents or strangers influence the communication they have with health professionals [25,30,36]. Young people with cystic fibrosis have been reported to feel that 13–16 years was the best time for them to be seen independently [18]. There is often a discrepancy between health care provider and parent as to when young people with SHCN should start to be seen independently [11]. It is important to remember that none of us are truly independent and our aim for these young people should be one of shared management and optimizing their interdependence (e.g. allowing the young person to *choose* who is in the consultation) [25].

Generic health

In view of the recognized long-term morbidities of transplantation in terms of premature arteriosclerosis, hyperlipidemia and osteoporosis, generic health issues such as substance use, nutrition and exercise should not be ignored. This is particularly pertinent during adolescence, which is the time when adult health-promoting behaviors often become established. Young people with chronic illnesses have been reported to have more age-related health concerns (e.g. weight, sexual health) compared with their healthy peers [37] and have more serious and diverse concerns than perceived by their health care providers [38].

Experimentation is part of "normal" adolescent psychosocial development but becomes concerning when it evolves into risk-taking behavior. A history of substance misuse has been reported in young people who are nonadherent with medication and hence an important (albeit at times difficult) aspect of history taking [39]. Pediatricians who usually see younger patients may not appreciate that even preadolescents may have specific health concerns and may be already involved in risky behaviors [40]. Conversely, a delay in onset of risk-taking behaviors has been observed in teenagers with cystic fibrosis and sickle cell disease [41], suggesting the provision of anticipatory guidance for such behaviors is important for both pediatric and adult providers.

Greater levels of exercise are associated with well-being and long-term functioning in patients with chronic conditions [42] and are to be encouraged when feasible, particularly in the light of the concerns of the morbidity of the inactivity of today's youth generally. A further issue is the importance of weight-bearing exercise for young people on steroid therapy in view of the risk of premature osteoporosis post-transplant [43].

Sexual health issues for young people with transplants include all the usual concerns of their peers, which accompany the development of a sexual identity. In addition, they also have to deal with the reciprocal influences of puberty and chronic illness and/or transplantation, teratogenic drug therapy, effects on fertility, heredity issues and physical limitations. Chronically ill adolescents are reported to be as sexually active as their healthy peers but are also at increased risk of negative outcomes of such behavior (e.g. sexually transmitted infections [STIs] and sexual abuse) [44]. The former are of particular concern if the patient remains on immunosuppressive drugs, yet are often forgotten with avoidance of pregnancy being the usual (and only) consideration. Differential attitudes between sexual health counseling for male and female patients with respect to protection against STIs may also be prevalent, with male patients potentially ignored [45]. Despite young people with chronic illnesses wanting sexual health information [25,46,47], they do not always receive it, especially if their condition has impacted on their school attendance and access to school-based sex and relationship education. Nixon *et al.* [46] reported 87% of adolescents with cystic fibrosis (median age 15 years) and 78% of their mothers had had no discussion regarding sexual health with their specialists. Approximately half of young adults with renal transplants reported they would have welcomed some counseling or advice about sexual health including contraception, relationships, fertility and pregnancy [32]. Merzel *et al.* [36] reported that young people rarely initiated such discussions and the latter was facilitated by the absence of parents and a health professional comfortable with such discussions.

It is important to provide information about contraception. Although barrier methods are the safest, there is a high failure rate. It is safe for girls to take a low-dose estrogen/progesterone contraceptive pill or to take the "morning after pill" [48]. However, chronic liver disease or therapy can cause delayed puberty which may begin after a successful transplant. Most immunosuppressive drugs are not teratogenic and do not affect fertility. Many girls develop menorrhagia post-transplant and specific advice from a gynecologist trained in managing contraception and pregnancy in patients on immunosuppressive drugs is particularly useful [49].

Mental health

Mental health is an important component of transitional care, although psychosocial issues can vary with the primary diagnosis (e.g. adolescents with cystic fibrosis and transplants did not appear to have reduced self-esteem unlike pediatric kidney transplant recipients) [50]. Coping with teasing and/or bullying, side-effects of drugs on body image and disclosure issues are important issues to address with the young person during adolescence and transition [25,51]. Patients with different types of disease require different psychosocial services as they await transplant, with those patients who have had disease since birth faring better than those with later onset disease [51,52]. Transplantation itself may be associated with a reduction in the prevalence of depressive symptomatology [52,53], although it can remain significant [52].

Coping with teasing or bullying as well as disclosure issues are important issues to address with the young person during adolescence and transition. Transplant recipients may be particularly vulnerable because of their altered appearance as a result of disease or medication, or because of time lost from school. Disclosure is an important lifelong issue whether it refers to disclosing details of the chronic condition or therapy to a friend, significant other or potential employer. Exploring and developing coping strategies for disclosure with a health professional can help the young person gain in confidence in this arena.

Vocational issues

An important component of future-focused transitional care is the asking the simple question – "What do you want to do when you leave school?" even if the answer is "Don't know!" Despite the tremendous success of transplantation in terms of life expectancy, lower levels of employment have been reported in adult survivors of a pediatric dialysis and transplant program [31]. Unemployment was associated with lower educational performance [31], which in turn has been reported to be related to poorer self-esteem [54]. Increased school absence is one possible explanation [55], but further prospective studies are needed to determine the etiology of unemployment in young people in order to improve this important aspect of quality of life.

Two recent studies [56,57] indicate that health-related quality of life was nearly normal, so full employment is possible but needs to be encouraged. However, measurement of intelligence quotient (IQ) is a little lower in transplant recipients, but whether this is because of the prolonged pretransplant illness or the result of long-term immunosuppression is unknown [58,59], but may affect educational and employment potential.

A useful concept to consider in such research is *vocational readiness*. Vocational readiness is not only related to educational achievement but also to prior work experience, expectations of both the young person, their family and their health professional, psychological factors (e.g. self-esteem, extent of knowledge about career services and community resources) as well as society's attitudes towards disability. All these aspects need to be considered by professionals involved in transitional care, some of whom need training in this area [60].

A useful clinical tool for clinical consultations with adolescents is HEADS (Home Education Activities Drugs Sex), which ensures the important topics (including those discussed above) are covered [61].

Unfortunately, in certain health care systems, financial aspects of care are a concern of young people with chronic conditions as they transfer into adult care [22,62] and will need to be addressed in transition programs in some countries. Service resource issues and cost effectiveness are also areas that have yet to be definitely and objectively studied, despite their importance.

Adherence issues

In any discussion regarding nonadherence in adolescence, it is important to reflect on what young people with chronic diseases have to face day-to-day. They often face long-term therapeutic regimens and they often have to continue medication even when they feel well. Many drug regimens also required regular monitoring in accordance with the course of the disease. These factors potentially lead to restrictions on leisure time, personal freedom, spontaneity and peer interactions. Nonadherent behavior may be the only control mechanism open to the young person or be a simple wish to

be heard and to take an active role in the decision-making process. Self-medication is an important aspect of becoming an independent young adult but it must be seen in the context of shared decision making, self-care and self-management [63]. Experimentation is a normal part of adolescent development and may be practiced by the self-medicating adolescent. However, in the post-transplantation period, nonadherence can be associated with morbidity and even mortality of transplant recipients [64,65], and particularly of late graft loss [66].

It is important to decriminalize nonadherence in the clinic setting and rather than asking "Have you been taking your tablets every day," ask "When was the last time you forgot to take your medication."

The parent/caregiver perspective

One of the basic tenets of a transitional care program is that it is inclusive of the family, not exclusive. Family connectedness, family role models, family concern for the well-being of the child and autonomy at home are all factors that foster resilience in the young person and should be encouraged and affirmed [67], especially during adolescence and transition. Conversely, lack of parental support at this time has been associated with negative outcomes (e.g. greater nonadherence to medication) [39].

The challenge of negotiating the appropriate extent of parental involvement is an integral component of adolescent health, whatever the specialty. Parental overprotectiveness has been reported in several studies of adolescents with transplants [50,68–70], as in other chronic illnesses [24]. Durst *et al.* [50] reported that parental overprotectiveness remained an ongoing challenge for adolescents with cystic fibrosis following lung transplant, despite the patient's age and the time since transplantation. Overprotective parenting was also one reason given for their unemployment status by young adult survivors on the European Dialysis and Transplant Association (EDTA) registry [68]. Geenen *et al.* [11] reported a significant discrepancy between the perceived age for commencing self-management skills training between parents of young people with special health care needs and their health care providers. One cause of this protectiveness lies in the continuous balancing of the risks of infection and rejection versus the benefits of living a normal life – often parents' and adolescents' views will differ on each side of this debate! Meeting the transitional care needs of the parents of young people has been emphasized in the recent major policy documents on both sides of the Atlantic [2,3]. Transitional care programs therefore need to support and prepare parents for transition and transfer including developing an understanding of adolescent development in the context of chronic illness, their own important dynamic role in the process, provision of advice about negotiation of boundaries and informational resources and support services available for parents both within the hospital and the local community.

	Pediatric	Adult
Age-related factors	Growth and development; future focused	Senescence
Focus	Family	Individual
Approach	Paternalistic Proactive	Collaborative Reactive
Communication style	Vertical > horizontal	Horizontal
Diagnostic style	Cognitive but with restrained diagnostic enthusiasm	Cognitive
Shared decision-making	With parent	With patient
Management plans	Prescriptive	Collaborative
Dealing with poor adherence	More assistance	More tolerance
Procedural pain management	Lower threshold for active input	Higher threshold for active input
Tolerance of immaturity in patient	Higher	Lower
Coordination with education and social services	Integral	Less emphasis
Care provision	Interdisciplinary	Multidisciplinary
Numbers of patients per doctor	Fewer	Greater

Table 55.3 The different cultures of pediatric and adult health care.

Health care providers

When considering the perspective of the health care providers, the "cultural" differences between pediatric and adult health care need to be acknowledged and respected as has been well-reviewed by Rosen [71]. Table 55.3 details some such differences, acknowledging that neither represents a gold standard. For adolescents with chronic conditions, some aspects of both cultures will be appropriate for some patients, some of the time.

Adolescent health care, including transitional care, is of particular interest with respect to communication skills of professionals as it is the only age group when health professionals are not communicating directly with adults. Communication and counseling skills are influenced by a range of practical, attitudinal and behavioral factors that warrant consideration during development of adolescent services (e.g. duration and frequency of contact, gender, perceived attitudes towards adolescents, communication skills of both the adolescent and the professional, presence of others, type of information needed, and perceived lack of interest in the wider impact of the chronic illness on the part of the professional) [30,45,61]. Time is particularly important as clinic consultation times are often longer in pediatric care than adult care [72]. However, health professionals may perceive they spend more time with adolescents in consultations than they actually do [33,73]. Time is needed

to facilitate seeing the young person independent of their parents, exploration of their "hidden agendas," health promotion opportunities, and self-advocacy skills training in addition to addressing the needs of the parents.

The pediatric provider perspective

The pediatric team are integral to the start of transition, which some say should start on the day of diagnosis [74], and to the preparation for eventual transfer to adult care. However, timing of transition events (including transfer) is multifactorial and depends not only on chronologic age but also on maturity, current medical status, adherence, independence, self-advocacy skills, preparation, readiness of the young person and availability of an appropriate adult specialist. The use of individualized transition plans [5] are advocated by both young people [25,27] and professionals [2–5,24] to ensure the process of transition is as seamless and coordinated as possible.

Pediatric providers need to acknowledge that they are not primarily skilled in adult medicine and are unlikely to be able to provide age and developmentally appropriate health care for their patients during adulthood. Just as the parents find it difficult to let go, so may the pediatric team, particularly if they have been involved in the care of the young person since early childhood. The paternalistic and family-centered approach of pediatrics may unknowingly hamper the development of self-advocacy in adolescents and is less likely to provide confidential services and opportunity for the young person to be seen separately from the parents [45,75].

During transition, while the pediatric team are preparing the young person for adult care, they must guard against portraying the adult services as being "inferior" rather than "different" to the pediatric service. Ideally, the pediatric team need to objectively inform young people of the differences between the services and nurture the skills required to negotiate both systems. For this, pediatric providers need to learn about the respective adult services and the realities of the patient perspective. Liaison staff who work in both pediatric and adult settings are a potential means for success in this aspect of transition.

Transitional care can be further hampered by a lack of professional confidence in the adult team to look after childhood onset conditions. Development of combined clinics and/or young adult clinics with both pediatric and adult team members is one method of nurturing such collaboration while at the same time providing age and developmentally appropriate care for young people during late adolescence and early adulthood. Several studies have reported greater satisfaction with transfer models where the young person has the opportunity to meet the adult team prior to transfer [14–17,20,25]. Such collaboration is also key when there are potential research implications to loss of study cohorts on transfer. Knowledge of outcomes will be of relevance to both pediatric and adult providers.

The adult perspective

One major issue for some specialties is that there may be no experienced adult team in late effects of transplantation available locally. Furthermore, the adult team may have no training in looking after childhood onset and/or congenital disease. Adult specialists may assume such diseases are the same as their adult counterparts and forget disease-specific differences (e.g. primary diagnoses, type of graft, donor population, post-transplant complications) in addition to a longer potential life span in which to develop complications (e.g. osteoporosis, atherosclerosis, renal failure). They may also feel that pediatric care is too paternalistic, have higher expectations for learning, personal choice, self-care and independent follow-up and be reluctant to acknowledge the process of transition. Adult services may be less interdisciplinary and more fragmented than their pediatric counterparts. Just as pediatricians call for age and developmentally appropriate care for children and adolescents, adults with childhood onset disease have the right to appropriate adult-focused health care. For some specialties, this will require workforce planning as there may not be adult physicians familiar with these "new" diseases. For many specialties, development of formal training in adolescent health and transitional care to address

the areas detailed above, is required in both pediatric and adult postgraduate curricula.

CONCLUSIONS

To date, much of the research and service development in transitional care has been made in the pediatric and adolescent sectors and there is now a need to continue the impetus into adult-centered care so that transition becomes the normal, expected, planned and desired outcome of pediatric care. A respectful acknowledgement of differences in practice philosophies and style between pediatric and adult teams is imperative for successful transitional care, an area of transplantation ripe for further research. It is to be hoped that close collaboration of professionals working in pediatrics, adolescent health and adult medicine with these young people will enhance the current evidence base for the future.

ACKNOWLEDGMENT

JEMcD is an Arthritis Research Campaign (www.arc.org.uk) Clinical Senior Lecturer in Pediatric and Adolescent Rheumatology.

REFERENCES

1 Blum RW, Garell D, Hadgman CH, *et al.* Transition from child-centred to adult health-care systems for adolescents with chronic conditions: a position paper of the Society for Adolescent Medicine. *J Adolesc Health* 1993;**14**:570–6.

2 American Academy of Pediatrics. A consensus statement on health care transitions for young adults with special health care needs. *Pediatrics* 2002;**110**(Suppl):1304–6.

3 Department of Health. *Getting the Right Start: National Service Framework for Children.* Standard for Hospital Services, April 2003.

4 Royal College of Paediatrics and Child Health. *Bridging the Gap: Health Care for Adolescents.* June 2003. (www.rcpch.ac.uk)

5 Royal College of Nursing. *Adolescent Transition Care: Guidance for Nursing Staff.* London, 002313 (publication code) 2004. (www.rcn.org.uk)

6 Rosen DS, Blum RW, Britto M, Sawyer SM, Siegel DM. Society for Adolescent Medicine. Transition to adult health care for adolescents and young adults with chronic conditions: position paper of the Society for Adolescent Medicine. *J Adolesc Health* 2003;**33**:309–11.

7 Reiss J, Gibson R. Health care transitions: destinations unknown. *Pediatrics* 2002;**110**(Suppl):1307–14.

8 Scal P. Transition for youth with chronic conditions: primary care physicians' approaches. *Pediatrics* 2002;**110**:1315–21.

9 Suris JC, Michaud PA, Viner R. The adolescent with a chronic condition. Part I: developmental isssues. *Arch Dis Child* 2004;**8**: 938–42.

10 While A, Forbes A, Ullman R, Lewis S, Mathes L, Griffiths P. Good practices that address continuity during transition from child to adult care: syntheses of the evidence. *Child: Care, Health and Development* 2004;30:5:439–52.

11 Geenen SJ, Powers LE, Sells W. Understanding the role of health care providers during the transition of adolescents with disabilities and special health care needs. *J Adolesc Health* 2003;32:225–33.

12 Scal P, Evans T, Blozis S, Okinow N, Blum R. Trends in transition from pediatric to adult health care services for young adults with chronic conditions. *J Adolesc Health* 1999;24:259–64.

13 Peter N, Ginsburg K, Forke C, Schwarz D. Transition from pediatric to adult care: the internists' perspective. *J Adolesc Health* 2003;32:150.

14 Boyle MP, Farukhi Z, Nosky ML. Strategies for improving transition to adult cystic fibrosis care, based on patient and parent views. *Pediatr Pulmonol* 2001;32:428–36.

15 Steinkamp G, Ullrich G, Muller C, Fabel H, von der Hardt. Transition of adult patients with cystic fibrosis from paediatric to adult care: the patients' perspective before and after start-up of an adult clinic. *Eur J Med Res* 2001;6:85–92.

16 Landaw LI. Cystic fibrosis: transition from pediatric to adult physician's care. *Thorax* 1995;50:1031–2.

17 Nasr SZ, Campbell C, Howatt W. Transition program from paediatric to adult care for cystic fibrosis patients. *J Adolesc Health* 1992;13:682–5.

18 Zack J, Jacobs CP, Keenan PM, *et al.* Perspectives of patients with cystic fibrosis on preventive counselling and transition to adult care. *Pediatr Pulmonol* 2003;36:376–450.

19 Flume PA, Anderson DL, Hardy KK, Gray S. Transition programs in cystic fibrosis centers: perceptions of pediatric and adult program directors. *Pediatr Pulmonol* 2001;31:443–50.

20 Kipps S, Bahu T, Ong K, *et al.* Current methods of transfer of young people with type 1 diabetes to adult services. *Diabet Med* 2002;19:649–54.

21 Orr DP, Fineberg NS, Gray DL. Glycemic control and transfer of health care among adolescents with insulin dependent diabetes mellitus. *J Adolesc Health* 1996;18:44–7.

22 Telfair J, Myers J, Drezner S. Transfer as a component of the transition of adolescents with sickle cell disease to adult care: adolescent, adult and parent perspectives. *J Adolesc Health* 1994;15:558–65.

23 Telfair J, Ehiri JE, Loosier PS, Baskin ML. Transition to adult care for adolescents with sickle cell disease: results of a national survey. *Int J Adolesc Med Health* 2004;16:47–64.

24 Shaw KL, Southwood TR, McDonagh JE. Developing a programme of transitional care for adolescents with juvenile idiopathic arthritis: results of a postal survey. *Rheumatology* 2004;43:211–9.

25 Shaw KL, Southwood TR, McDonagh JE on behalf of the British Paediatric Rheumatology Group. User perspectives of transitional care for adolescents with juvenile idiopathic arthritis. *Rheumatology (Oxford)* 2004;43(6):770–8.

26 McDonagh JE, Southwood JE, Shaw KL. Unmet adolescent health training needs for rheumatology health professionals. *Rheumatology* 2004;43:737–43.

27 Shaw KL, Southwood TR, McDonagh JE. Transitional care for adolescents with juvenile idiopathic arthritis: results of a Delphi study. *Rheumatology* 2004;43:1000–6.

28 Chamberlain MA, Rooney CM. Young adults with arthritis: meeting their transitional needs. *Br J Rheumatol* 1996;35:84–90.

29 Kyngas HA. Patient education: perspective of adolescents with a chronic disease. *J Clin Nurs* 2003;12:744–51.

30 Beresford B, Sloper P. Chronically ill adolescents' experiences of communicating with doctors: a qualitative study. *J Adolesc Health* 2003;33:172–9.

31 Reynolds JM, Morton MJ, Garralda ME, Postlethwaite RJ, Goh D. Psychosocial adjustment of adult survivors of a paediatric dialysis and transplant programme. *Arch Dis Child* 1993;68:104–10.

32 Brook G, Hunt J, Johnson A, Reed J. Supporting the child and family. In: Kelly DA, ed. *Diseases of the Liver and Biliary Disease in Children*, 2nd edn. Oxford: Blackwell Publishing, 2004: 1–16.

33 Schubiner H, Eggly S. Strategies for health education for adolescent patients: a preliminary investigation. *J Adolesc Health* 1995;17:37–41.

34 McPherson A. Primary health care and adolescence. In: MacFarlane A, ed. *Adolescent Medicine*. London: Royal College of Physicians, 1996: 33–41.

35 Cheng TL, Savageau JA, Sattler AL, DeWitt TG. Confidentiality in health care: a survey of knowledge, perceptions and attitudes among high school students. *JAMA* 1993;269:1404–7.

36 Merzel CR, Vandevanter NL, Middlestadt S, *et al.* Attitudinal and contextual factors associated with discussion of sexual issues during adolescent health visits. *J Adolesc Health* 2004;35:108–15.

37 Carroll G, Massarelli E, Opzoomer A, *et al.* Adolescents with chronic disease: are they receiving comprehensive health care? *J Adolesc Health Care* 1983;4:261–5.

38 Kowpak M. Adolescent health concerns: a comparison of adolescent and health care provider perceptions. *J Am Acad Nurse Pract* 1991;3:122–8.

39 Lurie S, Shemesh E, Sheiner PA, *et al.* Nonadherence in pediatric liver transplant recipients: an assessment if risk factors and natural history. *Pediatr Transplant* 2000;4:200–6.

40 Millstein SG, Irwin CE, Adler NE, *et al.* Health risk behaviours and health concerns among young adolescents. *Pediatrics* 1992;89:422–8.

41 Britto MT, Garrett JM, Dugliss MAL, *et al.* Risky behaviour in teens with cystic fibrosis or sickle cell disease: a multicentre study. *Pediatrics* 1998;101:250–4.

42 Stewart AL, Hays RD, Wells KB, *et al.* Long-term functioning and well-being outcomes associated with physical activity and exercise in patients with chronic conditions in the Medical Outcomes Study. *J Clin Epidemiol* 1994;47:719–30.

43 Rodino MA, Shane E. Osteoporosis after organ transplantation. *Am J Med* 1998;104:459–69.

44 Suris JC, Resnick MD, Cassuto N, Blum RW. Sexual behaviour of adolescents with chronic disease and disability. *J Adolesc Health* 1996;19:124–31.

45 Britto MT, Rosenthal SL, Taylor J, Passo MH. Improving rheumatologists screening for alcohol use and sexual activity. *Arch Pediatr Adolesc Med* 2000;154:478–83.

46 Nixon GM, Glazner JA, Martin JM, Sawyer SM. Female sexual health in cystic fibrosis. *Arch Dis Child* 2003;88:265–6.

47 Sawyer SM, Roberts KV. Sexual and reproductive health in young people with spina bifida. *Dev Med Child Neurol* 1999;41:671–5.

48 Sucato G, Murray P. Gynecologic issues of the adolescent female solid organ transplant recipient. *Pediatr Clin North Am* 2003;**50**:1521–42.

49 Radley-Smith R, Wray J. Depression in pediatric patients before and 1 year after heart or heart-lung transplantation. *J Heart Lung Transplant* 2004;**23**:1103–10.

50 Durst CL, Horn MV, MacLaughlin EF, *et al.* Psychosocial responses of adolescent cystic fibrosis patients to lung transplantation. *Pediatr Transplant* 2001;**5**:27–31.

51 Radley-Smith R, Wray J. Depression in pediatric patients before and 1 year after heart or heart-lung transplantation. *J Heart Lung Transplant* 2004;**23**:1103–10.

52 Burker EJ, Carels RA, Thompson LF, Rodgers L, Egan T. Quality of life in patients awaiting lung transplant: cystic fibrosis versus other end stage lung diseases. *Pediatr Pulmonol* 2000;**30**: 453–60.

53 Baum M, Freier C, Freeman K, Chinnock RE. Developmental outcomes and cognitive functioning in infant and child heart transplant recipients. *Progr Pediatr Cardiol* 2000;**11**:159–63.

54 Morton MJ, Reynolds JM, Garralda ME, Postlethwaite RJ, Goh D. Psychiatric adjustment in end-stage renal disease: a follow-up study of former paediatric patients. *J Psychosom Res* 1994;**38**: 293–303.

55 Eiser C. *Growing Up with a Chronic Disease*. London: Kingsley, 1993.

56 Alonso EM, Neighbors K, Mattson C, *et al.* Functional outcomes of pediatric liver transplantation. *J Pediatr Gastroenterol Nutr* 2003;**37**:155–60.

57 Bucuvalas JC, Britto M, Krug S, *et al.* Health-related quality of life in pediatric liver transplant recipients: a single-center study. *Liver Transplant* 2003;**9**:62–71.

58 Krull K, Fuchs C, Uurk H. Neurocognitive outcome in pediatric liver transplant recipients. *Pediatr Transplant* 2003;**7**:111–8.

59 Quist E, Pihko H, Fagerudd P, *et al.* Neurodevelopmental outcome in high-risk patients after renal transplantation in early childhood. *Pediatr Transplant* 2002;**6**:53–62.

60 Bateman BJ, Finlay F. Long term medical conditions: career prospects. *Arch Dis Child* 2002;**87**:291–2.

61 McDonagh JE. Growing up and moving on: transition from pediatric to adult care. *Pediatr Transplant* 2004;**8**:1–9.

62 White PH. Access to health care: health insurance considerations for young adults in special health care needs/disabilities. *Arch Pediatr Adolesc Med* 1996;**150**:692–8.

63 Tomlin S, Saunders D. Pharmaceutical care: improving practice for children in hospital. *Paediatr Nurs* 2001;**13**:25–9.

64 Molmenti E, Mazariegos G, Bueno T. Noncompliance after paediatric liver transplantation. *Transplant Proc* 1999;**31**:408.

65 Watson AR. Non-compliance and transfer from paediatric to adult transplant unit. *Pediatr Nephrol* 2000;**14**:469–72.

66 Sudan D. Causes of late mortality in pediatric liver transplant. *Ann Surg* 1998;**227**:289–95.

67 Patterson J, Blum RJ. Risk and resilience among children and youth with disabilities. *Arch Pediatr Adolesc Med* 1996;**150**: 692–8.

68 Ehrich JHH, Rizzoni G, Broyer M, *et al.* Rehabilitation of young adults during renal replacement therapy in Europe. 2. Schooling, employment and social situation. *Nephrol Dial Transplant* 1992;**7**:573–8.

69 Sexson S, Rubenow J. *Psychiatric Aspects of Organ Transplantation: Transplants in Children and Adolescents*. New York: Oxford University Press, 1992.

70 Gold L, Kirkpatrick B, Fricker F, Zitelli B. Psychosocial issues in pediatric organ transplantation: parent's perspective. *Pediatrics* 1986;**77**:738–44.

71 Rosen D. Between two worlds: bridging the cultures of child health and adult medicine. *J Adolesc Health* 1995;**17**:10–6.

72 Robertson LP, McDonagh JE, Southwood TR, Shaw KL. Growing up and moving on. A multicentre UK audit of the transfer of adolescents with juvenile idiopathic arthritis (JIA) from paediatric to adult centred care. *Ann Rheum Dis* 2006;**65**:74–80.

73 Jacobson LD, Wilkinson C, Owen PA. Is the potential of teenage consultations being missed? A study of consultation times in primary care. *Fam Pract* 1994;**11**:296–99.

74 White PH. Success on the road to adulthood: issues and hurdles for adolescents with disabilities. *Rheum Dis Clin North Am* 1997;**23**:697–707.

75 Akinbami LJ, Gandhi H, Cheng TL. Availability of adolescent health services and confidentiality in primary care practices. *Pediatrics* 2003;**111**:394–401.

Index

Note: Page numbers in *italic* refer to figures and/or tables separate from the corresponding text

Plate sections face pages 224 & 225 and 384 & 385